BLOOD IN CONTACT WITH NATURAL AND ARTIFICIAL SURFACES

ANNALS OF THE NEW YORK ACADEMY OF SCIENCES
Volume 516

BLOOD IN CONTACT WITH NATURAL AND ARTIFICIAL SURFACES

Edited by Edward F. Leonard, Vincent T. Turitto, and Leo Vroman

The New York Academy of Sciences
New York, New York
1987

Cover (soft cover only): *A pen-and-ink drawing by Leo Vroman depicting the stretching of an artificial (top) and an endothelial (bottom) surface in the presence of plasma. As Dr. Vroman writes in his contribution to this volume, "The apparent simplicity of the interaction of plasma and endothelial surface is maintained by the complexity of the substrate. The complexity of the interaction of plasma and polymer surface is caused by the simplicity of the substrate." (For details,* *see pp. 300–305.)*

Library of Congress Cataloging in Publication Data

Blood in contact with natural and artificial surfaces / edited by
Edward F. Leonard, Vincent T. Turitto, and Leo Vroman.
p. cm. — (Annals of the New York Academy of Sciences, ISSN 0077-8923; v. 516)
Based on a conference held by the New York Academy of Sciences on Nov. 12–14, 1986, in New York, N.Y.
Includes bibliographies and index.
1. Blood—Coagulation—Congresses. 2. Biocompatibility—Congresses. 3. Blood vessel prosthesis—Congresses. 4. Thrombosis—Congresses. I. Leonard, Edward F. II. Turitto, Vincent T. III. Vroman, Leo, 1915– . IV. New York Academy of Sciences. V. Series.
[DNLM: 1. Biocompatible Materials—congresses. 2. Blood—congresses. 3. Blood Vessel Prosthesis—congresses. 4. Surface Properties—congresses. W1 AN626YL v. 516 / WH 100 B65535 1986]
Q11.N5 vol. 516
[QP93.5]
500 s—dc19
[612'.115]
DNLM/DLC
for Library of Congress 87-34318
CIP

SP
Printed in the United States of America
ISBN 0-89766-427-2 (cloth)
ISBN 0-89766-428-0 (paper)
ISSN 0077-8923

ANNALS OF THE NEW YORK ACADEMY OF SCIENCES

Volume 516
December 28, 1987

BLOOD IN CONTACT WITH NATURAL AND ARTIFICIAL SURFACES[a]

Honorary Conference Chair
THEODORE H. SPAET

Editors and Conference Organizers
EDWARD F. LEONARD, VINCENT T. TURITTO, AND LEO VROMAN

CONTENTS

[a]This volume is the result of a conference entitled Blood in Contact with Natural and Artificial Surfaces, which was held by the New York Academy of Sciences on November 12–14, 1986, in New York, NY.

Theme II. Blood Elements at Surfaces

PART I. PLASMA SYSTEMS

Theme IV. The Study of Phenomena *in Vivo* and *ex Vivo*

Part I. Methods of Assessing Thrombosis

Part II. Thrombogenesis on Prosthetic Surfaces

Financial assistance was received from:

- ADVANCED CARDIOVASCULAR SYSTEMS, INC.
- EASTMAN KODAK COMPANY
- GAMBRO, INC.
- W. L. GORE & ASSOCIATES
- HEALTH-CARE INSTRUMENT AND DEVICES INSTITUTE
- HOECHST-ROUSSEL PHARMACEUTICALS, INC.
- LILLY RESEARCH LABORATORIES
- NATIONAL HEART, LUNG AND BLOOD INSTITUTE-NATIONAL INSTITUTES OF HEALTH
- NATIONAL MEDICAL CARE
- ORGANON TEKNIKA CORPORATION
- SANDOZ CORPORATION
- SCHERING-PLOUGH CORPORATION
- SEARLE RESEARCH AND DEVELOPMENT
- TRAVENOL LABORATORIES

Blood in Contact with Artificial Surfaces: Where Have We Been and Where Are We Going?

A Modest Proposal

THEODORE H. SPAET

Division of Hematology
Department of Medicine
Montefiore Division of the Albert Einstein College of Medicine
Bronx, New York 10467

Ten years ago I launched the predecessor of this meeting with the metaphor that we are all blind men characterizing an elephant by palpation.[1] Who would deny that we still are? But we have since encountered parts of the beast that we had never before imagined. As is so often the case with our general discipline, each step forward expands the horizon and reveals a multitude of new avenues to traverse. The present view of hemostasis and the interaction of its components with the normal and altered vessel wall, and the many consequences of replacing this biological structure with an artificial device, would be virtually unrecognizable to the biologist of 1976.

At the time we wondered how we could best get our message to the public so that congressional support of our work would yield adequate funding. Now, the potential of organ or tissue transplant is aired daily in the mass media and by the standard modes of scientific communication. In fact, many now consider it a right to receive a new heart or allegedly suitable substitute. These considerations aside, the remainder of this meeting will be devoted to the knowledge we have accumulated since last we met. I now plan to concentrate on what I see as the current state-of-the-art in certain selected and critical areas.

Perhaps the most apparent change in our view of hemostasis is that we now consider the various reactions of the plasma clotting factors to occur almost exclusively on surfaces. These are surfaces on the vessel wall and on the formed elements of the blood. Few important reactions take place in bulk, and it is now clear that the precise placement required for portions of complex molecules and their associated cations with each other is too unlikely to be attributable to random encounter by diffusion. Instead, a surface affixes a reactant, which in turn enables others to gather in appropriate order, with a flowing system, to yield the final molecular complex. In our previous meeting, this general principle was suggested by a few "radical" investigators[2,3]; now it is routinely accepted,[4] and the detailed reactions have been largely clarified.

The basis for the localization of lesions, however, is less clear. How, exactly, does vessel size and original structure affect the pathogenesis of the lesions? The role of von Willebrand factor has been illuminated considerably, most significantly by identification of the multimeric system and the critical participation of the largest-size multimers in the interaction of platelets with the vessel wall,[5] and also the still evolving question as to whether this class of proteins is required in the first place for the initial platelet adhesion reaction. The theoretical impact of flow properties such as viscosity and velocity has often been discussed,[6] but has it been definitively related to human disease? The participating clotting factors no longer have a need for names, or even

1976

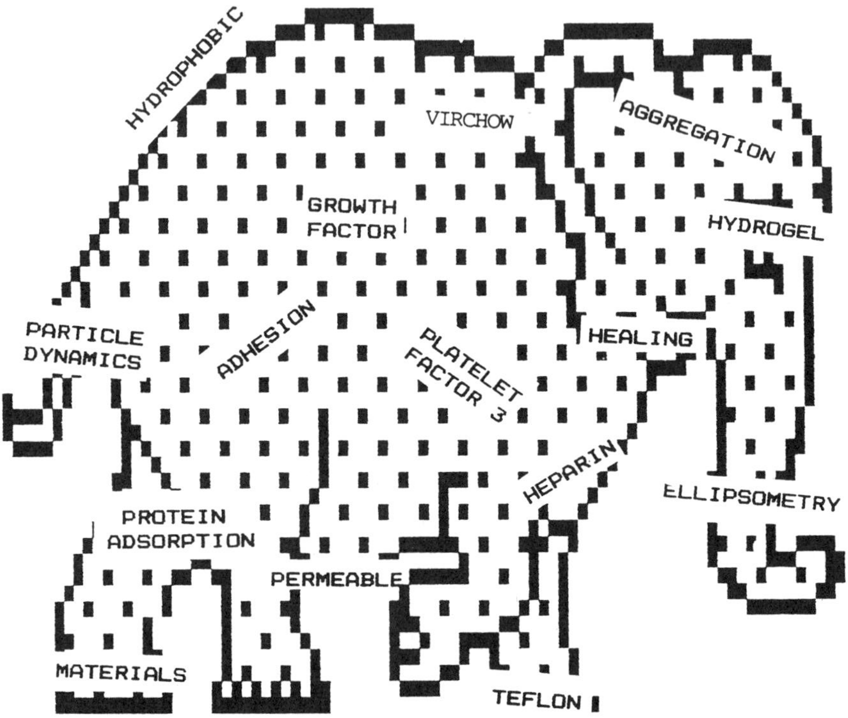

numbers. The chemistry of almost all of them has advanced to the point of total sequencing,[7] with *in vitro* synthesis following rapidly.[8] The biochemistry of the reacting surface, the vessel wall, and its relation to its counterparts on platelets and leukocytes will be covered in considerable detail as this meeting evolves, and I expect it will prove to be a jigsaw puzzle (elephant?) in which many areas show a recognizable picture, whereas others require primary definition or drastic modification. Of particular interest is how agents from the platelets are released to make their way to the reactive components within smooth muscle cells and elicit a proliferative response. I should like to interject my perhaps pedantic insistence on use of the term "mitogens" instead of the irresponsible generality "growth factors." Indeed, the vessel wall may thicken as a consequence of increased smooth muscle size (hypertrophy) or increased numbers of cells (hyperplasia); it may also thicken with deposits of intercellular material of various types (arteriosclerosis when the deposit is primarily connective tissue, atherosclerosis when cholesterol and other lipids and calcium deposits predominate). Mitogens typically produce hyperplasia.

A topic that has never been suitably addressed is the relationship between *in vitro* and animal studies and the application of these studies to human disease. The vast majority of my own data was derived from rabbits with an occasional rat or two thrown in. The results we obtained were certainly of more interest to veterinarians than to our clinical colleagues. (I am reminded of a clinical presentation given at a Federation meeting, when they were held in Atlantic City, during which was overheard the remark, "That is all very well, but how does it apply to the rat?") At the risk of being controversial, I assert that the final prize in this business is something that leads to a health benefit.

At the same time, I am suspicious of "directed" research, whereby incentives are given to promote narrow work directed at a specific disease category. Professor Leonard has generated here a reasonable balance between the theoretical, the experimental, and the practical; it is possible to satisfy our intellectual appetites and also to save lives. I thus hope that each of you may step out of your daily professional role and try, at least, to perceive a reasonable view of the larger picture. Particular attention should be given to ascertaining how well one's own piece of the action matches with the rest. I recognize that many of you have cosmic schemes; I suspect that each is an example of elephantizing.

What does the future hold? There are two categories: what one predicts, and what one would like to see. I expect there will continue to be pressure from various special interest groups seeking to promote their own pet projects. The campaign for this or that ailment is all too familiar, and Congress too frequently responds in an emotional rather than a scientifically prudent manner. It would be interesting to ascertain the health benefits that have stemmed from directed as opposed to investigator-oriented research. In any event, the unusual study that is guided by special insight should be nurtured in order to foster creativity. There are some signs of a burgeoning in this area; may they flourish!

I further anticipate that, in the near future at least, it will be more difficult to obtain funding for truly creative endeavors, and the hope for exciting innovation and breakthroughs will have to depend more upon countries other than ours. Competition from the military and from mass health care seems to be eating into the medical

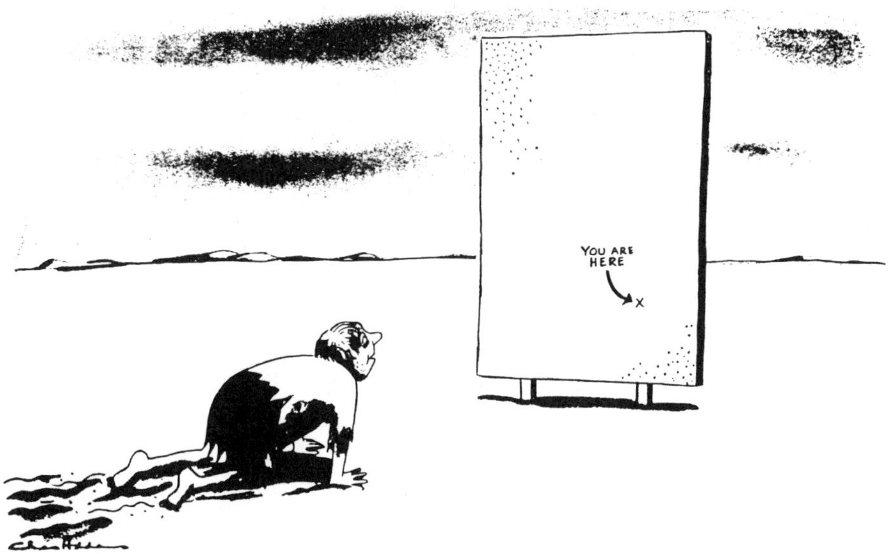

Drawing by Chas. Addams; © 1974
The New Yorker Magazine, Inc.

research budget. Additionally there will probably be an inordinate degree of concentration on the practical aspects of heart and vessel transplantation and installation of artificial prostheses before the biology of these procedures is adequately understood. Will these sessions put such matters into proper perspective? What does a surface have to be to be "physiological," and can this actually be synthesized by other than the appropriate cell *in vivo?* The evidently unique plasticity of biological material contributes to its ability to avoid the formation of traps for potentially thrombogenic blood components. The surgical interfacing of synthetic with biological structures has always presented difficulties, and continues to do so; attention to these reactions should be fruitful. Perhaps the adverse reaction can be postponed by some temporary measure that would allow a normal healing reaction to supervene, thus allowing such an interface to achieve permanence. Above all, we must restrain the impulse to rush in with a device before the consequences of its implantation are clear.

Let us return to the elephant. Perhaps there are now a fortunate few (our chairpersons included) who can perceive its totality, even if only dimly. Certainly it has demonstrated a thick skin wherever palpated, but we now have the instrumentation to explore its interior, and even to characterize its workings. In addition we can be sure that there is enough detail still hidden to keep us busy for the remainder of our working lives.

REFERENCES

1. Spaet, T. H. 1977. Blood and biomaterials: A glimpse at the elephant. Ann. N.Y. Acad. Sci. **283:** 2.
2. Ratnoff, O. D. & H. Saito. 1977. Coagulation factors and the role of surface in their activation. Ann. N.Y. Acad. Sci. **283:** 88.
3. Hemker, H. C., M. J. Lindhout & C. Vermeer. 1977. Blood coagulation factors at phospholipid surfaces. Ann. N.Y. Acad. Sci. **283:** 104.
4. Mann, K. G. 1984. Membrane-bound enzyme complexes in blood coagulation. Prog. Hemostas. Thromb. **7:** 1.
5. Hoyer, L. W. & J. R. Shainoff. 1980. Factor VIII-related protein circulates in normal human plasma as high molecular weight multimers. Blood **55:** 1056.
6. Copley, A. L. & G. V. F. Copley, Eds. 1983. Ann. N.Y. Acad. Sci. **416:** 1–761.
7. Davie, E. W. The blood coagulation factors: Their CDNase, genes, and expression. *In* Hemostasis and Thrombosis. R. W. Colman & J. Hirsh, Eds. In press.
8. Kane, W. H. & E. W. Davie. 1986. Molecular cloning of a cDNA coding for the human factor Va light chain (abstract). Circulation **74**(4, Part 2): 410.

Vascular Endothelium: Nature's Blood-Compatible Container[a]

MICHAEL A. GIMBRONE, JR.

Vascular Research Division
Department of Pathology
Brigham and Women's Hospital
Harvard Medical School
Boston, Massachusetts 02115

INTRODUCTION

Vascular endothelium, the continuous, single-cell-thick lining of the cardiovascular system, constitutes Nature's blood-compatible container. As long as blood stays within this container, it remains fluid and can perform its essential transport and communication functions unimpeded. Simple contact of blood with a nonendothelial surface, however, is sufficient to trigger platelet activation and the coagulation cascade. If unchecked, this normally adaptive hemostatic response can lead to various pathologic sequelae, including thrombosis, vascular occlusion, and ischemic tissue injury.

During the last decade, our understanding of the physiologic mechanisms that normally act to maintain the integrity of the endothelial lining, as well as the pathophysiologic stimuli that can mediate its injury or dysfunction, has expanded at a rapid rate. Particularly relevant to the theme of this volume is the emerging concept of the vascular endothelium as a *dynamic regulator* of hemostasis and thrombosis.[1]

ENDOTHELIAL HEMOSTATIC-THROMBOTIC BALANCE: EVOLUTION OF THE CONCEPT

The importance of the vascular lining for the maintenance of blood fluidity was appreciated as early as 1856 by Rudolph Virchow and formed part of his classic triad of predisposing factors for pathologic thrombosis.[2] Subsequently, this "nonthrombogenic" behavior of the vascular lining was shown, in part, to be a reflection of the failure of the endothelial cell surface to activate the plasma coagulation system or to induce platelet adhesion. Until recently, this property was considered to be more passive than active, *i.e.*, the endothelial lining was viewed as a sort of insulation, preventing blood from interacting with more reactive subendothelial tissues. With the discovery that endothelial cells can synthesize prostacyclin,[3] the most potent naturally occurring inhibitor of platelet aggregation, a more active "antithrombotic" role for endothelium became apparent.

With the increasing awareness of the functional complexities of endothelium, our appreciation of its multiple roles in hemostasis and thrombosis has also evolved. The

[a]Research in the author's laboratory was supported primarily by grants from the National Institutes of Health.

current working concept[1] is that the vascular endothelial lining is the locus of a multi-factorial "hemostatic-thrombotic balance" involving both "antithrombotic" and "prothrombotic" influences (FIG. 1). Thus, in addition to its major influence on platelet function, endothelium also appears to be a pivotal element in the coagulation and fibrinolytic systems. Many of these functions appear to be "anti"-thrombotic in nature. Thus, several of the "natural anticoagulant mechanisms,"[5] including the heparin-antithrombin mechanism, the protein C-thrombomodulin mechanism, and the tissue plasminogen activator mechanism, are endothelial-associated. In addition to these "antithrombotic" functions, the endothelial cell also appears capable of active "prothrombotic" behavior. Not only does it synthesize adhesive cofactors such as von Willebrand factor, fibronectin and thrombospondin, and procoagulant factors such as factor V, but it also provides a surface on which procoagulant factors can be assembled and activated. It has been suggested that these endothelial functions represent a mechanism for the localization of clot-promoting activity near the surface of an injured vessel wall and thus efficient hemostatic plug formation.[4] As discussed below, it is also

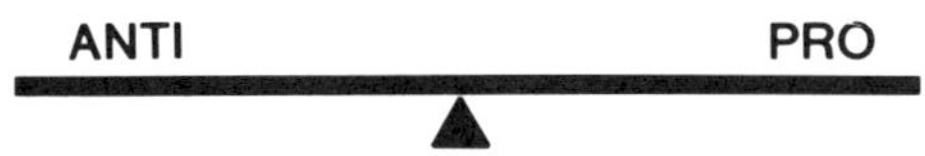

PROSTACYCLIN	PLATELET-ACTIVATING FACTOR
THROMBOMODULIN	TISSUE FACTOR
HEPARIN-like MOLECULES	COAGULATION FACTOR(S): Synthesis, Binding, Activation
Ecto-ADPase	von WILLEBRAND FACTOR: Synthesis, Secretion
t-PA, UROKINASE	t-PA INHIBITOR

FIGURE 1. The endothelial hemostatic-thrombotic balance. These various endothelial-associated factors and functions contribute to a dynamic physiologic antagonism or "balance" that determines the status of local hemostatic-thrombotic activity. (From Gimbrone.[1] Reprinted with permission from Churchill Livingstone.)

apparent that the endothelial cell can be "activated" to express surface-available tissue factor, in the absence of overt cellular injury, through the action of immune-inflammatory mediators such as interleukin-1 and noxious stimuli such as endotoxin.

Thus, the endothelial cell appears capable of playing a number of roles, both "pro"- and "anti"-hemostatic-thrombotic, that are relevant to the maintenance of normal blood fluidity, adaptive hemostatic reactions, and pathologic thrombosis. The challenge, as considered in the next section, is to better understand the stimuli that help regulate these various functions and potentially can provoke "endothelial dysfunction."

ENDOTHELIAL DYSFUNCTION: POTENTIAL ROLE IN THROMBOSIS

It has long been appreciated that frank denudation of the endothelial lining is sufficient to initiate thrombosis. As noted above, with the realization that the endothelial cell is a dynamic, interactive element in the hemostatic mechanism, it is now becoming apparent that the functional status of the vascular lining may be as important as anatomic integrity. This is especially true since many of the relevant surface and metabolic properties of endothelium are inducible, rather than constitutive, and thus are subject to physiologic regulation and potentially pathologic derangement.

The potential for vascular endothelium to undergo reversible phenotypic modulation to a nonadaptive functional state can be termed "endothelial dysfunction."[6] This might entail the loss of normal nonthrombogenic surface functions, as manifested by increased platelet adherence and/or activation of intrinsic or extrinsic coagulation pathways, or a serious "systems imbalance" between endothelial-dependent procoagulant and anticoagulant mechanisms. The net result conceivably could be manifest as an acute, localized thrombotic event; a more chronic, systemic thrombotic tendency; or disease of the vessel wall per se, as in atherosclerosis.[6] To date, most investigations of endothelial dysfunction in hemostasis and thrombosis have focused primarily on altered prostacyclin production by diseased blood vessels in experimental animals and in patients undergoing vascular surgery.[3] However, useful insights into other mechanisms and potential pathophysiologic stimuli for endothelial dysfunction have also been forthcoming from *in vitro* studies, as illustrated by the following examples.

Viral, Chemical, and Hemodynamic Influences

Transformation of cultured human endothelial cells, as accomplished by transfection of SV40 viral DNA fragments,[7] results in a marked change in the morphologic organization of the endothelial monolayer and a dramatic increase in their adhesivity for human blood platelets.[8,9] This increased platelet reactivity does not appear to be due to alterations in arachidonic acid metabolism or to the generation of thrombin. Further, the addition of pharmacological quantities of prostacyclin does not abolish the increased surface adhesive interaction of platelets with the virally altered endothelial cell surface. Cultured bovine aortic endothelial cells treated with chemical mutagens also show increased adhesivity for platelets,[10] and analogous changes in leukocyte sticking are observed when animal and human endothelial cells are acutely infected with certain pathogenic viruses.[12] Interestingly, chronic (24–48 hour) exposure of cultured endothelial monolayers to fluid shear stresses *in vitro,* comparable to those encountered under physiologic conditions of laminar blood flow *in vivo,* can induce increased endothelial cell adhesivity for blood elements such as platelets,[12] without morphologically detectable injury.

The mechanisms by which these diverse stimuli—viral, chemical, and mechanical—act to alter the normally nonadhesive endothelial surface have not yet been defined, but qualitative and quantitative changes in extracellular matrix production, as well as apical-basal cell surface polarity,[13] may be involved. In addition to their implications for hemostasis and thrombosis, transient interaction of platelets and leukocytes with an apparently intact endothelial lining *in vivo* may constitute an efficient mechanism for the transfer of labile mediators and growth factors to the vessel wall.

Cytokines as Regulators of Endothelial Hemostatic-Thrombotic Balance

Endothelial surface properties can also be dramatically altered, both structurally and functionally, through the action of immunoregulatory cytokines and other humoral mediators.[14–17] Especially noteworthy is the recent discovery, by Bevilacqua and coworkers,[18–20] that interleukin-1 (IL-1) and related cytokines can induce cell surface expression of a tissue factor-like procoagulant activity in human vascular endothelial cells. Thus, cultured monolayers of human endothelial cells (isolated from either umbilical veins or adult arteries and veins), which normally express negligible levels of surface-available procoagulant activity, develop a highly clot-promoting surface after 1–4 hours treatment with human monocyte-derived or recombinant IL-1. This dramatic change in the nonthrombogenic surface properties of endothelium appears to involve the de novo synthesis and cell surface expression of a tissue factor-like molecule, which catalyzes the generation of thrombin via a factor VIIa and X-dependent mechanism. In contrast to previously reported *in vitro* "injury" models of tissue factor expression,[21] endothelial cell damage is not morphologically or biochemically detectable after IL-1 treatment. This mechanism for tissue factor expression helps to explain previous reports of the development of procoagulant activity by endothelial cells when they were cocultured with peripheral blood leukocytes,[22] and suggest that interactions between leukocytes (monocytes and lymphocytes) and endothelium may actively contribute to fibrin generation at sites of immune-inflammatory reactions. Furthermore, human endothelial cells are stimulated to produce IL-1 by gram-negative endotoxins,[23,24] agents that can also induce tissue factor expression in these cells. Taken together, these findings suggest an active and complex role for vascular endothelium in the pathogenesis of disseminated intravascular coagulation associated with endotoxemia.

In addition to the induction of tissue factor-like procoagulant activity, IL-1 and the related cytokine tumor necrosis factor (TNF) also appear to modulate other components of the coagulation and fibrinolytic mechanisms. For example, IL-1 can influence endothelial fibrinolytic activity through a two-pronged mechanism involving decreased production of tissue plasminogen activator and increased production of plasminogen activator inhibitor.[25–27] The net effect of these processes would be to foster the maintenance of fibrin once it has been generated via the procoagulant mechanism. Recent studies also suggest that several other components of the "endothelial hemostatic-thrombotic balance," including thrombomodulin,[28] platelet-activating factor,[29] and prostacyclin,[30] can be significantly influenced by interleukin-1 and other cytokines. Thus, a complex picture is emerging, in which the endothelial lining may be playing a pivotal role in the balance of anticoagulant and procoagulant mechanisms under the influence of immune-inflammatory mediators.

PATHOPHYSIOLOGIC IMPLICATIONS AND FUTURE DIRECTIONS

The working concept, outlined above, of a dynamically regulated endothelial hemostatic-thrombotic balance has several important pathophysiologic implications and indicates a number of future research directions. The first, and perhaps most dramatic, is that the normally nonthrombogenic lining of the heart and peripheral vasculature can be provoked to become actively clot-promoting. Identification of the stimuli for this form of endothelial dysfunction, and their antecedents, should provide new insights into the pathogenesis of certain forms of thrombotic vascular disease. A second implication is that the vascular lining functions as an integrator of multiple stimuli, originating locally or delivered through the bloodstream, which are then transduced into a complex temporal and spatial pattern of response. Better understanding of endothelial signal transduction mechanisms thus might permit a more rational approach to systemic or local anticoagulant therapy. A third implication is that the detection of functionally altered endothelium *in vivo* will require new and innovative approaches. Further description of "endothelial activation antigens,"[17,31] the expression of which can be correlated with defined functional changes such as hyperadhesiveness for leukocytes[18,19,32] or enhanced immune reactivity,[33] should be helpful in this regard. In addition, development of noninvasive methods of assessing endothelial dysfunction, both systemically and locally, is clearly needed. A final implication, especially relevant to the theme of this volume, is that the endothelial hemostatic-thrombotic balance might be seriously perturbed by transplantation of this tissue into an unfavorable environment. Such "transplantation" may occur in the context of the actual allografting of an organ, the transposition of a venous segment into the arterial system, or the seeding of a vascular prosthesis with isolated endothelial cells.[34] Given the widespread current and proposed clinical applications of such approaches, a major challenge for future research is how best to monitor endothelial function in these settings, and avoid or offset potentially dysfunctional stimuli.

In conclusion, the recent appreciation of the highly evolved mechanisms underlying the blood container function of endothelium represents an exciting new chapter in vascular pathobiology. Further study of these mechanisms should contribute significantly to our understanding of vascular endothelium in health and disease.

ACKNOWLEDGMENTS

The author wishes to acknowledge his colleagues and collaborators, in particular, Drs. M.P. Bevilacqua, R.S. Cotran, P.F. Davies, and J.S. Pober, who contributed to various of the studies summarized here, and to thank Ms. C. Curtis for preparation of the manuscript.

REFERENCES

1. GIMBRONE, M. A., JR. 1986. Vascular endothelium: Nature's blood container. *In* Vascular Endothelium in Hemostasis and Thrombosis (Chap. 1). M. A. Gimbrone, Jr., Ed.: 1–13. Churchill Livingstone. Edinburgh.
2. VIRCHOW, R. 1856. Phlogose und Thrombose in Gefessystem. *In* Gesammelte Adhandlungen zur Wissenschaftlichen Medicin. Meidinger Sohn and Company. Frankfurt-am-Main. pp. 458–463.
3. WEKSLER, B. B. & E. A. JAFFE. 1986. Prostacyclin and the endothelium. *In* Vascular Endothelium in Hemostasis and Thrombosis (Chap. 3). M. A. Gimbrone, Jr., Ed.: 40–56. Churchill Livingstone. Edinburgh.
4. NAWROTH, P. P. & D. M. STERN. 1986. Endothelial cells as active participants in procoagulant reactions. *In* Vascular Endothelium in Hemostasis and Thrombosis (Chap. 2). M. A. Gimbrone, Jr., Ed.: 14–39. Churchill Livingstone. Edinburgh.
5. ROSENBERG, R. D. & J. S. ROSENBERG. 1984. Natural anticoagulant mechanisms. J. Clin. Invest. **74:** 1–6.
6. GIMBRONE, M. A., JR. 1986. Endothelial dysfunction and the pathogenesis of atherosclerosis. Atherosclerosis VII. N. H. Fidge & P. J. Nestel, Eds.: 367–369. Elsevier Science Publishers. New York.
7. GIMBRONE, M. A., JR. & G. C. FAREED. 1976. Transformation of cultured human vascular endothelium by SV40 DNA. Cell **9:** 685–693.
8. CURWEN, K., M. A. GIMBRONE, JR. & R. I. HANDIN. 1980. In vitro studies of thromboresistance: The role of prostacyclin (PGI_2) in platelet adhesion to cultured normal and virally transformed human vascular endothelial cells. Lab. Invest. **42:** 366–374.
9. GIMBRONE. M. A., JR. & M. R. BUCHANAN. 1982. Interactions of platelets and leukocytes with vascular endothelium. Ann. N. Y. Acad. Sci. **401:** 171–183.
10. ZETTER, B. R., L. K. JOHNSON, M. A. SHUMAN & D. GOSPODAROWICZ. 1978. The isolation

of vascular endothelial cell lines with altered cell surface and platelet-binding properties. Cell **14:** 501–507.

11. MacGregor, R. R., H. M. Friedman, E. J. Macarak & N. A. Kefalides. 1980. Virus infection of endothelial cells increases granulocyte adherence. J. Clin. Invest. **65:** 1469–1477.
12. Dewey, C. F., Jr., M. A. Gimbrone, Jr., S. R. Bussolari & P. F. Davies. 1981. The dynamic response of vascular endothelial cells to fluid shear stress. J. Biomech. Eng. **103:** 177–185.
13. Muller, W. A. & M. A. Gimbrone, Jr. 1986. Plasmalemmal proteins of cultured vascular endothelial cells exhibit apical-basal polarity: Analysis by surface-selective iodination. J. Cell Biol. **103(6):** 2389–2402.
14. Pober, J. S. & M. A. Gimbrone, Jr. 1982. Expression of Ia-like antigens by human vascular endothelial cells is inducible in vitro: Demonstration by monoclonal antibody binding and immunoprecipitation. Proc. Natl. Acad. Sci. U.S.A. **79:** 6641–6645.
15. Pober, J. S., M. A. Gimbrone, Jr., R. S. Cotran, C. S. Reiss, S. J. Burakoff & K. A. Ault. 1983. Ia expression by vascular endothelium is inducible by activated T-lymphocytes and human gamma interferon. J. Exp. Med. **157:** 1339–1353.
16. Pober, J. S., T. Collins, M. A. Gimbrone, Jr., R. S. Cotran, J. Gitlin, W. Fiers, C. Clayberger, A. Krensky, S. J. Burakoff & C. S. Reiss. 1983. Lymphocytes recognize human vascular endothelial and dermal fibroblast Ia antigens induced by recombinant immune interferon. Nature **305:** 726–729.
17. Pober, J. S., M. P. Bevilacqua, D. L. Mendrick, L. A. Lapierre, W. Fiers & M. A. Gimbrone, Jr. 1986. Two distinct monokines, interleukin 1 and tumor necrosis factor, each independently induce biosynthesis and transient expression of the same antigen on the surface of cultured human vascular endothelial cells. J. Immunol. **136:** 1680–1687.
18. Bevilacqua, M. P., J. S. Pober, G. R. Majeau, R. S. Cotran & M. A. Gimbrone, Jr. 1984. Interleukin 1 (IL-1) induces biosynthesis and cell surface expression of procoagulant activity in human vascular endothelial cells. J. Exp. Med. **160(2):** 618–623.
19. Bevilacqua, M. P., J. S. Pober, M. E. Wheeler, R. S. Cotran & M. A. Gimbrone, Jr. 1985. Interleukin-1 (IL-1) activation of vascular endothelium: Effects of procoagulant activity and leukocyte adhesion. Am. J. Pathol. **121:** 393–403.
20. Bevilacqua, M. P., J. S. Pober, G. R. Majeau, W. Fiers, R. S. Cotran & M. A. Gimbrone, Jr. 1986. Recombinant tumor necrosis factor induces procoagulant activity in cultured human vascular endothelium: Characterization and comparison with the actions of interleukin 1. Proc. Natl. Acad. Sci. U.S.A. **83:** 4533–4537.
21. Maynard, J. R., B. E. Dreyer, M. B. Stemerman & F. A. Pitlick. 1977. Tissue factor coagulant activity of cultured human endothelial cells and smooth muscle cells and fibroblasts. Blood **50:** 387.
22. Lydberg, T., K. S. Galdal, S. A. Evensen & H. Prydz. 1983. Cellular cooperation in endothelial cell thromboplastin synthesis. Brit. J. Haematol. **53:** 85.
23. Wagner, C. R., R. M. Vetto & D. R. Burger. 1985. Expression of I-region-associated antigen (Ia) and interleukin 1 by sub-cultured human endothelial cells. Cell Immunol. **93:** 91–104.
24. Libby, P., J. M. Ordovas, K. R. Auger, A. H. Robbins, L. K. Birinyi & C. A. Dinarello. 1986. Endotoxin and tumor necrosis factor induce interleukin-1 gene expression in adult human vascular endothelial cells. Am. J. Pathol. **124:** 179–185.
25. Bevilacqua, M. P., R. R. Schleef, M. A. Gimbrone, Jr. & D. J. Loskutoff. 1986. Regulation of the fibrinolytic system of cultured human vascular endothelium by interleukin 1. J. Clin. Invest. **78:** 587–591.
26. Nachman, R. L., K. A. Hajjar, R. L. Silverstein & C. A. Dinarello. 1986. Interleukin 1 induces endothelial cell synthesis of plasminogen activator inhibitor. J. Exp. Med. **163:** 1595–1600.
27. Emeis, J. J. & T. Kooistra. 1986. Interleukin 1 and lipopolysaccharide induce an inhibitor of tissue-type plasminogen activator in vivo and in cultured endothelial cells. J. Exp. Med. **163:** 1260–1266.
28. Nawroth, P. P., D. A. Handley, C. T. Esmon & D. M. Stern. 1986. Interleukin 1 induces endothelial cell procoagulant while suppressing cell-surface anticoagulant activity. Proc. Natl. Acad. Sci. U.S.A. **83:** 3460–3464.

29. BUSSOLINO, F., F. BREVIARIO, C. TETTA, M. AGLIETTA & E. DEJANA. 1986. Interleukin 1 stimulates platelet-activating factor production in cultured human endothelial cells. J. Clin. Invest. **77:** 2027.
30. ROSSI, V., F. BREVIARIO, P. GHEZZI, E. DEJANA & A. MANTOVANI. 1985. Prostacyclin synthesis induced in vascular cells by interleukin 1. Science **229:** 174–176.
31. COTRAN, R. S., M. A. GIMBRONE, JR., M. P. BEVILACQUA, D. MENDRICK & J. S. POBER. 1986. Induction and detection of a human endothelial activation antigen *in vivo*. J. Exp. Med. **164(2):** 661–666.
32. BEVILACQUA, M. P., M. E. WHEELER, J. S. POBER, W. FIERS, D. L. MENDRICK, R. S. COTRAN & M. A. GIMBRONE, JR. 1987. Endothelial-dependent mechanisms of leukocyte adhesion: Regulation by interleukin 1 and tumor necrosis factor. *In* Leukocyte Emigration and Its Sequelae. H. Movat, Ed.: 79–93. Karger. Basel.
33. POBER, J. S., T. COLLINS, M. A. GIMBRONE, JR., P. LIBBY & C. S. REISS. 1986. Inducible expression of class II major histocompatibility complex antigens and the immunogenicity of vascular endothelium. Transplantation **41(2):** 141–146.
34. LIBBY, P., L. K. BIRINYI & A. D. CALLOW. 1987. Functions of endothelial cells related to seeding of vascular prostheses: The unanswered questions. *In* Endothelial Seeding in Vascular Surgery. M. B. Herring, & J. Glover, Eds.: 17–35. Grune and Stratton. Orlando, FL.

Thrombogenic and Nonthrombogenic Biological Surfaces

J. F. MUSTARD,[a] H. M. GROVES,[a]
R. L. KINLOUGH-RATHBONE,[a] AND M. A. PACKHAM[b]

[a]*Department of Pathology*
McMaster University
Hamilton, Canada

[b]*Department of Biochemistry*
University of Toronto
Toronto, Canada

Normal blood vessels are characteristically nonthrombogenic. When blood vessels are injured, the formed elements of the blood, such as platelets, accumulate and take part in hemostasis, thrombosis, and some forms of acute inflammatory reactions, particularly those involving the microcirculatory bed. When thrombosis occurs in the larger arteries of humans, it is almost invariably associated with atherosclerosis and a break in the lining over an atherosclerotic plaque. An important question is how long such a site remains thrombogenic.

Many studies that have examined the thrombogenic and nonthrombogenic characteristics of surfaces have been done in young experimental animals with normal vessels and the findings should not necessarily be extrapolated to events that occur in older humans. Other studies have been done using cultured endothelial cells that are not subjected to the physical forces that occur *in vivo* and whose subendothelial matrix is not cushioned and possibly conditioned by medial smooth muscle cells.

ENDOTHELIUM

The endothelium of normal vessels is a nonthrombogenic, blood-compatible surface. The reasons for the nonthrombogenicity of the lining of blood vessels are complex, but are probably related to the surface properties of the endothelium, its ability to neutralize thrombin, and its ability to produce plasminogen activator that converts plasminogen to plasmin which lyses any fibrin that might form in the circulation.

Antithrombin III contributes to the anticoagulant properties of the endothelium by becoming associated with heparin-like glycosaminoglycans that act as high affinity binding sites for it on the endothelium.[1,2] The antithrombin III reacts with thrombin to form a complex as a result of which both thrombin and antithrombin III are inactivated. As well as inhibiting thrombin, antithrombin III also inhibits factor Xa and possibly also factors IXa, XIa, and XIIa.[3,4] Protein C also plays a major role in regulating coagulation through its selective inhibition of factors V and VIII.[5] The endothelium provides a surface receptor, thrombomodulin, to which thrombin binds avidly. As a result of this, thrombin activates protein C which in turn inactivates the coagulation factors Va and VIIIa. Protein C requires another protein, protein S, to express optimal functional activity; protein S acts as a cofactor, forming a 1:1 complex with protein C. This complex requires the presence of a negatively charged phospholipid surface and Ca^{2+} to give the maximum rate of inactivation of factor Va.[6]

Endothelial cells also produce plasminogen activators that can convert circulating plasminogen to plasmin which causes fibrinolysis. In addition, endothelial cells have been shown to produce inhibitors of plasminogen activators[7,8] so that the extent to which fibrinolysis occurs depends upon the balance between activation and inhibition of fibrinolysis. Activated protein C stimulates fibrinolysis[9] and a recent report indicates that it may exert this effect by interacting with the inhibitors of plasminogen activators elaborated by the endothelium and decreasing their capacity to interact with the plasminogen activators;[10] this loss of inhibitory effect leads to enhancement of fibrinolysis.

Deficiencies of antithrombin III, protein C, or protein S or impairment of fibrinolysis have been associated with thrombotic tendencies of varying severity in a number of individuals.[11,12] Although these occur almost exclusively in the venous circulation, clinical complications that may be attributable to arterial thrombosis have been reported in a few individuals with a deficiency in protein C.[11,13,14]

When the endothelium is altered it may lose its nonthrombogenic characteristics, but the extent to which this occurs varies under different conditions. For example, it has been observed in experiments in animals that endothelial cells that have been extensively damaged and whose luminal surface remains in contact with flowing blood do not appear to be thrombogenic.[15] The abluminal surface of these cells is highly reactive to circulating platelets, however, and it may be that the collagen, elastin, fibronectin and some glycosaminoglycans of the intima, or elaborated by the endothelial cells, contribute to these properties that make the underside of the endothelium "proadhesive." A number of factors have been implicated as causes of endothelial cell injury, including lipids, bacteria, endotoxin, viruses, homocystine, and high concentrations of blood glucose,[16,17] but the evidence concerning whether they are able to alter the endothelium sufficiently to make it thrombogenic is inconclusive. Endothelium that has been altered because of exposure to the constituents of cigarette smoke either *in vivo* or *in vitro* becomes attractive to platelets.[18] It is not clear, however, whether platelets found in association with the endothelium under these conditions are directly in contact with the endothelium or whether there has been separation of the endothelial cells that leads to the adhesion of platelets to matrix proteins; the aggregates that form in this way may be in contact with the endothelium without necessarily being adherent to it.

White cells can adhere to the endothelium and can cross the endothelial cell barrier. Harlan[19] has recently reviewed the factors influencing white cell adhesion to the endothelium. Under some conditions, including acute inflammatory reactions and vessel injury, there is an increase in the number of white cells that adhere to the endothelium and there is some indication that more injured white cells adhere to damaged endothelial cells than to normal endothelial cells. Bevilacqua and his colleagues[20,21] have shown in studies with cultured endothelium that human monocyte-derived interleukin-1 can stimulate the synthesis and surface expression of tissue factor-like procoagulant activity. These workers have also shown that interleukin-1 acts on human endothelial cells and increases their adhesive properties for polymorphonuclear leukocytes, monocytes, and related cell lines.[22] This could lead to the ongoing production of tissue factor and the promotion of coagulation at injury sites as well as the recruitment of platelets to form thrombi.

The relevance to thrombosis of changes in the properties of the endothelium are not clear. Congenital defects in plasma proteins that interact with the endothelium (such as protein C) are associated with an increased incidence of venous thrombosis.

Although it seems probable that the effects of tissue necrosis factor, interleukin-1, or endotoxin may play a significant part in thrombotic events that occur in the microcirculation in association with inflammation, there is as yet no evidence that they change the properties of the endothelium in arteries.

SUBENDOTHELIUM

When the endothelium is lost from the surface of a blood vessel, subendothelial structures are exposed to the flowing blood. These include collagen, microfibrils around elastin, and amorphous subendothelial connective tissue.[23,24] Blood platelets rapidly adhere to these exposed subendothelial structures. The extent to which platelets adhere to the subendothelial matrix and the sequence of events that is initiated depends largely upon the severity of the injury. When the endothelium is removed from a medium or large artery by passage of a balloon catheter, platelets rapidly adhere to the subendothelium and form a carpet on the subendothelial structures.[23,25–27] Occasionally, however, segments of the vessel appear morphologically to be denuded of endothelium, but few platelets adhere to the structures that are exposed.[27] In some studies, methods for inducing injury have been developed that remove small areas of endothelium from the surface of vessels.[28] These techniques usually involve bringing a flexible nylon filament into contact with the luminal surface of an artery and removing a zone of endothelium without affecting the media. Some platelets adhere to the freshly exposed surface, but this is not always extensive because fibrillar collagen and microfibrils are not exposed.

Under conditions of laminar flow, coagulation does not seem to contribute to the reaction of platelets with the injury site produced by passage of a balloon catheter, probably because activated coagulation factors are rapidly removed by the flowing blood. Thus, fibrin is rarely seen on the surface of a de-endothelialized vessel.[27] Where flow is not laminar or where there has been severe damage to a vessel, for example medial smooth muscle cell injury, thrombin generated at the injury site can contribute to the development of platelet-fibrin thrombi. This can come about because of activation of both the extrinsic and intrinsic pathways of coagulation. The intrinsic pathway can be initiated when factor XII comes into contact with collagen exposed at the injury site.[29,30] Platelets stimulated with either collagen or ADP activate factor XII in the presence of kallikrein and high molecular weight kininogen.[31] The extrinsic pathway is activated by tissue factor and the expression of tissue factor activity appears to require only cell surface trauma.[32] Smooth muscle cell trauma could occur with some forms of vessel injury.

Of the subendothelial constituents exposed, only collagen[33] and microfibrils in the presence of von Willebrand factor[34] are able to cause the platelets to release their granule contents and activate the arachidonic acid pathway leading to the formation of thromboxane A_2. Thromboxane A_2, released ADP, and serotonin cause platelet aggregation, and act together in a synergistic manner.[35] When platelets are stimulated by these aggregating agents, their normally nonthrombogenic surface is altered, fibrinogen receptors become available on the membrane,[36] and the platelets can adhere to each other and to platelets that are already adherent to the damaged vessel wall. However, platelet aggregates do not form on the surface unless blood flow is disturbed so that materials released from platelets and the activated platelets can accumulate. On the surface of platelets that have released granule contents, phospholipid becomes available and accelerates two steps of the intrinsic coagulation pathway leading to thrombin generation.[37] Thrombin not only induces further platelet aggregation, release of granule contents, and thromboxane A_2 formation, it converts fibrinogen to fibrin. Polymerizing fibrin presents a surface to which platelets adhere although they do not adhere to fully polymerized fibrin[38] if the thrombin has been removed by blood flow or neutralized by antithrombin III. Thus, fibrin changes from a thrombogenic to a nonthrombogenic surface as it polymerizes.

Extensive studies have been done on the adherence of platelets to collagens of different types. Vessel walls contain collagen types I, III, IV, and V. Type I is found mainly in the adventitia but has also been detected in the media and subendothelium. Types III and V collagen are present in the subendothelium; types IV and V are mainly in the basement membrane.[24] Platelets adhere to types I, III and IV collagen; type V appears to be nonthrombogenic.[39]

Many studies have been done with experimental animals and with the Baumgartner flow chamber to assess the contribution of plasma proteins to platelet adhesion to the subendothelium exposed by passage of a balloon catheter. At the high shear rates that occur in capillaries and small arterioles, von Willebrand factor promotes platelet adhesion to the subendothelium,[40,41] although this protein has no apparent effect on adhesion at the low shear rates that are characteristic of larger arteries or veins. Experimental work by Stel and colleagues[42] has shown that von Willebrand factor in the subendothelium makes some contribution to platelet adhesion, but that absorption of the protein from plasma (or release from the alpha granules of adherent platelets) is required to support the adhesion of normal numbers of platelets. The importance of von Willebrand factor in hemostasis is well recognized, but its possible role in thrombosis at stenotic lesions that are subjected to high shear rates has received little attention. Although von Willebrand factor can bind to the surface of activated platelets,[43,44] it does not do so in the presence of normal concentrations of fibrinogen.[45,46]

The role of fibronectin in platelet adhesion to damaged vessels has been less thoroughly studied. Fibronectin is an adhesive protein known to bind to almost everything with which it comes in contact, including collagen, fibrinogen, and activated platelets.[47] There are three possible sources of fibronectin: it is synthesized by endothelial cells and is present in large amounts in the subendothelium; plasma contains fibronectin; and the alpha granules of platelets also contain fibronectin. As with von Willebrand factor, however, the binding of fibronectin to activated platelets is inhibited by fibrinogen.[48] At high shear rates, fibronectin in the subendothelium promotes platelet adhesion when the endothelium has been removed.[49]

Thrombospondin is another adhesive protein found in platelet alpha granules, endothelial cells, smooth muscle cells, fibroblasts, monocytes and macrophages.[50,51] Its role in stabilizing platelet aggregates is related to its lectin-like activity. The ability of thrombospondin to bind to type V collagen, which occurs in the subendothelium, and to activated platelets, points to a possible role in platelet adhesion at injury sites. This multifunctional protein with binding sites for many substances has been shown to be present on the surface of atherosclerotic vessels.[52]

One of the distinctive characteristics of an injury that results in the accumulation of a layer of platelets on the vessel wall is that after a short time these platelets present an essentially nonthrombogenic surface to the blood and further platelet accumulation does not occur.[25] Experimentally, this has been shown to take place within 10 minutes of the initial injury in rabbits.[27] The explanation is not clear, but it may be that the receptors on the surface of the platelets that are adherent to the vessel wall are no longer capable of interacting with circulating platelets, and that the circulating platelets themselves are not being altered sufficiently to be able to adhere to the platelets adherent to the wall. In rabbits, the platelets are gradually lost from the subendothelium and very few remain at 4 days;[27] the denuded surface is nonthrombogenic. Thus, in rabbits, after the subendothelium has passed through an acute thrombogenic phase, it becomes essentially a nonthrombogenic surface. The mechanisms producing this change are not established, but it appears most likely that it will be found to be mediated through vessel wall alterations involving either enzymatic effects on the surface materials or the synthesis of materials such as proteoglycans by the vessel wall. The change in thrombogenicity is not due to increased PGI_2 production since the surface becomes nonthrombogenic when PGI_2 formation is inhibited by administration of aspirin.[53] In addition, the ability of the de-endothelialized vessel wall to form PGI_2 is greatly diminished.[54] It seems unlikely that the loss of the reactivity of the vessel wall can be attributed to the absorption of plasma proteins at the injury sites because this should take place immediately. Thus the way in which the injured vessel wall gradually changes to a nonthrombogenic surface is not established. There may be species differences in the rate and extent to which this occurs.

If platelets are prevented from adhering to the subendothelium of rabbits for a period of 8 hours by the infusion of PGI_2, when the infusion is stopped, very few platelets accumulate on the surface.[55] This observation indicates that the subendothelial surface gradually becomes nonthrombogenic even if there are no platelets on it.

The practical application of these observations about the development of nonthrombogenic surfaces is clearly in the prevention of occlusion of vascular grafts in humans. Observations of the pattern of platelet accumulation on vascular grafts is to some extent compatible with the observations from experimental work in animals.[56,57] However, one of the features of bypass grafts is that the initial platelet accumulation may be much slower than on an artery from which the endothelium has been removed with a balloon catheter. The reason for the delay may be that the endothelium is not lost until some time after the graft is in place and then the exposed surface requires more time until it becomes relatively nonthrombogenic.

INJURED NEOINTIMA

The interaction of the components of the blood with diseased arteries is obviously more complex than with an injured normal vessel. One experimental approach to this problem has been to examine the effect of injury to the neointima that forms in an artery following removal of the endothelium.[25,26,58] This neointima is composed of smooth muscle cells whose surface forms a nonthrombogenic lining of the blood vessel. The response of the blood to an injured neointima is strikingly different from the response to exposure of the subendothelium. Small platelet-fibrin thrombi form in association with the damaged smooth muscle cells. However, the loss of the reactivity of this surface parallels in many ways that of the exposed subendothelium. Shortly after the initial platelet-fibrin thrombus forms on the vessel wall, the surface becomes relatively nonreactive to further platelet accumulation.[25,58] In addition, if the accumulation of platelets on the surface is inhibited by infusion of PGI_2 for 8 hours, very few platelets adhere to the surface when the infusion is terminated.[55] It is apparent that this surface, like the exposed subendothelium, eventually becomes nonreactive, indicating that the activation of coagulation leading to thrombin formation does not persist indefinitely. It may be that the injured smooth muscle cells are altered or lost from the surface so that there is no longer a tissue factor stimulus for the generation of thrombin. Thus, it appears that a neointima composed of smooth muscle cells is a nonthrombogenic surface and in addition, after it is injured, it becomes acutely thrombogenic for a brief period and rapidly again becomes a nonthrombogenic surface.

In areas where the smooth muscle cells are removed by the second injury, platelets adhere in a single layer to the exposed connective tissue matrix in a manner that is similar to their adherence to the subendothelium following a single injury with a balloon catheter.[58]

REPEATED VESSEL WALL INJURY

Repeated damage to the vessel wall such as that caused by an indwelling aortic catheter produces a surface that continues to be reactive to platelets.[25] In addition, platelet survival is shortened under these conditions because of the increased turnover of platelets on the repeatedly damaged surface. It seems likely that the platelets that are freed from an injury site on a vessel wall may have been released through the action of proteolytic enzymes that hydrolyze membrane glycoproteins that are involved in adhesion. These enzymes may include plasmin, leukocyte elastase, and proteolytic enzymes released by the platelets themselves. It has been shown experimentally that removal of platelet membrane glycoproteins by treatment with plasmin shortens platelet survival[59] and that administration of the antifibrinolytic agent epsilon aminocaproic acid reduces platelet turnover and prolongs platelet survival in animals with indwelling aortic catheters.[60]

ATHEROSCLEROTIC LESIONS

In medium to large arteries there is a clear association of thrombosis with advanced atherosclerosis. The constituents of atherosclerotic plaques are quite different from those of the subendothelium or injured smooth muscle cells and materials from plaques have been shown to be thrombogenic.[16] Characteristically, clinically important arterial thrombi occur primarily on ruptured atherosclerotic plaques.[61,62] Extensive thrombus formation occurs only in regions where there is disturbed flow and eddy formation, such as in stenotic regions,[63] and extensive thrombosis can be found in aneurysms.[64]

In the management of arterial thrombosis, it is essential to understand the progression from thrombogenicity to nonthrombogenicity of surfaces that are not covered with endothelium as well as to consider ways in which the endothelium may be injured or removed. Possibly human atherosclerotic lesions that have lost their endothelial covering may be nonthrombogenic in some circumstances, but injurious materials, such as those in cigarette smoke, may make these surfaces reactive. In stenosed vessels, it may be that the shear effect of blood flow may render such surfaces thrombogenic.

ENDARTERECTOMY AND ANGIOPLASTY

There is only limited evidence available from human studies about the effect of injury on diseased vessels. Endarterectomy is one of the procedures carried out by surgeons in which success is probably dependent upon the fact that the surfaces do become nonthrombogenic quickly and if the blood flow pattern is fairly normal, the risk of an occlusive thrombus forming is limited.[65] The only experimental evidence available about the reactivity of a vessel that has been subjected to endarterectomy comes from a study in cats in which the injured area became nonthrombogenic within about six hours.[66] Angioplasty is another procedure in which a diseased vessel is severely injured by dilation of an atherosclerotic lesion with a balloon, breaking the plaque open and exposing all of its constituents. Despite the exposure of the thrombogenic material in the plaque, if a normal flow pattern is restored, occlusive thrombi rarely form.[67,68] Again, the surfaces appear to become nonreactive over a relatively short period of time.

PERIPHERAL VASCULAR DISEASE

In investigations in which indium-111–labeled platelets have been infused into humans with peripheral vascular disease, the infusion of PGI_2 to inhibit platelet aggregation at an active lesion has resulted in the lesion becoming nonreactive in terms of further platelet accumulation.[69]

VENOUS THROMBOSIS

Virchow[70] proposed that thrombi occur in vessels as a result of damage to the blood vessels, stasis of blood, and activation of coagulation. There is little doubt that the combination of stimulation of coagulation and stasis or severely restricted blood flow can lead to thrombus formation in veins.[71,72] Thus, the high incidence of venous thrombosis associated with immobilization and tissue trauma, such as occurs postoperatively, may be largely attributable to this mechanism. Many venous thrombi in the lower limbs appear to begin in valve pockets.[73,74] Since platelet aggregates tend to occur in association with vessel injury, vessel injury may be involved in the initiation of these thrombi. However, experimental studies of the role of vessel injury in venous thrombosis are controversial. In early experiments in rats, Robertson and his colleagues[75] demonstrated that external pressure on veins, combined with stasis, produced thrombosis. A number of other investigators have also used the combination of stasis and vessel injury to cause thrombosis.[76–78] In contrast, Thomas and his associates[72] could not demonstrate that injury of the jugular vein of rabbits, with stasis, led to thrombosis. It is possible that one explanation for the differences in results is the type of injury and the relation between the injury and stasis. In the experiments of Thomas and his colleagues,[72] stasis was induced at least 5 minutes after injury, whereas in most of the other studies, stasis and injury were concurrent. Since injury sites can become nonthrombogenic, at least in arteries,[25] it may be that in the experiments of Thomas and his coworkers[72] the surface became nonthrombogenic before stasis was induced.

CONCLUSIONS

All of these observations indicate that our concept of nonthrombogenic surfaces has to be extended to biological surfaces other than the normal endothelium. Clearly, the subendothelium after its initial response is relatively nonthrombogenic, a smooth muscle cell-rich intima that forms following endothelial injury is nonthrombogenic, and an injured smooth muscle cell surface which is initially acutely thrombogenic will, with time, also become nonthrombogenic.

These observations have practical applications in clinical procedures such as arterial grafting, endarterectomy, and angioplasty. Although the damage is extensive with these procedures, it may be possible to avoid extensive thrombosis until the surfaces have time to become nonreactive. In conjunction with prevention of thrombus formation during the period immediately after injury, it is essential that normal blood flow be restored to prevent the formation of occlusive thrombi at stenotic lesions. For example, although streptokinase may open a blocked coronary artery, when the infusion of streptokinase is stopped an occlusive thrombus may reform if blood flow is abnormal.[79] If, however, the lesion is dilated with a catheter and more normal flow patterns are restored, even though the surface may initially be thrombogenic, an occlusive thrombus will not form. This indicates that the most effective approach to preventing thrombosis may be to restore more normal flow patterns rather than to attempt to reduce the thrombogenicity of the blood vessel surface. Tailoring drugs or inhibitory agents to prevent arterial thrombosis during the acute period until the vessel becomes nonreactive may be more important than trying to design drugs that act over a longer period of time. More research is necessary to determine the thrombogenic role of the vein wall in venous thrombosis.

REFERENCES

1. Rosenberg, R. D. & J. S. Rosenberg. 1984. J. Clin. Invest. **74:** 1–6.
2. Gallagher, J. T., M. Lyon & W. P. Stewart. 1986. Biochem. J. **236:** 313–325.
3. Abilgaard, U. 1979. *In* The Physiological Inhibitors of Coagulation and Fibrinolysis. D. Collen, B. Wiman & M. Verstraete, Eds.: 19–29. Elsevier/North-Holland Biomedical Press. Amsterdam.
4. Barrowcliffe, T. W. & D. P. Thomas. 1981. *In* Haemostasis and Thrombosis. A. L. Bloom & D. P. Thomas, Eds.: 712–724. Churchill Livingstone. London.
5. Esmon, C. T. & N. L. Esmon. 1984. Semin. Thromb. Hemostas. **10:** 122–130.
6. Walker, F. J. 1984. Semin. Thromb. Hemostas. **10:** 131–138.
7. Loskutoff, D. J. & T. S. Edgington. 1977. Proc. Natl. Acad. Sci. U.S.A. **74:** 3903–3907.
8. Loskutoff, D. J. & T. S. Edgington. 1981. J. Biol. Chem. **256:** 4142–4145.
9. Comp, P. C. & C. T. Esmon. 1981. J. Clin. Invest. **68:** 1221–1228.
10. Sakata, Y., S. Curriden, D. Lawrence, J. H. Griffin & D. J. Loskutoff. 1985. Proc. Natl. Acad. Sci. U.S.A. **82:** 1121–1125.
11. Broekmans, A. W. 1985. Haemostasis **15:** 233–240.
12. Rodgers, G. M. & M. A. Shuman. 1986. Am. J. Hematol. **21:** 419–430.
13. Griffin, J. H., B. Evatt, T. S. Zimmerman, A. J. Kleiss & C. Wideman. 1981. J. Clin. Invest. **68:** 1370–1373.
14. Horellou, M. H., J. Conard, R. M. Bertina & M. Samama. 1984. Br. Med. J. **289:** 1285–1287.
15. Johnson, R. C., R. S. Crissman & L. J. DiDio. 1979. Lab. Invest. **40:** 183–193.
16. Packham, M. A. & J. F. Mustard. 1986. Semin. Hematol. **23:** 8–26.
17. Mustard, J. F., M. A. Packham & R. L. Kinlough-Rathbone. 1986. *In* Haemostasis and Thrombosis. 2nd edit. A. L. Bloom & D. P. Thomas, Eds.: 1073–1088. Churchill Livingstone. New York.
18. Pittilo, R. M., I. J. Mackie, P. M. Rowles, S. J. Machin & N. Woolf. 1982. Thromb. Haemostas. **48:** 173–176.
19. Harlan, J. M. 1985. Blood **65:** 513–525.
20. Bevilacqua, M. P., J. S. Pober, G. R. Majeau, R. S. Cotran & M. A. Gimbrone, Jr. 1984. J. Exp. Med. **160:** 618–623.
21. Bevilacqua, M. P., J. S. Pober, R. S. Cotran & M. A. Gimbrone, Jr. 1985. *In* Mononuclear Phagocytes. Characteristics, Physiology and Function. R. Van Furth, Ed.: 747–752. Martinus Nijhoff. Boston, Dordrecht, and Lancaster.
22. Bevilacqua, M. P., J. S. Pober, M. E. Wheeler, R. S. Cotran & M. A. Gimbrone, Jr. 1985. J. Clin. Invest. **76:** 2003–2011.
23. Baumgartner, H. R. & R. Muggli. 1976. *In* Platelets in Biology and Pathology, Vol. 1. J. L. Gordon, Ed.: 23–60. North-Holland Biomedical Press. Amsterdam.

24. PACKHAM, M. A. & J. F. MUSTARD. 1984. *In* Progress in Hemostasis and Thrombosis, Vol. 7. T. H. Spaet, Ed.: 211–288. Grune & Stratton. Orlando, FL.
25. KINLOUGH-RATHBONE, R. L., M. A. PACKHAM & J. F. MUSTARD. 1983. Arteriosclerosis **3:** 529–546.
26. STEMERMAN, M. B. 1973. Am. J. Pathol. **73:** 7–26.
27. GROVES, H. M., R. L. KINLOUGH-RATHBONE, M. RICHARDSON, S. MOORE & J. F. MUSTARD. 1979. Lab. Invest. **40:** 194–200.
28. REIDY, M. A. 1985. Lab. Invest. **53:** 513–520.
29. WILNER, G. D., H. L. NOSSEL & E. C. LEROY. 1968. J. Clin. Invest. **47:** 2608–2615.
30. NIEWIAROWSKI, S., R. K. STUART & D. P. THOMAS. 1966. Proc. Soc. Exp. Biol. Med. **123:** 196–200.
31. WALSH, P. N. 1985. Semin. Hematol. **22:** 178–186.
32. NEMERSON, Y. & R. BACH. 1982. *In* Progress in Hemostasis and Thrombosis, Vol. 6. T. H. Spaet, Ed.: 237–261. Grune & Stratton. New York.
33. BAUMGARTNER, H. R., R. MUGGLI, T. B. TSCHOPP & V. T. TURITTO. 1976. Thromb. Haemostas. **35:** 124–138.
34. LEGRAND, Y. J., F. FAUVEL, B. ARBEILLE, D. LEGER, H. MOUHLI, N. GUTMAN & J. P. MUH. 1986. Lab. Invest. **54:** 566–573.
35. KINLOUGH-RATHBONE, R. L. & J. F. MUSTARD. 1986. *In* Platelet Responses and Metabolism, Vol. 1. H. Holmsen, Ed.: 193–207. CRC Press. Boca Raton, FL.
36. PEERSCHKE, E. I. B. 1985. Semin.Hematol. **22:** 241–259.
37. JACKSON, C. M. & Y. NEMERSON. 1980. Ann. Rev. Biochem. **49:** 765–811.
38. NIEWIAROWSKI, S., E. REGOECZI, G. J. STEWART, A. F. SENYI & J. F. MUSTARD. 1972. J. Clin. Invest. **51:** 685–700.
39. PARSONS, T. J., D. L. HAYCRAFT, J. C. HOAK & H. SAGE. 1986. Thromb. Res. **43:** 435–443.
40. TURITTO, V. T. & H. R. BAUMGARTNER. 1982. *In* Hemostasis and Thrombosis. Basic Principles and Clinical Practice. R. W. Colman, J. Hirsh, V. J. Marder & E. W. Salzman, Eds.: 364–379. J. P. Lippincott. Philadelphia.
41. SAKARIASSEN, K. S., P. A. BOLHUIS & J. J. SIXMA. 1979. Nature **279:** 636–638.
42. STEL, H. V., K. S. SAKARIASSEN, P. G. DE GROOT, J. A. VAN MOURICK & J. J. SIXMA. 1985. Blood **65:** 85–90.
43. FUJIMOTO, T. & J. HAWIGER. 1982. Nature **297:** 154–156.
44. PLOW, E. F., R. P. MCEVER, B. S. COLLER, V. L. WOODS, JR., G. A. MARGUERIE & M. H. GINSBERG. 1985. Blood **66:** 724–727.
45. PIETU, G., G. CHEREL, G. MARGUERIE & D. MEYER. 1984. Nature **308:** 648–649.
46. SCHULLEK, J., J. JORDAN & R. R. MONTGOMERY. 1984. J. Clin. Invest. **73:** 421–428.
47. RUOSLAHTI, E., E. G. HAYMAN & M. D. PIERSCHBACHER. 1985. Arteriosclerosis **5:** 581–594.
48. PLOW, E. F., G. A. MARGUERIE & M. H. GINSBERG. 1985. Blood **66:** 26–32.
49. HOUDIJK, W. P. M. & J. J. SIXMA. 1985. Blood **65:** 598–604.
50. LAWLER, J. 1986. Blood **67:** 1197–1209.
51. SILVERSTEIN, R. L., L. L. K. LEUNG & R. L. NACHMAN. 1986. Arteriosclerosis **6:** 245–253.
52. WIGHT, T. N., G. J. RAUGI, S. M. MUMBY & P. BORNSTEIN. 1985. J. Histochem. Cytochem. **33:** 295–302.
53. DEJANA, E., J.-P. CAZENAVE, H. M. GROVES, R. L. KINLOUGH-RATHBONE, M. RICHARDSON, M. A. PACKMAN & J. F. MUSTARD. 1980. Thromb. Res. **17:** 453–464.
54. ELDOR, A., D. J. FALCONE, D. P. HAJJAR, C. R. MINICK & B. B. WEKSLER. 1981. J. Clin. Invest. **67:** 735–741.
55. GROVES, H. M., R. L. KINLOUGH-RATHBONE & J. F. MUSTARD. 1986. Arteriosclerosis **6:** 189–195.
56. FUSTER, V. & J. H. CHESEBRO. 1985. Circulation **72**(Suppl. V): 65–70.
57. DEWANJEE, M. K., M. TAGO, M. JOSA, V. FUSTER & M. P. KAYE. 1984. Circulation **69:** 350–356.
58. GROVES, H. M., R. L. KINLOUGH-RATHBONE, M. RICHARDSON, L. JØRGENSEN, S. MOORE & J. F. MUSTARD. 1982. Lab. Invest. **46:** 605–612.

59. GREENBERG, J. P., M. A. PACKHAM, M. A. GUCCIONE, M. L. RAND, H.-J. REIMERS & J. F. MUSTARD. 1979. Blood **53:** 916–927.
60. WINOCOUR, P. D., R. L. KINLOUGH-RATHBONE, M. RICHARDSON & J. F. MUSTARD. 1983. J. Clin. Invest. **71:** 159–164.
61. CHANDLER, A. B., I. CHAPMAN, L. R. ERHARDT, W. C. ROBERTS, C. J. SCHWARTZ, D. SINAPIUS, D. M. SPAIN, S. SHERRY, P. M. NESS & T. L. SIMON. 1974. Am. J. Cardiol. **34:** 823–833.
62. DAVIES, M. J. & A. THOMAS. 1984. N. Engl. J. Med. **310:** 1137–1140.
63. GERTZ, S. D., G. URETSKY, R. S. WAJNBERG, N. NAVOT & M. S. GOTSMAN. 1981. Circulation **63:** 476–486.
64. FRANCIS, C. W., R. E. MARKHAM, JR. & V. J. MARDER. 1984. Blood **63:** 1216–1224.
65. EUGENE, J., S. J. MCCOLGAN, M. E. POLLOCK, M. HAMMER-WILSON, E. W. MOORE-JEFFRIES & M. W. BERNS. 1985. J. Surg. Res. **39:** 31–38.
66. PIEPGRAS, D. G., T. M. SUNDT, JR. & P. DIDISHEIM. 1976. Stroke **7:** 248–254.
67. BLOCK, P. C., R. K. MYLER, S. STERTZ & J. T. FALLON. 1981. N. Engl. J. Med. **305:** 382–385.
68. STEELE, P. M., J. H. CHESEBRO, A. W. STANSON, D. R. HOLMES, JR., M. K. DEWANJEE, L. BADIMON & V. FUSTER. 1985. Circ. Res. **57:** 105–112.
69. FITSCHA, P., J. KALIMAN & H. SINZINGER. 1984. Biomed. Biochim. Acta **43:** 5403–5408.
70. VIRCHOW, R. 1856. *In* Gesammelte Abhandlungen zur Wissenschaftlichen Medicin. Meidinger Sohn. Frankfurt.
71. WESSLER, S. 1962. Am. J. Med. **33:** 648–666.
72. THOMAS, D. P., R. E. MERTON, R. D. WOOD & D. J. HOCKLEY. 1985. Br. J. Haematol. **59:** 449–457.
73. SEVITT, S. 1978. *In* Venous Problems. J. J. Bergan & J. S. T. Yao, Eds. Year Book Medical Publications. Chicago.
74. MCLACHLIN, J. & J. C. PATERSON. 1951. Surg. Gynecol. Obstet. **93:** 1–8.
75. ROBERTSON, H. R., J. R. MOORE & W. A. MERSEREAU. 1959. Can. J. Surg. **3:** 5–16.
76. DAY, T. K., S. V. COWPER, V. V. KAKKAR & K. G. A. CLARK. 1977. Thromb. Haemostas. **37:** 477–483.
77. KELTON, J. G., J. HIRSH, C. J. CARTER & M. R. BUCHANAN. 1978. J. Clin. Invest. **62:** 892–895.
78. ANDERSON, M. C. & T. W. SHIELDS. 1962. Surgery **51:** 347–350.
79. O'NEILL, W., G. C. TIMMIS, P. D. BOURDILLON, P. LAI, V. GANGHADARHAN, J. WALTON, JR., R. RAMOS, N. LAUFER, S. GORDON, M. SCHORK & B. PITT. 1986. N. Engl. J. Med. **314:** 812–818.

Activation of Endothelial Cells[a]

UNA S. RYAN

School of Medicine
University of Miami
Miami, Florida 33101

INTRODUCTION

The disposition of blood in contact with natural or artificial surfaces is the outcome of interactions between the components of blood with specific recognition sites on the endothelium or lack of such specific signaling. Endothelial cells of all vascular beds provide a dynamic interface for interaction with substrates and formed elements arriving via the blood and for interaction with the underlying layers of the vascular wall.[1] We will focus particularly on pulmonary endothelium since pulmonary endothelial cells are strategically situated both for regulation of the quality of systemic arterial blood and for transduction of blood-borne signals that may affect vascular tone.[2] However, it is the same anatomic location that makes pulmonary endothelium an immediate target of vascular injury in a wide range of conditions. Thus, it may be appropriate to consider some of the interactions between blood-borne cells and molecules with the endothelial surface and to examine how these may be modified by signals likely to occur during vascular injury or as a result of implantation of vascular prostheses. Endothelial cells of the pulmonary circulation are now known, both from *in vivo* and *in vitro* studies, to be highly active and capable of selectively metabolizing blood-borne substrates including peptides, biogenic amines, prostaglandins, and adenine nucleotides, and of degrading a variety of drugs and anesthetics to spare the systemic circulation.[3] In addition, pulmonary endothelial cells possess receptors for a spectrum of agonists and hemostatic factors. The receptor-mediated responses of endothelial cells include release of substances that affect vascular tone and blood fluidity. Thus, the presence or absence of endothelium determines (via endothelium-dependent substances) whether the outcome of interaction with, for example, platelet products, results in vasospastic or vasodilatory responses of the vascular wall.[4] In addition endothelial cells engage in complex interactions with neutrophils and complement components that have important bearing on inflammatory processes.[5] The activities of pulmonary endothelium are not limited to constitutive properties that depend on an intact monolayer. Endothelial cells are also capable of inducible functions, thus they can respond to stimuli in ways that alter their hemostatic and immunologic potential and that alter their shape and behavior.[6] Many of these responses can be viewed as *activation* phenomena and involve increased migration, division, and phagocytosis.[7] Endothelial activation responses seem to involve changes in intracellular calcium levels and alterations in adenylate cyclase and protein kinase.[8,9]

[a]This work was supported by grant nos. HL 21568 and HL 33064 from the National Institutes of Health and by grant no. 814 from the Council of Tobacco Research, U.S.A., Inc.

INTERACTIONS WITH CIRCULATING VASOACTIVE SUBSTANCES

Endothelial cells of the pulmonary circulation are constantly exposed to vasoactive substances arriving as central venous blood is converted to arterial blood. For example, in the less than 3 seconds required for blood to transit the pulmonary capillary bed, bradykinin is hydrolyzed to yield inactive products and angiotensin I is converted to angiotensin II.[10] The enzyme responsible for these reactions is a dipeptidyl carboxypeptidase (EC 3.4.15.1), known both as angiotensin-converting enzyme and kininase II. Thus, as a result of interaction with an endothelial cell-bound enzyme, a blood pressure lowering substance is removed and a potent hypertensive substance is released into the systemic arterial circulation for distribution to target organs. When angiotensin-converting enzyme (ACE) was shown to be localized on the surface of pulmonary endothelial cells[11] it indicated that endothelial cells were capable of active metabolic reactions (FIG. 1).

It is now known that endothelial cells can process a wide range of endogenous polypeptides, including bradykinin, the angiotensins, substance P, and vasopressin.[10] In addition, pulmonary endothelial cells possess surface enzymes such as carboxypeptidase N that can metabolize another group of excitatory polypeptides, the anaphylatoxins, during passage through the lung.[12]

Prostaglandins, and related lipids derived from arachidonic acid, are selectively cleared by the lungs, prostaglandins of the E and F series being removed,[13] while PGA and PGI_2 are not degraded.[14,15] Leukotrienes C_4 and D_4 appear to be inactivated.[16] The fate of circulating amines in the pulmonary circulation depends on transport from the vascular space and/or intrapulmonary metabolism.[17] Norepinephrine and 5-hydroxytryptamine are rapidly taken up into endothelial cells and degraded by monoamine oxidase and other enzymes. On the other hand several amines, similar in structure, are neither taken up nor metabolized within the pulmonary circulation; thus both epinephrine and dopamine escape degradation during intrapulmonary transit.[17]

The adenine nucleotides are substances likely to be released into the circulation during shock or thrombosis. ATP, ADP, and AMP are each cleared quantitatively during passage through the lungs by pulmonary endothelial enzymes that have been localized cytochemically to endothelial caveolae.[18,19] Adenosine formed during degradation is then taken up by endothelial cells.[20,21]

There are a number of other endothelial surface enzymes that process substrates arriving in the blood that are not normally considered vasoactive substances. For example, carbonic anhydrase of pulmonary endothelial cells facilitates the release of CO_2 and helps to maintain blood pH. All in all interactions between blood-borne substrates and the endothelial surface have great impact on target organs at a distance and on homeostasis in general. These functions appear to occur constantly in normal healthy endothelium but clearly are compromised if the endothelium is absent or damaged or if the quantities of substances arriving in mixed venous blood overwhelm the pulmonary endothelial enzymes available for processing. Conditions that reduce the pulmonary vascular surface area either by the absence of endothelial cells or by vascular occlusion would be expected to result in impaired processing. Both situations may pertain in the case of vascular grafts. So far, there have been no attempts made to imbue artificial prostheses with endothelial processing properties.

INTERACTIONS WITH HEMOSTATIC FACTORS

The direct apposition of endothelium with the blood makes it ideally suited to affect blood fluidity and in turn to bear the brunt of coagulation episodes both as a

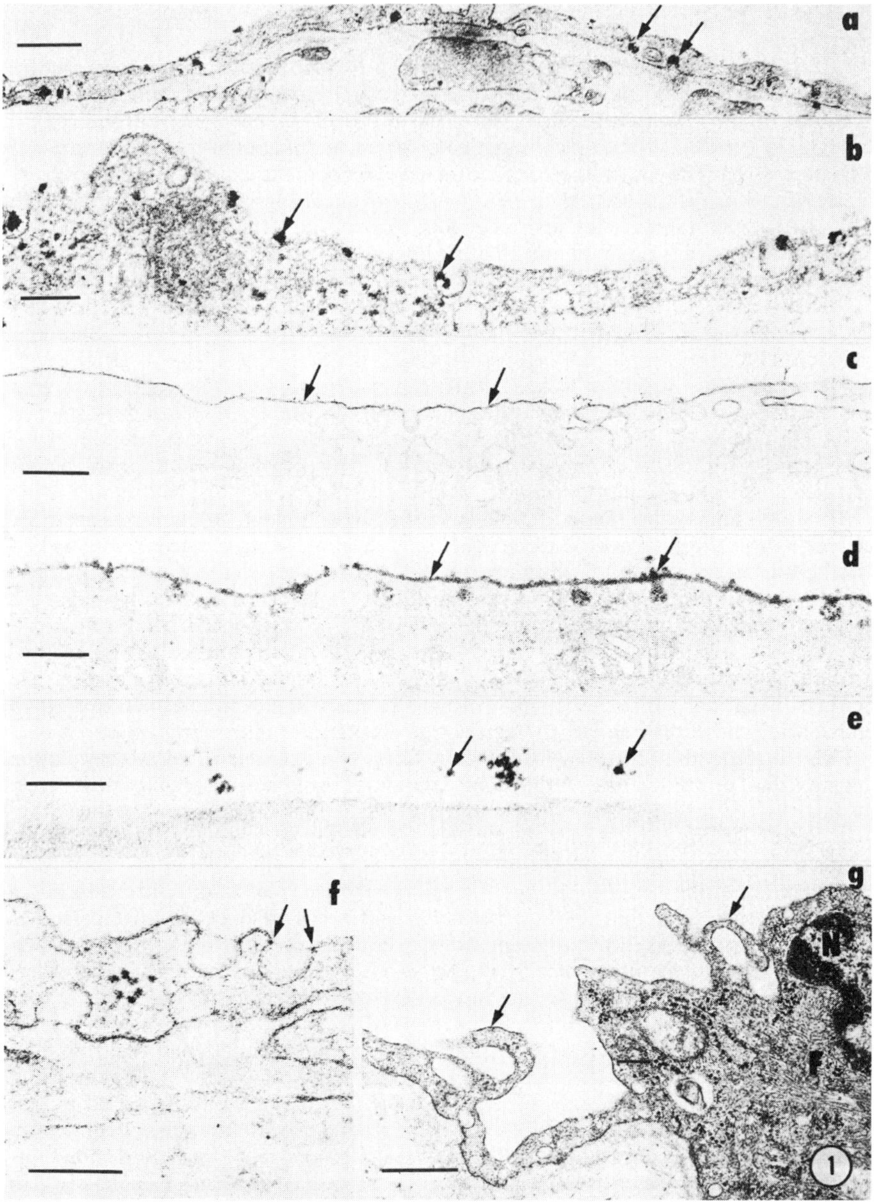

FIGURE 1. Enzymes of the endothelial plasma membrane and associated caveolae. (**a**) Cytochemical localization of ATPase on a capillary endothelial cell of fixed rat lung incubated with lead nitrate and ATP. Reaction product, indicating sites of ATPase activity, is specifically localized in caveolae *(arrows)*. *Bar* = 0.2 μm. (**b**) Cytochemical localization of 5′-nucleotidase activity on caveolae facing the vascular lumen *(arrows)*. *Bar* = 0.1 μm. (**c**) Immunocytochemical localization of ACE on a pulmonary endothelial cell in culture. Cells were incubated unfixed with antibodies to ACE, then with a secondary antibody conjugated to peroxidase. The peroxidase

result of occlusion and as a result of the actions of substances released by platelets and leukocytes.

Normally the endothelium is antithrombogenic, in part as a consequence of its ability to synthesize and release PGI_2 and its surface ADPase.[21,22] The hemostatic potential of the pulmonary endothelium is highly regulated (for review see ref. 23).

Recent studies indicate that endothelial cells become procoagulant when exposed to bacterial endotoxin, thrombin, or interleukin-1.[24–26] The procoagulant activity is due to the increased synthesis and expression of thromboplastin (tissue factor, factor III), which can initiate blood coagulation via both the extrinsic and intrinsic pathways.[27,28] It potentiates the factor-VIIa-mediated cleavage of factor X to factor Xa (extrinsic pathway), and of factor IX to factor IXa (intrinsic pathway). The latter appears to be the primary role for thromboplastin in endothelial cells.[29] In the presence of factor VIII, factor IXa further activates factor X. Factor Xa, formed via either pathway, then converts prothrombin to thrombin in a reaction that requires factor V. Thrombin converts soluble fibrinogen to insoluble fibrin, activates platelets, and inhibits vessel wall fibrinolytic activity.[30,31]

The endothelial surface provides all of the factors necessary for these procoagulant mechanisms to proceed. Thus, endothelial cells not only express thromboplastin activity, but also possess specific binding sites for factors VII, IX, and X, and synthesize factor V.[32] Factors IX and X bound to the endothelial cell surface can be readily activated to factors IXa and Xa, respectively, and prothrombin can be activated on the endothelial surface by factor Xa.[29,33,34]

In contrast to their lack of procoagulant activity, resting pulmonary endothelial cells possess marked fibrinolytic activity. This is due to their ability to synthesize and secrete plasminogen activators (tissue-plasminogen activators and urokinases).

Endotoxin dramatically suppresses the fibrinolytic activity of bovine pulmonary arterial endothelial cells.[35] Like the thromboplastin-stimulating effects of endotoxin, the fibrinolytic suppressive effects are slow in onset, and are seen with low concentrations of endotoxin. The endotoxin-induced inhibitor has an approximate molecular mass of 50 kDa, and is relatively labile,[36] distinguishing it from the unusually stable plasminogen activator inhibitor reported in bovine aortic endothelial cells.[37]

Thus, the hemostatic potential of the pulmonary endothelium results from a

moiety was reacted with 3,3′-diaminobenzidine in the presence of $H_2 2O_2$. The electron-dense reaction product indicating sites of immunoreactive ACE *(arrows)* is localized along the plasma membrane, including caveolae. *Bar* = 0.2 μm. **(d)** Immunocytochemical localization of CPN. Bovine pulmonary artery endothelial cells were incubated with antibodies to bovine plasma CPN and then treated as in **c.** Reaction product is on the plasma membrane and associated caveolae *(arrows)*. *Bar* = 0.2 μm. **(e)** Immunocytochemical localization of carbonic anhydrase. Bovine pulmonary endothelial cells were incubated with antibodies to carbonic anhydrase, then with secondary antibodies conjugated to ferritin. Sites of reactivity *(arrows)* are localized on the plasma membrane; the ferritin tag is restricted by a layer approximately 100Å thick. *Bar* = 0.5 μm. **(f)** Part of a capillary endothelial cell of a rat lung prepared for electron microscopy by standard techniques. Caveola membranes appear to be of unit membrane construction, whereas the diaphragm is composed of a single lamella. Dense knobs at junctions of diaphragm with caveola membrane and plasma membrane *(arrows)* may represent a skeletal rim or ring of beads, which could help to maintain patency of the stoma and integrity of the diaphragm. Some substructural beading of caveolae membranes can be seen. *Bar* = 0.1 μm. **(g)** Portion of an endothelial cell with its nucleus (*N*). Fibrillar strands (*F*) are present in the subnuclear cytoplasm. Endothelial projections *(arrows)* occur both on the main body of the cell and on the tenuous peripheral portions. *Bar* = 10 μm. (From Ryan and Ryan.[3] Reprinted with permission from *Circulation.*)

complex balance between active factors that have opposing biological actions and between active factors and specific inhibitors.

The dual effects of endotoxin on procoagulant and fibrinolytic activity would render the endothelial surface thrombogenic, and could contribute to the disseminated intravascular coagulation and fibrin deposition seen in severe sepsis or in the local occlusion characteristic of failed implants. In addition to its effects on hemostatic potential, endotoxin causes structural and metabolic changes in pulmonary endothelial cells and an increase in permeability of the endothelial layer.[38]

INTERACTIONS WITH COMPLEMENT AND IMMUNE COMPONENTS

As described above, the endothelium in a quiescent state is antithrombogenic but can be induced to become procoagulant. Similarly, normal endothelium is immunologically privileged[39] but can be stimulated to express Fc and C3b receptors by infection with viruses, and by exposure to endotoxin, white cell lysates, trypsin, or antibodies to endothelial enzymes (such as ACE and CPN) in the presence of complement.[6,40,41]

From the above studies, we speculated that circulating immune complexes with or without bound complement (C) components may initiate or contribute to the pulmonary inflammatory response once pulmonary endothelial cells have been altered, exposing the C3b and Fc-IgG receptors. The ability of lysates of PMN white blood cells and two viruses capable of infecting endothelial cells to unmask these receptors is likely to be of pathophysiologic significance. First, white blood cells activated by an anaphylatoxin such as C5a (a small peptide released from the activated fifth component of complement)[42] or by immune complexes[43] are known to marginate and attach to endothelial cells *in vivo.*[44] Secondly, endothelial cells infected with certain viruses acquire the capacity to bind PMNs, and the PMNs thus bound become adherent for other PMNs.[45] White blood cell aggregates might be expected to unmask receptors on endothelial cells. The stagnant or reduced blood flow caused by the mechanical blockage by white cell aggregates and emboli would favor binding of immune complexes with or without bound C components. In turn, endothelial cell-bound immune complexes would provide further stimuli for complement activation and complement-linked immune lysis. Presumably, this series of reactions would be most likely to occur under conditions of reduced blood flow such as in small diameter or occluded grafts.

This concept became even more plausible when we were able to show that normal undamaged bovine pulmonary endothelial cells have receptors for Clq, the binding portion of the first component of complement (FIG. 2).[46] The binding of ^{125}I-labeled Clq was dose-dependent, reversible, and saturable. The binding occurred via the collagenous portion of the molecule as was shown by two different protocols; first, purified ^{125}I-labeled Clq heads did not bind to the cells, and second, cell-bound native ^{125}I-labeled Clq was removed after treatment of the cells with collagenase at 37°C. Macromolecular C1 did not bind to the cells. In addition, rosettes were formed between endothelial cells incubated first with native Clq followed by sheep erythrocytes sensitized with specific IgG antibody (EA). This indicated that the Clq tails were bound to receptors and the globular heads were free to bind the Fc-IgG on the erythrocytes. Without pretreatment of the cells with Clq, no rosettes were formed since undamaged cells have no Fc receptors.[14,40]

Binding of circulating immune complexes to pulmonary endothelium via the Clq ligand-receptor and activation of complement and other inflammatory pathways could result in exposing the C3b and Fc-IgG receptors. This would enhance the binding to the endothelial cells of other immune complexes and eventually the influx of PMNs. As a result, inflammation and tissue damage would be expected to occur. Thus, it is quite feasible that the overall pathophysiologic effects of circulating immune complexes would have as their origin the endothelial cell-bound immune complexes.[12,41]

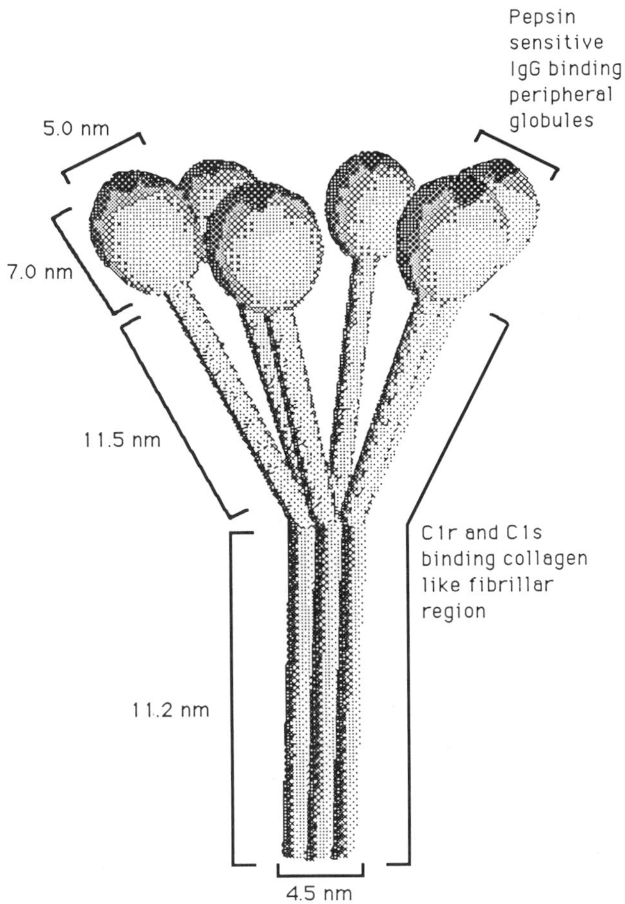

FIGURE 2. A pictorial representation of the structure of Clq. The six globular heads contain the binding sites for immunoglobin. The collagen-like portion is located in the stem-like tail region and bears the Clr and Cls binding sites.

INTERACTIONS WITH NEUTROPHILS

Endothelial cells do not normally interact with circulating unstimulated neutrophils and even when neutrophils marginate under physiologic conditions they do not cause vascular damage. On the contrary, activated neutrophils produce a spectrum of products, including proteolytic enzymes and reactive oxygen species, which have the potential to damage the endothelial layer. In collaborative studies[47] we showed that human blood neutrophils stimulated by a variety of agents have cytotoxic effects on bovine pulmonary artery endothelial cells. Effective agonists included immune complexes, opsonized zymosan, and 12-*O*-tetradecanoyl phorbol acetate. Unstimulated human neutrophils and neutrophils stimulated with *N*-formyl-methionyl-leucyl-phenylalanine or with platelet-activating factor failed to induce significant killing even though secretory release of lysosomal enzymes occurred. In comparing the effects of the different agonists, endothelial cell killing showed a better correlation with the production of H_2O_2 than with the generation of O_2^-. Endothelial cell killing by stimulated human neutrophils was inhibited by catalase but not by soybean trypsin inhibitor or superoxide dismutase. Killing was also inhibited by two scavengers (*N*,*N*-dimethylthiourea and D-mannitol) of hydroxyl radical and by deferoxamine mesylate, an iron-chelator. Iron-saturated deferoxamine mesylate was significantly less effective in protecting the endothelial cells against killing. Agents that were protective against endothelial cell killing did not interfere with the generation of O_2^- in stimulated neutrophils. These results suggest that leukocyte-induced endothelial cell killing *in vitro* can be induced by some but not all agonists for neutrophils and that the killing is oxygen-dependent and may be directly due to hydroxyl radical production. In subsequent studies[48] it appeared that the source of iron necessary for conversion of H_2O_2 to hydroxyl radical (via the Fenton reaction) is provided by the endothelial cells themselves. Thus endothelial cells can participate actively in the inflammatory response and contribute to reactions that are self-damaging.

INTERACTIONS WITH SMOOTH MUSCLE CELLS

Not only do endothelial cells interact with cellular and molecular stimuli on the blood front, they also interact with the underlying smooth muscle layers. These interactions are both structural and biochemical and there is no information on the production or fate of endothelial-derived factors on endothelialized vascular prostheses.

Myoendothelial junctions (FIG. 3) occur in a number of pulmonary vessels and are frequent in small pulmonary arteries and venules. They can consist of projections either from the endothelial cell (FIG. 3) or from the smooth muscle cell (FIG. 4). The function of these structural interactions is not known, nor is it known if they play any role in endothelium-dependent smooth muscle actions. Nevertheless, many vasodilators have been shown to act indirectly on blood vessels via release of endothelial-derived relaxing factor (EDRF).[49] Indirect evidence suggests that the release of EDRF is dependent on calcium of extracellular origin.[50,51] However, the majority of the intracellular calcium signal induced by ATP, thrombin, and bradykinin is due to release of intracellular calcium. Since the efflux of calcium is a good indicator of intracellular calcium release whereas calcium influx is a good indicator of the importance of extracellular calcium in a physiological process, we set out to determine the dose-response relationship for ^{45}Ca fluxes during release of EDRF from cultured endothelial cells.[52]

As shown previously,[53] endothelial cells cultured on microcarriers[54] are capable of releasing EDRF, which can be measured by bioassay on de-endothelialized vascular smooth muscle. We have found[52] that the release of EDRF in response to bradykinin is accompanied by an increase in the influx of calcium and by an increase in the efflux of calcium. The similarity in the dose-response relationship between the calcium efflux and the release of EDRF suggests that these processes are linked in some way. The similar efflux of calcium evoked by bradykinin in the presence and absence of

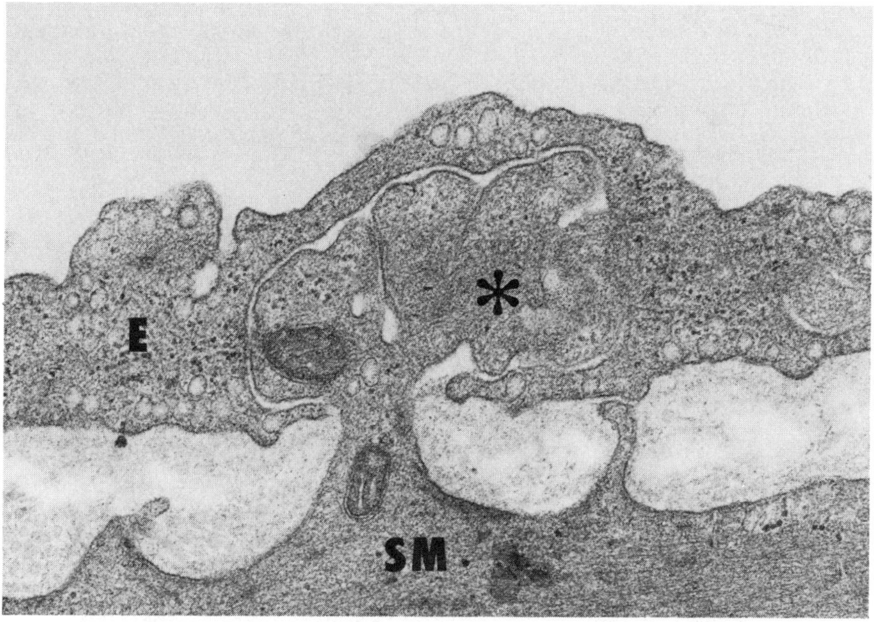

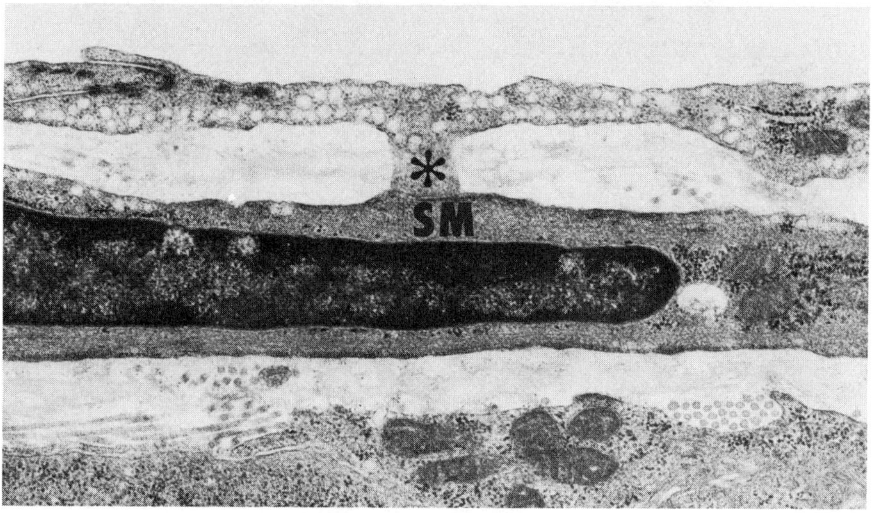

FIGURE 3. Electron micrograph of a myoendothelial junction from a small pulmonary artery (approximately 210 μm in diameter). The smooth muscle cell (*SM*) extends a projection (*) that indents the endothelial cell (*E*). Magnification: 37,000×.

FIGURE 4. Endomyothelial junction from a small pulmonary artery. In contrast to FIGURE 3, an endothelial cell process (*) protrudes to make close contact with the underlying smooth muscle layer (*SM*). Magnification: 25,000×.

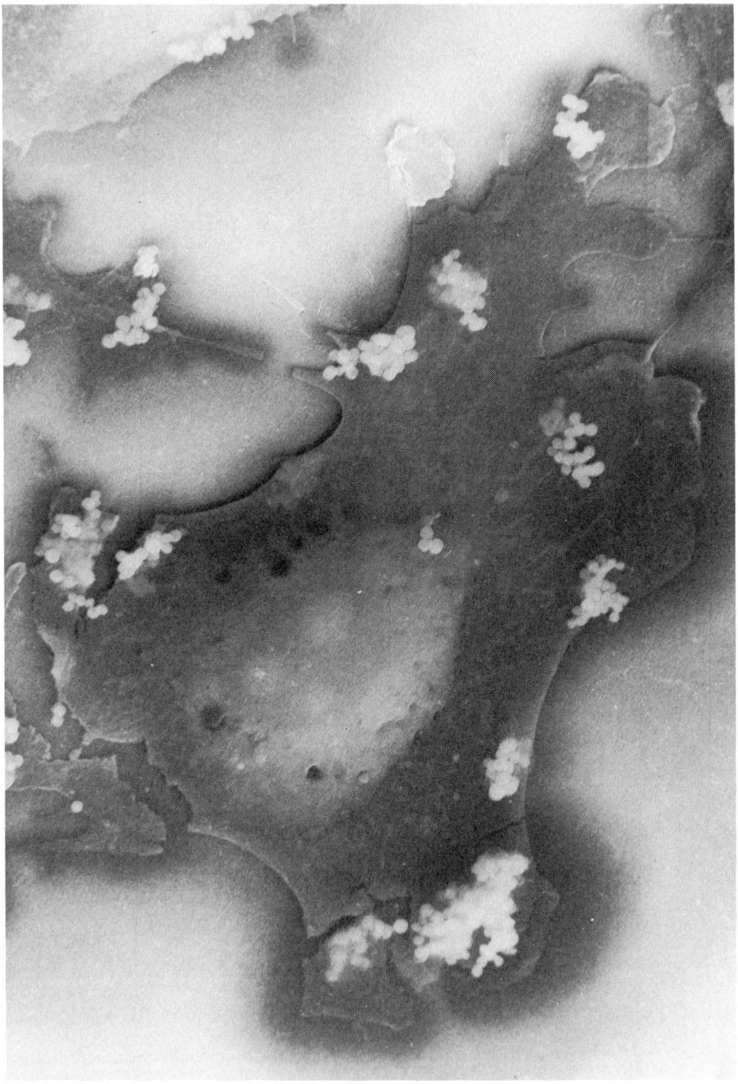

FIGURE 5. Scanning electron micrograph showing binding (15 min) of *Staphylococcus aureus* to the surface of a pulmonary endothelial cell but not to the surrounding culture flask. Magnification: 2800×.

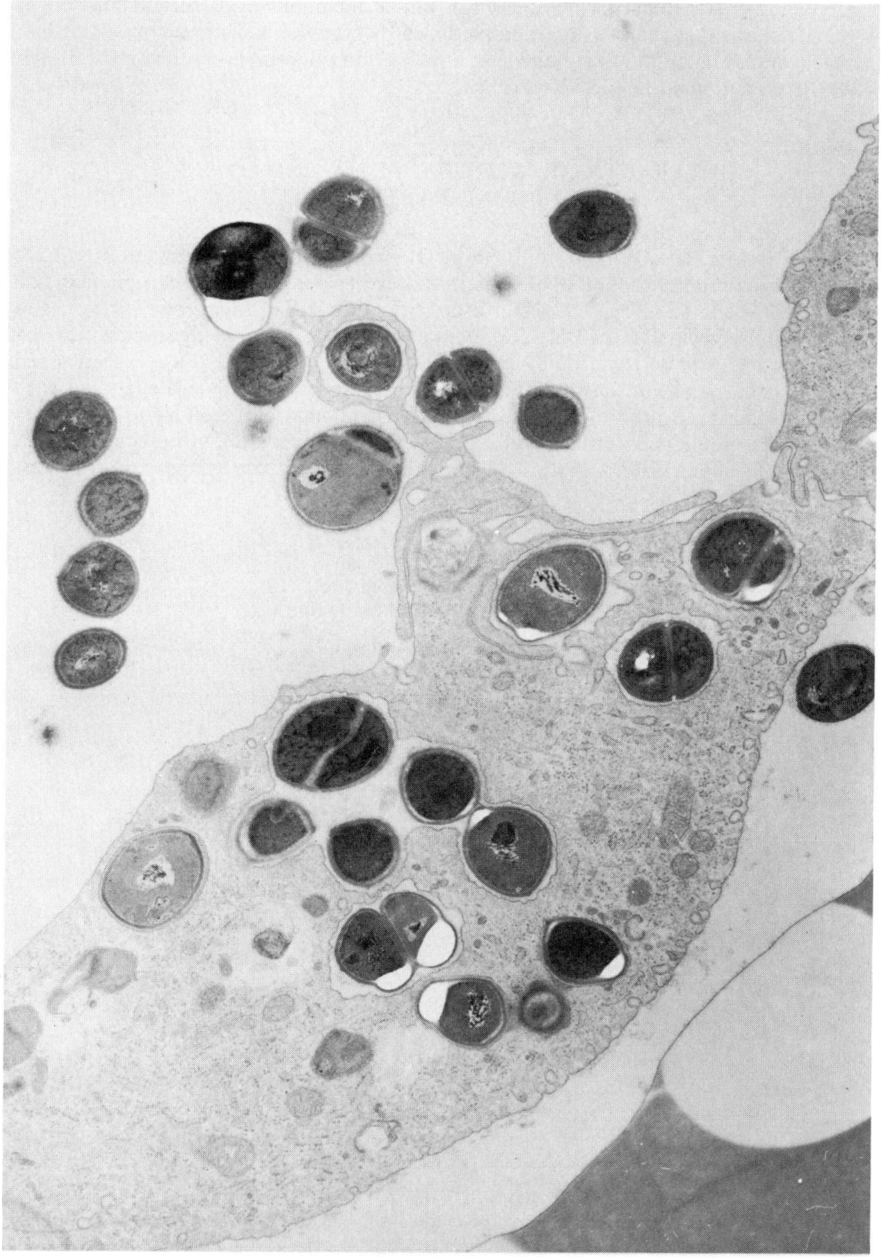

FIGURE 6. Transmission electron micrograph showing engulfment of *Staphylococcus aureus* by membrane flaps and internalization within pulmonary endothelial cell. Magnification: 19,500×.

extracellular calcium would suggest that the release of intracellular calcium is not triggered by the increased calcium influx but is mediated by a second messenger system. It seems that the calcium influx induced by bradykinin is more important than the intracellular calcium release and that it may be an essential prerequisite for EDRF release from pulmonary endothelial cells.

INTERACTIONS WITH BACTERIA AND OTHER BLOOD-BORNE PARTICULATES

Although one does not normally think of endothelium as phagocytic, we have shown that pulmonary endothelial cells in culture (passages 9–12) can phagocytize polystyrene beads (5–20 μ), cholesterol crystals, heat-killed *S. aureus* (0.2 μ), and fixed swelled red cells (10 μ). Both confluent and dividing cultures ingest particles in a time-dependent manner. Within 30 minutes, *S. aureus* are bound (FIG. 5), entrapped by pseudopodia, and internalized (FIG. 6). After 7 hours the cells are engorged with bacteria (>9 per cell profile). Recognition and entrapment of a bacterium appears to elicit further pseudopod activity and bacteria frequently are taken up consecutively and internalized as clusters. Within 12 hours lysosomal activity is apparent. Fluores-

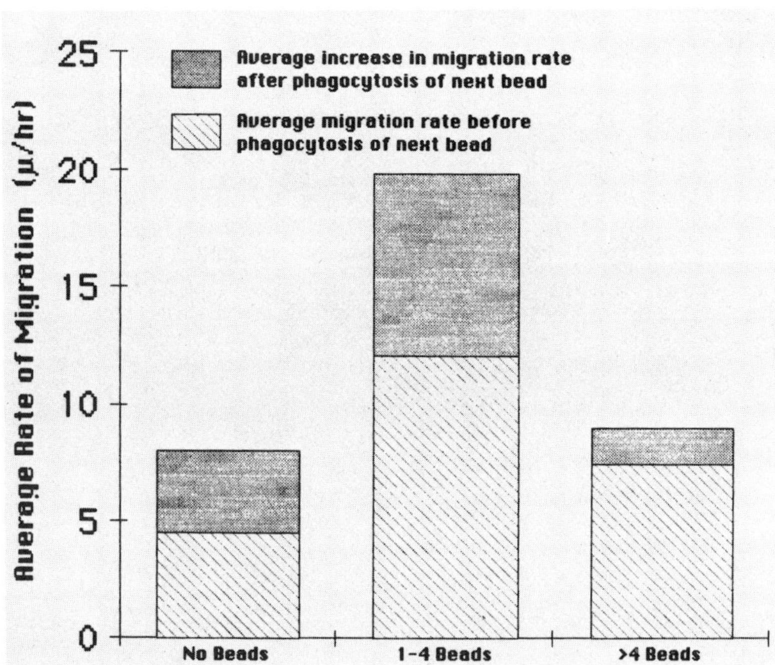

FIGURE 7. This figure illustrates the average increase in the rate of migration of an endothelial cell after the phagocytosis of another bead. Cells are categorized by number of beads initially ingested. Those cells initially containing no beads experience a significant "acceleration," and those that had ingested 1–4 beads before phagocytosis of another tend to undergo an even greater increase in migration rate. As endothelial cells collect more beads the increase in migration rate is less, as suggested by the small acceleration experienced by cells with more than 4 beads.

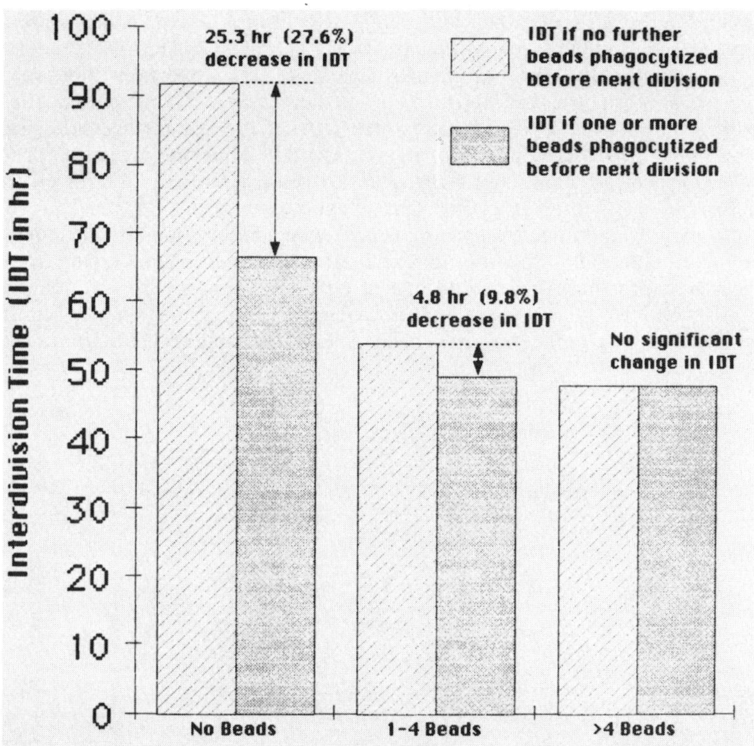

FIGURE 8. Effect of phagocytosis on interdivision time (IDT). The wounded monolayer assay was used. This bar graph reveals the effects of phagocytosis after wounding on the interdivision time of endothelial cells in three bead categories (based on number of beads initially ingested). Noticeably, those endothelial cells initially containing no beads experience a sharp decrease in the IDT after phagocytosis. For cells containing 1–4 beads, the IDT is shortened, but to a lesser extent, and those with more than 4 beads show only a negligible change in IDT. It is significant that cells not associated with beads before or after wounding have IDTs that, on the average, are nearly double the IDTs of cells that phagocytize at least one bead through the course of the experiment (92 vs. 52 h).

cent staining of mitochondria, cytoskeleton, and Golgi apparatus with monoclonal antibodies indicates marked intracellular rearrangement to accommodate ingested particles.

We have measured parameters of division and migration behavior previously using time-lapse cinematography.[55] We now have developed a system for time-lapse video recording of endothelial cells that can be interfaced with a Southern Micro Instruments Micro-comp PM interactive system and software. The data are analyzed by Quiktrak, a computer program written in this laboratory.[56] The program can (1) print several statistical reports relating the data from various perspectives of analysis; (2) print genealogy charts for each cell with its relation to its clone members; (3) print a trace of the cells migration pattern; and (4) create data files that can be interfaced with Lotus 1-2-3 and other spreadsheet and graphical software packages available.

Through the use of this system we can define the parameters of endothelial activation in terms of migratory and replicative ability. Phagocytosis appears to stimulate both endothelial cell migration (FIG. 7), division (FIG. 8), and further phagocytic activity (FIG. 9). At division, particles are apportioned between the daughter cells. Normally, endothelial cells do not express Fc receptors, but after phagocytosis they show a positive rosette assay with IgG-coated erythrocytes (EA 7S), indicating that Fc receptors have become unmasked.[6,7] Thus phagocytosis appears to activate this aspect of endothelial cells as well. Even low wall shear stresses prevent phagocytosis of particles, suggesting that phagocytosis may be a mechanism that comes into play in obstructed vessels or vessels where injury has altered recognition between endothelium and blood-borne particulates. In conditions following implantation of vascular prostheses one might expect partial occlusion with little flow giving opportunities both for phagocytosis and subsequently for immune complex binding.

Like professional phagocytes, endothelial cells are capable of discriminating on the

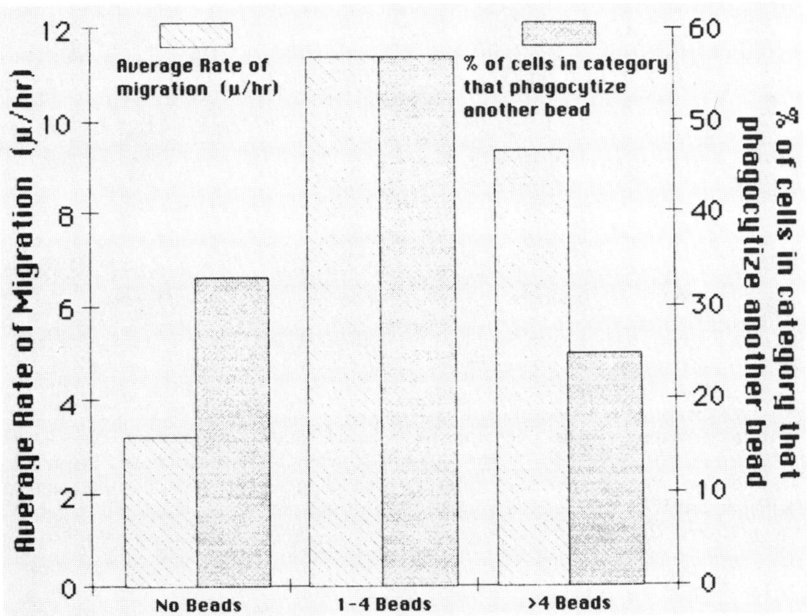

FIGURE 9. This figure shows both the average rate of migration of endothelial cells and their propensity to phagocytize beads, each as a function of the number of beads initially inside the cells. The average migration rate of cells with 1–4 beads is over three times greater than those with no beads, suggesting an activation mechanism. Though cells appear to slow down as they collect relatively large numbers of beads, their migration rates are still larger than those without beads. In addition, cells tend to phagocytize more beads "per capita" if they already contain a few beads, while those that have no beads have a lesser tendency to begin phagocytosis, and those that contain many beads have even a lesser such tendency. The graphic correlation between migration rates and propensities to phagocytize beads suggests that those cells that move about more are likely to encounter and absorb more beads. Qualitatively this correlation is valid in part, although cells with 1–4 beads appear much more "aggressive" than others when viewed in time-lapse. [Note: In determining the percentage of cells in each category that phagocytizes another bead, those cells that were within 10 h of division were excluded from the statistics, as they had insufficient time to encounter and ingest another bead.]

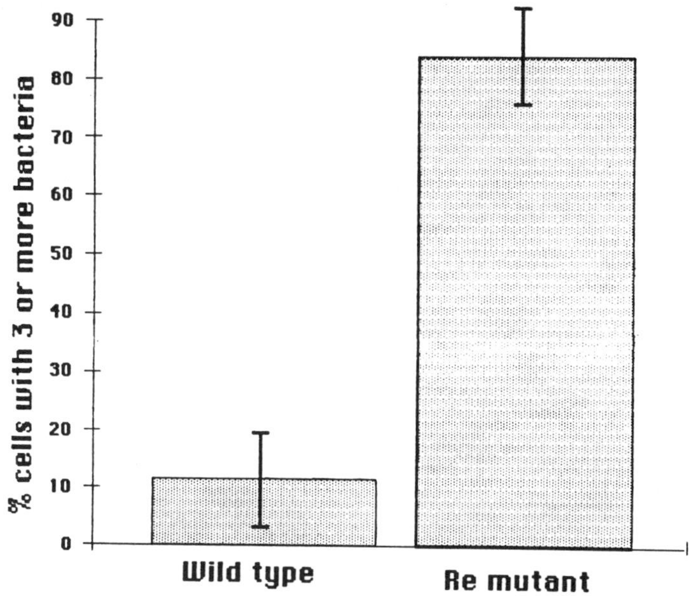

FIGURE 10. Phagocytosis of *S. minnesota* by pulmonary endothelial cells. The wild type (S form) is not phagocytized to any great extent, while the Re mutant binds and undergoes phagocytosis. Fifteen-minute incubation time, no serum, 10 bacteria per cell.

basis of surface molecules. For example, in contrast to the S-form of *Salmonella minnesota,* its Re mutant binds to endothelial cells and the binding triggers an oxidative burst that can be measured as superoxide anion (O_2^-) release.[57] Pulmonary endothelial cells show a clear discrimination between the wild and mutant forms in terms of binding and uptake (FIG. 10). However, triggering of an oxidative burst may not result in effective bacterial killing. Other studies[58,59] have demonstrated that endothelial cells are able to generate and secrete O_2^-. The signal transduction mechanism of O_2^- release by endothelial cells appears to involve synergistic effects of protein kinase C and Ca^{2+} mobilization.[57,59] These findings are of particular interest since we have found that the effects of platelet-activating factor on endothelial cells may also include β-adrenergic receptor desensitization and a mechanism involving C-kinase.[9] It appears that both Ca^{2+} influx and activation of C-kinase are required for eliciting full physiologic responses from pulmonary endothelial cells.

CONCLUSION

It is clear from the foregoing that there are a number of stimuli, including phagocytosis, that can activate endothelium. In addition to activation of hemostatic and immunologic mechanisms, endothelium can be induced to secrete proteases in response to angiogenic stimuli.[60] Furthermore, the activation process involves behavioral changes (increase in division and migration rates) that may be important in the replicative phase during the resolution of vascular damage and during endothelialization of vascular grafts. It is not yet known whether all aspects of endothelial activation occur concomitantly; nevertheless, they share some common mechanisms of cellular signal transduction.

Clearly, when the endothelium is absent, as in the implantation of an artificial biomaterial, both the constitutive and inducible functions are lost. However, even during re-endothelialization a number of situations could arise that would be expected to alter the normal interactions of endothelial cells with blood-borne vasoactive substances and to alter the communication systems between endothelium and other cell types. New probes, such as monoclonal antibodies to activated endothelial cells, should lead to improved understanding of modulations of endothelial structure, function, and behavior.

ACKNOWLEDGMENTS

It is a pleasure to thank Carlos Diaz-Silveira for typing the manuscript.

REFERENCES

1. Ryan, U. S. 1986. Pulmonary endothelium: A dynamic interface. Clin. Invest. Med. **9:** 124–132.
2. Ryan, U. S. 1982. Structural bases for metabolic activity. Ann. Rev. Physiol. **44:** 223–239.
3. Ryan, U. S. & J. W. Ryan. 1984. Cell biology of pulmonary endothelium. Circulation **70:** III-46–III-62.
4. Vanhoutte, P. M. & D. S. Houston. 1985. Platelets, endothelium and vasospasm. Circulation **72:** 728–734.
5. Warren, J. S., P. A. Ward & K. J. Johnson. 1987. Mechanisms of damage to pulmonary endothelium. *In* Pulmonary Endothelium in Health and Disease. U. S. Ryan, Ed. Marcel Dekker. New York. pp. 107–120.
6. Ryan, U. S. 1986. Metabolic activity of pulmonary endothelium: Modulation of structure and function. Ann. Rev. Physiol. **48:** 263–277.
7. Ryan, U. S., G. Maxwell, B. Olazabal, M. Hart & L. Mayfield. 1986. Endothelial Cell Phagocytosis and Activation. FASEB **45:** 217 (Abstr. 366).
8. Johns, A., U. S. Ryan & C. Van Breemen. 1987. Bradykinin induced calcium fluxes and EDRF release in cultured endothelial cells. Circulation. In press.
9. Grigorian, G. Yu., S. M. Danilov & U. S. Ryan. 1986. Alteration in β-adrenergic stimulation of pulmonary endothelial adenylate cyclase after treatment with PAF, U46619 and PMA. Circulation **74** (Suppl., Part 2): II-241 (Abstr. 962).
10. Ryan, U. S. 1985. Processing of angiotensin and other peptides by the lungs. *In* Handbook of Physiology: The Respiratory System 1 (Chap. 10). A. P. Fishman & A. B. Fisher, Eds.: 351–364. American Physiological Society. Bethesda, MD.
11. Ryan, U. S., J. W. Ryan, C. Whitaker & A. Chiu. 1976. Localization of angiotensin converting enzyme (kininase II). II. Immunocytochemistry and immunofluorescence. Tissue Cell **8:** 125–146.
12. Ryan, U. S. & J. W. Ryan. 1983. Endothelial cells and inflammation. *In* Clinics in Laboratory Medicine, Vol. 3. P. A. Ward, Ed.: 577–599. W. B. Saunders. Philadelphia.
13. Ferreira, S. H. & J. R. Vane. 1967. Prostaglandins. Their disappearance from and release into the circulation. Nature **216:** 868–873.
14. McGiff, J. C., N. A. Terrango, J. C. Strand, J. B. Lee, A. J. Lonigro & K. K. F. Ng. Selective passage of prostaglandins across the lung. Nature **216:** 762–766.
15. Dusting, G. J., S. Moncada & J. R. Vane. 1978. Recirculation of prostacyclin (PGI_2) in the dog. Br. J. Pharmacol. **64:** 315–320.
16. Piper, P. J., J. R. Tippins, M. N. Samhoun, H. R. Morris, G. W. Taylor & C. M. Jones.

1981. SRS-A and its formation by the lung. Bull. Eur. Physiopathol. Resp. (Clin. Resp. Physiol.) **17:** 571–583.
17. GILLIS, C. N. & B. R. PITT. 1982. The fate of circulating amines within the pulmonary circulation. Ann. Rev. Physiol. **44:** 269–281.
18. SMITH, U. & J. W. RYAN. 1971. Pinocytotic vesicles of the pulmonary endothelial cell. Chest **59:** 12s–15s.
19. RYAN, J. W. & U. SMITH. 1971. Metabolism of adenosine-5-monophosphate during circulation through the lungs. Trans. Assoc. Am. Physicians **84:** 297–306.
20. PEARSON, J. D., J. S. CARLTON, A. HUTCHINGS & J. L. GORDON. 1978. Uptake and metabolism of adenosine by pig aortic endothelial and smooth muscle cells in culture. Biochem. J. **170:** 265–271.
21. CRUTCHLEY, D. J., U. S. RYAN & J. W. RYAN. 1980. Effects of aspirin and dipyridamole on the degradation of adenosine diphosphate by cultured cells derived from bovine pulmonary artery. J. Clin. Invest. **66:** 29–35.
22. CRUTCHLEY, D. J., J. W. RYAN, U. S. RYAN & G. H. FISHER. 1983. Bradykinin-induced release of prostacyclin and thromboxanes from bovine pulmonary artery endothelial cells. Studies with lower homologs and calcium antagonists. Biochim. Biophys. Acta **751:** 99–107.
23. CRUTCHLEY, D. J. 1987. Hemostatic potential of the pulmonary endothelium. *In* The Pulmonary Circulation in Health and Disease. J. A. Will, C. A. Dawson, E. K. Weir & K. Buckner, Eds.: 351–361. Academic. Orlando, FL.
24. COLUCCI, M., G. BALCONI, R. LORENZET, A. PIETRA, D. LOCATI, M. B. DONATI & N. SEMERARO. 1983. Cultured human endothelial cells generate tissue factor in response to endotoxin. J. Clin. Invest. **71:** 1893–1896.
25. BROX, J. H., B. OSTERUD, E. BJORKLID & J. W. FENTON. 1984. Production and availability of thromboplastin in endothelial cells: The effects of thrombin, endotoxin and platelets. Br. J. Haematol. **57:** 239–246.
26. BEVILACQUA, M. P., J. S. POBER, G. R. MAJEAU, R. S. COTRAN & M. A. GIMBRONE. 1984. Interleukin-1 (IL-1) induces biosynthesis and cell surface expression of procoagulant activity in human vascular endothelial cells. J. Exp. Med. **160:** 618–623.
27. NEMERSON, Y. & F. A. PITLICK. 1972. The tissue factor pathway of blood coagulation. Prog. Hemostas. Thromb. **1:** 1–37.
28. OSTERUD, B. & S. I. RAPAPORT. 1977. Activation of factor IX by the reaction product of tissue factor and factor VII: Additional pathway for initiating blood coagulation. Proc. Natl. Acad. Sci. U.S.A. **74:** 5260–5264.
29. STERN, D. M., P. NAWROTH, D. HANDLEY & W. KISIEL. 1985. An endothelial cell-dependent pathway of coagulation. Proc. Natl. Acad. Sci. U.S.A. **82:** 2523–2527.
30. LOSKUTOFF, D. J. 1979. Effect of thrombin on the fibrinolytic activity of cultured bovine endothelial cells. J. Clin. Invest. **64:** 329–332.
31. GELEHRTER, T. D. & R. SZNYCER-LASZUK. 1986. Thrombin induction of plasminogen activator-inhibitor in cultured human endothelial cells. J. Clin. Invest. **77:** 165–169.
32. CERVENY, T. J., D. N. FASS & K. G. MANN. Synthesis of coagulation factor V by cultured aortic endothelium. Blood **63:** 1467–1474.
33. STERN, D. M., M. DRILLINGS, W. KISIEL, P. P. NAWROTH, H. L. NOSSEL & K. LAGAMMA. Activation of factor IX bound to cultured bovine aortic endothelial cells. Proc. Natl. Acad. Sci. U.S.A. **81:** 913–917.
34. RODGERS, G. M. & M. A. SHUMAN. Prothrombin is activated on vascular endothelial cells by factor Xa and calcium. Proc. Natl. Acad. Sci. U.S.A. **80:** 7001–7005.
35. CRUTCHLEY, D. J., L. B. CONANAN & U. S. RYAN. 1985. Endotoxin induction of a plasminogen activator inhibitor in bovine pulmonary artery endothelial cells. Fed. Proc. **44:** 1844 (Abstr. 8369).
36. CRUTCHLEY, D. J. & L. B. CONANAN. 1986. Endotoxin induction of an inhibitor of plasminogen activator in bovine pulmonary artery endothelial cells. J. Biol. Chem. **261:** 154–159.
37. LOSKUTOFF, D. J., J. A. VAN MOURIK, L. A. ERICKSON & D. LAWRENCE. 1983. Detection of an unusually stable fibrinolytic inhibitor produced by bovine endothelial cells. Proc. Natl. Acad. Sci. U.S.A. **80:** 2956–2960.

38. MEYRICK, B. O., U. S. RYAN & K. L. BRIGHAM. 1986. Direct effects of *E coli* endotoxin on structure and permeability of pulmonary endothelial monolayers and the endothelial layer of intimal explants. Am. J. Pathol. **122:** 140–151.
39. RYAN, U. S., D. R. SCHULTZ, P. DEL VECCHIO & J. W. RYAN. 1980. Endothelial cells of bovine pulmonary artery lack receptors for C3b and for the Fc portion of immunoglobulin G. Science **208:** 748–749.
40. RYAN, U. S., D. R. SCHULTZ & J. W. RYAN. 1981. Fc and C3b receptors on pulmonary endothelial cells: Induction by injury. Science **214:** 557–559.
41. SCHULTZ, D. R. & U. S. RYAN. 1987. Complement and immunoglobin ligand-receptors on pulmonary endothelial cells. *In* Endothelial Cells. U. S. Ryan, Ed. CRC Press. Boca Raton, FL.
42. HUGLI, T. E. & J. H. MULLER-EBERHARD. 1978. Anaphylatoxins C3a and C5a. Adv. Immunol. **26:** 1–53.
43. WARD, P. A. 1979. Immune complex injury of the lung. Am. J. Pathol. **97:** 85–91.
44. HENSON, P. M., K. MCCARTHY, G. L. LARSEN, R. O. WEBSTER, P. C. GICLAS, R. B. DREISIN, T. E. KING & J. O. SHAW. 1979. Complement fragments, alveolar macrophages, and alveolitis. Am. J. Pathol. **97:** 93–105.
45. MACGREGOR, R. R., H. M. FRIEDMAN, E. J. MACARAK & N. A. KEFALIDES. 1980. Virus infection of endothelial cells increases granulocyte adherence. J. Clin. Invest. **65:** 1469–1477.
46. ZHANG, S. C., D. R. SCHULTZ & U. S. RYAN. 1986. Receptor-mediated binding of Clq on pulmonary endothelial cells. Tissue Cell. **18:** 13–18.
47. VARANI, J., S. E. G. FLIGIEL, G. O. TILL, U. S. RYAN & P. A. WARD. 1985. Pulmonary endothelial cell killing by human neutrophils: Possible involvement of hydroxyl radical. Lab. Invest. **53:** 656–663.
48. GANNON, D. E., J. VARANI, G. O. TILL, U. S. RYAN, R. H. SIMON & P. A. WARD. 1986. Source of iron in neutrophil-mediated killing of endothelial cells. Am. Rev. Resp. Dis. **133:** A262 (Abstr. 01052).
49. FURCHGOTT, R. F. 1984. Ann. Rev. Pharmacol. Toxicol. **24:** 175–197.
50. EDWARDS, D. H., T. M. GRIFFITH, A. H. HENDERSON, M. J. LEWIS & A. C. NEWBY. 1985. Br. J. Pharmacol. **85:** 344P (Abstr.).
51. SINGER, H. A. & M. H. PEACH. 1982. Hypertension **4** (Suppl. 2): II-19–25.
52. JOHNS, A., R. A. KHALIL, U. S. RYAN & C. VAN BREEMEN. 1987. Endothelium-derived relaxing factor. *In* Endothelial Cells. U. S. Ryan, Ed. CRC Press. Boca Raton, FL. In press.
53. COCKS, T. M., J. A. ANGUS, J. H. CAMPBELL & G. R. CAMPBELL. 1985. Release and properties of endothelium-derived relaxing factor (EDRF) from endothelial cells in culture. J. Cell. Physiol. **123:** 310–320.
54. RYAN, U. S., M. MORTARA & C. WHITAKER. 1980. Methods for microcarrier culture of bovine pulmonary artery endothelial cells avoiding the use of enzymes. Tissue Cell **12:** 619–635.
55. RYAN, U. S., M. ABSHER, B. M. OLAZABAL, L. M. BROWN & J. W. RYAN. 1982. Proliferation of pulmonary endothelial cells: Time-lapse cinematography of growth to confluence and restitution of monolayer after wounding. Tissue Cell **14:** 637–649.
56. RYAN, U. S. & L. J. MAYFIELD. 1986. Video analysis of endothelial cells genealogy, migration and division. J. Tissue Cult. Methods **10:** 55–60.
57. RYAN, U. S. & P. M. SELVARAJ. Unpublished results.
58. ROSEN, G. M. & B. A. FREEMAN. 1984. Detection of superoxide generated by endothelial cells. Proc. Natl. Acad. Sci. U.S.A. **81:** 7269–7273.
59. MATSUBARA, T. & M. ZIFF. 1986. Superoxide anion release by human endothelial cells: Synergism between a phorbol ester and a calcium ionophore. J. Cell. Physiol. **127:** 207–210.
60. GROSS, J. L., D. MOSCATELLI & D. B. RIFKIN. 1983. Increased capillary endothelial cell protease activity in response to angiogenic stimuli in vitro. Proc. Natl. Acad. Sci. U.S.A. **80:** 2623–2627.

Adhesion of Blood Platelets to the Extracellular Matrix of Cultured Human Endothelial Cells

JAN J. SIXMA, PATRICIA F. E. M. NIEVELSTEIN, JAAP-JAN ZWAGINGA, AND PHILIP G. DE GROOT

Department of Hematology
University Hospital
3511 GV Utrecht, the Netherlands

INTRODUCTION

One of the most crucial steps in the formation of a hemostatic plug is adhesion of blood platelets to the denuded and exposed connective tissue of the vessel wall upon injury. When this adhesion is decreased as in the Bernard-Soulier syndrome or in von Willebrand's disease, a severely prolonged bleeding time ensues. Increase of platelet adhesion may be even more important, because it may offer an explanation as to why a limited injury to the vessel wall may occasionally lead to the exaggerated hemostatic reaction causing thrombosis.

The study of the process of platelet adhesion and of local thrombus formation has long been hampered by the limitations of *in vivo* experimentation in animals. The introduction by Baumgartner and his associates of a perfusion system in which an everted vessel segment was exposed to standardized flow provided a convenient *in vitro* model.[1-3] When first introduced, rabbit aorta was used as blood vessel. More recently, to avoid problems introduced by species differences, human vessels were employed, first postmortem renal arteries and later umbilical arteries because of their more general availability and reproducible wall thickness.[4,5]

The use of everted vessels as model for injured vessel walls has a number of disadvantages. The removal of the endothelium, whether it is carried out by ballooning or by exposure to air, followed by mounting it inside out on the central rod, may damage the subendothelium. A potentially more important problem is that the time between obtaining a vessel segment from the intact animal or umbilical cord and using it for perfusion studies is sometimes long, and this may result in denaturation of certain vessel wall components. In practice these disadvantages may not be very important, because gentle handling and experience may minimize the damage, and even prolonged storage at 4°C has been shown not to influence platelet adhesion.

A more important limitation of the use of blood vessels, however, is that it does not allow the study of the variability of the subendothelium as a function of the exposure of endothelium to various physiologic conditions and/or stimuli. Another problem with denuded vessel segments is that it is difficult to relate the binding of specific proteins to the vessel wall and their subsequent functional role in platelet adhesion, because, perhaps due to the stretching associated with mounting the vessel inside out on a rod, the vessel wall may act as a sponge, and proteins may bind to many irrelevant sites in deeper layers of the vessel wall.

Neither of these limitations (the problems of damage and variable storage times) is encountered when the connective tissue matrix of cultured vessel wall cells is used as a model of the vessel wall for the study of platelet adhesion. Because this model is a further abstraction from the *in vivo* situation, it is important to consider to what extent such a model reflects what is happening in the body.

It is the purpose of this paper to discuss the use of the connective tissue matrix of human endothelial cells (endothelial cell matrix, ECM) for the study of platelet adhesion. We will show that adhesion to this matrix has many features in common with the adhesion to the vessel wall, we will highlight the advantages of the use of ECM, and we will point out where the ECM differs from the vessel wall in its properties to generate platelet adhesion.

THE PERFUSION SYSTEM

A special perfusion chamber is required to study platelet adhesion to ECM. Several chambers have been developed for this purpose.[7] The chamber developed by Sakariassen in our laboratory, which was used in the studies reported here, is shown in FIGURE 1. An extensive description of the characteristics of this chamber has been published.[9] More recently an adaptation of this chamber, containing two knobs instead of one, has been made. The advantage is that duplicate results are obtained with a single perfusion and that increased sensitivity is obtained for measuring changes in plasma components generated by the contact with the ECM (fibrinopeptide A, PGI_2, etc.). A further advantage is that the influence of upstream phenomena such as local thrombin formation or PGI_2 production on downstream platelet adhesion can be studied. Extensive testing under nonthrombogenic conditions has shown that platelet adhesion to the glass coverslip at the upstream knob shows no significant difference from that at the downstream knob. With a very thrombogenic surface, platelet deposition decreases along the glass coverslip. This phenomenon, for which the term axial dependence was coined, was found in the case of platelet adhesion to fibrillar collagen type I.[10] It is caused either by exhaustion of platelets in the boundary layer due to their massive participation in the thrombus formation or by disturbance of the boundary layer by the large thrombi. Platelet adhesion was also diminished at the second knob in such a situation.

The original perfusion chamber as described had a height of 1 mm, allowing the study of platelet adhesion up to shear rates of 1000 s^{-1}. For the study of platelet adhesion at higher shear rates up to 2000 s^{-1}, a chamber with a height of 0.6 mm was developed. For shear rates above 2000 s^{-1}, a chamber with a slit of 0.4 mm was developed but special precautions had to be taken to prevent increased turbulence at such a narrow slit.[11]

CULTURED ENDOTHELIAL CELLS AND THEIR REMOVAL

Endothelial cells to be used for platelet adhesion studies are grown on standard glass coverslips covered with gelatin. The gelatin was routinely fixed with 0.5% glutaraldehyde. As a rule human umbilical vein cells were cultured in a medium consisting of RPMI-1640 (Gibco, U.K.) substituted with 20% pooled human serum and antibiotics. Usually confluent cells from the third passage were used. Such cells can be directly exposed to flowing blood in the perfusion chamber up to shear rates of 300 s^{-1} for more than 2 hours without appreciable damage. Also short-time exposure to shear rates of 1300 s^{-1} can be performed without harm to the endothelial cell monolayer. No systematic study has been performed, as yet, on the resistance of endothelial cells to shear forces, but as we will discuss later, exposing the cells to shear may have profound influence on the ECM produced.

Ideally, removal of endothelial cells should be performed in such a way that complete removal of the cells occurs without harm to ECM, but also without extraction of material from the matrix that may influence platelet adhesion. Several methods used for removal of the cells are summarized in TABLE 1, and the reactivity of the

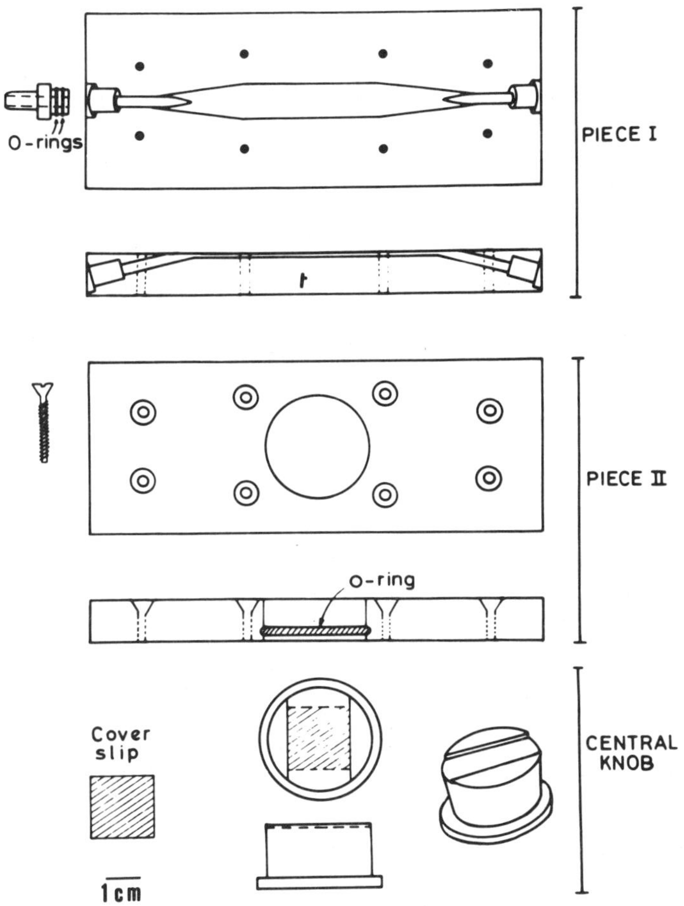

FIGURE 1. Schematic drawing of the parallel plate rectangular perfusion chamber, according to Sakariassen.[9]

remaining matrix on platelet adhesion is shown. All three methods caused similar adhesion in studies with whole normal blood, although the values with NH_4OH tended occasionally to be somewhat lower. Freeze-thawing was also compared in another experiment, and this gave results similar to EDTA or Triton X 100 (results not shown). This is surprising, because studies by Buchanan *et al.*[12,13] have demonstrated that endothelial cells produce a lipoxygenase product 13-hydroxy-octadecadienoic acid

TABLE 1. Effect of Removal Technique for Endothelial Cell on Platelet Adhesion

Removal Technique	Platelet Adhesion (% Coverage)
0.1 M NH_4OH, 30 min	32.5
0.1% Triton X 100, 30 min	43.8
50 mM EDTA, 37°C, 30 min	48.5

Mean of duplicate experiments. Perfusion time: 5 min; shear rate: 1300 s^{-1}.

(13-HODE) with an inhibitory effect on platelet adhesion, and this product is present in the extracellular matrix. Because it is a lipophilic product, treatment with Triton X-100 and NH_4OH will cause extraction, whereas EDTA and freeze-thawing will not influence its presence. Whether our results may be taken to indicate that the role of 13-HODE is less in flowing blood than in a static system remains to be determined. Currently experiments are being performed in collaboration with Dr. M. R. Buchanan in which the 13-HODE content of the matrix after removal of the endothelial cells is measured and related to platelet adhesion found with these ECMs.

The results shown in TABLE 1 were obtained with whole blood containing sufficient von Willebrand factor (vWF) to support platelet adhesion. The vWF content of the matrix is thus not critical for adhesion. Direct measurement, however, shows that treatment of the matrix with 0.1 M NH_4OH may cause partial extraction of vWF from the ECM (TABLE 2). These data indicate that this method of removal should not be used under conditions in which the vWF content is critical for platelet adhesion. In practice, the vWF content in the ECM after NH_4OH treatment is usually more or less sufficient for adhesion.

ADHESION OF PLATELETS

Evaluation of platelet adhesion to endothelial cells and to ECM can be performed in three different ways: (1) Platelets can be radiolabeled with ^{51}Cr or with ^{111}In and platelet adhesion can be estimated by counting the radioactivity present on the glass coverslip after perfusion. (2) More direct estimation can be performed by fixing the cells with glutardialdehyde followed by staining with May Grunwald-Giemsa. Evaluation is subsequently performed by morphometry on en face preparations with a specially constructed eye piece or with an automated method using an image analyzing system. Estimation of platelet adhesion to ECM of normal cultured endothelial cells with radiolabeled platelets and by direct en face evaluation shows good correlation, indicating that little platelet aggregate formation has occurred on the ECM. When aggregates are present, as is the case under special conditions, the surface coverage can

TABLE 2. Effect of Removal Technique on vWF in Matrix

Removal Technique	vWF Content ($ng/10^6$ Cells)
0.1 M NH_4OH, 30 min	9.2 ± 1.8
0.1% Triton X 100, 30 min	32.4 ± 0.8
50 mM EDTA, 37°C, 30 min	28.7 ± 2.1
Freezing-thawing	21.1 ± 0.7

Mean ± SD (n = 3). Results obtained by ELISA.

still be estimated by the en face method but no data are obtained on the size or height of the aggregates. Moreover, with large aggregates the estimation of surface coverage becomes inaccurate because the actual attachment of the basis of a large thrombus may be smaller than its maximal size as seen from above. (3) The most exact estimation of the way in which platelets adhere to ECM is performed on cross-sectioned material. For this purpose, ECM has to be embedded. Glass coverslips can be used for this purpose but the glass has to be etched away, a laborious technique. Equally good results and much easier preparation of the material has been obtained with Thermanox® (Miles, Naperville, IL) coverslips.[11] Endothelial cells grow well on such coverslips when these are covered with gelatin. Separation between the epon-embedded ECM and the coverslip is attained by heating the embedded coverslip followed by rapid cooling in liquid nitrogen, which causes separation between the epon

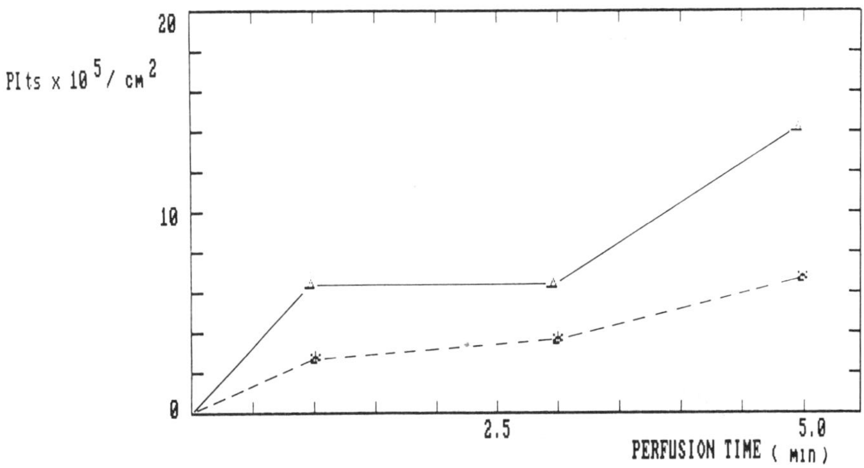

FIGURE 2. The effect of treatment of endothelial cells with acetyl salicylic acid (10 μM during 30 min) on platelet adhesion. Perfusion was for 5 min at 800 s^{-1} with reconstituted whole blood. Platelets had been labeled with ^{111}In. Platelet adhesion is given in $10^5/cm^2$. The cells are not completely confluent as is evident from the relatively high platelet adhesion; * = treatment without acetyl salicylic acid; Δ = treatment with acetyl salicylic acid.

layer and the Thermanox because of the difference in shrinkage between the two materials caused by the change in temperature. The epon-embedded ECM is then evaluated for platelet contact, spreading, and thrombus formation as described by Baumgartner *et al.*[1–3]

When confluent endothelial cells are exposed to flowing blood, little or no platelet adhesion is observed. When endothelial cells are not confluent, platelet adhesion occurs to ECM between the cells. This adhesion is partially inhibited by the prostacyclin, which is formed by the endothelial cells, as may be deduced from the increase in adhesion observed when endothelial cells have been treated with acetyl salicylic acid (FIGURE 2).

The time course of platelet adhesion to ECM is shown in FIGURE 3. Platelet adhesion is more or less linear with time for the first 5 minutes. Almost complete coverage is attained after 10 minutes of perfusion. Morphologically, the platelets are

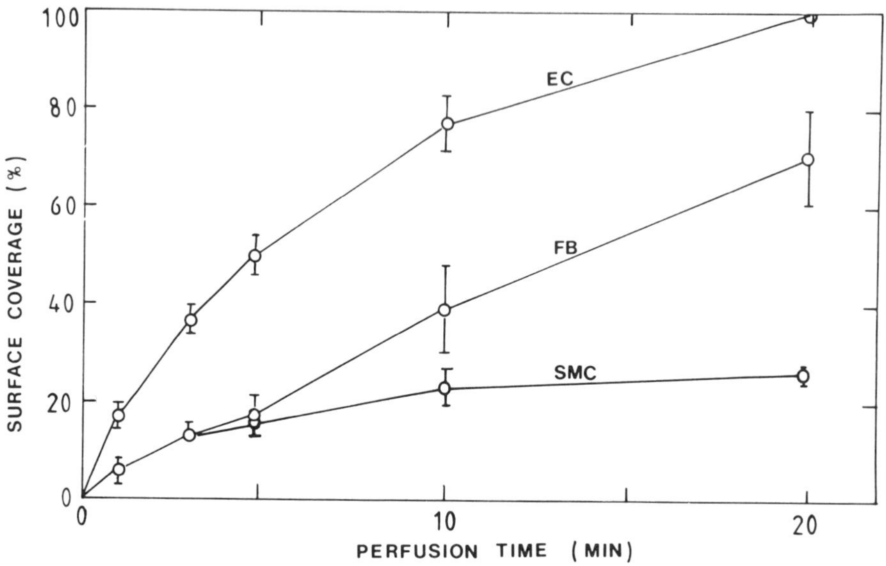

FIGURE 3. Time course of platelet adhesion to ECM, FBM, and SMCM, at 1300 s^{-1}. Evaluation of platelet adhesion was performed on en face preparations using an image analyzer (Quantimet 720, Imanco, Royston, U.K.). Platelet adhesion is expressed as percentage of the surface covered with platelets. Adhesion on SMCM is relatively low, because platelets are less spread out than on the other surfaces.

spread on the surface with little or no aggregate formation under normal conditions. Early on during the perfusion, there is preference for platelet adhesion along unidentified fibrillar structures in ECM. The shear rate dependence of adhesion of platelets to ECM is shown in FIGURE 4. Platelet adhesion increases up to a shear rate of 800 s^{-1} and then levels off or decreases slightly.

COMPARISON WITH THE MATRIX OF SMOOTH MUSCLE CELLS AND FIBROBLASTS

Platelets also adhere to the matrix of cultured smooth muscle cell (SMCM) obtained from umbilical arteries and to the matrix of cultured fibroblasts (FBM) obtained from fetal lung tissue. Platelet adhesion to the SMCM is difficult to quantitate, because the SMCM varies in thickness and adhering platelets often cannot be observed well. This variation in thickness may also influence the local shear rate, particularly so when narrow slits are used in order to attain a high shear rate. More accurate estimation of actual platelet adherence can be obtained with the use of radiolabeled platelets, and this is allowed because little or no aggregation formation occurs on SMCM. FBM is of uniform thickness, and en face evaluation gives reliable and reproducible results. Comparison of platelet adhesion from whole citrated blood to the various matrices is shown in FIGURE 3. Adhesion to SMCM and FBM is lower than to ECM, but the adhesion to SMCM may be underestimated in morphometric experiments on en face preparations. Platelets on SMCM tend to be less spread out than on ECM. The pattern of adhesion on FBM is similar to that to ECM. Platelets are spread out and show little aggregate formation. Preliminary recent data indicate that the pattern of adhesion to FBM may depend on the passage of the cell with more extensive adhesion and aggregate formation on early passage cells.

Platelet adhesion to SMCM and to FBM has a similar dependence on vWF and on fibronectin as adhesion to ECM and also similar platelet surface glycoproteins are involved (data not shown). The use of SMCM and of the much more easily studied FBM is particularly advantageous for the investigation of the contribution of exogenous vWF to platelet adhesion, because neither matrix contains vWF itself.

ROLE OF ADHESIVE PROTEINS

In previous studies with human umbilical arteries and with isolated collagen type I and III obtained from the wall of these arteries, a requirement for vWF and for fibronectin was found.[14–16] Vessel wall vWF was responsible for 40% of platelet adhesion and plasma vWF was required for optimal adhesion.[17,18] For fibronectin, the quantity present in the vessel wall was sufficient, because omission of fibronectin from the perfusate had no effect on platelet adhesion and the contribution of fibronectin was only demonstrable with the use of inhibitory polyclonal antibodies.[15] Studies on the role of vWF and fibronectin on platelet adhesion to ECM have also been performed.[19] The data for fibronectin are summarized in FIGURE 5. In contrast to the vessel wall, inhibition of platelet adhesion is seen with fibronectin-free plasma, indicating that fibronectin in the ECM is not quite sufficient for platelet adhesion. Profound inhibition was seen when a combination of fibronectin-free plasma and preincubation of ECM with antifibronectin antibodies was used. Inhibition in the ECM system was seen at a shear rate of 300 s^{-1}, lower than observed in the vessel wall system. Such differences

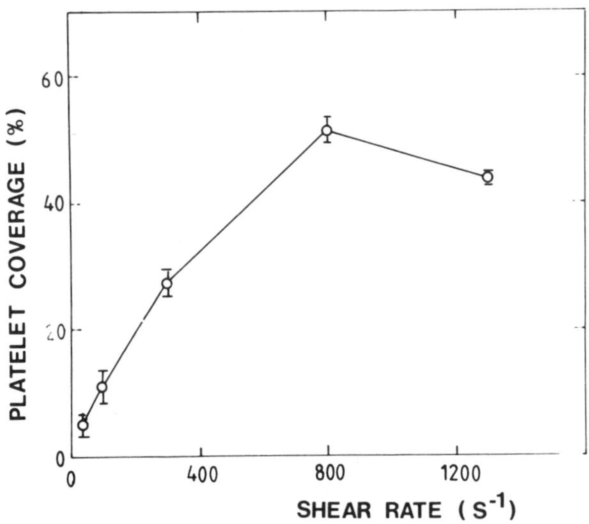

FIGURE 4. Effect of shear rate on platelet adhesion to ECM. Perfusion was for 5 min with whole citrated blood.

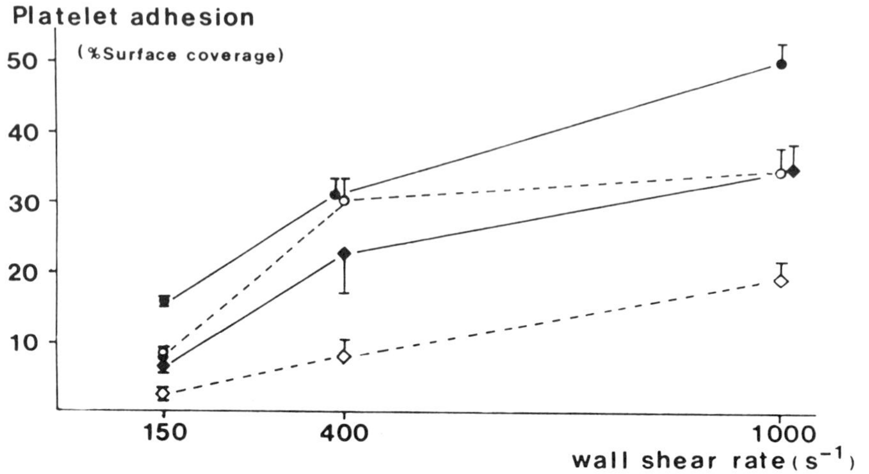

FIGURE 5. Role of fibronectin in platelet adhesion to ECM at different shear rates. Platelet perfusion was with reconstituted whole blood for 5 minutes; ● = normal blood. ○ = fibronectin-free plasma; ♦ = preincubation of the matrix with anti-fibronectin $F(ab)_2$ and perfusion with normal blood; ◇ = preincubation of the matrix and perfusion with fibronectin-free plasma. Details of the experiment have been reported elsewhere.[19]

may be due to the different types of collagen present at the different surfaces.[20] The data for vWF are summarized in TABLE 3. As in the vessel wall system, platelet adhesion has a complete dependence on vWF, but with ECM there is no need for plasma vWF. As mentioned before, the concentration of vWF is influenced by the removal procedure for the endothelial cells and lower concentrations of vWF are encountered when 0.1 M NH_4OH has been used. In that case dependence on plasma vWF may be observed.

Platelet adhesion to ECM is not dependent on thrombospondin, as was demon-

TABLE 3. Platelet Adhesion (% Surface Coverage) to Extracellular Matrix of Human Vascular Endothelial Cells: Effect of Preincubation with Anti-vWF

		Wall Shear Rate, s^{-1}			
ECM	Perfusate	100	300	800	1300
−	−	11.0 ± 2.1	26.0 ± 4.1	51.7 ± 1.5	45.0 ± 1.0
+	−	12.9 ± 2.0	25.4 ± 6.2	51.0 ± 4.0	34.1 ± 4.7
−	+	8.4 ± 1.0	17.2 ± 3.2	5.9 ± 2.9*	5.8 ± 2.8*
+	+	11.0 ± 1.3	24.4 ± 2.4	7.0 ± 2.2	2.6 ± 1.0*

The extracellular matrix (ECM) of human vascular endothelial cells was preincubated for 60 min at room temperature with CLB-RAg 35, a monoclonal antibody against the platelet-binding domain of the vWF molecule.[26] Ascites fluid was diluted 1:500 in PBS. The perfusate was preincubated with CLB-RAg 35 (ascites) for 10 min at 37°C at a 1:500 dilution in plasma. Perfusion was performed for 5 min with anticoagulated whole blood at the indicated wall shear rates. After perfusion the matrices were fixed and stained, and the percentage surface coverage determined by morphometrical evaluation. Values are the mean ± SEM; $n = 3$.

*$p < 0.001$, compared with perfusion without CLB-RAg 35 preincubation.

strated with a range of antibodies against it.[19] This does not exclude the possibility that thrombospondin has a modulating role by influencing the adhesion to other substances.

Little is known about the contribution of other substances in the ECM to platelet adhesion. Preliminary data with polyclonal antibodies against various components have suggested that laminin, collagen type VI, and nidogen may be involved.[21] ECM also synthesizes collagen type III, and this substance has been shown to support platelet adhesion when applied as an isolated substance to a glass coverslip.[19] Adhesion to collagen type III was dependent on vWF and fibronectin and this suggested that collagen type III might be the substance to which both proteins bind in ECM. Experiments with ECM from endothelial cells in which the formation of collagen had been prevented, however, showed that vWF under these conditions was still deposited in fibrillar structures together with fibronectin.[22] Direct binding of vWF to fibronectin was demonstrated under specific conditions.[23] From these data, it was suggested that vWF in the ECM involved in platelet adhesion was not associated with collagen, but direct evidence for this conclusion was lacking. Recently, we could demonstrate with monoclonal antibodies against vWF that the binding of vWF to ECM and to SMCM does not involve collagen, but rather another, as yet unidentified, substance.[24] It seems unlikely that this substance should be fibronectin. Studies with isolated collagen type I and III have demonstrated that vWF and fibronectin act independently,[16] and direct studies of binding of vWF to fibronectin using an ELISA-type setup showed no binding of vWF to fibronectin. A more likely candidate for the binding site of vWF may be a proteoglycan. It has been shown that vWF contains a heparin-binding site,[25] but the most recent data indicate that this binding site is located on a different part of the molecule than the epitope for the monoclonal antibody inhibiting vWF binding to ECM.[24,26]

ROLE OF MEMBRANE GLYCOPROTEINS IN PLATELET ADHESION TO ECM

The role of platelet membrane glycoproteins in the adhesion of platelets to ECM has been studied with monoclonal antibodies against some of these membrane glycoproteins and with platelets possessing a deficiency of relevant glycoproteins. The effect of a monoclonal against glycoprotein Ib (GP Ib) is shown in FIGURE 6. Platelet adhesion is inhibited down to a shear rate of 50 s^{-1}, whereas a monoclonal inhibiting the interaction of vWF with platelets has a less pronounced effect. This may indicate that GP Ib has another role in platelet adhesion, apart from serving as the binding site for vWF. Studies with platelets of a patient with Glanzmann's thombasthenia showed some decrease in platelet adhesion at higher shear rates, but this effect was not strong, and similar to the inhibition in platelet adhesion to the vessel wall seen in citrate blood.[27,28]

DETERMINANTS OF PLATELET ADHESION TO ECM

Studies of platelet adhesion to ECM have mostly been performed with ECM derived from human umbilical vein endothelial cells. Preliminary data obtained with ECM from human aortic endothelial cells or cells from the right atrium obtained from a patient undergoing heart transplantation are shown in TABLE 4. Platelet adhesion to the ECM of adult aorta cells was somewhat decreased, but exogenous vWF was not

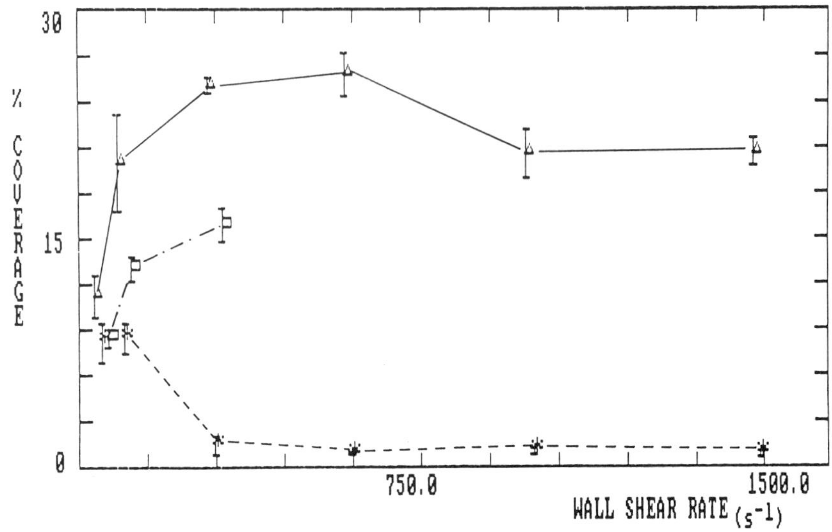

FIGURE 6. Effect of a monoclonal antibody against GP Ib (6D1, courtesy of Dr. B. Coller, SUNY at Stony Brook, Stony Brook, NY) and a monoclonal antibody against vWF (CLB-RAg 35, courtesy of Dr. J. A. van Mourik, Amsterdam) on platelet adhesion to ECM at different shear rates. Perfusion time was 5 min. The monoclonal antibodies were added as ascites at a dilution of 1:100 to the plasma: Δ = no addition; * = anti GP Ib; □ = anti vWF 35. Previous studies had shown that ascites by itself had no effect at this dilution.

required. The ECM of adult atrial cells was only studied with a human albumin solution. It is thus at present unknown whether extra exogenous vWF may have an enhancing effect. Further detailed studies are required to indicate whether the decrease in platelet adhesion to adult aorta is a general phenomenon or caused by accidental culture conditions. It will also be of interest to look at capillary endothelium.

Cultured endothelial cells differ from endothelial cells *in vivo* in that they have not been exposed to flow. Experiments in which endothelial cells were grown and maintained under flow conditions showed major differences in the morphology and

TABLE 4. Effect of Origin of ECM on Adhesion

	Platelet Adhesion	
	Normal Plasma	Human Albumin
Original endothelial cell matrix from:		
Adult aorta	16.9	25.9
Adult atrium	—	38.6
Umbilical vein	80.0[a]	50.0[a]

Platelet adhesion is expressed as percent coverage except for the umbilical vein, where data with indium-111 labeling are presented. Previous data have indicated platelet coverage correlates well with number of adhering platelets in $10^5/cm^2$.

[a]Mean of duplicate experiments. Shear rate 1300 s^{-1}, 5 min.

cytoskeletal organization of the cells.[29] Exposure to flow also appeared to have a major role in the composition of the various proteoglycans that were released from endothelial cells and deposited into the ECM.[30] It therefore seems likely that culturing endothelial cells under flow will strongly affect the adhesive properties of the ECM, but direct data are lacking.

Perhaps one of the most interesting and important variables influencing the reactivity of ECM is the effect of various stimuli on the endothelial cells. An example is the effect of thrombin. Thrombin has been shown to increase PGI_2 production; it causes release of vWF from the Weibel-Palade bodies and also increases the release of tissue plasminogen activator. Short-time exposure of endothelial cells to thrombin causes an increase in reactivity of the ECM.[31] One would expect this to be due to an increase in vWF, but direct estimation of vWF in the matrix shows no increase in local concentration. More prolonged exposure of endothelial cells to thrombin causes a decreased reactivity of the ECM and this decreased reactivity is paralleled by a diminished concentration of both vWF and fibronectin in the matrix. Preincubation of the ECM with vWF restores the reactivity completely. An effect similar to that seen with thrombin exposure is also observed with phorbol myristate acetate, which also causes release of vWF.[31] Short-term exposure gave increased adhesion, and long-term exposure also caused a decrease in the reactivity of the ECM. This was due to decreased concentration of vWF in the ECM. One would expect a diminished synthesis of vWF, but this has not been borne out by radiolabel studies and quantitation of mRNA for vWF in the endothelial cells. Two alternatives exist: increased breakdown or altered routing of recently synthesized vWF.

Stimulation of endothelial cells with interleukin-1, a stimulatory peptide secreted by monocyte-macrophages, but under special conditions also by endothelial cells themselves, also caused diminished reactivity of ECM due to a decrease in vWF. In this case, however, the decrease was due to diminished synthesis as was evident from the decrease in steady-state levels of mRNA encoding for vWF found in the cells.[32]

Effects such as these may become important in understanding some of the effects of, for instance, infection on tendency to thrombosis. Full understanding of all these effects is at present not possible, as too few of the variables are known as yet. The stimulation of endothelial cells with interleukin-1 is a case in point. Decrease in vWF causes diminished reactivity, but this is probably more than overcome *in vivo* by the increase in tissue thromboplastin formation by the endothelial cells, which is also secreted towards the ECM. Preliminary studies from our laboratory using a thrombosis model indicate that this greatly increases the thrombogenicity of the ECM.[33]

CONCLUSION: ECM AS MODEL FOR THE VESSEL WALL

Endothelial cell matrix has recently been used extensively for the study of platelet adhesion.[9,19,24,35] As shown above, many variables important for the interaction of platelets with subendothelium can be studied with the ECM. The system also has the advantage that the effect of perturbation of endothelial cells on their subsequent thrombogenicity can be studied easily. The question arises, however, as to the extent to which ECM may serve as model for the vessel wall. As demonstrated above, platelet adhesion to ECM and adhesion to the vessel wall are similarly dependent on vWF, fibronectin, and on platelet membrane glycoproteins. There are some differences, however, which are worthy of note. The shear rate dependence of the effect of vWF and fibronectin on platelet adhesion is less pronounced with ECM: *i.e.,* presence or absence of these two proteins still has an effect on platelet adhesion at relatively low shear rates.

Another difference is that in contrast to the vessel wall, ECM contains sufficient vWF and not enough fibronectin for optimal adhesion, whereas the reverse is true for the vessel wall. An important issue deserving more study with respect to the use of the matrix of cultured cells is the effect of the passage of the cells and the question of how long the cells have been allowed to stay in confluence before the matrix was harvested. For bovine smooth muscle cells, it was recently pointed out that these cells produce very little collagen while proliferating rapidly. Collagen production became much more prominent once confluence had been reached.[34]

REFERENCES

1. BAUMGARTNER, H. R. & R. MUGGLI. 1976. Adhesion and aggregation: Morphological demonstration and quantitation in vivo and in vitro (Chap. 1.) *In* Platelets in Biology and Pathology. J. L. Gordon, Ed.: 23–60. North-Holland. Amsterdam.
2. BAUMGARTNER, H. R., R. MUGGLI, T. B. TSCHOPP & V. T. TURITTO. 1976. Platelet surface properties and platelet function. Thromb. Haem. **35:** 124–138.
3. TSCHOPP, T. B. & H. R. BAUMGARTNER. 1975. Physiological experiments in hemostasis and thrombosis. Br. J. Haem. **31:** 221–229.
4. SAKARIASSEN, K. S., P. A. BOLHUIS & J. J. SIXMA. 1979. Adhesion of human blood platelets to human artery subendothelium is mediated by FVIII-VWF bound to subendothelium. Nature **279:** 636–638.
5. SAKARIASSEN, K. S., M. CATTANEO, A. VAN DEN BERG, Z. M. RUGGERI, P. M. MANNUCCI, & J. J. SIXMA. 1984. DDAVP enhances platelet adherence and platelet aggregate growth on human artery subendothelium. Blood **64:** 229–236.
6. GRABOWSKI, E. F., K. K. HERTER & P. DIDISHEIM. 1976. Human vs. dog platelet adhesion to cuprophane under controlled conditions of whole blood flow. J. Lab. Clin. Med. **88:** 368–374.
7. MUGGLI, R., H. R. BAUMGARTNER, T. B. TSCHOPP & H. KELLER. 1980. Automated microdensitometry protein assay as a measure for platelet adhesion and aggregation on collagen coated slides under controlled and flow conditions. J. Lab. Clin. Med. **95:** 195–207.
8. PARSONS, I. J., D. L. HAYCRAFT, J. C. HOAK & H. SAGE. 1986. Interaction of platelets and purified collagens in a laminar flow model. Thomb. Res. **43:** 435–443.
9. SAKARIASSEN, K. S., P. A. M. M. AARTS, PH.G. DE GROOT, W. P. M. HOUDIJK, & J. J. SIXMA. 1983. A perfusion chamber developed to investigate platelet interaction in flowing blood with human vessel wall cells, their extracellular matrix and purified components. J. Lab. Clin. Med. **102:** 522–535.
10. BAUMGARTNER, H. R. & K. S. SAKARIASSEN. 1985. Factors controlling thrombus formation on arterial lesions. Ann. N. Y. Acad. Sci. U.S.A. **454:** 162–177.
11. SAKARIASSEN, K. S., R. MUGGLI & H. R. BAUMGARTNER. 1987. Measurements of platelet interaction with components of the vessel wall in flowing blood. *In* Methods in Enzymology. J. Hawiger *et al.,* Eds. Academic Press. Orlando, FL. In press.
12. BUCHANAN, M. R., R. W. BLUTT, Z. MAGAS, J. VAN RIJN, J. HIRSH & D. J. NAZIR. 1985. Endothelial cells produce a lipoxygenase derived chemorepellent which influences platelet/endothelial cells interactions: Effect of aspirin and salicylate. Thromb. Haem. **53:** 306–311.
13. BUCHANAN, M. R., TH.A. HAAS, M. CAGARDE & M. GUICHARDANT. 1985. 13-Hydroxyoctadecadienoic acid is the vessel wall chemorepellant factor, LDX. J. Biol. Chem. **360:** 16056–16059.
14. WEISS, H. J., H. R. BAUMGARTNER, T. B. TSCHOPP, V. T. TURITTO & D. COHEN. 1978. Correction of factor VIII of the impaired platelet adhesion to subendothelium in von Willebrand's disease. Blood **51:** 267–279.
15. HOUDIJK, W. P. M. & J. J. SIXMA. 1985. Fibronectin in artery subendothelium is important for platelet adhesion. Blood **65:** 598–604.
16. HOUDIJK, W. P. M., K. S. SAKARIASSEN, P. F. E. M. NIEVELSTEIN & J. J. SIXMA. 1985.

Role of factor VIII-von Willebrand factor and fibronectin in the interaction of platelets in flowing blood with monomeric and fibrillar human collagen types I and III. J. Clin. Invest. **75:** 531–540.

17. Stel, H. V., K. S. Sakariassen, Ph.G. de Groot, J. A. van Mourik & J. J. Sixma. 1985. Von Willebrand factor in the vessel wall mediates platelet adherence. Blood **65:** 85–90.
18. Turitto, V. T., H. J. Weiss, T. S. Zimmerman & I. I. Sussman. 1985. Factor VIII/von Willebrand factor in subendothelium mediates platelet adhesion. Blood **65:** 623–631.
19. Houdijk, W. P. M., Ph.G. de Groot, P. F. E. M. Nievelstein, K. S. Sakariassen & J. J. Sixma. 1986. Von Willebrand factor and fibronectin but not thrombospondin are involved in platelet adhesion to the extracellular matrix of human vascular endothelial cells. Arteriosclerosis **6:** 24–33.
20. Sage, H., E. Crouch & P. Bornstein. 1979. Collagen synthesis by bovine aortic endothelial cells in culture. Biochemistry **18:** 5433–5442.
21. De Groot, Ph.G., M. Ottenhof-Rovers, M. Dziadek, R. Timpl & J. J. Sixma. 1985. Nidogen is present in the extracellular matrix of human endothelial cells and is involved in platelet adhesion to this matrix. Thromb. Haem. **54:** 231.
22. Wagner, D. D., M. Urban-Pickering & V. J. Marder. 1984. Von Willebrand protein binds to extracellular matrices independently of collagen. Proc. Natl. Acad. Sci. U.S.A. **81:** 471–475.
23. Hormia, M., V. P. Lehto & I. Virtanen. 1983. Factor VIII-related antigen, a pericellular matrix protein of cultured human endothelial cells. Exp. Cell Res. **149:** 483–497.
24. De Groot, Ph.G., M. Ottenhof-Rovers, J. A. van Mourik & J. J. Sixma. Binding site of von Willebrand factor in the vessel wall which mediates platelet adhesion is not collagen. Submitted.
25. Bockenstedt, P., J. M. Greenberg, & R. I. Handin. 1986. Structural basis of von Willebrand factor binding to glycoprotein I and collagen. J. Clin. Invest. **77:** 743–749.
26. Sixma, J. J., J. A. van Mourik, K. S. Sakariassen, H. V. Stel, D. W. der Maur, R. J. Hamer, & Ph.G. de Groot. 1984. Functional domains in von Willebrand factor. Recognition of discrete tryptic fragments by monoclonal antibodies that inhibit interaction of von Willebrand factor with platelets and with collagen. J. Clin. Invest. **74:** 736–744.
27. Sakariassen, K. S., P. F. E. M. Nievelstein, B. S. Coller & J. J. Sixma. 1986. The role of glycoprotein Ib and IIb-IIIa in platelet adherence to human artery subendothelium. Br. J. Haematol. **63:** 681–691.
28. Weiss, H. J., V. T. Turitto & H. R. Baumgartner. 1986. Platelet adhesion and thrombus formation on subendothelium in platelets deficient in glycoproteins IIb-IIIa and Ib and storage α granules. Blood **67:** 322–331.
29. Dewey, C. F., S. R. Bussolari, M. A. Gimbrone & P. F. Davies. 1981. The dynamic response of vascular endothelial cells to fluid shear stress. J. Biomech. Eng. **103:** 177–185.
30. Grimm, J., R. Keller & Ph.G. de Groot. Laminar flow induces cell polarity and leads to rearrangement of proteoglycan metabolism in endothelial cells. Submitted.
31. De Groot, Ph.G., J. H. Reinders & J. J. Sixma. 1987. Perturbation of human endothelial cells by thrombin or PMA changes the reactivity of their extracellular matrix towards platelets. J. Cell Biol. **104:** 697–704.
32. De Groot, Ph. G., C. Verwey, P. P. Nawroth, H. de Boer, D. M. Stern, & J. J. Sixma. 1987. Interleukin-1 inhibits the synthesis of von Willebrand factor in endothelial cells which results in a decreased reactivity of their matrix towards platelets. Arteriosclerosis. In press.
33. Zwaginga, J. J., Ph.G. de Groot & J. J. Sixma. PMA perturbation of endothelial cells increases thrombin formation in flowing blood together with platelet aggregation on their matrix. Br. J. Haematol. In press.
34. Stepp, M. A., M. S. Kindy, C. Franzblau & C. E. Sonenshein. 1986. Complex regulation of collagen expression in cultured bovine aortic smooth muscle cells. J. Biol. Chem. **261:** 6542–6547.
35. Vlodarsky, I., A. Eldor, E. Hyam, R. Atzmon & Z. Fuks. 1982. Platelet interaction with the extracellular matrix produced by cultured endothelial cells: A model to study the thrombogenecity of isolated subendothelial basal lamina. Thromb. Res. **28:** 179–191.

Role of Platelet Membrane Glycoproteins and Von Willebrand Factor in Adhesion of Platelets to Subendothelium and Collagen

KJELL S. SAKARIASSEN,[a] EDITH FRESSINAUD,[b]
JEAN-PIERRE GIRMA,[b] DOMINIQUE MEYER,[b]
AND HANS R. BAUMGARTNER[c]

[a]*Department of Pathology*
University of Washington
Seattle, Washington 98105

[b]*Hôpital de Bicetre*
Paris, France

[c]*Pharma Research*
F. Hoffmann-La Roche
Basel, Switzerland

INTRODUCTION

Adhesion of platelets to sites of vascular lesions is one of the initial events of primary hemostasis and thrombosis.[1,2] A number of factors, including glycoproteins (GPs) in the platelet membrane,[3–9] connective tissue components in the vessel wall,[10–16] proteins[14,17–19] and ions[20,21] in plasma, and the blood shear rate at the vessel wall control this interaction.[1,7,8,14,16,19,21,22]

Development of *in vitro* perfusion systems that allowed exposure of arterial subendothelium[23] and other surfaces[24] to flowing blood and to partially reconstituted blood[12,18,21] provided new insights into the mechanism of platelet adhesion. Some of these experiments were designed to help define roles of platelet membranes and plasma constituents in the adhesion mechanism, and were performed with: (1) blood from patients with deficiencies in platelet GPs[4,7–9] or von Willebrand factor (vWF)[8,14,17,18,25]; (2) perfusates of selected purified proteins in a human albumin solution (HAS) instead of plasma[12,13,16,18,21,25]; (3) blood from normals with the addition of monoclonal antibodies directed against various GPs[6–8] or specific plasma proteins[14,26,27]; and (4) perfusates consisting of normal blood with the addition of a synthetic dodecapeptide of residues 400–411 of the γ-chain of fibrinogen.[28] Other perfusion experiments were designed to identify components in the vessel wall that were able to interact with platelets. These experiments used arterial subendothelium that was either digested with various enzymes[10,11] or treated with polyclonal and monoclonal antibodies directed against subendothelial proteins.[13–16] In addition, artificial surfaces were constructed of the pericellular matrix of cultured vascular cells and of purified connective tissue components on glass or plastic coverslips.[12,24] These and other approaches led to the recognition of a variety of factors involved in platelet adhesion, including GPIa,[9] GPIb,[3–8] and GPIIb/IIIa[7,8] in platelet membranes; vWF[17–19] and divalent cations in plasma[20,21]; collagen,[10] fibronectin (FN),[12,16] and vWF in subendothelium[14,15]; as well as the unambiguous role played by the shear rate.[22,23]

In this paper we have focused on the role of platelet GPs, particularly GPIb and GPIIb/IIIa, as receptors for vWF in the process of binding platelets to collagen.

MATERIALS AND METHODS

Deficiencies of Platelet GPs

Deficiencies of platelet GPIa, GPIb, and GPIIb/IIIa from patients suffering from bleeding diatheses were established by two-dimensional electrophoresis of platelet proteins labeled by ^{125}I with iodogen, and by 3–30% polyacrylamide gel electrophoresis of SDS-solubilized platelets.[29,30] Characterizations of patients and platelets were previously given.[8,9,31]

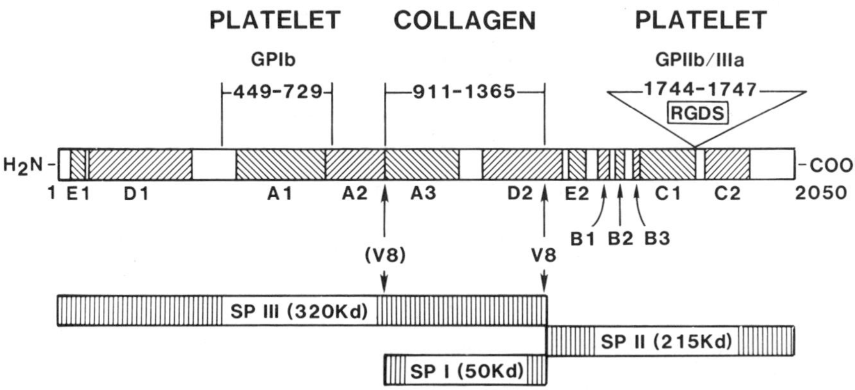

FIGURE 1. Schematic illustration of structure-function relationships for the subunit of mature vWF[34,46–49] and the proteolytic fragments SPI, SPII, and SPIII.[33,34] The subunit consists of 2050 amino acids, with serine and lysine in positions 1 (amino terminal) and 2050 (carboxy terminal), respectively. *Hatched areas* indicate internal sequence duplication (A1–E2). The domains binding to GPIb (449–729), to collagen (911–1365), and to GPIIb/IIIa (1744–1747) are indicated. The two principal sites of *S. aureus* V-8 protease cleavage are indicated (*V8*). The less susceptible site was located between A2 and A3. SPI, SPII, and SPIII are also indicated, together with their corresponding M_r.[5]

vWF and Proteolytic vWF Fragments

Von Willebrand factor was purified from factor VIII concentrates.[32] Proteolytic vWF fragments SPI, SPII, and SPIII were generated by digestion of purified vWF with *S. aureus* V-8 protease[33,34] (FIGURE 1). The fragments were purified according to the method in Girma *et al.*[33] SPI has an apparent molecular weight (M_r) of 50 kilodaltons (kDa), possesses a binding domain for collagen, and is localized to the midportion of the vWF subunit. SPII has M_r 215 kDa, possesses a binding domain for platelet GPIIb/IIIa, and is part of the carboxy-terminal segment of the vWF subunit.

SPIII has M_r 320 kDa, possesses binding domains for platelet GPIb and collagen, and is part of the amino-terminal segment of the vWF subunit.

Monoclonal Antibodies and γ_{FIB} 400–411 Peptide

Roles of platelet GPs and various domains of vWF in the adhesion mechanism were probed by a series of experiments with several monoclonal antibodies (MAbs). MAb 6D1[35] binds to GPIb, and MAb 10E5[36] and MAb EDU3[37] bind to GPIIb/IIIa. MAb 6D1 and MAb 10E5 were provided by Dr. B. S. Coller, and MAb EDU3 was provided by Dr. R. Vilella. MAbs directed against vWF included MAb H9, which inhibits binding of vWF to GPIb in the presence of the antibiotic ristocetin; MAb 9, which inhibits binding of vWF to GPIIb/IIIa of ADP- or thrombin-stimulated platelets; MAb B202, which inhibits binding to vWF to collagen; and MAb 4, which binds to vWF, but apparently does not affect any known function of vWF. Detailed characterization of each antibody was previously reported.[27,34]

The role of GPIIb/IIIa in adhesion was also investigated with a synthetic dodecapeptide. This peptide, γ_{FIB} 400–411, has a primary structure identical to the carboxy terminal of the γ-chain of fibrinogen.[38] The sequence of the peptide is:

His-His-Leu-Gly-Gly-Ala-Lys-Gln-Ala-Gly-Asp-Val.

Binding of vWF, FN, and fibrinogen to GPIIb/IIIa of ADP- and thrombin-stimulated platelets is inhibited by γ_{FIB} 400–411.[38,39]

Perfusion Chambers

Annular perfusion chambers[23] were used to expose subendothelium of human umbilical arteries[40] to flowing citrated blood. These chambers consist of a central rod surrounded by a cylinder. An everted arterial segment is mounted on the rod, and the gap between the subendothelial surface and the cylinder allows blood to pass over the surface. A wide range of shear rates can be obtained by varying the width of the gap and/or varying the blood flow rate.

Parallel-plate perfusion chambers[24] were used to expose collagen fibrils to flowing citrated blood and reconstituted perfusates.[41] These chambers consist of a rectangular flow slit with a coverslip holder holding a plastic coverslip which can be coated with various components. Purified type III collagen[41] or Horm collagen (Hormon Chemie, Munich, FRG) was spray coated on plastic coverslips ($\simeq$30 μg/cm^2),[24,42] allowed to air dry, and placed into the coverslip holder, which subsequently was positioned into the chamber and exposed to flowing blood. In some experiments, coverslips coated with type III collagen were incubated with vWF, SPI, SPII, SPIII, and Tris-HCl, as previously described.[41] A wide range of shear rates can be obtained by varying the height of the flow slit and/or varying the blood flow rate.

Perfusates and Perfusions

Blood from patients and healthy individuals was anticoagulated with 1/10 vol 110 mM trisodium citrate (20 mM in plasma). Reconstituted blood was prepared from washed platelets, washed erythrocytes, and plasma.[43] In some experiments with reconstituted blood, plasma was replaced by a human albumin solution (HAS).[41]

MAbs or γ_{FIB} 400–411 were added to perfusates prior to the perfusions. Perfusions were carried out at 37°C at preselected flow rates (shear rates) by recirculating perfusates from a reservoir for 5 min.[23,43]

Quantitation of Platelet-Surface Interactions

Platelet-surface interactions were quantified by morphometric evaluation of semithin sections.[1] This method measures percent of surface coverage with platelets (platelet adhesion) and also the percent of surface coverage with thrombi more than 2.5 μm in height. Platelet adhesion can be further differentiated into percent of surface coverage with platelets making contact with the surface (contact platelets) and percent of surface coverage with platelets spread out on the surface (spread platelets). Platelets making contact with the surface have not spread out, and only a small portion of the platelet membrane is actually interacting with the surface.

RESULTS AND DISCUSSION

Roles of GPIa, GPIb, and GPIIb/IIIa in platelet adhesion were investigated through the use of blood from patients with these GP deficiences, and through MAbs directed against GPIb and GPIIb/IIIa. The significance of vWF binding to GPIb, to GPIIb/IIIa, and to collagen in the process of platelet adhesion was studied with MAbs that specifically inhibit these interactions, and using proteolytic fragments of vWF possessing one or two of the domains binding to the respective components. For further elucidation of the role of GPIIb/IIIa in platelet adhesion, γ_{FIB} 400–411, which inhibits binding of vWF, FN, and fibrinogen to GPIIb/IIIa of ADP- or thrombin-stimulated platelets,[38,39] was included as an additional probe.

Deficiencies of Platelet GPIa, GPIb, and GPIIb/IIIa

The mandatory need for GPIb in adhesion of platelets to arterial subendothelium and collagen fibrils was demonstrated more than a decade ago.[3–5] However, recent data have indicated roles for GPIa[9] and GPIIb/IIIa[7,8] in adhesion as well.

Platelets deficient in GPIa do not demonstrate any spreading on subendothelium at shear rates that prevail in large arteries (300 s^{-1}) or in microcirculation (1800 s^{-1}) (FIGURE 2B). Deficiency of GPIIb/IIIa impairs the spreading of platelets also, but at microcirculatory shear rates only, and much less severely than deficiency of GPIa (FIGURE 2B). Platelets deficient in GPIIb/IIIa spread out less than platelets from healthy subjects, and they do not overlap neighboring platelets, as do normal platelets, but keep themselves surrounded by small rims of denuded subendothelium. However, both GP deficiencies result in more platelets making contact with the subendothelium than in the normal state (FIGURE 2A), indicating that GPIa and GPIIb/IIIa are not involved in the initial attachment of platelets to the surface but in the spreading. Deficiency of GPIb appears, on the contrary, to prevent the initial attachment of platelets, as contact platelets are only occasionally encountered on the subendothelium (FIGURE 2A).

A second striking feature of GPIIb/IIIa-deficient platelets is their lack of aggregation on the subendothelium (FIGURE 2C). In addition, these platelets do not aggregate in response to ADP, thrombin, or collagen in the aggregometer device.[44] The

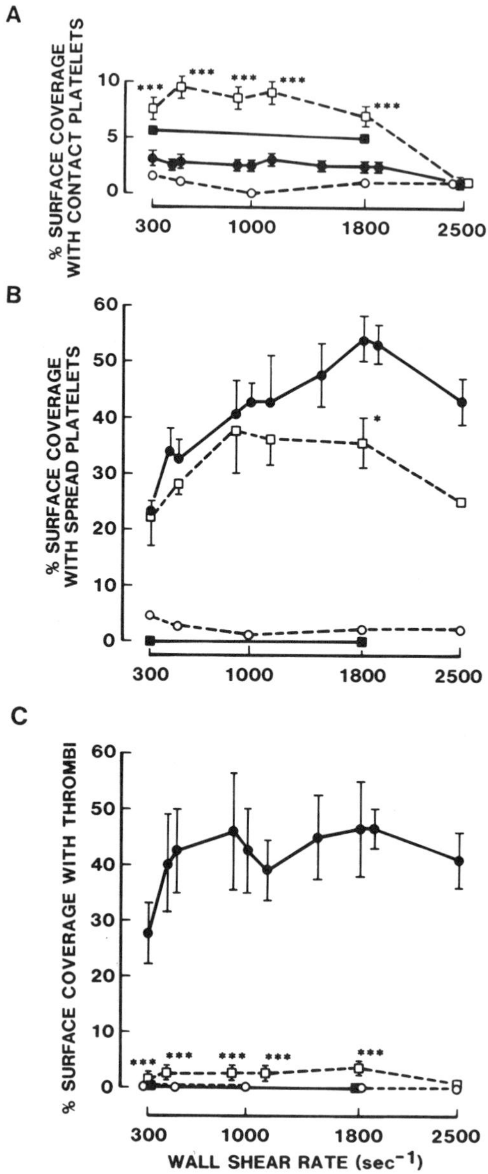

FIGURE 2. Effect of GP deficiencies on platelet-subendothelium interactions following 5-min perfusions at shear rates ranging from 300 to 2600 s^{-1}. Platelet adhesion was evaluated as (**A**) contact platelets and (**B**) spread platelets. (**C**) Platelet aggregates were evaluated when deposited platelet masses were higher than 2.5 μm. Citrated blood was perfused from one patient with GPIa deficiency (■——■), two patients with GPIb deficiency (○– –○), four patients with GPIIb/IIIa deficiency (□– –□), and nine normal individuals (●——●). Values for GPIIb/IIIa deficiency and normals represent mean ± SE, with the exception of the value of GPIIb/IIIa deficiency at 2500 s^{-1}, which represents the average for two patients. Values for GPIa and GPIb represent average values from determinations on three and two different occasions, respectively. $^{*}p < 0.05$, $^{***}p < 0.001$, Student's t-test, relative to the respective values for normals.

gross impairment of platelet adhesion in GPIa and GPIb deficiencies prevents study of aggregation because adhesion within the normal range is a prerequisite for proper investigation of platelet-platelet cohesion in our flow models.[1,45] However, previously published data have shown that the hallmark of GPIa-deficient platelets is lack of response to collagen, while aggregation occurs normally with other agonists.[31] GPIb-deficient platelets also have normal platelet aggregation, although these platelets fail to agglutinate in the presence of the antibiotic ristocetin.[44]

MAbs against GPIb and GPIIb/IIIa

MAbs directed against GPIb and GPIIb/IIIa have been raised by several groups of investigators. To our knowledge, antibodies against GPIa have not yet been produced. However, the available antibodies offer unique panels of probes to localize and

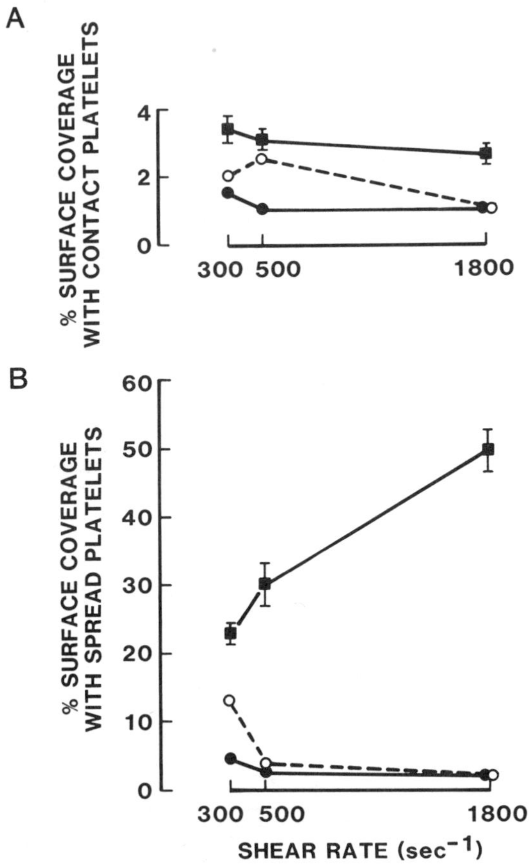

FIGURE 3. Effect of anti-GPIb MAb 6D1 on adhesion of platelets to subendothelium when added to citrated blood from normal subjects. Platelet adhesion was evaluated as (**A**) contact platelets and (**B**) spread platelets. Perfusates consisting of citrated blood from two patients with GPIb deficiency (●——●), citrated blood from two normals with added MAb 6D1 (○– –○), and from four normals (■——■) were perfused for 5 min at shear rates of 300, 500, and 1800 s^{-1}. Values for normals represent mean ±SE, whereas values for patients with GPIb deficiency and values for normal blood with the addition of MAb 6D1 represent the average of two determinations.

characterize domains on GPs involved in various functions and to substantiate the roles of GPs in adhesion. We have taken advantage of the latter possibility by utilizing MAbs against GPIb and GPIIb/IIIa.

Addition of MAb 6D1,[35] a MAb directed against GPIb, to blood from normal subjects reproduces the poor adhesion observed in blood from patients with GPIb deficiency (FIGURES 3A and 3B). MAb 6D1 virtually abolishes the initial attachment of platelets and their subsequent spreading on subendothelium, particularly at shear rates above 500 s^{-1} that prevail in small- and middle-sized arteries. The effect of MAb 6D1 in normal blood confirms the observations with GPIb-deficient blood, and emphasizes the importance of GPIb at high shear rate in the initial attachment of platelets to subendothelium.

Addition of MAb 10E5[36] or MAb EDU3,[37] MAbs directed against GPIIb/IIIa, to blood from normal subjects decreases spreading of platelets at high shear rate (1800 s^{-1}) only, similar to blood with GPIIb/IIIa-deficient platelets (FIGURE 4B). However, the inhibitory effect of MAb EDU3 is significantly more pronounced than the average decrement of the group of patients ($p < 0.05$; Student's t-test). Increased surface

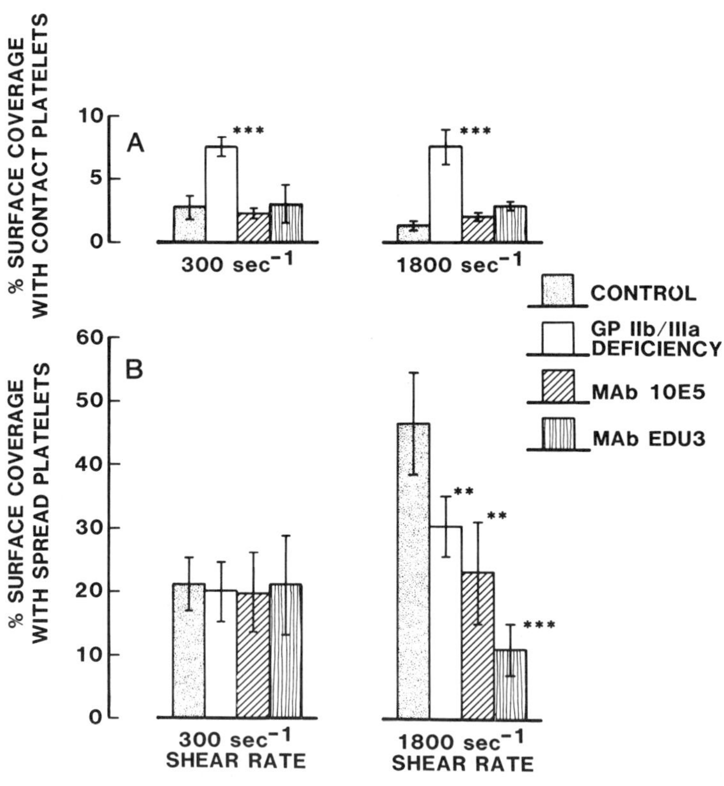

FIGURE 4. Effects of anti-GPIIb/IIIa MAb 10E5 and MAb EDU3 on adhesion of platelets to subendothelium when added to citrated blood from normal subjects. Platelet adhesion was evaluated as (**A**) contact platelets and (**B**) spread platelets following 5-min perfusions at shear rates of 300 and 1800 s^{-1}. Values represent mean ± SE; $n = 3$. $^{**}p < 0.01$; $^{***}p < 0.001$, Student's t-test, relative to the respective values for the controls.

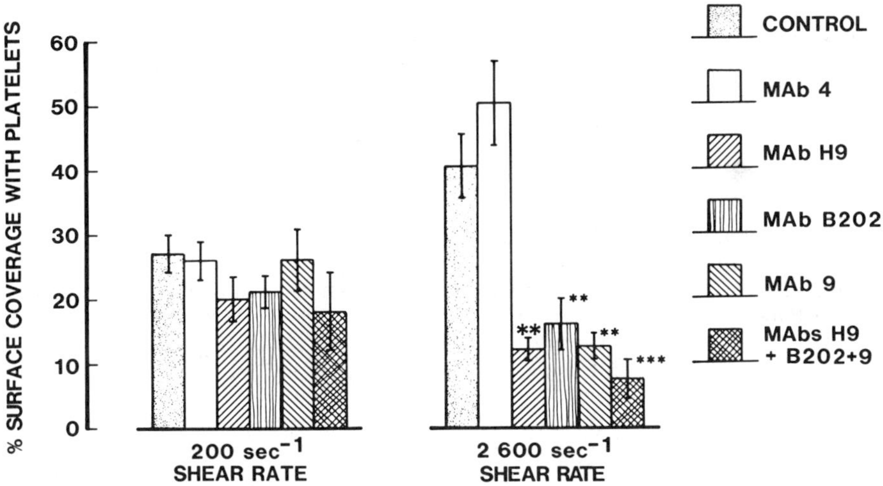

FIGURE 5. Effects of anti-vWF MAb H9, MAb 9, and MAb 202 on adhesion of platelets to Horm collagen when added to citrated blood from normal subjects. Platelet adhesion was evaluated as the sum of contact and spread platelets following 5-min perfusions at shear rates of 200 and 2600 s^{-1}. Values represent mean ± SE; $n = 3$. $^{**}p < 0.01$; $^{***}p < 0.001$, Student's *t*-test, relative to the respective values for the controls.

coverage with contact platelets, as in GPIIb/IIIa-deficient blood, is not noted in the presence of any MAb (FIGURE 4A). However, both MAbs inhibit platelet aggregation on subendothelium, similar to GPIIb/IIIa-deficient platelets, and they substantiate the surprising finding that GPIIb/IIIa is involved in platelet adhesion. Further evidence for involvement of GPIIb/IIIa in adhesion is presented in the following sections.

Binding of vWF to GPIb, GPIIb/IIIa, and Collagen

The complete amino acid sequence of the mature vWF protein was recently determined by direct analysis of stretches of the vWF protein[46] and from cDNA clones.[47–49] The vWF subunit has at least three different domains that bind to GPIb, GPIIb/IIIa, and collagen, respectively (FIGURE 1). These domains were recognized by identification of proteolytic vWF digests with MAbs directed against vWF[33,34,50,51] and by perfusion studies with proteolytic fragments of vWF.[41]

The importance of these domains in platelet-collagen adhesion was investigated by anti-vWF MAbs that block the binding between vWF and platelets and between vWF and collagen. Collagen-coated surfaces were chosen in these and other perfusion experiments where vWF-mediated platelet adhesion was studied because platelet adhesion is also mediated by subendothelial vWF-related protein,[14,15] which otherwise could lead to misinterpretation of the data. MAbs that block binding of vWF to GPIb (MAb H9), to GPIIb/IIIa (MAb 9), and to collagen (MAb B202) inhibit adhesion in normal blood by about 70% each (FIGURE 5). However, inhibition occurs only at high shear rate (2600 s^{-1}). Simultaneous addition of all three MAbs to normal blood inhibits adhesion by slightly more, about 80%. The dramatic effects of these MAbs on platelet adhesion and on binding of vWF to platelets and to collagen indicate that GPIb and GPIIb/IIIa function as receptors for vWF in the process of bridging platelets to collagen. Furthermore, the results imply that vWF is required for both the initial attachment and the subsequent spreading of platelets on collagenous surfaces, and not in initial attachment alone[52] or in spreading alone,[53] as previously reported.

γ_{FIB} *400–411*

Experimental evidence for a role of GPIIb/IIIa in platelet adhesion is based on observations with platelets deficient in GPIIb/IIIa (FIGURE 2), with MAbs directed against GPIIb/IIIa (FIGURE 4), and with MAb 9 (FIGURE 5), which inhibits adhesion by blocking the interaction of vWF with GPIIb/IIIa. A synthetic dodecapeptide of residues 400–411 of the carboxy terminal of the γ-chain of fibrinogen, γ_{FIB} 400–411,[38] also inhibits binding of vWF and of FN and fibrinogen to GPIIb/IIIa of ADP- and thrombin-stimulated platelets.[38,39]

Addition of γ_{FIB} 400–411 to citrated blood from normals impairs adhesion of platelets to collagen, but only at microcirculatory shear rate (FIGURE 6). A concentration of 300 μM in plasma is needed to achieve this effect, and higher concentrations do not enhance the inhibition. These data are in accordance with a role for GPIIb/IIIa as a receptor for vWF, FN, and/or fibrinogen in platelet adhesion. However, in view of the inhibitory effect on platelet adhesion by MAb 9 (FIGURE 5) through its inhibition of binding of vWF to GPIIb/IIIa, the data suggest that γ_{FIB} 400–411 affects adhesion by inhibiting the GPIIb/IIIa-vWF interaction.

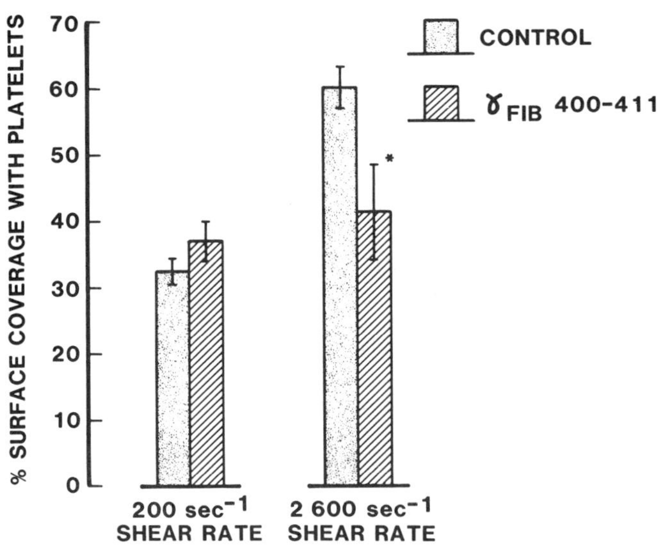

FIGURE 6. Effect of γ_{FIB} 400–411, a synthetic peptide of residues 400–411 of the carboxy terminal of the γ-chain of fibrinogen, on the adhesion of platelets to purified collagen type III when added to citrated blood from normal subjects. Platelet adhesion was evaluated as the sum of contact and spread platelets following 5-min perfusions at shear rates of 200 and 2600 s^{-1}. Values represent mean ± SE; $n = 3$. *$p < 0.05$, Student's t-test, relative to the respective values for the controls.

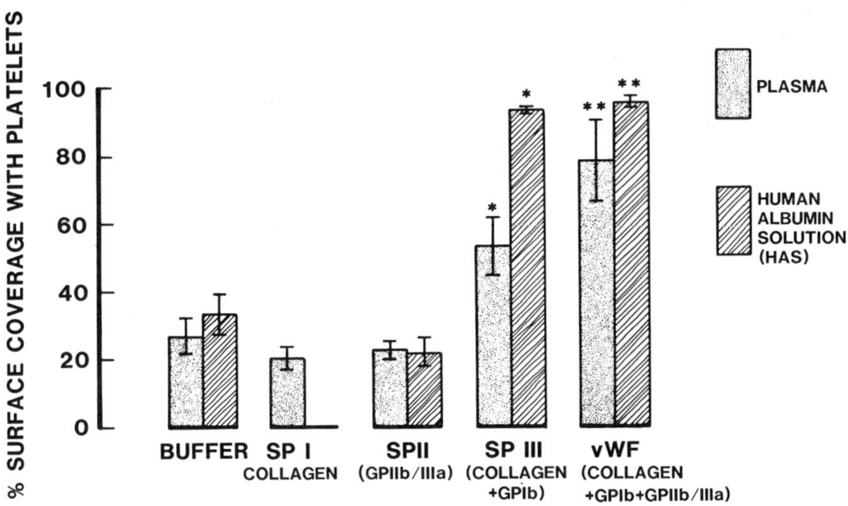

FIGURE 7. Effects on platelet adhesion to purified type III collagen following incubation of collagen coats with vWF, the proteolytic vWF fragments SPI, SPII, and SPIII, or buffer only. Domains of SPI, SPII, SPIII, and vWF binding to GPIb, GPIIb/IIIa, or collagen are indicated. 5-min perfusions were performed at 2600 s^{-1} shear rate with reconstituted perfusates with plasma, or with HAS[41] instead of plasma. Values represent mean ± SE; $n = 3$. $^{*}p < 0.05$; $^{**}p < 0.01$, Student's t-test, relative to the respective values for collagen coats incubated with buffer (Tris-HCl, pH 7.4). Collagen coats incubated with SPI were exposed to reconstituted blood with plasma only.

Von Willebrand Factor Domains Binding to GPIb, GPIIb/IIIa, and Collagen

Preparation and isolation of three proteolytic fragments of the vWF subunit possessing one or two domains binding to GPIb, GPIIb/IIIa, or collagen were recently achieved[33] (FIGURE 1). *S. aureus* V-8 protease was used to digest vWF into fragments that were named SPI, SPII, and SPIII.

Incubation of these unique fragments with purified collagen fibrils and subsequent exposure to reconstituted blood shows that only SPIII, which possesses binding domains for GPIb and collagen, mediates platelet adhesion (FIGURE 7). The apparent independence of GPIIb/IIIa may be masked by vWF-related protein released from platelet α-granules,[54] implying that SPIII mediates initial attachment of platelets to collagen, followed by activation of platelets and binding to α-granular vWF to GPIIb/IIIa and subsequent mediation of spreading of platelets on collagen fibrils. The other vWF fragments, SPI and SPII, which possess binding domains for collagen and for GPIIb/IIIa, respectively, do not mediate adhesion. The effects of these vWF fragments on platelet-collagen adhesion emphasize the need for specific domains of the vWF molecule binding to platelet and to vessel wall, and confirm the concept of vWF functioning as a bridge or glue between platelet and vessel wall.[18]

SUMMARY

Development of *in vitro* perfusion systems and quantitative methods to evaluate various aspects of platelet-surface interactions have helped to elucidate some complex interactions in platelet adhesion and platelet-platelet cohesion. The importance of platelet GPs in these interactions was soon evident, and rapid progress in biochemistry and immunology has made it possible to study the roles of these GPs in more detail. From our studies, which made use of platelets with GP deficiencies, MAbs, purified vWF, proteolytic fragments of vWF, a synthetic peptide, and *in vitro* perfusion systems, it appeared that GPIb and GPIIb/IIIa function as receptors for vWF, which binds platelets to connective tissue at sites of vascular lesions (FIGURE 8). More detailed information about these interactions is expected in the near future when bioengineered products are available for testing in flow models and in other experimental approaches.

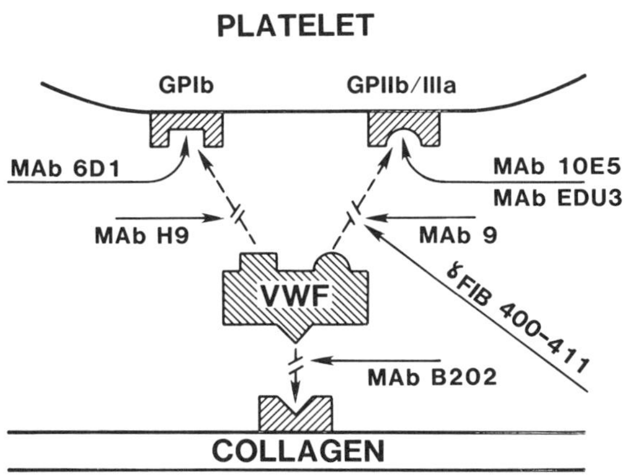

FIGURE 8. Schematic illustration of interactions between various domains of vWF with collagen and with GPIb and GPIIb/IIIa in platelet-collagen adhesion. MAbs inhibiting the different interactions between vWF, platelet, and collagen, and MAbs binding to GPIb and GPIIb/IIIa are indicated. Inhibition of binding of vWF to GPIIb/IIIa by γ_{FIB} 400–411 is also indicated. It is noted that γ_{FIB} 400–411 inhibits binding of FN and fibrinogen to GPIIb/IIIa as well.

ACKNOWLEDGMENTS

We thank Dr. Russell Ross for supporting these studies, Drs. Jerry S. Powell and Steven Leytus for many suggestions, and Mary Hillman for help in manuscript preparation.

REFERENCES

1. BAUMGARTNER, H. R. & R. MUGGLI. 1976. Adhesion and aggregation: Morphological demonstration and quantitation in vivo and in vitro. *In* Platelets in Biology and Pathology. J. L. Gordon, Ed.: 23–60. Elsevier/North Holland Biomedical Press. New York.
2. SIXMA, J. J. & J. WESTER. 1977. The haemostatic plug. Semin. Hematol. **14:** 265–299.
3. CAEN, J. P. & S. LEVY-TOLEDANO. 1973. Interaction between platelets and von Willebrand factor provides a new scheme for primary haemostasis. Nature, New Biol. **244:** 159–160.

4. WEISS, H. J., T. B. TSCHOPP, H. R. BAUMGARTNER, I. I. SUSSMAN, M. M. JOHNSON & J. J. EGAN. 1974. Decreased adhesion of giant (Bernard Soulier) platelets to subendothelium. Further implications on the role of the von Willebrand factor in hemostasis. Am. J. Med. **57:** 920–925.
5. TOBELEM, G., S. LEVY-TOLEDANO, R. BREDOUX, H. MICHEL, A. NURDEN & J. P. CAEN. 1976. New approach to determination of specific functions of platelet membrane sites. Nature **263:** 427–428.
6. RUAN, C., G. TOBELEM, A. MCMICHAEL, L. DROUET, Y. LEGRAND, L. DEGOS, N. KIEFFER, J. LEE & J. P. CAEN. 1981. Monoclonal antibody to human platelet glycoprotein I. II. Effect on human platelet function. Br. J. Haematol. **49:** 511–519.
7. WEISS, H. J., V. T. TURITTO & H. R. BAUMGARTNER. 1986. Platelet adhesion and thrombus formation on subendothelium in platelets deficient in glycoproteins IIb-IIIa, Ib, and storage granules. Blood **67:** 322–330.
8. SAKARIASSEN, K. S., P. F. E. M. NIEVELSTEIN, B. S. COLLER & J. J. SIXMA. 1986. The role of platelet membrane glycoproteins Ib and IIb-IIIa in platelet adherence to human artery subendothelium. Br. J. Haematol. **63:** 681–691.
9. NIEUWENHUIS, H. K., K. S. SAKARIASSEN, W. P. M. HOUDIJK, P. F. E. M. NIEVELSTEIN & J. J. SIXMA. 1986. Deficiency of platelet membrane glycoprotein Ia associated with a decreased platelet adhesion to subendothelium: A defect in platelet spreading. Blood **68:** 692–695.
10. BAUMGARTNER, H. R. & C. HAUDENSCHILD. 1972. Adhesion of platelets to subendothelium. Ann. N.Y. Acad. Sci. **201:** 22–36.
11. FAUVEL, F., M. E. GRANT, Y. J. LEGRAND, H. SOUCHON, G. TOBELEM, D. S. JACKSON & J. P. CAEN. 1983. Interaction of blood platelets with a microfibrillar extract from adult bovine aorta: Requirement for von Willebrand factor. Proc. Natl. Acad. Sci. U.S.A. **80:** 551–554.
12. HOUDIJK, W. P. M., K. S. SAKARIASSEN, P. F. E. M. NIEVELSTEIN & J. J. SIXMA. 1985. Role of factor VIII-von Willebrand factor and fibronectin in the interaction of platelets in flowing blood with monomeric and fibrillar human collagen types I and II. J. Clin. Invest. **75:** 531–540.
13. HOUDIJK, W. P. M. & J. J. SIXMA. 1985. Fibronectin in artery subendothelium is important for platelet adhesion. Blood **65:** 598–604.
14. STEL, H. V., K. S. SAKARIASSEN, PH. G. DE GROOT, J. A. VON MOURIK & J. J. SIXMA. 1985. von Willebrand factor in the vessel wall mediates platelet adherence. Blood **65:** 85–90.
15. TURITTO, V. T., H. J. WEISS, T. ZIMMERMAN & I. I. SUSSMAN. 1985. Factor VIII/von Willebrand factor in subendothelium mediates platelet adhesion. Blood **65:** 823–828.
16. HOUDIJK. W. P. M., PH. G. DE GROOT, P. F. E. M. NIEVELSTEIN, K. S. SAKARIASSEN & J. J. SIXMA. 1986. Subendothelial proteins and platelet adhesion: von Willebrand factor and fibronectin, not thrombospondin, are involved in platelet adhesion to extracellular matrix of human vascular endothelial cells. Arteriosclerosis **6:** 24–33.
17. TSCHOPP, T. B., H. J. WEISS & H. R. BAUMGARTNER. 1974. Decreased adhesion of platelets to subendothelium in von Willebrand's disease. J. Lab. Clin. Med. **83:** 296–300.
18. SAKARIASSEN, K. S., P. A. BOLHUIS & J. J. SIXMA. 1979. Human blood platelet adhesion to artery subendothelium is mediated by factor VIII-von Willebrand factor bound to the subendothelium. Nature **279:** 636–638.
19. BAUMGARTNER, H. R., T. B. TSCHOPP & D. MEYER. 1980. Shear rate dependent inhibition of platelet adhesion and aggregation on collagenous surfaces by antibodies to human factor VIII/von Willebrand factor. Br. J. Haematol. **44:** 127–139.
20. BAUMGARTNER, H. R., R. MUGGLI, T. B. TSCHOPP & V. T. TURITTO. 1975. Platelet adhesion, release and aggregation in flowing blood: Effects of surface properties and platelet function. Thromb. Haemostas. **35:** 124–138.
21. SAKARIASSEN, K. S., M. OTTENHOF-ROVERS & J. J. SIXMA. 1984. Factor VIII-von Willebrand factor requires calcium for facilitation of platelet adherence. Blood **63:** 996–1003.
22. TURITTO, V. T. 1982. Blood viscosity, mass transport and thrombogenesis. *In* Progress in Hemostasis and Thrombosis. T. H. Spaet, Ed.: 139–177. Grune & Stratton. New York.
23. BAUMGARTNER, H. R. 1973. The role of blood flow in platelet adhesion, fibrin deposition, and formation of mural thrombi. Microvasc. Res. **5:** 167–179.

24. SAKARIASSEN, K. S., P. A. M. M. AARTS, PH. G. DE GROOT, W. P. M. HOUDIJK & J. J. SIXMA. 1983. A perfusion chamber developed to investigate platelet interaction in flowing blood with human vessel wall cells, their extracellular matrix, and purified components. J. Lab. Clin. Med. **102:** 522–535.
25. SAKARIASSEN, K. S., M. CATTANEO, A VAN DER BERG, Z. M. RUGGERI, P. M. MANNUCCI & J. J. SIXMA. 1984. DDAVP enhances platelet adherence and platelet aggregate growth on human artery subendothelium. Blood **64:** 229–236.
26. STEL, H. V., K. S. SAKARIASSEN, B. J. SCHOLTE, E. C. I. VEERMAN, TH. H. VAN DER KWAST, PH. G. DE GROOT, J. J. SIXMA & J. A. VAN MOURIK. 1984. Characterization of 25 monoclonal antibodies to factor VIII-von Willebrand factor: Relationship between ristocetin-induced platelet aggregation and platelet adherence to subendothelium. Blood **63:** 1408–1415.
27. MEYER, D., H. R. BAUMGARTNER & T. S. EDGINGTON. 1984. Hybridoma antibodies in human von Willebrand factor. II. Relative role of intramolecular loci in mediation of platelet adhesion to the subendothelium. Br. J. Haematol. **57:** 609–620.
28. SAKARIASSEN, K. S., P. HADVARY, D. GILLESSEN & H. R. BAUMGARTNER. 1985. The dodecapeptide gamma 400–411 fibrinogen inhibits platelet adhesion to human collagen fibrils. Thromb. Haemostas. **54:** 230.
29. O'FARRELL, P. H. 1975. High resolution two-dimensional electrophoresis of proteins. J. Biol. Chem. **250:** 4007–4027.
30. SIXMA, J. J. & M. E. SCHIPHORST. 1980. Identification of ectoproteins of human platelets. Combination of radioactive labelling and two-dimensional electrophoresis. Biochim. Biophys. Acta. **603:** 70–83.
31. NIEUWENHUIS, H. K., J. W. N. AKKERMAN, W. P. M. HOUDIJK & J. J. SIXMA. 1985. Human blood platelets showing no response to collagen fail to express surface glycoprotein Ia. Nature **318:** 470–472.
32. CHOPEK, M. W., J. P. GIRMA, K. FUJIKAWA, E. W. DAVIE & K. TITANI. 1986. Human von Willebrand factor: a multivalent portion composed of identical subunits. Biochemistry **25:** 3146–3155.
33. GIRMA, J. P., M. W. CHOPEK, K. TITANI & E. W. DAVIE. 1986. Limited proteolysis of human von Willebrand factor by Staphylococcus aureus V-8 protease: Isolation and partial characterization of a platelet-binding domain. Biochemistry **25:** 3156–3163.
34. GIRMA, J. P., M. KALAFATIS, G. PIETU, J. M. LAWERGNE, M. W. CHOPEK, T. S. EDGINGTON & D. MEYER. 1986. Mapping of distinct von Willebrand factor domains interacting with platlet GPIb and GPIIb/IIIa and with collagen using monoclonal antibodies. Blood **67:** 1356–1366.
35. COLLER, B. S., E. I. PEERSCHKE, I. E. SCUDDER & C. A. SULLIVAN. 1983. Studies with a murine monoclonal antibody that abolish ristocetin induced binding of von Willebrand factor to platelets: Additional evidence in support of GPIb as a platelet receptor for von Willebrand factor. Blood **61:** 99–110.
36. COLLER, B. S., E. I. PEERSCHKE, I. E. SCUDDER & C. A. SULLIVAN. 1983. A murine antibody that completely blocks the binding of fibrinogen to platelet produces a thromboasthenic-like state in normal platelets and binds to glycoproteins IIb and/or IIIa. J. Clin. Invest. **72:** 325–338.
37. VILELLA, R., T. LOZANO, F. MILA, L. BORCHE, G. ERCILLA, T. ORDINAS & J. VIVES. 1984. An antiplatelet monoclonal antibody that inhibits ADP and epinephrine-induced aggregation. Thromb. Haemostas. **51:** 1–4.
38. KLOCZEWIAK, M., S. TIMMONS, J. LUKAS & J. HAWIGER. 1984. Platelet receptor recognition site on human fibrinogen. Synthesis and structure-function relationship of peptides corresponding to the carboxy-terminal segment of the γ-chain. Biochemistry **23:** 1767–1774.
39. PLOW, E. J., A. H. SROUJI, D. MEYER, G. MARGUERIE & M. H. GINSBURG. 1984. Evidence that three adhesive proteins interact with a common recognition site on activated platelets. J. Biol. Chem. **259:** 5388–5391.
40. SAKARIASSEN, K. S., J. D. BANGA, PH. G. DE GROOT & J. J. SIXMA. 1984. Comparison of platelet interaction with subendothelium of human renal and umbilical arteries and the extracellular matrix produced by human venous cells. Thromb. Haemostas. **52:** 60–64.
41. SAKARIASSEN, K. S., E. FRESSINAUD, J. P. GIRMA, H. R. BAUMGARTNER & D. MEYER.

1986. Mediation of platelet adhesion to fibrillar collagen in flowing blood by a proteolytic fragment of human von Willebrand factor. Blood **67:** 1515–1518.

42. MUGGLI, R., H. R. BAUMGARTNER, T. B. TSCHOPP & H. KELLER. 1980. Automated microdensitometry and protein assays as a measure for platelet adhesion and aggregation on collagen-coated slides under controlled flow conditions. J. Lab. Clin. Med. **9:** 195–203.
43. SAKARIASSEN, K. S., R. MUGGLI & H. R. BAUMGARTNER. 1986. Measurements of platelet interaction with components of the vessel wall in flowing blood. *In* Platelets: Methods in Enzymology. J. J. Hawiger, Ed. Academic. New York. In press.
44. HARDISTY, R. M. & J. P. CAEN 1981. Disorders of platelet function. *In* Haemostasis and Thrombosis. A. L. Bloom & D. P. Duncan, Eds.: 300–320. Churchill Livingstone. Edinburgh.
45. BAUMGARTNER, H. R. & K. S. SAKARIASSEN. 1985. Factors controlling thrombus formation on arterial lesions. Ann. N. Y. Acad. Sci. **454:** 162–177.
46. TITANI, K., S. KUMAR, K. TAKIO, L. H. ERICSSON, R. D. WADE, K. ASHIDA, K. A. WALSH, M. W. CHOPEK, J. E. SADLER & K. FUJIKAWA. 1986. Amino acid sequence of human von Willebrand factor. Biochemistry **25:** 3171–3184.
47. SHELTON-INLOES, B. B., K. TITANI & J. E. SANDLER. 1986. cDNA sequences for human von Willebrand factor reveal five types of repeated domains and five possible protein sequence polymorphisms. Biochemistry **25:** 3164–3171.
48. SADLER, J. E., B. B. SHELTON-INHLOES, J. M. SOARCE, J. M. HARLAN, K. TITANI & E. W. DAVIE. 1985. Cloning and characterization of two cDNAs coding for human von Willebrand factor. Proc. Natl. Acad. Sci. U. S. A. **82:** 6394–6398.
49. VERWEIJ, C. L., P. J. DIERGAARDE, M. HART & H. PANNEKEOK. 1986. Full-length von Willebrand factor (vWF) cDNA encodes a highly repetitive protein considerably larger than the mature vWF subunit. EMBO J. **5:** 1839–1847.
50. SIXMA, J. J., K. S. SAKARIASSEN, H. V. STEL, W. P. M. HOUDIJK, D. W. IN DER MAUR, R. J. HAMER, PH. G. DE GROOT & J. A. VAN MOURIK. 1984. Functional domains on von Willebrand factor. Recognition of discrete tryptic fragments by monoclonal antibodies that inhibit interaction of von Willebrand factor with platelets and collagen. J. Clin. Invest. **74:** 736–744.
51. HOUDIJK, W. P. M., M. E. SCHIPHORST & J. J. SIXMA. 1986. Identification of functional domains on von Willebrand factor by binding of tryptic fragments to collagen and to platelets in the presence of ristocetin. Blood **67:** 1498–1503.
52. TURITTO, V. T., H. J. WEISS & H. R. BAUMGARTNER. 1983. Decreased platelet adhesion on vessel segments in von Willebrand's disease: A defect in initial platelet attachment. J. Lab. Clin. Med. **102:** 551–564.
53. BOLHUIS, P. A., K. S. SAKARIASSEN, H. J. SANDER, B. N. BOUMA & J. J. SIXMA. 1981. Binding of Factor VIII-von Willebrand factor to human arterial subendothelium precedes increased platelet adherence and enhances platelet spreading. J. Lab. Clin. Med. **97:** 568–576.
54. FRESSINAUD, E., D. BARUCH, C. ROTSCHILD, H. R. BAUMGARTNER & D. MEYER. 1986. Platelet von Willebrand factor: Evidence for its involvement in platelet adhesion to collagen. Blood. In press.

Summary

Endothelium and Subendothelium

JAMES M. ANDERSON

Departments of Pathology, Macromolecular Science, and Biomedical Engineering
Case Western Reserve University
Cleveland, Ohio 44106

In 1977, the New York Academy of Sciences published the proceedings of the conference on the Behavior of Blood and Its Components at Interfaces (*Annals of the New York Academy of Sciences,* Vol. 283, L. Vroman and E.F. Leonard, Eds.). Theodore H. Spaet, in his overview of these proceedings, suggested that one of the goals of the conference was to provide a scientific basis and foundation for the successful development of blood-compatible biomaterials. While it can be argued that that specific goal has yet to be attained, it is clear that the breadth and depth of our knowledge of the ideal blood-compatible material, *i.e.,* the vascular endothelium, has greatly increased and provided us with valuable insights and perspectives on the behavior of blood and its components at interfaces. Furthermore, it is clear from studies on natural surfaces that contact blood that new perspectives and approaches to the development of synthetic blood-compatible materials are available to biomaterial scientists.

One of the major goals of this conference has been the presentation of new information, data, hypotheses, and theories in interdisciplinary areas in the continuing search for blood-compatible biomaterials. The first theme of the conference was "Surfaces That Contact Blood." The preceding five papers dealt comprehensively with thrombogenic and nonthrombogenic biological surfaces, with special emphasis on the endothelium and subendothelium.

Over the past decade, great strides have been made in understanding and appreciating the dynamic role of the endothelium in controlling blood interactions. In the 1970s, much information was acquired on the active role played by endothelium in controlling coagulation, anticoagulation, and thrombosis. From the perspective of blood-compatible biomaterials, the endothelium in general was thought to be the passive, non-blood-clotting cellular surface lining the vessels of the body. It served an additional function as a permeability barrier to the transport of macromolecules and cells. Its identifiable properties were that it was passive, non-blood clotting, and semipermeable. These constituted the characteristics scientists attempted to incorporate into their own studies on the research and development of blood-compatible biomaterials. As is seen in this volume, these concepts are changing and the dynamic and active role of the endothelium is becoming apparent. The emergence of new concepts on the role of endothelium is reflected in two ways in this volume: first, in the extent and depth of new knowledge that has been accumulated on the role of endothelium in contact with blood, and, secondly, in the integration of these new concepts into the research and development of new blood-compatible biomaterials.

The emerging concept of the vascular endothelium as a dynamic regulator of homeostasis and of thrombosis was presented by Michael Gimbrone. In his paper, special emphasis is placed on appreciating the endothelial homeostatic-thrombotic balance with its anticoagulant and procoagulant endothelial-associated factors and functions. The concept of soluble mediators acting on endothelium to alter functional surface properties was presented.

In discussing thrombogenic and nonthrombogenic biological surfaces, J. Frazer Mustard extended the concept of nonthrombogenic surfaces to biological surfaces other than the normal vascular endothelium. In particular, the alteration of the subendothelium from a thrombogenic to a relatively nonthrombogenic surface after injury was presented. The role played by the endothelium in the regulation of the quality of systemic arterial blood and the transduction of blood-borne signals to the components of the vasculature was presented by Una Ryan. Activation of endothelial cells and the interaction of endothelium with mediators including complement and white cells certainly provides new avenues for the biomaterials scientist to explore.

It is obvious that experimental design and methodology may influence experimental results in investigating surface interactions with blood. Jan Sixma discussed the limitations of *in vivo* experimentation in animals and presented new methods to investigate platelet adhesion to human endothelial cells. The role of platelet membrane glycoproteins and von Willebrand factor in the adhesion of platelets to subendothelium and collagen was presented by Kjell Sakariassen.

Although great strides have been made in the last decade in research on the role and function of vascular endothelium, we must remain cautious in our utilization of this information and continue to ask difficult questions regarding the use of vascular endothelium as a model for blood-compatible materials. Questions still remain and must be addressed if true blood-compatible biomaterials are to be developed and utilized in clinical practice. For example, do species differences exist and, if so, what are the similarities and differences among mammalian, nonhuman primate, and human endothelium? In considering potential sites of application, are there differences in human arterial, venous, and capillary endothelium? Although these and other important questions remain unanswered, knowledge gained over the past 10 years has provided us with new and valuable insights on the behavior of blood and its components at interfaces. The knowledge gained on endothelial cells and their dynamic activity as well as on the subendothelium has resulted in new perspectives and approaches to the development of synthetic blood-compatible materials. The incorporation of this new knowledge into the research and development of blood-compatible biomaterials is a challenge for the next decade.

Selected Methods of Investigation for Blood-Contact Surfaces[a]

R. E. BAIER

Health-Care Instruments and Devices Institute (HIDI)
State University of New York at Buffalo
Buffalo, New York 14214

INTRODUCTION

Many techniques are available for determining the surface properties of various materials proposed for contact with flowing blood. Not all are equally suitable for determining those material surface properties most relevant to their end-use condition. This is particularly the case when implants or other blood-contacting medical devices must be characterized in their sterile (about-to-be-placed) conditions. Certainly all of the vagaries of fabrication, packaging, sterilization, and (often) long-term storage must be accounted for.

In this paper, emphasis will be placed on methods confirmed over the past decade to be directly applicable to the surfaces of artificial, that is, synthetic, materials. They are equally suitable for biosynthetics, that is, nonliving materials of originally natural origin, and for harvested blood vessels, heart valves, or tissue tubes both before and after preservation, storage, or implantation. These characterization methods can qualify the material surface parameters, before their first blood exposure, as at least meeting minimum requirements for safety and effectiveness. Demonstration of surface properties within established, predetermined ranges for various materials would allow their immediate exposure (presuming their sterility and lack of toxicologic factors) to contact with human blood to achieve the goals of the prosthetic designer and operating surgeon.

IDENTIFICATION OF THE MOST IMPORTANT SURFACE PARAMETERS

Most of the direct blood compatibility tests for diverse biomaterials, as practiced over the pioneering period of 1964 through 1974 and even later, were complicated and difficult to dignify with quantitative end points. One such test, the vena cava ring implant trial (popularized by Dr. Vincent Gott and his followers), did yield a significant body of important correlating data for the predominantly physicochemical methods reiterated here.[1]

It was first observed at a prior convocation of blood materials research specialists that three natural divisions of the surface qualities of potential implant materials or

[a]Financial support of this work from the National Heart, Lung, and Blood Institute under contract no. N01–HB–3–2953 is gratefully acknowledged.

prosthetic devices were obvious, namely, their surface textures (or degrees of roughness), their surface charges (or electrochemical potentials), and their surface chemistries (or thermodynamic free energies).[2] Each major group of parameters has had its champions in the research community.

In the course of early investigations of the influence of each of these parameters, unfortunately often in confusing combinations, the most important biological determinant of the fitness and suitability of various materials for even short-term contact with human blood (with or without added anticoagulants) was considered to be the tendency for attachment of blood platelets.[3] Platelet distress as a result of that attachment, and growth of platelet aggregates into occluding pyramidal mounds of white thrombi in lakes of fibrin and entrapped erythrocytes, reflected the general character of thrombogenic surfaces.[4]

Careful inspection of the sequence of this deposition process revealed first a primary, spontaneously and immediately deposited, film of plasma proteins. This is the "surface conditioning" event that transduces the properties of all foreign surfaces to the level at which platelet attachment and subsequent aggregation with arriving cellular neighbors is efficient.[5,6]

An early observation that has not yet been properly appreciated by developers of new blood-contacting materials was that simple enumeration of the attached platelets was an insufficient and often quite misleading indicator of the passivity or reactivity of these materials towards the facing, flowing blood milieus.[7] Rather, the response of the first randomly attached population of blood platelets to the transducing "conditioning film" of (usually fibrinogen dominated) plasma proteins on these materials is the key to discrimination of that property called "thromboresistance."

One promising method that does seem able to reflect this quality directly is the measurement of spread surface areas for the first attached platelet population within a few minutes of their first exposure to the freshly placed foreign material surface.[8,9] Platelet spreading, and thrombogenesis, are reflective of the differing degrees of denaturation of the deposited protein precursor films, including those of fibrinogen.[10,11]

There remains considerable debate about the actual composition of the interfacial blood "conditioning films" at the time they are most effective in associating randomly arriving particulate matter with their own surfaces, and thus with the emplaced foreign material. There is no doubt as to their reality and general uniformity, indeed their requirements, as precursors to such bioadhesion. The generality of this observation extends even to objects in the sea, where their spontaneous coating with obviously differently composed but nonetheless similarly functioning macromolecular films is known to precede all practical events of biodeterioration, such as those initiated by bacterial adhesion, algal spore settling, or attachment of the larval forms of barnacles and tubeworms.[12,13]

It has been demonstrated for materials in contact with flowing blood, as well as in contact with other diverse biofluids, ranging from saliva to culture media to saline waters of the open ocean, that in some cases the uniformity and/or permanence of attachment of these biofilms (not yet including particulate matter such as cells or their fragments) is temporary and imperfect.[14,15] Thus, the lack of secure attachment of these primary "conditioning films" is the key feature separating thromboresistant or otherwise bioabhesive materials from the larger body of thrombogenic and bioadhesive substances available for exposure to diverse biological milieus. It is the task of "selection" among the many available characterization techniques to identify the most relevant of the surface descriptors—texture, charge, chemistry—that can predict best these "conditioning film" and cell attachment processes.

EXAMINATION OF SURFACE TEXTURE

It has often been held that surface roughness or other topographical irregularities of emplaced biomaterials are most responsible for adverse events of blood coagulation or induction of thrombosis. It is now generally accepted, however, that surfaces that do not contain gross roughness features or extreme textural heterogeneities (that is, with roughness element dimensions exceeding a micrometer or so in breadth or depth) are not a priori unsuitable for direct contact with flowing blood if care is taken first to "wet out" or liquid-fill the cracks, fissures, and valleys (or other air bubble nucleating cul-de-sacs that might be present initially).

For a long time there was a widely held notion that the silica filler components of common medical grade silicone rubber were the offending fragments that induced blood gelation in contact with such materials, whether through the coagulative or thrombosthetic pathway. This has been convincingly disproved by results with pure filler-free polydimethylsiloxane overlayers and the observation that it is really the microroughness (and air bubble nucleation therein) that triggers untoward biological events leading to blood clot formation. That is, the inappropriate surface quality that was discovered was that of the retained air-blood interface,[16,17] a long-known insulting interface for sensitive blood proteins,[18] and not the more benign and passive low-surface-energy polymers. The major problem of the latter materials is their associated hydrophobicity, which makes elimination of entrapped air bubbles (or nuclei for air bubble formation) very difficult.

A significant proof of the tolerability of even extreme surface roughness when that surface is fully discharged of its gaseous pockets is provided by the common medical hydrogels, such as radiation-polymerized coatings of poly(hydroxyethyl methacrylate) (PHEMA). These water loving and therefore easily wettable materials have extraordinary surface topographies that would certainly entrap vast quantities of air if it were not for their significant hydrophilicities.[19–21]

Thus, it is more a material's surface chemistry, as it influences events of wetting, spreading, and adhesion of even the suspending aqueous phase for most biological particles, that is significant for predicting and/or controlling biocompatibility than is that material's intrinsic surface roughness or texture. For that reason, aside from light microscopic inspection of biomaterials surfaces for gross imperfections or irregularities, which should always be done in concert with inspections for the presence of inadvertent particulate matter or debris,[18] there is no surface textural technique among the recommended "selected methods" required for meeting the minimum essential requirements of good biomaterials practice.

DETERMINATION OF SURFACE ELECTRICAL PARAMETERS

A convincing early suggestion was that surface charge was the primary physical or chemical feature of blood contact material surfaces that correlated with their demonstration of thromboresistance. It was postulated that the surface charge of "compatible" materials should be clearly net negative, or their electrochemical potentials should be on the negative, corrosive end of the electromotive series. This hypothesis had the merit of immediate visualization of how a net-negative prosthesis might simply repel the demonstrably negative particles and macromolecules of all known flowing biological fluids.

Unfortunately, a large and regularly reproduced body of information, which has wasted considerable time and intellectual and financial resources, now exists to show that such a simplistic approach to biomaterials design or selection is in error. The major confounding assumption in coming to the simple conclusion that negative surfaces will repel net negative bioparticles was that the intervening space was filled with a neutral or insulating void rather than the high ionic strength, salty (dead short) milieus that comprise all real biofluids. Thus, in experiments that involved the measurement of streaming potential, surface potential, and surface charge, the conclusion was reached by using well-calibrated methods to provide voltage clamping, calculate the zeta potentials, and account for secondary electronic phenomena that surface electrical properties of materials to be brought into contact with blood or other salty aqueous fluids have very little to do with preventing biological adhesion.[18,22,23]

Indeed, there is growing current evidence that any state of surface electrification will be associated with greater rather than lesser accumulations of biological debris on such surfaces, with an obvious accentuation of adhesive induction by net positive surfaces. Positively charged surfaces can beneficially interact, where that is desired, with the intrinsically negative biomass once that organic matter has actually come into the adhesive zone of interaction of the foreign material.

Here again there is a decision that can be taken. That is, as interesting as such parameters might be, there is no requirement to include any particular surface electrical or electrochemical charge determining test among the "selected methods" recommended as minimum standards for good biomaterials practice.

DETERMINATIONS OF SURFACE CHEMISTRY

Surface chemical determinations set out to answer two key questions: What is actually at the surface of an in-place prosthetic device or foreign material? What interactions will it have with the biological phase it contacts?

Surface Spectroscopy

It is obviously crucial to know the actual chemical composition of the material within that outermost micrometer or so of a material brought into contact with as fragile and reactive a substance as human blood. Methods of bulk analysis, including the common spectroscopies and diffraction techniques, are generally inadequate for this task. Yet a method known and widely available, based on more than twenty years of routine practice in laboratories around the world, is fully capable of giving that information quickly and inexpensively for materials in their actual end-use states.

The method is called multiple attenuated internal reflection infrared spectroscopy. It allows the production of both qualitative and (within single spectra) quantitative comparisons of the abundance of all those substances which have covalent chemical bonds. Thus, polyethylene compounds whose superficial phases are modified by inadvertent oxidation during processing, poly(vinyl chloride) tubing plasticized and inadvertently surface-enriched with phthalate compounds, and sterile objects bearing potentially disadvantageous residues from the sterilizing procedure can all be segregated from the purer, cleaner, or otherwise more desirable lots for ultimate surgical use.

The special capability of this method for determination of at least the average surface compositions of such complicated materials as the intimal zones of harvested, fixed, or otherwise stabilized blood vessels provides a good case in point.[24–26] Here, particularly, as also in the case of leaflets of bioprosthetic heart valves, it is important to know that the tanning or preservative compounds are not free or in excess at the tissue surface that will contact flowing blood, where they might trigger thrombotic and perhaps local necrotic consequences. The technique is also good for identifying the average surface compositions of bioprosthetic blood vessels such as those generally known as Sparks mandril grafts, with special attention to the demonstration that excess amounts of lipids which predispose to secondary mineralization are not present.

It has long been known that this method can be applied to tissues in their naturally hydrated states, or as modified with various plasticizing or therapeutic reagents. The method is used in routine inspections of the qualities of living human skin *in situ*.[27,28] Use of the method for determination of the bioreactive (chemical) qualities of the capsules produced by nature adjacent to (and sometimes in strong adhesive liaison with) implanted biomaterials have often been reported.[29,30] An interesting finding is that even tissue sources as different as those of muscle and subdermal fat will, in essence, react similarly to implant materials of otherwise constant properties (which can be controlled as a method to either prevent or induce biological adhesion). Implant degradation in the biological environment can also be followed by this technique.[31,32]

Elemental Analysis

One major deficiency of the infrared spectroscopic technique, whether by traditional transmission methods or the internal reflection method just discussed, is that it is blind to ionically bonded compounds (such as simple salt, sodium chloride) or specific scale-forming elements (such as calcium or magnesium),[23] or implant metal constituents (like cobalt or chromium). Thus, it is of significant benefit to a proper material characterization if it can be inspected by some technique such as energy dispersive X-ray analysis or electron microprobe methods for the determination of the elemental constituents that may be inadvertently enriched in the surface zone. Recognizing that energy-dispersive X-ray analysis is most easily used in combination with scanning electron microscopy, it is for this reason (as well as for the gain in extra information about surface textural qualities) that scanning electron microscopy and energy dispersive X-ray analysis are strongly recommended characterization techniques for those specimens that will not be rendered irrelevant to their end-use condition by exposure to the vacuum chamber of the instruments used.

Surface Reactivity

If we know the general chemical composition of the material's interfacial region by infrared spectroscopy using the surface-sensitive multiple attenuated internal reflection technique and the elemental enrichments for atomic numbers 12 and greater by energy-dispersive X-ray analysis, it remains only to identify a method capable of revealing the outermost atomic constitution or molecular arrays on that material which will dictate all further interactions with sensitive environments including blood.

The required final technique is the time-honored method of contact angle measurements using a large series of highly purified, well-calibrated and well-characterized liquids of diverse type.[34] Perhaps the worst error in this regard would be to respect this recommendation only in part, determining the contact angles of only one type of liquid (usually water, salt solutions, or water-alcohol mixtures) while ignoring the larger variety of wetting liquids available. The analyst should certainly include some simple mineral oils or more complex polar aromatic reagents that can reveal more fundamental and important surface-specific information than can the limited hydrophilic-hydrophobic ratio so often quoted.

Indeed, as discussed earlier in the surface textural comparison of medical grade silicone rubber and PHEMA hydrogels, these two materials of opposite hydrophobicities have both been reported to exhibit benign short-term interactions with flowing blood or other biological phases (although their long-term behaviors may be quite undesirable on the basis of imbibation of biological matter into their loose bulk phases). It is, of course, of the utmost importance to know the wetting, spreading, and adhesive tendencies of any material about to be brought into contact with flowing blood. Knowledge of the specific reactive potential for aqueous fluid encounters is a reasonable subcategory of that desirable characterization. More important, however, is the development of a full "wettability profile" by the use of a large enough variety of test fluids of a broad enough range of intrinsic surface tensions (energies) that the true critical interactions (as empirically developed using the critical surface tension as one useful parameter, for instance) can be determined.[35–37]

For bioprosthetic materials in particular, it is very likely that easy water wettability will be displayed by materials that are otherwise illustrated to be of remarkably low surface free energy.[38] They will not support wetting, spreading, and adhesion by contacting phases lacking extremely high hydrogen bonding and solvating characteristics. It is important to know that contact angle values of the sort required can be determined directly on hydrated surfaces if that is desirable. Thus, they can be used as immediate, effective, quality control parameters (with the aid of sterile diagnostic fluids) at the surgical table when and if desired by the operating surgeon for confirmation of the surface properties of an implement about to be implanted.

Necessity for Multiparameter Characterization

It is necessary to point out that contact angle techniques alone are insufficient to reveal the entire range of surface chemistries that will be encountered (and should be documented) prior to blood contact with any material. As an example, intrinsically high surface free energy materials—surgical stainless steel, cobalt-chromium-molybdenum alloys, ceramics and glasses of all types—all have very similar critical surface tensions when free of organic contaminating overlayers. The conclusion would be drawn from contact angle measurements on any of these that their blood reactivity would be similar, and this would be confirmed over the short run. No proper inferences could be drawn from the contact angle data alone about the possible migration and secondary interaction of corroding-eroding segments of these materials into the biological surrounding area.

It is clear, therefore, that the combination of (1) internal reflection infrared spectroscopy, which characterizes predominantly the organic qualities of a foreign material interface, (2) energy dispersive X-ray analysis, which illustrates the elemental and particularly inorganic composition of that same superficial zone, and (3) contact angle measurements, which are exquisitely sensitive to the outermost constitution and organization of those constituents at the true reactive interface, may be required to adequately characterize a material at, at least, the level of its being safe and effective for blood contact applications (when it is also known to be sterile and free of leachable toxicants by independent tests).

These selected methods are recommended along with the decade-old advice of our colleague, Dr. John Autian, regarding biomedical devices: "When used as intended, they should behave as intended."

SOURCES OF ILLUSTRATIVE DATA

It is the technical judgment of this author that the described methods, especially as they are simple and direct, are *in combination* sufficient to characterize surfaces of new materials (or often-used, but previously uncharacterized materials) for fitness and suitability prior to their contact with flowing human blood.[39,40] The required or desired features of the surface laboratory in which these tests are best done[41] and schematic illustrations of the practice of these techniques have been provided in published forms elsewhere. It is particularly useful to consult a recently published handbook on biomedical materials evaluation for specific illustrations of the utility of these characterization methods[42] and of available primary reference standards[43] against which these methods and all others considered should be calibrated.

CONCLUSION AND FORECAST

The "selected methods" described here, and many others, have been applied for two decades now by the author and coworkers to an amazing diversity of biomaterials proposed for blood contact uses. The conclusion has been drawn that characterization of the surface chemistry of the materials, taken to include the interfacial composition, organization, and outermost atomic array, is the most critical requirement of all with regard to understanding, predicting, and properly controlling the interactions of materials with flowing human blood[44,45] (in clinical circumstances) during the acute periods when these surface properties are clearly more important than secondary bulk interactions which may ultimately determine an implant's longer-term success.

In this regard, for those desiring production of material surfaces associated with the minimum blood reactivity, minimum thrombosis, and minimum biological adhesion, the cumulative results of this surface characterization approach strongly indicate that the most favorable surfaces are those exhibiting critical surface tensions in the range between 20 and 30 dynes per centimeter, independently of the intrinsic degree of hydrophilicity or hydrophobicity of those materials. Given the fabrication of synthetic blood-contact materials de novo, it is the safer and more direct approach (to design) to have those surfaces, within the preferred critical surface tension range, also dominated by dispersive and van der Waal's forces and to minimize the presence of polar sites.

Conversely, for those many situations in which strong biological anchorage, reaction, adhesion, or induction of adjacent cellular activity might be desired, the recommendation would be to develop materials having critical surface tensions in the range of 35–40 dyn/cm, with a high proportion of polar interactive sites present at their interfaces.

All biomaterials producers and users should be acutely aware that both types of materials might be considered "biocompatible" when limited to use in their specifically intended circumstances—that is, as passive or, alternatively, reactive inserts—but that materials that are "biocompatible" with tissue and bone are not "biocompatible" with blood, and vice versa.

SUMMARY

It is imperative that operating personnel and regulatory agencies have secure, advance, and accurate knowledge of the true surface properties of materials to be contacted with flowing blood. The actual devices must be characterized in their sterile, immediate pre-exposure states. Although very sensitive electronic instrumental analysis techniques are available, the requirements for small specimens exposed to high vacuums and energetic beams hinder their use with practical prosthetic implants. Thus, it remains important that classical estimation of the "wettability" of nonphysiologic materials by simple contact angle measurements can document their real surface qualities in the condition and environment of their intended application. These data, acquired quickly and nondestructively, together with confirming laboratory results from internal reflection infrared spectroscopy, scanning microscopy, and X-ray analysis, are the most useful indicators of material safety and effectiveness for blood contact uses. Experience has shown that the critical surface tensions of materials, determined from contact angle measurements in air rather than underwater, are generally predictive of the tenacity of bioadhesion at their boundaries with blood and other living tissues. Overall, it is now recommended that the surface chemistry of all implant materials be characterized before any exposure to flowing blood, as a minimum requirement of good practice.

ACKNOWLEDGMENTS

Significant contributions to the concepts discussed in this paper have been made by the author's colleagues Anne Meyer, Vito DePalma, Dennis Goupil, and Edward Gasiecki. The author is especially grateful for the opportunity to share these concerns with other members of the Columbia University Biomaterials Seminar over the past two decades. The manuscript was very professionally prepared by Nancy Veihdeffer.

REFERENCES

1. BAIER, R. E., V. L. GOTT & A. FURUSE. 1970. Surface chemical evaluation of thromboresistant materials before and after venous implantation. Trans. Am. Soc. Artif. Int. Organs **16:** 50–57.
2. BAIER, R. E. 1972. The role of surface energy in thrombogenesis. Bull. N.Y. Acad. Med. **48:** 257–272.
3. DUTTON, R. C., R. E. BAIER, R. L. DEDRICK & R. L. BOWMAN. 1968. Initial thrombus formation on foreign surfaces. Trans. Am. Soc. Artif. Organs **14:** 57–62.
4. DUTTON, R. C., A. J. WEBER, S. A. JOHNSON & R. E. BAIER. 1969. Microstructure of initial thrombus formation on foreign materials. J. Biomed. Mater. Res. **3:** 13–23.
5. BAIER, R. E. & R. C. DUTTON. 1969. Initial events in interactions of blood with a foreign surface. J. Biomed. Mater. Res. **3:** 191–206.
6. BAIER, R. E., R. C. DUTTON & V. L. GOTT. 1970. Surface chemical features of blood vessel walls and of synthetic materials exhibiting thromboresistance. *In* Surface Chemistry of Biological Systems. M. Blank, Ed.: 235–260. Plenum. New York.
7. SHOEN, F. 1971. Discussion. Fed. Proc. **30:** 1647.
8. BAIER, R. E., V. A. DEPALMA, D. W. GOUPIL & E. COHEN. 1985. Human platelet spreading on substrata of known surface chemistry. J. Biomed. Mater. Res. **19:** 1157–1167.
9. BAIER, R. E. & A. E. MEYER. 1984. Surface chemistry and physics relevant to platelet interactions with prosthetic devices and other biomaterials. *In* Blood Platelet Function and Medicinal Chemistry. A. Lasslo, Ed.: 175–177. Elsevier Biomedical. New York.
10. MEYER, A. E., V. A. DEPALMA, D. W. GOUPIL & R. E. BAIER. 1986. Human fibrinogen adsorption onto surface-energy-controlled substrata. Bioelectrochem. Bioenerg. **16:** 27–41.
11. BAIER, R. E. 1987. Interfacial biophysics of proteins. Paper presented at the 192d National Meeting of the American Chemical Society.
12. BAIER, R. E. 1984. Initial events in microbial film formation, *In* Marine Biodeterioration:

Interdisciplinary Study. J. D. Costlow & R. C. Tipper, Eds.: 57–62. Naval Institute Press. Annapolis, MD.
13. BAIER, R. E. 1980. Substrata influences on adhesion of microorganisms and their resultant new surface properties. *In* Adsorption of Microorganisms to Surfaces. G. Bitton & K. C. Marshall, Eds.: 59–104. John Wiley & Sons. New York.
14. BAIER, R. E. 1982. Conditioning surfaces to suit the biomedical environment: Recent progress. J. Biomech. Eng. **104:** 257–271.
15. BAIER, R. E., A. E. MEYER, V. A. DEPALMA, R. W. KING & M. S. FORNALIK. 1983. Surface microfouling during the induction period. J. Heat Trans. **105:** 618–624.
16. WARD, C. A. & T. W. FOREST. 1976. On the relation between platelet adhesion and the roughness of a synthetic biomaterial. Ann. Biomed. Eng. **4:**184–207.
17. WARD, C. A., B. RUEGSEGGER, D. STANGA, W. ZINGG & M. A. HERBERT. 1977. Relation of proteins, platelets, and gas nuclei in adhesion to a synthetic material. Am. J. Physiol. **233:** H100–H105.
18. NATIONAL HEART, LUNG, AND BLOOD INSTITUTE WORKING GROUP. 1985. Guidelines for blood-material interactions. Appendices 5–10. NIH Publication No. 85–2185. U.S. Department of Health and Human Services, Public Health Service, National Institutes of Health. Bethesda, MD.
19. RATNER, B. D. & A. S. HOFFMAN. 1976. Synthetic hydrogels for biomedical applications. *In* Hydrogels for Medical and Related Applications. ACS Symposium Series No. 31. J. D. Andrade, Ed.: 1–36. American Chemical Society. Washington, DC.
20. SILBERBERG, A. 1976. The hydrogel-water interface. *In* Hydrogels for Medical and Related Applications. ACS Symposium Series No. 31, J. Andrade, Ed.: 198–205. American Chemical Society. Washington, DC.
21. ANDRADE, J. D., R. N. KING & D. E. GREGONIS. 1976. Probing the hydrogel/water interface. *In* Hydrogels for Medical and Related Applications. ACS Symposium Series No. 31. J. Andrade, Ed.: 206–224. American Chemical Society. Washington, DC.
22. DEPALMA, V. A. 1976. Correlation of surface electrical properties with initial events in bioadhesion. Ph.D. thesis, State University of New York at Buffalo, Buffalo, NY.
23. DEPALMA, V. A. 1980. Apparatus for zeta potential measurement of rectangular flow cells. Rev. Sci. Instrum. **51:** 1390–1395.
24. BAIER, R. E., C. K. AKERS, S. PERLMUTTER, H. DARDIK, I. DARDIK & M. WODKA. 1976. Processed human umbilical cord veins for vascular reconstructive surgery. Trans. Am. Soc. Artif. Intern. Organs **22:** 514–524.
25. BAIER, R. E., C. K. AKERS, J. R. NATIELLA, M. A. MEENAGHAN & J. WIRTH. 1980. Physicochemical properties of stabilized umbilical vein. Vasc. Surg. **14:** 145–157.
26. SHAPIRO, R. I., F. B. CERRA, J. K. HOFFMAN & R. E. BAIER. 1978. Surface chemistry characteristics of human umbilical vein used as chronic canine arteriovenous fistulas. Artif. Organs **2:** 301–304.
27. BAIER, R. E. 1978. Noninvasive, rapid characterization of human skin chemistry *in situ*. J. Soc. Cosmet. Chem. **29:** 283–306.
28. BAIER, R. E., A. E. MEYER & R. W. BESSETTE. 1986. Noninvasive measures of tissue viability. Proceedings of the Eighth Annual Conference of the IEEE/Engineering in Medicine and Biology Society. IEEE. New York. pp. 1837–1839.
29. BAIER, R. E. & A. E. MEYER. 1983. Surface energetics and biological adhesion. *In* Physicochemical Aspects of Polymeric Coatings. K. L. Mittal, Ed.: 895–909. Plenum. New York.
30. BAIER, R. E., A. E. MEYER, J. R. NATIELLA, R. R. NATIELLA & J. M. CARTER. 1984. Surface properties determine bioadhesive outcomes: Methods and results. J. Biomed. Mater. Res. **18:** 337–355.
31. BAIER, R. E. & W. M. ABBOTT. 1978. Comparative biophysical properties of the flow surfaces of contemporary vascular grafts. *In* Graft Materials in Vascular Surgery. H. Dardik, Ed.: 79–103. Symposia Specialists. Miami, FL.
32. DARDIK, H., I. M. IBRAHIM, B. SUSSMAN, M. KAHN, M. SANCHEZ, S. KLAUSNER, R. E. BAIER, A. E. MEYER & I. I. DARDIK. 1984. Biodegradation and aneurysm formation in umbilical vein grafts. Ann. Surg. **199:** 61–68.
33. TOMSON, M. B. & G. H. NANCOLLAS. 1978. Mineralization kinetics: A constant composition approach. Science **200:** 1059–1060.

34. Zisman, W. A. 1964. Relation of the equilibrium contact angle to liquid and solid constitution. Adv. Chem. Ser. **43:** 1–51.
35. Baier, R. E. & W. A. Zisman. 1970. Wettability and multiple attenuated internal reflection infrared spectroscopy of solvent-cast thin films of polyamides. Macromolecules **3:** 462–468.
36. Baier, R. E. & W. A. Zisman. 1970. The influence of polymer conformation on the surface properties of poly(gamma-methyl L-glutamate) and poly(benzyl glutamate). Macromolecules **3:** 70–79.
37. Baier, R. E. & G. I. Loeb. 1971. Multiple parameters characterizing interfacial films of a protein analogue, polymethylglutamate. *In* Polymer Characterization: Interdisciplinary Approaches. C. D. Craver, Ed.: 79–96. Plenum. New York.
38. Baier, R. E. 1978. Physical chemistrv of the vascular interface: Composition, texture, and adhesive quality. *In* Vascular Grafts. P. N. Sawyer & M. J. Kaplitt, Eds.: 76–107. Appleton-Century-Crofts. New York.
39. Baier, R. E., G. I. Loeb & G. T. Wallace. 1971. Role of an artificial boundary in modifying blood proteins. Fed. Proc. **30:** 1523–1538.
40. Baier, R. E. 1982. Physical chemistry of blood-surface interface. *In* Biologic and Synthetic Vascular Prostheses. J. C. Stanley, Ed.: 83–99. Grune and Stratton. New York.
41. Baier, R. E. 1985. Surface laboratory: Its essentials and fundamentals. Biomater., Med. Dev., Artif. Organs **12:** 113–126.
42. Baier, R. E. & A. E. Meyer. 1986. Surface Analysis. *In* Handbook of Biomaterials Evaluation. A. F. von Recum, Ed.: 97–108. Macmillan. New York.
43. Meyer, A. E. 1986. Reference materials. *In* Handbook of Biomaterials Evaluation. A. F. von Recum, Ed.: 131–139. Macmillan. New York.
44. Baier, R. E. 1977. The organization of blood components near interfaces. Ann. N.Y. Acad. Sci. **283:** 17–36.
45. Baier, R. E. 1983. Surface chemical factors presaging bioadhesive events. Ann. N.Y. Acad. Sci. **416:** 34–57.

Influence of Endogenous Albumin Binding on Blood-Material Interactions[a]

R. C. EBERHART, M. S. MUNRO, J. R. FRAUTSCHI,
M. LUBIN,[b] F. J. CLUBB, JR., C. W. MILLER,[c]
AND V. I. SEVASTIANOV[d]

Departments of Surgery and Pathology
University of Texas Health Science Center at Dallas
Dallas, Texas 75235

[b]*Telectronics, Inc.*
Englewood, Colorado 80112

[c]*College of Veterinary Medicine*
Colorado State University
Fort Collins, Colorado 80523

[d]*Institute of Transplantology and Artificial Organs*
Moscow, Union of Soviet Socialist Republics

BACKGROUND

Albumin coatings have long been thought to passivate the plastic surfaces of artificial organs.[1-3] However, few *in vivo* experiments of long duration designed to evaluate this approach have been reported,[4] and clinical evidence has been merely anecdotal. We have studied the passivating tendencies of spontaneously adsorbed albumin *in vitro,* and have found adsorption from solution to provide only sparse coverage.[5] While a preadsorbed layer of albumin inhibits the subsequent adsorption of fibrinogen, a potentially thromboresistive effect, this albumin is easily desorbed in a fluid shear field.[6] Methods to immobilize albumin on the surface prior to implantation have been developed,[1,3,7] but the thromboresistive effect is thought to be transitory, owing to the ultimate denaturation of the adsorbate. Munro proposed a method of binding that allows a renewable albumin buffer layer to form between polymer and blood. This paper reviews the technique and the results of blood and plasma studies, all of which support Munro's hypothesis.

Noting that albumin in whole blood has a high affinity for circulating free fatty acids, Munro proposed the covalent binding to polymer surfaces of 16 or 18 carbon alkyl chains.[8] These chains would mimic the nonpolar structure of the saturated fatty acids and thus might develop a strong hydrophobic interaction with albumin. While the chain-terminating ionic group of the ionized fatty acid does not exist in this case, the hydrophobic bond might suffice to retain albumin, and also permit its removal upon denaturation. The hydrophobic bond is thought to occur in a region where a number of extended helices with long hydrophobic strips have been postulated. The alkyl chain would align with one or more hydrophobic strips. It might stabilize the tertiary (bulk) structure of the bound albumin and thus preserve its inert character in

[a]This work was supported in part by grants from the USPHS (no. HL 28690), the American Heart Association, Texas Affiliate, and Telectronics.

bulk, insofar as surface-activated defenses are concerned. Upon denaturation of the albumin the characteristic alignment of its hydrophobic strips would be lost. Without the chain-terminating ionic group found in the fatty acids to maintain its bond to the substrate, the albumin would desorb. However the (covalently bound) surface alkyl group would remain, able to interact with other functional albumin molecules. The surface albumin layer might thus be maintained indefinitely.

How might an albumin layer so formed inhibit the activation of various blood-borne host defenses? Two mechanisms appear to be possible: (1) prevention of the surface contact-initiating step, due to blockage of surface active sites, and (2) complexing of surface contact-activated material, most likely plasma proteins, with the surface-bound albumin.

Munro *et al.*[9] observed that albumin binds avidly on C_{18}-alkylated polyurethane surfaces. Binding rose with the increase in surface concentration of alkyl groups.[8] C_{18}-alkylated polyurethane surfaces incubated with equal concentrations of albumin and fibrinogen showed a significant decrease in fibrinogen binding.

Similar experiments with albumin : gamma globulin showed no inhibitory effect on globulin fraction adsorption, nor would one be expected, because of competition for the alkyl sites by hydrophobic patches on the surface of gamma globulin.[9] Subsequent experiments demonstrated that the fibrinogen adsorption-inhibiting effect was proportional to the additional albumin bound at the surface alkyl sites.[10] The influence of fluid shear on the organization of albumin on the polyurethane surface was examined by a double antibody immunolabel technique.[11] Albumin was shown to bind within 60 seconds on the alkylated surface, whereas binding on controls was sparse and slow. Albumin binding to the alkylated surface was unaffected by the imposition of a high fluid shear field, which significantly reduced binding to controls. When high concentrations of adsorbed albumin were obtained on control surfaces in prolonged static incubation, they were quickly desorbed following the application of a high shear field. In contrast, albumin was retained on alkylated surfaces given the same treatment. The albumin affinity enhancing effect was demonstrated for a number of other polymers,[12–15] suggesting that the treatment method is broadly applicable.

COMPLEMENT SYSTEM PASSIVATION

Activation of complement proteins C3 and C5 is known to occur upon exposure of cellulosics, polyesters, and other polymers to whole blood, with adverse effects in hemodialysis, cardiopulmonary bypass, and other procedures.[16,17] Since a surface contact activation process has been postulated to account for this effect, we investigated the influences of albumin binding on the activation of C3 and C5. Following Tingey's related work with polyester,[18] regenerated cellulose (Cuprophan, ENKA) was grafted with poly-4-vinyl pyridine (P4VP).[15] Albumin bound extensively to long-chain P4VP-grafted Cuprophan, but not to short-chain-grafted material (TABLE 1). While albumin binding to C_{16}-alkylated P4VP (C_{16}P4VP) was not significantly greater than its binding to P4VP-grafted Cuprophan, its retention following exposure to a moderate fluid shear field, 1200 inverse seconds, was significantly greater than was the case for the unalkylated material.

Activation of C3 and C5 was tested by the radioimmunoassay method of Wagner and Hugli,[19] indicating little activation of C5 for any material, but a significant decrease in C3 activation only for the C_{16}P4VP-treated Cuprophan (TABLE 2). This suggests that the albumin bound to the alkylated surface may have been retained in a conformation, possibly stabilized by the hydrophobic interaction, which blocked the

TABLE 1. Albumin Retention

	Saline Wash	Fraction Retained from NaOH/ETOH Wash
Control	1.0	0.26 ± 0.02
P4VPs	1.10 ± 0.27	0.15 ± 0.08
P4VP1	3.82 ± 0.50^a	0.26 ± 0.03
C_{16}-P4VP1	4.20 ± 1.20^a	0.70 ± 0.01^a

[a] $p < 0.05$ with respect to control.

activation of C3. In contrast the albumin bound (spontaneously) to the P4VP-grafted material was unable to block surface active sites, or was conformationally altered so that C3 activation was enabled. The C3a-inhibiting effect of the alkylated material appears to be clinically significant in its own right, but perhaps more importantly, it suggests that the conformation of the albumin adsorbate, not merely its mass, is an important consideration in determining its biocompatibility.

THROMBORESISTANCE

The thromboresistance of C_{18}-alkylated surfaces was evaluated in a series of canine studies employing a small diameter arterial graft model. Wire-reinforced 4- and 5-mm diameter polyetherpolyurethane tubes (Biomer, Ethicon) were alkylated by the one-step octadecyl isocyanate method.[9,10] Using standard surgical exposure techniques, the tubes were implanted bilaterally at femoral arterial sites. The first series employed a short, 30-minute blood exposure in order to assess the influence of this treatment on the well-known massive thrombotic response within 1 hour in the dog. Tubes were filled with saline, having received no prior exposure to any biological material, and the cut artery was gently sleeved over the tube, in order to minimize implant time. Cross clamps were released and following the specified period of exposure to flowing whole blood the arteries were reclamped, and the tubes were quickly removed and gently flushed with saline. No clot was recovered from either control or alkylated grafts. Following 24-h fixation in 3% glutaraldehyde solution, grafts were sliced axially.

No adherent thrombotic material was observed on any alkylated graft. In contrast, the bilateral control grafts were all covered with a massive mural thrombus. SEM examination revealed that the control grafts contained numerous platelet aggregates as well as a complete mural fibrin network. In contrast, no fibrin or platelet thrombi were seen on the alkylated surfaces, although singly adherent platelets and leukocytes were seen (FIGURES 1a and 1b).[10] Since alkylated but otherwise unmodified surfaces were

TABLE 2. Complement Activation

	C3a (μg/ml)	C3a Reduction (% of Control)
Control	67.7 ± 16.6	100.0
P4VPs	61.1	91.1
P4VP1	50.5 ± 18.0	74.1
C_{16}-P4VP1	25.7 ± 6.3^a	37.2^a

[a] $p < 0.05$ with respect to control.

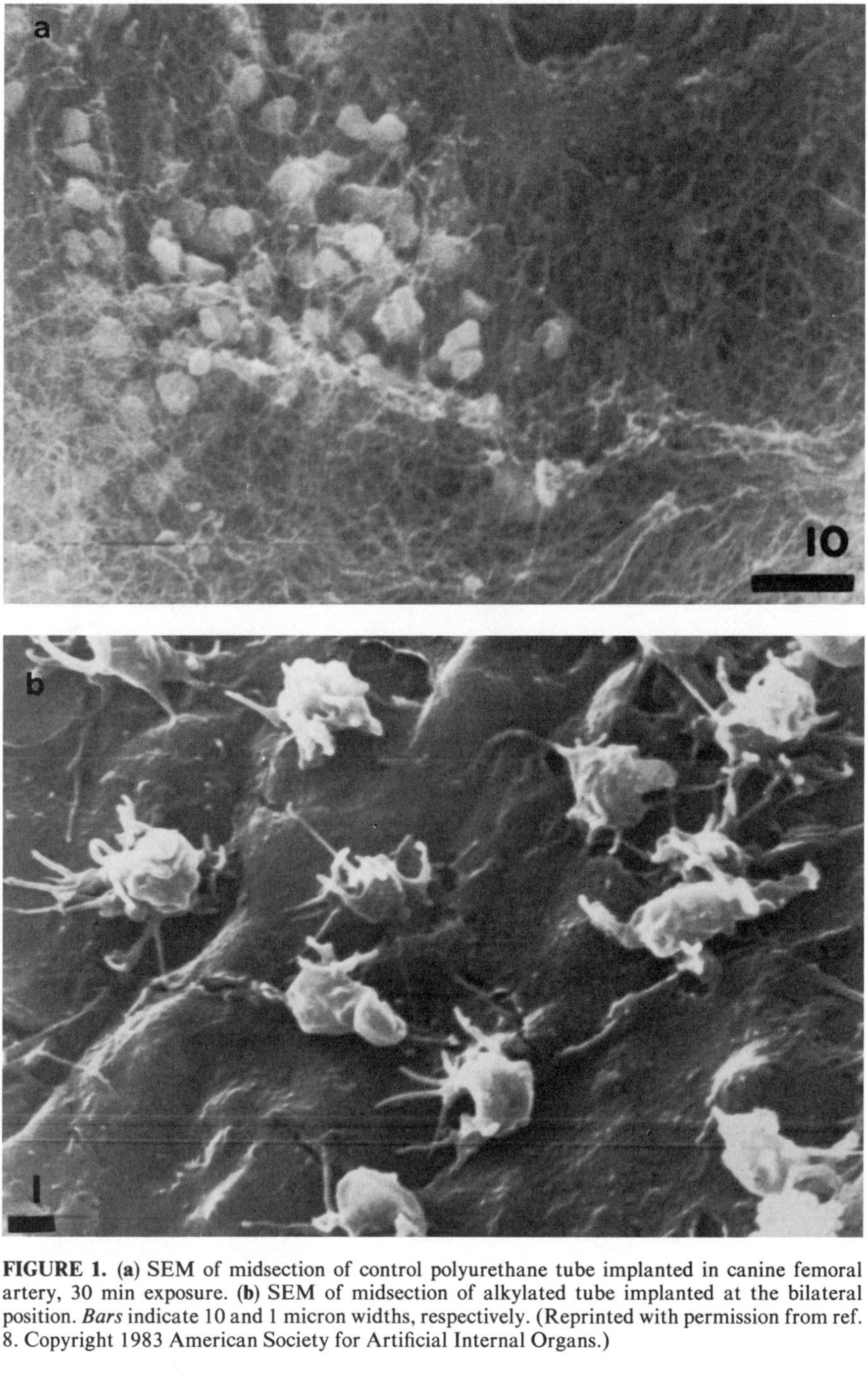

FIGURE 1. (**a**) SEM of midsection of control polyurethane tube implanted in canine femoral artery, 30 min exposure. (**b**) SEM of midsection of alkylated tube implanted at the bilateral position. *Bars* indicate 10 and 1 micron widths, respectively. (Reprinted with permission from ref. 8. Copyright 1983 American Society for Artificial Internal Organs.)

exposed to the bloodstream, it follows that some blood-borne substance, possibly albumin adherent at the alkyl sites, prevented thrombus formation.

These results were supported in 2-, 4-, and 20-hour implantation series in which the vessels were sewn to the arteries, employing running suture technique. The results of the 2- and 4-hour series supported the shorter term findings, although some thrombotic material had embolized from the control tubes, and occasional thrombi were observed on the derivatized surfaces. In the 20-hour series ^{125}I-labeled fibrinogen was infused via a venous catheter immediately following the grafting procedure. Uptake of labeled fibrinogen occurred quickly in the control graft, as measured with a portable gamma counting system (FIGURE 2).[10] In contrast, labeled fibrinogen accumulated much more slowly on the walls of the alkylated tubes, originally appearing at the anastomoses, and subsequently filling in the graft. The accumulations were significantly lower on treated surfaces than on controls at the termination of the experiment. The initial fibrinogen deposits may have occurred at the suture lines in response, at least in part, to leakage of procoagulant and platelet activating substances from the cut ends of the arteries. Two animals had tubes implanted bilaterally for extended periods, 47 and 80 days. In both cases the alkylated and control vessels were thrombosed at explantation. These results might be expected in light of the observed early buildup of fibrinogen at the suture line. The finding of significant thromboresistance in the early period should, however, not be overlooked. The small vascular graft model may be unduly restrictive, since release

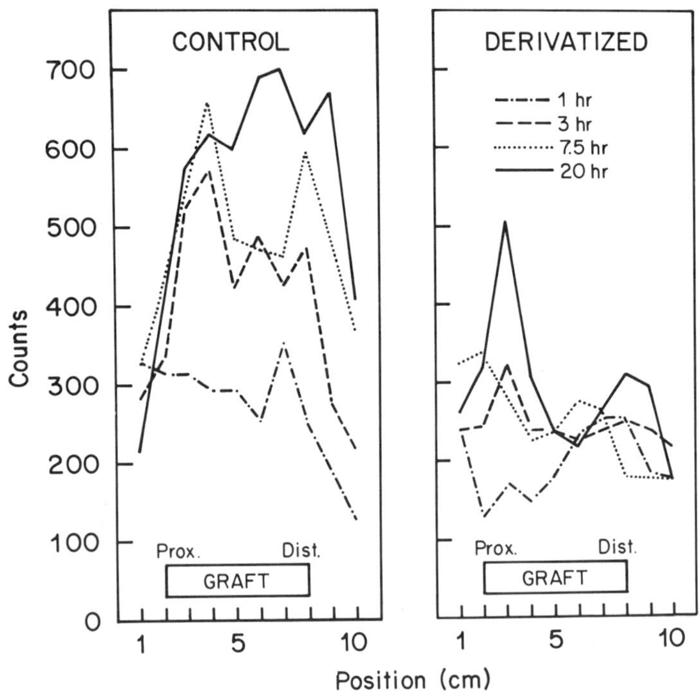

FIGURE 2. Canine ^{125}I-labeled fibrinogen uptake on control and C_{18}-alkylated polyurethane tubes at bilateral femoral arterial sites. (Reproduced with permission from ref. 10. Copyright 1983 American Society for Artificial Internal Organs.)

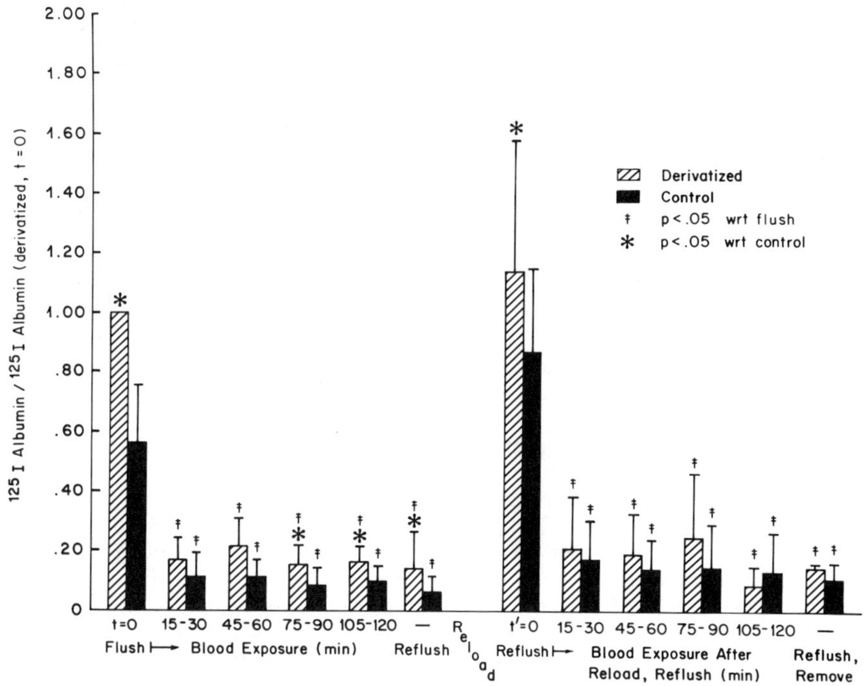

FIGURE 3. Albumin retention on C_{18}-alkylated and control polyurethane tubes at bilateral femoral arterial sites for two sequential blood exposure periods; reincubation with albumin following saline flush at 2 hours. (Reproduced with permission from *Artificial Organs*.[20] Copyright 1987 Raven Press.)

of tissue thromboplastin, collagen contact, and other thrombus-promoting effects would be initiated at the anastomoses.

ALBUMIN BINDING IN PLASMA AND BLOOD

The kinetics of albumin binding and retention to surfaces exposed to flowing blood were examined in the same canine femoral arterial model.[20] Grafts treated in the same way were implanted bilaterally, using the sleeving technique. Proximal and distal branch vessels were cannulated, to allow infusion of ^{125}I-labeled pooled canine albumin, reconstituted from the lyophilized protein. Following a 20-minute incubation, grafts were gently flushed with saline and only then were cross clamps released. Periodic scans of the tube-artery system indicated that significantly more albumin bound to the C_{18}-alkylated Biomer tubes than to the bilateral controls prior to blood exposure (FIGURE 3). Upon exposure to flowing whole blood approximately 80% of the preadsorbed albumin was quickly desorbed, although statistically significant differences of bound labeled albumin were retained for much of the 2-hour period of blood flow. To investigate the possible uptake of substances from blood which might interfere with the albumin-alkyl chain interaction, a second period of blood exposure was planned. The arteries were again cross-clamped, the grafts gently flushed with saline, and then reincubated with the labeled albumin solution. Significant differences in albumin readsorption between the alkylated and control grafts were observed at this time, although in comparison with the first exposure period it was noted that more albumin bound to the control surface (FIGURE 3). This suggested that other material(s) had accumulated on the control surface, possibly including IgG, which could complex with albumin.[21] Absence of increased albumin binding on the derivatized surface at this second incubation, compared with the first incubation period, suggested that no binding or complexing of endogenous substances with the alkylated surface was occurring. The added albumin was interpreted to be in the form of a loosely held layer[22,23] on top of the albumin held by hydrophobic interaction. Upon release of arterial cross clamps that loosely held layer was again desorbed, as it had been in the first blood exposure period. In this second period there were no significant differences in retained labeled albumin between derivatized and control surfaces. The results, while not conclusive, are consistent with the hypothesis of avid binding of albumin to the alkylated surface, with no further binding of that albumin to other biological material.

An instructive experimental mistake was made that supports the idea that albumin binds directly out of blood to the C_{16}- or C_{18}-alkylated surface. In one of the albumin preincubation studies blood was inadvertently allowed into the alkylated tube prior to perfusion with the radiolabeled albumin solution. The experiment was completed without further error; results indicated a significant decrease in binding of labeled albumin that persisted throughout the blood exposure, the following albumin incubation, and the second blood exposure periods. Repeat tests confirmed the finding. When dilute whole blood was similarly exposed to the control tube there was no reduction in subsequent labeled albumin binding (FIGURE 4).[20] In view of the high concentration of albumin in blood relative to other proteins, it is likely that endogenous albumin was

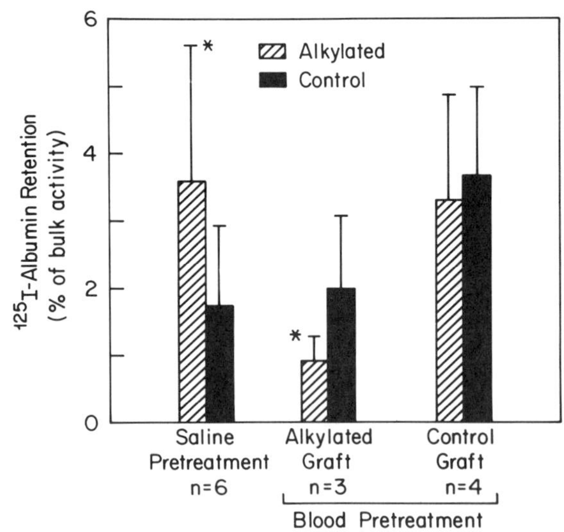

FIGURE 4. Effects of saline and blood pretreatment on uptake of canine ^{125}I-labeled albumin on polyurethane tubes implanted at bilateral femoral arterial sites. $*p < 0.05$ with respect to control.

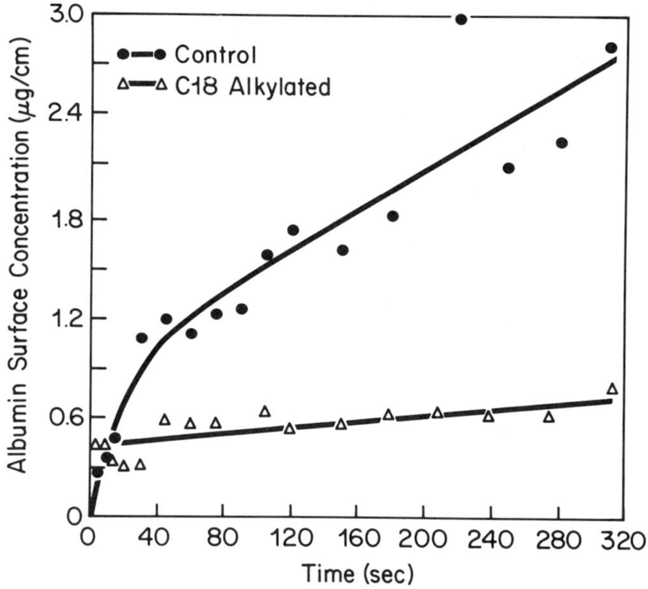

FIGURE 5. Albumin adsorption kinetic profiles on control and C_{18}-alkylated polyurethane (CCS Urethane) films, using human serum spiked with ^{125}I-labeled human serum albumin. Curves are calculated according to the method described in Sevastianov *et al.*[25]

preferentially bound at the alkyl sites during the dilute blood exposure, which did not exchange with the labeled albumin upon its subsequent introduction. While a definitive experiment is yet to be done, evidence collected to date strongly supports that conclusion.

Adsorption of albumin from plasma was measured by the kinetic method of Sevastianov *et al.*[24] Human serum albumin (Reanal) was labeled with ^{131}I by the Chloramine T method. The labeled albumin was added to human plasma in 5–7% concentration. Samples were incubated in labeled plasma for the specified time period. Following incubation, samples were washed three times in saline, and the gamma emissions measured with a well-type counter (Berthold 8F 5300). The specific activity of the labeled plasma was 100 cpm/μg; the relative measurement error was 10–15% with a confidence interval of 0.9. Biomer films alkylated by the one-step octadecyl isocyanate method were rapidly coated with albumin in an apparent substrate-specific reaction (FIGURE 5). In contrast, albumin bound to controls at an initially slower rate, although by 15 seconds the albumin concentration had surpassed that on the derivatized surface. The kinetic model developed by Sevastianov *et al.*[25] was fit to the data (FIGURE 5 and TABLE 3). The results indicated that irreversible albumin adsorption was favored on the alkylated surface, even though more albumin ultimately bound to controls. This suggested that albumin bound to the derivatized surface existed in a configuration that inhibited the binding or complexing of additional albumin, in support of the albumin retention study conducted in whole blood (see above).

A study of fibrinogen adsorption was also carried out in Sevastianov's laboratory. Cohn I fraction human fibrinogen (Sigma) was labeled with ^{125}I, remixed with human plasma, incubated with C_{18}-alkylated Biomer samples, and analyzed as described above. Less fibrinogen adsorbed to the alkylated polymer than to control at 5 minutes

TABLE 3. Adsorption/Desorption Rate Constants (CCS Urethane Exposed to Plasma)

	k_1	k_4	K_3	K_6	$\beta = \frac{k_1 K_3}{k_4 K_6}$
Albumin					
Control	0.041	0.052	0.0123	0.0063	1.55
C_{18} Alkylated	0.746	0.718	0.0018	0.0008	2.28
Fibrinogen					
Control	0.088	0.063	0.0072	0.0070	1.43
C_{18} Alkylated	0.153	0.136	0.0075	0.0074	1.13

MODEL: $[A]$ Dissolved protein concentration at the surface
$[P]$ Concentration of irreversibly adsorbed protein
$[D]$ Concentration of desorbing protein
C_0 Bulk protein concentration

$$\frac{d[A]}{dt} = -k_1[A]$$

$$\frac{d[P]}{dt} = k_2[A] + K_3 - k_4[D]$$

$$\frac{d[D]}{dt} = k_5[A] + K_6 - k_4[D]$$

$$t = 0 \quad [A] = C_0, \quad [P] = [D] = 0$$

(FIGURE 6). The adsorption rate constant was also moderately lower (TABLE 3). The substantial reduction in fibrinogen binding observed in the two-protein (albumin-fibrinogen) binding study described earlier was not observed to the same degree in this plasma study. A definitive explanation for the difference in results is not available at this time; however, some interesting speculations can be offered. Equal and dilute bulk concentrations of the two proteins were used in the solution study, which provided greater influence at the surface to fibrinogen, yet much less adsorbed to the alkylated surface. Fibrinogen displacement by high molecular weight kininogen and other trace plasma proteins, known to begin at approximately two minutes in plasma,[26] may not have occurred due to the absence of these proteins, although relatively impure fibrinogen fractions were used in this solution study. In the plasma study, fibrinogen could be displaced by trace proteins, if the surface were capable of supporting such interactions. That might not be possible on the alkylated surface, if the bulk conformation for the adsorbed albumin were retained. Such suppression by spontaneously bound albumin on the control surface may not have been possible if its conformation was altered upon adsorption. This might also be indirect evidence for inhibition of the surface contact activation of the plasminogen system by the albumin buffer layer on the alkylated surface, although the experiment was too short (5 min) to allow full activation of that system.[27]

PROLONGED IMPLANTATION STUDY

An extended-term implant study of the performance of six different polymer surface treatments has recently been carried out for posible application to a sensing-pacemaker catheter.[28] The basic implant structure was a fixed-tip endocardial pacing lead, 4F × 60 cm (OSCOR Medical) insulated with 4F-80A polyether polyurethane (Pellethane 2363-80A, Upjohn). Five of the six surface treatments were applied to this insulator. The remaining system was insulated with 6.5F-70A silicone rubber tubing (Vesta Inc.). Surface treatments are listed in TABLE 4. Note that one is a bulk additive, incorporated into the polyurethane prior to a special extrusion which provides a very smooth surface. Each lead was cut into two sections. The section without the corkscrew tip was dipped at both ends in a polyurethane solution made with reagent grade tetrahydrofuran or silicone rubber solution, as appropriate; this segment was subsequently implanted in the inferior vena cava. The cut end of the other segment was similarly treated, but the corkscrew tip and proximal 3 cm was neither dipped nor surface treated, and thus served as a control. The surface of the bulk additive treatment catheter was approximated to this condition by dipping in the polyurethane solution. All devices were washed in 70% methanol and sterilized with ethylene oxide, except for the Hydromer coated devices, which were treated with approximately 3 Mrad gamma irradiation.

Fourteen-month-old colony bred female beagles (11 kg, LRE Inc.) were acclimatized in pairs for 2 weeks to outdoor runs. Animals were prepared for aseptic surgery, employing standard techniques.[28] Blunt dissection and cautery were employed to minimize surgical trauma. The devices were introduced into the inferior vena cava (IVC) via the left femoral vein, placing the tip 5–8 cm below the diaphragm. Devices were introduced into the right ventricle via the right external jugular vein, fixing the corkscrew into the apical endocardium. All devices were sutured in place at the entry site, excess implant material was trimmed, and the ends were buried subcutaneously. Following radiographic verification of catheter position the wounds were closed in

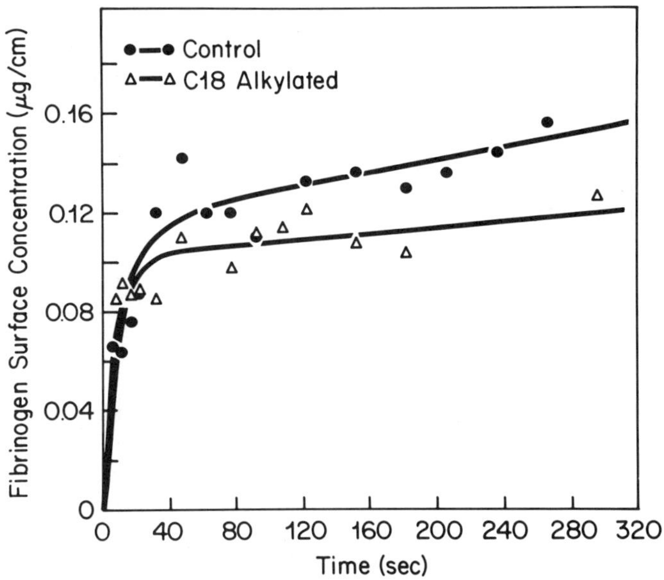

FIGURE 6. Fibrinogen adsorption kinetic profiles on control and C_{18}-alkylated polyurethane (CCS Urethane) films, using human serum spiked with ^{125}I-labeled human fibrinogen. Curves are calculated according to the method described in Sevastianov *et al.*[25]

TABLE 4. Catheter Treatments for 17-Week Implant Study

	Source	Bulk Polymer	Surface Treatment
Control	Upjohn	Pellethane-2363-80A[a]	none
UT	University of Texas Health Science Center	Pellethane-2363-80A	C_{18} alkylation
MER	Mercor, Inc.	Pellethane + <3% proprietary amphipathic additive	none
102	Biomaterials International	Pellethane 2363-80A	high polyether content polyurethane
CAR	Carmeda	silicone rubber	heparin
HYD	Hydromer, Inc.	Pellethane 2363-80A	polyvinylpyrrolidone
103	Biomaterials International	Pellethane 2363-80A	60% higher polyether content polyurethane

[a]No helical tip.

layers. Fasting venous blood samples were drawn biweekly and analyzed for erythrocyte and differential leukocyte numbers, leukocyte count, platelet numbers, prothrombin time, activated partial thromboplastin time, albumin and fibrinogen concentrations, and serum electrolytes. Prior to explantation, animals were anesthetized, systemically heparinized, and exsanguinated by axillary arteriotomy. The relevant vasculature was exposed and a complete lengthwise venotomy and ventriculotomy was performed. Following saline rinse, specimens were photographed *in situ,* removed and rephotographed, and then fixed in buffered formalin (Poly/Lem, Polysciences Inc.). Heart, lungs, and all major pulmonary arteries were examined for thromboemboli;

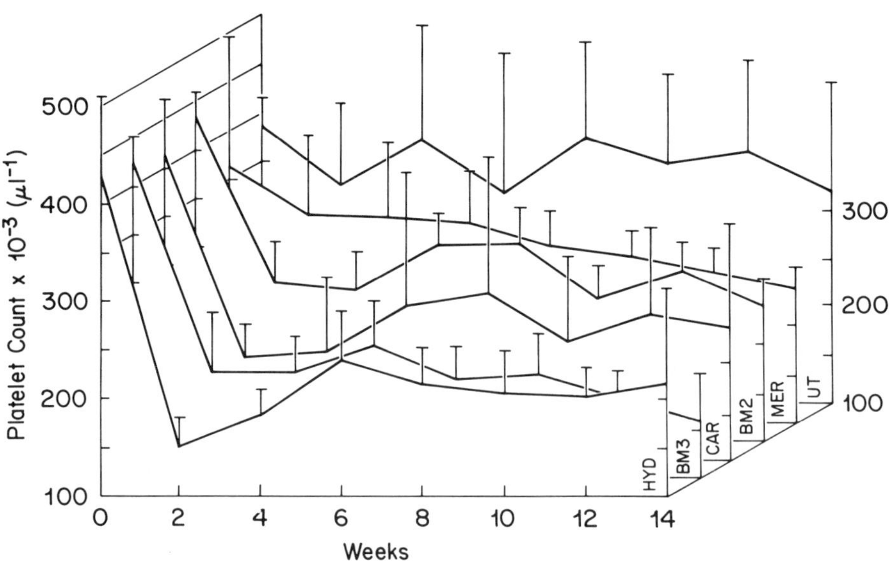

FIGURE 7. Circulating platelet count during period of implantation. *Bars* represent standard deviations; $n = 5$ for all groups as indicated. See text for details.

none were found. For microscopic evaluation, sample segments 2.5 cm long were taken 6 cm distal to the sealed IVC tip and 4 cm proximal to the RV helix. For light microscopy, 0.5 cm segments were halved longitudinally, dehydrated in ethanol, and embedded in methacrylate. One-micron-thick sections were obtained and stained with either hematoxylin and eosin or a modified Carstair's stain for platelets. For SEM, 0.5 cm segments were halved longitudinally, dehydrated through graded acetones, and

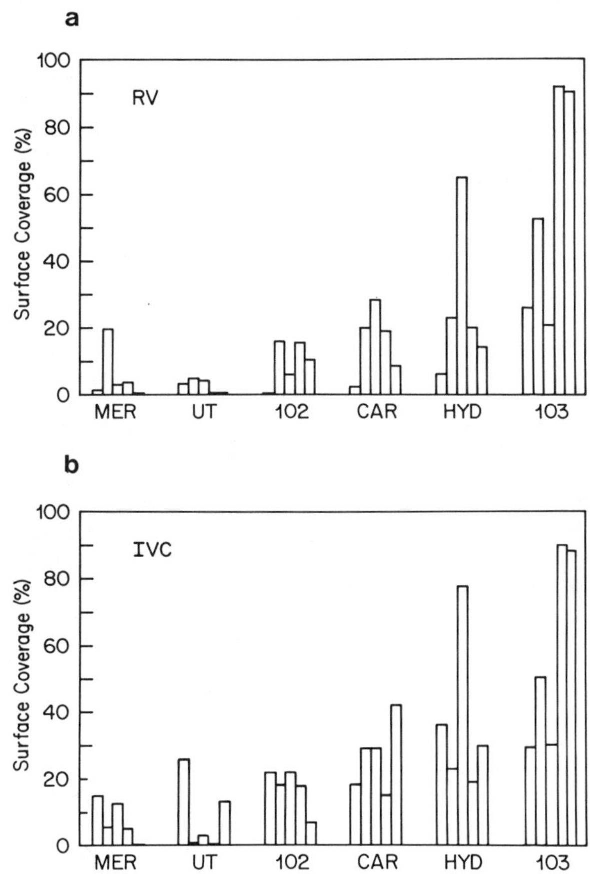

FIGURE 8. (**a**) Surface coverage of catheters implanted in the right ventricle for 17 weeks. (**b**) Surface coverage of catheters implanted in the inferior vena cava for 17 weeks. Coverage determined by planimetry of enlarged photographs. See TABLE 4 for surface treatments and text for details. (Reproduced with permission from Lubin *et al.*[28] Copyright 1986 Futura Publishing Co.)

CO_2 critical point dried. Samples were then mounted on aluminum slabs and coated with gold palladium.

Six animals each received two treated catheters: one each at IVC and RV positions. One animal from each group was sacrificed at 8 weeks to check that no unusual reactions were taking place. The remaining five animals in each group were sacrificed at 17 weeks. All samples were coded, in order that all personnel involved in catheter implantation, animal handling, and surface analysis be unaware of surface treatment. Two animals received sham operations and were followed along with the other groups. After 17 weeks, these animals received "control" polyurethane tubes from the same lot, which were dip-sealed and sterilized but otherwise untreated; these tubes were introduced into the IVC via the contralateral vein and the two animals were maintained an additional eight weeks. Circulating platelet count decreased moderately throughout the implant period for the control group and the alkylated catheter group; decreases for all other groups were much larger (FIGURE 7). This is the one remarkable trend in blood parameters. Little variation in serum electrolytes and coagulation parameters was observed between treatment groups over the 17-week implantation period.

The fraction of the catheter surface encased in tissue, as observed by macroscopic photography, was measured in duplicate by planimetry; results are shown in FIGURES 8a and 8b. Although group ranking was similar, RV implants generally performed better than IVC implants. Three surface treatments, MER, UT, and 102, gave better results by this measure; adherent material was generally limited to the distal half of the catheters in these cases. The three surface treatments with poorer results were observed to have adherent material over the entire length of the catheters. Thrombus on the distal sections of all catheters is expected, since the vein was tied off distal to the insertion site, producing a region of almost stagnant blood up to the vessel branching. Endocardial and valvular lesions were found in the hearts, and endothelial lesions were found in the SVC and IVC of all animals: these were unrelated to the surface treatment. The control dogs had catheters without helical tips and wire cores and showed much less evidence of endothelial trauma in the 8-week implantation. No endocardial cellular proliferations were observed in the left ventricle.

SEM and light microscopic evaluation reiterated the gross analysis and the comparative rankings (FIGURES 9–11). Surface roughening was seen to some degree on all implanted, and nonimplanted but treated samples, compared to untreated controls. The group rankings of biological coatings also applied, in general, to the degree of surface roughening. The gross and microscopic examination of the untreated control samples showed them to be at least as low in adherent material coverage as the best treated samples.

Energy dispersive X-ray spectrometry (EDAX) indicated several of the materials with more prevalent biological coatings also developed calcium-rich deposits. The bulk additive treatment (MER) yielded the least mineralization of the surface. The alkylated surface treatment (UT) came next in rank. The third-ranked treatment in terms of biological coating, 102, developed a pronounced subsurface mineralization, which pushed up the surface.

It was concluded that surface roughness rather than surface treatment was the primary factor influencing growth of a biological layer on these catheters. The improved surface finish and the amphipathic bulk additive probably both contributed to the improved performance of the Mercor catheters. Mild solvent swelling may have improved the surface finish of the alkylated catheters, but solvent evaporation was not controlled to that end. The more probable explanation for the improved performance of the catheters with surface C_{18} alkylation treatment is related to the creation of an endogenous albumin buffer layer.

Additional study is necessary to verify these results. In particular it is necessary to generate a 17-week implant group, with the control catheters being stiffened, with attached helical tips, in order to test the concept that the smooth surface finish of these samples may alone account for the long-term differences in blood compatibility. In

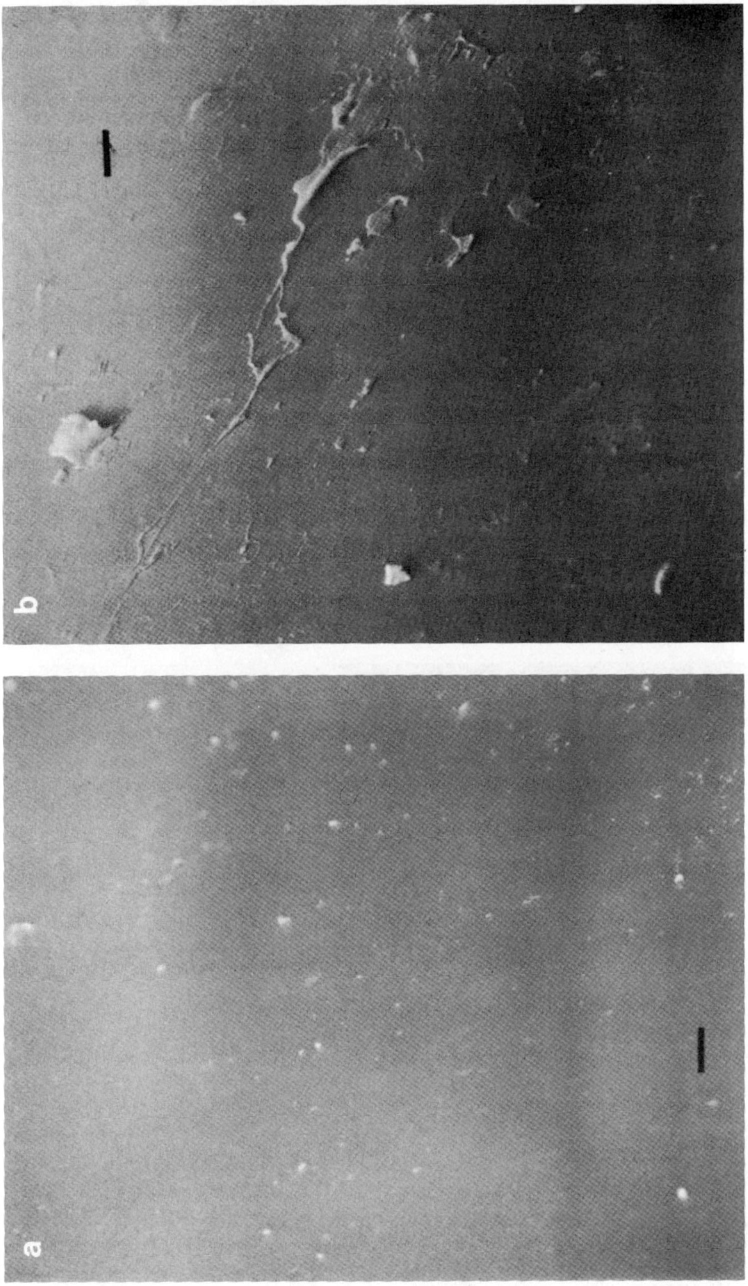

FIGURE 9. SEM of C_{18}-alkylated catheter. **(a)** Prior to implantation. **(b)** Segment from right ventricle (17-week implantation). *Bar* = 10 μm. See text for details.

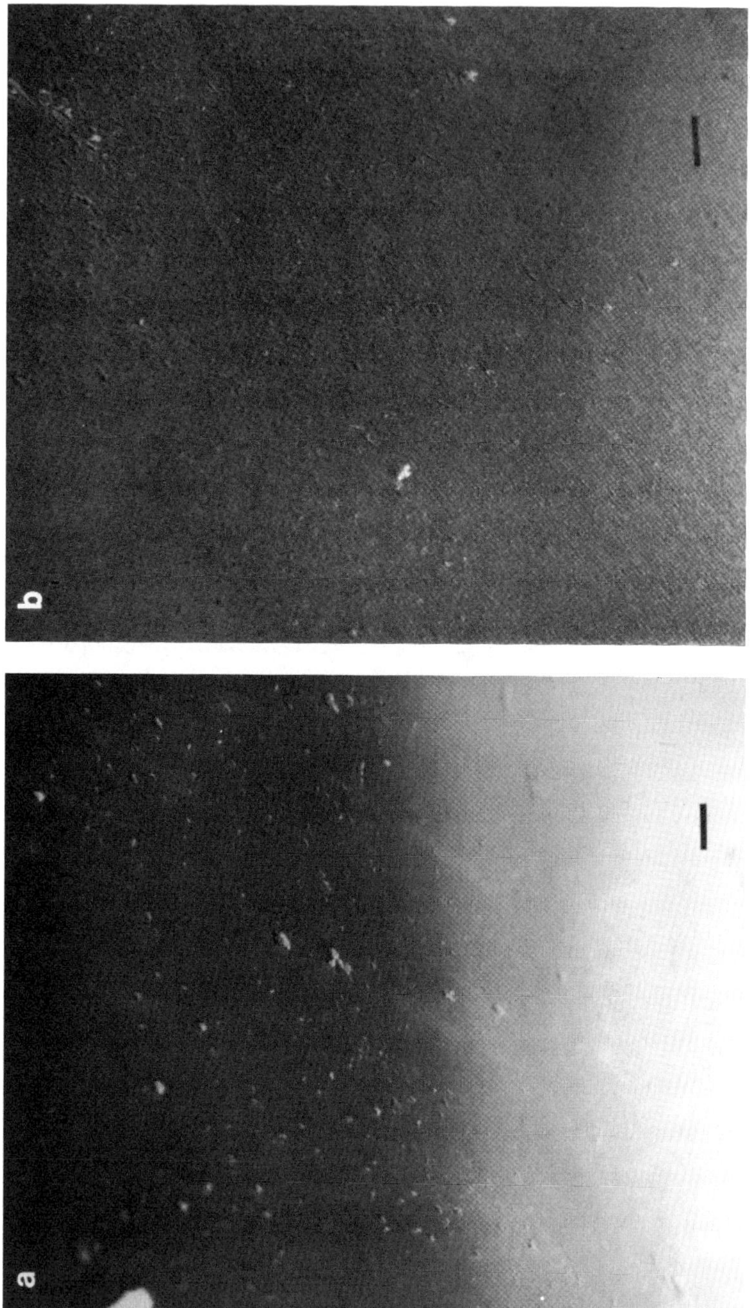

FIGURE 10. SEM of Mercor treated catheter. **(a)** Prior to implantation. **(b)** Segment from right ventricle (17-week implantation). *Bar* = 10 μm. See text for details.

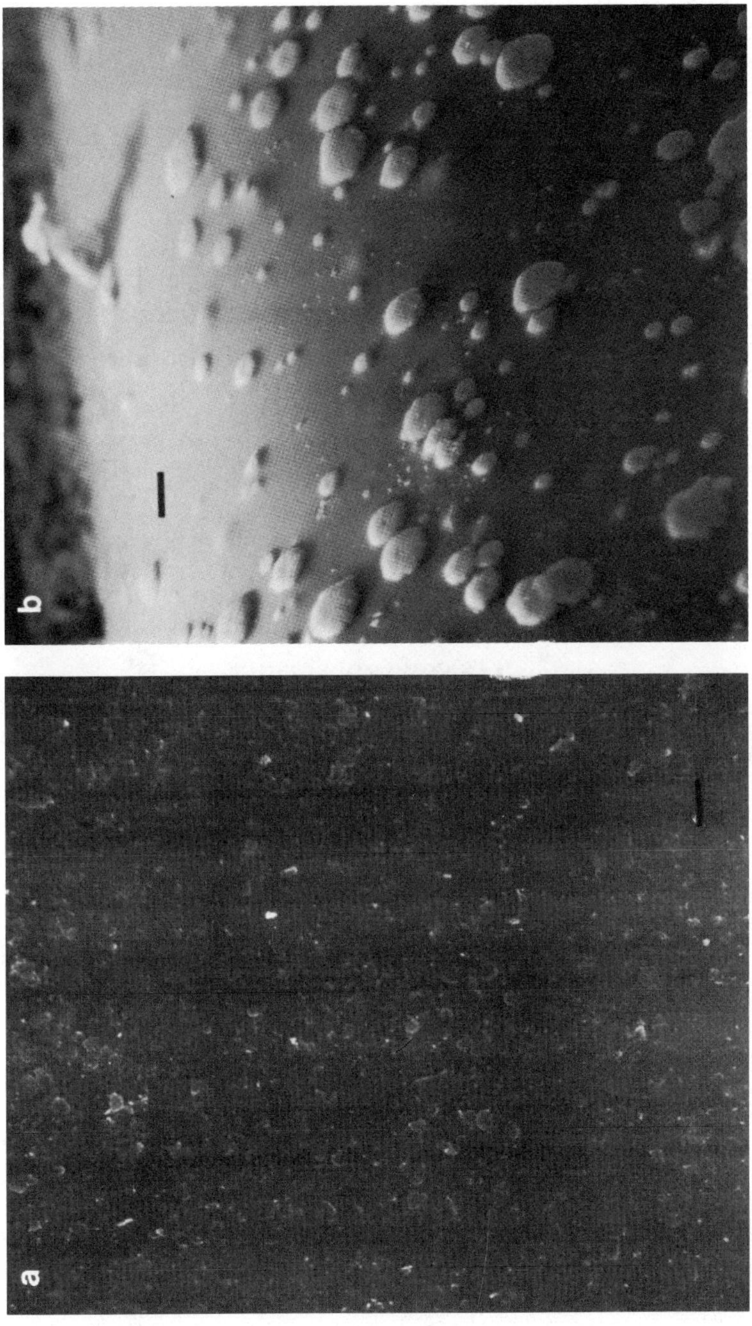

FIGURE 11. SEM of catheter 102 (Biomaterials International). **(a)** Prior to implantation. **(b)** Segment from right ventricle (17-week implantation). *Bar* = 10 μm. See text for details.

terms of the observed differences in performance (adherent coating, platelet consumption, and mineralization) the alkylated catheters ranked the highest.

These results are consistent with the findings of the shorter term experiments, all suggesting that the endogenous albumin layer adsorbed on C_{18}-alkylated surfaces inhibits surface active processes which would otherwise adversely affect the blood-contacting material and its host.

SUMMARY

A method has been developed to enhance the albumin affinity of a number of medical polymers, based on alkylation of the surface with straight-chain 16- or 18-carbon alkyl groups. This method has been demonstrated to induce the rapid binding of albumin from single and binary protein solutions, from plasma, and apparently, from whole blood. The bound albumin resists fluid shear or chemically induced desorption. Fibrinogen adsorption is inhibited *in vitro* and *in vivo*. Complement protein C3 activation from plasma is inhibited. Fibrin formation and platelet aggregation is inhibited in short-term *in vivo* experiments. Long-term catheter implant studies suggest that the C_{18} alkylation is more effective than most, if not all, currently available treatments for the retention of a clean, biocompatible, blood-contacting surface. No data have been obtained to date that conflict with the hypothesis that a renewable albumin layer, so formed, blocks the adsorption or conformational alteration of plasma proteins that otherwise might initiate or participate in various host defenses.

ACKNOWLEDGMENTS

The technical assistance of Nancy Maki, Geraldine Williams and Jayna Stegner is appreciated. The contributions of many graduate students who have participated in this research, including Fertac Bilge, Kevin Tingey, Samuel Riccitelli, Robert Schlatterer, Jay Hendrix, and Mark Rainbow, is gratefully acknowledged.

REFERENCES

1. Chang, T. M. S. 1969. Removal of endogenous and exogenous toxins by a microencapsulated adsorbent. Can. J. Physiol. Pharmacol. **4:** 10–43.
2. Lyman, D. J., L. C. Metcalf, D. Albo, Jr., K. F. Richards & J. Lamb. 1974. The effect of chemical structure and surface properties of synthetic polymers on the coagulation of blood. III. In vivo adsorption of proteins on polymer surfaces. Trans. Am. Soc. Artif. Intern. Organs **20:** 474–478.
3. Imai, Y., K. Tajima & Y. Nose. 1971. Biolized material for cardiovascular prosthesis. Trans. Am. Soc. Artif. Intern. Organs **17:** 6–31.
4. Guidoin, R. G., M. W. King, J. Awad, L. Martin, D. Domurado, M. Marois, M. F. Sigot-Luizard, C. Gosselin, K. Gunasekera & D. Gagnon. 1983. Albumin coated and critical point dried polyester prostheses as substitutes in the thoracic aorta of dogs. Trans. Am. Soc. Artif. Intern. Organs **29:** 290–295.
5. Eberhart, R. C., L. Prokop, J. Wissinger & M. Wilkov. 1977. Observation of albumin deposits on Teflon surfaces. Trans. Am. Soc. Artif. Intern. Organs **23:** 134–139.
6. Eberhart, R. C., M. E. Lynch, F. H. Bilge, J. F. Wissinger, M. S. Munro, S. R. Ellsworth & A. J. Quattrone. 1982. Protein adsorption on polymers: Visualization, study of fluid shear and roughness effects, and methods to enhance albumin binding. *In* Biomaterials: Interfacial Phenomena and Applications, Advances in Chemistry, Vol. 199. S. L. Cooper & N. A. Peppas, Eds. American Chemical Society. Washington, D.C.

7. HOFFMAN, A. S., G. SCHMER, C. HARRIS & W. G. KRAFT. 1972. Covalent binding of biomolecules to radiation grafted hydrogels on inert polymer surfaces. Trans. Am. Soc. Artif. Intern. Organs **18:** 10–17.
8. MUNRO, M. S. 1986. Alkyl substituted polymers with enhanced thromboresistance. Ph.D. thesis, University of Texas Health Science Center at Dallas, Dallas, TX.
9. MUNRO, M. S., A. J. QUATTRONE, S. R. ELLSWORTH, P. KULKARNI & R. C. EBERHART. 1981. Alkyl substituted polymers with enhanced albumin affinity. Trans. Am. Soc. Artif. Intern. Organs **27:** 499–503.
10. MUNRO, M. S., R. C. EBERHART, N. J. MAKI, B. E. BRINK & W. J. FRY. 1983. Thromboresistant alkyl derivatized polyurethanes. asaio J. **6:** 65–75.
11. RICCITELLI, S. D., R. G. SCHLATTERER, J. A. HENDRIX, G. B. WILLIAMS & R. C. EBERHART. 1985. Albumin coatings resistant to shear induced desorption. Trans. Am. Soc. Artif. Intern. Organs **31:** 174–180.
12. FRAUTSCHI, J. R., M. S. MUNRO, D. R. LLOYD & R. C. EBERHART. 1983. Alkyl derivatized cellulose acetate membranes with enhanced albumin affinity. Trans. Am. Soc. Artif. Intern. Organs **29:** 242–244.
13. TINGEY, K. G., J. R. FRAUTSCHI, D. R. LLOYD & R. C. EBERHART. 1986. Alkylated polyethylene terephthalate with enhanced albumin affinity. Trans. Soc. Biomater. **9:** 125.
14. FRAUTSCHI, J. R. & R. C. EBERHART. 1987. Improved blood compatibility of alkylated Cuprophan. Trans. Soc. Biomater. In press. **10:** 125.
15. MUNRO, M. S., A. J. QUATTRONE, S. R. ELLSWORTH & R. C. EBERHART. 1985. Alkyl Substituted Polymers Having Enhanced Albumin Affinity. U. S. Patent #4,530,974.
16. CRADDOCK, P. R., J. FEHR, K. L. BRIGHAM, R. S. KRONENBERG & H. S. JACOB. 1977. Complement and leukocyte-mediated pulmonary dysfunction in hemodialysis. N. Engl. J. Med. **296(14):** 769–774.
17. CHENOWETH, D. E., S. W. COOPER, T. E. HUGLI, R. W. STEWART, E. H. BLACKSTONE & J. W. KIRKLIN. 1981. Complement activation during cardiopulmonary bypass. N. Engl. J. Med. **304(9):** 497–502.
18. TINGEY, K. G. 1985. Synthesis, Analysis, and Albumin Adsorption Properties of Alkylated Poly-4-Vinyl-Pyridine Grafted Polyethylene Terephthalate. M.S. thesis, University of Texas, Austin, TX.
19. WAGNER, J. L. & T. E. HUGLI. 1984. Radioimmunoassay for anaphylatoxins: A sensitive method for determining complement activation products in biological fluids. Anal. Biochem. **136(1):** 75–88.
20. EBERHART, R. C., M. S. MUNRO, G. O. BRIDGES, P. V. KULKARNI, W. A. SHANNON, JR., B. E. BRINK & W. J. FRY. 1987. Albumin adsorption and retention on alkyl derivatized polyurethane vascular grafts. Artif. Organs **11(5)**.
21. SHARMA, N. C., S. F. MOHAMMED, H. Y. K. CHUANG & R. B. MASON. 1981. Albumin-IgG complexes in human serum and plasma that inhibit blood platelet adhesion. Proc. Natl. Acad. Sci. **78:** 7750–7755.
22. LOK, B. K., Y. L. CHENG & C. R. ROBERTSON. 1983. Total internal reflection fluorescence: A technique for examining interactions of macromolecules with solid surfaces. J. Coll. Int. Sci. **91:** 87–102.
23. RAINBOW, M. R., S. ATHERTON & R. C. EBERHART. 1987. Fluorescence lifetime measurements using total internal reflection fluorimetry: Evidence for a conformational change in albumin adsorbed to quartz. J. Biomed. Mater. Res. **21(5):** 539–555.
24. SEVASTIANOV, V. I., Z. M. BELOMESTNAIA & N. K. ZIMIN. 1983. In vitro assessment of hemocompatible properties of polymers. Artif. Organs **7(1):** 126–133.
25. SEVASTIANOV, V. I., A. V. VOLKOV, O. N. RODIN & L. I. VALUEV. 1981. Kinetics of the early stages of protein adsorption on the surface of polymer materials. Doklad. Akad. Nauk SSSR. **260:** 383–386.
26. VROMAN, L. & A. L. ADAMS. 1980. Interaction of high molecular weight kininogen, factor XII, and fibrinogen in plasma at interfaces. Blood **55:** 156–159.
27. BRASH, J. L. & J. A. THIBODEAU. 1986. Identification of proteins adsorbed from human plasma to glass bead columns: Plasmin induced degradation of adsorbed fibrinogen. J. Biomed. Mater. Res. **20(9):** 1263–1275.
28. LUBIN, M., T. NAPPHOLZ, C. W. MILLER, R. WRIGLEY & J. F. CLUBB, JR. 1986. Chronic antithrombogenic biomaterials screen. Pace **9(6,II):** 1154–1159.

Modification of Material Surfaces to Affect How They Interact with Blood[a]

ALLAN S. HOFFMAN

Center for Bioengineering
and
Chemical Engineering Department
University of Washington
Seattle, Washington 98195

When a foreign biomaterial contacts blood the first measurable response in the initial seconds to minutes is the adsorption of proteins. This is followed by platelet, white blood cell, and red blood cell interaction. The initial cell interactions are most likely mediated by the character and composition of the initially deposited protein layer. There are many important material properties and system factors that can influence the protein adsorption and subsequent cell interactions at the biomaterial-biological interface (TABLE 1). It is probable that in static or low flow situations the surface composition most strongly influences the composition and organization of the initial adsorbed protein layer. In higher flow environments the surface molecular motions and topography (smoothness or roughness) may become more important in influencing blood responses. It can be concluded that the polymeric material surface will have a significant if not dominant influence on initial blood-interactions, whether it be through its composition, molecular motions, or topography. At longer times the porosity, the sorption of water or lipids, and the compliance of the material can become important factors in the material-blood interactions in both low and high flow regimes.

Many different techniques have been utilized to modify polymer surfaces in order to improve their resistance to thrombosis and embolization. These techniques may be separated into two major categories: physicochemical and biological. TABLE 2 identifies the various approaches that have been taken over the past 30 years. The most common chemical surface modification technique has been to radiation graft copolymerize selected monomer compositions.[1,2] This may be followed by bonding of antithrombogenic or fibrinolytic agents onto the reactable groups introduced in the graft copolymer.[1–4] Plasma gas discharge (or radio frequency glow discharge, RFGD) has more recently emerged as another interesting and unique way to modify biomaterial surfaces.[2,5–8] TABLE 3 compares these two surface modification processes. It can be seen that despite some similarities these processes are fundamentally very different.

Examples of physicochemical surface modifications are given in TABLE 4. A wide variety of hypotheses have led investigators to study these different surface chemistries shown in the table.

Hydrophobic coatings composed of silicon- and fluorine-containing polymers as well as polyurethanes have been studied because of the relatively good clinical performances of Silastic, Teflon, and polyurethane polymers in cardiovascular implants and devices. Filler-free silicone rubber has been used to reduce potential

[a]The author would like to acknowledge the generous support of his research program by the Johnson & Johnson Company and the support of NIH-NHLBI grant no. HL 33229-02, specifically for research on blood-material interactions.

TABLE 1. Important Biomaterial Properties Influencing Acute and Chronic Responses of Blood to Foreign Materials

I. Biomaterial surface
   A. Chemical composition (polar/apolar, acid/base, H-bonding, ionic charges, immobilized biomolecules)
   B. Molecular motions (polymer chain ends, loops and their flexibility)
   C. Topography (roughness, porosity, imperfections, gas microbubbles)
   D. Domains (distributions of any of the above in the surface)

II. Acute and chronic
   A. Water ("bound" vs. "structured" vs. "free")
   B. Ions (*e.g.*, calcium ion; acidic or basic ions; local pH; electrochemical reactions)
   C. Lipids
   D. Sugars, glycosaminoglycans (GAGs)
   E. Amino acids, peptides, proteins (composition and organization)
   F. Changes in the above with time

III. Bulk absorption, desorption
   A. Absorption from the biologic space (water, ions, lipids, sugars, amino acids)
   B. Desorption of additives or impurities (plasticizers, stabilizers, unreacted monomers, oligomers)
   C. Desorption of breakdown products (biodegradation, erosion or corrosion byproducts)

complications of surface-exposed silica filler particles in Silastic.[9] Polymeric fluorocarbon coatings deposited from a tetrafluoroethylene gas discharge have been found to greatly enhance resistance to both acute thrombotic occlusion and embolization in small-diameter Dacron grafts.[10,11] Polyurethanes have also been synthetically modified and/or fabricated under different conditions in attempts to optimize the hard segment : soft segment ratio and composition at the polymer surface.[12–14] Certain lipophilic surfaces have been proposed to selectively bind albumin, producing a passivating protein layer.[15] Complement activation has been reduced by esterifying -OH groups in cellulosic dialysis membranes.[16]

Hydrophilic coatings have also been popular because of their low interfacial tension in biologic environments. Hydrogels as well as various combinations of

TABLE 2. Biomaterial Surface Modification Techniques

I. Physicochemical
   A. Physical deposition of coating
   B. Chemical modification
   C. Graft copolymerization
      1. Radiation
      2. Photochemical
      3. Chemical
   D. Plasma gas discharge
      1. Etching (ablation)
      2. Deposition

II. Biological
   A. Pre-sorption of proteins
   B. Drug, enzyme immobilization
   C. Cell seeding
   D. Preclotting

TABLE 3. Comparison of Biomaterials Coating Processes

RFGD Polymer Deposition	Radiation Graft Copolymerization
RFGD at low pressure	γ, β at ambient pressure
organic vapor onto solid	liquid monomer onto solid (inert atm.) OR preirradiate solid in air, then contact liquid monomer + cocatalyst (inert atm.)
free radical reactions	free radical reactions
thin, cross-linked, smooth conformal coating	variable thickness and roughness, copolymer coating
unpredictable chemistry	predictable chemistry

hydrophilic and hydrophobic monomers have been studied on the premise that there will be an optimum polar : dispersion force ratio which best matches that on the surfaces of the most passivating proteins and which therefore will be recognized as a passive surface.[1,2,17] Some researchers have suggested that the polar and apolar surface components should be distributed in specific domain structures for optimum blood responses.[18] Polyethylene oxide coated surfaces have been found to resist protein adsorption and cell adhesion and have therefore been proposed as potential "blood compatible" coatings.[19]

A variety of surfaces have been synthesized which either contain positive, cationic charges capable of ionically bonding heparin,[3,20,21] or which resemble the anticoagulant heparin.[20] This leads us to the area of biological surface modification. Examples of this approach to polymer surface modification are listed in TABLE 5.

Many different groups have studied immobilization of heparin, heparin analogues and heparin-prostaglandin or heparin-fibrinolytic enzyme conjugates[3,4,20–22] (FIG. 1). A major point of contention has been whether slow leakage of heparin is needed for it to be effective as an immobilized antithrombogenic agent, since this action could be hindered by being "coated over" with an adsorbed layer of more common proteins such as albumin and fibrinogen.[23,24]

Albumin-coated surfaces have been studied because surfaces that resisted platelet

TABLE 4. Examples of Physicochemical Surface Modifications

1. Physical deposition of coatings
   Polyurethanes, FFSR, cationic soaps, polyethylene oxides
2. Chemical modification
   Heparin-like groups, lipophilic groups, polyethylene oxides, -OH blocking esters
3. Graft copolymerization
   Hydrogels, polyelectrolytes, hydrophilic/hydrophobic copolymers, lipophilic groups
4. Plasma gas discharge
   Silanes, fluorocarbons

TABLE 5. Examples of Biological Surface Modifications

1. Presorption of proteins Albumin, fibronectin
2. Drug, enzyme immobilization Heparin, prostaglandins, enzymes
3. Cell seeding Endothelial cells
4. Preclotting Fresh whole blood

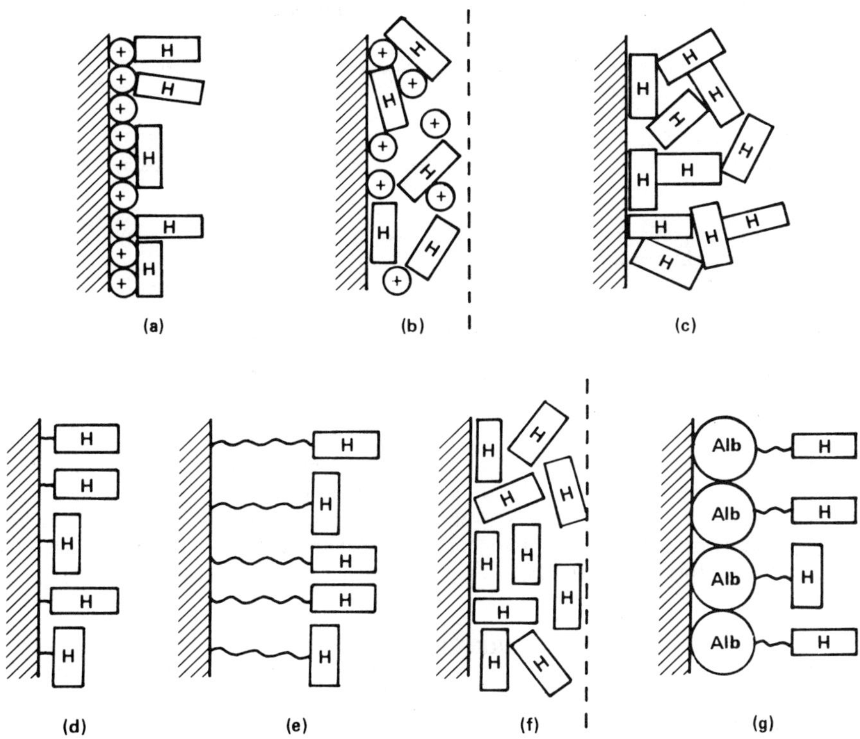

FIGURE 1. Various methods for heparinization of surfaces: (**a**) heparin bound ionically on positively charged surface; (**b**) heparin ionically bound polymer used as coating on a substrate polymer; (**c**) heparin cross-linked surface; (**d**) heparin-immobilized surface; (**e**) heparin immobilization via spacer arms; (**f**) heparin-dispersed hydrophobic polymers (heparin released via diffusion); (**g**) heparin-albumin conjugate-coated surface.[21]

adhesion *in vitro* were noted to adsorb albumin preferentially.[25] Fibronectin coatings have been used prior to *in vitro* endothelial cell seeding, which is being investigated as a method to prepare a surface *in vivo* which most resembles that of the natural blood vessel lumen.[26]

Fibrinolytic enzymes and various prostaglandins have also been immobilized by themselves in order to take advantage of their unique fibrin dissolution or antiplatelet aggregation actions, respectively.[4,21] Once again, an implied premise is that such immobilized biomolecules will not be coated over by a layer of proteins and lose biological activity.

As the reader will realize, almost every biological modification discussed so far involves some type of physicochemical surface modification as a first step. A number of such sequential surface modification processes are shown in TABLE 6.

Finally, one "biological modification" which is commonly used in the clinic is to preclot porous vascular grafts or patches with the patient's own blood.[27] The implant may or may not be surface-modified (before preclotting) according to the methodologies reviewed here, although it usually has no special surface modification.

TABLE 6. Some Sequential Surface Modification Processes for Polymeric Biomaterials

First step		Second step
1. Deposit cationic soap or radiation graft polycation	→	ionically adsorb heparin
2. Radiation graft hydrogel or chemically modify surface or gas discharge treatment	→	chemically immobilize biomolecule
3. Deposit lipophilic groups (chemically or via radiation grafting)	→	hydrophobically adsorb albumin
4. Deposit fibronectin	→	seed with endothelial cells ←
5. Gas discharge treatment	→	preferential fibronectin adsorption (→ seed with endothelial cells)

In summary, polymeric biomaterial surfaces have been modified by a wide variety of techniques, chemistries, and biochemistries in order to improve their performance in contact with blood. The great diversity of approaches is a reflection both of the relative lack of understanding plus the great complexity of the processes of thrombosis and embolization at foreign interfaces.

REFERENCES

1. HOFFMAN, A. S. 1981. Radiation processing in biomaterials: A review. Radiat. Phys. Chem. **18(1):** 323.
2. HOFFMAN, A. S. 1984. Adv. Polym. Sci. **57:** 141–157.
3. LEININGER, R. I. *et al.* 1968. Blood compatible plastics. Ann. N. Y. Acad. Sci. **146:** 11.
4. HOFFMAN, A. S. *et al.* 1972. Covalent binding of biomolecules to radiation-grafting hydrogels on inert polymer surfaces. Trans. Am. Soc. Artif. Intern. Organs **18:** 10.
5. YASUDA H. & M. GAZICKI. 1982. Biomedical applications of plasma polymerization of plasma treatment of polymer surfaces. Biomaterials **3:** 68.
6. CHAWLA, A. S. 1986. Plasma polymerization and plasma modification of surfaces for

biomaterial applications. *In* Polymeric Biomaterials. E. Piskin & A. S. Hoffman, Eds: 221. M. Nijhoff. Dordrecht, The Netherlands.

7. GOMBOTZ, W. R. & A. S. HOFFMAN. 1987. Gas discharge techniques for modification of biomaterials. *In* Critical Reviews in Biocompatibility. D. Williams, Ed. CRC Press. Boca Raton, FL. In press.
8. OSADA, Y. *et al.* 1984. Plasma-initiated solution polymerization and its application to immobilization of enzymes. J. Appl. Polym. Sci., Appl. Polym. Symp. **38:** 45–54.
9. KOLOBOW, T. *et al.* 1977. Blood compatibility of silicone rubbers without silica fillers in the spiral-coiled membrane lung. J. Biomed. Mater. Res. **11:** 471–481.
10. GARFINKLE, A. G. *et al.* 1984. Effects of a TFE flow discharge on patency of small diameter dacron vascular grafts. Trans. Am. Soc. Artif. Intern. Organs **30:** 432–439.
11. HOFFMAN, A. S. *et al.* 1986. The importance of vascular graft surface composition as demonstrated by a new gas discharge treatment for small diameter grafts. *In* Vascular Graft Update. H. Kambic, A. Kantrowitz & P. Sung, Eds. ASTM. Philadelphia.
12. SA DE COSTA, V. *et al.* 1983. Polyurethanes as biomaterials: Assessment of blood compatibility. *In* Polymers in Medicine. Polymer Science and Technology, Vol. 23. E. Chiellini & P. Giusti, Eds.: 231. Plenum. New York.
13. HANSON, S. R. *et al.* 1982. Evaluation of artificial surfaces using the baboon arteriovenous shunt model. *In* Biomaterials 1980. G. D. Winter, D. F. Gibbons & H. Plenk, JR., Eds.: 519–530. Wiley and Sons. Chichester, UK.
14. LELAH, M. D. & S. L. COOPER. 1986. Polyurethanes in medicine. CRC Press. Boca Raton, FL.
15. MUNRO, M. S. *et al.* 1983. Thromboresistant alkyl derivatized polyurethanes. asaio J. **6(2):** 65–75.
16. CHENOWETH, D. E. 1984. Complement activation during hemodialysis: Observations, mechanisms and implications. *In* Artificial Organs, Vol. 8. No. 3. Raven Press. pp. 281–287.
17. HOFFMAN, A. S. *et al.* 1984. Unusual biological interactions at radiation graft copolymer interfaces. *In* Progress in Artificial Organs: 1983, Vol. 2. K. Atsumi, M. Maekawa & K. Ota, Eds.: 819–824. ISAO Press No. 204. Cleveland, OH.
18. OKANO, T. *et al.* 1981. Effect of hydrophilic and hydrophobic microdomains on mode of interaction between block polymer and blood platelets. J. Biomed. Mater. Res. **15:** 393–402.
19. MORI, Y. *et al.* 1982. A new antithrombogenic material with long polyethyleneoxide chains. Trans. Am. Soc. Artif. Intern. Organs **28:** 459–463.
20. WHIFFEN, J. D. *et al.* 1964. Heparin application to graphite coated intravascular prosthesis. Surgery **56:** 404–412.
21. KIM, S. W. & J. FEIJEN. 1985. Surface modification of polymers for improved blood compatibility. *In* CRC Critical Reviews in Biocompatibility, Vol. I., Issue 3. D. Williams, Ed.: 229–260. CRC Press. Boca Raton, FL.
22. JOZEFOWICZ, M. & J. JOZEFONVICZ. 1985. New approaches to anticoagulation: Heparin-like biomaterials. asaio J. **8:** 218–222.
23. FALB, R. D. *et al.* 1967. Studies on the stability and protein adsorption characteristics of heparinized polymer surfaces by radioisotope labeling techniques. J. Biomed. Mater. Res. **1:** 239.
24. LAGERGREN, H. *et al.* 1968. Preparation and evaluation of ‘nonthrombogenic’ surfaces. J Thorac. Cardiovasc. Surg. **56:** 381–387.
25. KIM, S. W. *et al.* 1974. Platelet adhesion to polymer surfaces. Trans. Am. Soc. Artif. Intern. Organs **20:** 449–455.
26. VAN WACHEM, P. B. *et al.* 1985. Interaction of cultured human endothelial cells with polymeric surfaces of different wettabilities. Biomaterials **6:** 403–408.
27. YATES, S. G. *et al.* 1978. The preclotting of porous arterial prostheses. Ann. Surg. **188:** 611–622.

The Search for Thromboresistance Using Immobilized Heparin

R. LARSSON,[a] O. LARM,[b] AND P. OLSSON[c]

[a]*Pharmacia AB*
S-751 82 Uppsala, Sweden

[b]*Carmeda AB*
S-113 47 Stockholm, Sweden

[c]*Department of Experimental Surgery*
Karolinska Hospital
S-104 01 Stockholm, Sweden

INTRODUCTION

The search for artificial thromboresistant surfaces based on the use of heparin started with surface-precipitated complexes of heparin and various cationic surfactants.[1,2] The drawback of these surfaces was that they were not stable in the blood environment. Stabilization of such a complex with glutaraldehyde offered a promising solution to this problem,[3] at a time when several reports appeared in the literature describing unsuccessful attempts to prepare stable heparin surfaces by covalent binding.[4,5] The stabilized ionic heparin surface provided a valuable tool with which to gain insight into some of the crucial requirements for thromboresistance.[6,7] These, primarily, comprised the prevention of platelet adhesion and the inactivation of thrombin via a process consisting of adsorption of thrombin and inhibition in the presence of plasma inhibitors.

These requirements were validated by experimental[7–10] and clinical studies.[11,12] Later, heparinized surfaces were prepared by covalently coupling heparin via an end group.[13] The mechanism of the mode of action of surface-immobilized heparin that had evolved during the previous studies was substantiated.[13] This communication reviews the more recent *in vitro* and *in vivo* studies performed with end-point attached heparin. Two practical applications will also be briefly described.

METHOD OF PREPARATION

Heparin is a linear sulfated polysaccharide with alternating 1,4-linked uronic acid and glucosamine residues. Heparin exerts its main blood-anticoagulant effect by binding to the plasma protein antithrombin (AT), thereby potentiating the inhibitory effect of AT on plasma serine proteases.[14] Only about one third of the molecules in a commercial preparation of heparin bind with high affinity to AT.[15–17] These molecules contain a specific AT-binding pentasaccharide sequence,[18,19] and any alteration of a functional group in a residue in this sequence destroys the AT-binding capacity of heparin. An essential feature of the new method was that it did not affect the AT-binding sequence.[13] Heparin was partially degraded with nitrous acid, yielding fragments with reactive aldehyde groups at the reducing terminal residues (2,5-anhydro-D-mannose) that could be covalently linked in aqueous solution via reductive amination using sodium cyanoborohydride. The molecular weights of the partially degraded fragments were in the range of 5000–8000 daltons.

The primary amine groups were introduced by different methods depending on the supporting substrate. In the most frequently used procedure, polyethyleneimine (PEI) was adsorbed onto a negatively charged surface. In a typical experiment, low-density polyethylene (PE) tubing was negatively charged by treatment with concentrated sulfuric acid containing potassium permanganate (2 g/l), whereby sulfate groups were introduced onto the hydrophobic PE surface, as verified by ESCA (electron spectroscopy for chemical analysis).[20–22] The cationic polymer PEI was then irreversibly adsorbed onto the negatively charged surface. Attempts to elute surface adsorbed PEI by incubation with 1% sodium dodecylsulfate, 4 M guanidine-HCl, 5 M sodium hydroxide, or 3 M sodium chloride were unsuccessful. Apart from being used as a matrix for end-point-attached heparin, surface-adsorbed PEI could also be utilized as a model for preparing heparin surfaces with different characteristics.[13]

TABLE 1. Amounts of Surface-bound Heparin Available for Binding to Thrombin after Exposure to a Thrombin/Albumin Solution

	Type of Rinsing Before Exposure to Thrombin		
Type of Surface	H_2O	Buffer pH 9, Saline	Plasma Saline
Multi-point, unmodified heparin (ionic)	0.75 ± 0.04	0.75 ± 0.04	0.79 ± 0.05
End-point, unmodified heparin (ionic)	0.00	0.00	0.00
End-point, modified heparin (covalent)	0.87 ± 0.05	0.90 ± 0.04	0.90 ± 0.07

Heparin was exposed to thrombin/albumin solution (10 NIH units/ml, 4% albumin) for 15 minutes. Results are expressed as estimated units of surface-bound thrombin per cm^2. Thrombin activity was determined with the aid of a chromogenic substrate, S, 2238 ($n = 9$).

Type I: End-Point Attachment

PEI was dissolved in borate buffer pH 9 to give a final concentration of 0.1 mg/ml. The negatively charged PE surface was exposed to the PEI solution for 10 minutes at room temperature, rinsed with water, and then exposed to a solution of partially degraded heparin (consult ref. 13 for details). The final rinsing procedure included incubation in borate buffer pH 9 for 5 minutes followed by rinsing with water.

Type II: Multi-Point Attachment

PEI was dissolved in water to give a final concentration of 0.1 mg/ml and pH adjusted to 3 with hydrochloric acid. PE surfaces ($KMnO_4/H_2SO_4$, 2 mg/ml) were treated with PEI solution and heparin as above. The classification of these two types of surfaces into end-point or multi-point attachment, respectively, was based on the striking difference in the strengths of their ionic binding of heparin. This was demonstrated by incubating the two PEI surfaces with nondegraded heparin dissolved in saline (0.2 mg/ml) and the pH adjusted to 3.5. After incubating for 2 hours at 50°C, the test surfaces were rinsed with water. One group was further rinsed with borate buffer, pH 9, in order to remove any heparin not firmly attached and one group was rinsed with borate buffer and further incubated with plasma. Surface-bound heparin was assessed by measuring the amount of thrombin activity that could be bound to the surfaces (cf. below). As shown in TABLE 1, the immobilized heparin could not be eluted from the type II surface irrespective of whether it was ionically or covalently bound, whereas the type I surface with ionically bound heparin was highly unstable and, in fact, lost its heparin upon exposure to the thrombin solution (cf. ref. 13).

A possible explanation to these phenomena, partly supported by ESCA studies,[21] would be that PEI adsorbed at pH 3 acquires a configuration that imposes steric restrictions on the attached heparin molecules so that these are irreversibly held by multi-point ionic bonds. PEI adsorbed at pH 9 apparently does not impose such restrictions. Hence, only the terminal covalent bond would hold the molecule in place, which indeed should provide for a true end-point attachment.

ADSORPTION AND INHIBITION OF THROMBIN AND FACTOR Xa

The vascular endothelium constitutes a surface that rapidly inactivates thrombin.[23,24] Early studies using artificial surfaces with immobilized heparin or heparin-like substances also identified surface-catalyzed inhibition of thrombin as a crucial nonthrombogenic principle.[6,7] A number of negatively charged surfaces bound thrombin upon exposure to the enzyme dissolved in saline containing 4% albumin, whereas no binding could be detected on unmodified PE. The surface-bound thrombin showed enzymatic activity against a synthetic amidolytic substrate but also against fibrinogen.[6] There was a striking difference, however, between the various sulfated surfaces when the degree of thrombin inhibition was measured after exposure of the thrombin-loaded surfaces to defibrinogenated plasma or solutions containing purified AT. Only the surfaces containing immobilized heparin were found to loose surface-bound thrombin activity completely. The enzymatic activity of thrombin adsorbed on other sulfated surfaces could not be effectively inhibited.[6] Even multipoint attachment of heparin resulted in a surface which retained surface-bound thrombin activity during prolonged exposure to defibrinogenated plasma.[13] Classification of the test surfaces into thrombogenic or thromboresistant on the basis of the degree of thrombin inhibition correlated with the performance in a canine arteriovenous shunt model[7,8] or a Chandler loop model *in vitro* using nonanticoagulated blood (TABLE 2).

TABLE 2. Chandler Loop Rotation of Non-anticoagulated Human Blood for Thirty Minutes

Type of Surface	Number of Adhering Platelets ($\times 10^{-3}/cm^2$) Determined by Bioluminescence after Rinsing	Platelet Count ($\times 10^{-9}/l$) in Blood after Rotation
Polyethylene	4960 ± 744	complete clot
Multi-point heparin	25 ± 8	complete clot
End-point heparin	8 ± 3	259 ± 29, not different from preexperimental value

PE tubings with an inner diameter of 1.8 mm and a length of 100 cm, filled with blood to two thirds of their volume, were used. If not clotted, the blood aliquots were poured into 3.8% sodium citrate in the proportions 9:1 for a platelet count ($n = 9$).

A number of studies have demonstrated a striking similarity between the heparinized surface and the vascular endothelium with respect to adsorption and inhibition of

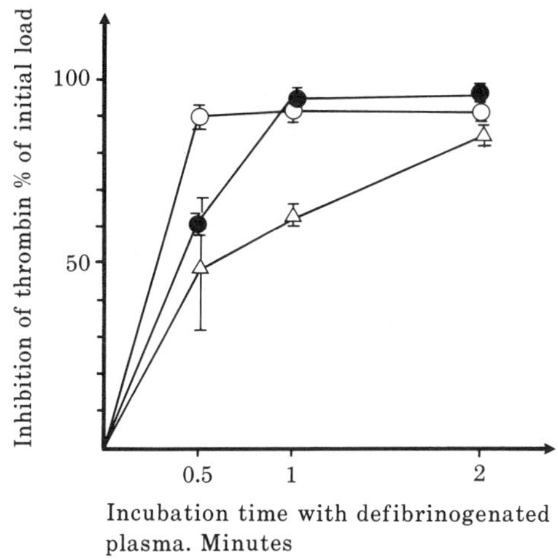

FIGURE 1. Inhibition rates of surface-bound thrombin activity after exposure to heat-defibrinogenated plasma, as a function of incubation time: ○ = endothelium of porcine aorta; ● = end-point attached heparin surface; △ = glutaraldehyde-stabilized ionic heparin surface.

thrombin.[24–27] In an experiment designed for a direct comparison,[27] the heparin surface prepared by end-point attachment exhibited a rate of inhibition of surface-bound thrombin that approached that of the vascular endothelium. The rate of inhibition at the stabilized ionic heparin surface was less (FIG. 1.).

A further series of experiments was designed to elucidate possible mechanisms for the rapid inhibition of thrombin on the heparin surface prepared by end-point attachment.[28] Binding of AT to the heparin surface was demonstrated by measuring the loss of AT activity in plasma or a Tyrode solution containing purified AT (AT/Tyrode), respectively, when rotated in a Chandler loop. Considerably more AT disappeared from the Tyrode solution than from plasma (TABLE 3). Heparin surfaces preexposed to either plasma, AT/Tyrode, or without any preexposure were next exposed as before to thrombin dissolved in saline/4% albumin. The decreases in thrombin activity from the solutions were similar irrespective of the type of preexposure, and there was no difference in the surface-bound thrombin activity recovered (TABLE 4). Hence, the AT molecules preadsorbed to the immobilized heparin were unable to inhibit thrombin. Rapid inhibition occurred, however, when the thrombin-loaded surfaces were subsequently exposed to solutions containing AT. The rate of

TABLE 3. AT Content in Plasma or AT/Tyrode before and after Exposure to Unmodified Polyethylene and Heparin-Coated PE (End-Point)

Type of Surface	AT Content in Plasma before Rotation	AT Content in Plasma after Rotation	AT Content in Tyrode before Rotation	AT Content in Tyrode after Rotation
Polyethylene	1.01 ± 0.01	0.98 ± 0.01 $p < 0.001$	0.76 ± 0.05	0.68 ± 0.06 $p < 0.001$
Polyethylene with end-point-attached heparin	1.01 ± 0.01	0.87 ± 0.02	0.76 ± 0.05	0.00

A total surface area of 50 cm² was exposed to 0.5 ml of AT solution for 1 hour by rotation in Chandler loops. The AT content was assayed as heparin cofactor activity with the aid of a chromogenic substrate ($n = 4$).

TABLE 4. Chandler Loop Rotation of Thrombin, Dissolved in Saline Supplemented with 4% Albumin, in PE Tubings Modified with End-Point-Attached Heparin

Medium Used for Preexposure	Thrombin Activity in Solution before Rotation (NIH Units)	Loss of Thrombin Activity during Rotation (NIH Units)	Loss of Thrombin Activity Calculated to Corresponding Surface-bound Activity per cm^2 (NIH Units $\times 10^3/cm^2$)	Recovered Surface-bound Thrombin Activity (Est. Units $\times 10^3/cm^2$)
No preexposure	10.0 ± 0.25 ($n = 7$)	8.9 ± 0.36 ($n = 7$)	0.36	0.20 ± 0.02 ($n = 7$)
Platelet-free human plasma	10.0 ± 0.25 ($n = 7$)	9.2 ± 0.65 ($n = 7$)	0.37	0.19 ± 0.01 ($n = 7$)
AT/Tyrode	10.0 ± 0.05 ($n = 5$)	9.38 ± 0.08 ($n = 5$)	0.38	0.19 ± 0.01 ($n = 5$)

Thrombin activity in solution and surface-bound thrombin activity after rotation and rinsing with saline was determined by means of a chromogenic substrate. The heparin coated tubings were preexposed to plasma or AT/Tyrode or tested without any preexposure.

inhibition decreased considerably when the concentration of AT in plasma was reduced by dilution with saline/4% albumin (FIG. 2).

The capacity of surfaces prepared by end-point attachment of heparin to inactivate factor Xa were also investigated.[29] When the heparinized surface was tested without any prior exposure to plasma or AT, no binding of factor Xa was noted as measured by loss of factor Xa in the exposed solution (factor Xa, Kabi AB, Stockholm, Sweden, 1.78 nkat/ml dissolved in Tris buffer containing 4% albumin, volume/surface area = 1 ml/28 cm^2). Preexposure of the heparinized surfaces to plasma or AT, however, resulted repeatedly in a total loss of factor Xa activity from the exposed solutions until a point was reached where there was no further loss. When unmodified PE was likewise preexposed no measurable loss of factor Xa activity in the exposed solutions was observed. When the heparin surface had reached the point where there was no further loss of factor Xa from the exposed solution, the capacity of the surface to bind factor Xa could be fully restored by exposing the surface to plasma or AT. In contrast to the experiments with thrombin, no surface-bound amidolytic activity could be detected.

FIGURE 2. Inhibition of surface-bound thrombin activity on end-point-immobilized heparin as influenced by the concentration of AT in plasma (varied by dilution with 4% albumin in saline); ○ = undiluted plasma; ● = plasma diluted 1:2; △ = plasma diluted 1:4; ⊗ = statistically different, $p < 0.001$. The heparin tubings were preexposed to plasma (c.f. TABLE 4; $n = 4$).

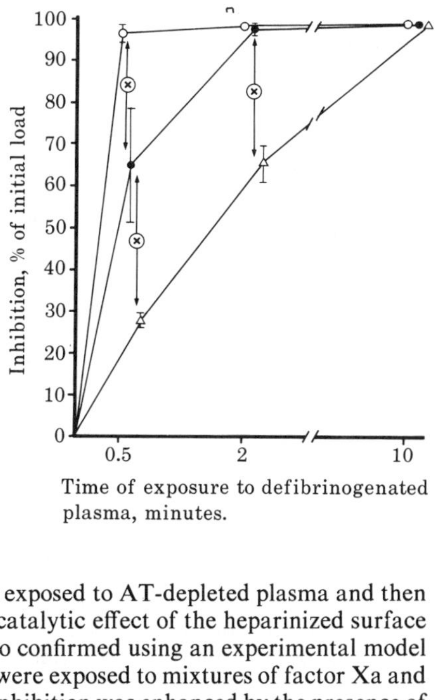

Furthermore, if the heparin surface was first exposed to AT-depleted plasma and then a factor Xa solution, there was no loss. The catalytic effect of the heparinized surface on the rate of inhibition of factor Xa was also confirmed using an experimental model in which unmodified and heparin-coated PE were exposed to mixtures of factor Xa and AT for different periods of time. The rate of inhibition was enhanced by the presence of immobilized heparin.[29]

In conclusion, these experiments indicate that AT interacts with end-point immobilized heparin in a specific mode whereby serine proteases such as thrombin and factor Xa are rapidly inactivated.

COMPATIBILITY OF HEPARINIZED SURFACES WITH BLOOD CELLS

Surfaces prepared by end-point attachment of heparin were tested for compatibility with different blood cellular systems *in vitro*. Poly(methyl methacrylate) (PMMA) was used as a reference to a commonly used biomaterial (*e.g.*, intraocular lens, IOL).

TABLE 5. Activation of Human Granulocytes

Type of Surface	Relative Light Units
PMMA	7009 ± 1468
	($p < 0.001$)
Heparin-coated PMMA	252 ± 31

Activation is expressed in relative light units (chemiluminescence) provoked by exposure to unmodified or heparin-coated PMMA.

Activation of Granulocytes

The generation of the free radical superoxide (O_2^-) by granulocytes is an important reaction in the inflammatory response.[30] The release of superoxide and other reactive metabolites of oxygen can be determined by Luminol-dependent chemiluminescence. Human granulocytes were isolated from heparinized venous blood by dextran sedimentation and Ficoll-Hypaque centrifugation. The cell suspension was kept on ice and used within 3 hours. The final cell concentration was approximately 10^6 cells/ml. Phorbol myristate acetate (PMA), which is a recognized inducer of respiratory burst, was used to check each cell preparation. Unmodified or heparin-coated beads of PMMA (200 μm, 100 mg) were mixed with 100 μl of cell suspension and 400 μl of Luminol diluted 1:50 with phosphate-buffered saline (PBS) containing magnesium and calcium. The test tube, prewarmed at 37°C, was immediately placed in a Luminometer and the relative light intensity recorded. With unmodified PMMA the light intensity gradually rose, reaching a plateau within 10 minutes. Only very low light intensity was recorded when heparin-coated beads were tested. In TABLE 5 the relative light intensities recorded after 10-minute incubation are shown.

Outgrowth of Macrophages

Human venous blood was defibrinated and supplemented with 0.38 M EDTA. The monocytes were then separated by hyperosmotic density gradient centrifugation with equal volumes of Nycodenz and 1.47% NaCl. The cells were washed once in PBS and resuspended in RPMI medium containing 1% glutamine and 1% Gibco Antibiotic Antimycotic Solution. A total of 20,000 cells in 25 μl medium were seeded onto the plane surface of unmodified or heparin-coated IOLs. The cells were allowed to sediment for 2 hours at 37°C, 5% CO_2. After addition of 0.5 ml medium, the lenses were incubated for 5–7 days. On the second day, the medium was exchanged for RPMI medium supplemented with 1% glutamine, 10% FCS, 10% supernatant from a T-cell hydridoma culture, and 1% Gibco solution.

TABLE 6. Semiquantitative Estimations of the Number of Macrophages Present on an Unmodified or Heparin-coated PMMA Surface after Incubation in Cell Culture

Type of Surface	Score
PMMA	3.75 ± 0.34
	($p < 0.001$)
Heparin-coated PMMA	1.31 ± 0.26

Incubation was in human monocyte cell culture for 5–7 days. Scores were obtained by three independent observers ($n = 4$).

After incubation the surface-attached cells were stained immunohistochemically by macrophage-specific antibodies (OKMI). The macrophages were also identified by staining for nonspecific esterase.

The number of cells on the test surfaces was estimated semiquantitatively using a scale from zero to five graduated into 11 steps. The unmodified PMMA surface was normally covered by a layer of evenly distributed discrete cells. The number of macrophages detected on the heparin-coated surface was significantly reduced (TABLE 6).

Platelet Adhesion

Platelet adhesion and activation is a fundamental process in wound healing and thrombosis. The synthesis of prostacyclin by the endothelial cells is presumably of considerable importance in preventing the platelets from sticking to the vascular endothelium.[31] Platelet adhesion is also effectively prevented by surface-immobilized heparin,[8,13] as well as other sulfated glycosaminoglycans (GAGs),[7] which is interesting in view of the fact that the glycocalyx coating of the endothelial cells contains sulfated GAGs.[32,33] The following experiments were performed to assess the degree of platelet

TABLE 7. Blood Cell Adhesion on Intraocular Lenses (Unmodified PMMA or Heparin-coated PMMA)

Type of Surface	Surface Concentration of ATP (μmol × 10^6/cm^2)
PMMA	120 ± 52
	($p < 0.001$)
Heparin-coated PMMA	0.3 ± 0.1

Blood cell adhesion on intraocular lenses after 1-hour exposure to human citrated blood is expressed as relative surface concentration of ATP. Results were obtained by testing six lenses of each type on three occasions using separate blood donors.

adhesion on unmodified and heparin-coated PMMA after exposure to human citrated or non-anticoagulated blood.

Unmodified and heparin-coated IOLs were mounted via their loops (haptics) onto stoppers fitting to polystyrene test tubes (10 × 55 mm) such that the lenses could not adhere to the wall of the test tube. Each test tube was partly filled with 1 ml of fresh human citrated blood (3.8% trisodium citrate in the proportions 9:1), and put on a vertical rotating table for 1 hour. Each lens was then rinsed five times in fresh portions of saline and then immediately placed in 0.7 ml of a buffer (20 M Tris HCl, 2 mM EDTA, pH 7.75) in order to extract adenosine triphosphate (ATP) from the surface-attached cells.

Some lenses were prepared for phase-contrast microscopy by using the same rinsing procedure. The lenses were then fixed in 2% buffered glutaraldehyde, rinsed with water, incubated for 30 minutes with Giemsa stain solution, rinsed with water, and dried. The same procedure was adapted when nonanticoagulated blood was used except for the following points. Blood was withdrawn using a heparin-coated cannula and sampling tube. The test tube and stopper used for testing the lens were also coated with heparin. The test procedure was started immediately after withdrawal of blood. Using citrated blood, there was a more than 100-fold reduction in ATP recovered from the heparin-coated surface compared to the unmodified PMMA surface (TABLE 7).

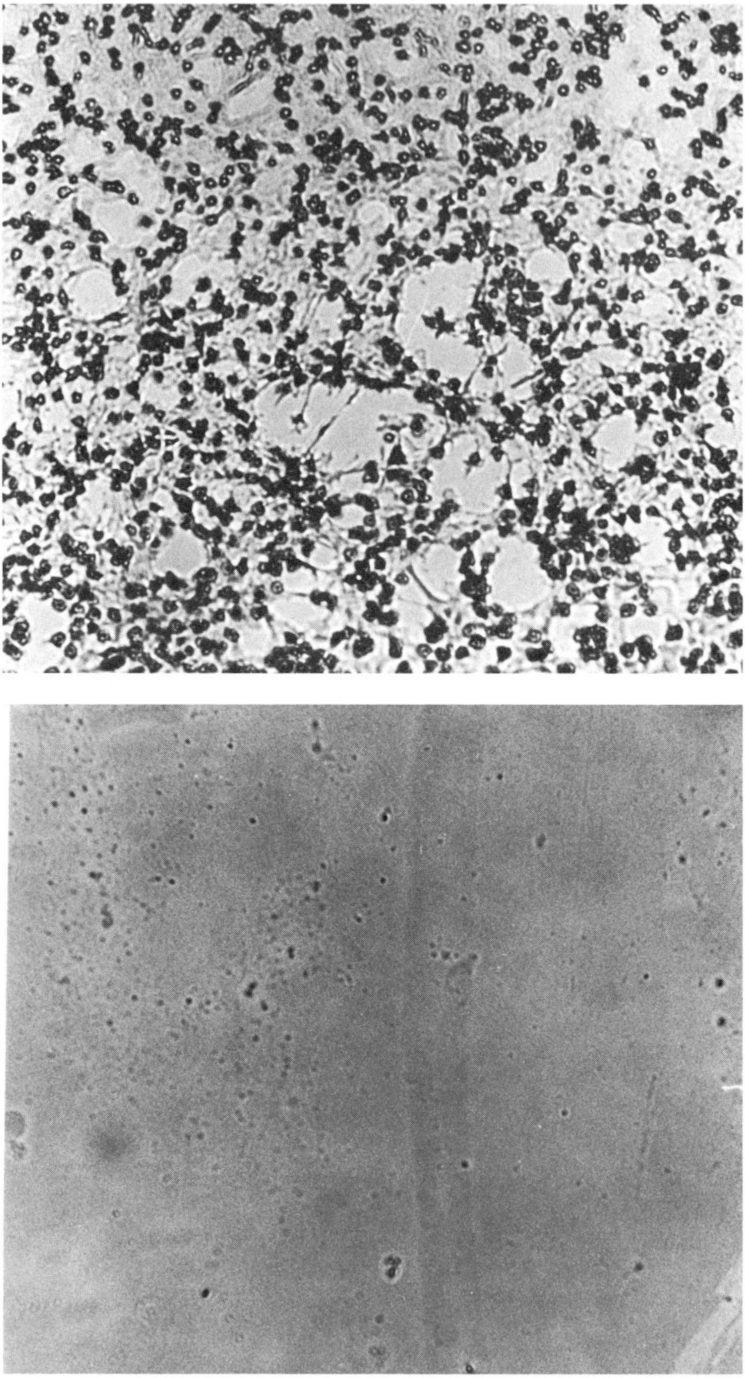

FIGURE 3. Phase-contrast microscopy of a PMMA lens (*right*) and a heparin-coated lens (*left*) after exposure to human citrated blood for 60 minutes. Magnification: 600×.

Examination of the test surfaces in a phase-contrast microscope fully confirmed these figures. Representative photos are shown in FIG. 3. The unmodified surface was normally completely covered by a dense layer of cells, mostly platelets, whereas the heparin-coated surface was almost totally devoid of cells. Occasionally a few erythrocytes could be spotted on the otherwise clean heparin surface. When non-anticoagulated blood was used, the thrombogenic reaction was markedly amplified on the PMMA surface, which was now completely surrounded by a macroscopical blood clot, which made it meaningless to record the ATP content. The heparin-coated surface remained indistinguishable from the heparin surface tested with citrated blood as judged by ATP content and microscopy.

IN VIVO STABILITY

The long-term stability *in vivo* of the heparinized surface was investigated by implanting tubular PE segments prepared by end-point attachment of heparin in the aorta of pigs.[35] The implants were left in place for up to four months. After being removed, the capacity of the implanted specimens to adsorb and inhibit thrombin was compared with the corresponding heparinized controls that had not been implanted. As seen in TABLE 8, the functional characteristics of the implanted surfaces, as reflected by their capacity to adsorb and inhibit thrombin, were virtually unchanged after 4 months implantation. This would indicate that the implanted specimens had not been exposed to any significant heparin degrading activity. Furthermore, the results support the view that the surface-immobilized heparin is regenerative in respect to capacity for enzyme inactivation and, hence, does not become passivated by, *e.g.*, an enzyme-inhibitor complex.[6,36]

TABLE 8. Stability of End-Point-Attached Heparin as Reflected by the Capacity of the Surface to Adsorb and Inhibit Thrombin after Four-Months Implantation in the Pig Aorta

Type of Surface	Adsorbed Surface-bound Thrombin Activity before AT contact (Est. Units/cm^2)	Remaining Surface-bound Thrombin Activity after Contact with Defibrinogenated Plasma for 30 Seconds (Est. Units/cm^2)
Nonimplanted heparin surface	0.43 ± 0.08	0.10 ± 0.03
Heparin surface after 4 months implantation	0.43 ± 0.10	0.02 ± 0.01

PRACTICAL APPLICATIONS

Intraocular Lenses

At present, almost all intraocular lenses implanted clinically have an optic part made of PMMA and haptics of either polypropylene or PMMA. Although such IOLs have been used extensively with good clinical results, it has become evident with the increasing number of implantations that many patients develop slight acute inflammation which in some cases might proceed into a persistent postoperative uveitis.[37] These events are likely to coincide with a partial and transient breakdown of the barrier between blood and aqueous humour. To further improve the biocompatibility of PMMA, lenses with PP haptics were modified with end-point attached heparin. Examination by ESCA revealed that the characteristic ester carbon peak of PMMA was absent, indicating complete coverage.[38] Unmodified and heparin-coated PMMA lenses were compared by implanting twelve lenses of each type in a total of twenty-four rabbits. Details of the operating procedure and clinical and histological examinations will be published elsewhere. Clinical examination using the slit lamp revealed a significant difference after 3 weeks implantation in terms of cellular overgrowth on the optic part of the lens. This difference was also confirmed by removing the lenses, fixation in 1% buffered formalin, and staining for nonspecific esterases. As seen in TABLE 9, the heparin-coated lenses showed significantly fewer cells on their surfaces than PMMA.

Extracorporeal Elimination of Carbon Dioxide Using a Surface-Heparinized Veno-Venous Bypass System

The heparin surface was tested in an assembled extracorporeal system for carbon dioxide elimination in the dog.[39] Three types of hollow fiber oxygenators were

TABLE 9. Image Analysis of Cell Growth on the Central Part of IOLs

Type of Surface	Covered Area % of Total
PMMA	30.0 ± 8.3
	($p < 0.001$)
Heparin-coated PMMA	7.1 ± 1.6

Image analysis was performed after 3 weeks implantation in the rabbit eye. An interactive computerized image analysis system was used ($n = 12$).

furnished with the heparin surface: Capiox II (Terumo Corp., Tokyo, Japan), Bentley BOS-CM 40 (American Bentley, Irvine, CA), and William-Harvey HF-4000 (Bard Inc., Billerica, MA), all having a surface area of 4 m^2 or more. The gas exchange capacity of the oxygenators did not change during the experiments. In the experimental model (anaesthetized dogs), blood was pumped at an approximate rate of 500 ml/min with the aid of nonocclusive roller pumps from the inferior caval vein to a jugular vein. In a loop from this master line, blood was recirculated with the aid of another pump at a flow rate of 2 to 4 liter per min through the membrane oxygenator. The air flow through the oxygenator and the carbon dioxide concentration on the outlet side were determined. The extraction of carbon dioxide was sufficient to keep the animals apnoeic during the extracorporeal circulation, which lasted for 24 to 27 hours. Oxygenation was achieved by passive oxygen diffusion from a catheter placed at the carina level. To prevent atelectasis, the lungs were inflated with a low air volume every second minute. Despite the complex experimental setup, the procedure was remarkably easy to perform in comparison with the use of nonsurface heparinized equipment and systemic heparinization. Circulation parameters and blood gases remained unchanged throughout the experimental period. The condition of the animals was perhaps best demonstrated by the fact that spontaneous breathing commenced within 60 seconds after discontinuation of the extracorporeal circulation. There was no measurable release of heparin and the coagulation time was normal. The concentration of fibrinopeptide A (FPA) in plasma rose gradually up to the slightly elevated level of 50 nmol/l at the end of the bypass session. The platelet count remained essentially unchanged until the last hours when a drop of about 30% was observed. Whether this late decline was surface-induced or due to traumatization of blood in the pumps or to other factors remains to be clarified. The cannulae, tubings, and the hollow fiber part of all the oxygenators were found to be free from visible clotting after rinsing. In each type of oxygenator, however, minor clots had formed. The common feature of these clot-inducing areas was unfavorable hydrodynamic conditions causing stagnation of blood. Although the experiments demonstrated that extracorporeal circulation for carbon dioxide removal can be maintained without systemic heparinization, it is quite clear that the design of membrane gas exchangers and other devices for extracorporeal circulation needs to be modified to utilize fully the advantageous properties of the heparin coating.

REFERENCES

1. GOTT, V. L., J. D. WHIFFEN & R. C. DUTTON. 1963. Heparin bonding on collodial graphite surfaces. Science **142:** 1297–1298.
2. ERIKSSON, J. C., G. GILLBERG & H. LAGERGREN. 1967. A new method for preparing non-thrombogenic plastic surfaces. J. Biomed. Mater. Res. **1:** 301–312.
3. LAGERGREN, H. R. & J. C. ERIKSSON. 1971. Plastics with a stable monolayer of cross-linked heparin. Trans. Am. Soc. Artif. Intern. Organs **17:** 10–12.
4. MERRILL, E. W., E. W. SALZMAN, P. S. L. WONG, T. P. ASHFORD, A. H. BROWN & W. G. AUSTEN. 1970. Polyvinyl-alcohol-heparin hydrogel "G". J. Appl. Physiol. **29:** 723–730.
5. HOFFMAN, A. S., G. SCHMER, C. HARRIS & W. G. KRAFT. 1972. Covalent bonding of biomolecules to radiation-grafted hydrogels on inert polymer surfaces. Trans. Am. Soc. Artif. Intern. Organs **18:** 10–16.
6. LARSSON, R., P. OLSSON & U. LINDAHL. 1980. Inhibition of thrombin on surfaces coated with immobilized heparin and heparin-like polysaccharides: A crucial non-thrombogenic principle. Thromb. Res. **19:** 43–54.
7. LARSSON, R. & U. LINDAHL. 1979. Platelet adhesion and activation of coagulation at surfaces with heparin and heparin-like substances. Proceedings of the Second Meeting of the International Society of Artificial Organs, New York. Artif. Organs **3**(Suppl.).
8. LARSSON, R., J. C. ERIKSSON, H. LAGERGREN & R. OLSSON. 1979. Platelet and plasma coagulation compatibility of heparinized and sulphated surfaces. Thromb. Res. **15:** 157–167.
9. NILSSON, E., G. EDVALL, R. LARSSON & P. OLSSON. 1981. Polarographic pO_2 sensors with heparinized membranes for *in vitro* and continuous *in vivo* registration. Scand. J. Clin. Invest. **41:** 557–563.
10. NILSSON, E., G. EDVALL, R. LARSSON & P. OLSSON. 1982. Continuous intraarterial pO_2 monitoring with a surface heparinized catheter electrode. Scand. J. Clin. Invest. **42:** 331–338.
11. ELDH, P. & B. JACOBSSON. 1974. Heparinized vascular catheters. A clinical trial. Radiology **111:** 289–292.
12. NILSSON, E. & C. ARNANDER. 1984. Long-term monitoring of arterial pO_2 in burned patients. Clin. Physiol. **4:** 13–21.
13. LARM, O., R. LARSSON & P. OLSSON. 1983. A new non-thrombogenic surface prepared by selective covalent binding of heparin via a reducing terminal residue. Biomat. Med. Devices Artif. Organs. **11:** 161–174.
14. ROSENBERG, R. D. & P. S. DAMUS. 1973. The purificiation and mechanism of action of human antithrombin-heparin cofactor. J. Biol. Chem. **248:** 6490–6505.

15. LAM, L. H., J. E. SILBERT & R. D. ROSENBERG. 1976. The separation of active and inactive forms of heparin. Biochem. Biophys. Res. Commun. **69:** 570–577.
16. HÖÖK, M., I. BJÖRK, J. HOPWOOD & U. LINDAHL. 1976. Anticoagulant activity of heparin: separation of high activity and low activity heparin species by affinity chromatography on immobilized antithrombin. FEBS Lett. **66:** 90–93.
17. ANDERSSON, L.-O., T.W. BARROWCLIFFE, E. HOLMER, E. A. JOHNSON & G. E. C. SIMS. 1976. Anticoagulant properties of heparin fractioned by affinity chromatography on matrix bound antithrombin III and by gel filtration. Throm. Res. **9:** 575–583.
18. THUNBERG, L., G. BÄCKSTRÖM & U. LINDAHL. 1982. Further characterization of the antithrombin-binding sequence in heparin. Carbohydr. Res. **100:** 393–410.
19. CASU, B., P. ORESTE, G. TORRI, G. ZOPPETTI, J. CHOAY, J.-C. LORMEAU, M. PETITOU, & P. X. SINAŸ. 1981. The structure of heparin oligosaccharide fragments with high anti-(factor X_a) activity containing the minimal antithrombin III binding sequence. Biochem. J. **197:** 599–609.
20. LARSSON, R., J. C. ERIKSSON & P. OLSSON. 1979. The effects of surface localized sulphate groups on the clotting time in plasma. Thromb. Res. **14:** 941–952.
21. LARSSON, N., P. STENIUS, J. C. ERIKSSON, R. MARIPUU & B. LINDBERG. 1982. ESCA studies on sulphated polyetylene surfaces modified by adsorption of polyethyleneimine and colloidal silica particles. J. Colloid Interface Sci. **90:** 127–136.
22. ERIKSSON, J. C., C. G. GÖLANDER, A. BASZKIN & L. TER-MINASSIAN-SARAGA. 1984. Characterization of $KMnO_4/H_2SO_4$-oxidized polyethylene surfaces by means of ESCA and $^{45}Ca^{2+}$ adsorption. J. Colloid Interface Sci. **100:** 381–392.
23. LOLLAR, P. & W. G. OWEN. 1980. Clearance of thrombin from circulation in rabbits by high-affinity binding sites on endothelium. Possible role in the activation of thrombin by antithrombin III. J. Clin. Invest. **66:** 1222–1230.
24. SWEDENBORG, J., M. DRYJSKI & P. OLSSON. 1983. Inactivation of thrombin by the aortic endothelium. Thromb. Haemostas. **50:** 635—638.
25. DRYJSKI, M., R. LARSSON, P. OLSSON & J. SWEDENBORG. 1983. Effect of glycosaminoglycans and antithrombin III on uptake and inhibition of thrombin by the vascular wall. Thromb. Res. **32:** 355–363.
26. SWEDENBORG, J., M. DRYJSKI, S. FREBELIUS & P. OLSSON. 1985. Uptake and inactivation of thrombin on rabbit aortic endothelium studied with two different substrates. Thromb. Haemostas. **54:** 828–832.
27. ARNANDER, C., M. DRYJKSI, R. LARSSON, P. OLSSON & J. SWEDENBORG. 1986. Thrombin uptake and inhibition on endothelium and surfaces with a stable heparin coating: A comparative *in vitro* study. J. Biomed. Mater. Res. **20:** 235–246.
28. PASCHE, B., K. KODAMA, O. LARM, P. OLSSON & J. SWEDENBORG. 1986. Thrombin inactivation on surfaces with covalently bonded heparin. Thromb. Res. **44:** 739–748.
29. KODAMA, K., O. LARM, P. OLSSON, B. PASCHE & J. SWEDENBORG. In preparation.
30. DAHINDEN, C. A., J. FEHR & T. E. HUGLI. 1983. Role of cell surface contact in the kinetics of superoxide production by granulocytes. J. Clin. Invest. **72:** 113–121.
31. MONCADA, S., A. G. HERMAN, E. A. HIGGS & J. R. VANE. 1977. Differential formation of prostacyclin (PGX or PGI_2) by layers of the arterial wall. An explanation for the anti-thrombotic properties of the vascular endothelium. Thromb. Res. **11:** 323–344.
32. BUONASSISI, V. & M. ROOT. 1975. Enzymatic degradation of heparin-related mucopolysaccharides from the surface of endothelial cell cultures. Biochim. Biophys. Acta **385:** 1–10.
33. NAKAZAWA, K. & K. MURATA. 1975. Acid glycosaminoglycans in three layers on human aorta. Their different constitution and anticoagulant function. Arterial Wall **2:** 203–211.
34. OLSSON, P., B. BLOMBÄCK, H. LAGERGREN, R. LARSSON & M. TOMIKAVA. 1978. Interaction of platelets with surface-bound or conjugated fibrinogen. *In* Recent Progress in Blood Coagulation and Thrombosis Research. Bibl. Haematol. (Basel) No. 44. Karger. Basel. pp. 134–138.
35. ARNANDER, C., D. BAGGER-SJÖBÄCK, S. FREBELIUS, R. LARSSON & J. SWEDENBORG. 1987. Long-term stability *in vivo* of a thromboresistant heparinized surface. Biomaterials. In press.
36. GOOSEN, M. F. A. & M. V. SEFTON. 1982. Invalidation of concerns with long-term use of

heparin: Thrombin/antithrombin III interactions. Trans. Am. Soc. Artif. Intern. Organs **28:** 451–455.

37. Apple, D. J., J. M. Craythorn, R. J. Olson, L. E. Little, J. B. Lyman, J. J. Reidy & K. Loftfield. 1984. Anterior segment complications and neovascular glaucoma following implantation of a posterior chamber intraocular lens. Ophtalmology **91:** 403–419.
38. Lindberg, B. & R. Larsson. Unpublished results.
39. Bindslev, L., J. Gouda, K. Inacio, K. Kodama, H. Lagergren, O. Larm, E. Nilsson & P. Olsson. 1986. Extracorporeal elimination of carbon dioxide using a surface-heparinized veno-venous bypass system. Trans. Am. Soc. Artif. Intern Organs. In press.

Nonthrombogenic Bioactive Surfaces[a]

S. W. KIM, H. JACOBS, J. Y. LIN, C. NOJORI,
AND T. OKANO

Department of Pharmaceutics
University of Utah
Salt Lake City, Utah 84112

INTRODUCTION

Fibrin formation and platelet aggregation are the two main mechanisms governing hemostasis in animals. The two mechanisms are separate, yet synergistic, in controlling bleeding and providing a defense mechanism against vascular injury and foreign surfaces.

Fibrin formation involves activation of the intrinsic coagulation cascade. The cascade is initiated by plasma proteins adsorbing onto an activating surface (*e.g.*, polymers, negatively charged collagen, or activated platelet membranes). Various proteolytic enzymes are involved in the cascade, leading to the conversion of prothrombin to thrombin. Thrombin then converts fibrinogen to fibrin monomers that are subsequently cross-linked to form a fibrin network (clot).[1]

Platelet aggregation and adhesion are initiated by exposure of blood to activating agents, such as polymer surfaces, sublayer structures of injured vasculature (microfibrils, basement membranes or collagen), established fibrin clots, or various chemicals (ADP, seritonin). Platelets attach to surfaces, then activate and contract to release the contents of their intracellular granules (ADP and ATP). These agents stimulate further platelet aggregation to ultimately form a platelet plug and release platelet factors.[2]

Fibrin formation and platelet aggregation are controlled by heparin and prostaglandins, respectively. Heparin is an effective antithrombotic agent for certain conditions. Its interactions with antithrombin III (ATIII) and prevention of fibrin clot formation are well documented.[1,3] Prostaglandins (PGI_2, PGE_1, and PGD_2) interact with membrane-bound platelet receptors to inhibit platelet adhesion and aggregation.[2,4]

Many research groups have demonstrated release of heparin from various polymer surfaces, including Teflon (PTFE),[5] polyvinyl alcohols,[6] and several other surfaces.[7–10] In clinical trials, the results showed a decrease in fibrin formation; however, a significant number of platelets had adhered and aggregated on the surfaces.

Heyman *et al.*[11] studied the *in vitro* and *in vivo* release phenomena of heparin using implanted catheters in dogs. They were able to correlate the *in vitro* release rate with the biocompatibility of the device in short-term experiments. It also confirmed the minimal release rate described by Tanzawa,[12] which allowed minimal thrombus formation on the surface.

The prevention of platelet surface activation can be controlled by the release of

[a]This research was supported by NIH grant no. HL-20251.

prostaglandins in a monolithic device. This has been extensively studied by many researchers, including McRea *et al.*[13,14] They investigated the *in vitro* stability and release of prostaglandin I_2 (PGI_2) and prostaglandin E_1 (PGE_1) from various polymer substrates. The findings were that these agents were stable in the matrix and retained their bioactivity when released. An *ex vivo* study by Lin *et al.*[15] investigated the platelet reaction to PGE_1 released from an arteriovenous shunt (A-V) fabricated from polyurethane. The results showed that the released PGE_1 was active and the surface concentrations were sufficient to prevent extensive coverage of the surface by activated platelets. Also, Jansen *et al.*[16] investigated the effectiveness of coating heart valve leaflets with PGE_1 in an *in vivo* calf model. The scanning electron micrograph (SEM) photographs confirmed that the released drug prevented any significant platelet aggregates on the surface.

Heparin and PGE_1 have been combined together in a polymer matrix[17] and the release of each drug monitored. Different release rates, diffusion mechanisms, and microdomains were found to be associated with each drug. This can be attributed to the difference in molecular weight, hydrophobicity, and charge density between heparin and PGE_1.

The alternate approach, taken by many researchers, to make polymer surfaces less thrombogenic is to covalently immobilize these agents on the polymer surface. This approach has the theoretical advantage of having the agents permanently attached to the surface and it does not have the limitations of device depletion due to loss of the drug.

Ebert *et al.*[18] and Heyman *et al.*[19] have tested the *in vitro* and *in vivo* effectiveness of immobilized heparin surfaces using hydrophobic spacer groups (carbon numbers 2 to 12). The *in vitro* experiments indicated that heparin immobilized via a C-12 spacer significantly prolonged the clotting times in APTT evaluations. The *in vivo* experiments, however, showed no correlation between spacer length and clotting times, yet all heparin-immobilized polyurethane surfaces showed significantly less thrombus as compared to control.

An important observation in the above studies was that for any given system, the drug used affected only its particular pharmacological response, *i.e.*, the heparinized surfaces showed decreases in fibrin formation and activation of platelets, while the PGE_1 surfaces showed reduced platelet aggregation, with no affect on fibrin deposition. This led researchers to investigate the combining of bioactive agents to prevent both fibrin formation and platelet activation.

An approach studied by Hennick *et al.*[20] was to covalently bind heparin to human albumin and preadsorb this conjugate onto polymer surfaces. This method utilized the fact that albumin preadsorbed onto surfaces reduced platelet adhesion,[21] while heparin was able to interact with ATIII, preventing thrombus formation. The investigators found that the heparin-albumin conjugate significantly reduced both the amount of fibrin formation and the extent of platelet aggregation. This indicated that it is possible to prevent both mechanisms of thrombogensis by a macromolecule.

Another approach taken by Jacobs *et al.*[22] was to form a covalent bond between PGE_1 and heparin. This procedure was to create a macromolecule utilizing a dual pharmacological approach to inhibit fibrin formation with heparin and simultaneously inhibit platelet aggregation with PGE_1. The results showed that the bioactivity of heparin has been retained, while the PGE_1 has reduced activity.

This paper will deal with our current progress in the controlled release of several bioactive agents (PGE_1, heparin, and the PGE_1-heparin conjugate) as well as the immobilization of heparin and the PGE_1-heparin conjugate onto a model surface using hydrophilic (polyethylene oxide) spacer groups.

PGE_1-HEPARIN CONJUGATE

A covalently bonded conjugate of commercial grade heparin and PGE_1 was synethesized to apply a dual pharmacological approach to inhibit fibrin formation and prevent platelet aggregation.[22] The compound was synthesized using a modified mixed carbonic anhydride method of amide bond formation between the carboxylic acid moiety of PGE_1 and a primary amine group on heparin. Quantitation of free amine groups on heparin was made by spectroscopically (UV) measuring a TNBS-heparin adduct formed. Quantitation of PGE_1 coupling was measured by spectroscopically monitoring a base-catalyzed degradation product of PGE_1, PGB_1, and extrapolating the data to PGE_1-HEP (PGB_1-HEP). Contamination experiments were performed to ensure that the influence of PGE_1 on platelet aggregation was from the conjugate, and not free (unbound) PGE_1. $[^{14}C]PGF_2\alpha$ was used to monitor the extent of any unconjugated prostaglandin after purification.

Bioactivity tests on the conjugates (APTT and platelet aggregation) confirmed that the antithrombic activity of heparin was maintained. Also, aggregation experiments were performed on a mixture of PGE_1 and heparin to determine any influence that these high doses of heparin may have on platelet responsiveness. The bioactivity of PGE_1 as measured by ADP-induced platelet aggregation had decreased, but was still active, and there was no effect of heparin on the responsiveness of platelets or PGE_1.

This decrease in activity was attributed to the reaction conditions, which may have caused degradation of PGE_1, or to steric interference of PGE_1 attached to heparin preventing efficient interaction with the membrane-bound (platelet) receptors.

As described, the PGE_1-heparin conjugate was able to inhibit fibrin formation and reduce platelet aggregation as a macromolecule *in vitro*. A major concern in using PGE_1 systemically is the severe side effects of toxicity of PGE_1 on cardiac tissue and on the pheripheral vascular resistance. The PGE_1, coupled to heparin, may show less toxicity on these cardiac and venous tissues when coupled to a macromolecule. This may be a result of different sites of distribution, metabolism, and effects on receptor sites of the conjugate as compared to pure PGE_1.

As mentioned, the *in vitro* release of PGE_1 and heparin are different, and the control of optimum release rates for both agents may be difficult to achieve. The conjugate would show release data more like heparin, in its release characteristics, and would be simpler to monitor.

Likewise, in the immobilized system, it would be more efficient to couple a macromolecule with dual functions to the surface than to couple each agent separately. This is especially important with a chemically unstable molecule such as PGE_1.

IMMOBILIZATION OF BIOACTIVE AGENTS

The objective of these studies was to investigate the effects of immobilizing heparin and the PGE_1-heparin conjugate onto a model surface using hydrophilic spacer groups.

The material chosen in the initial studies was Reacti-Gel 6X (Pierce Chem. Co.). This surface is a cross-linked agarose bead ($\approx 100\ \mu$ dia.) with a carbonyldiimidazole-derivatized surface. This activating group reacts readily with primary amines to form stable urethane bonds.

The spacer groups chosen were diamino-terminated polyethylene oxide polymers, with molecular weights of 400, 1000 (1 k) and 4000 (4 k) (Japan Fat and Oils Company). Also, diaminoethane (C-2) was used as a control to immobilize the agents directly onto the surface.

TABLE 1. *In Vitro* Evaluation of Heparin and PGE_1-Heparin Immobilized Spacer Surfaces

Spacer Group	COLUMN A Quantitation of Spacer Groups (μmoles NH/ml Bead)	COLUMN B Quantitation of Immobilized Heparin and PGE_1-Heparin (mg/ml Bead)	COLUMN C Thrombin Time Heparin Activity (Units/ml Bead)	COLUMN D Factor Xa Heparin Activity (Units/ml Bead)
Heparin				
C-2	23.4	0.213	0.85	0.56
400	4.2	0.190	0.96	1.04
1k	7.1	0.217	1.20	2.32
4k	0.76	0.086	1.10	1.26
PGE_1-Heparin				
C-2	23.4	0.163	0.99	0.84
400	4.2	0.186	1.28	1.56
1k	7.1	0.228	1.33	1.84
4k	0.76	0.117	1.10	1.64

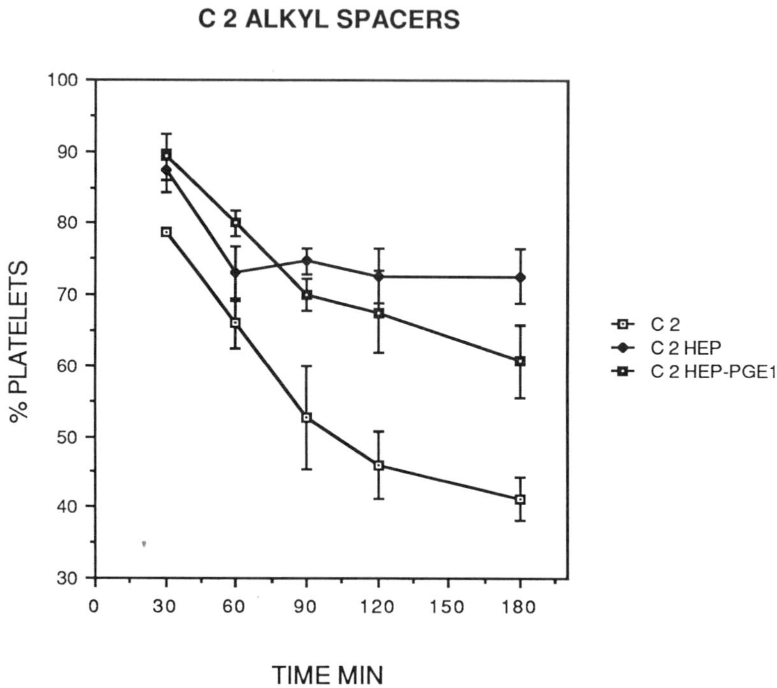
C 2 ALKYL SPACERS
100
90
80
70
60
50
40
30
% PLATELETS
0
30
60
90
120
150
180
TIME MIN
C 2
C 2 HEP
C 2 HEP-PGE1

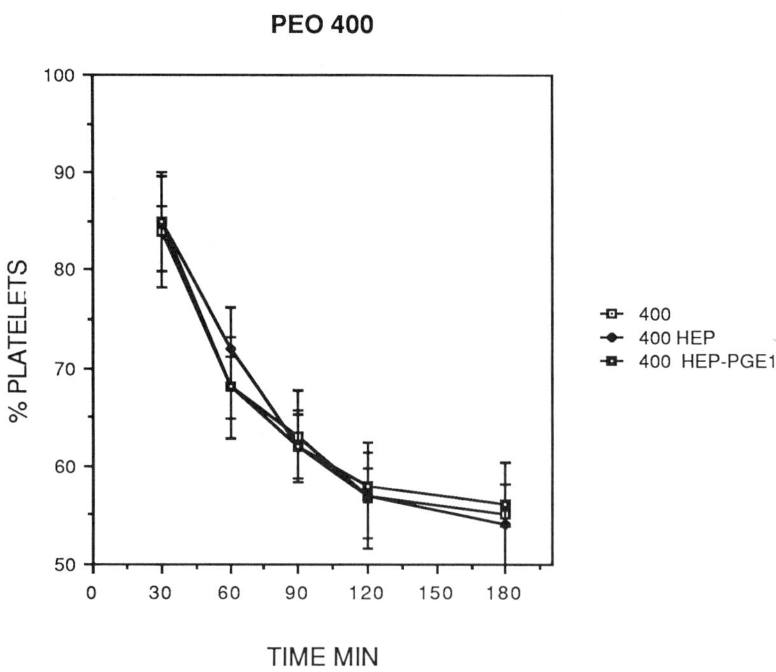
PEO 400
100
90
80
70
60
50
% PLATELETS
0
30
60
90
120
150
180
TIME MIN
400
400 HEP
400 HEP-PGE1

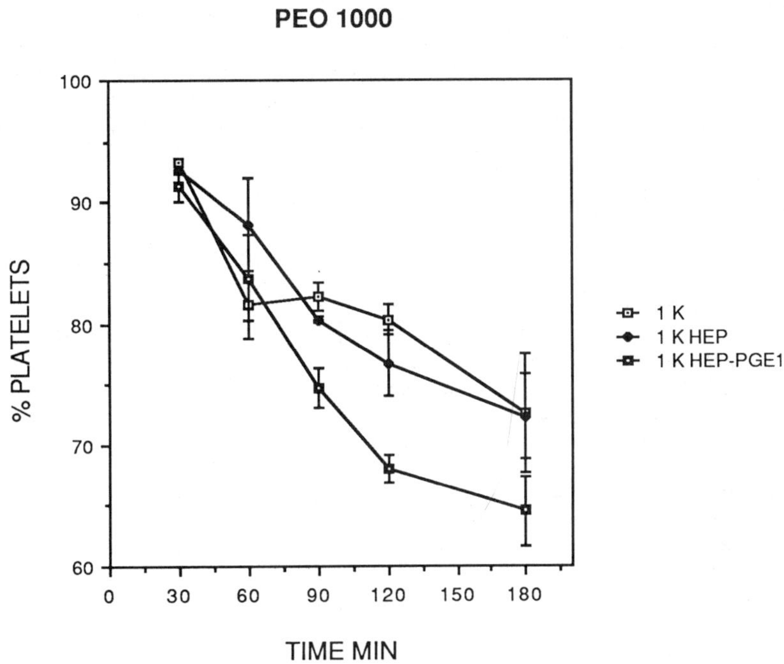

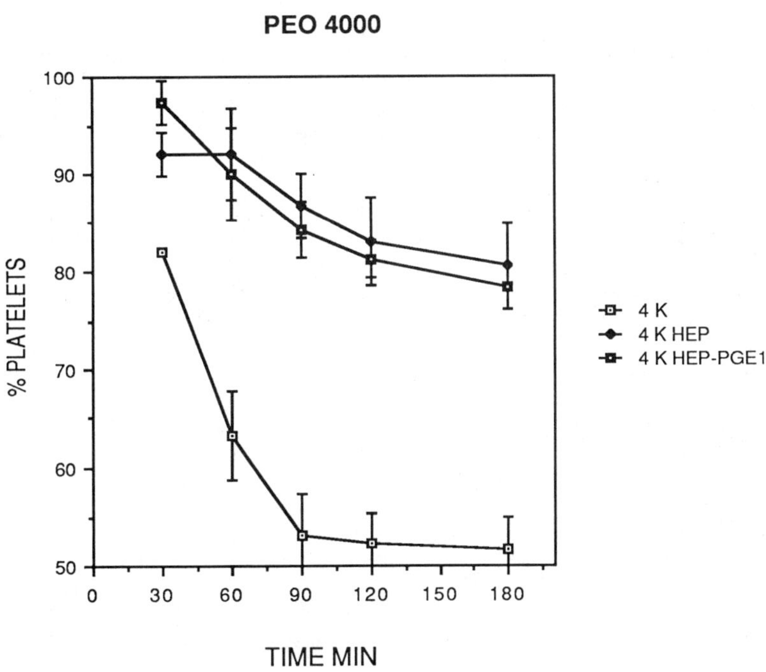

FIGURES 1–4. Platelet adhesion studies comparing spacer groups, heparin-spacer, and PGE_1-heparin spacer systems.

The procedure to immobilize the spacers to the surface was recommended by the manufacturer.[23] A desired weight for each of the specific spacer groups, representing a 10 molar excess of amine groups, was dissolved in a carbonate buffer and the pH adjusted to 10. The beads were added to the spacer solution and rotated for 24 hours at room temperature. The spacer immobilized beads were then washed extensively with distilled water, 1 M NaCl, and finally water. The beads were stored in a PBS buffer until further used.

Quantitation of spacer coupling was achieved using a picric acid derivatization of primary amines.[24] The specific spacer beads were washed in acetone to remove water and any unreacted spacer groups. The spacer beads were then washed with 0.05 M picric acid/acetone solution, followed by extensive washing with acetone and water to remove all of the unbound picric acid. *N,N*-diisopropylethylamine was added to the picric-acid-derivatized spacer beads, and washed with acetone. The collected washings were diluted with acetone, and the absorbance determined at 378 nm (extinction coefficient of 16,800 $1/\text{mole} \times \text{cm}^2$). The amount of picric-diisoproplyethylamine displaced from the beads represents the amount of free amines on the spacer bead surface. The results of this procedure are presented in TABLE 1, Column A.

Commercial grade heparin (Diosynth, 190 U/mg) and PGE_1-heparin conjugate were immobilized to the individual spacer beads using a water-soluble carbodiimide. The goal was to form an amide bond between the carboxylic group on heparin and the primary amine group of the spacer. Care was taken to derivatize only 20% of the carboxylic groups on the heparin molecule. Ebert *et al.*[25] determined that up to 20% of the carboxylic groups on heparin can be derivatized with no loss in bioactivity.

Based on the amount of primary amines available on the beads, heparin was added to represent a 5 molar excess of carboxylic groups (1.7 μmoles COOH/mg heparin). The heparin was dissolved in distilled water and the pH adjusted to 4.5. Ethyl-3-(3-dimethylaminopropyl) carbodiimide (EDC) was used in a concentration to activate 20% of the carboxylic groups on heparin. The specific spacer beads and the appropriate amount of heparin were mixed together, and portions of the EDC solution added over a 30 minute period while rotating the slurry. After all of the EDC had been added, the pH was adjusted to 4.5, and the reaction proceeded for 24 hours at room temperature. An identical procedure was used to immobilize the PGE_1-heparin conjugate to each of the spacer beads.

Quantitation of heparin and PGE_1-heparin conjugate immobilization was achieved using the toluidine blue chromogenic determination.[26] This procedure utilizes a dye depletion reaction of heparin and toluidine blue. The toluidine blue solution was added to a volume of packed beads, mixed, and finally centrifuged at 200 g for 5 minutes. The absorbance of the supernatant solution was measured at 631 nm and compared to a standard curve of known concentrations of heparin and toluidine blue solution. The results of this procedure are shown in TABLE 1, Column B.

The above quantitation of heparin and PGE_1-heparin immobilization onto the specific spacer beads does not depict the bioactivity of the immobilized drug, only the physically bound amount. The specific bioactivity of the drugs can be determined by various bioactivity tests, including thrombin time measurements and the inactivation of factor Xa. These tests clearly reveal the biological activity of immobilized heparin or the heparin molecule of the PGE_1-heparin conjugate.

The species used in these determinations were New Zealand white rabbits. This was chosen since the bioactivity of the PGE_1-heparin conjugate and previous release studies were performed on this model. The blood was obtained as previously described,[22] and separated to obtain platelet-rich (PRP) and platelet-poor plasma (PPP).

The determination of thrombin times involves adding a specific amount of

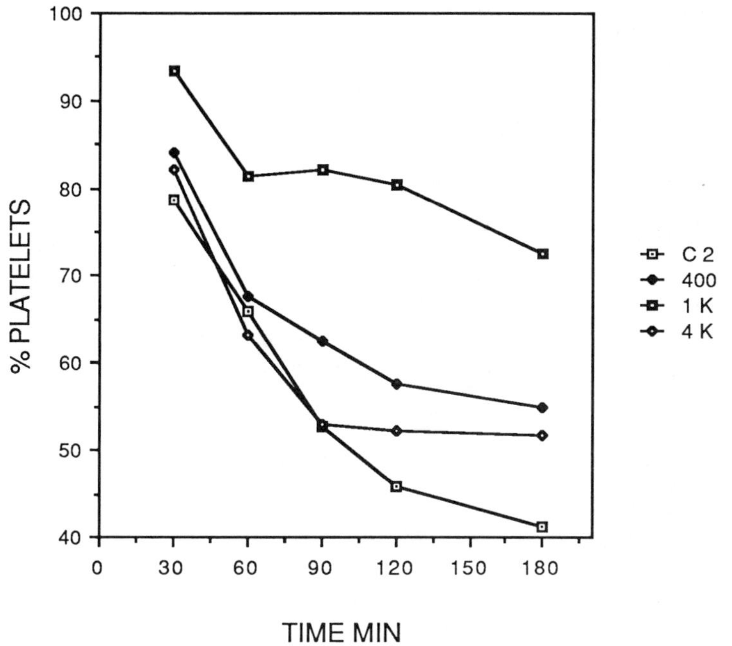

FIGURE 5. Platelet adhesion studies comparing only the spacer groups.

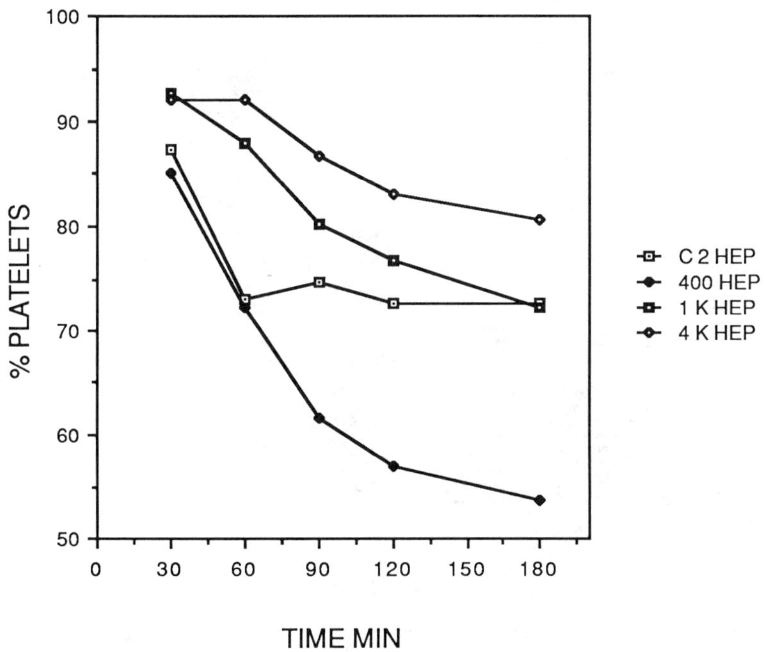

FIGURE 6. Platelet adhesion studies comparing the heparin-spacer immobilized groups.

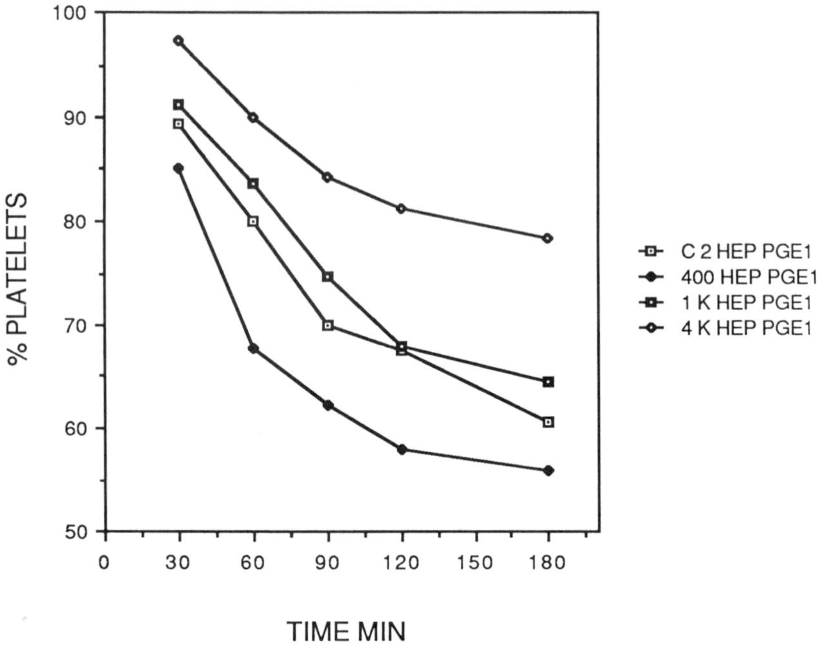

FIGURE 7. Platelet adhesion studies comparing the PGE_1-heparin-spacer immobilized groups.

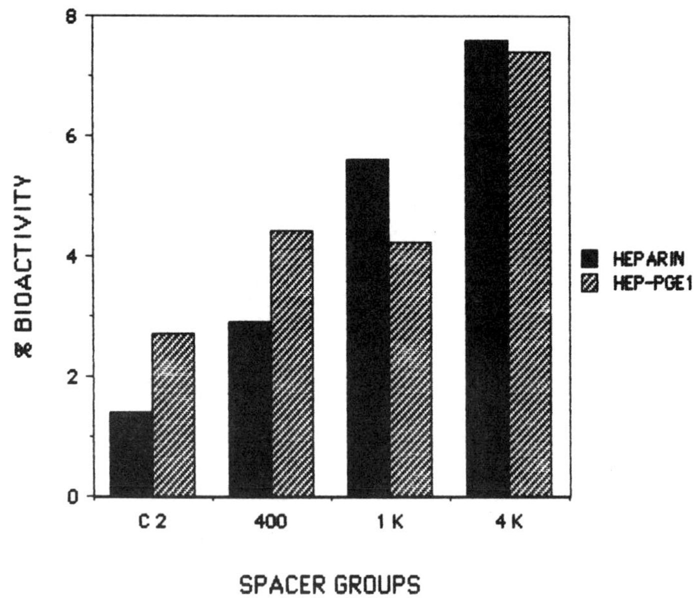

FIGURE 8. Percent bioactivity using factor Xa based on activity determined by inactivation of factor Xa versus toluidine blue quantitation.

thrombin to heparinized plasma and noting the time for a fibrin clot to form. The heparinized plasma is made up into concentrations ranging from 0 to 0.3 units heparin per ml PPP. A standard curve of clotting time versus heparin concentration can be constructed.

The specific heparin and PGE_1-heparin conjugate immobilized beads were incubated in PPP for 15 min at 37°C while being rotated. An aliquot was added to a fibrometer cup and thrombin (15 units/ml) was added. The time for a clot to form (mechanical end point) in the fibrometer (FibroSystem) was noted and compared to the standard curve to determine the equivalent amount of heparin activity. The results from this experiment are found in TABLE 1, Column C.

The inactivation of factor Xa is a chromogenic assay supplied by Helena Labs. The procedure involves adding an excess amount of antithrombin III (ATIII), a known

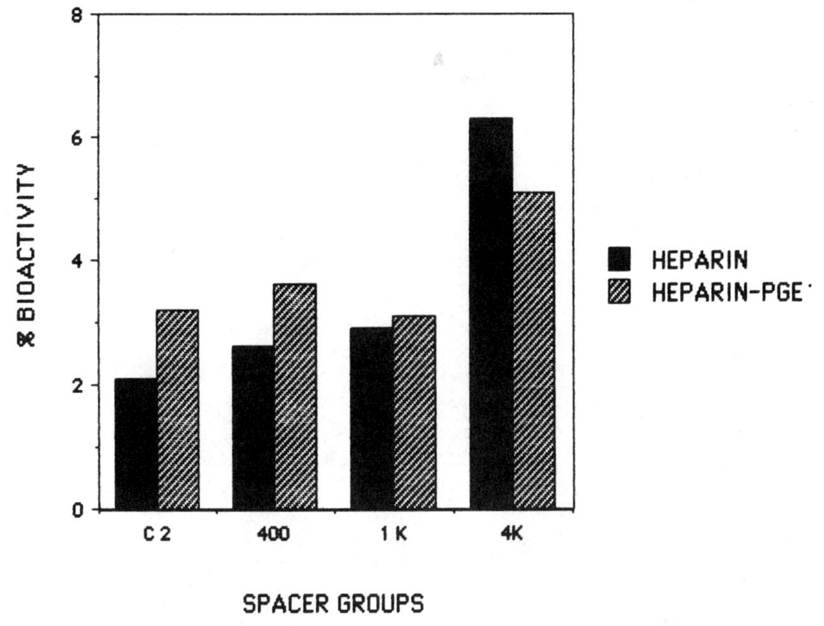

FIGURE 9. Percent bioactivity using thrombin times, based on activity determined by thrombin times versus toluidine blue quantitation.

amount of factor Xa, and a varying amount of heparin. The heparin and ATIII form a complex which binds and inactivates factor Xa. Any excess factor Xa in the solution is then able to cleave a substrate (S2222) to yield a chromogenic peptide. The absorbance is inversely proportional to the amount of heparin in solution and a standard curve is generated using known heparin concentrations.

The heparin and PGE_1-heparin immobilized beads were evaluated for the bioactivity of the immobilized agent by this procedure. A volume of the beads were suspended in a buffer and ATIII (10 U/ml) was added. This suspension was incubated at 37°C for 3 minutes, after which factor Xa (7 nKat/ml) was added. This was incubated for 30 seconds at 37°C and S2222 was added. After 180 seconds, 50% acetic acid was added to quench the reaction. The absorbance of the supernatant solution was determined at

405 nm and extrapolated to the standard curve to obtain the specific heparin activity. The results of this procedure are listed in TABLE 1, Column D.

All of the immobilized beads were investigated for platelet adhesion to the beads in a static *in vitro* experiment. A low platelet count (90,000/mm^3) was used to increase the surface area to platelet ratio. The beads and PRP were gently rotated in a syringe at 37°C in a water bath. An aliquot of the suspension was removed at specified time intervals and the platelet number was determined on a Coulter Counter. All of the immobilized heparin and PGE$_1$-heparin spacer beads were evaluated by this procedure. The results are shown in FIGURES 1 through 7.

The conjugate and heparin have been immobilized on the bead surface with hydrophilic spacer groups. The thrombin times and factor Xa assays indicated that the immobilized heparin and the heparin associated with the conjugate are biologically active. The comparison of activities showed that spacer length does not dramatically influence bioactivity. However, we can define a percent bioactivity as the ratio of heparin activity as determined by factor Xa or thrombin times divided by quantitation by toluidine blue assay. This comparison shows a spacer length effect among the different spacer groups as shown in FIGURES 8 and 9, with the 4-k heparin and conjugate system having the highest percent bioactivity.

The evaluation of the PGE$_1$ contribution to the conjugate in the immobilized system are inconclusive. As shown in FIGURES 1–4, there appeared to be more platelets adhered to the PGE$_1$-heparin immobilized beads than to the heparin surfaces. However, these experiments did not differentiate between reversibly and irreversibly bound platelets, and there was a specific binding site on the platelet receptor site for PGE$_1$. Further experiments to monitor cyclic AMP, a direct effect of prostaglandin interaction with platelets, are planned.

CONTROLLED RELEASE A-A SHUNTS

The biological efficacy of heparin, PGE$_1$, and the PGE$_1$-heparin conjugate were evaluated in a controlled release system using an arterio-arterial (A-A) bypass shunt model. The A-A bypass was used in place of A-V bypass due to lower blood flow rate through the shunts.

The controlled release systems were composed of each drug uniformly dispersed into a hydrophilic polyurethane (Toyobo Company, Japan) solution. Heparin and the conjugate (30% wt/wt drug in polymer) were initially dissolved in foramide before addition to the polymer solution. A 10% wt/wt PGE$_1$/polymer solution was formed by dissolving PGE$_1$ into DMF, then mixing the solution into polymer-DMF solution. The drug/polymer solutions were diluted to 1% wt/wt concentration and applied to the lumen of polyurethane tubings with multiple coatings.

The femoral artery of the rabbit was catheterized as a blood sample port, and the carotid artery was exposed and ligated. The shunt was interposed across the ligated section and the flow rate adjusted by a tourniquet at the outflow (superior side of

TABLE 2. Occlusion Time Results of Various A-A Shunt Experiments

Occlusion Time	Mean (h)	Range (h)
Control (hydrophilic polyurethane)	0.60	0.50–0.67
Heparin (30% loading)	3.75	3.00–5.40
PGE$_1$ (1% loading)	>10	>10
Conjugate (30% loading)	≈ 10	$8 > 10$ h >10

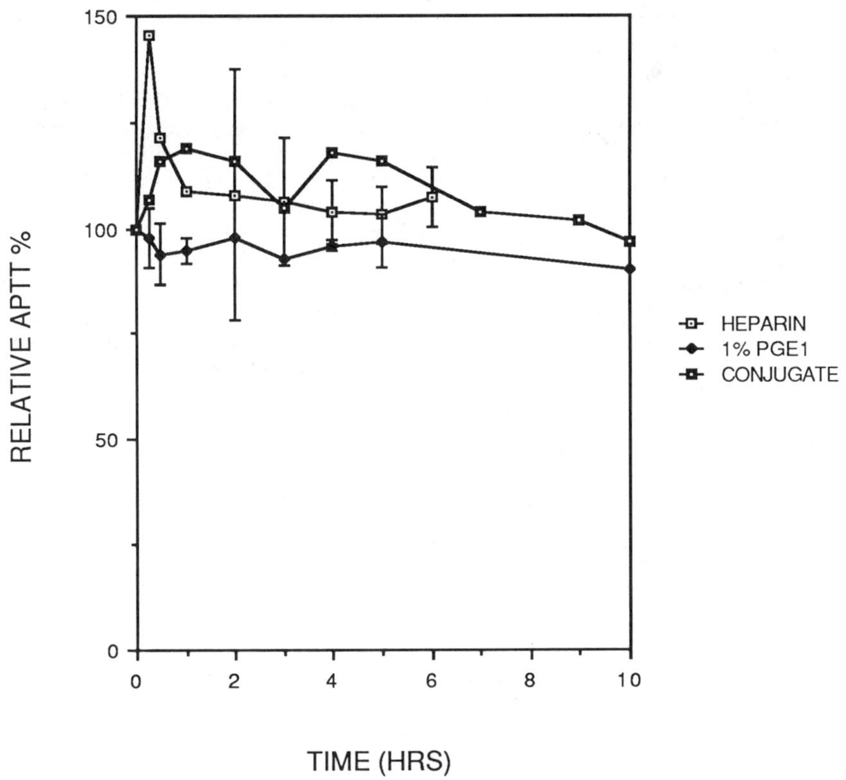

FIGURE 10. Relative APTT of systemic blood during the A-A shunt experiments.

carotid). The blood flow was monitored by an ultrasonic flowmeter with a 2 mm cross-sectional probe (Transonic System, Ithaca, NY).

Blood samples were taken at timed intervals to measure APTT, platelet number, hematocrit, and platelet aggregation for systemic effects of the shunts and its released agents. The experiments were terminated at occlusion of the shunt as indicated by flow meter measurements, or at 10 hours.

The occlusion times for the test shunts are shown in TABLE 2. At the same loading dose, the conjugate shunts had a longer patency time than heparin shunts. The PGE_1 shunts did not occlude for the duration of the experiments; however, the effective PGE_1 concentrations of the PGE_1 shunts were approximately 200 times that of the conjugate shunts.

The results of the systemic monitoring of APTT are shown in FIGURE 10. The control and PGE_1 shunts had no effect on prolonging APTT. The heparin shunts showed prolonged APTT at 15- and 30-minute sampling times, which extrapolated to less than 0.1 U/ml heparin concentration in the tested plasma. The APTT decreased to normal values after 1 hour. The increase in APTT can be attributed to the initial burst effect of heparin released from the surface. If the shunts were soaked and flushed for 15 minutes prior to surgical insertion, the prolongation of systemic APTT was not seen. The flushed shunts had an occlusion time of 3 h versus 5 h for shunts not flushed. All conjugate shunts were soaked and flushed prior to shunt insertion. The APTT did not vary above normal values.

The control shunts showed decreased platelet counts at 15 and 30 minutes. No values beyond 30 minutes were measured. The platelet numbers varied between 80% and 120% of initial count values for all shunts. The heparin shunts showed a decrease in platelet counts at 15 and 30 minutes which returned to normal counts at 1 hour and beyond. The PGE_1 and conjugate shunts did not show any decrease in platelet counts at 15 and 30 minutes. These results are summarized in FIGURE 11.

The normal hematocrit values of healthy male New Zealand white rabbits, between 5 and 6 pounds, had a range of 38–40%. All test rabbits maintained their hematocrit values at these levels for the duration of the experiments.

The control and heparin shunts did not affect the *in vitro* measurement of ADP-induced platelet aggregation. The platelets totally aggregated, and heparin enhancement of aggregation was not detected. The PGE_1 and conjugate shunts showed a suppression of platelet aggregation in that the aggregation curves showed an initial aggregation followed by deaggregation of platelets. Additional ADP did not cause further aggregation and this phenomenon lasted throughout the duration of the shunt experiments.

After occlusion, the thrombi in the shunts were flushed out with PBS and fixed with glutaraldehyde for scanning electron microscopy, as shown in FIGURE 12. The control and heparin shunts had similar platelet morphologies on their surfaces. The

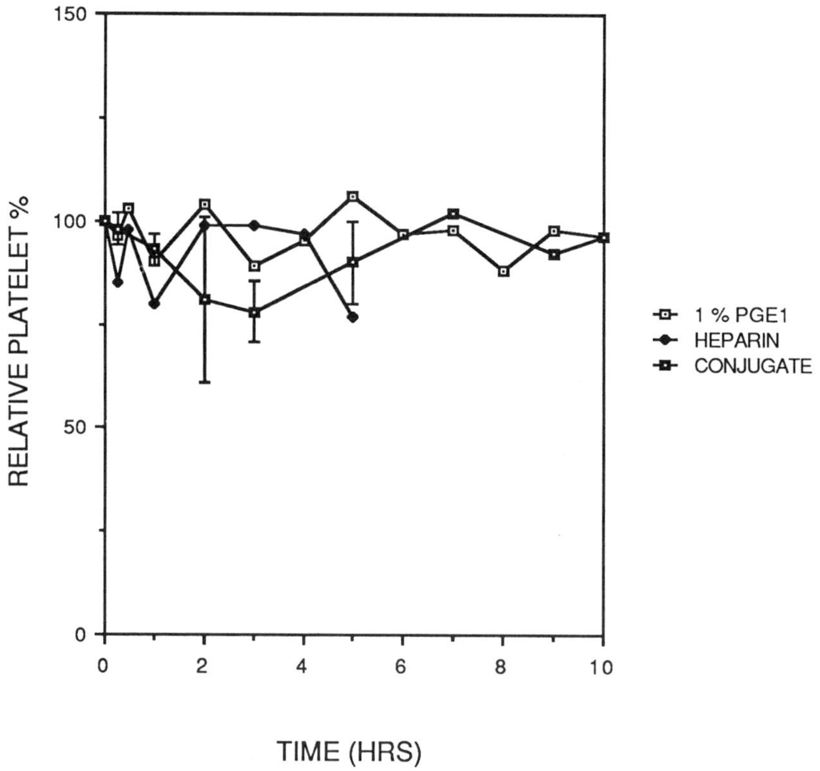

FIGURE 11. Relative platelet numbers during the A-A shunt experiments.

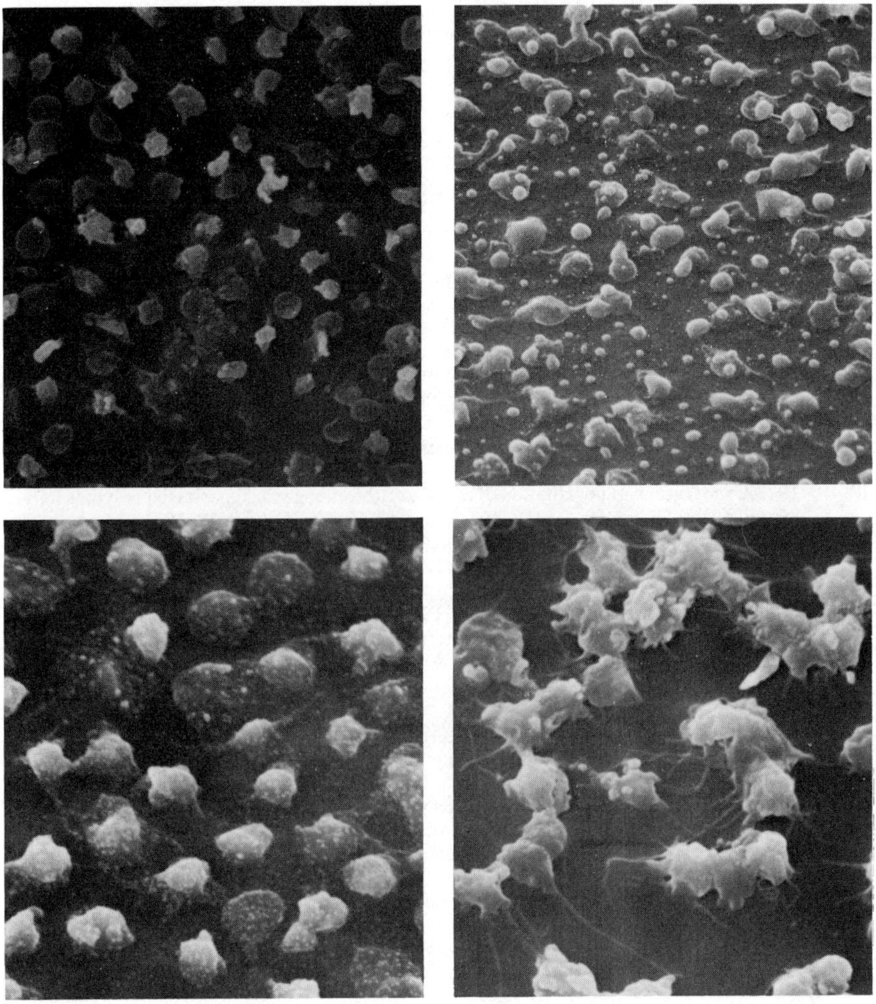

FIGURE 12. SEM of test shunts at the end of the experiments. *Above left,* PGE_1-heparin conjugate (magnification: 2000×). *Above right,* PGE_1 (2000×). *Below left,* heparin (4000×). *Below right,* hydrophilic polyurethane control (4000×).

adhered platelets were extensively activated, with pseudopods. The PGE_1 and conjugate shunts had round-shaped platelets and are reversibly activated.

REFERENCES

1. BIGGS, R. & K. DENSON. 1976. Inhibitors of blood coagulations. *In* Human Blood Coagulation, Haemostasis and Thrombosis. 2d edit. R. Biggs, Ed.: 143–167. Blackwell Scientific Publications. London.
2. AIKEN, J. 1984. Prostaglandins. J. Cardiovasc. Pharmacol. **6:** 5413–5420.

3. DAMUS, P. S., M. HICKS & R. B. ROSENBERG. 1977. Anticoagulant action of heparin. Nature **246:** 355–357.
4. WHITTLE, B., S. MONCADA & J. R. VANE. 1978. Comparisons of the effect of PGI_1 and PGD_2 on platelet aggregation in different species. Prostaglandins **16:** 373–388.
5. PLATE, G., L. HOLLIER & P. GLOVICZKI. 1984. Overcoming failure of venous vascular prostheses. Surgery **96(3):** 503–510.
6. GOOSEN, M., & M. SEFTON. 1983. Properties of heparin-poly(vinyl alcohol) hydrogel coating. J. Biomed. Mater. Res. **17(2):** 359–373.
7. NICHOLS, A., J. OWEN & B. GROSSMAN. 1984. Effect of heparin bonding on catheter-induced fibrin formation and platelet activation. Circulation **70(5):** 843–850.
8. MORI, Y., S. NAGOAKA & Y. MASUBUCHI. 1978. The effects of released heparin from heparinized hydrophilic polymer (HRSD) on the process of thrombus formation. Trans. Am. Soc. Intern. Organs **24:** 736–745.
9. BENNENGARD, K., I. CURELARU & B. GUSTAUSSON. 1982. Material thrombogenicity in central venous catheterization. Acta Anaesthesia Scand. **26(2):** 112–120.
10. LAMBRECHT, L., B. YOUNG & D. MOSHER. 1981. Transient thrombus deposition in chitosan-heparin coated polyethylene. Trans. Am. Soc. Artif. Int. Organs **27:** 380–385.
11. HEYMAN, P., C. S. CHO, J. C. MCREA, D. BOLSEN & S. W. KIM. 1985. Heparinized polyurethanes: *In vitro* and *In vivo* studies. J. Biomed. Mater. Res. **19:** 419–436.
12. TANZAWA, H., Y. MORI, N. HARUMIYA, H. MIAMA, M. HORI, N. OHSHIMA & Y. IDEZUKI. 1973. Preparation and evaluation of a new antithrombogenic heparinized polymer for use in cardiovascular system. Trans. Am. Soc. Artif. Intern. Organs **19:** 188–194.
13. MCREA, J. C. & S. W. KIM. 1978. Characterization of controlled release of prostaglandin from polymer matries for thrombus prevention. Trans. Am. Soc. Artif. Intern. Organs **24:** 746.
14. MCREA, J. C., C. D. EBERT & S. W. KIM. 1981. Prostaglandin releasing polymers: Stability and efficacy. Trans. Am. Soc. Artif. Intern. Organs **27:** 511.
15. LIN, J. Y., T. OKANO, L. DOST, J. FEIJEN & S. W. KIM. 1985. Prevention of platelet contact activation by prostaglandin E_1 released from polyurethane surfaces. Trans. Am. Soc. Artif. Intern. Organs **31:** 468.
16. JANSEN, J., J. M. GRAVELINK, S. W. KIM, W. J. KLOFF & H. REUL. 1987. New polyurethane trileaflet valves: Performance and blood compatibility. Proc. ESAO. In press.
17. KIM, S. W., C. EBERT, J. LIN & J. MCREA. 1983. Nonthrombogenic polymers. Asaio J. **6:** 76–87.
18. EBERT, C. D. & S. W. KIM. 1982. Immobilized heparin: Spacer arm effects on biological interactions. Thromb. Res. **26:** 43–57.
19. HEYMAN, P. & S. W. KIM. 1985. Blood compatibility of heparinized polyurethanes. Makromol. Chem. Suppl. **9:** 119–124.
20. HENNICK, W., J. FEIJEN, C. EBERT & S. W. KIM. 1983. Covalently bound conjugates of albumin and heparin: Synthesis, fractionation and characterization. Thromb. Res. **29:** 1–13.
21. HENNICK, W., L. DOST, J. FEIJEN & S. W. KIM. 1983. Interaction of albumin heparin conjugate preadsorbed surfaces with blood. Trans. Am. Soc. Artif. Intern. Organs **29:** 200–205.
22. JACOBS, H., & S. W. KIM. 1986. *In vitro* bioactivity of a synthesized prostaglandin E_1-heparin conjugate. J. Pharm. Sci. **75:** 172.
23. HANDBOOK AND GENERAL CATALOGS 1986–1987. Pierce Chemical Company. Rockford, Ill.
24. LEE, C. C. Y. & G. M. LOUDON. 1979. Qualitative determination of amino groups on derivatized controlled glass surfaces: A comparison of methods. Anal. Biochem. **94:** 60–64.
25. EBERT, C. D., E. S. LEE, J. DENERIS & S. W. KIM. 1982. The anticoagulant activity of derivatized and immobilized heparins. *In* Biomaterials: Interfacial Phenomena and Application. Adv. Chem. Ser. **99.** American Chemical Society. Washington, D.C.
26. SMITH, P. K., A. K. MALLIA & G. T. HERMANSON. 1980. Colormetric method for the assay of heparin content in immobilized heparin preparations. Anal. Biochem. **109:** 466–473.

Endothelial Linings in Prosthetic Vascular Grafts

WILLIAM E. BURKEL,[a] LINDA M. GRAHAM,[b] AND JAMES C. STANLEY[b]

[a]Department of Anatomy and Cell Biology
[b]Department of Surgery
The University of Michigan
Ann Arbor, Michigan 48109

Of all the animals so far studied, man is the only one known to be incapable of healing prosthetic vascular grafts with its own natural endothelium. Consequently there has been considerable effort in the 30 or so years since the first prosthetic grafts became available either to find truly nonthrombogenic artificial materials or to enhance the body's own natural healing processes in order to provide blood-compatible devices. It has been known from the days of the earliest prosthetic grafts that the fibrin-platelet coagulum that typically lines them is an adequate surface only for grafts of 8 mm i.d. or greater. Unfortunately, the need for smaller prostheses is equal to or greater than that for the large. In the early days, emphasis in graft development was focused on different materials, such as nylon, Dacron, Teflon, tanned bovine carotid arteries, or umbilical veins as conduits.

Paralleling the work with prosthetic vessels was the development of the artificial heart and the desire to provide blood-compatible linings for these devices. The idea of cell or tissue fragment seeding of prostheses in order to provide pseudointimal linings originated because of its applicability to artificial hearts (see ref. 2 for a review of this early work). Our own work in this area began with artificial hearts as well, under the auspices of the National Heart, Lung, and Blood Institute and the Artificial Heart Program. At that time the emphasis was on developing microfiber substrates upon which to grow pseudointimal linings and on finding a cell or tissue type that would provide a blood-compatible surface. In order to develop these materials and methods the prosthetic devices were fabricated into nonporous urethane tubes lined with a microfiber scaffold and of a size that could be tested by interposition in the abdominal aorta of a dog (FIG. 1). The cells were introduced into the prostheses and cultivated *in vitro* until a pseudointima developed.[3] The progress was slow; materials were not very cell compatible, and the cells that were easily grown *in vitro* were thrombogenic. However, in the late 1970s several developments occurred that made cell-lined vascular grafts a practical reality. First, we and other groups of investigators finally learned how to isolate and grow adult endothelial cells. Second, we switched from the troublesome microfiber grafts to commercially available vascular prostheses (FIG. 2). Third, a new group of investigators[4] discovered that scrapings from the intima of cutaneous veins, seeded into grafts in clotted blood and then immediately implanted into dogs, would produce endothelial linings in these vessels. With these developments research on endothelial cell seeding greatly increased. In the last few years endothelial cell seeding techniques have developed rapidly to the point where clinical reports of success with the method are beginning to appear[5] (for a complete review, see refs. 6 and 7). In the following pages we will briefly describe the method and the current status of research in this area. This presentation is not meant to be exhaustive, but to highlight some of the more important observations as well as questions still to be answered.

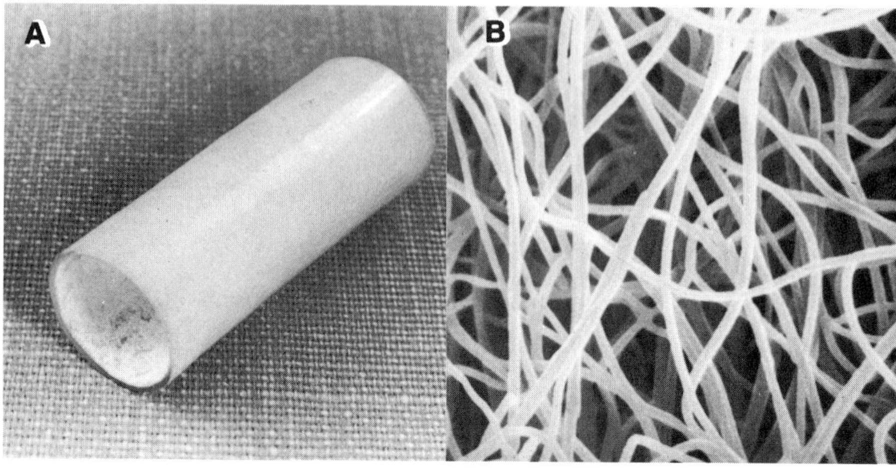

FIGURE 1. (**A**) Urethane tube lined with nonwoven polypropylene microfiber like that used in early seeding experiments (shown actual size). (**B**) SEM micrograph of microfiber lining; magnification: 1000×.

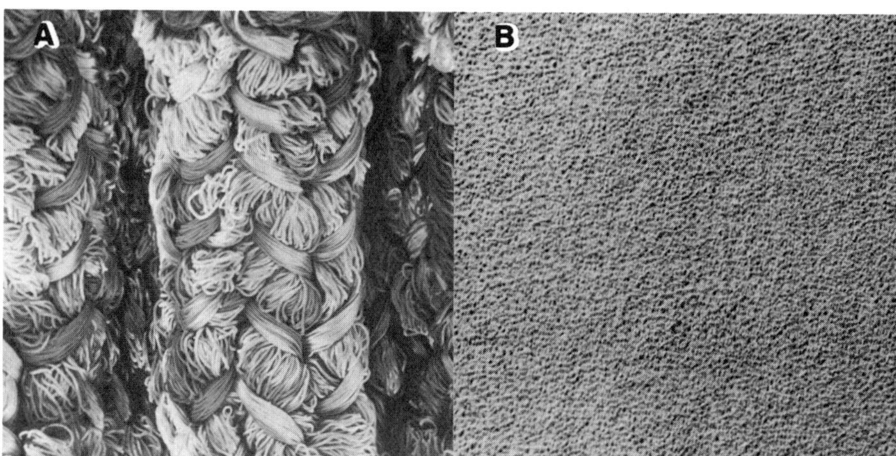

FIGURE 2. (**A**) Surface of a clinically used knitted Dacron, velour, crimped graft; magnification: 25×. (**B**) Surface of expanded Teflon (ePTFE) graft at the same magnification as **A;** note the relative smoothness.

THE METHOD

Endothelial Cell Isolation

Most commonly, endothelial cells (EC) are isolated from subcutaneous veins using proteolytic enzymes. In dogs external jugular veins are isolated, removed, and everted over stainless steel rods[8] in order to prevent exposure of nonendothelial cells to the

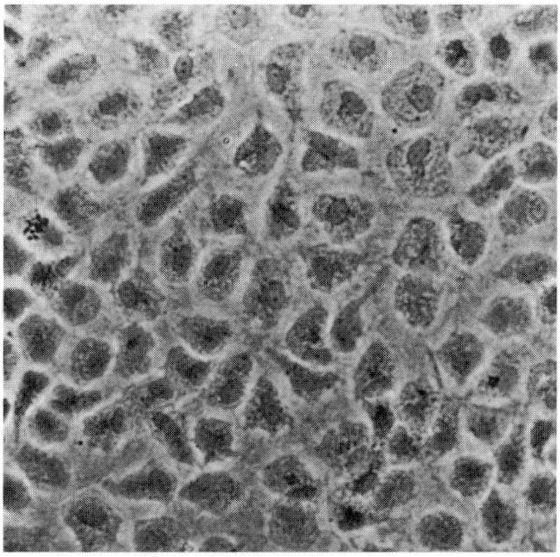

FIGURE 3. Phase contrast micrograph of typical canine venous endothelial cells in tissue culture; magnification: 300×.

enzymes. After washing in calcium- and magnesium-free Hanks' balanced salt solution (CMF-HBSS), the veins are incubated successively in 0.1% trypsin-0.125% EDTA, pH 8, and 0.5% collagenase (CLS type II), pH 8, each for 10 minutes at 37°C. The rods are then spun in Medium·199 (M199) to dislodge the EC and the exfoliated cells washed in M199 in preparation for graft seeding or tissue culture (FIG. 3).

A good cell harvest will yield 1.0–1.5 × 10^6 cells from a 10 × 0.5 cm segment of vein.

Endothelial Cell Seeding

The EC, either immediately after isolation or after *in vitro* cultivation, are seeded into vascular grafts which have been precoated with autologous blood or some other adhesive, such as fibronectin.[9–11] With Dacron grafts, which are usually porous, the cells are suspended in 0.5 ml of M199 and mixed with 10 to 15 ml of whole blood, the

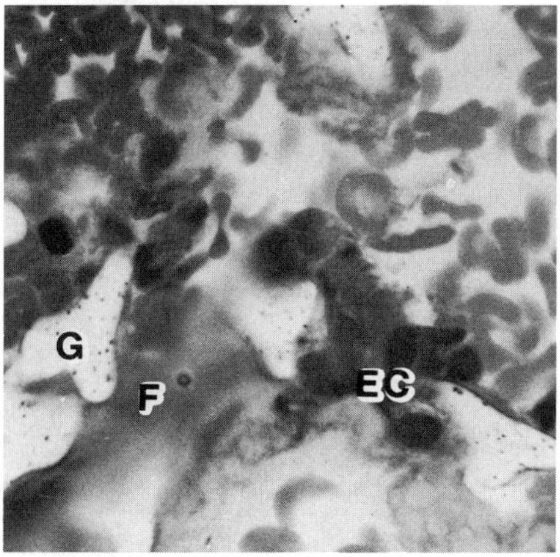

FIGURE 4. Photomicrograph of a section of a Dacron graft seeded with endothelial cells; *EC*, endothelial cells; *G*, graft fiber; *F*, fibrin. Magnification: 600×.

distal end of the graft clamped, and the cell-blood mixture injected into the graft, as for preclotting. The blood is forced through the graft wall filtering out the endothelial cells, which are thus seeded into the interstices (FIG. 4).[9,12] With grafts that are nonporous to blood, such as expanded Teflon (ePTFE), the cells are mixed with a small amount of tissue culture medium, injected into the graft, which has been pretreated with blood or some other adhesive, the ends clamped, and the graft left to sit horizontally.[13] Periodic rotation of the graft during the seeding process allows for even distribution of cells. If blood has been used in the seeding process, the grafts are flushed with a small amount of heparinized blood.[19] The grafts are implanted in the experimental animal using standard surgical procedures, with care taken to prevent dessication. In experiments using EC that have been cultivated prior to seeding,[9] the procedures are the same following trypsinization of the culture flasks to obtain a cell suspension. As an alternative, grafts may be cultivated *in vitro* after seeding in order to obtain a confluent endothelial lining prior to implantation. The methods used are similar to those described in ref. 2. This procedure may be more useful for grafts placed in small vessels or in the venous circulation,[14] which with low flow are more susceptible to thrombosis.

A variety of graft types have been used for EC seeding studies, such as knitted Dacron, with or without velour surface, crimped or noncrimped, externally supported or not. Expanded Teflon grafts are seeded equally well, whether of standard or greater than standard porosity. Sites for implantation and testing of the seeded grafts have included: thoracoabdominal bypass grafts, infrarenal, aortoiliac, iliac, iliofemoral, femoral, and carotid arteries as well as inferior vena cava. Small diameter grafts (<6 mm i.d.), whether seeded or not, have usually required pharmacological intervention to maintain early patency.[14]

RESULTS

Endothelialization (healing) of the graft surface proceeds rapidly after graft implantation, the rate depending upon the number of cells that are seeded and how tightly adherent they are to the graft surface. Small clusters of EC, appearing much like colonies of cells in a tissue culture flask, are visible on the graft surface between 1 and 4 days (FIGS. 5 and 6).[12] These cells grow rapidly and by 14 days as much as 75% of the graft surface is covered with endothelium (FIG. 7). Within the next month the remainder of the surface becomes covered with EC (FIG. 8). Initially this neointima is a monolayer of cells (FIG. 9), but with time subendothelial smooth muscle cells appear to form a layer of variable thickness (FIG. 10) depending upon the graft type and length of implantation.[15] The lining cells display all of the characteristics of endothelium, including cobblestone morphology and tight intercellular junctions,[15] Weibel-Palade bodies,[16] the presence of factor-VIII-related antigen[17] (FIG. 11), nonthrombogenicity,[18] and lack of platelet adhesion and production of prostacyclin (PGI_2).[19] In addition, platelet serotonin levels[19] and platelet survival return to normal significantly faster in seeded grafts.[20,21]

Nonseeded grafts, in contrast, become lined with a fibrin-platelet coagulum shortly after implantation that is frequently several hundred micrometers in thickness and which may persist indefinitely (FIG. 12). Eventually most nonseeded porous grafts in experimental animals heal from cells growing into the graft as pannus from the natural vessel, from tissue surrounding the graft, or perhaps from circulating EC spontaneously seeded from the bloodstream.

These results have been duplicated in both large (>6 mm i.d.) and small diameter

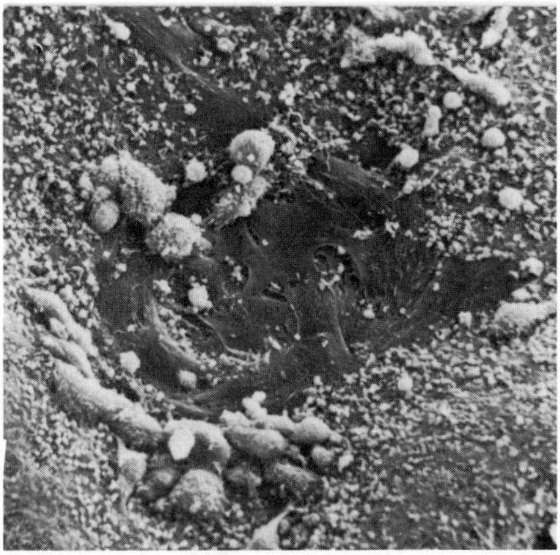

FIGURE 5. SEM micrograph of a cluster of EC on a Dacron graft shortly after implantation; magnification: 400×.

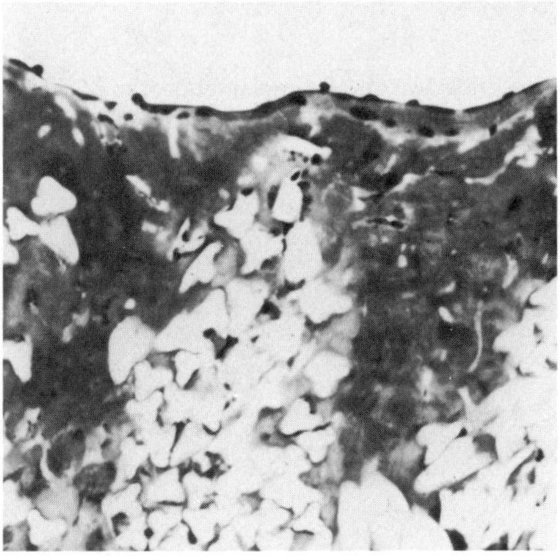

FIGURE 6. Light micrograph of a seeded Dacron graft 4 days after implantation; the cells have begun to form a monolayer on the surface; magnification: 200×.

(<6 mm i.d.) arterial grafts as well as venous grafts. In addition, EC seeding has been shown to be effective in man[5] as well as baboons[22] and rhesus monkey.[23]

DISCUSSION

Cell Sources

As pointed out earlier, a wide variety of tissue sources were initially evaluated[2] in attempts to find a cell type that was readily available, easily isolated, and that possessed the necessary nonthrombogenic characteristics. The obvious choice for lining grafts was the endothelial cell, but routine methods for obtaining large quantities of cells necessary for seeding had not been developed. The publication of a routine method

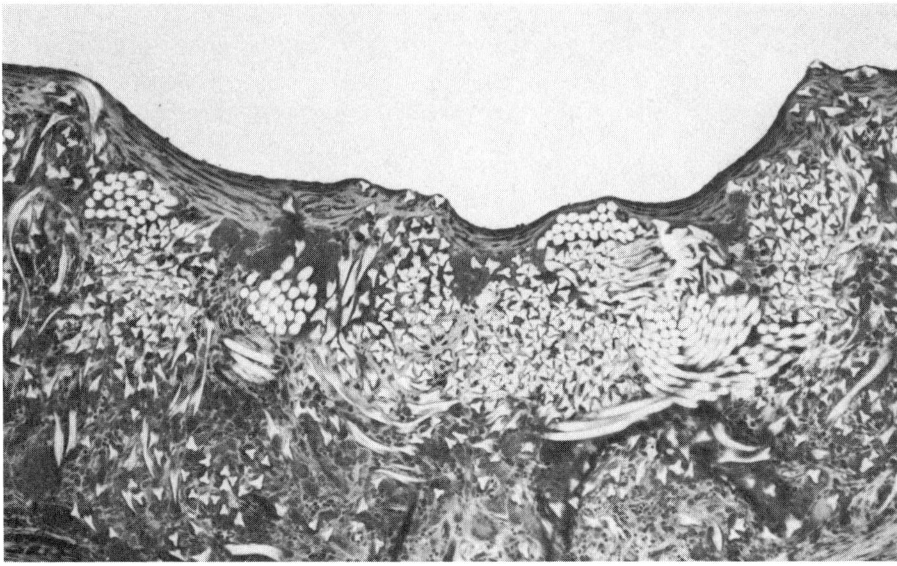

FIGURE 7. Light micrograph of a seeded Dacron graft 2 weeks postimplantation; the EC lining and subjacent smooth muscle are well developed; magnification: 100×.

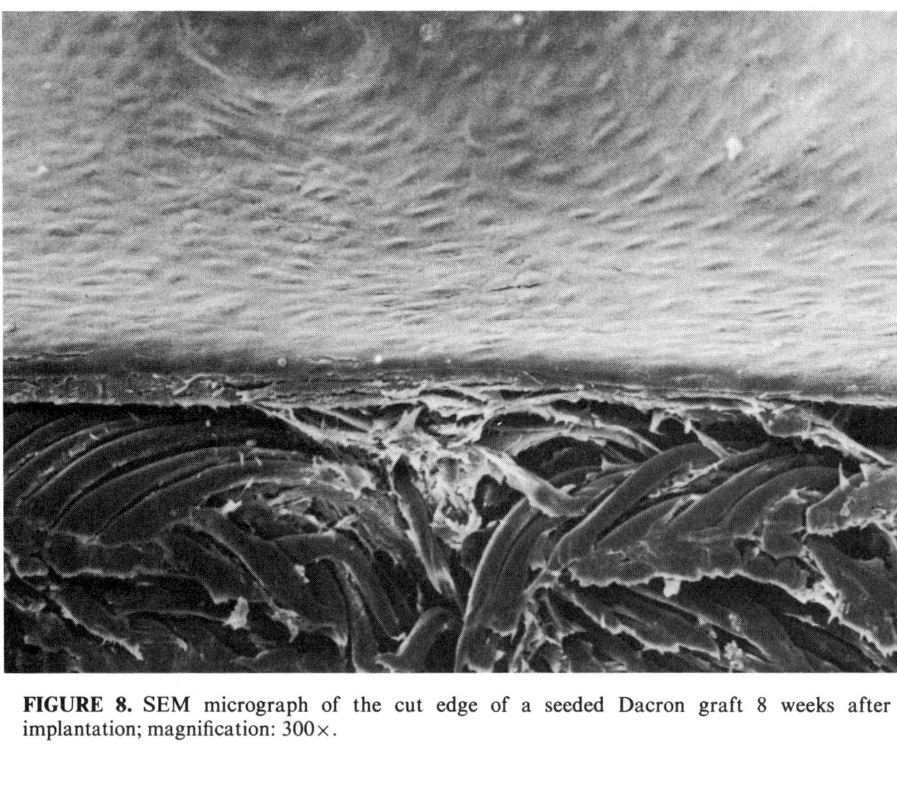

FIGURE 8. SEM micrograph of the cut edge of a seeded Dacron graft 8 weeks after implantation; magnification: 300×.

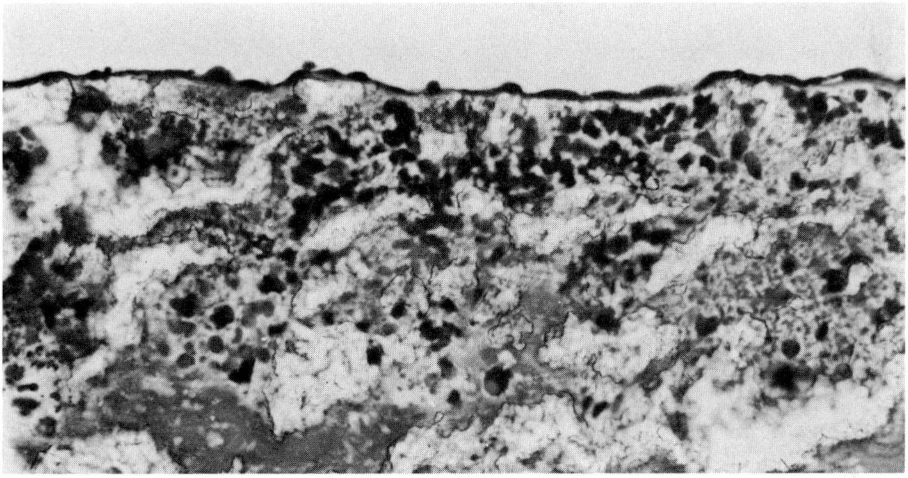

FIGURE 9. Light micrograph of a seeded a PTFE graft 1 month after implantation; the EC are in a monolayer; magnification: 300×.

for obtaining EC from human umbilical veins by Jaffe *et al.*[24] spurred interest in this cell type. With the demonstration that the method could be modified to harvest bovine aortic EC,[25] two models were available and *in vitro* research flourished. While adequate to harvest embryonic and bovine EC, these methods worked only poorly on adult vessels and the adult EC derived were difficult to grow in culture.

In addition, to prevent rejection, autologous EC were needed for seeding the grafts. Over the next few years the above methods were successfully modified to isolate adult EC from several different types of animals and vessels, including: human iliac arteries; human and bovine pulmonary arteries and veins; porcine aortas, inferior vena cavas, and pulmonary veins; rabbit aortas and marginal ear vessels; guinea pig aortas and

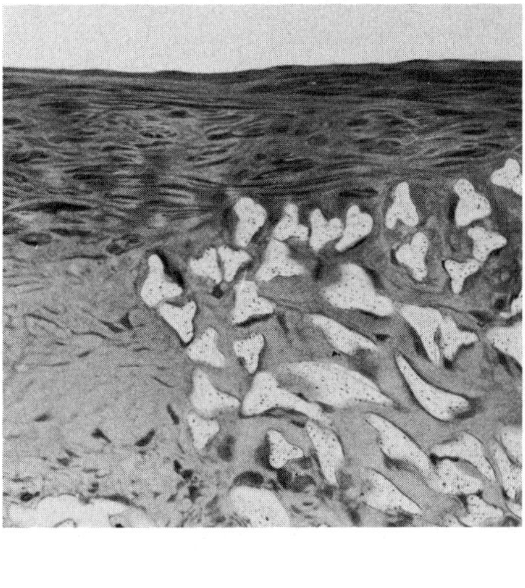

FIGURE 10. Light micrograph of a seeded Dacron graft at 1 year. The original monolayer lining has thickened considerably due to growth of the underlying smooth muscle cells; magnification: 150×.

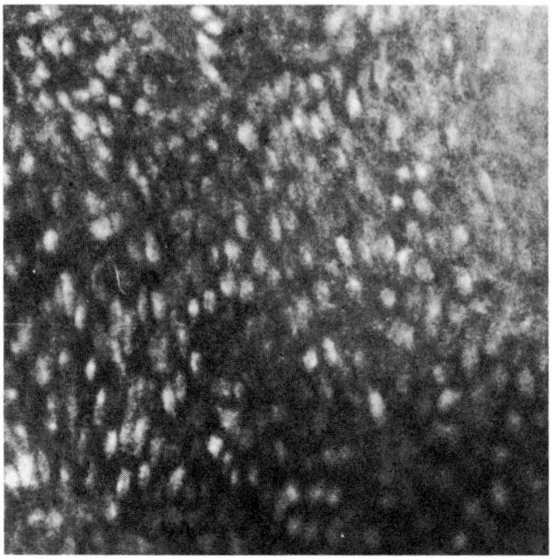

FIGURE 11. Fluorescence micrograph of a seeded Dacron graft stained for factor-VIII-related antigen and photographed by epi-illumination. The white dots are clusters of stained factor VIII in individual cells; magnification: 100×.

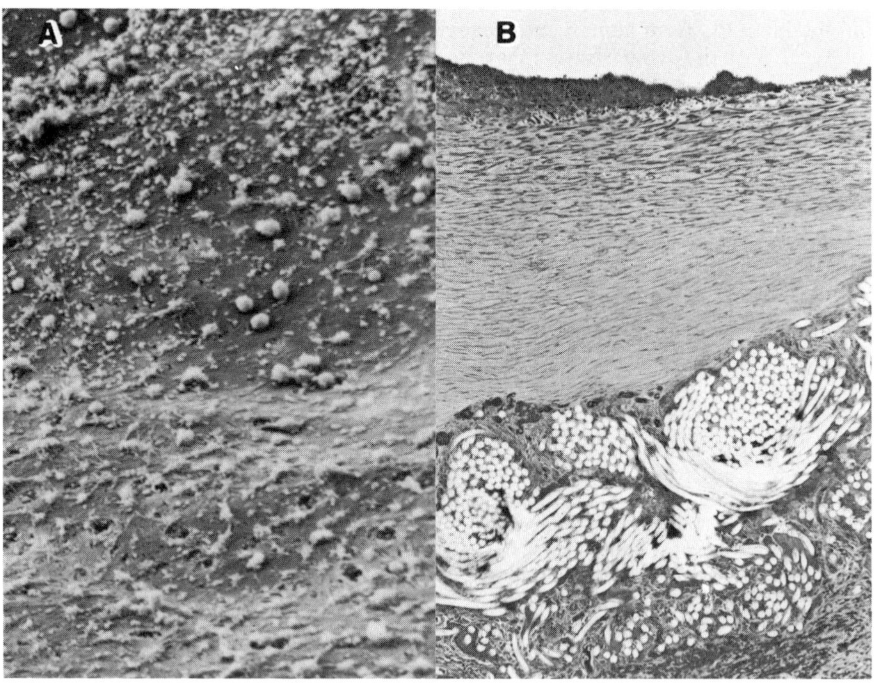

FIGURE 12. (**A**) SEM micrograph of a nonseeded Dacron graft 1 month after implantation, and (**B**) light micrograph of a similar graft 6 months after implantation. The surface of both is composed of a fibrin platelet coagulum. Magnifications: (**A**) 800×; (**B**) 150×.

portal veins; and canine jugular veins and aortas (see ref. 26 for further discussion). Of most importance for graft seeding purposes were methods that could be applied to adult subcutaneous veins that are expendable and potentially useful for clinical application of the seeding technique. Most experiments involving graft seeding have been done with canine jugular veins, a model for human saphenous vein, which is the current choice for clinical application.

While subcutaneous veins such as saphenous can provide large numbers of cells (potentially 1×10^5 cells/cm^2 of vein surface), microvascular EC from adipose tissue is even more abundant (potentially 1×10^6 cells per gram of fat) as well as expendable. With this quantity of cells it may be possible to seed enough cells at the time of implantation to line the graft completely.[27,28] While abundant cells are available from microvasculature, there is a possibility of considerable contamination of the isolates with perivascular or smooth muscle cells. The effect of these cells on the ultimate fate of a seeded graft is unknown.

Recently, mesothelial cells derived from omentum have been used for graft seeding and have been found to produce an intimal lining similar to endothelium.[29] These cells produce large amounts of PGI_2, possess fibrinolytic activity, and do not adhere platelets. Like microvasculature from fat, mesothelial cells are abundant and easily isolated, thus sparing subcutaneous veins for possible coronary bypass if necessary. No long-term studies of grafts seeded with these cells have been done, however.

It has been reported that grafts seeded with nonautologous EC give rise to endothelial linings.[30–32] Considering the known antigenic nature of EC, it seems unlikely that the cells lining these grafts could be from the donor. Grafts were examined only at 2 months postimplantation, more than long enough for spontaneous healing to occur.

Endothelium has been observed in the middle of nonseeded grafts used as controls as early as 2 weeks.[12] Until it has been proved that the cells lining these grafts were actually from the donor, these reports must be viewed with some skepticism. It seems possible, however, that something in the inoculum, such as growth factors from the donor cells (before their loss), could have hastened healing.

Cell Isolation

The earliest and most common methods of isolating EC have been through the use of proteolytic enzymes that attack either the cell junctions or substrate to which the cells are attached. Jaffe *et al.*[24] used collagenase injected into cannulated umbilical veins. While this works well for easily detached EC, it works less well for adult vessels, particularly canine. Rapid perfusion of fluids through the vessel helps in removing cells, but for dog vessels we prefer a method that offers even more agitation or shearing forces to dislodge cells.[8] This is accomplished by everting the vein over a stainless steel rod, suturing it in place, and then after incubation in the enzyme solutions, spinning it with a stirring motor while submerged in M199. Although collagenase has been widely used experimentally, there has been some concern raised about its clinical use since it may contain undesirable DNases.

Other enzymes, such as trypsin without EDTA, chymotrypsin, pronase, and elastase have been used with less success. The neutral protease Dispase (grades I or II) has been suggested by the manufacturer to be good for cell isolation. Thilo *et al.*[33] used it for umbilical vein cells with good results.

Mechanical removal of EC from vessels with steel wool pledgets was used by Herring *et al.*[4] in their early seeding studies. Most likely smooth muscle cells from the tunica media of the veins were removed as well, however, and this method would appear to give mixtures of cell types that may be undesirable. Ryan[34] has long advocated the use of mechanical removal of EC either through gentle scraping of the vessels or by using polystyrene beads.

While these mechanical methods preserve cell surface coatings and receptors on EC, their use does not seem practical for EC seeding.

The isolation of microvascular endothelium from fat requires collagenase digestion of minced tissue and a series of filtering and sedimentation steps to get capillary fragments.[27] While the method produces large quantities of cells, the procedure is somewhat more lengthy than that used for large vessel endothelium; mixtures of EC, pericytes, and smooth muscle are likely and this may therefore be less desirable. Mesothelium from omentum, in contrast, was removed by collagenase digestion and can be done quite rapidly, but may have the same contamination problems.

Seeding of Grafts

Application of EC to the grafts has been done in a variety of ways. In their first report of successful endothelial cell seeding Herring *et al.*[4] mixed the cells with whole blood that was used to preclot the grafts.

Subsequently several other investigators have used this method on both large-and small-diameter Dacron and ePTFE grafts.

When using this method with Dacron grafts, the cells are trapped in the interstices of the graft wall and 50–75% of the cells remain in the graft when blood flow is restored.[35,36] Grafts of ePTFE are not usually preclotted, since they are relatively impermeable to blood, but introducing cells into the grafts using blood as an initial adhesive produces a healing in the grafts at a rate comparable to that of Dacron even though only 3–4% of the initial inoculum remains after blood flow is restored.[11] Since the rate of healing depends upon the number of cells in the graft per unit area that contributes to the endothelial lining and large numbers of cells may not be available for clinical seeding, it is important that all of the cells introduced into the graft remain.

To accomplish this, two things are necessary: (1) to get the cells to the graft surface, and (2) to provide a suitable substrate to which the cells can tenaciously attach. Simple settling of cells on the surface by gravity is the simplest method, but is slow and even distribution is difficult to obtain. Introducing cells in blood and trapping them in a clot also works, but many cells are lost when blood flow is restored since the cells are not really attached to the graft itself. Forcing the cells against the graft surface by centrifugal force quickly provides almost 100% cell attachment,[3] but is somewhat impractical for long small-diameter or bifurcated grafts. Although much work has been done on cell adhesives for grafts, little work has been done on getting the cells directly on the surface and evenly distributed.

Providing the best surface for cell attachment has been a goal since the earliest days of seeding.[2] Clearly the reason that recent EC seeding on standard Dacron[4,9] and ePTFE[15] is successful is that the cells do not come directly in contact with the graft, but with blood proteins coating the graft. This has been shown in studies on EC adhesion with Dacron[27] and ePTFE,[37] where bare grafts gave poor adhesion while coatings of collagens, or plasma,[27] or fibronectin[37] greatly increased cell retention. In addition, the DNA content of EC attached to bare ePTFE decreased with time, indicating a lack of cell proliferation.[38] On ePTFE grafts coated with glucosaminoglycan-keratin cell adhesion was promoted, but like the naked graft cells showed minimal proliferation.[39]

Sentissi[38] reported that EC seeded on ePTFE coated with fibronectin and type I collagen gave good growth and were highly resistant to shear in an *in vitro* shunt. In *in vivo* studies, Koeveker *et al.*[41] found that fibrin glue, used to make grafts impermeable, provided a poorer surface for EC healing than did whole blood coatings.

Extracellular matrices similar to those underlying natural endothelium would seem intuitively to be the best graft coatings.[27] Dacron grafts coated with a combination of interstitial collagens (types I/III) and amnion-derived basement membrane (collagen type IV) gave firm adherence to 70% of seeded cells within 30 min. Interestingly, grafts treated with platelet-rich plasma alone gave similar attachment in only 10 min.

In *in vivo* studies with ePTFE grafts, Ramalanjoana *et al.*[11] found that 47% of EC attached to grafts coated with fibronectin in comparison to 19.8% on grafts in which cells were seeded in blood. When implanted in the carotid artery, fibronectin did not prevent cell loss within the first 30 min, but at 24 hours six times as many cells were present in the coated compared to the noncoated grafts (21.3 vs. 3.4%). Despite the increase in cell adhesion by coatings with extracellular matrix proteins, the loss of 80% of the seeded cells leaves much room for improvement, and much work still needs to be done on both coatings and seeding methods.

If all of the seeded cells remained attached to the grafts they would heal in a matter of days instead of weeks as is now the case.

There is no agreement on the best physical design of a graft for EC seeding, with some[6] advocating less porous and others[42] more porous grafts. There does seem to be general agreement that a relatively smooth surface is better.[43] The graft material seems to be less important than the surface coating. With current knowledge of extracellular matrix proteins and growth factors, it should be possible in the near future to design a graft ideally suited to endothelial cell seeding.

The addition of EC growth factors to graft surfaces to enhance healing may also be desirable. Greisler *et al.*[44] have recently reported attempts to bond endothelial cell growth factor (ECGF) to biomaterials. Heparin-bonded biomaterials have been available for several years. It is of interest that fibronectin binds heparin as well. Heparin has been shown to be synergistic with ECGF in promoting EC growth,[45] and in addition inhibits smooth muscle cell proliferation.[46] Smooth muscle growth in the body of grafts may be of little consequence, but it has been implicated in the development of anastomotic intimal hyperplasia (IH), said to be the cause of late failure in small diameter grafts. Why IH occurs is not known, but it has been suggested that platelet adhesion with subsequent release of platelet-derived growth factor (PDGF) stimulates the smooth muscle to proliferate. Antiplatelet drugs have been reported to decrease IH in experimental animals, but their efficacy in man remains to be proved.[47] It is clear that antiplatelet drugs are necessary to maintain patency in small diameter grafts in the short term.[48] Aspirin and dipyridamole have been the most commonly used, but other cyclooxygenase and thromboxane synthetase inhibitors have been used as well. The most effective appears to be aspirin alone, although the reasons are unclear.[49,50] Whether the rapid endothelialization of grafts by seeding will reduce IH has not been proved. It has been shown that EC continue to turn over and smooth muscle cells continue to proliferate at anastomoses even after grafts are healed.[51] It has been suggested that this is due to chronic EC injury. It has been shown that smooth muscle cells secrete growth factors acting on neighboring smooth muscle cells and that normal EC produce a heparin-like inhibitor of smooth muscle proliferation.[52] It has been suggested that injured EC may be incapable of secreting this inhibitor, and the result is IH.[50]

It is clear that EC seeding has dramatically improved small diameter graft patency in both animals[48] and man[5] in the short term. Whether it will improve the long-term failure rate is unknown at this point. In the long run the solution to small vessel grafting will most likely be a combination of better grafts, enhancement of healing by seeding or other means, as well as pharmacological intervention.

REFERENCES

1. LIOTTA, D., C. W. HALL, A. VILLANUEVA, R. M. O'NEAL & M. E. DEBAKEY. 1966. A permanent autologous lining for implantable blood pumps. Cardiovasc. Res. Cent. Bull. **4:** 69–80.
2. BURKEL, W. E. & R. H. KAHN. 1976. Cell-lined, nonwoven microfiber scaffolds as a blood interface. Ann. N. Y. Acad. Sci. **283:** 419–442.
3. KAHN, R. H., W. E. BURKEL & V. P. PERRY. 1974. Homeostatic and mass culture technology. J. Natl. Cancer Inst. **53:** 1471–1477.
4. HERRING, M. B., A. GARDNER & J. GLOVER. 1978. A single-staged technique for seeding vascular grafts with autogenous endothelium. Surgery **84:** 498–504.
5. HERRING, M. B., R. S. COMPTON, D. R. LEGRAND, A. L. GARDNER, D. L. MADISON & J. L. GLOVER. 1987. Early experiences with endothelial seeding on PTFE femoral popliteal bypasses: A randomized study. J. Vasc. Surg. Submitted.
6. STANLEY, J. C., W. E. BURKEL, L. M. GRAHAM & B. LINDBLAD. 1985. Endothelial cell seeding of synthetic vascular prostheses. 1985. Acta Chir. Scand. Suppl. **529:** 17–28.
7. GRAHAM, L. M., J. C. STANLEY & W. E. BURKEL. 1986. Endothelial seeding of synthetic vascular grafts. *In* Endothelial Cells. U. Ryan, Ed. CRC Press. Boca Raton, FL.
8. FORD, J. W., W. E. BURKEL & R. H. KAHN. 1981. Isolation of adult canine venous endothelium for tissue culture. In Vitro **17:** 44–50.
9. GRAHAM, L. M., D. W. VINTER, J. W. FORD, R. H. KAHN, W. E. BURKEL & J. C. STANLEY. 1980. Endothelial cell seeding of prosthetic vascular grafts. Early experimental studies with cultured autologous canine endothelium. Arch. Surg. **115:** 929–933.
10. GRAHAM, L. M., D. W. VINTER, J. W. FORD, R. H. KAHN, W. E. BURKEL & J. C. STANLEY. 1980. Immediate seeding of enzymatically derived endothelium in Dacron vascular grafts. Arch. Surg. **115:** 1289–1294.
11. RAMALANJOANA, G., R. F. KEMPCZINSKI, J. E. ROSENMAN & E. B. SILBERSTEIN. 1986. The effect of fibronectin coating on endothelial cell kinetics in polytetrafluoroethylene grafts. J. Vasc. Surg. **3:** 264–272.
12. BURKEL, W. E., D. W. VINTER, J. W. FORD, R. H. KAHN, L. M. GRAHAM & J. C. STANLEY. 1981. Sequential studies of healing in endothelial seeded vascular prostheses: Histologic and ultrastructure characteristics of graft incorporation. J. Surg. Res. **30:** 305–324.
13. GRAHAM, L. M., W. E. BURKEL, J. W. FORD, D. W. VINTER, R. H. KAHN & J. C. STANLEY. 1982. Expanded polytetrafluoroethylene vascular prostheses seeded with enzymatically derived and cultured canine endothelial cells. Surgery **91:** 550–559.
14. HERRING, M. B., A. GARDNER, P. PEIGH, D. MADISON, S. BAUGHMAN, J. BROWN & J. GLOVER. 1984. Patency in inferior vena cava grafting: Effects of graft material, size, and endothelial seeding. J. Vasc. Surg. **1:** 877–887.
15. BURKEL, W. E., J. W. FORD, D. W. VINTER, R. H. KAHN, L. M. GRAHAM & J. C. STANLEY. 1982. Fate of knitted Dacron velour vascular grafts seeded with enzymatically derived autologous canine endothelium. Trans. Am. Soc. Artif. Intern. Organs **28:** 178–184.
16. HERRING, M. B., R. DILLEY, R. A. JERSILD, L. BOXER, A. GARDNER & J. GLOVER. 1979. Seeding of arterial prostheses with vascular endothelium. The nature of the lining. Ann. Surg. **190:** 84–90.
17. DILLEY, R., M. B. HERRING, L. BOXER, A. GARDNER & J. GLOVER. 1979. Immunofluorescent staining for factor VIII-related antigen: A tool for study of healing in vascular prostheses. J. Surg. Res. **27:** 149–155.
18. SCHMIDT, S. P., T. J. HUNTER, W. V. SHARP, G. S. MALINDZAK & M. M. EVANCHO. 1984. Endothelial cell-seeded four millimeter Dacron vascular grafts: Effects of blood flow manipulation through the grafts. J. Vasc. Surg. **1:** 434–441.
19. CLAGETT, G. P., W. E. BURKEL, J. B. SHAREFKIN, J. W. FORD, H. HUFNAGEL, D. W. VINTER, R. H. KAHN, L. M. GRAHAM, & J. C. STANLEY & P. W. RAMWELL. 1984.

Platelet reactivity in vivo in dogs with arterial prostheses seeded with endothelial cells. Circulation **69:** 632–639.

20. SHAREFKIN, J. B., C. LATKER, M. SMITH, D. CREUSS, C. P. CLAGETT & N. M. RICH. 1982. Early normalization of platelet survival by endothelial seeding of Dacron arterial prostheses in dogs. Surgery **92:** 385–383.
21. WHITEHOUSE, W. M. JR., T. W. WAKEFIELD, D. W. VINTER, J. W. FORD, D. P. SWANSON, J. H. THRALL, J. W. FROELICH, L. E. BROWN, W. E. BURKEL, L. M. GRAHAM & J. C. STANLEY. 1983. Indium-111-oxine labeled platelet imaging of endothelial cell seeded Dacron thoracoabdominal vascular prostheses in a canine model. Trans. Am. Soc. Artif. Intern. Organs **29:** 183–187.
22. SHEPARD, A. D., J. ELDRUP-JORGENSEN, E. M. KEOUGH, T. F. FOXHALL, K. RAMBERG, R. J. CONNOLLY, W. C. MACKEY, V. GARVIS, K. R. AUGER, P. LIBBY, T. F. O'DONNELL & A. D. CALLOW. 1986. Endothelial seeding of small-caliber synthetic grafts in the baboon. Surgery **99:** 318–325.
23. BURKEL, W. E., L. M. GRAHAM & J. C. STANLEY. Unpublished results.
24. JAFFE, E. A., R. L. NACHMAN, C. G. BECKER & C. R. MINICK. 1972. Culture of human endothelial cells derived from human umbilical cord veins. Circulation **46**(Suppl. II): 252.
25. BOOYSE, F. M., B. J. SEDLAK & M. E. RAFELSON, JR. 1975. Culture of arterial cells. Characterization and growth of bovine aortic cells. Thromb. Diath. Haemorrh. **34:** 825–839.
26. JAFFE, E. A. 1984. Tissue culture of endothelial cells. *In* Biology of Endothelial Cells. E. A. Jaffe, Ed.: 1–13. Martinus Nijhoff. Boston.
27. JARRELL, B. E., S. K. WILLIAMS, L. SOLOMON, L. SPEICHER, E. KOOLPE, J. RADOMSKI, R. A. CARABASI, D. GREENER & F. E. ROSATO. 1986. Use of an endothelial monolayer on a vascular graft prior to implantation. Ann. Surg. **203:** 671–678.
28. PEARCE, W. H., R. B. RUTHERFORD, T. WHITEHALL *et al.* 1987. Successful endothelial seeding using omentally derived microvascular endothelial cells. J. Vasc. Surg. **5:** 203–206.
29. CLARKE, J. M., R. M. PITTILO, L. J. NICHOLSON, N. WOOLF & A. MARSTON. 1984. Seeding Dacron arterial prostheses with peritoneal mesothelial cells: A preliminary morphological study. Br. J. Surg. **71:** 492–494.
30. HOLLIER, L. H., R. J. FOWL, C. F. HECK, K. A. WINTER, D. N. FASSE & M. P. KAYE. 1986. Are seeded endothelial cells the origin of neointima on prosthetic vascular grafts? J. Vasc. Surg. **3:** 65.
31. PENNELL, R. C., L. H. HOLLIER, E. SOLIS & M. P. KAYE. 1986. Xenograft seeding of Dacron grafts in dogs. J. Surg. Res. **40:** 332.
32. ZAMORA, J. L., L. T. NARARRO, C. L. IVES, D. G. WEILBAECHER, Z. R. GAO & G. P. NOON. 1986. Seeding of arteriovenous prostheses with homologous endothelium. J. Vasc. Surg. **3:** 860–866.
33. THILO, D. G. S., S. MULLER-KUSEL, D. HEINRICH, I. KAUFER & E. WEISS. 1980. Isolation of human venous endothelial cells by different proteases. Artery **8:** 259–266.
34. RYAN, U. S. 1984. Culture of pulmonary endothelial cells on microcarrier beads. *In* Biology of Endothelial Cells. E. A. Jaffe, Ed.: 34–50. Martinus Nijhoff. Boston.
35. SHAREFKIN, J. B., C. LATHER, M. SMITH & N. M. RICH. 1983. Endothelial cell labelling with indium-111-oxine as a marker of cell attachment to bioprosthetic surfaces. J. Biomed. Mater. Res. **17:** 345–357.
36. GRAHAM, L. M., J. V. FORD, D. W. VINTER, J. C. STANLEY & W. E. BURKEL. 1984. Endothelial cell adherence to Dacron vascular prostheses: Optimization of seeding technique. Trans. Am. Soc. Artif. Intern. Organs **13:** 26.
37. SEEGER, J. M. 1985. Improved endothelial cell seeding density after flow exposure in fibronectin-coated grafts. Surg. Forum **36:** 450–452.
38. SENTISSI, J. M., K. RAMBERG, T. F. O'DONNELL, R. J. CONNOLLY & A. D. CALLOW. 1986. The effect of flow on vascular endothelial cells grown in tissue culture on polytetrafluoroethylene grafts. Surgery **99:** 337–343.
39. SOBINSKIE, K. R., P. FLANIGAN, A. WINDRA, J. P. MEYER & J. J. CASTRONUOVO. 1984. Glucosaminoglycan-keratin coating enhances endothelial cell growth rate on seeded vascular prostheses. Surg. Forum **35:** 435–436.

40. MACARAK, E. J. & P. S. HOWARD. 1983. Adhesion of endothelial cells to extracellular matrix proteins. J. Cell Physiol. **116:** 76–86.
41. KOEVEKER, G. B., K. H. PETZKE, M. BORG & K. NEBENDAHL. 1986. Reduction of thrombogenicity in small-diameter vascular prostheses seeded with autologous endothelial cells. Thorac. Cardiovasc. Surg. **34:** 49–51.
42. KEMPCZINSKI, R. F., J. E. ROSENMAN, W. H. PEARCE, L. R. ROEDERSHEIMER, Y. BERLATZKY & G. RAMALANJAONA. 1985. Endothelial cell seeding of a new PTFE vascular prosthesis. J. Vasc. Surg. **2:** 424–429.
43. HERRING, M. B., R. DILLEY, A. GARDNER & J. GLOVER. 1980. The effects of crimping on the healing of prosthetic arterial grafts. J. Cardiovasc. Surg. **21:** 596.
44. GREISLER, H., J. KLOSAK, J. DENNIS, D. KIM, W. BURGESS & T. MACIAG. 1986. Endothelial cell growth factor (ECGF) attachment to biomaterials. Trans. Am. Soc. Artif. Intern. Organs **15:** 25.
45. THORNTON, S. C., S. M. MUELLER & E. M. LEVINE. 1983. Human endothelial cells: Use of heparin in cloning and long-term serial cultivation. Science **222:** 623–625.
46. CASTELLOT, J. J., R. D. ROSENBERG & M. J. KARNOVSKY. 1984. Endothelium, heparin, and the regulation of vascular smooth muscle growth. *In* The Biology of Endothelial Cells. E. A. Jaffe, Ed.: 118–128. Martinus Nijhoff. Boston.
47. CLOWES, A. W. 1986. The role of aspirin in enhancing arterial graft patency. J. Vasc. Surg. **3:** 381–385.
48. STANLEY, J. C., W. E. BURKEL, J. W. FORD, D. W. VINTER, R. H. KAHN, W. W. WHITEHOUSE & L. M. GRAHAM. 1982. Enhanced patency of small-diameter, externally supported Dacron iliofemoral grafts seeded with endothelial cells. Surgery **92:** 994–1005.
49. ALLEN, B. T., J. A. LONG, M. J. WELCH, K. T. HOPKINS, G. A. SICARD & R. E. CLARK. 1983. Effect of aspirin therapy and its withdrawal on control and endothelial seeded grafts. Surg. Forum **34:** 470–472.
50. GRAHAM, L. M., J. C. STANLEY & W. E. BURKEL. 1986. Influence of endothelial cell seeding and antiplatelet drugs on patency of prosthetic vascular grafts. *In* Endothelialization of Vascular Grafts. R. Fasol, Ed. Karger. Basel. In press.
51. CLOWES, A. W., T. R. KIRKMAN & M. CLOWES. 1986. Mechanisms of arterial graft failure. II. Chronic endothelial and smooth muscle cell proliferation in healing polytetrafluoroethylene prostheses. J. Vasc. Surg. **3:** 877–884.
52. CASTELLOT, J. J., M. L. ADDONZIO, R. ROSENBERG & M. J. KARNOVSKY. 1981. Cultured endothelial cells produce a heparin-like inhibitor of smooth muscle cell growth. J. Cell. Biol. **90:** 372–379.

Thrombosis on Endothelializable Protheses

STUART K. WILLIAMS AND BRUCE E. JARRELL

Department of Surgery
Jefferson Medical College
Philadelphia, Pennsylvania 19107

INTRODUCTION

The study of artificial vascular graft interactions with blood elements has revealed a complex group of events occurring within the lumen. In most small diameter polymer grafts, these events result in progressive luminal occlusion secondary to either thrombus within the midgraft region or cellular hyperplasia at the anastomotic regions.[1,2] In grafts implanted into humans, it has been observed that endothelial cells fail to line the majority of the lumenal surface. A number of investigators have hypothesized that if a stable endothelial cell monolayer could be established on a graft, patency rates in small diameter grafts might improve. This endothelial lining would function as not only a nonthrombogenic surface, but also as an active antithrombogenic surface with metabolic activities that replicate exactly a native artery wall. Efforts to establish an endothelial cell lining on prosthetic devices have focused both on stimulation of native spontaneous endothelialization processes and the transplantation of autologous cells to the surface of a vascular graft.[3–5]

Implantation of vascular grafts in animal species other than man results in a degree of spontaneous endothelialization.[1] Variable rates of spontaneous endothelialization have been observed and are believed to result from three possible mechanisms. First, endothelium on a native blood vessel can migrate across the anastomosis onto artificial surfaces.[4] This process is slow in all species and rarely extends more than 2 cm from the anastomostic site. Second, microvascular endothelium can migrate through the porous graft interstices, reach the surface, and proliferate to create an endothelialized surface.[6] The rate of transinterstitial ingrowth appears variable between animal species, but it appears that currently used grafts implanted in humans will not endothelialize by this process. Finally, blood-borne cells adhere to the surface of implanted grafts and proliferate to create an endothelial surface.[7] Minimal data exist concerning the potential of this process for spontaneous endothelialization, and again, no reports of this form of spontaneous endothelialization have been reported in man.

Alternatively, several investigators have evaluated procedures to establish endothelial cell monlayers on grafts by transplanting endothelium onto the surface of the grafts. Two procedures have evolved to create endothelialized surfaces and are presented in TABLE 1. Endothelial cell seeding represents the incorporation of endothelial cells within a clot on a graft surface or direct seeding onto the surface. The density of cells is generally low, necessitating the proliferation of endothelium to create a confluent endothelial monolayer. An alternate procedure is the establishment of an endothelial cell monolayer on a vascular graft prior to its implantation.[8] This procedure is known as sodding or *in vitro* endothelialization and differs from seeding technologies in several important respects. Seeding procedures utilize minimal cell numbers (due to availability), which are placed within plasma or blood, and subsequently preclotted within and on the graft surface. The resulting luminal surface exists as a highly thrombogenic fibrin meshwork. On the other hand, sodding utilizes a large number of cells to establish an endothelial cell monolayer on the luminal surface of a graft. Thus at the time of implantation the luminal surface presents an actively antithrombogenic surface.

The immediate establishment of an antithrombogenic endothelial monolayer prior to graft implantation is a methodological goal of our laboratory. Several factors must be considered before this goal can be achieved. The source of endothelial cells, as well as the effects of cell isolation procedures and the effects of culture, if necessary, must be evaluated. Factors that affect cell-to-surface interactions must be defined. Inherent within this study is the determination of the effect of artificial polymers and polymer treatments on endothelial cell association. When a full understanding of the interaction between endothelial cells and surfaces is achieved a clinically acceptable endothelialized graft surface may be feasible.

The creation of an endothelializable vascular graft is hampered by the lack of a suitable polymeric surface for endothelial cell association. We must overcome this problem by masking this hostile cell surface with a substrate that stimulates cell attachment. Lessons from natural surfaces begin to suggest that a surface with affinity for endothelium and inherent nonthrombogenic characteristics may be achievable.

TABLE 1. Comparison of Endothelial Cell Seeding and Sodding Techniques

	Seeding (EC in Plasma Clot)	Sodding (EC in Culture Medium)
EC location	within clot	upon surface
Critical adherence variable	clot-to-graft interaction	EC-to-graft interaction
Cell density	low	high
Method of monolayer formation	growth and migration	attachment and spreading—no growth

MATERIAL AND METHODS

Isolation and Culture of Human Endothelial Cells

Endothelial cells (ECs) were isolated from vascular tissue procured from brain-dead, heart-beating cadaver renal donors and were cultured according to our previously published procedures.[9,10] In the present study, ECs from adult human iliac veins were used. Briefly, cells were isolated from a fresh iliac vein by treating the luminal surface with collagenase (Worthington Type I; Worthington Diagnostic Systems, Inc., Freehold, NJ) and grown in 25 cm^2 tissue culture flasks precoated with gelatin (1%) in culture medium (medium 199, 20% heat-inactivated fetal calf serum, 90 μg/ml heparin [porcine], and 20 μg/ml endothelial cell growth factor [ECGF]). Population doublings were calculated during culture by the formula PD = $\log^2$ (number of cells harvested per number of cells seeded $\times$ attachment efficiency) and summed to give the cumulative population doublings (CPDs). The EC identity of cultures was established using criteria previously reported,[9] and included positive staining for factor-VIII-related antigen, cobblestone morphology, and the expression of EC-specific prostaglandin and angiotensin-converting enzyme activity.

Isolation of Human Adult Microvascular ECs

Human perinephric or omental fat was obtained from brain-dead, heart-beating cadaver organ donors or patients undergoing unrelated surgical procedures in accordance with Institutional Review Board protocol. The fat was mechanically minced and placed in sterile 50-ml screw cap Erlenmeyer flasks containing 10 ml of Dulbecco cation-free (DCF) buffer, pH 7.4, with collagenase (Worthington type I; Cooper, Biomedical, Malver, PA), 4 mg/ml, and bovine serum albumin (BSA, Sigma type V; Sigma Chemical Co., St. Louis, MO), 4 mg/ml. The flasks were incubated for 25 minutes at 37°C with gentle agitation. The contents of the flask were centrifuged at 200 ×g for 7 minutes. The pellet was washed twice in DCF buffer containing 0.1% BSA and spun for 3 minutes at 200 ×g.

The resultant pellet was resuspended in 45% Percoll (Pharmacia Fine Chemicals, Piscataway, NJ) in DCF and centrifuged at 20,000 ×g for 20 minutes at 4°C. The tufts of capillary EC were in a milky-white layer at the top of the density gradient with vessel fragments and cellular debris in the pellet. The capillary ECs were washed twice in DCF-BSA buffer at 200 ×g for 3 minutes. The tufts were resuspended in medium 199 with 20% fetal calf serum (Hazeltown Research Laboratories, Denver, PA). The identification of ECs in the primary isolate is based primarily on morphologic examination by phase-contrast microscopy. Primary isolates, plated at high density and subjected to primary culture, exhibited positive staining for factor-VIII-related antigen and displayed angiotensin-I-converting enzyme activity.

Graft Surface Preparation

Cooley graft-woven low-porosity Dacron fabric (supplied by Meadox Medicals, Oakland, NJ) was serially washed in acetone, 8.5% H_3PO_4 and 1 N NaOH; this was followed by extensive washing with double-distilled H_2O. After drying, it was placed in a Harrick plasma cleaner (Harrick Industry, Ossining, NY) for 10 minutes at 10^{-4} torr in an air atmosphere. A 2.5 by 5 cm segment of the graft material was prepared for substrate coating and EC seeding.

Dacron Treatment with Platelet-Rich Plasma

Platelet-rich plasma (PRP) was prepared from fresh anticoagulated whole blood from normal human donors. PRP was mixed with 50 mmol/l $CaCl_2$ just before graft treatment. The PRP was then placed onto the graft material immobilized in a seeding chamber, as will be described. Once treated with PRP, the fibrin clot was permitted to form at 37°C on the graft surface. The excess clot was then removed, and the graft surface was washed with culture medium before EC seeding.

Preparation of Human Basement Membrane Native Matrix Surfaces

A surface of human basement membrane components was prepared using fresh human placenta.[11,12] All procedures were performed under sterile conditions. The inner amnionic membrane was gently separated manually from chorion, washed three times with sterile distilled H_2O, and incubated with 1 mM *N*-ethylmaleimide for 1 hour at 4°C. The amnion was then incubated in 4% deoxycholate solution for 2 hours at 36°C. This procedure loosened the epithelial cells from underlying basement membrane and facilitated the denudation of the epithelial cell layer with the addition of gentle agitation using a rubber policeman. The underlying basement membrane was exposed and served as a surface for EC seeding. Prepared amnion was preserved until graft preparation in complete culture media (M199, 20% heat-inactivated FCS, 90 mg/ml L-glutamine) supplemented with 1200 μg/ml penicillin-streptomycin and 4 μg/ml Fungizone. Prior to use, the amnionic membranes were incubated for a minimum of 2 hours in culture media.

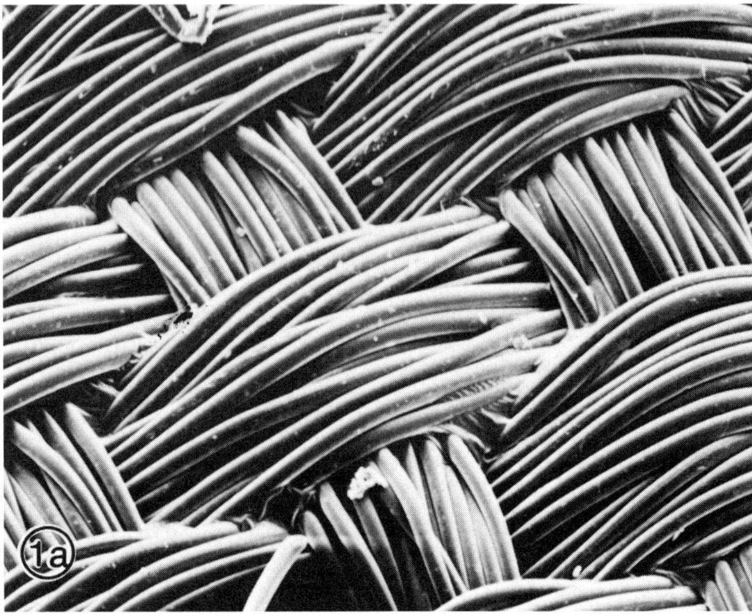
1a

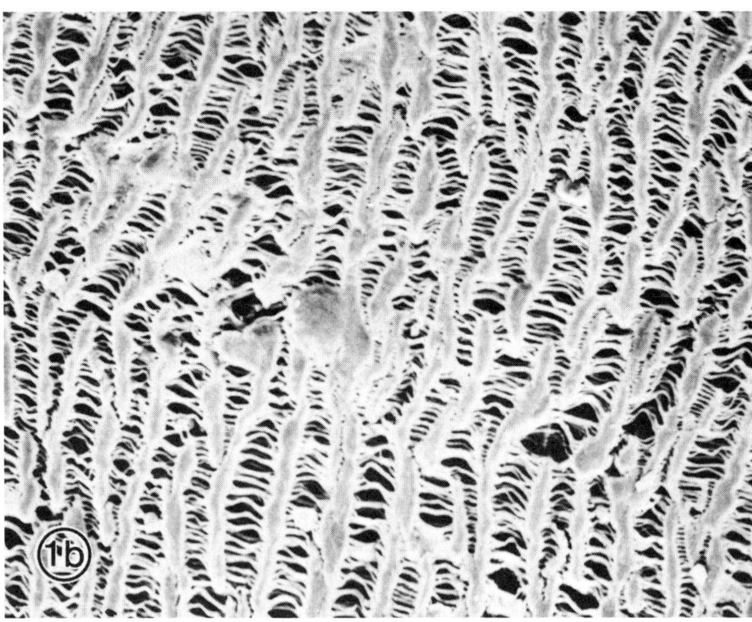
1b

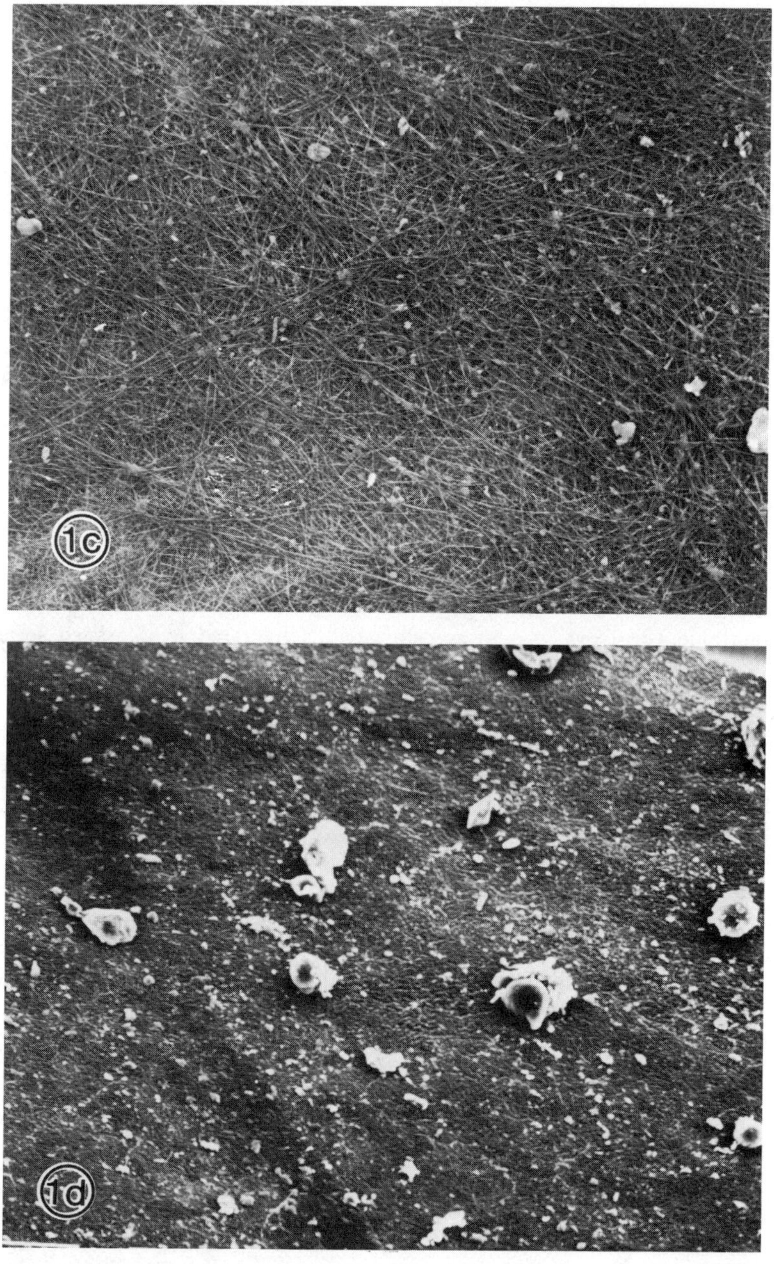

FIGURE 1. Scanning electron micrographs illustrating the morphology of currently used endothelialized surfaces. **(a)** Untreated dacron. **(b)** Untreated expanded teflon. **(c)** Dacron treated with fibrin. **(d)** Dacron treated with amnion. The amnion is immobilized such that the basement membrane surface is towards the lumen.

Collagen Preparation

Heterologous interstitial collagen types I and III were prepared from human placenta following the procedures of Madri.[13] Briefly, minced and freeze-dried placenta was pepsin-digested and a collagen fraction was solubilized with 0.5 M acetic acid. Types I and III collagen were precipitated with 1.4 M NaCl, and the precipitate was collected and dialyzed extensively against buffer. The white flocculent collagen was used either immediately or freeze-dried and stored at −20°C until use.

Scanning Electron Microscopy

Seeded graft surfaces were fixed with 1% glutaraldehyde for 1 hour, 3% glutaraldehyde for 2 hours, washed three times (20-minute period) with Tyrodes cacodylate buffer (pH 7.4), and dehydrated in a graded series of acetone. The grafts, still immobilized within plastic rings, were critical-point dried and coated with gold palladium. Mounted samples were examined in a Phillips scanning electron microscope.

Transmission Electron Microscopy

Glutaraldehyde fixed tissue was osmicated, dehydrated in a graded series of acetone, and embedded in Spurr Resin. Sections were then obtained with a diamond knife (Diatome, LKB, Switzerland) and examined in a Zeiss EM-9 electron microscope (Carl Zeiss, Federal Republic of Germany).

RESULTS

Several surfaces were evaluated for their ability to support the attachment and spreading of human adult endothelial cells (HAEC). These surfaces included raw dacron (FIG. 1a), raw expanded teflon (FIG. 1b), fibrin-coated dacron (FIG. 1c), and amnion-coated dacron (FIG. 1d). These surface represent a wide range of textures and protein composition as well as surfaces with varying degrees of inherent thrombogenicity. Subsequent treatment of these surfaces with HAEC resulted in significant variations in cell association. Raw dacron and expanded teflon presented a surface quite hostile to HAEC adherence (FIG. 2), with only focal adherence of cells. The pretreatment of dacron with either fibrin (FIG. 3a) or interstitial collagen (FIG. 3b) further stimulated EC adherence, however cell-cell interaction was often interrupted by gaps.

Human amnion was used as a substitute for the basement membrane upon which HAEC normally adhere. When HAEC were incubated with amnion-treated dacron, we observed a time-dependent association of cells with the surface (FIGS. 4a–c). By 1 minute (FIG. 4a) shear-resistant cell attachment had occurred; however, the cells remained round and were not physically attached to the surface. Within 10 minutes on amnion (FIG. 4b), cellular projections were observed on the basal surface of the cell in close apposition to the amnion surface. By 30 minutes (FIG. 4c) cells were observed spread over the entire amnion surface attached basally to the amnion and to each other through immature junctions.

DISCUSSION

The optimal vascular graft would display characteristics identical to a native blood vessel. With the development of new polymer chemistry technologies it is now possible to reproduce physical characteristics of the native blood vessel such as compliance and suturability; however, the "living" nature of natural vessels may not be attainable with

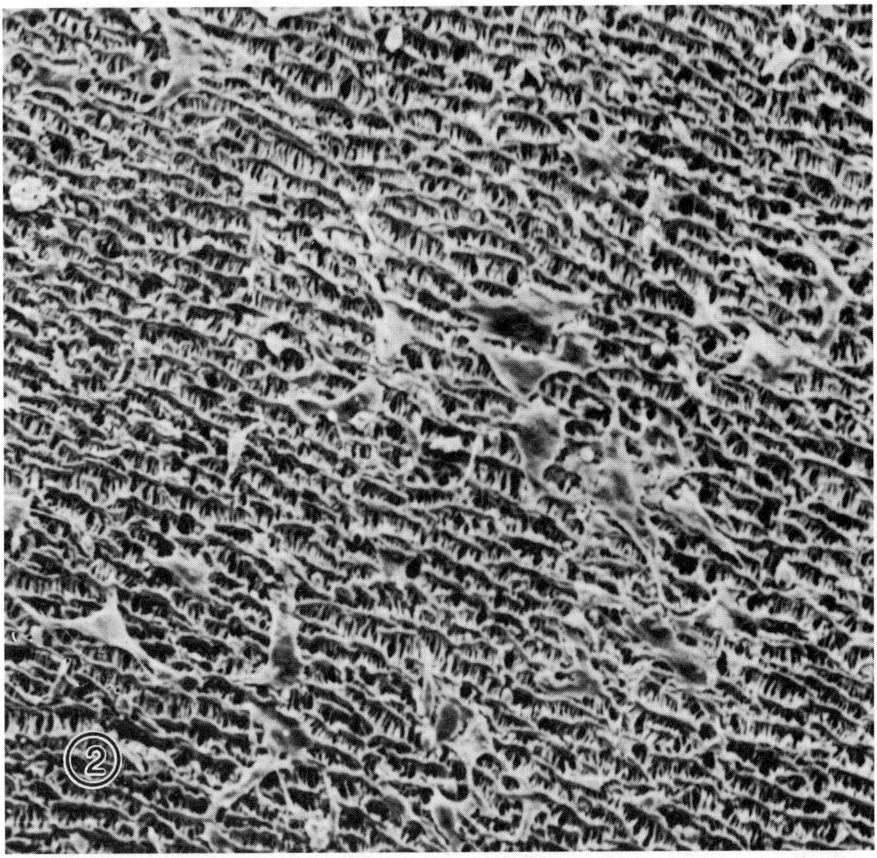

FIGURE 2. Untreated polymer surfaces represent a poor substrate for human adult endothelial cell adherence as illustrated in this scanning electron micrograph of an HAEC-treated expanded teflon graft.

polymers. For this reason, polymeric grafts can only hope to achieve nonthrombogenic status with only questionable possibilities of possessing renewable antithrombogenic characteristics. We have embarked on studies on improving the long-term survival of vascular grafts by accepting as a goal inherently nonthrombogenic polymers with surfaces that can be endothelialized with the patient's own endothelial cells prior to implantation.

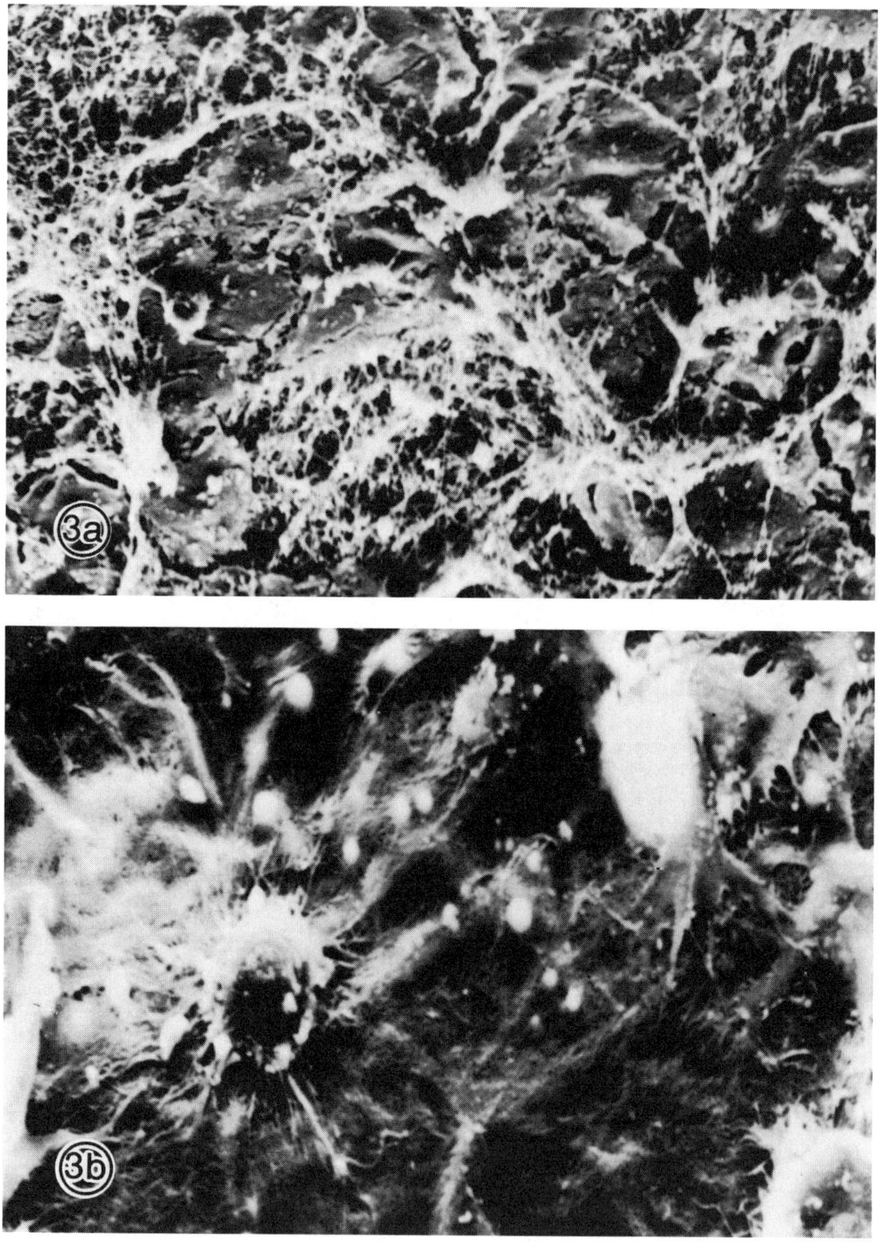

FIGURE 3. The adherence of human endothelium can be stimulated by treating the surface with proteins such as (**a**) fibrin or (**b**) collagen. However, these scanning electron micrographs illustrate the poor cell-to-cell interaction.

Source of Autologous Endothelium: Microvessels

A major problem in graft endothelialization has been the past inability to procure large quantities of HAEC for the treatment of polymeric surfaces. Our initial studies were directed towards expanding cultures of human-derived EC derived from small segments of patients' native blood vessels. This expansion was made possible by the discovery that heparin and endothelial cell growth factor dramatically stimulated the growth of EC derived from human adult blood vessels.[9,10] With large quantities of cultured HAEC we began to study the interaction of human EC with artificial grafts.[14] However, several problems existed in using cultured cells for treating vascular grafts clinically. These problems included: (1) The use of cultured cells would require 1 to 3 weeks to produce enough cells to endothelialize a graft. (2) Not all patients' blood vessels yielded cells and not all of the HAEC isolated would proliferate. (3) Cell culture introduces many variables, including the effect of nonautologous serum, growth factors, and viruses on cells. (4) Cell culture must be performed outside the operating room.

We subsequently have found an alternative source of HAEC in human microvascularized fat. These microvascular endothelial cells (microvessels, since they are derived from arterioles, venules, and capillaries) can easily be isolated in large quantities ($>10^6$ cells/g fat) from the patient's own fat. With an easily obtainable source of autologous EC we have subsequently turned our attention to polymers and polymer surface treatments that will support rapid endothelial cell adherence. In addition, the surface must also permit the maintenance of a stable, regeneratable endothelial cell monolayer.

Endothelial Cell Adherence to Polymers and Substrates

The initial evaluations of HAEC interaction with untreated polymers resulted in the expected result that currently available grafts do not support HAEC adherence. Since graft manufacturers developed polymers that would resist cellular activation and attachment, the lack of endothelial cell association was not surprising. Obviously the polymeric surface must be altered in some way to facilitate EC association.

Several avenues of investigation have resulted from this line of reasoning, leading investigators to attempt to develop either polymer treatments that will (1) facilitate endothelial cell ingrowth from the anastomoses, (2) stimulate transinterstitial (through the graft) capillary microvessel migration and growth, or (3) support endothelial adherence and spreading. If a vascular graft could be developed that would support spontaneous endothelialization through rapid pannus ingrowth or capillary transinterstitial ingrowth, long-term graft survival might be extended. However, these processes require at a minimum days, and most likely weeks, before a confluent EC layer is obtained. We therefore have focused on developing either a polymer treatment or a new polymer that supports the rapid adherence and spreading of HAEC to create an immediate monolayer at the time of graft implantation.

The easiest solution to overcome the poor EC adherence to currently available graft polymers is to treat the surface with a protein(s) that has known affinity for endothelium. The proteins currently used are fibronectin, collagens, laminin, glycosoaminoglycans, components of the extracellular matrix upon which endothelium normally rests. Fibronectin has received the greatest attention due to the well-characterized cell binding domains in this molecule.[15] These polymer treatments have indeed stimulated both human and nonhuman cell adherence to grafts.[14,16] Initial work in our laboratory indicated that collagen (interstitial types I and III) supported the

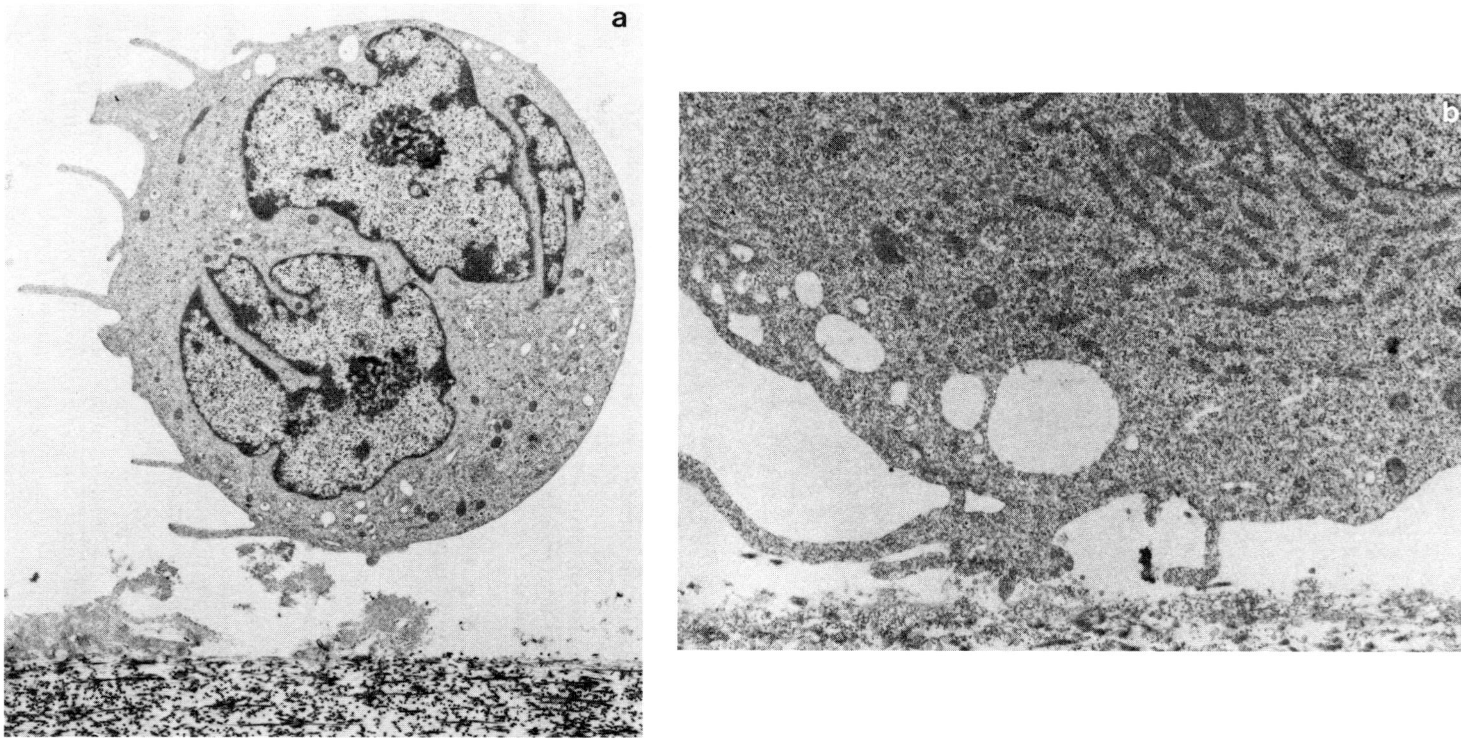
a
b

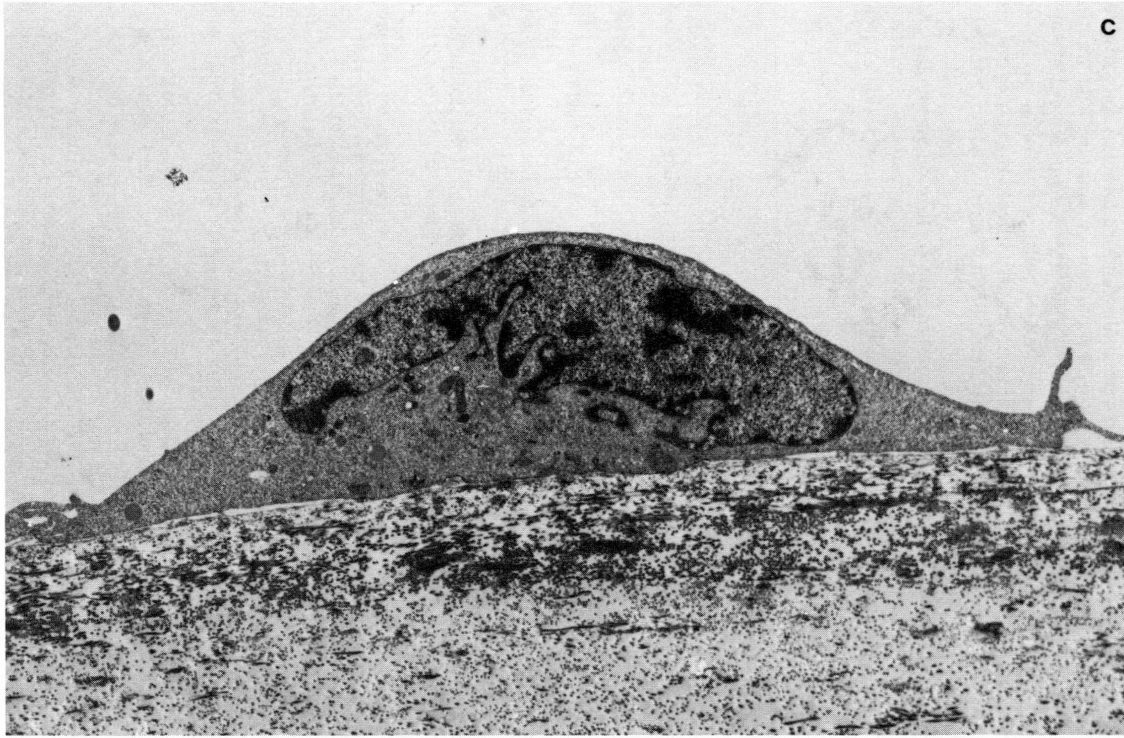

FIGURE 4. Human amnion provides an excellent surface for the rapid adherence of human endothelial cells. Transmission electron micrographs illustrate the interaction of HAEC with amnion following **(a)** 1 minute, **(b)** 5 minutes, and **(c)** 30 minutes of incubation.

greatest quantitative adherence of cells.[12] However, we began to consider that not only the number of endothelial cells attached but also their morphology was of extreme importance. Furthermore, the functional status of the endothelium must also be considered. The rapid establishment of a confluent monolayer would be meaningless if the cells exhibited procoagulant activity.[17]

In an attempt to mimic the native surface upon which endothelial cells adhere, we have utilized the basement membrane surface of human amnion. The amnion is annealed to Dacron covalently, producing a stable surface. This basement membrane supports rapid adherence of human adult endothelial cells, permitting a monolayer of endothelium to be achieved within 1 hour. These results indicate that an antithrombogenic surface can be rapidly achieved on a treated polymer surface within a time frame necessary for the operating room.

The development of a renewable, antithrombogenic surface on a vascular graft is the major goal in the development of a blood-compatible prosthetic surface. The formation of an endothelial cell monolayer on vascular grafts is one solution to creating this antithrombogenic surface.

REFERENCES

1. Clowes, A. W., A. M. Gown, S. R. Hanson & M. A. Reidy. 1985. Mechanisms of arterial graft failure. I. Role of cellular proliferation in early healing of PTFE prostheses. Am. J. Pathol. **118:** 43–54.
2. Sauvage, L., K. Gerger, S. Wood, S. Yates, J. Smith & P. Mansfield. Interspecies healing of porous arterial prosthesis. Arch. Surg. **109:** 698–705.
3. Pennell, R. C., L. H. Hollier, E. Solis & M. P. Kaye. 1986. Xenograft seeding of dacron grafts in dogs. J. Surg. Res. **40:** 332–339.
4. Graham, L., W. Burkel, W. Ford, D. Vinter, R. Kahn & J. Stanley. 1980. Immediate seeding of enzymatically derived autologous canine endothelium in dacron velour vascular grafts. Arch. Surg. **115:** 1298.
5. Belder, T. A., S. P. Schmidt, L. J. Falkow & W. L. Sharp. 1982. Endothelial cell seeding of small-diameter vascular grafts. Trans. Am. Soc. Artif. Intern. Organs **28:** 173–177.
6. Clowes, A. W., T. R. Kirkman & M. A. Reidy. 1986. Mechanisms of arterial graft healing: Rapid transmural capillary ingrowth provides a source of intimal endothelium and smooth muscle in porous PTFE prostheses. Am. J. Pathol. **123:** 220–230.
7. Mackenzie, J. R., M. Huckett, C. Topuzlu & D. J. Tibbs. 1968. Origin of arterial prosthesis lining from circulating blood cells. Arch. Surg. **97:** 879–885.
8. Jarrell, B., S. Williams, L. Solomon, L. Speicher, E. Koolpe, J. Radomski, R. Carabasi, D. Greener & F. Rosato. 1986. Use of an endothelial monolayer upon a vascular graft prior to implantation: Temporal dynamics and compatibility with the operating room. Ann. Surg. **293(6):** 671–678.
9. Jarrell, B., S. Shapiro, S. Williams, R. Carabasi, E. Levine, S. Mueller & S. Thornton. 1984. Human adult endothelial cell growth in culture. J. Vasc. Surg. **6:** 757.
10. Thornton, S., S. Mueller & E. Levine. 1983. Human endothelial cells: Cloning and long-term serial cultivation employing heparin. Science **222:** 623.
11. Liotta, L., C. Lee & D. Morakis. 1980. New method for preparing large surfaces of intact human basement membrane for tumor invasion studies. Cancer Lett. **11:** 141–52.
12. Baker, K. S., S. K. Williams, B. E. Jarrell, et al. 1985. Endothelialization of human collagen surfaces with human adult endothelial cells. Am. J. Surg. **150:** 197–200.
13. Madri, J. A. & S. K. Williams. 1983. Capillary endothelial cell cultures: Phenotypic modulation by matrix components. J. Cell. Biol. **97:** 153–165.
14. Williams, S., B. Jarrell, L. Friend, J. Radomski, R. Carabasi, E. Koolpe, S. Mueller, S. Thornton, T. Marinucci & E. Levine. 1985. Adult human endothelial cell compatibility with prosthetic graft material. J. Surg. Res. **38:** 618.

15. GRINNEL, F. & T. PHAN. 1985. Platelet attachment and spreading on polystyrene surfaces. Dependence on fibronectin and plasma concentration. Thrombosis Res. **39:** 165–171.
16. RAMALANJAONA, G., R. KEMPCZINSKI, J. ROSENMAN, C. DOUVILLE & E. SILBERSTEIN. The effect of fibronectin coating on endothelial cell kinetics in polytetrafluoroethylene grafts. J. Vasc. Surg. **3(2):** 264–272.
17. STERN, D., M. DRILLINGS, W. KISIEL, D. HANDLEY, M. DRILLINGS & J. BARTOS. 1984. A coagulation pathway on bovine aortic segments leading to generation of factor Xa and thrombin. J. Clin. Invest. **74:** 1910–22.

Plasma Protein Adsorption: The Big Twelve[a]

J. D. ANDRADE[a] AND V. HLADY[b]

[a]*Department of Bioengineering*
University of Utah
Salt Lake City, Utah 84112
[b]*Institut Ruder Boskovic*
Zagreb, Yugoslavia

INTRODUCTION

FIGURE 1 presents a protein adsorption complexity spectrum and in schematic form suggests that proteins vary greatly in complexity. The simplest include the insulin dimer, lysozyme, and myoglobin, whose X-ray crystallographic, three-dimensional structures are well-known and whose function is generally well understood. The structures of such proteins can be imaged and manipulated using modern computer graphics algorithms and equipment. Through careful consideration of the surface chemistry of such proteins and by appreciation that the surface chemistry is far from uniform on a protein particle (there are different "faces," each with different interaction potentials with specific surfaces or interfaces), one can develop estimates or hypotheses as to optimum interaction orientations for such model proteins at model interfaces. This approach has been very fruitful in the study of the adsorption of chicken and human lysozyme at model surfaces,[1,2] as well as in studies of the adsorption of myoglobin on model surfaces and the interaction of the adsorbed protein with specific monoclonal antibodies.[3]

Most of the plasma proteins, however, are considerably more complex. Their detailed three-dimensional structures are not known. For example, the plasma immunoglobulins vary greatly, particularly their Fab portions and variable regions, because of their wide and varied specific antigen binding characteristics. Although the structure of fibrinogen is fairly well-known,[4] the detailed three-dimensional structure of even the major domains is not yet available.

The problem increases in complexity if one considers multicomponent solutions, particularly multicomponent solutions of complex proteins, such as serum or plasma and tears, because one now has a variety of proteins all interacting with the surface in a competitive fashion, and interacting with each other, both on the surface and in the bulk solution.

FIGURE 1 also includes a complexity axis for the surface or interface. One can consider that the simplest interface available is probably the air-water interface. Much of what we know of protein adsorption and protein behavior at interfaces is taken from Langmuir Blodgett monolayer studies.[5,6] Studies at liquid-liquid, particularly oil-water, interfaces have also provided much information and such interfaces are

[a]This work has been partially supported by the National Institutes of Health, the National Science Foundation, the Office of Naval Research, the University of Utah Center for Biopolymers at Interfaces, and the R. Boskovic Institute.

extremely useful model systems.[7,8] One can directly monitor the kinetics of adsorption, the spreading characteristics of the adsorbed proteins, conformational changes, and two-dimensional ordering-structuring by Langmuir Blodgett and interfacial tension methods.[7,8]

The surface of an amorphous, homogenous homopolymer, such as poly(methyl methacrylate) (PMMA) or poly(dimethyl siloxane) (PDMSO), could also be considered relatively simple. One must remember, however, that such surfaces may not be truly rigid, particularly the surfaces of elastomers, such as PDMSO, because of the

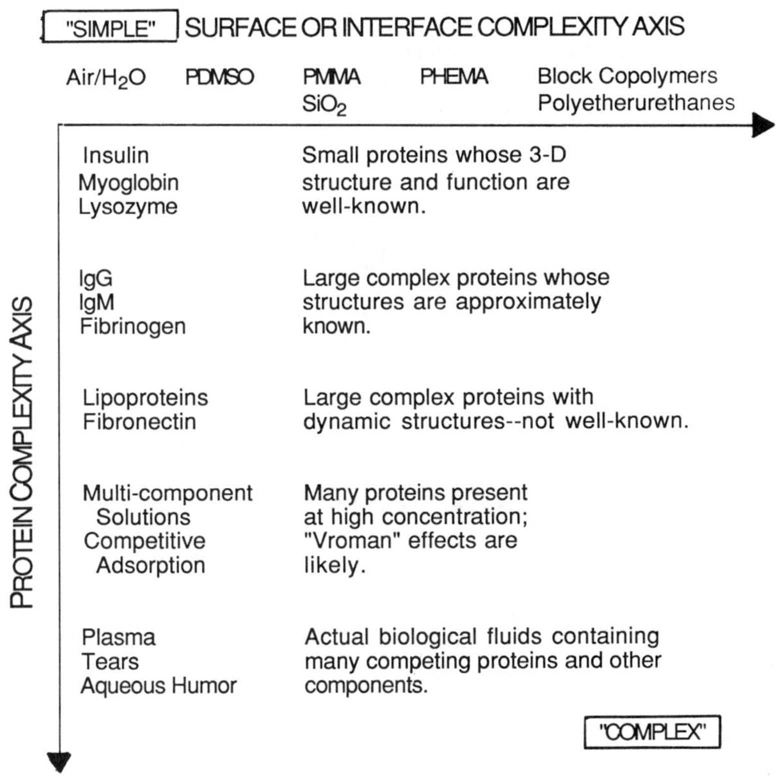

FIGURE 1. A protein adsorption complexity matrix. The upper left represents "simple" systems; the lower right shows highly complex systems. A solid surface complexity axis runs from left to right; the protein complexity axis runs from top to bottom. See text for abbreviations and details.

mobility of polymer chains and segments at room and body temperature. In addition, the intrinsic mobility and dynamics of proteins themselves suggest that very complex interactions and even interpenetrations may occur. Even for a rigid surface, such as PMMA, the amphiphilic nature of the polymer's hydrophilic ester group and the hydrophobic backbone can result in slight water uptake, and even side-chain orientation or reorientation at the polymer-water interface.[9] Virtually all polymer surfaces are dynamic. Methods are available for at least qualitatively characterizing the nature of the surface in air and underwater and even the dynamics of surface restructuring in going from one environment to another.[9]

As one continues along the material surface complexity axis (FIGURE 1), one eventually gets to such complex surfaces as block copolyetherurethanes, the most widely used materials for cardiac assist devices.[10] Such materials may have two or more phases and interphases present in the bulk structure and at the surface. Bulk and surface morphology are dependent on processing history, as well as on specific polymer chemistry. In addition, there is some evidence that the more hydrophobic phase tends to dominate the surface in air or vacuum, while the more hydrophilic phase tends to dominate it in an aqueous environment.[10] There is also concern that because of the dynamics of such elastomers, particularly due to the mobility of the soft segment phase, the water-equilibrated surface may restructure in order to optimally equilibrate with an adsorbed protein film—that is, the surface in water may change during the protein adsorption process as a result of the protein microenvironment with which it is now trying to equilibrate.

Although the situation in FIGURE 1, particularly at the bottom right, would appear to be quite complex, the situation at the top left is indeed relatively simple and is beginning to become qualitatively, even quantitatively, understood.

Most of what we know about protein adsorption is summarized in FIGURE 2, a general kinetic model for the process, assuming a one component protein solution for simplicity. A protein of bulk concentration, C_o, diffuses to and collides with the interface. At time zero initial contact occurs. If the interaction forces are sufficient, the protein stays on the surface for a certain residence time, probably in the range of milliseconds to seconds. Air-water interface studies have shown that a minimum contact area is required, which probably relates to the magnitude of the hydrophobic

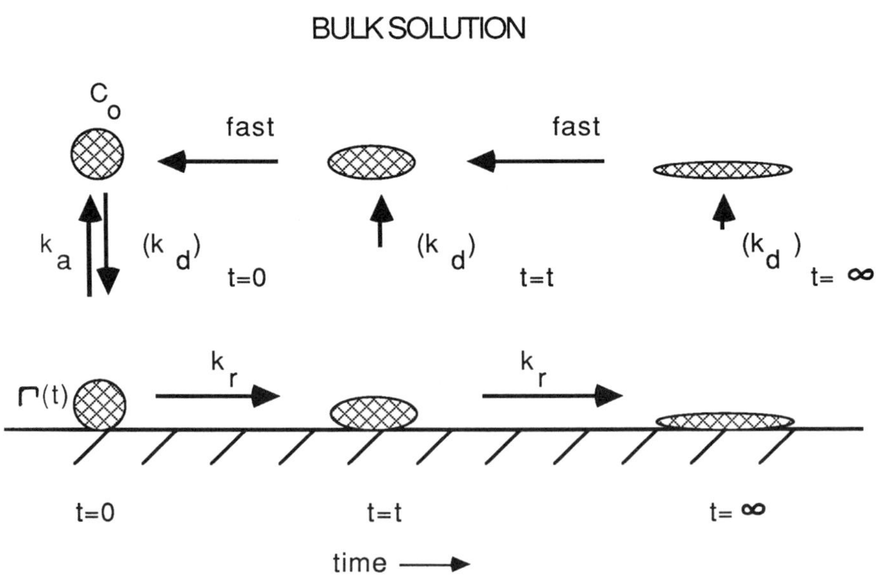

FIGURE 2. A kinetic protein adsorption model based in part on the ideas of Lundstrom, Walton, and Jennissen.[15,21–24] C_o is the bulk protein concentration; Γ is the surface concentration, which is a function of time t; k_a is the on-rate constant and $k_d(t)$ are the off-rate constants, which are a function of contact time (residence time).

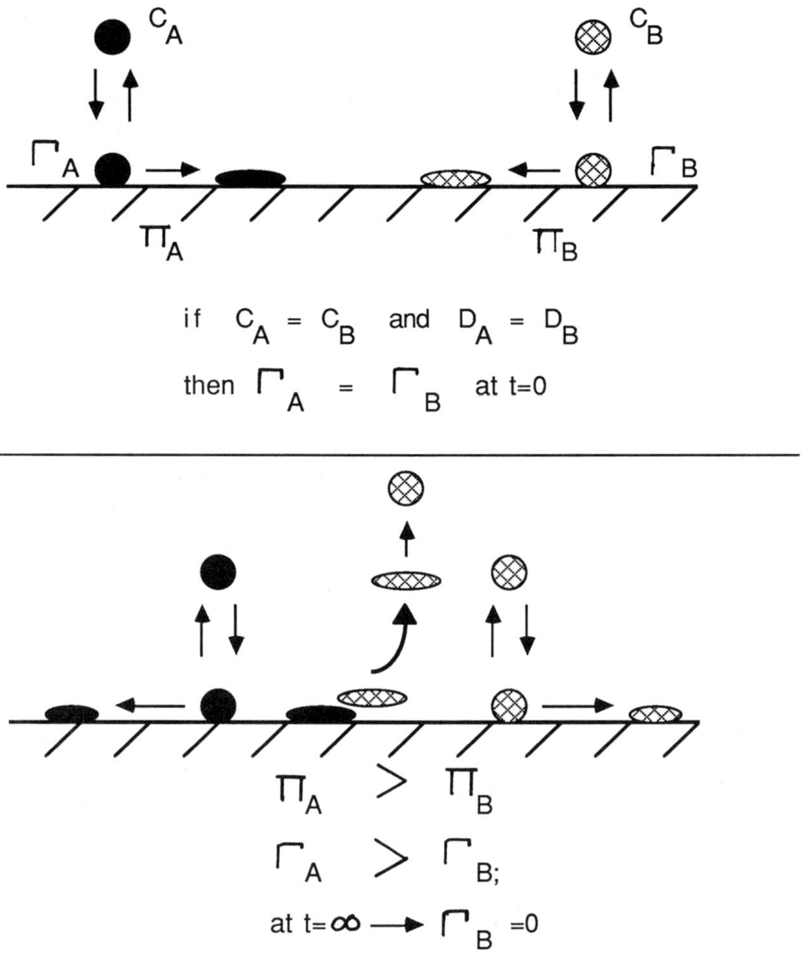

FIGURE 3. The competitive surface spreading hypothesis (from Bagnall.[8]) *Top:* Two proteins, *A* and *B*, have the same bulk concentration and diffusion coefficients and therefore have the same surface concentration (Γ) at $t = 0$ (initial contact). If the spreading pressure (π) of one is greater than the other, then eventually the protein with the larger π will dominate the interface. Here we show that A displaces B, since $\pi_A > \pi_B$.

interaction required for initial stabilization of the protein-surface complex.[5,11] The protein can desorb at this stage; an appropriate desorption rate constant is indicated in FIGURE 2.

While on the surface, the protein may begin a surface denaturation process, which is probably related to its intrinsic conformational lability. This is also related to the fact that globular proteins are only marginally stable,[12] and an energy of 5–15 kcal/mole is sufficient to denature them in normal buffer solutions.[11–13] Therefore, the interactions with the surface, particularly interactions of a hydrophobic nature, significantly affect the solution equilibrium of the protein.[11]

There may be a strong configurational entropy driving force in going from the globule to a more extended state, particularly if the extended state can be accommodated by maintaining a degree of hydrophobic interaction comparable to that provided by the globular state. Hydrophobic interaction can, of course, be provided, in part, by interactions with a partially hydrophobic surface. Dill has modeled and considered the configurational entropy aspects of globular protein structure,[12] as well as of hydrophobic surfaces containing alkyl chains—such as those commonly used in chromatography.[14]

A distorted or extended protein is generally less soluble in solution; thus, one expects the desorption tendency to decrease, allowing for increased binding and/or surface denaturation. Desorption of the protein is therefore a function of its residence time on the surface. With increasing contact times the probability for desorption decreases, as indicated in FIGURE 2. Assuming that the adsorption process does not result in any covalent bond changes in the protein molecule, the model then also assumes that if a denatured or partially denatured protein does desorb, it rapidly renatures to the equilibrium globular state. This portion of the model is controversial, as there is evidence in the literature that some desorbed proteins are permanently changed[15,16] due to covalent bond changes during the process.

Competitive adsorption in two component systems has been modeled by Cuypers *et al.*[17] His results suggest that the "Vroman effect"[18,19] is predicted by a competitive adsorption model which allows an exponential decrease in the affinity constant with increasing occupancy of the surface, similar to the classical Langmuir treatments of adsorption which incorporate a lateral interaction and variable surface site energy term.[20]

The effect of a surface-induced conformational change has been treated in a preliminary way by the models developed by Lundstrom *et al.*,[21–23] in which two states are considered: the initial state at time = 0, and the "equilibrium" state at long contact times, $t = \infty$. Lundstrom's models, which to date have been published only for single component solutions, nicely predict and explain adsorption behavior of labile globular proteins in single component systems.

FIGURE 3 begins to ask the question of what happens during a competitive adsorption process and is based on the ideas of Bagnall[8] and Jennissen,[24] who showed that the surface denaturation or accommodation process is dependent on the number and type of neighbors. If two different proteins have adsorbed next to each other, one is generally more labile or conformationally adaptable to the interface than the other. We can say that one "spreads" at the interface more effectively than the other. We can consider a spreading constant for such a protein, analogous to the solid-vapor and solid-liquid spreading constants so commonly used in classical surface chemistry.[20] One would expect that the spreading characteristics would be related to the solution denaturability[13] of the protein, and particularly to its behavior at water-air and water-oil interfaces.[5–8] Clearly, the more "surface active" protein would spread more effectively and may displace the other protein from the interface. This is another mechanism by which the Vroman effect can be explained. Clearly, the next step is to develop a model which incorporates the ideas of Cuypers,[17] Lundstrom,[21–23] and Bagnall,[8] but generalized for complex multicomponent systems.

THE BIG TWELVE

Blood plasma, however, consists of far more than one or two proteins. High-resolution, two-dimensional electrophoresis shows over 150 bands from plasma. It has been estimated that a typical cell has over 5000 different proteins! We have chosen to consider only those proteins in plasma that are expected to compete effectively for the interface in the initial collision or contact process, *i.e.,* those which are present at sufficient plasma concentration to be considered major constituents. We have chosen to consider only those proteins generally present in plasma at about 1 mg/ml or higher concentration. The twelve such proteins are shown in FIGURE 4 and described in TABLE 1. FIGURE 4 somewhat schematically separates the proteins by electrophoretic mobility and sedimentation coefficient, *i.e.,* by net charge and size, respectively. Albumin is clearly the major constituent, followed by IgG. The high- and low-density lipoproteins are also major components. The properties of these twelve proteins are summarized briefly and qualitatively in TABLE 1. TABLE 2, based on a simple diffusion limited mass transport view, asks the question, "When does the next protein arrive?"[25] or "Who gets there first?"

Clearly, protein collisions with the surface are dominated by albumin. Seven times as many albumin molecules as IgG molecules strike the surface, and a thousand times more albumin molecules than IgM molecules strike the surface. So it is certainly reasonable and predictable that the surface would be largely populated at or near time zero by albumin, assuming that there is sufficient interaction between albumin and the surface to lead to a reasonable residence time.[26] About one in seven of the collisions with the surface involves IgG. If IgG has a greater affinity or greater spreading pressure at the surface than does albumin, then the spreading IgG molecule may tend to displace some of the preadsorbed albumin from the surface. Thus, although the surface is rich in albumin initially, one may find that the concentration shifts to IgG with increasing time. One could also argue that, although fibrinogen may occupy 1 in 150 or so of the sites at time zero, the sites it does occupy are particularly stable and perhaps it is "irreversibly" adsorbed. Assuming that the affinity constant for albumin is not high, occasionally an albumin molecule will desorb. Although the now vacant surface site is seeing a collision frequency continually dominated by albumin, if a molecule of fibrinogen collides with that site, the adsorptive interaction, with its much higher affinity constant, will be longer lived and more stable than if albumin had collided with the vacant site.

Thus, there are two approaches to the Vroman effect. One can assume no conformational change, but essentially a surface occupancy lateral interaction model, such as that developed by Cuypers,[17] or one can assume a surface denaturation model, such as that being developed by Lundstrom.[21–23] Clearly, both are important, and both are occurring, not only for the Big Twelve discussed in TABLES 1 and 2, but for the other 150 or more protein constituents in plasma.

Nevertheless, we now know enough to begin to develop models, at least for two and three component systems. When those match the excellent, competitive adsorption data now becoming available,[19] we can, using more sophisticated mathematical and computer techniques, extend them to many components and parameters. A key problem is obtaining parameters which reflect or at least relate to the interaction energy at time 0, the surface denaturability, and perhaps the interaction energy at very long times.

We must know the nature of the solid interface. Polyurethanes are probably too complex at this stage for truly fundamental understanding. The best models are the column chromatography supports used for protein separation. Here the highly hydrophilic, nonionic nature of agarose and related matrices provide only very low energy interactions with proteins. Basically, such interactions prove to be weak and highly reversible, and therefore protein mixtures pass through such columns with little or no retention. By derivatizing agarose supports with low-density ionic, hydrophobic, or charge-transfer groups, one now imparts an interaction mechanism. The protein, depending on its structure and repertoire of surface functional groups, interacts with

TABLE 1. Properties of the "Big 12"—Plasma Proteins Whose Concentration is >1 mg/ml[a]

Protein	Plasma Concentration g/l = mg/ml	Plasma Concentration μmol	Molecular Weight	Diffusion Coefficient ($10^{-7}cm^2/s$)	Electrophoretic Mobility and Net Charge	$CD^{1/2}$	Carbohydrate (%)	Sialic Acid (%)
Albumin	40	600	66,000	6.1	α, −19	1500	0	0
IgG	8–17	53–113 100*	150,000	4.0	α_2–γ_3	200	2.9	0.3 1.6 M/M
LDL	4.0	2	2,000,000	2.0	β	3	—	—
HDL	3	18	170,000	4.6	α_1	39	—	—
α-Macroglobulin	2.7	3.3	725,000	2.4	α_2	5	8.4	1.8 48 M/M
Fibrinogen	2–3	6–9 7.5*	340,000	2	β_2, −26	11	2.5	0.6 4–8 M/M
Transferrin	2.3	30	77,000	5.0	β_1	67	5.9 (2 chains) biantennary	1.4 variable 4 M/M
α-Antitrypsin	2	40	(51,000) 54,000 (45,000)	5.2	α_1	91	14 content variable, biantennary	3.6 6 M/M (variable)
Haptoglobins	2.0 1.6–3.0 1.2–2.6	20 8–15 3–6.6	100,000 200,000 400,000	1-1 } 4.7 1-2 } (monomer) 2-2 }	α_2	43	20 (in β-chain) bi- & triantennary	5.3
C3	1.6	9	180,000	4.5	β_2	19	2.7	0.01
IgA	1–4	7–27 15*	150,000	4	α_2–γ_3	30	7.5	1.8 9 M/M
IgM	0.05–2	0.06–2 1*	900,000	2.6	β_2–γ_3	1.6	11.8	1.3 42 M/M

[a]Data are from refs. 43 and 44. Numbers used for calculation of $CD^{1/2}$ are indicated by *asterisks*.

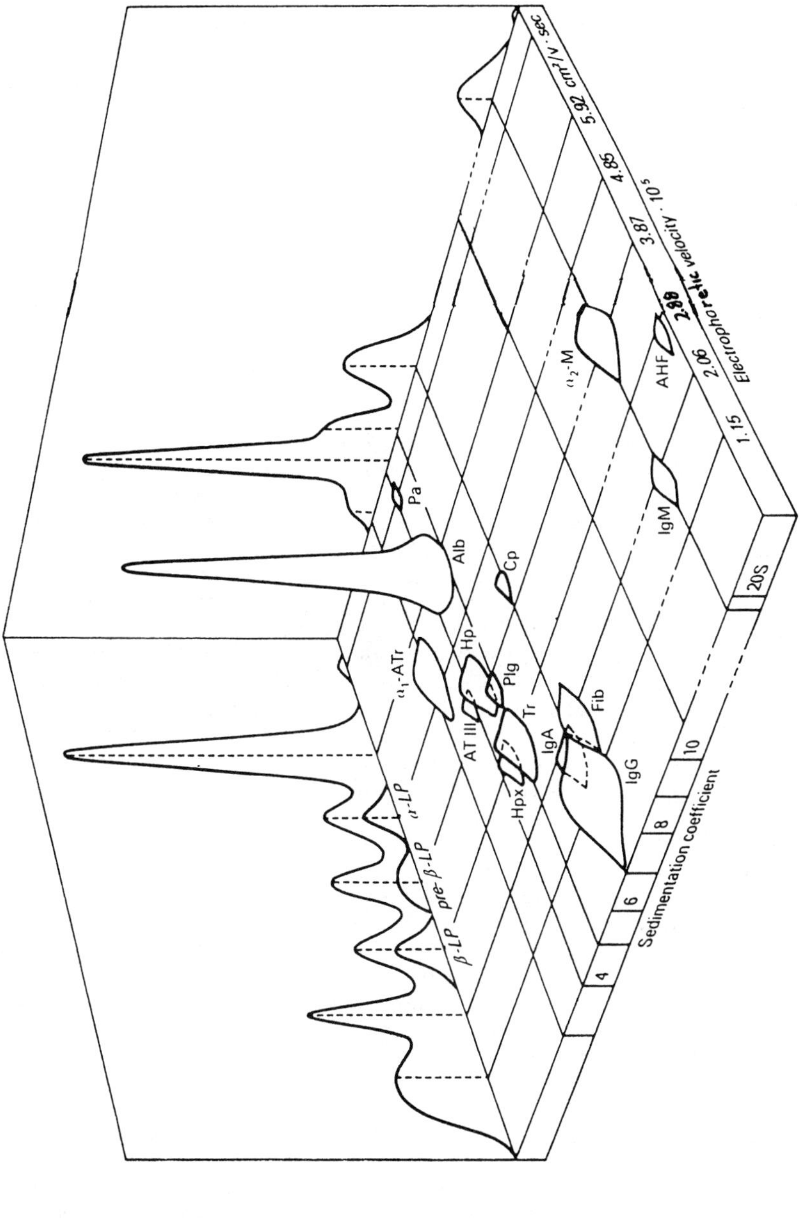

FIGURE 4. The major plasma protein constituents (based on ref. 27).

TABLE 2. Plasma Concentrations (C) and Diffusion Coefficients (D) for the Big 12 in Plasma (Data from TABLE 1)[a]

Protein	C (μmol/l)	D (10^{-7} cm^2/s)	$C\sqrt{D}$
Albumin	~600	6.1	1500
IgG	~100	4.0	200
α-Antitrypsin	~40	5.2	91
Transferrin	~30	5.0	67
Haptoglobin 1-1	~20	4.7	43
HDL	~18	~4.6	39
IgA	~15	4.0	30
Complement 3	~9	4.5	19
Fibrinogen	~7.5	2.0	11
α-Macroglobulin	~3.3	2.4	5
LDL	~2	~2.0	3
IgM	~1	~2.6	1.6

[a]Rate of arrival of protein molecules at the interface $dn/dt = C(D/\pi t)^{1/2}$.

the immobilized ligand on the agarose particle and is "retained." The adsorption is reversible if the interaction energy is not too high and if the number of interaction points per protein molecule is not greater than one. After the appropriate residence time the protein molecule is desorbed and goes on down the column, where it interacts with another ligand and another particle, stays for a moment, is released, and goes on. This process continues, and for a column of particular length, packing or support, and protein concentration and mixture, leads to a residence time or retention time in the column. This retention time is an empirical measure of the interaction energy or the affinity constant and the residence time of each adsorption event.

It is relatively straightforward to rank proteins on the basis of their interaction with hydrophobically derivatized agarose, so-called hydrophobic chromatography supports. This was done a decade ago by Hofstee.[28] One can do the same with cationic and anionic derivatized columns to get a measure of electrostatic interaction. As the hydrophobic and electrostatic interactions are probably the two dominant ones, because most of the hydrogen bonding possibilities are swamped by the 55-M concentration of water in aqueous solutions and even in blood plasma, one can characterize the intermolecular interaction potential for a protein interacting with chromatographic supports.

One must also apply what is known about the structure of the protein. If its three-dimensional structure is known, as discussed earlier for lysozyme, insulin, and myoglobin, then one should do graphics modeling and attempt to predict the optimum orientation of the protein for interaction with certain model surfaces. Structural information is available, even for the big plasma proteins, particularly fibrinogen,[4] where the charge distribution and the different domains and fragments are well-known, the four carbohydrate residues are precisely located, and where one can begin to guess as to what might be the orientation of the molecule on certain types of surfaces.

One possibly important feature of plasma proteins, which has been largely ignored in consideration of their interfacial properties, is the fact that virtually all of them are glycoproteins and contain carbohydrate chains, generally terminated with negatively charged sialic acid residues. Although Kim and coworkers[29] studied the adsorption of desialylated immunoglobulins and fibrinogen many years ago, there has been little consideration of the role of carbohydrates. This is probably because the major carbohydrate-containing proteins in plasma, which make up half or so of the Big Twelve (TABLE 1), have been largely ignored by the blood compatibility and surface chemistry community.

TABLE 3 briefly summarizes the glycoprotein and sialic acid composition of plasma proteins. The haptoglobins, for which very little adsorption data is available,[32] contain 20% carbohydrate. Unfortunately, the structure of the haptoglobins is not well-known and indeed they constitute a family of proteins rather than being a distinct, homogenous molecule, such as albumin. Two important protease inactivators, α-antitrypsin and α-macroglobulin, also have high glycoprotein contents. Transferrin, an iron-binding protein, is also fairly rich in carbohydrate. The adsorption characteristics of α-macroglobulin and transferrin have been studied by Young and Cooper.[33] There has been virtually no work on haptoglobin adsorption[32] or on antitrypsin, IgM, or complement C3. The extensive study by Young did show that the adsorption of macroglobulin and transferrin is apparently not of very high affinity. Although there could be many reasons for this, it does lead one to suggest that perhaps proteins with high carbohydrate contents, particularly if that carbohydrate is more or less uniformly distributed on the surface of the molecule, might enhance the solubility of the molecule and mask hydrophobic amino acid residues on its surface, thereby decreasing its adsorption at hydrophobic interfaces. Kim's study showed that desialylated fibrinogen did not influence fibrinogen adsorption,[29] probably because the carbohydrate in fibrinogen is located in the coiled-coiled region near the disulfide knot and on the β-chain in the terminal domains. There is apparently no carbohydrate on the γ-chain or the more extended, and probably more surface-active, α-chain. Also, the total carbohydrate in fibrinogen is relatively low.[4]

The role of carbohydrate in adsorption, which we call the "glycoprotein hypothesis," is probably only important for haptoglobin and antitrypsin. The carbohydrate in IgM is localized and not uniformly distributed around the molecule. Macroglobulin has such a unique dimeric structure that its adsorption will probably prove to be dependent on its unique structure and/or shape in solution.

FIGURE 5 illustrates the structure and composition of the plasma lipoproteins. We have included HDL, particularly HDL 3, and LDL 1 and 2 in the Big Twelve previously discussed (TABLE 1). There is evidence from at least two groups that the lipoproteins have unique and important adsorption properties.[35–37] Breemhaar *et al.* have shown preferential adsorption of high-density lipoprotein onto hydrophobic supports, including a demonstration of the Vroman effect with LDL, HDL, and fibrinogen mixtures.[35] We have shown that LDL adsorption from single component solutions increases significantly when going from 20° to 37°C on elastomers, but not on

TABLE 3. Carbohydrate and Sialic Acid Composition of Major Plasma Proteins (from Refs. 30, 31)

Protein	Percent CHO	Percent Sialic Acid
Haptoglobin	~20	5.3
α-Antitrypsin	~14	3.6
IgM	~12	1.3
α-Macroglobulin	~8.4	1.8
Transferrin	~5.9	1.4
IgG	~2.9	0.3
C3	~2.7	0.01
Fibrinogen	~2.5	0.6
Albumin	~0	0

rigid supports.[36] This leads to the hypothesis that the lipid phase transition in LDL, which occurs in the vicinity of 37°C, may be important in controlling the adsorption properties and perhaps the surface denaturability of such proteins. We have also shown that the adsorption of LDL and HDL from single component solutions onto rigid hydrophobic and hydrophilic supports suggests a reaction-limited process for both classes of lipoproteins adsorbed on hydrophobic supports, but adsorption on hydrophilic surfaces is diffusion limited.[37] One could draw the hypothesis that the lipoproteins may therefore be undergoing significant conformational alteration on the hydrophobic supports. Although there is not very much data on lipoproteins, their dynamic structure and their very high lipid content suggests a major role in the plasma adsorption process.

CLASS	SIZE Å	DENSITY gm/ml	S_f (1.063)	PLASMA CONC. mg/100ml
CHYLOMICRONS				0 to 50
VLDL	700	0.96	400	
LDL_1	400	1.019	12	225
LDL_2	200	1.063	0	350
HDL_2	120	1.125		100
HDL_3	75	1.21		200
$VHDL_1$		1.25		10
$VHDL_2$	?	>1.25		?

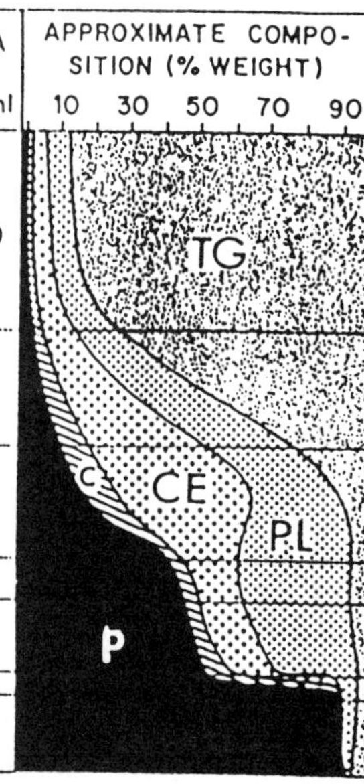

FIGURE 5. Schematic distribution of the major classes of plasma lipoproteins according to their flotation in the analytical ultracentrifuge. *TG* = triglycerides; *PL* = phospholipids; *CE* = cholesterol esters; *C* = cholesterol; *P* = apoprotein (from ref. 34).

SURFACE DENATURABILITY

In addition to the on- and off-rate constants, which can be derived as described above, one should have a measure of the ability of the protein molecule to denature at the interface as a function of time. Such information is very difficult to get at solid-liquid interfaces, although, in principle, some of the surface-sensitive spectroscopic techniques can provide some such information. For example, ATR-FTIR studies of the adsorption of a single component protein from dilute solutions can provide evidence of conformational change as a function of time at the interface.[38] Total internal reflection fluorescence also provides evidence for changes with time at the interface,[39] but such techniques are specialized, difficult to quantitate, and difficult to interpret in terms of actual structural changes. Also, they are substrate limited and even substrate specific due to the optical properties required for the total internal reflection condition. Some such information is also available via ellipsometry in terms of changes in the refractive index and thickness of the adsorbed layer as a function of contact time (see refs. 17 and 21).

We feel that a more fruitful approach may be to study the behavior of proteins at water-air, water-oil, water-fluorocarbon liquid, and water-siloxane liquid interfaces, using the standard, proven, and inexpensive surface and interfacial tension techniques.[6–8,20] With such techniques, one can measure the spreading pressure through the decrease in surface or interfacial tension of various individual proteins. One can also measure the temperature dependence of interfacial processes. Although this does not relate directly to the interface between a biomedical material and plasma, it helps characterize the interfacial activity of the various protein species of interest. One can develop an empirical parameter and use it as a coefficient or exponent in the appropriate terms in the equations. The problem is to get such data (chromatographic and interfacial activity data) for the proteins of interest. Although some such data is available in the literature, it is generally very protein specific, and there is no compilation of information on the interfacial activity of plasma proteins. If such data were available, the modeling and simulation of the Vroman effect and other complex interfacial processes could actually be straightforward.

CONCLUSIONS

We offer the following conclusions:

1. FIGURE 6 suggests that the early stages of adsorption (very short contact times) are functions of the particular chemistry of the surface, the particular three-dimensional structure and orientation of the protein, and the number of species and their concentration. In addition, adsorption at short contact times is also a function of occupancy and lateral interactions, as modeled so nicely by Cuypers.[17] We suggest that the time-dependent conformational adaptation to the surface, as modeled by Lundstrom,[21–23] is related to the bulk solution denaturation tendencies of the protein, including thermal denaturation, denaturation in urea or guanidinium chloride solutions, and denaturation in solutions of different pH. We further suggest that surface and interfacial tension measurements of proteins at water-air, water-oil, and other water-liquid interfaces will be useful measures of protein surface activity at the solid-water interface.
2. We suggest that lipoproteins are very important in the adsorption process and in the Vroman effect, due in part to their structural and compositional dynamics, particularly on hydrophobic elastomeric surfaces, where one might expect some interpenetration of protein and lipid components with the polymer chains.[36]
3. It is known that the presence of carbohydrates in proteins both masks and protects the proteins from proteolytic attack and helps improve their solubility, as well as providing stabilization of conformation.[30,31] It is therefore reasonable to suggest that proteins with high carbohydrate contents, particularly if the carbohydrate is more or less uniformly distributed over the protein, may show little adsorption or interaction with hydrophobic or with negatively charged supports.
4. At equilibrium adsorption will be dominated by proteins with the following characteristics: large molecular weight and large size, which suggests a large number of potential contact points with the surface; readily denaturable or

conformationally labile, permitting the protein to readily accommodate to the microenvironment of the interface; and low carbohydrate content, or at least significant regions of the molecule which are free of carbohydrate, because of the possible masking effect of carbohydrate at hydrophobic and/or negatively charged surfaces.

Although it is clear that fibrinogen is not necessarily the equilibrium species in plasma, it has the attributes described above. It is low in carbohydrate and what carbohydrate it does have is localized. It is conformationally quite labile and indeed has very high interfacial activity and spreading pressure. It is large and asymmetric and can have very large contact areas. It has a fairly asymmetric charge distribution,

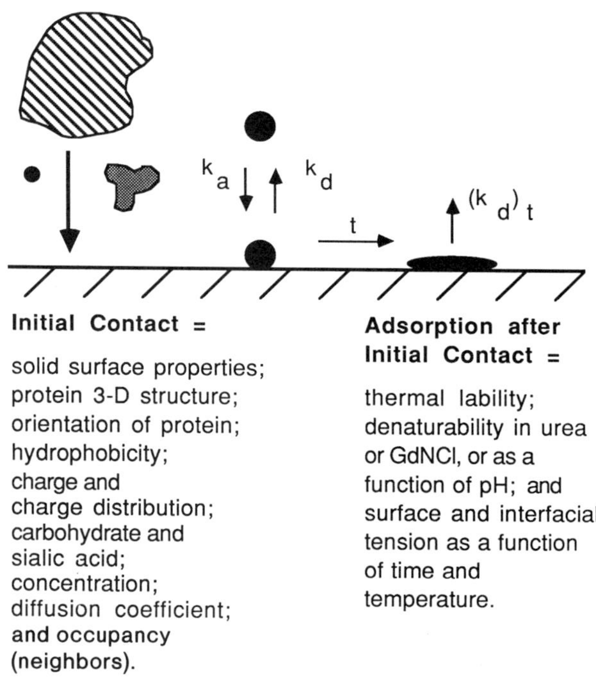

FIGURE 6. The key parameters involved in the initial contact phase of adsorption (left side) and in the time-dependent surface and protein "denaturation" processes (right side).

as well as significant hydrophobicity, so it can interact successfully with a wide variety of interfaces.

CAUTION

We have assumed throughout the discussion that there are no covalent changes imposed on the molecules prior to, during, or after the adsorption process. Clearly, the work of Brash and others demonstrates that covalent bond changes can indeed occur.[16] Certainly plasma has a variety of active proteases and protease inhibitors, which change in concentration depending on local needs and processes. Clearly the conformational adaptation to the surface which we have described may make a molecule more or less susceptible to proteolysis or to other chemical processes. Indeed, the very act of interacting with certain types of surfaces could, in part, direct covalent chemistries, such as possibly the interaction of C3 with nucleophilic surfaces.[40] The surface activation models, which are being developed by Sefton,[41] Mann,[42] and coworkers, coupled with the modeling and simulation suggested here, will be an important next step in attempting to treat truly practical blood-material interfaces.

SUMMARY

We have discussed the general principles of protein adsorption at solid-liquid interfaces from single component and multicomponent solutions, based on qualitative kinetic models that include mass transport considerations, initial interaction energies, surface-dependent conformational changes, and possible desorption processes. We have surveyed plasma protein components greater than one milligram per milliliter in concentration, which we call "The Big Twelve." We considered their size, concentration, diffusion coefficient, structure and function, and methods of estimating their "surface denaturability" by using bulk solution measures of denaturation and conformational change. We have suggested that the role of the carbohydrate moieties in plasma proteins may have some bearing on their adsorption properties. We further suggest that lipoproteins, because of their lipid phase transition and conformational lability at body temperature, may tend to dominate the adsorption process, particularly on mobile elastomeric polymer surfaces. We suggest that detailed consideration of the structure and characteristics of each of the proteins involved is necessary in order to begin to understand plasma adsorption processes. Detailed characterization and understanding of the solid surface in the aqueous and protein environments are also required.

ACKNOWLEDGMENTS

We acknowledge stimulating discussions with I. Lundstrom, H. Elwing, P. Cuypers, H. Jennissen, S. W. Kim, and others on these topics over the last several years.

REFERENCES

1. HANSEN, J., J. D. ANDRADE & K. ELY. 1987. J. Colloid Interface Sci. Submitted.
2. HORSELEY, D., J. HERRON, V. HLADY & J. D. ANDRADE. 1987. *In* Proteins at Interfaces—ACS Symposium Series, Vol. 343. T. A. Horbett & J. L. Brash, Eds. American Chemical Society. Washington, D.C.
3. DARST, S., C. R. ROBERTSON & J. A. BERZOFSKY. 1987. Biochemistry. In press.
4. DOOLITTLE, R. F. 1981. Sci. Am. Dec.: 126–135.
5. MACRITCHIE, F. 1978. Adv. Protein Chem. **32:** 283–326.
6. PHILLIPS, M. C. 1977. Chem. Ind. March 5: 170–176.
7. TORNBERG, E., Y. GRANFELDT & C. HAKANSSON. 1982. J. Sci. Food Agric. **33:** 904–917.
8. BAGNALL, R. D. 1978. J. Biomed. Materials Res. **12:** 203–217.
9. ANDRADE, J. D., D. E. GREGONIS & L. M. SMITH. 1985. *In* Surface and Interfacial Aspects of Biomedical Polymers, Vol. 1. J. D. Andrade, Ed.: 15–42. Plenum. New York.
10. LELAH, M. D. & S. L. COOPER. 1986. Polyurethanes in Medicine. CRC Press. Boca Raton, FL.

11. ANDRADE, J. D. 1985. *In* Protein Adsorption. J. D. Andrade, Ed.: 1–80. Plenum. New York.
12. DILL, K. A. 1985. Biochemistry **24:** 1501–1509.
13. PACE, C. N. 1975. CRC Crit. Rev. Biochem. **3:** 1–43.
14. DILL, K. A. 1987. J. Phys. Chem. In press.
15. SODERQUIST, M. E. & A. G. WALTON. 1980. J. Colloid Interface Sci. **75:** 386–392.
16. CHAN, B. M. C. & J. L. BRASH. 1981. J. Colloid Interface Sci. **84:** 263–265.
17. CUYPERS, P. A., G. M. WILLEMS, H. C. HEMKER & W. TH. HERMENS. 1987. This volume.
18. BRASH, J. L. 1987. This volume.
19. SLACK, S. M., J. L. BOHNERT & T. A. HORBETT. 1987. This volume.
20. ADAMSON, A. W. 1983. Physical Chemistry of Surfaces. 4th edit. Wiley. New York.
21. LUNDSTROM, I. 1985. Prog. Colloid Polymer Sci. **70:** 76–82.
22. LUNDSTROM, I. 1985. *In* Oral Interfacial Reactions of Bone. P. O. Glantz, S. A. Leach & T. Ericson, Eds. IRL Press. Oxford.
23. LUNDSTROM, I., B. IVARSSON, U. JONSSON & H. ELWING. 1987. *In* Polymer Surfaces and Interfaces. W. J. Feast & H. S. Munro, Eds. Wiley. New York.
24. JENNISSEN, H. P. 1986. J. Colloid Interface Sci. **111:** 570–586.
25. VROMAN, L. 1986. Trans. Soc. Biomater. **9:** 59.
26. DEBOER, J. H. 1968. Dynamical Character of Adsorption. 2d edit. Clarendon Press. Oxford.
27. ANDERSSON, L-O & R. LUNDEN. 1979. *In* Plasma Proteins. B. Blomback & L. A. Hanson, Eds.: 18–19. Wiley. New York.
28. HOFSTEE, B. H. J. 1979. Pure Appl. Chem. **51:** 1537–1548.
29. LEE, E. S. 1979. Ph.D. thesis, University of Utah, Salt Lake City, UT.
30. SHARON, N. 1984. Trends Biochem. Sci. **9:** 198–202.
31. SCHAUER, R. 1985. Trends Biochem. Sci. **10:** 357–360.
32. LOWE, R., V. HLADY, J. D. ANDRADE & R. A. VANWAGENEN. 1986. Biomaterials **7:** 41–44.
33. YOUNG, B. R. 1984. Ph.D. thesis, University of Wisconsin, Madison, WI.
34. SCANU, A. M. 1986. *In* Biochemistry and Biology of Plasma Lipoproteins. A. M. Scanu & A. A. Spector, Eds.: 1–10. Dekker. New York.
35. BREEMHAAR, W., E. BRINKMAN, D. J. ELLENS, T. BEUGELING & A. BANTJES. 1984. Biomaterials **5:** 269–274.
36. DONG, D. E., J. D. ANDRADE & D. L. COLEMAN. 1987. J. Biomed. Mater. Res. **21:** 683.
37. HLADY, V., J. RICKEL & J. D. ANDRADE. 1987. J. Colloid Interface Sci. Submitted.
38. PITT, W. G. & S. L. COOPER. 1987. *In* Proteins at Interfaces. ACS Symposium Series, Vol. 343. T. A. Horbett & J. L. Brash, Eds. American Chemical Society. Washington, D.C.
39. IWAMOTO, G. K., L. C. WINTERTON, R. S. STOKER, R. A. VANWAGENEN, J. D. ANDRADE & D. F. MOSHER. 1985. J. Colloid Interface Sci. **106:** 459–464.
40. CHENOWETH, D. L. This volume.
41. BASMADJIAN, D. & M. V. SEFTON. 1986. J. Biomed. Mater. Res. **20:** 633–651.
42. NESHEIM, M. E., R. P. TRACY & K. G. MANN. 1984. J. Biol. Chem. **259:** 1447–1453.
43. SCHULTZE, H. E. & J. J. HEREMANS. 1966. Molecular Biology of Plasma Proteins. Elsevier. Amsterdam.
44. BLOMBACK, B. & L. A. HANSON, Eds. Plasma Proteins. Wiley. New York. p. 79.

Spectroscopic Approaches to the Investigation of Interactions between Artificial Surfaces and Proteins[a]

ROBERT I. LEININGER,[b] TIMOTHY B. HUTSON,[c] AND ROBERT J. JAKOBSEN[d]

[c]*Battelle Columbus Division*
Columbus, Ohio 43201

[d]*Mattson Institute for Spectroscopic Research*
Columbus, Ohio

INTRODUCTION

Compatibility of an artificial surface with blood requires that the surface does not activate the coagulation system or induce any other harmful effects. Progress has been made towards compatible synthetic surfaces primarily through two approaches: synthesis of new polymers or modification of surfaces by the bonding of various bioactive agents. Both approaches have led to surfaces of improved compatibility, especially as to decreased thrombogenicity. The improvements have not been sufficient and the direction of research more recently has emphasized the study of blood-materials interactions in an attempt to provide a foundation for the synthesis of polymers suitable for long-time use in the cardiovascular system.

Of the many interactions of blood with a foreign surface, it is agreed that the first interaction is the adsorption of proteins and that further interactions of the blood are influenced, if not controlled, by the nature of the protein adsorbate. One cannot, however, assume that the first proteins adsorbed from blood forecast the compatibility of the surface. Displacement reactions have been shown to change the composition of the developing adsorbate (the so-called Vroman effect wherein adsorbed fibrinogen, Fb, is displaced by unidentified plasma components).[1] In addition, Brash[2] has reported on the analysis of the eluates from plasma adsorbates and a major portion of the eluates were found to be unidentified proteins other than the three major blood proteins.

The adsorption of proteins to quartz surfaces has been long known,[3,4] but the adsorption to candidate synthetic blood-contacting surfaces with the consequent modification of the surface properties was seen in 1964.[5,6] In this work it was found that protein adsorption patterns varied with the surface and the conclusion was drawn that a "knowledge of adsorption patterns can lead to an understanding of the mechanism of blood/surface interactions which in turn can lead to a knowledge of the surface characteristics needed for blood compatibility."[7]

Because of the agreement that the adsorption of proteins is both the first and also a very important blood-surface interaction, a large body of literature on protein adsorption has been amassed over the last 20 years. Entrance to this literature can be

[a]This work was supported in part by NHLBI grant no. HL–24015 and the Mattson Institute for Spectroscopic Research.

[b]Present address: 1973 Milden Rd., Columbus, OH 43221.

gained through the proceedings of several meetings, including this one, which have emphasized protein adsorption.[8,9]

Various methods have been used to study the adsorption of blood proteins on foreign surfaces. Most prominent has been the use of radiolabeled proteins, but other methods such as elution and subsequent identification and quantification of the adsorbed proteins, total internal reflectance fluorescence spectroscopy using either fluor-labeled proteins or the intrinsic fluorescence of the protein, the use of antisera to specific proteins, ellipsometry, microcalorimetry, depletion of solute, and direct weighing. The primary limitations of these methods are difficulties in (1) application to mixtures of proteins; (2) providing information on the adsorbate from essentially zero time to hours; (2) use under physiological conditions; and (d) detecting possible changes in protein structure effected by the combination of the adsorption process and the nature of the adsorbing surface.

It was because of the possibility of reducing these difficulties and thereby supplying

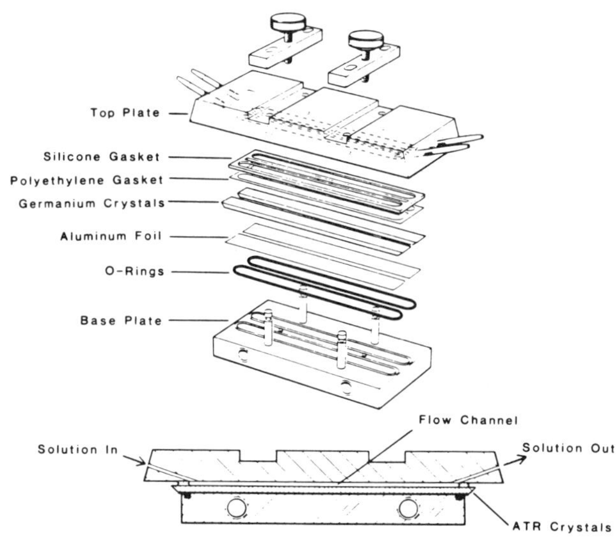

FIGURE 1. Dual flow cell.

additional information as to the effects of surface structure and composition on the adsorption of blood proteins that the use of attenuated total reflectance Fourier transform infrared spectroscopy (ATR/FT-IR) was investigated at Battelle. The following sections will present an overview of the instruments, accessories, procedures, and methods of data handling so far developed and the examples of the types of information obtained. A number of persons have taken part in this effort (see refs.).

METHODS

Equipment and Accessories

Because it was desired to study the adsorption of proteins under near physiological conditions, a dual channel flow cell was jointly designed by the Harrick Scientific Co.

and Battelle's Columbus Laboratory. This cell, shown in FIGURE 1, has two rectangular channels approximately 0.08 cm deep × 0.8 cm wide × 9.0 cm long. The flow channels are formed from rectangular germanium internal reflection elements (IRE) as the lower surfaces with the tops and sides machined from a poly(methyl methacrylate) block. The stainless steel base can slide so as to position either cell reproducibly in the interferometer. Gaskets are polyethylene and silicone films, with the former against the germanium to avoid any IR bands from the silicone film in contact with the germanium. Peristaltic pumps, valves, and reservoirs are arranged so that saline (or buffer) and protein solutions can be pumped through the cells sequentially at shear rates up to 2100 s^{-1} without exposure of the adsorbing surfaces to air. Static adsorption studies were made in either the flow cell or in a microcircle cell (Spectra-Tech, Inc.), which has the advantage of using volumes of solution as small as 20 μl.

In the development of these spectroscopic methods at Battelle, adsorptions have been done primarily on uncoated germanium, but polymer-coated surfaces formed by multiple dip coating or spin casting of filtered, dilute polymer solutions on the IRE have also been used. Thickness of the coatings is estimated to be $\leq$0.1 μM.

Spectrometers used for the flow studies have been Models FTS-10C or FTS-15 (Digilab, Inc., Cambridge, MA) equipped with high sensitivity, narrow range mercury-cadmium-telluride detectors and fast scan capability. Static adsorption experiments have also been made using a Sirius 100 (Mattson Instrument Co., Madison, WI).

Treatment of Spectral Data

The spectra obtained as a protein solution displaces a saline solution or buffer in a flow cell such as that shown in FIGURE 1 contain the contributions from the IRE, any polymer coating on the crystal, saline solution, adsorbing protein, plus the solute protein within the IR evanescent field. The latter is called the bulk contribution and unless the solute protein concentration is low, the bulk contribution may be greater than that of the adsorbed protein.

The steps necessary to resolve the original spectra into the individual spectra of the solute protein and the adsorbate are:

1. Ratio the 1640 cm^1 water band to a standard value in order to eliminate differences from run-to-run or cell-to-cell.
2. Perform baseline straightening.
3. Subtract the combined spectrum of the infrared crystal, gasket, polymer, and saline (or buffer). (This spectrum is that obtained before the protein solution is admitted into the cell.)

[NOTE: Steps 1 and 2 both involve subjective judgment. A computerized method has been developed[10] that simplifies these operations and makes comparisons of separate spectral experiments more valid.]

In all cases the spectra are co-added (up to the limits of the time resolution desired) to enhance the signal-to-noise ratio. Scale expansion is done to show the spectral detail desired in the absorbance ranges of interest. Using the 1550 cm^{-1} absorbance band as the indicator of the amount of protein, FIGURE 2 schematically shows the total protein seen in an experiment in which protein adsorbs to a near equilibrium value, the bulk protein is displaced by saline, and the original protein solution is again admitted and displaces the saline. The different periods in such an experiment can be described as:

AB: Period during which protein diffuses from the incoming protein solution into the region of the evanescent wave region and initial adsorption of protein begins.

BC: Period during which protein adsorbs until equilibrium or quasi-equilibrium both as to amount of protein and the composition of the adsorbate is reached.
CD: Period during which the bulk protein is displaced by the saline.
DE: Period during which the proteins in the incoming protein solution diffuse into the evanescent wave region and equilibrate with the bulk solution.

Derivation of Adsorbate Spectra

It is seen from FIGURE 2 that the protein represented in the region *CD* is the adsorbed protein because all of the bulk protein has been removed by the saline wash. As the bulk contribution is constant throughout the experiment, subtraction of the adsorbate contribution from the total protein contribution at the end of the adsorbing period gives the bulk contribution. Thus subtraction of this derived bulk contribution from the total at chosen intervals in the period *BC* yields spectra of the adsorbate at those times desired.

The period *AB* represents a different case because in the initial period the concentration of protein in the evanescent wave zone increases from zero to that protein concentration of the solution used (bulk). During this period, protein adsorption may also begin. However, if one considers the rise in protein concentration represented in the region *DE* in FIGURE 2, that rise is the result only of the diffusion of protein into the evanescent region as opposed to the rise in the region *AB* . Therefore, if the curve shown in region *DE* is subtracted from the same time period of region *AB*, the difference will be the formation of the protein adsorbate. These bulk and adsorbate spectra may, of course, be processed as desired by the usual derivatization and deconvolution procedures. FIGURES 3A and 3B show the diffusion of the protein into the evanescent region, the development of the adsorbate, and the total protein signal seen in the adsorption of Alb and IgG from solution.

Quantification of Protein Adsorbates

Methods for relating spectral data to the surface concentration have been developed through two approaches, which will be outlined here. In one case,[11] the procedure follows closely that used in the conventional radiolabeling methods except that a flow system has been used for both the adsorption and washing steps with the processes being followed spectroscopically. Adsorption can be stopped at serial intervals in order to obtain relation between peak heights and surface concentration. Washing is continued until the Amide II absorbance band at 1550 cm^{-1} is stable. (Other bands such as the 1400 cm^{-1} may also be used.) The infrared element is rinsed again after the cell is disassembled and the rinse solution checked for radioactivity. Before rinsing, the edges of the element are swabbed to determine if any of the tagged protein solution had leaked past the gaskets.

A simpler method not involving the use of radiolabeled proteins has been used by Pitt.[12] Known volumes of a dilute protein solution were spread on an IRE and dried. Areas under the band at 1550 cm^{-1} were measured and used to establish a linear calibration correlation between the peak area and the known surface concentration.

Identification and Quantification of Adsorbate Constituents

Classically, components of a mixture have been identified by use of one or more unique spectral features of the individual components. Examples of such features are

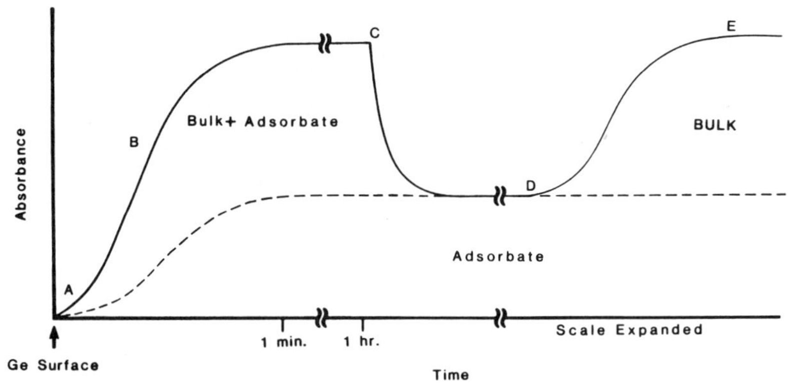

FIGURE 2. Schematic of the contributions of the bulk and the adsorbate to the spectra obtained during the adsorption of protein from solution.

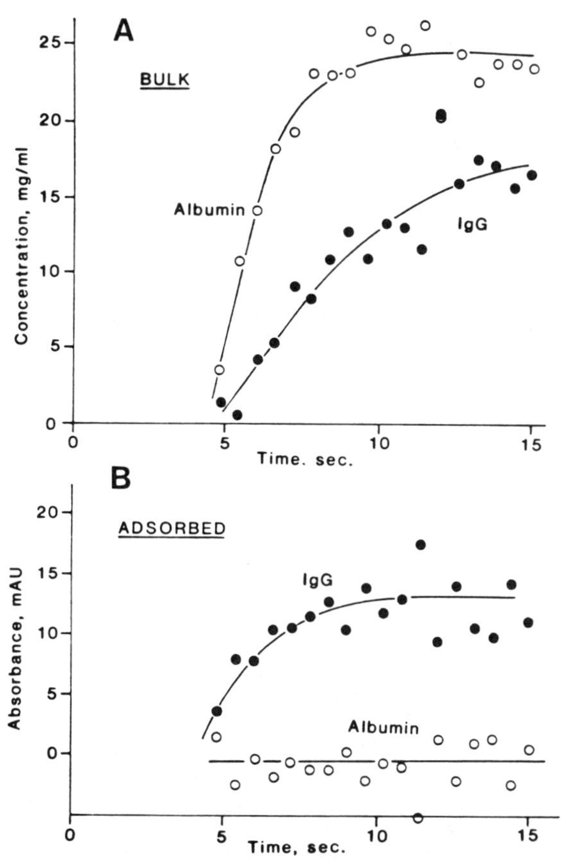

FIGURE 3. **(A)** Concurrent diffusion of albumin into the evanescent zone and formation of adsorbate. **(B)** Concurrent diffusion of IgG into the evanescent zone and formation of adsorbate.

unique absorbance bands, shoulders, band widths, band height ratios, and the like. In the case of proteins as seen in the spectra of albumin (Alb), IgG, and fibrinogen (Fb) in FIGURE 4, spectral features can be used to estimate the proportions in a binary mixture. In mixtures of three or more proteins, computer-aided methods become necessary. We have concentrated on the application of methods based on matrix algebra.[13] These methods are based on the comparison of absorbances at a number of wavelengths of known mixtures of the proteins of interest (training sets) with the absorbances of the unknown mixture at the same wavelengths. The known mixtures must include the components over the concentration ranges expected. The use of the "P" matrix allows

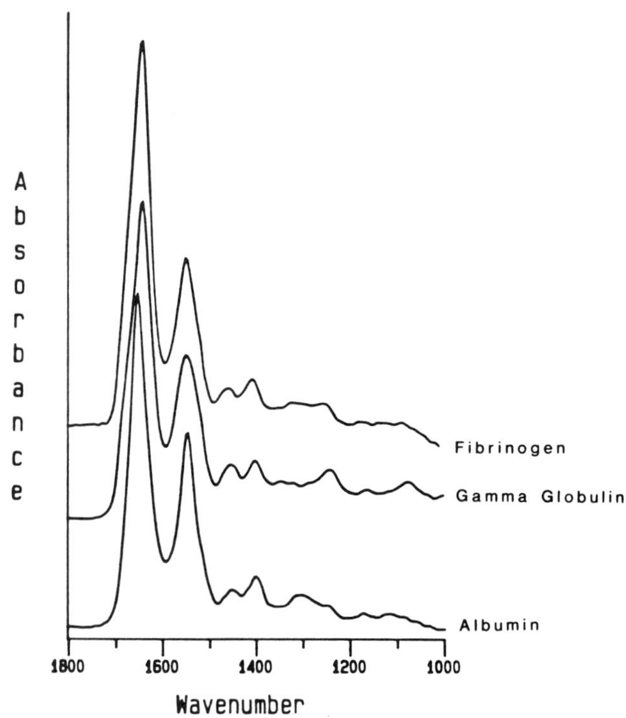

FIGURE 4. Spectra of albumin, IgG, and fibrinogen.

the treating of undefined impurities of "background" as an additional single component with the restriction that its composition remain constant. One may also use band intensity ratios, half bandwidths, or band areas instead of band intensities for comparison. Software is available for implementing these methods. To date application of these methods to determine the composition of adsorbates has been through the use of transmission spectra of mixtures of the proteins of interest in solution.[14] Because of the possible spectral changes induced by the adsorption it would be preferable to use training sets based on adsorbed proteins, but the difficulty of preparing mixed adsorbates with the needed ranges of compositions has precluded this step.

REPRESENTATIVE APPLICATIONS OF THE ABOVE TECHNIQUES

Determination of the Rates of Adsorption

In the case of single proteins, rates of adsorption are readily found by plotting the absorbance at 1550 cm^{-1} against time until an apparent equilibrium is reached. Time intervals plotted in the work referenced here have been as short as 0.8 seconds, which permitted the co-adding of four spectra. Thus, it is of especial value in the study of the early events such as in the adsorption of Alb and IgG on germanium as shown in FIGURE 4. Adsorbate spectra are derived by the sequence of spectral subtractions described earlier. Other rates that are of interest in this adsorption process can also be determined. Examples are rates of diffusion of the proteins from the solution into the evanescent wave region, desorption and conversion of a labile adsorbed species to a stable (and perhaps altered) form, competitive and replacement reactions, and conformational changes. In addition effects of such variables as shear rate, protein concentration, nature of surface, and the like can be determined. Reversibility of the adsorption can be determined by allowing the protein solution to flow for a chosen short period followed by displacement of the protein by saline or buffer. Such experiments[15] have shown that Alb when first adsorbed on germanium is readily desorbed by saline during the first 10–15 seconds after adsorption begins. IgG, however, appears irreversibly adsorbed essentially immediately (*i.e.,* within a few seconds).

This capability of FT-IR is especially useful in observing the very early events in the adsorption of proteins from blood or plasma. This is possible despite the complexity of the protein mixture because the first observable protein in the early period is Alb because of both its low molecular weight and abundance. This is followed by IgG, so that the interaction of those two proteins with the surface can be studied relatively free from other proteins. Also seen in the first few seconds was an unidentified glycoprotein which, based on its low molecular weight as shown by its rapid diffusion into the evanescent wave region, possibly was acid α_1-glycoprotein. However, this work[16] using an *ex vivo* blood source (sheep) predated development of the method to derive the individual bulk and adsorbate spectra of the very initial phase for individual study.

Quantification of Adsorbed Proteins

FIGURE 5 shows the correlation between the absorbance peak heights at 1550 cm^{-1} and surface concentration of Alb, IgG, and Fb as determined through the use of tagged proteins. Of note is the significant difference in slope among the proteins, although the difference between Alb and IgG is in accord with the extinction coefficients of the two proteins measured in transmission. There is no ready explanation available for the deviation of the slope of the Fb curve in relation to that expected from the Fb extinction coefficient.

No direct comparison of these results with the method of Pitt *et al.*[12] which was used with fibronectin (Fn) is available, although it should be noted that the Fb data are in approximate agreement with the results of Pitt if the high carbohydrate content of the Fn is considered as a diluent of the Fn protein. Both of these methods appear to have detection limits of at least 0.05 $\mu g/cm^{-1}$.

The use of these two IR techniques is limited to single proteins because of the variance of extinction coefficients even when the proteins do not contain major amounts of constituents such as lipids or carbohydrates, unless there is an independent measurement of the ratios of the different proteins in the adsorbate.

Competitive Adsorption

In the simplest case of competitive adsorption, that of adsorption from a binary solution, one can take advantage of readily seen spectral differences.[17] For example Alb, IgG, and Fb each show differences in the ratios of the heights of the 1400 cm^{-1} and 1450 cm^{-1} and of the 1320 cm^{-1} and 1230 cm^{-1} bands. Using these band ratios it has been seen that in the adsorption on Ge from a mixture of Alb and IgG the early adsorbate (5 minutes) was primarily Alb, but after 177 minutes IgG replaced the Alb until only a trace of Alb was present in the adsorbate. In the case of Alb and Fb, the results were similar except that the early adsorbate was richer in Alb and the final adsorbate contained no detectable Alb. The higher Alb content of the early adsorbate in the latter pair probably reflects the slower diffusion rate of the Fb compared to that of the IgG. With the third pair, IgG and Fb, both the early and late adsorbate contained only trace amounts of Fb. Thus it was seen that both IgG and Fb displaced the earlier adsorbing Alb, and that IgG, which reaches the surface earlier than does the Fb, is not displaced by the Fb.

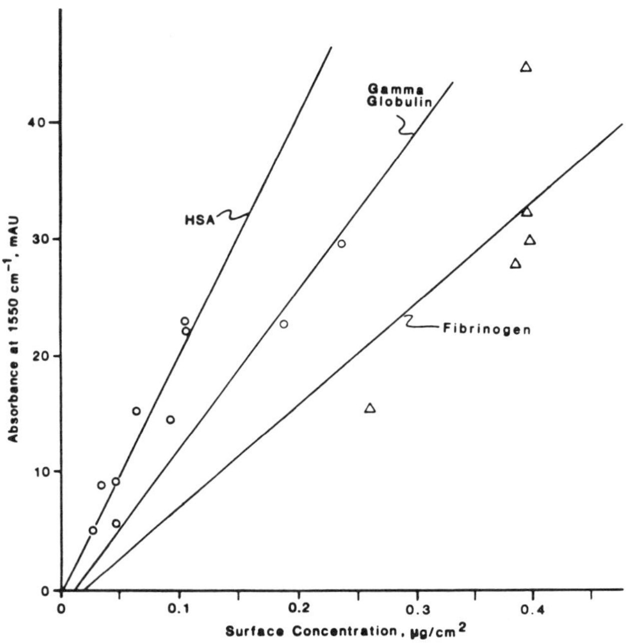

FIGURE 5. Relation of absorbance at 1550 cm^{-1} to surface concentration. (Adapted from ref. 8.)

It should be noted that Brash[2] found similar results with binary solutions of Alb and Fb adsorbing on glass and also found on glass that from a ternary solution of the three proteins, Fb dominated the adsorbate with lesser amounts of IgG and only trace amounts of Alb present.

The effect of the surface on the adsorbate composition forming from Alb/IgG

TABLE 1. Observed Frequencies (cm^{-1}) of Adsorbed Proteins on Surfaces

	IgG	Albumin
Germanium	1240	1320
Biomer	1240 + some 1270	1285
Alkylated cellulose	1240 + strong 1270	1315

solutions was investigated by Chittur *et al.*[18] Analyses of the adsorbates forming on Ge and a polyurethane were made by the P-matrix method and showed appreciably higher Alb contents (approx. 45%) on the latter surface compared to about 14% on Ge.

Effect of Adsorption on the Conformation of Proteins

No extensive study has been made of the effects of the nature of the adsorbing surface on the conformation of blood proteins, although it has been established that conformational changes do occur. Morrisey and Stromberg[19] in 1974 used transmission IR to measure the number of bonding points per molecule between Alb, prothrombin, and Fb and colloidal silica gel as a substrate and concluded that denaturation can result from adsorption. In early (unpublished) work at Battelle, frequency shifts were seen when Alb and IgG were adsorbed on Ge, Biomer, or alkylated cellulose (courtesy of Dr. R. C. Eberhart), as shown in TABLE 1. FIGURE 6 shows spectral differences between Alb, which has been adsorbed on Ge for 15 minutes, and the Alb in solution from which it adsorbed. The changes in the Amide III region indicate an increase in disordered structure (chain unfolding) and the broadening in the half-width of the Amide I band of the adsorbate indicates an increase in the bound water content. This latter change is in accord with the greater exposure to water of the interior of the adsorbed protein because of the chain unfolding, according to recent work relating

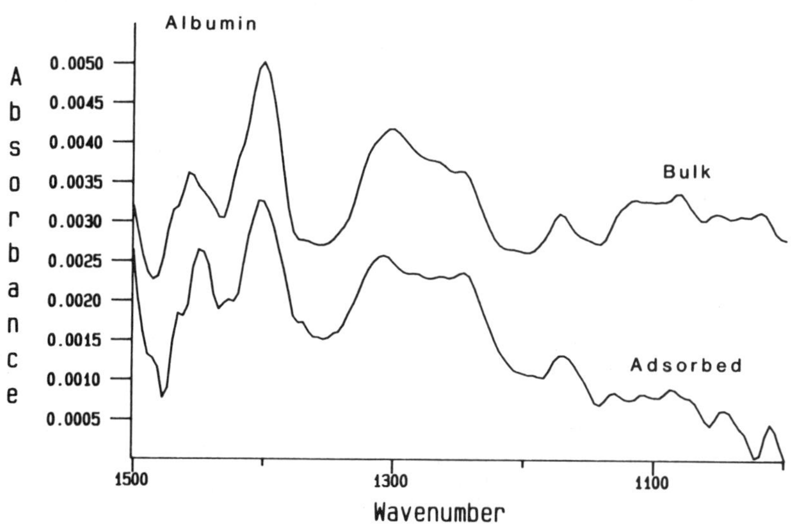

FIGURE 6. Spectra of solute and adsorbed albumin.

spectral changes to structural changes of a protein.[20] Recently, Pitt *et al.*[12] studied the adsorption of fibronectin on four polyurethane ureas and found that on the more hydrophobic polymers spectral changes were greater and that the first molecules to adsorb were more altered than those adsorbing later.

DISCUSSION

It is seen that at the present state of development, FT-IR spectroscopy can contribute to knowledge of interactions between blood and surfaces in two areas: (1) single proteins or mixtures of known proteins, and (2) adsorption of protein from whole blood or plasma onto different surfaces.

In the case of single proteins or mixtures of known proteins, IR can be used to determine, as affected by the nature of the adsorbing surface:

1. The rate and amount of adsorption of a single protein
2. Competitive adsorption from mixtures of known proteins
3. The reversibility of the adsorption process and the time for a newly adsorbed protein to become irreversibly adsorbed
4. The rate and degree of conformational change of the proteins after adsorption
5. The displacement of one adsorbed protein by another

In the case of protein adsorption from whole blood or plasma onto different surfaces, IR spectroscopy can be expected to:

1. Follow the course of protein adsorption in the very early phase when the primary constituents of the adsorbate are the low molecular weight, relatively high concentration proteins such as Alb, IgG, and acid α_1-glycoprotein
2. Determine the time needed for the adsorbate composition to reach at least a near equilibrium composition
3. Aid in the identification of proteins or classes of proteins that are minor constituents of plasma but are preferentially adsorbed and thereby concentrated in the substrate
4. Determine the comparative time needed and peak protein absorbance from blood or plasma before displacement reactions (Vroman effect) take place

It is seen that FT-IR spectroscopy provides a clear advantage over other methods in that the time scale of events can be examined in much greater detail. In addition, the capability of the method to detect changes in conformation caused by the adsorption process may be the most important capability because that change in proteins may be the controlling factor in the compatibility of a foreign surface with blood.

REFERENCES

1. Vroman, L., A. L. Adams, G. C. Fischer & P. C. Munoz. 1980. Interaction of high molecular weight kininogen, factor XII, and fibrinogen in plasma at interfaces. Thromb. Haemostas. **47:** 156–159.
2. Brash, J. L. 1987. Studies of protein adsorption at the solid-solution interface in relation to the blood-materials interactions. *In* Proteins at Interfaces: Physicochemical and Biochemical Studies. ACS Symposium Series, Vol. 343. J. L. Brash & T. A. Horbett, Eds. American Chemical Society. Washington, D.C.
3. Moyer, L. S. & M. H. Gorin. 1940. J. Biol. Chem. **133:** 605.
4. Horan, F. E., F. G. Hirsch, L. A. Wood & I. S. Wright. 1950. J. Clin. Invest. **29:** 202.

5. BECK, R. E., V. MIRKOVICK, P. G. ANDRUS & R. I. LEININGER. 1963. Apparatus for the determination of zeta potentials. J. Appl. Physiol. **18:** 1263–1265.
6. LEININGER, R. I., V. MIRKOVITCH, R. E. BECK, P. G. ANDRUS & W. J. KOLFF. 1964. The zeta potentials of some selected solids in respect to plasma and plasma fractions. Trans. Am. Soc. Artif. Organs **10:** 237–238.
7. LEININGER, R. I. 1965. Surface effects in blood-plastic compatibility. *In* Biophysical Mechanisms in Vascular Homeostasis and Intravascular Thrombosis. Philip Sawyer, Ed.: 288–297. Appleton-Century Crofts. New York.
8. COOPER, S. L. & N. PAPPAS, Eds. 1982. Biomaterials: Interfacial Phenomena and Applications. Adv. Chem. Ser. **199.**
9. BRASH, J. L. & T. A. HORBETT, Eds. Proteins at Interfaces: Physicochemical and Biochemical Studies. ACS Symposium Series, Vol. 343. American Chemical Society, Washington, D.C.
10. POWELL, J. R., F. M. WASACZ & R. J. JAKOBSEN. 1986. An algorithm for the reproducible spectral subtraction of water from the FT-IR spectra of proteins in dilute solution and adsorbed monolayers. Appl. Spectrosc. **40:** 239.
11. FINK, D. J., T. B. HUTSON, K. K. CHITTUR, R. I. LEININGER & R. M. GENDREAU. 1986. Quantitative surface studies of protein adsorption by infrared spectroscopy: II. Quantification of adsorbed and bulk proteins. Anal. Biochem. Submitted.
12. PITT, W. G., S. H. SPIEGELBERG & S. L. COOPER. 1986. Fourier transform infrared spectroscopy studies of the adsorption of fibronectin to polyurethane surfaces. *In* Proteins at Interfaces: Physicochemical and Biochemical Studies. ACS Symposium Series, Vol. 343. J. A. Brash & T. A. Horbett, Eds. American Chemical Society. Washington, D.C.
13. BROWN, C. W., P. F. LYNCH, P. F. OBREMSKI & D. S. LAVERY. 1982. Matrix representation and criteria for selecting analytical wavelengths for multicomponent spectroscopic analysis. Anal. Chem. **54:** 1472–1481.
14. CHITTUR, K. K., D. J. FINK, R. M. GENDREAU, R. J. JAKOBSEN & R. I. LEININGER. 1987. FT/IR studies of protein adsorption in flowing systems. *In* Proteins at Interfaces: Physicochemical and Biochemical Studies. ACS Symposium Series, Vol. 343. J. L. Brash & T. A. Horbett, Eds. American Chemical Society. Washington, D.C.
15. CHITTUR, K. K. Unpublished results.
16. WINTERS, S., R. M. GENDREAU, R. I. LEININGER & R. J. JAKOBSEN. 1982. Fourier transform infrared spectroscopy of protein adsorption from whole blood II. *Ex vivo* sheep studies. Appl. Spectrosc. **36:** 404–409.
17. LEININGER, R. I., D. J. FINK, R. M. GENDREAU, T. B. HUTSON & R. J. JAKOBSEN. 1983. Spectroscopic probes of blood-surface interaction. Trans. Am. Soc. Artif. Organs **19:** 152–158.
18. CHITTUR, K. K., D. J. FINK, R. I. LEININGER & T. B. HUTSON. 1986. FT-IR/ATR studies of protein adsorption in flowing systems: Approaches for bulk correction and compositional analysis of adsorbed and bulk proteins in mixtures. J. Colloid Interface Sci. **41:** 419–433.
19. MORRISEY, B. W. & R. R. STROMBERG. 1974. Conformation of adsorbed proteins by infrared: Bound fraction measurements. J. Colloid Interface Sci. **46:** 152–164.
20. JAKOBSEN, R. J. & F. M. WASACZ. 1987. FT-IR studies of the effects of the environment on the structure of adsorbed proteins. *In* Proteins at Interfaces: Physicochemical and Biochemical Studies. ACS Symposium Series, Vol. 343. J. L. Brash & T. A. Horbett, Eds. American Chemical Society. Washington, D.C.

Role of Fibrinogen in Activation of Platelets by Artificial Surfaces

EDWIN W. SALZMAN,[a] JACK LINDON,[a] GERALD McMANAMA,[a] AND J. ANTHONY WARE[b]

[a]*Department of Surgery*
[b]*Department of Medicine*
Beth Israel Hospital
and
Harvard Medical School
Boston, Massachusetts 02215

Activation of platelets by contact with artificial surfaces is a key event in the thromboembolic complications of prosthetic devices in contact with the blood,[1,2] but the mechanism of these events is not fully understood. It is known that a film of plasma protein adsorbs on artificial materials exposed to blood and that this event precedes interaction of the surface with blood cells.[3,4] A corollary of this thesis is that the blood cells do not react directly with the underlying surface but rather with the adsorbed protein coat. The composition of the protein film and the configuration of its molecular constituents must relay to the blood elements information describing the nature of the underlying surface.

Fibrinogen appears to be an important component of the adsorbed protein film and may be an essential player in the early events of platelet activation,[5,6] adsorbing preferentially on many surfaces in a concentration relatively higher than in the bulk plasma and participating in the platelet response to the prosthetic surface.[7–12]

Fibrinogen is now recognized as an indispensible element in platelet aggregation.[13,14] An early feature of activation of platelets by soluble agonists such as ADP or thrombin is exposure of specific membrane glycoproteins (GP IIb-IIIa), to which fibrinogen molecules bind with high affinity.[15,16] According to current dogma, the divalent fibrinogen molecule is necessary for the formation of connecting bridges between contiguous platelets, perhaps in conjunction with other "adhesive proteins,"[7,17] such as von Willebrand's factor, thrombospondin, or fibronectin. It should be noted that fibrinogen dissolved in plasma does not induce platelet aggregation but rather acts as a cofactor in the process. Fibrinogen normally circulates in peaceful coexistence with platelets without any obvious interaction. It is claimed that platelets have membrane receptors of low affinity for fibrinogen,[16–19] which would permit reversible interactions at physiologic fibrinogen concentrations, but the prevailing view is that it is only in the "activated" platelet (*i.e.*, the platelet stimulated by agonists such as thrombin or ADP) that fibrinogen forms a detectable complex with its glycoprotein membrane receptors, which are "masked" or otherwise unavailable in intact nonactivated circulating platelets.[20,22]

If adsorbed fibrinogen were involved in some way in platelet adhesion to surfaces, perhaps by bridging the gap between platelet and surface in a manner analogous to its action in platelet aggregation, an important question would be whether prior activation of the platelet would be required or whether interaction with adsorbed fibrinogen molecules might occur without preliminary alteration of the basal platelet. It has been suggested that fibrinogen molecules adsorbed on artificial surfaces undergo conformational changes that lead platelets to regard them as "foreign" and that might even be responsible for the progression from platelet adhesion to aggregation and secretion.[9,23–25]

We set out to study these events *in vitro* employing a series of polymers that vary in a systematic way in structure and in the degree of their interaction with platelets, namely the poly(alkyl methacrylates). We have previously reported[26] that platelet reactivity of this family of polymers increases with the length of the alkyl side chain.

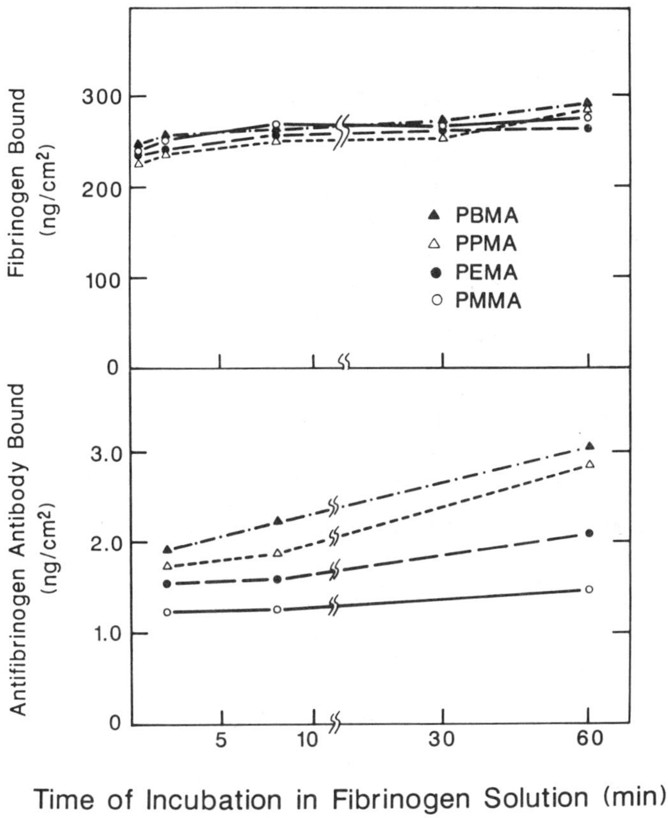

FIGURE 1. *Upper panel,* Concentration of ^{125}I-labeled fibrinogen on coverslips coated with various methacrylates after incubation in purified fibrinogen solution. There is no significant difference among the four materials tested. *Lower panel,* Binding of ^{125}I-labeled antifibrinogen antibody by methacrylate-coated coverslips after various periods of incubation in a solution of purified (unlabeled) fibrinogen, 250 μg/ml. (From Lindon *et al.*[28] Reprinted by permission from *Blood.*)

We found that removal of platelets from whole blood passed through a column of methacrylate beads varied from 30% for poly(methyl methacrylate) (PMMA) to 70% or greater for poly-*n*-butylmethacrylate (PBMA). In these experiments platelet reactivity resulted in activation of platelets in the column and led to a combination of platelet adhesion to the beads and subsequent platelet aggregation.[27] Secretion of platelet granule contents paralleled platelet retention.

We measured fibrinogen adsorption on coverslips coated with the polymers polymethyl, polyethyl, poly-*n*-propyl, and poly-*n*-butyl methacrylate (PMMA, PEMA, PPMA, and PBMA)[28] and more recently have studied the same phenomenon in columns loaded with beads coated with these polymers. Adsorbed fibrinogen was measured by two techniques: one that assessed the total quantity of the adsorbed protein spiked with ^{125}I-labeled fibrinogen[29,30] in solution in buffer or in plasma and a second that measured the adsorbed molecules that were detectable by ^{125}I-labeled antifibrinogen antibodies.[28] The adsorption of fibrinogen was carried out from purified solution[31] or from plasma and was saturable on these polymers at concentrations ranging from 50 to 100 μg/ml (FIGURE 1).

In contrast to studies reported in the literature, we found no correlation of total concentration of bound fibrinogen with platelet reactivity of the polymers. After incubation for an hour with 250 μg/ml of fibrinogen, the concentration of bound fibrinogen approximated 0.3 μg/cm^2 and was about the same for all the methacrylates in experiments in which coverslips were incubated with purified fibrinogen dissolved in buffer. If the surfaces were incubated in plasma, the concentration of adsorbed fibrinogen was about 0.2 μg/cm^2 and was likewise not correlated with platelet reactivity of the polymers.

On the other hand, when adsorbed fibrinogen was measured by exposing coverslips which had first been incubated with unlabeled fibrinogen in buffer or with plasma to radiolabeled polyclonal antibodies against human fibrinogen, the amount of antifibrinogen antibody bound was positively correlated with the platelet reactivity of the polymers (FIGURE 2). Bound antibody varied from 5.7 ± 0.4 ng/cm^2 on poly(methyl methacrylate) to 9.4 ± 0.8 ng/cm^2 on poly-*n*-butyl methacrylate after incubation with an antibody solution at a concentration of 1 μg/ml. These results suggest that platelet interaction with such polymers is more closely related to the portion of adsorbed fibrinogen that is antibody recognizable or "native" than to the total amount of fibrinogen adsorbed and, as a corollary, that adsorbed fibrinogen whose conformation

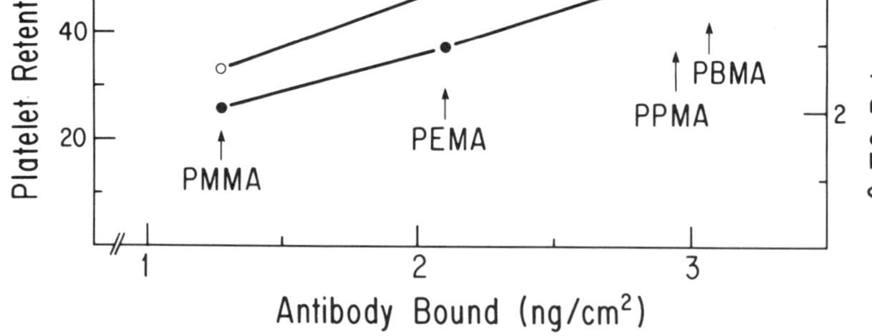

FIGURE 2. Correlation of binding of labeled antifibrinogen antibody on fibrinogen-coated coverslips with platelet retention and β-thromboglobulin release on passage of whole blood through bead columns coated with the same polymer.

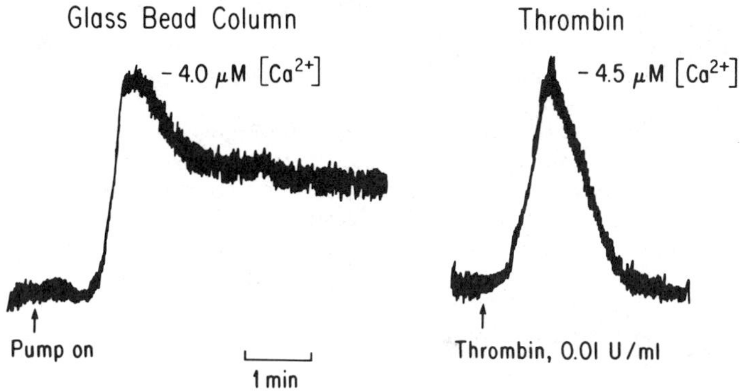

FIGURE 3. Elevation of ionized cytoplasmic calcium concentration in aequorin-loaded platelets in modified Tyrode's buffer containing 1 mM Ca^{2+} pumped through a glass bead column or exposed to thrombin (0.01 U/ml).

is altered by adsorption to the point that the molecule is not recognizable by the antibody is relatively unimportant in platelet-surface interactions.

Examination of other polymers in this context provided useful comparative information.[28] A series of polyacrylates ranging from poly(methylacrylate) (PMA) to poly(butylacrylate) (PBA) had increasing platelet reactivity with increasing length of the alkyl side chain, similar to the behavior of the methacrylates. However, in the case of the acrylates, both the total fibrinogen bound and the antibody-detectable fraction were correlated with platelet reactivity. This relationship also held for polystyrene and a commercially available polyurethane, Biomer. Thus, these data suggest that artificial surfaces might minimize their platelet reactivity either by holding to a minimum total adsorbed fibrinogen or, if they adsorb substantial quantities of fibrinogen, by changing its conformation to a form that is unrecognizable to antifibrinogen antibodies and presumably also unrecognizable to platelet receptors for fibrinogen.

The behavior of fibrinogen adsorbed from plasma or from purified fibrinogen solutions was similar. Vroman *et al.*[32] have described desorption of adsorbed fibrinogen by interaction with plasma components (particularly high molecular weight kininogen), but this phenomenon does not appear to have been a significant factor in these experiments, as there was no reduction of the total fibrinogen concentration on the surfaces with time. The fact that the polymers we studied were largely hydrophobic may account for the difference between our results and those of Vroman.

We considered the possibility that interaction of platelets with fibrinogen molecules adsorbed on surfaces in their "native" conformation might itself be a stimulus to platelet activation, perhaps by cross-linking or otherwise sterically affecting the glycoprotein receptors for fibrinogen on platelets (analogous to the "mobile receptor" hypothesis of Jacobs and Cuatrecasas[33]). Activation of platelets by such soluble agonists as thrombin or ADP is known to be accompanied by a rise in the concentration of ionized calcium in the cytoplasm (FIGURE 3).[34-36] We loaded platelets with the calcium-sensitive photoprotein aequorin by a technique we have previously described.[35] When platelets loaded with aequorin and suspended in a medium containing fibrinogen were passed through a column of glass beads, a rise in cytosolic calcium occurred, as indicated by the increase in aequorin light output. The pattern of the response resembled the effect of thrombin on platelet calcium. These results indicate that retention of platelets on the bead columns is truly an expression of activation of the platelets and not simply the result of adhesion of otherwise unreacting platelets. The experiments suggest that platelet responses to surface contact follow pathways otherwise shared by more conventional soluble agonists such as thrombin, ADP, and epinephrine.

An important issue is the apparent reactivity of fibrinogen adsorbed in its "native" state with platelets, whose GP IIb-IIIa receptors are conventionally regarded as unavailable unless the platelets have been subjected to prior activation. An explanation may perhaps be found in the work of Hornick and Karush,[37] who showed that interaction of molecules in solution with a multivalent ligand, in their case anti-DNP(2,4-dinitrophenol) antibodies, occurred with an association constant of 3.5×10^{-11} compared with 6×10^{-6} for monovalent association. Clearly, multivalency has the capacity to magnify enormously the total binding affinity of an adsorbant.[38] Under

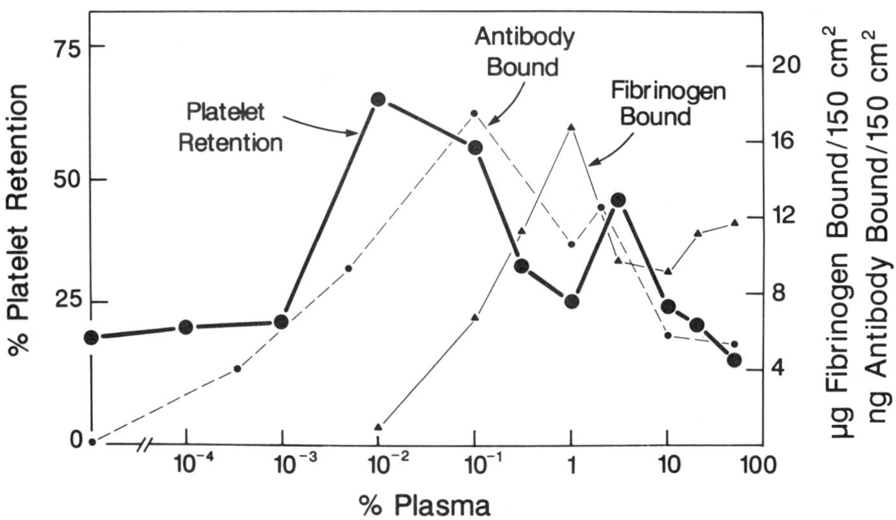

FIGURE 4. Retention of washed platelets suspended in modified Tyrode's buffer on PBMA bead columns following pretreatment of the column with platelet-free plasma in various dilutions. In parallel experiments a column was exposed to either a solution of ^{125}I-labeled fibrinogen or to unlabeled fibrinogen followed by ^{125}I-labeled antifibrinogen antibody for measurement respectively of total fibrinogen bound or antibody-recognizable fibrinogen bound by the surface.

the circumstances of our experiments, the monovalent ligand would be represented by fibrinogen in solution, which might react with very low affinity, perhaps undetectable by conventional techniques. When adsorbed on a surface, however, the immobilized fibrinogen would become a multivalent ligand, the affinity of whose interaction with platelet receptors would be substantially enhanced. The effect would be materially reinforced by the high concentration of fibrinogen that might be reached in an adsorbed film (for example, a surface coated with fibrinogen at a concentration of 1 $\mu g/cm^2$ has a local concentration equivalent to that of a 100 mM solution.[28]

The role of adsorbed fibrinogen in platelet reactions with an artificial surface was further examined by a preincubation of poly(methyl methacrylate) or poly(butyl methacrylate) bead columns with various dilutions of plasma and subsequently pumping a suspension of washed platelets through the column (FIGURE 4). Retention of platelets in the column varied, depending on the degree of dilution of the plasma in the precoating solution. Preliminary exposure of the bead column to whole plasma led to minimal retention of washed platelets on the column. The surface was essentially passivated. The opposite effect was observed when diluted plasma was employed, however; platelet activity was enhanced, maximal reactivity of the column being observed at concentrations of plasma between 0.01% and 0.1%. Measurement of the concentration of adsorbed fibrinogen that resulted from exposure of methacrylate polymers to such plasma dilutions revealed that the peak platelet reactivity did not correspond to the concentration of plasma at which fibrinogen adsorption was greatest (1%) but rather occurred at a plasma concentration at which total fibrinogen adsorption was very low and at which adsorption of "native" fibrinogen was at a maximum, as indicated by measurement using the labeled antibody technique. Thus, these experiments provided additional evidence implicating fibrinogen in its relatively unaltered conformation as an important participant in platelet interaction with surfaces.

We attempted to model the possible effects of a multivalent ligand composed of sterically constrained fibrinogen molecules in high local concentration by preparing soluble polymers of fibrinogen with these characteristics.[39] We first cross-linked fibrinogen with the cross-linking agent dimethyl suberimidate. By this technique we obtained soluble oligomers ranging in size from dimers to pentamers. Unfortunately these were inactive when added to platelet suspensions, producing no aggregation of the platelets and having no effect on aggregation induced by the addition of ADP with fibrinogen. Other polymers produced by cross-linking fibrinogen with activated factor XIII were likewise inert when added to a platelet suspension. The inactivity of these polymers probably resulted from the fact that lysine residues are involved in cross-linking proteins by either of these approaches and were therefore unavailable to take part in platelet-fibrinogen interactions. Agam and Livne[40] have provided evidence that reactions involving lysine residues are critical in the binding of platelets to fibrinogen, which according to several laboratories takes place at the carboxy-terminal end of the γ- and α-chains of the fibrinogen molecule.[17,41–44] These platelet-binding loci on the fibrinogen molecule are located in the D-domain, the terminal nodules in fibrinogen's trinodular structure.

We therefore prepared soluble polymers of fibrinogen cross-linked across the E-domain but sparing the critical D-domain platelet binding sites by incubating fibrinogen with divalent rabbit anti-human E-domain antibodies (Fab′2 fragments) from which the Fc portion had been removed to minimize nonspecific interactions with platelets.[45,46] These antibodies were prepared by affinity chromatography of polyvalent antifibrinogen antibodies using immobilized E fragments of plasmin-digested fibrinogen to remove selectively the anti-E species, which were then eluted from the column with a concentrated salt solution. Soluble polymers were produced by incubating the antibodies with fibrinogen at a molecular ratio of 2 to 1. Molecular weight of the polymers was difficult to determine because of their lability, but size exclusion chromatography suggested a molecular weight of at least 5 million.

Upon addition of this polymer to a suspension of gel-filtered platelets in buffer at 37°, brisk platelet aggregation and secretion of labeled serotonin occurred (FIGURE 5). The effect was concentration dependent and could be duplicated after a short lag period by addition of the components of the polymer but not by a mixture of fibrinogen with monovalent (Fab) fragments of the anti-E antibody or by fibrinogen or the Fab′2 fragments added separately. The response of platelets to the polymers was not simple agglutination (as might have been induced by a polycation such as polylysine[47]), as it was blocked by the metabolic inhibitors sodium azide and 2-deoxyglucose. The response was also blocked by antibodies directed against the platelet's glycoprotein receptors for fibrinogen (GP IIb-IIIa, inhibited specifically by the monoclonal antibody 10E5, obtained through the kindness of Dr. Barry Coller[48]) or by monovalent Fab fragments of antibodies against the D-domain of fibrinogen, the location of fibrinogen's platelet-reactive site.

The platelet response to soluble fibrinogen polymers appeared to involve ADP released from the platelet, for the platelet response was partially inhibited by ADP-scavenging enzyme systems (creatine phosphate, creatine phosphokinase[49]) or by blockade of the platelet's ADP receptor by 5′-fluorosulfonyl benzoyl adenosine (FSBA),[51] a relatively selective covalent inhibitor of the platelet's ADP receptor. Likewise, platelet metabolism of arachidonic acid to thromboxane A_2 appeared to occur in response to the fibrinogen polymer; the effects of the polymer on platelets were attenuated by cyclooxygenase inhibition by aspirin. Platelet aggregation induced by the soluble fibrinogen polymer was accompanied by release of serotonin, indicating further that the platelet response involved internal changes and not simply agglutination. This was further shown by studies employing platelets loaded with the calcium-sensitive indicator aequorin (FIGURE 6). An elevation of ionized cytoplasmic calcium

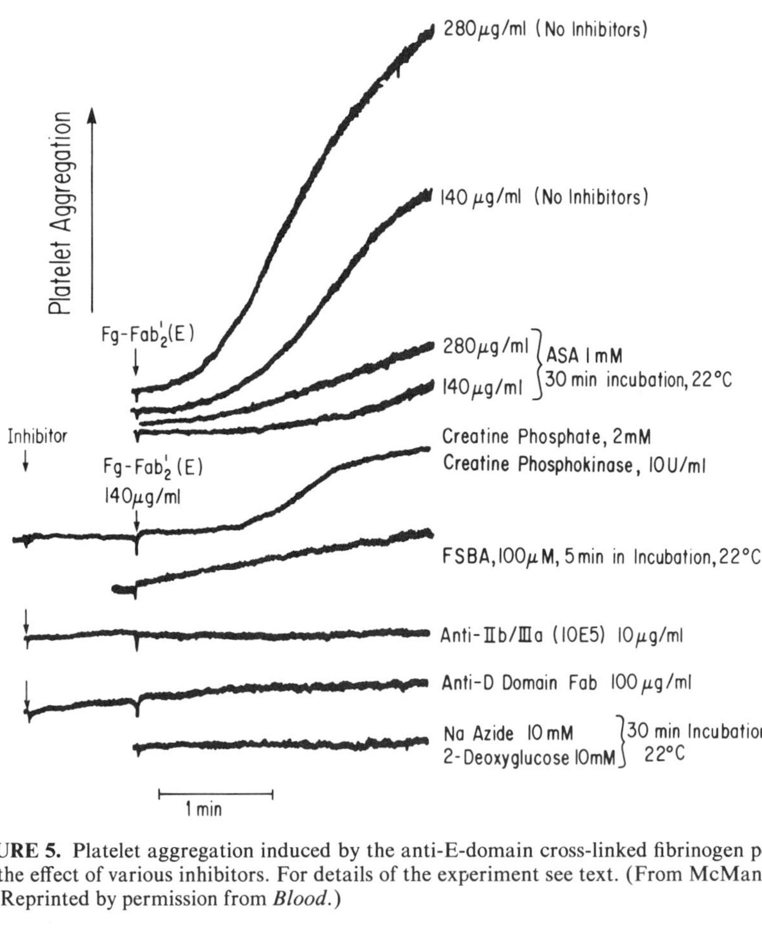

FIGURE 5. Platelet aggregation induced by the anti-E-domain cross-linked fibrinogen polymer and the effect of various inhibitors. For details of the experiment see text. (From McManama *et al.*[39] Reprinted by permission from *Blood.*)

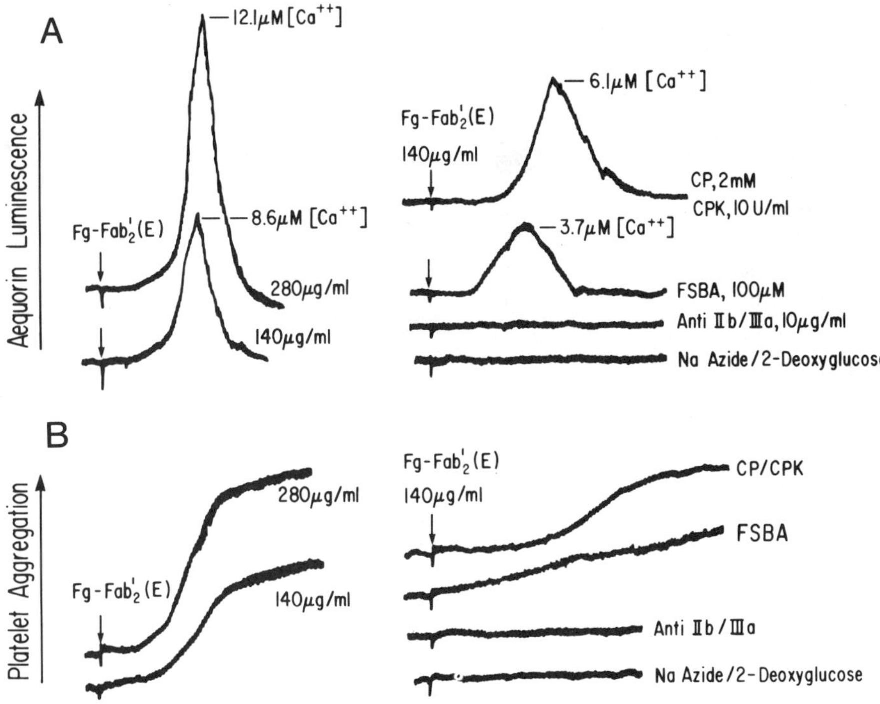

FIGURE 6. Aequorin-indicated elevation of (**A**) ionized cytoplasmic calcium concentration or (**B**) platelet aggregation induced by anti-E-domain fibrinogen polymer and their inhibition by various inhibitors. For details see text. (From McManama *et al.*[39] Reprinted by permission from *Blood.*)

was induced by reaction of platelets with the fibrinogen polymers. The calcium rise was eliminated by sodium azide and 2-deoxyglucose[51,52] and by the monoclonal antibody[48] against the glycoproteins IIb-IIIa (fibrinogen receptor) and was partially inhibited by FSBA and by the creatine phosphate and creatine phosphokinase (CP/CPK) enzyme system.

The mechanism by which reaction with the soluble fibrinogen polymer leads to changes in platelet cytosolic calcium concentration is not certain. There is evidence that glycoproteins IIb-IIIa in the platelet membrane, generally acknowledged to be the chief fibrinogen receptor on platelets, may also bind calcium and perhaps serve as a transmembrane calcium channel.[53] It is tempting to speculate (FIGURE 7) that the interaction of fibrinogen polymers (and possibly of fibrinogen adsorbed on surfaces) with these "fibrinogen receptors" might lead to a local zone of increased concentration of ionized calcium and thence to recruitment of secondary processes such as activation of membrane phospholipases, generation of the second messengers diacylglycerol and inositol triphosphate, more generalized elevation of cytoplasmic calcium, and ultimately to exposure of additional fibrinogen receptors leading to platelet aggregation. Further studies will be necessary to test this hypothesis and to assess the validity of the soluble fibrinogen polymer as a model for fibrinogen adsorbed on artificial surfaces.

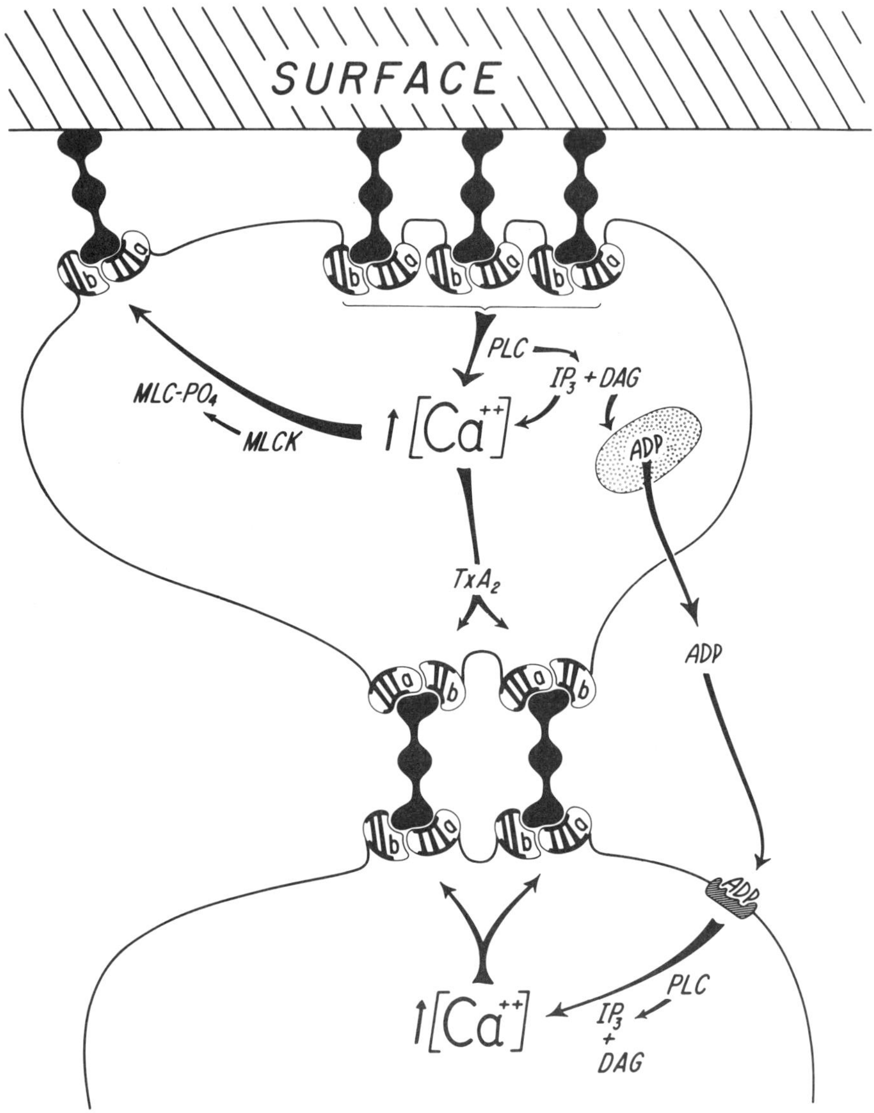

FIGURE 7. Hypothetical scheme of platelet activation by adhesion to fibrinogen-coated surfaces. Adsorbed fibrinogen, conformationally relatively intact, reacts with glycoprotein IIb-IIIa platelet receptors, masked and of low affinity, which by activation of phospholipase C and resulting generation of inositol trisphosphate and diacylglycerol leads to elevation of ionized cytoplasmic calcium concentration. This in turn activates myosin light-chain kinase leading to exposure of glycoprotein receptors of higher affinity, resulting in further fibrinogen binding and to adherence of additional platelets and formation of a platelet aggregate. The response may be enhanced by ADP secreted from the adherent platelets and by activation of calcium-sensitive phospholipase A_2 with resultant generation of thromboxane A_2.

REFERENCES

1. SALZMAN, E. W. & E. W. MERRILL. 1987. Interaction of blood with artificial surfaces. *In* Hemostasis and Thrombosis. 2d edit. R. W. Colman, J. Hirsh, V. J. Marder & E. W. Salzman, Eds.: 1335–1347. J. B. Lippincott. Philadelphia.
2. CLAGETT, G. P. Artificial devices in clinical practice. *In* Hemostasis and Thrombosis. 2d edit. R. W. Colman, J. Hirsh, V. J. Marder & E. W. Salzman, Eds. J. B. Lippincott. Philadelphia. pp. 1348–1365.
3. BAIER, R. E. & R. C. DUTTON. 1969. Initial events in interactions of blood with a foreign surface. J. Biomed. Mater. Res. **3:** 191–206.
4. SCARBOROUGH, D. E., R. G. MASON, P. G. DALLDORF & K. M. BRINKHOUS. 1969. Morphological manifestations of blood-solid interfacial reactions: A scanning and transmission electron microscopic study. Lab. Invest. **20:** 164–169.
5. PACKHAM, M. A., G. EVANS, M. F. GLYNN & J. F. MUSTARD. 1969. The effect of plasma proteins on the interaction of platelets with glass surfaces. J. Lab. Clin. Med. **73:** 686–697.
6. ZUCKER, M. B. & L. VROMAN. 1969. Platelet adhesion induced by fibrinogen adsorbed onto glass. Soc. Exp. Biol. Med. **131:** 318–320.
7. BRASH, J. L. & S. UNIYAL. 1979. Dependence of albumin-fibrinogen simple and competitive adsorption on surface properties of biomaterials. J. Polym. Sci. **66:** 377–389.
8. YOUNG, B. R., L. K. LAMBRECHT, D. F. MOSHER & S. L. COOPER. 1982. Plasma proteins: Their role in initiating platelet and fibrin deposition on biomaterials. Adv. Chem. Ser. **199:** 317–350.
9. NYILAS, E. & T. H. CHIU. 1978. Artificial surface/sorbed protein structure/hemocompatibility correlations. Artif. Organs. **2**(Suppl.): 56–62.
10. LEE, R. G., C. ADAMSON & S. W. KIM. 1974. Competitive adsorption plasma proteins onto polymer surfaces. Thromb. Res. **4:** 485–490.
11. HORBETT, T. A. & A. S. HOFFMAN. 1975. Bovine plasma protein adsorption onto radiation-grafted hydrogels based on hydroxyethyl methacrylate and N-vinyl-pyrrolidone. *In* Applied Chemistry at Protein Interfaces. R. E. Baier, Ed.: 230. American Chemical Society. Washington, D.C.
12. BRASH, J. L. 1977. Hydrophobic polymer surfaces and their interactions with blood. Ann. N.Y. Acad. Sci. **283:** 356–371.
13. CROSS, M. J. 1964. Effect of fibrinogen on the aggregation of platelets by adenosine diphosphate. Thromb. Diath. Haemorrh. **12:** 524–527.
14. NIEWIAROWSKI, S., A. Z. BUDZYNSKI & B. LIPINSKI. 1977. Significance of the intact polypeptide chains of human fibrinogen in ADP-induced platelet aggregation. Blood **49:** 635–644.
15. MARGUERIE, G. A., T. S. EDGINGTON & E. F. PLOW. 1980. Interaction of fibrinogen with its platelet receptor as part of a multistep reaction in ADP-induced platelet aggregation. J. Biol. Chem. **255:** 154–161.
16. PEERSCHKE, E. I., M. B. ZUCKER, R. A. GRANT, J. J. EGAN & M. M. JOHNSON. 1980. Correlation between fibrinogen binding to human platelets and platelet aggregability. Blood **55:** 841–847.
17. PLOW, E., A. H. SROUJI, D. MEYER, G. MARGUERIE & M. H. GINSBERG. 1984. Evidence that three adhesive proteins interact with a common recognition site on activated platelets. J. Biol. Chem. **259:** 5388–5391.
18. KORNECKI, E., S. NIEWIAROSKI, T. A. MORIMELLI & M. KLOCZEWIAK. 1981. Effects of chymotrypsin and adenosine diphosphate on the exposure of fibrinogen receptors on normal human and Glanzmann's thrombosthenic platelets. J. Biol. Chem. **256:** 5696–5701.
19. PEERSCHKE, E. I. & D. K. GALANAKIS. 1983. Binding of fibrinogen to ADP treated platelets. J. Lab. Clin. Med. **101:** 453–460.
20. MARGUERIE, G. A., E. F. PLOW & T. S. EDGINGTON. 1979. Human platelets possess an inducible and saturable receptor specific for fibrinogen. J. Biol. Chem. **254:** 5357–5363.
21. BENNETT, J. S. & G. VILAIRE. 1979. Exposure of platelet fibrinogen receptors by ADP and epinephrine. J. Clin. Invest. **64:** 1393–1401.

22. MUSTARD, J. F., M. A. PACKHAM, R. L. KINLOUGH-RATHBONE, D. W. PERRY & E. REGOECZI. 1978. Fibrinogen and ADP-induced platelet aggregation. Blood **52:** 453–466.
23. CHIU, T. H., E. NYILAS & L. R. TURCOTTE. 1978. Microcalorimetric and electrophoretic studies of protein sorption from plasma. Trans. Am. Soc. Artif. Intern. Organs **24:** 389–402.
24. TOMIKAWA, M., M. IWAMOTO, P. OLSSON, S. SODERMAN & B. BLOMBACK. 1980. On the platelet-fibrinogen interaction. Thromb. Res. **19:** 869–876.
25. CHAN, B. & J. L. BRASH. 1979. Interactions of human fibrinogen with glass surface. Thromb. Hemostas. **42:** 132.
26. BRIER-RUSSELL, D., E. W. SALZMAN, J. LINDON, R. HANDIN, E. W. MERRILL, A. K. DINCER & J. S. WU. 1981. In vitro assessment of interaction of blood with model surfaces: Acrylates and methacrylates. J. Colloid Interface Sci. **81:** 311–318.
27. LINDON, J. N., R. RODVIEN, D. BRIER, R. GREENBERG, E. MERRILL & E. W. SALZMAN. 1978. In vitro assessment of interaction of blood with model surfaces. J. Lab. Clin. Med. **92:** 904–915.
28. LINDON, J. N., G. MCMANAMA, L. KUSHNER, E. W. MERRILL & E. W. SALZMAN. 1986. Does the conformation of adsorbed fibrinogen dictate platelet interactions with artificial surfaces? Blood **68:** 355–362.
29. FRAKER, P. J. & J. C. SPECK. 1978. Protein and cell membrane iodinations with a sparingly soluble chloroamide, 1,3,4,6-tetrachloro-3a,6a-diphenylglycoluril. Biochem. Biophys. Res. Commun. **80:** 849–857.
30. KNIGHT, L. C., A. Z. BUDZYNSKI & S. A. OLEXA. 1981. Radiolabeling of fibrinogen using the Iodogen technique. Thromb. Haemostas. **46:** 593–596.
31. WANG, T. 1977. Human platelet morphology and ADP-induced aggregation response: Effect of plasma constitutents and apyrase. Ph.D. thesis, Massachusetts Institute of Technology. Cambridge, MA.
32. VROMAN, L., A. L. ADAMS, G. C. FISCHER & P. C. MUNOZ. 1980. Interaction of high molecular weight kininogen, factor XII, and fibrinogen in plasma at interfaces. Blood **55:** 156–159.
33. JACOBS, S. & P. CUATRECASAS. 1977. The mobile receptor hypothesis for cell membrane receptor action. Trends Biochem. Sci. December: 280–282.
34. RINK, T. J., S. W. SMITH & R. Y. TSIEN. 1982. Cytoplasmic free calcium in human platelets: Calcium thresholds and calcium-independent activation for shape change and secretion. FEBS Lett. **148:** 21–26.
35. JOHNSON, P. C., J. A. WARE, P. B. CLIVEDEN, M. SMITH, A. M. DVORAK & E. W. SALZMAN. 1985. Measurement of ionized calcium in blood platelets with the photoprotein aequorin. J. Biol. Chem. **260:** 2069–2076.
36. WARE, J. A., P. C. JOHNSON & E. W. SALZMAN. 1986. The effect of common agonists on cytoplasmic ionized calcium concentration in platelets: Measurement with Quin2 and aequorin. J. Clin. Invest. **77:** 878–886.
37. HORNICK, C. L. & F. KARUSH. 1969. The interaction of hapten-coupled bacteriophage OX174 with antihapten antibody. Israel J. Med. Sci. **5:** 163–170.
38. CROTHERS, D. M. & H. METZGER. 1972. The influence of polyvalency on the binding properties of antibodies. Immunochemistry **9:** 341–357.
39. MCMANAMA, G., J. N. LINDON, M. KLOCZEWIAK, M. A. SMITH, J. A. WARE, J. HAWIGER, E. W. MERRILL & E. W. SALZMAN. 1986. Platelet aggregation by fibrinogen polymers crosslinked across the E domain. Blood **68:** 363–371.
40. AGAM, G., R. LURIA, O. SHOHAT, A. DVILANSKY, U. SELIGSOHN & A. LIVNE. 1985. Lysine binding to activated human platelets and its similarity to fibrinogen binding. Biochim. Biophys. Acta **847:** 293–300.
41. HAWIGER, J., S. TIMMONS, M. D. KLOCZEWIAK, D. D. STRONG & R. DOOLITTLE. 1982. Gamma and alpha chains of human fibrinogen possess sites reactive with human platelet receptors. Proc. Natl. Acad. Sci. U.S.A. **79:** 2068–2071.
42. KLOCZEWIAK, M., S. TIMMONS & J. HAWIGER. 1982. Localization of a site interacting with human platelet receptor on carboxy terminal segment of human fibrinogen gamma chain. Biochem. Biophys. Res. Comm. **107:** 181–187.
43. KLOCZEWIAK, M., S. TIMMONS & J. HAWIGER. 1983. Recognition site for the platelet

receptor is present on the 15-residue carboxy terminal fragment of the gamma chain of human fibrinogen and is not involved in the fibrin polymerization reaction. Thromb. Res. **29:** 249–255.

44. Kloczewiak, M., S. Timmons, T. T. Lukas & J. Hawiger. 1984. Platelet receptor recognition site on human fibrinogen. Synthesis and structure-function relationship of peptides corresponding to the carboxy terminal segment of the gamma chain. Biochemistry **23:** 1767–1774.
45. Porter, R. R. 1959. The hydrolysis of rabbit gamma globulin and antibodies with crystalline papain. Biochem. J. **73:** 119–126.
46. Nisonoff, A., F. C. Wissler & L. N. Lipman. 1960. Properties of the major component of a peptide digest of rabbit antibody. Science **132:** 1770–1771.
47. Luscher, E. F., S. L. Pfueller & P. Massini. 1973. Platelet aggregation by large molecules. Ser. Haemat. **6:** 382–391.
48. Coller, B. S., E. I. Peerschke, L. E. Scudder & C. A. Sullivan. 1983. A murine monoclonal antibody that completely blocks the binding of fibrinogen to platelets produces a thrombasthenic-like state in normal platelets and binds to glycoproteins IIb and/or IIIa. J. Clin. Invest **72:** 325–338.
49. Packham, M. A., M. A. Guccione, J. P. Greenberg, R. L. Kinlough-Rathbone & J. F. Mustard. 1977. Release of ^{14}C-serotonin during initial platelet changes induced by thrombin, collagen, or A23187. Blood **50:** 915–926.
50. Bennett, J. S., G. Vilaire, R. F. Colman & R. W. Colman. 1981. Localization of human platelet membrane-associated actomyosis using the affinity label 5′-p-fluorosulfonylbenzoyl adenosine. J. Biol. Chem. **256:** 1185–1190.
51. Stibbe, J. & H. Holmsen. 1977. Effect of sodium azide on platelet function. Thromb. Haemorrh. **38:** 1042.
52. Verhoeven, A. J. M., M. E. Mommersteeg & J. W. N. Akkerman. 1985. Balanced contribution of glycolytic and adenylate pool in supply of metabolic energy in platelets. J. Biol. Chem. **260:** 2621–2624.
53. Brass, L. F. 1985. Ca^{2+} transport across the platelet plasma membrane. J. Biol. Chem. **260:** 2231–2236.

Distinctions and Correspondences among Surfaces Contacting Blood

EDWARD W. MERRILL

Department of Chemical Engineering
Massachusetts Institute of Technology
Cambridge, Massachusetts 02139

Those working on the front lines of molecular biology and in particular those concerned with "downstream processing" by affinity methods to separate proteins like interferon and tissue plasminogen activator from nondesired species have made us increasingly aware of the very specific ways[a] in which proteins can "recognize" and adhere to surfaces by special affinity ligand bonding, for example IgG onto bound protein A, and of the less specific ways, as suggested by the common phrase "nonspecific binding." In biotechnological downstream processing it may be possible to tolerate some nonspecific binding on affinity surfaces if the yield of specifically bound material is high and "pure," meaning that cyclic changes from coupling to decoupling solutions release intact the desired biopolymer while not releasing much nonspecifically bound biopolymer.

In the context of this symposium, we do not have open to us the possibility of wondering what the effects of changing the nature of the solution (drop pH to 3, raise NaCl to 1.0 molar, change to 2 normal urea, etc.) on the release of adsorbed proteins will be: we are stuck with blood plasma at pH 7.4 and ionic strength around 300 milliosmoles, and fixed limits of anions and cations.

Therefore the central question to us becomes, not in general what happens when some biopolymer in some mixture of biopolymers in some medium is in contact with some surface, but in particular what happens when the biopolymers of blood—the proteins and the enzyme clotting factors—in the plasma milieu come in contact with surfaces.

What does a biopolymer "do" upon contact with the surface? Rebound without change? Adsorb, but sparsely? Adsorb and form a close-packed layer? Adsorb and change conformation so as to become more active?

Thus whether or how plasma proteins adsorb to a surface becomes a central issue in addressing the problem of whether thrombosis ultimately occurs via the intrinsic system or via platelets.[b] In *simplest* terms there are only three scenarios:

1. The surface presented to blood adsorbs no biopolymers; platelets are not adsorbed or activated, thus thrombosis does not occur.
2. The surface actively adsorbs a "bland" biopolymer, albumin for instance, to the exclusion of all else, and thus presents to the blood a surface that does not activate platelets or set off the intrinsic clotting system.
3. The surface indiscriminately, or discriminately, adsorbs biopolymers, one or more of which when adsorbed cause platelet accumulation or trigger the intrinsic system.

[a]These concepts are discussed in ref. 1, especially in chapter 5.
[b]These concepts are discussed in refs. 2 and 4, in chap. 9 of ref. 5, and in chap. 8 of ref. 6.

Beyond these three simple possibilities, one must accept a fourth, that of the biologically active surface. This could mean a permeable surface from which heparin or prostaglandins are slowly released, thereby actively blocking steps in the thrombotic processes, or surfaces to which biologically active polymers are bound, notably (but not necessarily only) the active pentamer of heparin.

By *surface*[c] we mean that which is accessible to the biopolymer probes of blood. Therefore the thickness of the surface that controls behavior can be of the order of a few tens of angstrom units, and can be completely different from the bulk interior not accessed by the biopolymer.

It is in this conceptual framework that we reflect on categorizing schemes commonly considered relevant to surfaces that are used to collect materials, especially organic polymer materials, into families of "like" things. (TABLE 1).

According to the scheme presented in TABLE 1, all metals and all ceramics are solid and "hard" (high modulus). None fail to adsorb biopolymers when exposed to blood. Only chain macromolecules have the capacity to be "liquid," *i.e.,* to have their molecular substance in active Brownian motion at 37°C at a surface, with the consequences that (1) they are permeable, at least to small molecules, (2) they can interact with plasma biopolymers by adapting their structure (pillow effect), and (3) because of their liquid state the energy of adsorption might be less than a "solid" surface of the same composition. In the list of "liquid" materials we note two that seem to have a low degree of adsorption: PEG and the PTMO soft segment sequence of segmented polyurethanes (SPU). None of those in the list of hard surfaces, which would include crystalline PE and glassy polycarbonate, polystyrene, poly(methyl methacrylate), and polysulfone, is of low adsorptivity. Pyrolytic carbon is a special case: it appears under some high flow conditions to achieve a stable layer of protein.

TABLE 1. "Liquid" vs. "Solid" Surfaces

"Liquid"	"Solid"
poly(vinyl alcohol) (PVA), hydrated	pyrolytic carbon
ethylene propylene rubber (EPR)	polycarbonate
polyacrylamide gel	polysulfone
agarose gel	poly(vinyl chloride) (PVC)
poly(hydroxyethyl methacrylate) (PHEMA)	poly(methyl methacrylate) (PMMA)
soft segment of polyurethane (SPU)	hard segment of polyurethane
silicone rubber (PDMS)	silica
grafted alkanes	polyethylene, crystalline (PE)
poly(ethylene oxide) gel (PEO)	poly(ethylene oxide) crystalline (PEO)

Conclusion: Most "hard" (polycrystalline, glassy, metal, ceramic) surfaces adsorb biopolymers, and thrombosis eventuates.[d]

Is the surface "hydrophilic" or "hydrophobic"?[e] (See TABLE 2.) "Hydrophilicity" of polymers can be evaluated by combining the results of two experimental methods: interfacial tension against water, and swelling in water. If water persists in sitting on the test surface as "sessile drops" with a contact angle greater than 90°, and if insignificant swelling occurs, at equilibrium, the material is de facto hydrophobic (*e.g.,* PTFE, C_8 to C_{18} grafted alkanes, ethylene propylene rubber and polystyrene). I

[c] See the extensive discussion in ref. 3.
[d] Coating these surfaces puts them in a different category of course.
[e] Widely discussed in the literature. See ref. 2 and especially ref. 5.

emphasize that this must occur at equilibrium. Take, for example, PHEMA. When dried thoroughly water sits on it as a sessile drop and it expands slowly, but at equilibrium in a soft contact lens it holds around 50% water and a water drop readily spreads on it.

Of the hydrophobic polymers listed (and all others that could be listed) protein adsorption always ensues by hydrophobic[f] interaction and except in one case, thrombogenesis occurs, earlier or later, unless anticoagulants are used. The exception may be the surface to which albumin is densely bound to the exclusion of other plasma biopolymers, and thus also the alkane surfaces that bind albumin (studied by Eberhart[15]).

The remaining hydrophilic surfaces listed are all hydrogen bonding, but with widely different biopolymer adsorption properties.

Conclusion: Hydrophobic surfaces are generally adsorptive, and thus "bad," but hydrophilic surfaces are not in general nonadsorptive, thus not in general "good." The performances of these surfaces vary widely. Thus we must look more closely into "hydrophilicity" and its origins.

What makes a polymer surface hydrophilic? The synthetic polyelectrolytes, such as sulfonated styrene divinyl benzene, quarternary ammonium benzyl derivatives of

TABLE 2. "Hydrophilic" vs. "Hydrophobic" Surfaces

Hydrophilic	Hydrophobic
silica	silicone rubber
poly(vinyl alcohol)	ethylene propylene rubber
polyacrylamide (PAM)	polystyrene (PS)
agarose	polytetrafluoroethylene (PTFE)
poly(hydroxyethyl methacrylate)	polyethylene
cellophane	polypropylene
polyelectrolytes	
poly(ethylene oxide)	
poly(vinyl pyrrolidone) (PVP)	

the same, and cross-linked polyacrylic acid, are all "wet" and are by the criteria proposed hydrophilic. If not strongly cross-linked, they swell in water.

The synthetic polyanions, such as poly(styrene sulfonate), which should repel all plasma biopolymers if one believes that their negative charge and pH 7.4 is uniformly distributed over the biopolymer surface, are actively thrombogenic, as are the synthetic polycationic surfaces. These facts force us to accept the mosaic nature of charge on the biopolymer: there are more negative than positive charges (more fixed anions than fixed cations) but they are so arranged that cationic clusters on the biopolymer can bind to anionic surfaces, and vice versa (TABLE 3).[g]

Whole heparin, heparin fragments, and heparin-like synthetic materials, though polyelectrolytes, are studied for their activity toward antithrombin III and thus their ability to shift the kinetics of the reactions of thrombin and antithrombin III, thereby thwarting activation of fibrinogen. Such bound polyions cannot be said to be nonbinding to biopolymers. To the contrary, when effective they bind antithrombin III in a special way. Before dismissing polyelectrolytes out of hand, it is possible to imagine hydrophilic polymers containing some fixed ionic groups whose hydrophilicity depends

[f]See ref. 1, chapter 5, for a particularly good discussion.
[g]Again, refer to ref. 1, especially chapter 5.

TABLE 3. Electrically Charged Surfaces

Anionic Group	Cationic Group
sulfonate carboxyl sulfate	prim., sec., tert., quat. amine
poly(styrene sulfonate) (PSS)	poly(vinyl benzyl trimethyl ammonium chloride) (PVBTMAC) diethylaminoethyl cellulose (DEAE cellulose)

on hydrogen bonding interactions (the only other possible mode). The issue of hydrogen bonding deserves close scrutiny (TABLE 4).

The materials above the line in TABLE 4 are hydrogels, significantly swollen by water. The four below the line are obviously not hydrogels. In this list the mode of action by hydrogen bonding is indicated: the polymer may provide from its structure a hydrogen bonding proton capable of finding a receptor on a biopolymer, or it may provide an acceptor to which the proton of the biopolymer can bond, or both.

Polyurea shows both modes; it binds plasma biopolymers and is thrombogenic, as is polyvinyl alcohol, a hydrogen bond donor. PAM and agarose are used respectively for gel electrophoresis and support for gel chromatography, and are believed to have modest to low "nonspecific" bonding of biopolymers. Of the entire list the polyethers deserve most scrutiny because the virtually nonswellable PTMO, uncross-linked PPO containing 4% water at equilibrium, and PEO (PEG), which can swell to any degree in water depending on cross-link density, are all relatively nonadsorptive of plasma biopolymers. PEO (PEG) is by far the most nonadsorptive of any known polymer.[7,8] These polyether polymers can only act as H-bond acceptors. That this property alone is not sufficient is illustrated by PDMS. Only if spread as a very thin layer from chloroform solution onto water can water gain access to the siloxane, readily hydrolyzing it. On the other hand the silanol H of silica avidly binds to PDMS and to all plasma biopolymers at normal pH (7.4). Thus normally the surface of PDMS appears to a biopolymer as a layer of methyl, and therefore is hydrophobic.

Of the polymers that are hydrophilic because they are hydrogen bonding, PEG[7–9] as a hydrogel stands out above the others as closely approaching the condition of nonadsorption of plasma biopolymers. PNVP, like PEG, acts only as H-bond acceptor and is soluble without limit in water unless cross-linked, but adsorbs biopolymers

TABLE 4. Hydrogen Bonding: Donors and Acceptors

	H-Bond Donor	H-Bond Acceptor
Polyureas	>NH	>C=O
Polyurethanes	>NH	>C=O, —O—
Polyacrylamide		>C=O
Poly(vinyl alcohol)	—OH	
Cellophane	—OH	>C=O
Poly(vinyl pyrrol)		>C=O
Agarose	—OH	—O—
Poly(ethylene oxide) terminal	—OH (rare)	—O—
Silicone rubber		≡Si—O—Si≡
Silica	≡Si—OH	≡Si—O—Si≡
Poly(propylene oxide) (PPO)		—O—
Poly(tetramethylene oxide) (PTMO)		—O—

significantly. Agarose, like cellophane, is a polysaccharide with both donor and acceptor capability, but is considerably less adsorptive than cellophane. Thus we look for other similarities and differences that might account for these different responses. We can ask, for example, is the surface homogeneous or heterogeneous on a "colloidal" scale, *i.e.*, over distances of tens to hundreds of angstrom units? If the polymer contains two types of available surface, could a plasma biopolymer "sit" on one type or the other entirely, or would it have to straddle the two types?

All of the homopolymers listed in TABLE 5 (PE, PP, PAN, cellophane) have a crystalline phase as well as an amorphous phase, and nothing a priori excludes the possibility of the existence of crystalline material at the biopolymer surface. To the proposition that every crystalline polymer adsorbs plasma biopolymer, there appears to be no contrary evidence.[h] Even PEO, as a crystalline substance, significantly attracts platelets[10] and therefore must have adsorbed biopolymer. Of the list of heterogeneous surfaces (on a colloidal scale) the segmented polyurethanes are the most interesting because of the detailed studies that have been performed to determine what is at the surface. From these studies we know that the hard segment of segmented polyether polyureas as well as segmented polyether polyurethanes actively adsorb plasma biopolymer and thereafter accumulate platelets, whereas surfaces of these SPU in

TABLE 5. Homogeneity of the Surface: "Colloidal Scale"

Homogeneous	Heterogeneous
ethylene propylene rubber	polyethylene
poly(ethylene oxide) (gel)	polypropylene
	soft segment of polyurethane
	cellophane
	block copolymers
	polyacrylonitrile (PAN)

which only the polyether is found adsorb far less. Indeed if the polyether is PEG, the surface acts like a PEG hydrogel and adsorbs virtually no plasma biopolymer.[10]

Unplasticized PVC as well as PAN (as Orlon®, for example) adsorb plasma biopolymer strongly, but nothing new is to be learned since both are crystalline and glassy, and therefore solid, at 37°C. (Plasticized PVC is a completely different case since the "surface" is primarily a liquid, viz., the plasticizing solvent is usually 2-ethyl hexyl phthalate.)

Conclusion: It is impossible to demonstrate that any surface heterogeneous *at the colloidal scale does not adsorb plasma biopolymer. Amorphous sepharose (cross-linked) is far less adsorptive than cellophane; PEO as an amorphous hydrogel shows negligible adsorption, but does adsorb as a crystal. PDMS, although homogeneous, shows strong hydrophobic adsorption (already noted).*

So we turn to a finer scale of heterogeneity-homogeneity (TABLE 6). Now the question is whether, on a scale measured in a few angstrom units, we can learn something from heterogeneity of molecular groups. As a baseline consider PTFE and PE: all units are identical. Polypropylene consists of only two kinds, $-CH_2-$ and $-CH(CH_3)-$, as do the random copolymers of ethylene and propylene (EPR). This

[h] Note again the extensive data collected in ref. 3.

TABLE 6. Homogeneity of the Surface: Molecular-Atomic Scale

Homogeneous	Heterogeneous
polytetrafluoroethylene	poly(vinyl pyrrolidone)
polyethylene	poly(vinyl alcohol)
polypropylene	polyacrylamide
ethylene propylene rubber	polyelectrolytes
grafted alkanes	silicone rubber
	agarose
	poly(ethylene oxide)
	poly(propylene oxide)
	poly(tetramethylene oxide)

list could extend indefinitely but it is impossible to find any polymer that is homogeneous at this level and does not adsorb plasma biopolymer significantly. Only those having a surface of long alkane chains, which preferentially adsorb albumin, seem promising.[10] As we turn to those polymers in which two or more kinds of molecular groups are found, the list includes the polyelectrolytes already considered (whose biopolymer adsorption can be ascribed to ion pairing), PDMS (adsorption by hydrophobic interaction), and cellophane (whose crystalline content and H-bond donor capacity are probably most responsible for biopolymer binding). In comparing the low binding agarose with the high binding cellophane, we note that crystallinity is absent in agarose and H-bond donor capacity is reduced by cross-linking. H-bond-accepting ether linkages have a higher occurrence than in cellophane. Agarose represents a mixture of -C-O-C-, isolated -CH_2-, and -COH groups on a scale so fine that hydrophobic association (to the -CH_2-) is thwarted. By contrast poly(*N*-vinyl pyrrolidone) (PVP) has a sequence of -CH_2- units on the main chain next to four methylene units in the side ring, thus a sequence potentially capable of hydrophobic interaction despite the hydrophilicity of the amide group. Hydrogen bonding to the $>C = O$ of this amide group must be somewhat restricted in comparison with the accessibility of the ether oxygen of PEG to three molecules of water.

Comparison of PTMO, a principal component of medically useful polyurethane, with PNVP and with PDMS suggest that accessibility to, and ease of mixing with, the biopolymer in addition to the relative size of the hydrophobic part are important. Thus while the tetramethylene sequence of PTMO might involve hydrophobic adsorption, the interruption by -O- at each end makes this interaction far less possible than with the -CH_3 of PDMS or the ring of PVP. PEG represents that remarkable balance on a fine scale of hydrophobic -CH_2-CH_2- with hydrophilic -O- units, combined with noncrystallinity and hydration that offers very little to a plasma biopolymer to bind to. If it is to be hydrogen bond acceptance, the water next to the ether oxygen must be displaced. On the basis of fine scale mixture, the alternating -CH_2- and -O- units of

TABLE 7. Transformed Surfaces: Surface Composition Different from Bulk Composition

INTENTIONAL	
Ion plasma	add: $>C{=}O$, $>CF$
Radiation	add: grafted polymer
Activated (tresyl Cl, CDI)	add: heparin, biopolymer
ACCIDENTAL	
Heat, air, process	oxidized lubricant, "blooming" agents

Delrin® (polyformaldehyde) would be even better were it not for the fact that the material is hard, solid, and crystalline.

Finally we should reconsider polymers with transformed surfaces (TABLE 7). Among the accidentally transformed surfaces one has only to mention the spinning, drawing, or mold release lubricants found on thermally processed polymers, which are added internally in processing and not meant to improve the surface for some alternate use. Contact with protective wrappings will sometimes result in transfer of an ingredient in the wrapping to the polymer intended for biomaterial service. Nothing further need be said, except to note that the surface must be examined by XPS for the existence of such contaminants prior to evaluation of contact with plasma biopolymers.

The intentionally transformed surfaces[i] are more interesting. These are produced in a variety of ways, for example, "hydrophilization" of polystyrene culture dishes by exposure to an oxygen ion plasma, resulting in partial coverage of the surface by carbonyl and other H-bond participants. A variety of atoms may be added by ion plasmas:[12,13] amines from ammonia gas, fluoride from fluorine gas, etc. Usually some residue of the original polymer remains, so that the surface is mixed. Indeed this act may be turned around to produce a very clean surface of the original material by etching in an ion plasma of pure argon, which ablates the adventitious material noted above.

Radiation, either UV or high-energy electrons, can cause free radical grafting of a desired monomer to the surface, creating polymeric chains of the monomer and completely obliterating the original surface. *N*-vinyl pyrrolidone is the case of a monomer that can be readily grafted to a wide variety of supports. Although it leads to hydrophilic surfaces, it has the adsorptive properties toward plasma biopolymers of pure cross-linked PVP. Macromers such as PEG esters of methacrylic acid can be grafted by radical initiation (UV, electron, chemical) to a variety of mechanically useful support polymers (*e.g.*, PVC), totally transforming the surface to a layer seen by the protein as completely different. The studies of Nagaoka and associates[14] offer a particularly good example.

Finally we should consider more carefully those transformed surfaces that arise by "activation" of a surface group and subsequent covalent binding of a biopolymer. "Activation" of hydroxyl groups can be accomplished by hydrogen bromide, carbonyl diimidazole, and tresyl chloride, to name but three. The biopolymer is usually bound by one of its amine residues. Among common examples are agarose supports on which the bound biopolymer is an affinity ligand, for example an antibody IgG. These surfaces are used in affinity chromatograph packed bed because in general the affinity ligand can harvest out of a mixture a desired species while the support has relatively low nonspecific binding. In the context of biomaterials for contact with plasma, one looks to covalently fixed biopolymers that could function by binding a layer of albumin so densely as to prevent access of the plasma components that are connected with intrinsic clotting or platelet activation. An alternative would be to bind the biopolymer heparin but at a sufficiently low density and on long molecular leashes so that it maintains high activity toward antithrombin III and therefore can inactivate thrombin if antithrombin III is present. Poly(ethylene glycol) hydrogels constitute an excellent support, and provide a surface of bound heparin having tenfold greater activity than a surface of the same heparin bound at the same concentration to PVA.

To conclude this review of correspondences and differences, we see no clear single path of guidance but certain trends, notably that the surfaces having lowest protein

[i] Covered in many texts and references. See, for example, ref. 11.

binding and potentially useful from that point of view are not crystalline, not glassy, not hydrophobic, not molecularly homogeneous, but rather amorphous, solvated by water, nonelectrolytic, and H-bond accepting. Surfaces that bind protein include those that contain mobile hydrophobic groups (methyl, alkane chains). The latter, exploited by Eberhart,[15] attract albumin preferentially. These may be useful.

We should always keep in mind that nature has designed some of her plasma biopolymers to sit down on surfaces recognized as foreign and thereafter,[j] by one mode or another, calls for reinforcements, including platelets. In view of the recognitive sites on these plasma biopolymers—their very particular spatial arrangements—it is difficult to imagine any synthetic material surface that could escape recognition as foreign. In this respect PEG appears to keep a "low profile" for reasons alluded to before, and thus deserves continuing attention.

REFERENCES

1. WATSON, J. D., N. H. HOPKINS, J. W. ROBERTS, J. A. SEITZ & A. M. WEINER. 1984. Molecular Biology of the Gene, vol. 2. 4th edit. Benjamin/Cummings Publishing Company. Menlo Park, CA.
2. SALZMAN, E. W. & E. W. MERRILL. 1987. *In* Hemostasis and Thrombosis. 2d edit. R. W. Colman, J. Hirsh, V. J. Marder & E. W. Salzman, Eds. J. B. Lippincott. Philadelphia.
3. ANDRADE, J., Ed. 1985. Surface and Interfacial Aspects of Biomedical Polymers, Vol. 1: Surface Chemistry and Physics. Plenum. New York.
4. ANDRADE, J., Ed. 1985. Surface and Interfacial Aspects of Biomedical Polymers, Vol. 2: Protein Adsorption. Plenum. New York. NY.
5. HASTINGS, G. W. & P. DUCHEYNE, Eds. 1984. Macromolecular Biomaterials. CRC Press. Boca Raton, FL.
6. BORETOS, J. W. & M. EDEN, Eds. 1984. Contemporary Biomaterials. Noyes Publication. Park Ridge, NJ.
7. MERRILL, E. W. & E. W. SALZMAN. 1982. Polyethylene oxide as a biomaterial. J. Am. Soc. Artif. Int. Organs **6:** 60.
8. MERRILL, E. W., E. W. SALZMAN, K. A. DENNISON, S.-W. TAY & R. W. PEKALA. 1986. Nonadsorptive hydrogels for blood contact. *In* Progress in Artificial Organs 1985. Y. Nosé, C. Kjellstrand & P. Ivanovich, Eds. ISAO Press. Cleveland.
9. LING-CHENG, Y., S. A. DARST & C. R. ROBERTSON. 1987. Bovine serum albumin adsorption and desorption rates on solid surfaces with varying surface properties. J. Colloid Interface Sci. In press.
10. MERRILL, E. W., V. S. D. COSTA, E. W. SALZMAN, D. BRIER-RUSSELL, L. KUCHNER, D. F. WAUGH, G. TRUDEL III, S. STOPPER & V. VITALE. 1982. A critical study of segmented polyurethanes. Adv. Chem. Ser. **199.**
11. REMPP, P. & E. W. MERRILL. 1986. Polymer Synthesis. Chap. 10. Huthig & Wepf. Heidelberg.
12. SHEN, M., Ed. 1976. Plasma Chemistry of Polymers. Marcel Dekker. New York.
13. CLARK, D. T., A. DILKS & D. SHUTTLEWORTH. 1972. The Application of Plasmas to the Synthesis and Surface Modification of Polymers. *In* Polymer Surfaces. D. T. Clark & W. J. Feast, Eds. John Wiley & Sons. New York.
14. NAGOAKA, S., Y. MORI, H. TAKUCHI, K. YOKOTA, H. TANZAWA & S. NISHUMI. 1983. Polymer Preprints **24:** 67.
15. EBERHART, R. C., M. S. MUNRO, G. O. BRIDGES, P. V. KULKARNI & W. J. FRY. 1984. Albumin retention on C_{18} alkylated vascular grafts. *In* Biomaterials '84: Transactions. J. M. Anderson, Ed.: 97. Society for Biomaterials. Birmingham, AL.

[j] See the discussion in chapter 1 of ref. 1, and in refs. 2 and 4.

Summary

Artificial Surfaces

S. A. BARENBERG

E. I. du Pont de Nemours & Company
Wilmington, Delaware 19898

This session offered a wide-ranging investigation of the problems associated with using artificial substances, specifically polymers, for vascular prosthetic grafts. Given the variety of techniques and agents used to modify polymeric biomaterial surfaces, the session provided both an evaluation and a valuable overview of blood-contacting synthetic surface technology. *In vitro* and *in vivo* studies of surface preparations were reviewed. In addition, the papers contributed to a more complete understanding of the complexities of thrombosis and embolization when plasma reacts to artificial substances.

Many of the physical properties of polymers make them excellent candidates for vascular prosthetics. In practice, however, polymers create an environment hostile to blood, causing both thrombosis and embolization. In order to prevent such negative effects, prosthetics must be surfaced or seeded before implantation. At present a good surface either does not adsorb biopolymers, or it adsorbs only one "bland" biopolymer, like albumin. Otherwise, the adsorption process between plasma and the surface activates platelets and the intrinsic clotting system. We can look forward to development of a biologically active surface that blocks the thrombotic process. Research directed towards this goal will go beyond simple consideration of the stability of the surface substance. It will also take into account the speed with which the surface encourages adherence of endolethial cells, and the morphology of those cells.

Session panelists examined a number of existing and potential artificial surface substances and preparation techniques. These included use of the basement membrane surface of the human amnion annealed to Dacron, use of polyethylene glycol (PEG), end-point-attached heparin, albumin, fibronectin (in conjunction with endolethial seeding), endolethial cell seeding itself, and preclotting with the patient's blood prior to implantation (with or without a surface coating on the polymer). The existence of so many surface technologies is evidence of the complexity of the processes of thrombosis and embolization when plasma contacts foreign substances. It also demonstrates our lack of understanding of them. We know that some plasma biopolymers will bond and accumulate (clot) on foreign surfaces and therefore will recognize any synthetic surface as foreign. The chemistry of why and how they do that, however, remains quite unclear.

Two session reports in particular offered promising insight into the chemistry of the interaction of plasma and polymer prosthetics. Salzman *et al.* discussed the role of fibrinogen in activating platelet aggregation. Their work suggests that fibrinogen may bind calcium and in turn trigger clotting. Andrade and Hlady, in their work with the "Big Twelve" (plasma protein components with a concentration greater than one milligram per milliliter), suggest that carbohydrate moieties may affect adsorption properties. They also suggest that lipoproteins may dominate the adsorption process, especially when in contact with mobile elastomeric polymer surfaces. However, further research on the structure and characteristics of each involved protein is necessary to understand plasma adsorption.

The session also considered the technology available for studying blood protein adsorption and for determining the suitability of prosthetic materials in relationship to their end use. Promising work in the area of the adsorption process has been done at the Battelle Columbus Division using attenuated total reflectance Fourier transform infrared spectroscopy (ATR/FT-IR). FT-IR has few of the shortcomings of other methods presently utilized to study adsorption. With FT-IR it is possible to track the rate and amount of adsorption of a single protein, competitive adsorption from mixtures of known proteins, the course of protein adsorption from whole blood or plasma onto surfaces at its earliest phase, and a number of other processes that could not be tracked previously. Overall, FT-IR makes it possible to examine the time scale of events in far greater detail than the other methods researchers most frequently utilize. FT-IR makes it possible to spot changes in conformation caused by the adsorption process itself. Given that changes in proteins may be the controlling factor in the compatibility of blood with a foreign surface, this improvement over other methods of study is of no small importance.

R. E. Baier discussed the characterization methods used to qualify surface parameters in prosthetics and to determine whether these parameters meet minimum health and safety criteria. Dr. Beier argues that the characterization of the surface chemistry of biomaterials proposed for use in contact with blood is the most important requirement for understanding, predicting, and controlling the way these materials react to and interact with blood. Knowledge of these surface properties is of the utmost importance to the safe and proper end use of such biomaterials.

The widespread use of synthetic substances for vascular grafts, the relative "youth" of the process, and the equally relative newness of technologies to study blood adsorption all underscore the importance of research in the area of artificial vascular prosthetics. This session on artificial surfaces clarified many issues, brought together research reports on coating surfaces, and provided researchers with exposure to better methods for measuring blood adsorption. It was a step toward the unification of scientific and technical understanding of the complex interaction between blood and foreign surfaces.

The Fate of Fibrinogen following Adsorption at the Blood-Biomaterial Interface[a]

JOHN L. BRASH

Departments of Chemical Engineering and Pathology
McMaster University
Hamilton, Ontario L8S 4L7, Canada

INTRODUCTION

The formation of plasma protein layers occurs within seconds of blood contact with a foreign surface and thus "conditions" the surface for subsequent interactions, in particular cellular adhesion leading to thrombus formation. The sequence of blood-surface events is complex and although much has been learned in the recent past, our knowledge remains insufficient to permit such "control" of the sequence as would be implied in the realization of a nonthrombogenic surface.

FIGURE 1 shows a schematic of blood-surface events that incorporates the main features of current knowledge. Various sequences or "pathways" are distinguished, mainly as a pedagogic convenience. These pathways cannot be considered to be independent of each other, as indicated by the various interactions which occur between them. In addition the time interrelationships of the sequences are not at all clear.

Among the more recent findings a few should be mentioned specifically. It is now known that cellulosic hemodialysis membranes activate complement[1] and that this leads to transient white cell depletion. It seems unlikely that this phenomenon is relevant to thrombosis. Other types of surface are less active with respect to complement,[2] no doubt reflecting the different affinities of the surfaces for the complement proteins. Renewed recognition of the activation of the fibrinolytic system by surfaces, a phenomenon first reported several years ago,[3] has occurred[4] and has led to speculation that surfaces may possess fibrinolytic activity in the sense that they can catalyze the activation of plasminogen to plasmin independent of other activators or co-activators.

All the effects indicated in FIGURE 1 stem from the adsorbed protein layer previously mentioned. The composition of this layer is complex and is largely unknown. It is clear, however, that the layer composition varies from surface to surface and it seems likely that the differences in thrombogenicity among surfaces stem from protein layer differences. An aspect of the layer that has recently been recognized is its evolutive character. It has been hypothesized that proteins may replace one another at the surface in an ordered sequence,[5] and considerable evidence is now available to support at least a partial adoption of this view.[6-9] These transient phenomena have been designated the "Vroman effect" in recognition of Vroman's seminal contributions in

[a]Financial support of this work by the Medical Research Council of Canada and by the Heart and Stroke Foundation of Ontario is gratefully acknowledged.

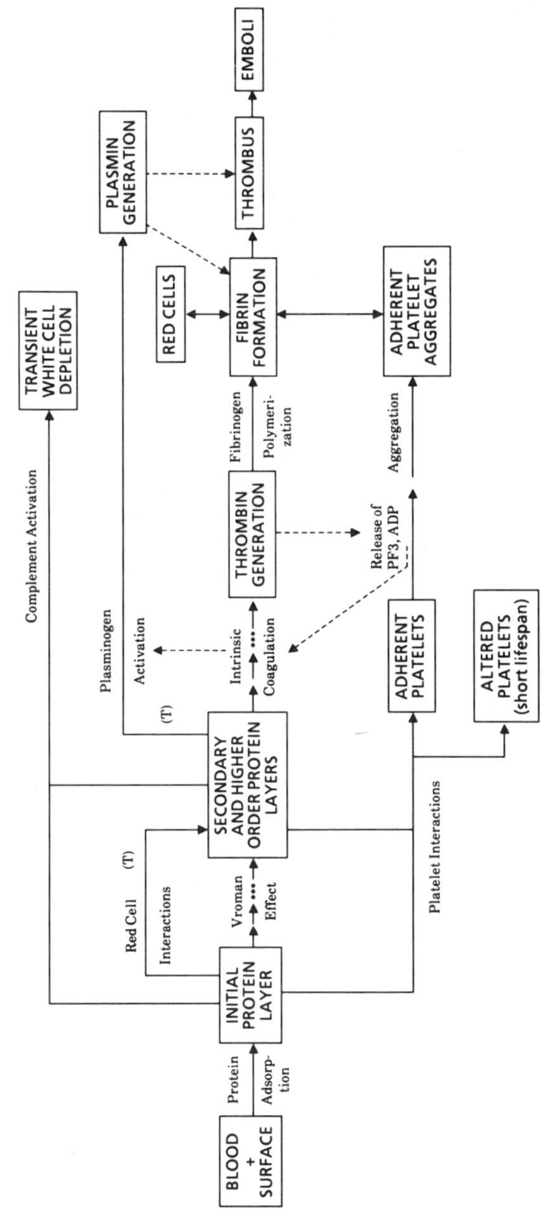

FIGURE 1. Sequence of events during blood-material interactions. The notation *T* indicates tentative.

this regard.[10-12] There is little doubt that they reflect competitive adsorption behavior in a situation where a large number of protein species are in competition for a limited number of surface sites. As indicated in FIGURE 1, it now seems appropriate to speak of initial, secondary, and perhaps higher-order protein layers.

The present communication summarizes the contributions made by our laboratory in the recent past to knowledge of the protein layer adsorbed from blood to foreign material (or biomaterial) surfaces. Our work has focused heavily on fibrinogen, partly for historical reasons,[13-17] but also because fibrinogen is a protein of high surface activity that plays an important role in early interactions of blood and solid surfaces. Our work may be conveniently discussed under two headings. First, we have performed quantitative studies of fibrinogen adsorption from plasma and blood. The variables examined are time and plasma or blood dilution. These studies bear on the displacement of initially adsorbed fibrinogen by other proteins. Second, we have carried out investigations of a more qualitative nature on the properties of the adsorbed protein layer at longer contact times. These studies provide indications of the generation of fibrinolytic activity at surfaces in contact with blood.

KINETICS OF EARLY FIBRINOGEN ADSORPTION FROM PLASMA AND BLOOD

In these studies, the surface specimens are tubing segments about 2.5 mm in diameter; the surface is therefore macroscopic. Fibrinogen (or other protein to be studied) is radioiodine-labeled and added to plasma as a tracer, thereby permitting a quantitative measure of fibrinogen adsorption to the surface. Of course the method must be validated for any system to be studied by showing that the labeled and unlabeled protein do not differ in adsorption behavior, *i.e.*, that the labeled protein truly acts as a tracer. This has proved to be true in the vast majority of systems we have studied[18] using either iodine monochloride or lactoperoxidase labeling methods.

Transient Adsorption of Fibrinogen as Revealed by Dependence on Time and Plasma Dilution: Basics of the Vroman Effect

An initial series of experiments was designed to measure the kinetics of adsorption of the abundant proteins albumin, IgG, and fibrinogen from normal citrate-anticoagulated plasma.[18] The surfaces used were glass, siliconized glass (as used in the coagulation laboratory), polyethylene, polystyrene and a number of segmented polyether urethanes, some hydrophilic (based on polyethylene oxide soft segments) and some hydrophobic (based on polypropylene oxide soft segments). Fibrinogen was not adsorbed to any significant extent on any of the hydrophilic surfaces (including glass) at contact times from 1 minute to 3 hours. On most of the hydrophobic surfaces, fibrinogen adsorption was transient and a maximum surface concentration occurred within the first minute of contact. After a few minutes most of the initially adsorbed firbrinogen had disappeared from the surface. Albumin and IgG showed conventional time dependence, *i.e.*, rapid adsorption to a "steady" value, in most cases considerably below full monolayer surface concentration.

The lack of fibrinogen in the layers present at longer times was surprising in view of the known preferential adsorption of this protein with respect to albumin and IgG.[19,20] The time dependence patterns of fibrinogen adsorption suggested that it was being displaced from the surface after a rapid initial adsorption, the rate of displacement being dependent on the type of surface. Of course Vroman *et al.*, using an immunochemical method of detection, had observed this behavior of fibrinogen several years earlier[10,11] but had been unable to distinguish between increasing immunochemical incompetence of adsorbed fibrinogen as a function of time and the actual departure of fibrinogen from the surface.

As already noted, we failed to detect fibrinogen on several surfaces, notably glass, within the early time limits of our experiment, namely about a minute. We hypothesized that fibrinogen displacement on these surfaces was too rapid for adsorption to be observed, and furthermore, that if, as had been suggested by Vroman *et al.*,[11] it was being displaced by trace proteins, its displacement should be slowed in diluted plasma. Thus initially adsorbed fibrinogen would, in sufficiently dilute plasma, remain on the

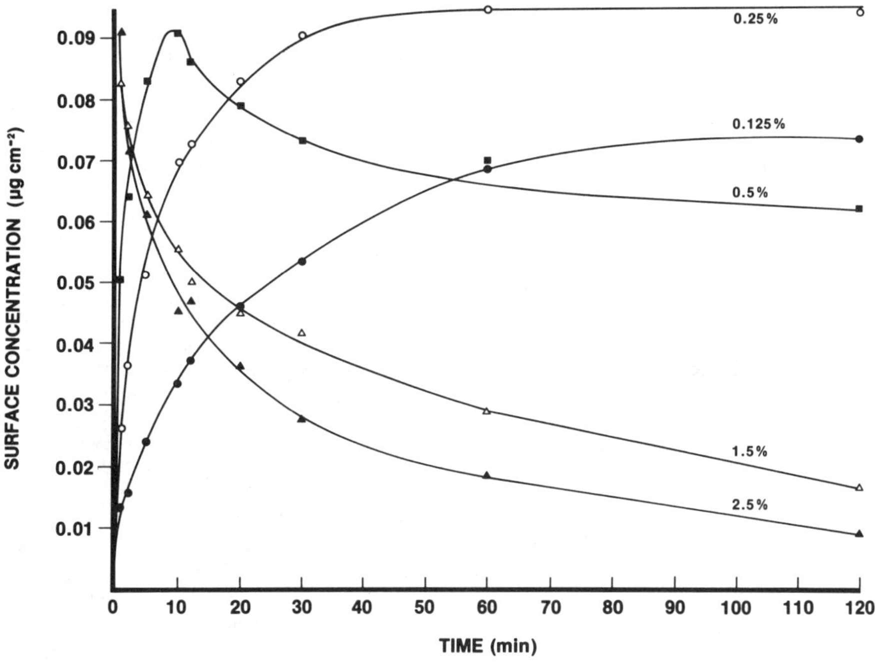

FIGURE 2. Kinetics of adsorption of fibrinogen to glass at varying plasma dilutions. Plasma concentrations are indicated on curves. (From Brash and ten Hove.[6] Reprinted with permission from *Thrombosis and Haemostasis.*)

surface longer than the 1 minute needed for detection. FIGURE 2[6] shows the time dependence of fibrinogen adsorption on glass from diluted plasma at several plasma dilutions ranging from 40 : 1 to 800 : 1. The data amply support the above hypothesis, and show that at higher dilutions more fibrinogen remains on the surface longer, and indeed that at sufficiently high dilution there is no displacement whatsoever. These data reflect what we now refer to as the Vroman effect. As is clear from FIGURE 2, the time and plasma concentration (or dilution) variables are interchangeable and plots of adsorption versus plasma concentration with time as a parameter also show maxima, with plasma concentration at maximum adsorption decreasing as the time increases.[7] Data of this type for a polyethylene surface and 5-minute adsorptions are shown in

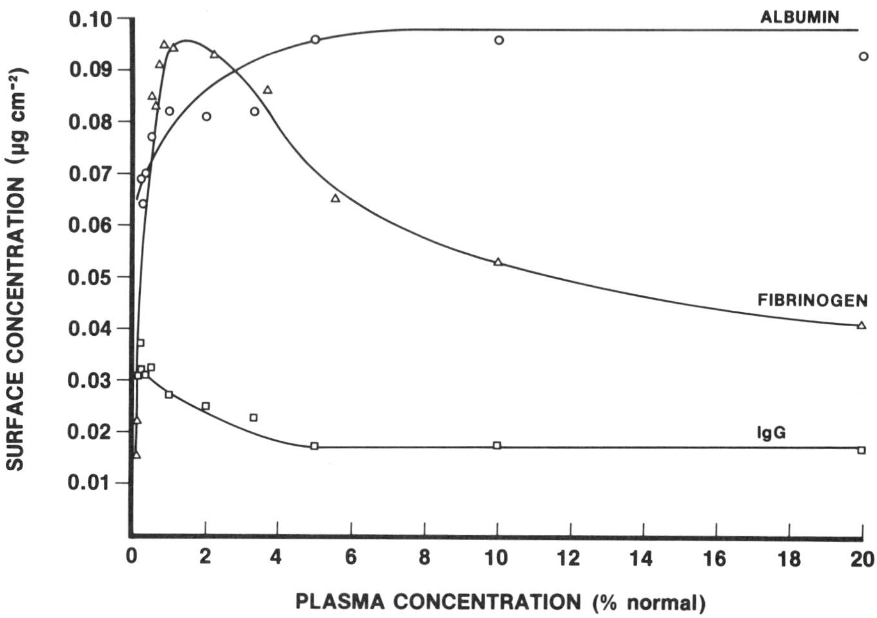

FIGURE 3. Adsorption of proteins to polyethylene from plasma as a function of plasma concentration. Plasma was diluted with isotonic tris, pH 7.35, and adsorptions were for 5 minutes. (From Brash and ten Hove.[6] Reprinted with permission from *Thrombosis and Haemostasis.*)

FIGURE 3. On this hydrophobic material it is clear that adsorbed fibrinogen is less readily displaced and thus that there is a surface-type dependence of the Vroman effect. IgG shows a "mild" Vroman effect, with the maximum adsorption occurring "earlier" than for fibrinogen, thus supporting the idea of an adsorption sequence IgG-fibrinogen. On the other hand, albumin adsorption on this surface (as on others) shows conventional concentration dependence, increasing onto a plateau at about 5% normal plasma concentration. There is thus no evidence that albumin adsorption is transient on this surface or that it is involved in any adsorption-displacement sequence of the type proposed by Vroman.[5]

Similar findings on fibrinogen adsorption from diluted plasma have been reported by Horbett,[8] Breemhaar *et al.*,[9] and more recently Lindon *et al.*[21] The Vroman effect is thus a well-established phenomenon in blood-material interactions. Grinnell and Feld[22] have reported maxima in the adsorption of fibronectin from serum as a function of dilution.

Phenomenology of the Vroman Effect: Variation with Fibrinogen Concentration in Plasma and with Surface Type

In follow-up studies[7,23,24] we have examined the effect of fibrinogen plasma concentration ranging from 10% to 200% of the average value, as well as the surface-type dependence of the Vroman effect. FIGURE 4 shows the effect of fibrinogen concentration on the 5-minute adsorption vs. plasma concentration curves for glass.

For these experiments a single plasma pool was defibrinated using a snake venom clotting enzyme, and fibrinogen was added back at varying final concentration. Thus all proteins other than fibrinogen remained at constant relative concentration. The peak height is seen to increase with increasing fibrinogen concentration while the peak position shifts progressively to lower plasma concentration. These variations reflect the effectiveness of fibrinogen in competitive adsorption in plasma, and were interpreted as showing that when the fibrinogen level is "average," about 50% of the surface may be covered with fibrinogen at the 5-minute adsorption maximum that occurs in plasma diluted 100 : 1. The decreasing portions of the curves are mathematically identical, in agreement with the view that this portion is determined by the concentration of the displacing species, which is the same in all cases. The initial slopes are proportional to the fibrinogen concentration as expected for a diffusion controlled adsorption (see below), obeying the equation

$$\Gamma = 2C\left(\frac{Dt}{\pi}\right)^{0.5}, \quad (1)$$

where Γ is the surface concentration, D is the diffusion coefficient, t is time, and C is the bulk concentration.

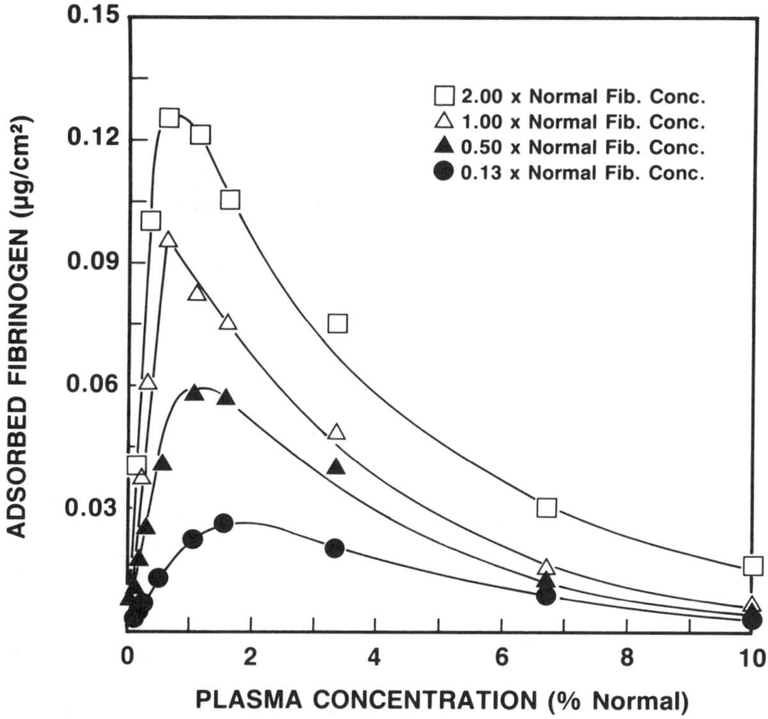

FIGURE 4. Five-minute adsorption "isotherms" for fibrinogen from plasma to glass using plasmas of widely varying fibrinogen concentration. (From Wojciechowski *et al.*[7] Reprinted with permission from the *Journal of Colloid and Interface Science*.)

It should be noted also that the surface concentrations of fibrinogen on glass at higher plasma concentrations are small but finite (0.01 to 0.02 $\mu g/cm^2$). This "long-term" residual fibrinogen turns out to be of considerable interest and is discussed in detail below (see PLASMIN-INDUCED LYSIS OF ADSORBED FIBRINOGEN).

With regard to surface-type dependence of the Vroman effect, FIGURE 5 shows data, again as surface concentration vs. plasma concentration at 5 minutes, for five different surfaces. The initial slopes of the curves are the same for all surfaces, reflecting, we believe, the fact that at low plasma concentrations the displacing proteins are ineffective, and the amount of fibrinogen adsorbed at short contact times is

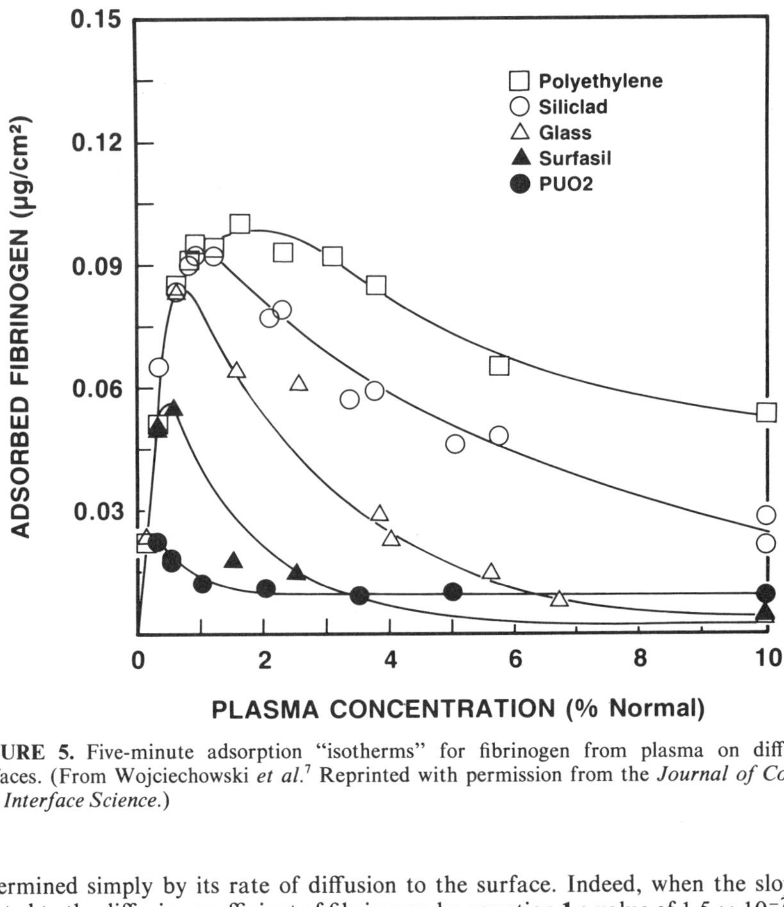

FIGURE 5. Five-minute adsorption "isotherms" for fibrinogen from plasma on different surfaces. (From Wojciechowski *et al.*[7] Reprinted with permission from the *Journal of Colloid and Interface Science.*)

determined simply by its rate of diffusion to the surface. Indeed, when the slope is related to the diffusion coefficient of fibrinogen by equation **1** a value of 1.5×10^{-7} cm^2 per second is obtained,[7] in good agreement with data from other methods. The peak heights and positions and the decreasing portions of the curves are strongly surface dependent. The decrease at higher plasma concentration reflects the displacement of fibrinogen by competing species and shows a correlation, though not a strong one, of increasing fibrinogen retention with increasing surface hydrophobicity.

With a series of segmented polyurethanes[23,24] we have found a very strong dependence of peak height on the polymer structural features, particularly the soft segment type. With polypropylene oxide as soft segment, the 5-minute adsorption vs. plasma concentration curves tend to flatten out as the molecular weight of the soft segment increases. With polyethylene oxide soft segments there appears to be no Vroman effect at all, and only a very low but constant level of fibrinogen adsorption is observed. Since the polyethylene-oxide-based materials are hydrophilic and hygroscopic, there may be a loss of adsorbed proteins during the rising procedure required to remove excess plasma prior to counting. Other workers, using *in situ* methods, have however also observed low levels of adsorption on polyethylene-oxide-based materials,[25] so that these surfaces may be truly nonadsorbing. Another material showing essentially no Vroman effect (in the range of dilutions studied), and a low level of fibrinogen adsorption, is cuprophan dialysis membrane.[26] We have also shown, however, that cuprophan adsorbs monolayer quantities of fibrinogen from single protein solutions. Thus it seems likely that a Vroman peak does occur on cuprophan but at very short times, and that extremely high dilutions of plasma would be required to observe any fibrinogen after 5 minutes. We will return to a discussion of these surface differences after considering the plasma components that are most likely responsible for fibrinogen displacement.

Mechanism of the Vroman Effect: Identification of Fibrinogen-displacing Proteins and Involvement of the Contact Phase of Intrinsic Coagulation

In collaboration with colleagues at Temple University in Philadelphia, we have carried out experiments to identify the proteins in plasma responsible for displacing initially adsorbed fibrinogen.[27,28] Based on the results of Vroman *et al.*[11,12] and Schmaier *et al.*,[29] the proteins of the contact phase of blood coagulation seemed likely candidates. These four proteins, factor XII, factor XI, prekallikrein, and high molecular weight kininogen (HMWK), participate in a complex sequence of reactions that initiates intrinsic plasma coagulation,[30,31] so that it is not unreasonable to expect that these proteins should have strong surface activity and should be involved in the early stages of blood-surface interactions.[32]

High molecular weight kininogen in particular should be highly surface active if the roles ascribed to it are correct. It is known that HMWK circulates in the blood as a 1 : 1 stoichiometric complex with both prekallikrein[33] and factor XI.[34] Its role as a cofactor of the contact phase is to transport these two proteins to the surface and to bind to the surface itself so that the complexes of factors XII, XI, and prekallikrein, necessary for coagulation to proceed, can be formed.[30,31,35]

Our studies of the contact phase proteins consisted of obtaining Vroman effect data (in the form of fibrinogen adsorption at 5 min versus plasma dilution) for plasmas congenitally deficient in the protein of interest. FIGURE 6 shows data for HMWK-deficient plasma compared to data for normal plasma on a glass surface. It is clear that the fibrinogen-displacing activity of HMWK-deficient plasma is greatly reduced although not zero. Reconstitution of HMWK-deficient plasma with purified HMWK tends to restore normal plasma behavior,[28] thus confirming that HMWK is a major fibrinogen-displacing protein. The same general trends were observed with polyethylene and siliconized glass surfaces.

Similar attenuation of fibrinogen displacement was observed for factor-XII-deficient plasma. We believe, however, that the action of factor XII is indirect in that it is required to convert prekallikrein to kallikrein, which in turn converts HMWK procofactor to HMWK active cofactor,[36] the form in which HMWK is fully active both in coagulation and fibrinogen displacement.

Data for fully contact-activated normal plasma (*i.e.*, plasma treated with dextran sulfate[37]) showed much-reduced fibrinogen displacement, whereas factor-XI-deficient plasma, treated in the same manner, showed a normal Vroman effect. From these observations we concluded that factor XIa destroys the ability of HMWK to displace fibrinogen, just as it destroys the coagulation cofactor activity of HMWK,[38] probably by extensive degradation of the HMWK light chain to inactive fragments.

We also considered the possibility that adsorbed fibrinogen might be enzymatically digested, and in the form of smaller fragments would be able to desorb more readily. Such a mechanism would also be consistent with an increased surface residence time at lower plasma concentrations. Plasmin in particular, which is known to be formed

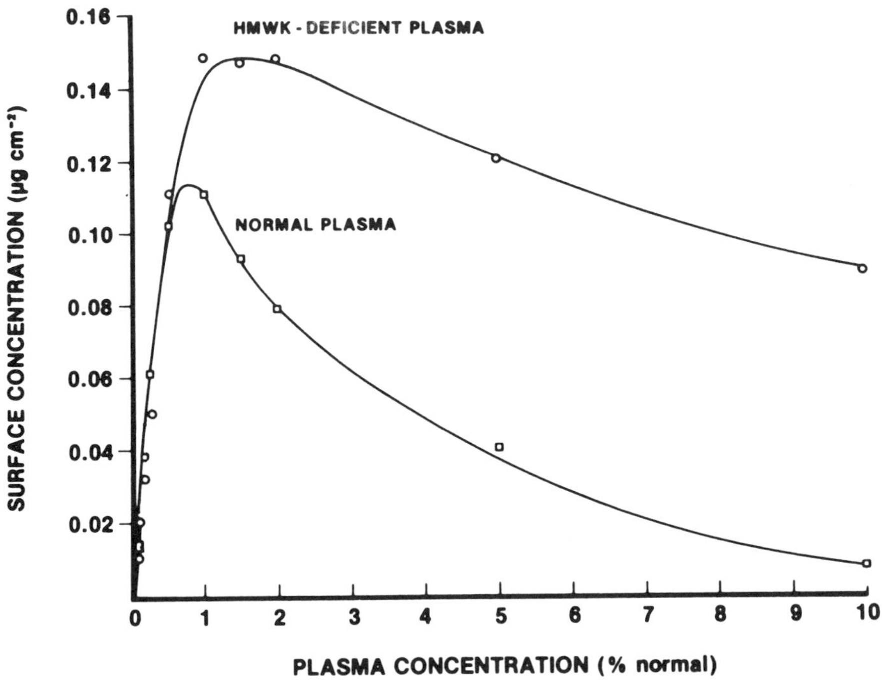

FIGURE 6. Five-minute adsorption "isotherms" for fibrinogen from plasma on glass: normal plasma vs. HMWK-deficient plasma.

during contact activation of plasma, was considered to be a prime candidate. We found, however, that for a glass surface fibrinogen adsorption from plasminogen-deficient plasma at 5 minutes as a function of plasma dilution is almost the same as from normal plasma. We therefore concluded that, at least for short contact times, fibrinogenolysis is not responsible for fibrinogen displacement. A similar observation was made by Schmaier *et al.*[29] Interestingly, we have shown in other experiments (see PLASMIN-INDUCED LYSIS OF ADSORBED FIBRINOGEN) that the small amounts of fibrinogen left on glass (and other surfaces) after the Vroman peak consist largely of plasmin-induced fragments. Enzymatic attack of adsorbed fibrinogen in plasma therefore does take place but is evidently much slower than the displacement reactions of the Vroman effect. Moreover, the fragments appear to be quite firmly bound and are only eluted at high ionic strength.

Possible Significance of the Vroman Effect with Respect to Thrombogenesis at Foreign Surfaces

The main conclusion of this study is that the displacement of adsorbed fibrinogen is strongly correlated with activation of the contact phase of coagulation, and depends in particular on the presence of active HMWK and factor XIIa. This conclusion is in agreement with the observations that, by and large, hydrophobic surfaces that are less procoagulant show a slower and less extensive fibrinogen displacement than a strongly procoagulant surface like glass. Possible explanations for these observations are: (1) fibrinogen is more strongly bound to hydrophobic surfaces and thus less readily displaced; (2) the concentration of active HMWK is smaller at hydrophobic surfaces, resulting in slower displacement of fibrinogen; (3) coagulation is less activated at hydrophobic surfaces because tightly held fibrinogen prevents access of contact factors to the surface where they can be activated. Regardless of which of these explanations is correct, and there may be an element of truth in all of them, it seems obvious that the Vroman effect reflects contact activation and that the plasma dilution experiment may, with development of a wide-enough data base, be usable as a simple, and above all, a high-precision quantitative measure of surface procoagulant activity.

With regard to the broader question of thrombogenesis at surfaces, involving platelets as well as coagulation, the significance of the Vroman effect is less clear. If the critical surface property is inertness toward coagulation, then fibrinogen retention, which probably prevents access of coagulation factors to the surface, may be desirable. On the other hand, if inertness to platelets is the most important property for nonthrombogenicity, and since adsorbed fibrinogen has been shown to be highly platelet reactive both *in vitro* and *in vivo,*[21,39-41] then rapid and complete displacement of fibrinogen would be desirable.

It should be mentioned finally that the Vroman effect has been studied mainly in plasma, and the question naturally arises whether the same phenomenon occurs in whole blood. Recent work in our laboratory[42] with freshly drawn citrate-anticoagulated human whole blood has shown that fibrinogen adsorption vs. blood dilution curves are the same as those obtained previously for plasma. This is true for several surfaces. Moreover, the curves are quantitatively identical. Therefore it may be concluded that this phenomenon is not influenced by red cells or platelets, in accord with expectations for an early blood-surface event. Cooper *et al.*[43] have observed a fibrinogen adsorption peak at times of less than a minute during *in vivo* contact of blood and a polymer surface (A-V shunts) in dogs. This is very likely a manifestation of the Vroman effect. The transient adsorption of fibrinogen is thus clearly relevant to blood-surface contact in clinical situations and merits further study in this regard.

PLASMIN-INDUCED LYSIS OF ADSORBED FIBRINOGEN

The conclusion of the studies described in this section, encapsulated in its title, has important implications for the development of nonthrombogenic surfaces. The work that led to this conclusion was motivated by a desire to know more about possible structural changes in proteins that could be induced by adsorption to a surface. The "story" therefore begins with studies of purified fibrinogen.

Lysis of "Purified" Fibrinogen Adsorbed from Single Protein Solutions

We found in preliminary studies[14] that fibrinogen eluted from glass showed a 50% loss of α-helicity relative to native fibrinogen and is thus significantly traumatized from a conformational standpoint. Other workers have shown losses of α-helicity to varying degrees for other proteins and surfaces.[44,45]

Using glass bead columns to provide a high surface-to-volume ratio, we then showed that fibrinogen eluted from the columns after 30 min to 3 h of contact was substantially degraded.[46] Moreover, the degradation products were shown, by SDS polyacrylamide gel electrophoresis, to be identical to those formed by the action of plasmin on fibrinogen.[47] We assumed that degradation was related to the presence of a trace of plasminogen in the fibrinogen preparation, and found indeed that when efforts were made to remove plasminogen (chromatography on DEAE cellulose[48] or sepharose-lysine[49]) degradation was reduced. EACA (ϵ-amino caproic acid), which inhibits fibrinogenolysis in solution by preempting the plasminogen binding site on fibrinogen, was not effective in preventing surface-induced fibrinogenolysis. Aprotinin, which inhibits plasmin directly by competitive binding,[50] was also without effect on the surface degradation reaction. These results show clearly that the same reaction occurring on a surface as opposed to in solution may behave very differently. In particular, for enzyme-substrate reactions, the binding required in solution may be unnecessary if suitable "apposition" on adjacent surface sites occurs. Also, for macromolecules such as proteins, which can be oriented in various ways on the surface, an active site on an adsorbed molecule may be relatively buried or relatively available, and again its availability for an adsorbed substrate may be different from that for a competitive inhibitor in solution.

When small amounts of plasminogen of the order of 0.1% were added to fibrinogen and the mixture was incubated on glass bead columns, surface degradation was virtually 100% (FIGURE 7).[46] On the other hand, samples of the same mixture incubated without glass beads in the buffers used to elute the columns were entirely intact, showing that the surface plays the central role in the degradation reaction.

The mechanism of this surface-induced degradation of fibrinogen is not yet clear. However, it is clear that plasminogen, even in the presence of an overwhelming excess of fibrinogen, is adsorbed to the surface (bands at 94,000 MW in FIGURE 7). The deliberately added plasminogen is known to be partly activated to plasmin,[46] and this too may be adsorbed. If so, the observed degradation in this experiment may be entirely due to this adsorbed preexisting plasmin. The role of the surface would then merely be to catalyze the plasmin-fibrinogen reaction (which does not occur in solution under the same conditions). On the other hand, it is not known whether the original fibrinogen preparation is contaminated with plasmin as well as plasminogen. If it is not, then plasmin must somehow be generated in the system. An interesting possibility in this regard is that adsorption of plasminogen may facilitate its conversion to plasmin or to a plasmin-like molecule with fibrinogen-lysing properties. Another possible mechanism is that contact factor contaminants, particularly factor XIIa, which are known to be plasminogen activators,[51] are responsible for the observed fibrinogen degradation via plasminogen activation at the surface. The relative merits of these tentative mechanisms will be discussed below in the light of column experiments with plasma.

Lysis of Fibrinogen Adsorbed from Plasma

Glass bead column experiments with plasma, similar to those using fibrinogen just discussed, were being conducted simultaneously with an entirely different goal in mind, namely to obtain more detailed information on the composition of the protein layer adsorbed from plasma. As discussed above, data obtained using radiolabeled fibrinogen, albumin, and IgG in plasma showed that these proteins could not account for more than a fraction of a monolayer based on known capacities of the surfaces for the individual proteins.[18] Therefore we assumed that the other proteins were being adsorbed in substantial amounts.

The plasma column experiments consisted of incubation, usually for 3 h, followed by elution using, in sequence, a mild (1 M tris buffer) and a strong (2% SDS in isotonic tris) eluent. SDS polyacrylamide gels were then run and attempts were made to identify the proteins in the eluates. FIGURE 8 shows a typical gel. As can be seen there

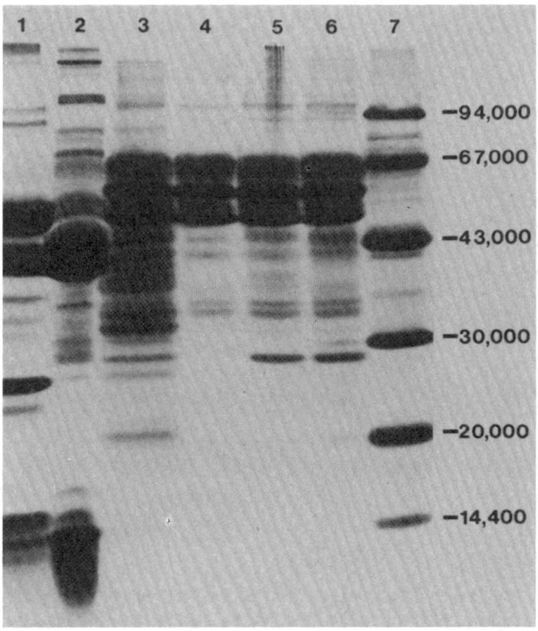

FIGURE 7. SDS-PAGE of fibrinogen incubated with 0.1% plasminogen after elution from glass bead column: lane 1, fibrinogen degradation products; lane 2, 1 M tris eluate; lane 3, SDS eluate; lane 4, fibrinogen; lane 5, fibrinogen incubated with 0.1% plasminogen in 1 M tris; lane 6, fibrinogen incubated with 0.1% plasminogen in SDS; lane 7, molecular weight standards. (From Brash *et al.*[46] Reprinted with permission from the *Journal of Biomedical Materials Research.*)

are many proteins in both the 1 M tris and SDS eluates, and we are still in the process of trying to identify many of them, particularly the strong band at 25,000 MW in the SDS eluate. For the 1 M tris eluate, positive reactions in Ouchterlony immunodiffusion assays were obtained for albumin, IgG, fibrinogen, and perhaps most significantly, plasminogen. The 1 M tris eluate can be seen to contain substantial amounts of plasmin-type FDP, similar to the fibrinogen single protein eluates already discussed. Therefore it appears that surface-catalyzed plasmin-type fibrinogen degradation also takes place in plasma.

Before discussing the mechanism of this degradation, it is perhaps pertinent to consider what appears to be a contradiction between the column experiments and the Vroman effect experiments using radiolabeled fibrinogen discussed above (see KINETICS OF EARLY FIBRINOGEN ADSORPTION FROM PLASMA AND BLOOD). The gels in FIGURE 8 appear to show that significant amounts of fibrinogen, either degraded (1 M tris) or intact (SDS), are adsorbed to glass from plasma after 3 hours, whereas the data on the Vroman effect indicate that only very small quantities of fibrinogen would remain on glass after just a few seconds of plasma contact. The contradiction is more apparent than real as the following argument should make clear. From glass bead column experiments using plasma "spiked" with radiolabeled fibrinogen, we found that the degraded fibrinogen (1 M tris eluate) and intact fibrinogen (SDS eluate) are present on the surface in a ratio of about 3 : 1. In addition the ratio of total protein in the 1 M tris and SDS peaks is about 1 : 9. If we assume that the fibrinogen contribution

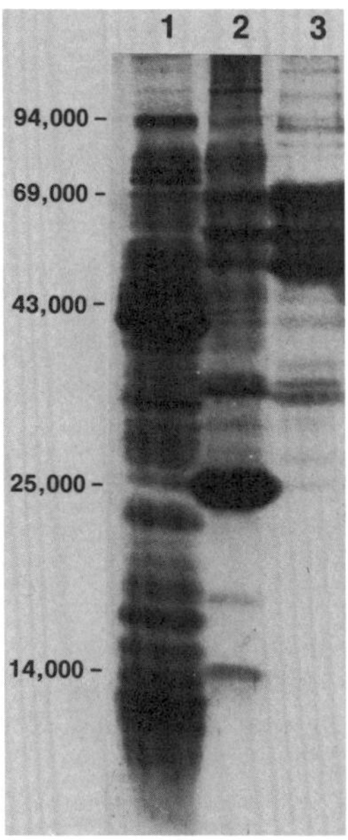

FIGURE 8. SDS-PAGE of proteins eluted from glass after contact with normal plasma: lane 1, proteins eluted by 1 M tris; lane 2, proteins eluted by SDS; lane 3, fibrinogen. (From Brash and Thibodeau.[4] Reprinted with permission from the *Journal of Biomedical Materials Research*.)

to the 1 M tris eluate is of the order of 30%, it may be estimated that fibrinogen contributes about 4% to the total adsorbed protein ($1.3 \times 30\%$ of 10%). If we assume, further, a monolayer surface concentration from plasma of about 0.5 $\mu g/cm^2$, then the surface concentration of fibrinogen based on material eluted from the column may be estimated as about 0.02 $\mu g/cm^2$, similar to the "residual" amount of fibrinogen observed in Vroman effect experiments.[6,7] Thus the contradiction or inconsistency is only apparent, and the fibrinogen observed in the column experiments is truly residual fibrinogen, *i.e.*, fibrinogen that has not been displaced during the Vroman effect. Clearly the sensitivity of the column experiment, with a high surface-to-volume ratio and gel detection of proteins, is much greater than that of the Vroman effect experiment.

When the glass bead column experiment was performed with factor-XII-deficient plasma, there was less fibrinogen degradation, and considerable intact fibrinogen appeared in the 1 M tris peak.[4] It was therefore concluded that part of the surface degradation of fibrinogen is due to the activation of adsorbed plasminogen by factor XIIa (probably also adsorbed). However, other mechanisms must also be involved since some FDP are still seen with factor-XII-deficient plasma. Again several possibilities seem worth considering:

1. Plasmin present in plasma is adsorbed and the surface merely catalyzes the degradation of adsorbed fibrinogen. This seems unlikely in that plasma inhibitors of plasmin, namely α_2-antiplasmin and α_2-macroglobulin, would rapidly inactivate any plasmin in the bulk phase.
2. Adsorbed plasminogen is converted to plasmin by the agency of the surface itself, independent of factor XII or other activators. Such a conversion may occur in two ways: (i) by forming "conventional" plasmin through cleavage of the Arg-560–Val-561 peptide bond in plasminogen,[52] the active site then being available for fibrinogen degradation; the role of the surface might simply be to "hold" the molecule in a strained conformation, thereby facilitating cleavage of the peptide bond or (ii) by forming a "plasmin-like" molecule through a conformational alteration in the adsorbed state that uncovers the active site without the need for peptide bond scission. Kichenin[53] has observed that purified plasminogen is adsorbed and becomes enzymatically active on the surface of modified polystyrenes without any cleavage of the molecule. Interestingly, we have shown (see below) that fibrinogen is degraded on the surface of these same polymers in contact with plasma.

Experiments are in progress to discriminate among these possible mechanisms. No conclusive results are as yet available.

Significance of Fibrinogen Lysis at Surfaces for the Development of Nonthrombogenic Surfaces

The implication in all of these observations on fibrinogen degradation is that surfaces may have inherent fibrinolytic as well as thrombogenic properties. In this connection it should be mentioned that the same phenomenon has been observed for several other surfaces. In particular we have detected FDP on the surfaces of various modified polystyrenes.[54] These materials contain sulfonate and glutamic acid sulfamide or arginine sulfamide groups, and have been shown to possess anticoagulant properties through adsorption of antithrombin III and heparin-like catalysis of the reaction of antithrombin III and thrombin.[55,56] They appear also to be capable of the same fibrinogen degradation reactions as glass, implying plasminogen adsorption and activation. Plasminogen adsorption has certainly been observed.[54] These materials are believed not to adsorb contact phase factors to any great extent, so that mechanisms involving direct surface activation of plasminogen may be more important.

Assuming in general that properties leading to fibrinolysis are attributable to surfaces, a valid approach to nonthrombogenicity may be to maximize these properties. Kusserow *et al.*[57] several years ago adopted an analogous approach by immobilizing urokinase on surfaces, and more recently Senatore *et al.*[58] have tried to incorporate urokinase into small diameter vascular grafts. The idea that emerges from the studies described in the present article, however, is that surfaces may have inherent plasminogen-activating capacity without the need for attachment of intrinsic plasminogen activators. The latter may be inactivated in the attached state or easily leached from the surface upon contact with blood.

ACKNOWLEDGMENTS

The author thanks his various coworkers who have contributed to the research described in this article. Their names can be found in the references.

REFERENCES

1. CRADDOCK, P. R., J. FEHR, A. P. DALMASSO, K. L. BRIGHAM & H. S. JACOB. 1977. Hemodialysis leukopenia: Pulmonary vascular leukostasis resulting from complement activation by dialyzer cellophane membranes. J. Clin. Invest. **59:** 879–888.
2. CHENOWETH, D. E. 1984. Biocompatibility of hemodialysis membranes. Evaluation with C3a anaphylatoxin radioimmunoassays. asaio J. **7:** 44–49.
3. RATNOFF, O. D. 1969. Some relationships among hemostasis, fibrinolytic phenomena, immunity and the inflammatory response. Adv. Immunol. **10:** 145–227.
4. BRASH, J. L. & J. A. THIBODEAU. 1986. Identification of proteins adsorbed from human plasma to glass bead columns: Plasmin-induced degradation of adsorbed fibrinogen. J. Biomed. Mater. Res. **20:** 1263–1275.
5. VROMAN, L. & A. L. ADAMS. 1986. Adsorption of proteins out of plasma and solutions in narrow spaces. J. Colloid Interface Sci. **111:** 391–402.
6. BRASH, J. L. & P. TEN HOVE. 1984. Effect of plasma dilution on adsorption of fibrinogen to solid surfaces. Thromb. Haemostas. **51:** 326–330.
7. WOJCIECHOWSKI, P., P. TEN HOVE & J. L. BRASH. 1986. Phenomenology and mechanism of the transient adsorption of fibrinogen from plasma (Vroman effect). J. Colloid Interface Sci. **111:** 455–465.
8. HORBETT, T. A. 1984. Mass action effects on the adsorption of fibrinogen from hemoglobin solutions and from plasma. Thromb. Haemostas. **51:** 174–181.
9. BREEMHAAR, W., E. BRINKMAN, D. J. ELLENS, T. BEUGELING & A. BANTJES. 1984. Preferential adsorption of high density lipoprotein from blood plasma onto biomaterial surfaces. Biomaterials **5:** 269–274.
10. VROMAN, L. & A. L. ADAMS. 1969. Identification of rapid changes at plasma-solid interfaces. J. Biomed. Mater. Res. **3:** 43–67.
11. VROMAN, L., A. L. ADAMS, G. C. FISCHER & P. MUNOZ. 1980. Interaction of high molecular weight kininogen, factor XII and fibrinogen in plasma at interfaces. Blood **55:** 156–159.
12. ADAMS, A. L., G. C. FISCHER, P. C. MUNOZ & L. VROMAN. 1984. Convex-lens-on-slide: A simple system for the study of human plasma and blood in narrow spaces. J. Biomed. Mater. Res. **18:** 643–654.
13. CHAN, B. M. C. & J. L. BRASH. 1981. Adsorption of fibrinogen on glass: Reversibility aspects. J. Colloid Interface Sci. **82:** 217–225.
14. CHAN, B. M. C. & J. L. BRASH. 1981. Conformational change in fibrinogen desorbed from glass surface. J. Colloid Interface Sci. **84:** 263–265.
15. SCHMITT, A., R. VAROQUI, S. UNIYAL, J. L. BRASH & C. PUSINERI. 1983. Interactions of fibrinogen with surfaces of varying charge and hydrophobic-hydrophilic balance. I. Adsorption isotherms. J. Colloid Interface Sci. **92:** 25–34.
16. BRASH, J. L., S. UNIYAL, C. PUSINERI & A. SCHMITT. 1983. Interaction of fibrinogen with solid surfaces of varying charge and hydrophobic-hydrophilic balance. II. Dynamic exchange between surface and solution molecules. J. Colloid Interface Sci. **95:** 28–37.
17. DE BAILLOU, N., P. DEJARDIN, A. SCHMITT & J. L. BRASH. 1984. Fibrinogen dimensions at an interface: Variations with bulk concentration, temperature and pH. J. Colloid Interface Sci. **100:** 167–174.
18. UNIYAL, S. & J. L. BRASH. 1982. Patterns of adsorption of proteins from human plasma onto foreign surfaces. Thromb. Haemostas. **47:** 285–290.
19. BRASH, J. L. & V. J. DAVIDSON. 1976. Adsorption on glass and polyethylene from solutions of fibrinogen and albumin. Thromb. Res. **9:** 249–259.
20. BRASH, J. L. & S. UNIYAL. 1979. Dependence of albumin-fibrinogen simple and competitive adsorption on surface properties of biomaterials. J. Polym. Sci. **C66:** 377–389.

21. LINDON, J. N., G. MCNAMANA, L. KUSHNER, E. W. MERRILL & E. W. SALZMAN. 1986. Does the conformation of adsorbed fibrinogen dictate platelet interactions with artificial surfaces? Blood **68:** 355–362.
22. GRINNELL, F. & M. K. FELD. 1982. Fibronectin adsorption on hydrophobic and hydrophilic surfaces detected by antibody binding and analyzed during cell adhesion in serum containing medium. J. Biol. Chem. **257:** 4888–4893.
23. HUDSON, C. B., J. L. BRASH & P. TEN HOVE. 1986. Adsorption of fibrinogen from plasma to segmented polyether-urethanes: Effect of soft segment. Trans. Soc. Biomaterials **9:** 122.
24. SANTERRE, P., C. B. HUDSON, P. TEN HOVE & J. L. BRASH. Unpublished results.
25. GOLANDER, C. G., S. JONSSON, T. VLADKOWA, P. STENIUS & J. C. ERIKSSON. 1986. Preparation and protein adsorption properties of photopolymerized hydrophilic films containing N-vinylpyrrolidone, acrylic acid or ethylene oxide units as studied by ESCA. Colloids and Surfaces. **21:** 149–165.
26. BRASH, J. L. & P. TEN HOVE. Unpublished results.
27. BRASH, J. L., C. F. SCOTT, P. TEN HOVE & R. W. COLMAN. 1985. Desorption of plasma fibrinogen from glass: Role of high molecular weight kininogen and factor XI. Trans. Soc. Biomater. **8:** 105.
28. BRASH, J. L., C. F. SCOTT, P. TEN HOVE, P. WOJCIECHOWSKI & R. W. COLMAN. 1987. Mechanism of transient adsorption of fibrinogen from plasma to solid surfaces: Role of HMWK, factor XII, factor XI, and plasminogen/plasmin. Submitted.
29. SCHMAIER, A. H., L. SILVER, A. L. ADAMS, G. C. FISCHER, P. C. MUNOZ, L. VROMAN & R. W. COLMAN. 1984. The effect of high molecular weight kininogen on surface-adsorbed fibrinogen. Thromb. Res. **33:** 51–67.
30. GRIFFIN, J. H. 1978. The role of surface-dependent activation of Hageman factor (factor XII). Proc. Natl. Acad. Sci. U.S.A. **75:** 1998–2002.
31. GRIFFIN, J. H. 1981. Surface-dependent activation of blood coagulation. *In* Interaction of the Blood with Natural and Artificial Surfaces. E. W. Salzman, Ed.: 134–170. Marcel Dekker. New York.
32. OGSTON, D. & B. BENNETT. 1978. Surface mediated reactions in the formation of thrombin, plasmin and kallikrein. Br. Med. Bull. **34:** 107–112.
33. MANDLE, R., R. W. COLMAN & A. P. KAPLAN. 1976. Identification of prekallikrein and high molecular weight kininogen as a complex in human plasma. Proc. Natl. Acad. Sci. U.S.A. **73:** 4179–4183.
34. THOMPSON, R. E., R. MANDLE & A. P. KAPLAN. 1977. Association of factor XI and high molecular weight kininogen in plasma. J. Clin. Invest. **60:** 1376–1380.
35. GRIFFIN, J. H. & C. G. COCHRANE. 1979. Recent advances in the understanding of contact activation reactions. Sem. Thromb. Haemostas. **5:** 254–273.
36. SCOTT, C. F., L. D. SILVER, M. SCHAPIRA & R. W. COLMAN. 1984. Cleavage of high molecular weight kininogen markedly enhances its coagulant activity: Evidence that this molecule exists as a procofactor. J. Clin. Invest. **73:** 954–962.
37. KLUFT, C. 1978. Determination of prekallikrein in human plasma: Optimal conditions for activating prekallikrein. J. Lab. Clin. Med. **91:** 83–95.
38. SCOTT, C. F., L. D. SILVER, A. D. PURDON & R. W. COLMAN. 1985. Cleavage of human high molecular weight kininogen by factor XIa in vitro. J. Biol. Chem. **260:** 10856–10863.
39. PACKHAM, M. A., G. EVANS, M. F. GLYNN & J. F. MUSTARD. 1969. The effect of plasma proteins on the interaction of platelets with glass surfaces. J. Lab. Clin. Med. **73:** 686–697.
40. WHICHER, S. J. & J. L. BRASH. 1978. Platelet-foreign surface interactions: Release of granule constituents from adherent platelets. J. Biomed. Mater. Res. **12:** 181–201.
41. YOUNG, B. R., L. K. LAMBRECHT, R. M. ALBRECHT, D. F. MOSHER & S. L. COOPER. 1983. Platelet-protein interactions at blood-polymer interfaces in the canine test model. Trans. Am. Soc. Artif. Int. Organs **29:** 442–446.
42. BRASH, J. L. & P. TEN HOVE. Unpublished results.
43. LELAH, M. D., T. G. GRAESEL, J. A. PIERCE, L. K. LAMBRECHT & S. L. COOPER. 1986. Ex vivo interactions and surface property relations for polyether urethanes. J. Biomed. Mater. Res. **20:** 433–468.

44. SODERQUIST, M. E. & A. G. WALTON. 1980. Structural changes in proteins adsorbed on polymer surfaces. J. Colloid Interface Sci. **75:** 386–397.
45. NORDE, W., F. MACRITCHIE, G. NOWICKA & J. LYKLEMA. 1986. Protein adsorption at solid-liquid interfaces: Reversibility and conformation aspects. J. Colloid Interface Sci. **112:** 447–456.
46. BRASH, J. L., B. M. C. CHAN, P. SZOTA & J. A. THIBODEAU. 1985. Degradation of adsorbed fibrinogen by surface generated plasmin. J. Biomed. Mater. Res. **19:** 1017–1029.
47. DOOLITTLE, R. F. 1981. Fibrinogen and fibrin. Sci. Am. **244**(Dec.): 126–135.
48. LAWRIE, J. S., J. ROSS & G. D. KEMP. 1979. Purification of fibrinogen and the separation of its degradation products in the presence of calcium ions. Biochem. Soc. Trans. **7:** 693–694.
49. DEUTSCH, D. G. & E. T. MERTZ. 1970. Plasminogen: Purification from human plasma by affinity chromatography. Science **170:** 1095–1096.
50. AUHAGEN, E. 1967. Chemistry and biochemistry of trasylol. *In* International Symposium on Drugs of Animal Origin. Ferro Edizioni. Milan. pp. 69–80.
51. GOLDSMITH, G., H. SAITO & O. D. RATNOFF. 1978. The activation of plasminogen by Hageman factor (factor XII) and Hageman factor fragments. J. Clin. Invest. **62:** 54–60.
52. LIJNEN, H. R. & M. D. COLLEN. 1982. Interaction of plasminogen activators and inhibitors with plasminogen and fibrin. Sem. Thromb. Haemostas. **8:** 2–10.
53. KICHENIN, V. 1986. Action de polystyrènes substitués sur certaines protéines plasmatiques, en particulier le plasminogène. Doctoral thesis, Université Paris-Nord and Centre National de Transfusion Sanguine, Paris, France.
54. BOISSON, C., J. L. BRASH & J. JOZEFONVICZ. Unpublished results.
55. FOUGNOT, C., J. JOZEFONVICZ, M. SAMAMA & L. BARA. 1979. New heparin-like insoluble materials. Part I. Ann. Biomed. Eng. **7:** 429–439.
56. BOISSON, C., D. GULINO, J. JOZEFONVICZ, A. M. FISCHER & J. TAPON-BRETAUDIERE. 1984. Antithrombic properties of insoluble modified polystyrene. Part I. Thromb. Res. **34:** 269–276.
57. KUSSEROW, B. K., R. LARROW & J. NICHOLS. 1971. The urokinase-heparin bonded synthetic surface possessing composite antithrombogenic and thrombolytic properties. Trans. Am. Soc. Artif. Int. Organs **17:** 1–5.
58. SENATORE, F., F. BERNATH & K. MEISNER. 1986. Clinical study of urokinase-bound fibrocollagenous tubes. J. Biomed. Mater. Res. **20:** 177–188.

The Effects of Surface Chemistry and Coagulation Factors on Fibrinogen Adsorption from Plasma[a]

STEVEN M. SLACK, JANICE L. BOHNERT, AND THOMAS A. HORBETT

Department of Chemical Engineering
and
Center for Bioengineering
University of Washington
Seattle, Washington 98195

INTRODUCTION

The exposure of foreign materials to blood results in the rapid coverage of their surfaces with a thin layer of adsorbed proteins.[1] The protein layer effectively shields the surface from direct contact with blood and is thought to mediate subsequent cellular interactions involved in thrombosis. Since the composition of the adsorbed layer differs considerably, depending on the nature of the material, the mechanisms governing protein adsorption from blood and other complex protein mixtures have been the focus of many recent investigations.[2,3] Insights derived from such adsorption studies may eventually reveal why surfaces differ in their ability to induce thrombosis and thus lead to the development of materials with improved blood compatibility.

Fibrinogen adsorption from undiluted plasma onto polyethylene and many other apolar materials is higher initially than at longer times, whereas it is low initially and rises to a constant value at longer times on hydroxyethyl methacrylate (HEMA) and certain other polar materials.[4,5] Furthermore, when adsorption is measured after a single contact time from plasma that has been diluted to various degrees, fibrinogen adsorption reaches a maximum at intermediate plasma concentrations.[6–8] These phenomena, reflecting apparent displacement of adsorbed fibrinogen, have been referred to as the "Vroman effect."[6] The plasma concentration at which maximal adsorption occurs also varies with substrate composition.[6,9] For example, maximum fibrinogen adsorption occurs at plasma concentrations of 0.1% on glass and 10% on polytetrafluoroethylene.[6] Since platelet consumption is induced at different rates by many of these materials when they are used as *ex vivo* shunts in baboons, a connection between fibrinogen adsorption and platelet consumption has been suggested.[5] In addition, fibrinogen adsorption onto glass from normal plasma and plasma lacking the clotting factor high molecular weight kininogen (HMWK) has been reported to differ markedly.[10,11] If differences in fibrinogen adsorption onto surfaces reflect differences in the degree of contact activation induced by these materials, then the observed platelet behavior may also correlate with fibrinogen adsorption because platelets are susceptible to activation by thrombin.

[a]The financial support of the National Heart, Lung and Blood Institute (grant nos. HL19419 and HL25951) is gratefully acknowledged.

This report describes the measurement of fibrinogen adsorption from plasma as a function of time and plasma dilution to a variety of chemically distinct surfaces. Fibrinogen adsorption from plasmas deficient in certain coagulation factors to polymers was also measured in an effort to determine whether these factors could exert a strong influence on fibrinogen adsorption to surfaces other than glass. Finally, fibrinogen displacement behavior similar to that observed from plasma is shown to occur in binary mixtures of fibrinogen with either albumin or hemoglobin. These studies suggest that displacement of fibrinogen from surfaces in plasma is not solely attributable to the action of clotting factors but instead reflects more general phenomena common to all protein mixtures.

MATERIALS AND METHODS

General

The buffer used in all protein adsorption studies was 0.01 M sodium citrate, 0.01 M sodium phosphate, 0.12 M sodium chloride, 0.02% sodium azide, pH 7.4 (CPBSz). Freshly drawn baboon blood or human blood anticoagulated with 10% (vol/vol) acid citrate dextrose (ACD, NIH Formula "A") was centrifuged at 314 × g, 4°C for thirty minutes. The plasma was recentrifuged at 31,400 × g, 4°C for thirty minutes to remove any remaining cells and then frozen at −70°C until use. Normal pooled human plasma and human plasmas deficient in prekallikrein, kininogens, and factor IX were purchased from George King BioMedical, Inc. (Overland Park, KS). The tetrapeptide to inhibit kallikrein activity, D-phenylalanyl-L-phenylalanyl-L-arginine chloromethylketone (Phe-Phe-Arg-CMK), was obtained from Calbiochem-Behring (San Diego, CA). Human plasma was used for all coagulation factor studies and baboon plasma for the remainder of the experiments, unless otherwise noted.

Plasma fibrinogen concentrations were measured spectrophotometrically from the redissolved, thrombin-induced clot.[12] Human and baboon fibrinogen were isolated from plasma with a polyethylene glycol, β-alanine reprecipitation procedure described previously.[13] The fibrinogen preparations were at least 90% clottable and were homogeneous as judged by SDS gel electrophoresis. Baboon hemoglobin was purified from lysed red blood cells using a published gradient elution, ion exchange technique.[14] The isolated hemoglobin was in the oxygenated form as shown by comparison of its spectra with published data.[15] Prothrombin was a gift from Professor Craig Jackson, Washington University, St. Louis. It was found to be extremely pure, as judged by SDS gel electrophoresis of the ^{125}I-labeled form, where a single, very narrow peak (molecular weight = 71,550) was observed. Purified lathyritic rat skin collagen was a gift of Professor Paul Bornstein, University of Washington, Seattle. Bovine albumin (crystallized) and bovine immunoglobin G (code 64-140, electrophoretically homogeneous) were obtained from Miles Laboratories, Inc. (Naperville, IL) and used as received.

Fibrinogen, prothrombin, collagen, and albumin were radiolabeled with ^{125}I (Amersham, Arlington Heights, IL) by the iodine monochloride technique.[16] Unreacted ^{125}I was separated from the proteins by gel exclusion chromatography (Bio-Gel P-4, Bio-Rad, Richmond, CA). In most cases the ^{125}I-labeled fibrinogen was also dialyzed overnight at 4°C against CPBSz to remove any loosely associated ^{125}I. The ^{125}I-labeled fibrinogen was stored at −70°C and used within 2 weeks of preparation.

Surfaces

Silicone rubber tubing (Silastic, 0.125 in. i.d., Medical Grade) was obtained from Dow Corning (Midland, MI), polyethylene tubing (nonradiopaque, 0.125 in. i.d.) from Clay Adams (Parsippany, NJ), and polyethylene and polytetrafluoroethlyene sheets (10 mil thick) from Cadillac Plastics (Seattle, WA). Glass surfaces (10 or 12 mm "Diamond" brand coverslips) were purchased from J.M. Freed Co. (Perkasie, PA). Polystyrene samples were cut from Leighton paddles provided by Corning Glass Works (Corning, NY). PEU #1 (Biomer) and PEU #3 (Pellethane) were received as gifts from Ethicon (Somerville, NJ); PEU #2 (Tecoflex) was a gift of ThermoElectron Co. (Waltham, MA). Other polyurethanes were gifts from our colleague Buddy D. Ratner. They were synthesized by end-capping hydroxy-terminated polyethers—poly(propylene glycol) (PPG), poly(tetramethylene glycol) (PTMG) or, for the hard segment model, dipropyleneglycol—with methylene diisocyanate (MDI) and chain-extending with ethylenediamine. PEU 1000 and PEU 2000 were chain-extended with perfluoro alkanediols, as described elsewhere,[17] and their soft segments consisted of PTMG of molecular weight 1000 and 2000, respectively. All PEUs were purified by precipitation and were centrifugally coated onto glass coverslips. Hydroxyethyl methacrylate (HEMA) and ethyl methacrylate (EMA) polymers were prepared as grafts onto polyethylene using techniques for synthesis and characterization described previously.[18]

The silicone rubber, polyethylene, polytetrafluoroethylene, and polystyrene surfaces were cleaned by soaking them (sometimes with sonication) for thirty minutes in a 0.1% Ivory soap solution followed by extensive rinsing in deionized water. The glass coverslips were cleaned similarly in a 4% Isopanasol (C.R. Callen Corp., Seattle, WA) detergent.

Adsorption

Fibrinogen adsorption was measured from plasma or binary protein solutions to which the ^{125}I-labeled protein had been added. The mixture was serially diluted with CPBSz to the desired concentrations. Surfaces were equilibrated in CPBSz for approximately 1 hour in 4 ml polystyrene cups (Evergreen Scientific, Los Angeles, CA). An equal volume of plasma or protein solution (at twice the desired concentration) was added to the cup. The solution was mixed by gentle repipetting and adsorption was allowed to occur for the desired time. Adsorption was terminated by dilution-displacement of the protein mixture with at least twenty volumes of buffer.[19] In some experiments surfaces were removed from the adsorbing solution with forceps and individually rinsed in four beakers of buffer. Unless otherwise specified, all adsorption experiments were carried out at 37°C for 2 hours.

The kinetic adsorption experiments were performed with a tubular flow apparatus.[5] A roller pump (Model 4504-0B-01, Drake Willock, Portland, OR) was used to maintain flow at 100 ml/min. The flow circuit consisted of the polymer to be tested and silicone rubber. Plasma containing ^{125}I-labeled fibrinogen was passed through the circuit for the desired amount of time followed by a 1-min rinse with CPBSz. The sample was removed, cut, and placed into counting vials.

The competitive protein adsorption studies were performed as follows. A series of solutions containing a single, constant concentration of the radiolabled protein and increasing concentration of competing, unlabeled proteins was made. The adsorption was then measured after equilibrating each of these solutions with the surfaces and rinsing as described. The adsorption was converted to percentage of maximum by dividing all adsorption values by the maximum adsorption observed in the experiment.

In all experiments the samples were rinsed again following an overnight soak at room temperature. Fibrinogen adsorption was calculated by dividing the retained radioactivity, corrected for background and decay, by the specific activity of the original protein solution and the known surface area of the sample. Triplicate data were averaged and the standard deviations computed. All data reported here represent adsorption after the overnight soak and rinse, unless noted otherwise.

RESULTS

Effect of Substrate Surface Chemistry

Fibrinogen adsorption from plasma onto glass, polyethylene (PE), and polytetrafluoroethylene (PTFE) reaches a maximum at intermediate plasma concentrations, but the magnitude and position of the maximum vary considerably among these materials.[6] Further measurements of adsorption were therefore made onto a variety of surfaces in an effort to learn more about the effect of surface type on fibrinogen adsorption from plasma.

The fibrinogen adsorption isotherms from plasma onto four hydrophobic but chemically distinct surfaces are illustrated in FIGURE 1. The maximum adsorption

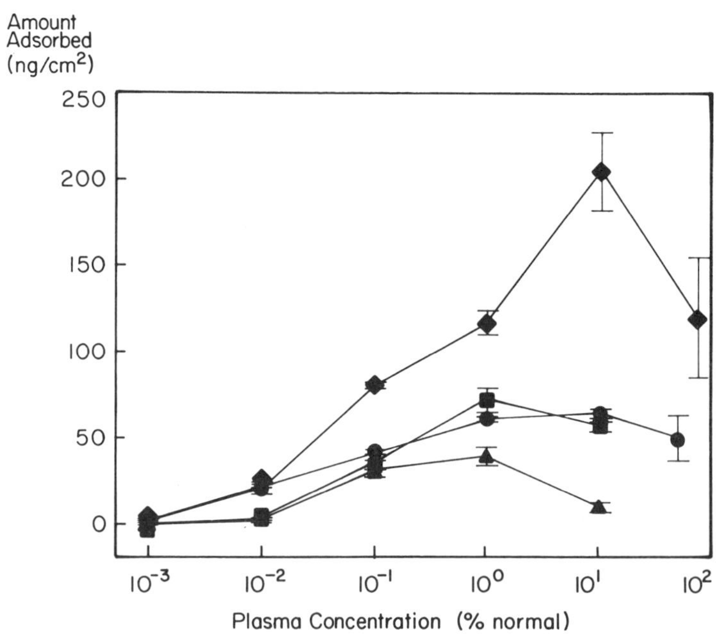

FIGURE 1. Fibrinogen adsorption from plasma: effect of substrate surface chemistry. Adsorption to silicone rubber (*triangles*), polyethylene (*squares*), polystyrene (*diamonds*), and polytetrafluoroethylene (*circles*) is shown.

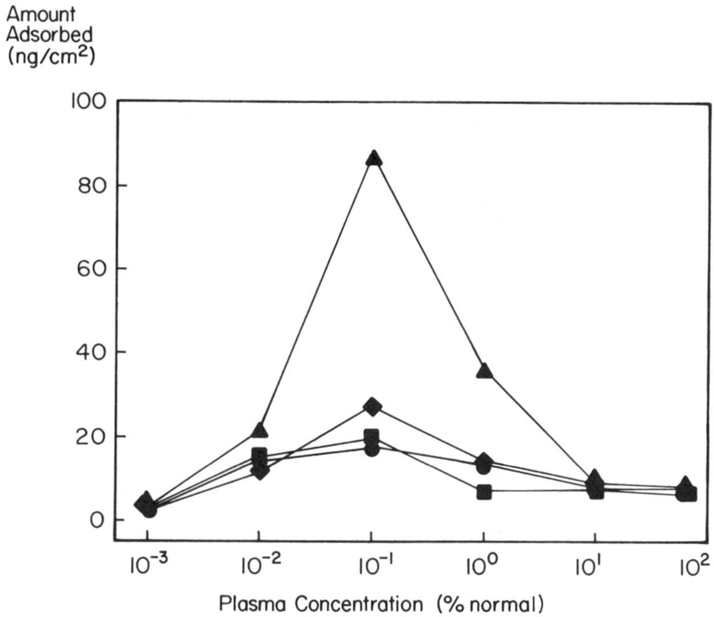

FIGURE 2. Fibrinogen adsorption from plasma onto polyurethanes. Adsorption to PEU PPG 1000 (*triangles*), PEU PPG 2000 (*squares*), PEU PTMG 1000 (*diamonds*), and PEU PTMG 2000 (*circles*) is shown. The coefficient of variation averaged 11.5%, 22.4%, 20.0%, and 30.4% for the data on PEU PPG 1000, PEU PPG 2000, PEU PTMG 1000, and PEU PTMG 2000, respectively.

observed for these polymers was in the following order: silicone rubber (40 ng/cm^2) < PE and PTFE (60 ng/cm^2 for both) < polystyrene (200 ng/cm^2). It should be noted that the polystyrene data represent initial adsorption and not "overnight soak" values (See MATERIALS AND METHODS). Nevertheless, only a small fraction of the initially adsorbed protein on other surfaces (usually <20%) comes off during the overnight soak. Thus, it appears that polystyrene adsorbed substantially more fibrinogen from plasma than the other surfaces compared in FIGURE 1. In addition, polystyrene and PTFE exhibited maximal adsorption at 10% plasma concentration whereas silicone rubber and polyethylene showed peak fibrinogen adsorption at 1% plasma concentration. The large differences in fibrinogen adsorption observed on these materials suggest that hydrophobicity, while an important property of surfaces, cannot fully account for the observed adsorption behavior.

Fibrinogen adsorption from plasma onto a series of polyurethanes was also measured (See FIGURES 2 and 3). In general, decreased adsorption occurred on polyurethanes containing more polyether soft segment. For instance, PEU PPG 1000 showed a maximum in fibrionogen adsorption of 90 ng/cm^2, PEU PPG 2000 showed 20 ng/cm^2, and PEU PTMG 2000 showed 15 ng/cm^2 (See TABLE 1). Similar effects of the soft segment component of fibrinogen adsorption have also been observed by others (J. Brash, personal communication). In contrast, the hard segment model adsorbed nearly 125 ng/cm^2 of fibrinogen at the peak. Despite this wide variation in the amount of fibrinogen bound to the different surfaces, the position of the maximum occurred at or near 0.1% plasma concentration for every surface except the hard segment model,

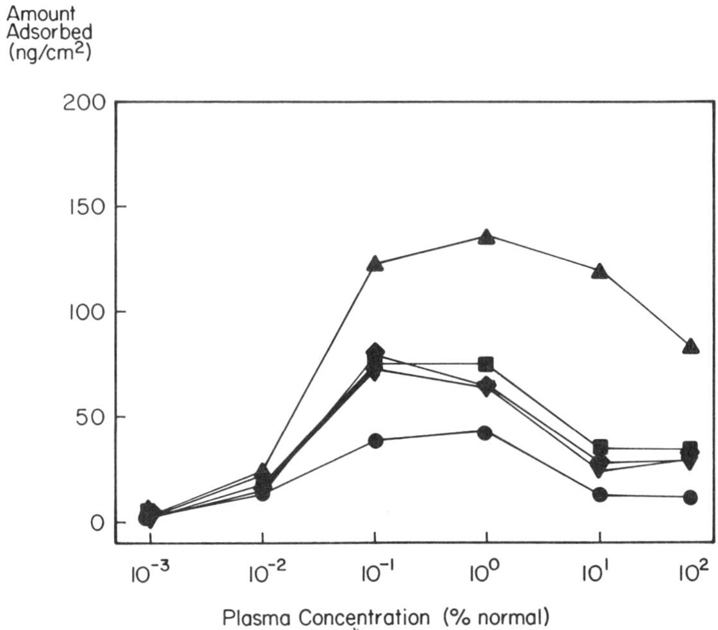

FIGURE 3. Fibrinogen adsorption from plasma to polyurethanes. Adsorption to the hard segment model (*triangles*), PEU 1000 (*squares*), PEU 2000 (*diamonds*), PEU #2 (Tecoflex, *circles*), and PEU #1 (Biomer, *upside-down triangles*) is shown. The coefficient of variation averaged 25.2%, 17.8%, 13.0%, 17.9%, and 17.7% for the data on the hard segment model, PEU 1000, PEU 2000, PEU #2, and PEU #1, respectively.

TABLE 1. Summary of Fibrinogen Adsorption from Plasma

Surface	Peak Plasma Concentration (%)	Adsorption Maximum (ng/cm^2)
Glass[a]	0.01–0.1	4–5
PEU PTMG 2000	0.01–0.1	15–20
PEU PPG 2000	~0.1	15–20
PEU PPG 1000	~0.1	80–90
PEU #2 (Tecoflex)	~0.1	70–80
Silicone rubber[b]	0.1–1.0	30–35
PEU #1 (Biomer)	~1.0	35–40
Polyethylene	~1.0	60–70
Hard segment model	~1.0	120–130
Polytetrafluoroethylene	~10.0	60–65
Polystyrene[c]	~10.0	190–210

[a]Overnight rinse performed with dilution-displacement technique.
[b]Data obtained with human plasma.
[c]No overnight soak and rinse.

PEU 1000 and PEU #1 (Biomer). Moreover, the fibrinogen adsorption isotherms from plasma onto silicone rubber and PEU # 1 (Biomer) were very similar despite the large differences in the compositions of the two polymers.

Effect of Coagulation Factors

Adsorption from Blood and Plasma

The adsorption of fibrinogen from plasma to many surfaces exhibits an unusual time dependence.[5] An example is shown in FIGURE 4. Fibrinogen adsorption from

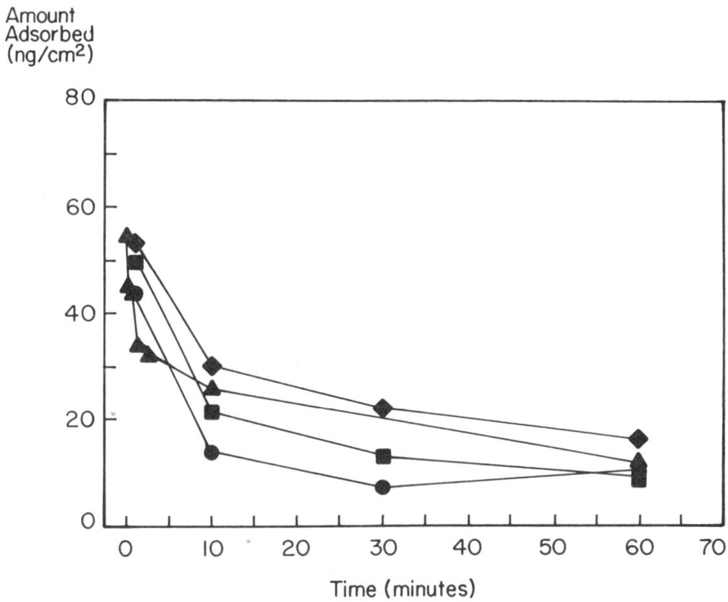

FIGURE 4. Fibrinogen adsorption kinetics from plasma and blood to various surfaces. Adsorption from plasma onto polyethylene (*triangles*) and from blood onto polyethylene (*squares*), silicone rubber (*diamonds*), and PEU #3 (Pellethane, *circles*) is shown. The coefficient of variation averaged 12.6%, 10.6%, 10.9%, and 25.3% for the data on polyethylene from plasma, polyethylene from blood, silicone rubber, and PEU #3 (Pellethane), respectively.

undiluted plasma onto PE reaches a maximum of 60–70 ng/cm^2 after 10 seconds and falls steadily to a surface concentration of 10–20 ng/cm^2 after 2 hours of exposure. The same behavior occurs when fibrinogen adsorbs from whole blood, also shown in FIGURE 4. Fibrinogen adsorption onto PE, silicone rubber, and PEU #3 (Pellethane) is initially high but decreases markedly after one hour of exposure, a phenomenon we refer to as "displacement."

Adsorption from BaSO$_4$-treated Plasma and Serum

The treatment of plasma with $BaSO_4$ removes the vitamin-K-dependent proteases (factors II, VII, IX, and X), only two of which factors (IX and X) participate solely in

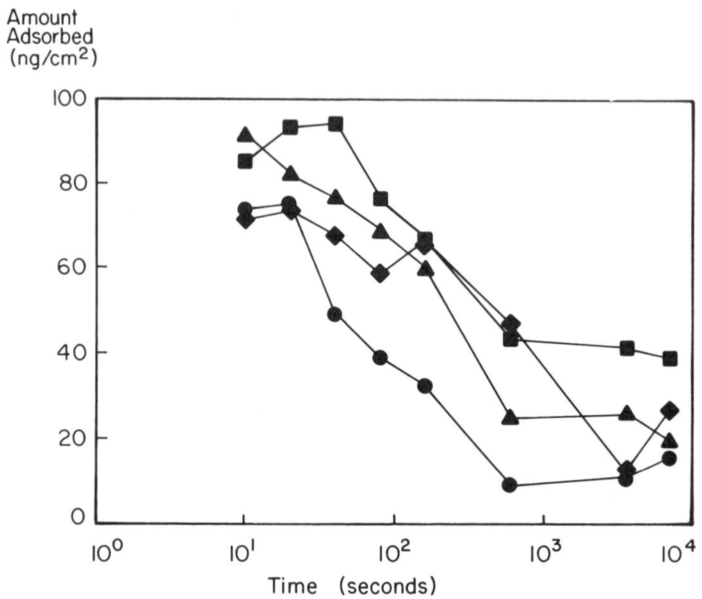

FIGURE 5. Fibrinogen adsorption kinetics to polyethylene: effect of plasma composition. Adsorption from normal (*triangles*), kininogen-deficient (*squares*), and $BaSO_4$-treated (*diamonds*) plasmas and from serum to which fibrinogen was added (*circles*) are shown. The coefficient of variation averaged 5.3%, 4.2%, and 8.6% for the data from normal, kininogen-deficient, and $BaSO_4$-treated plasmas, respectively, and 7.6% for serum to which fibrinogen was added.

the intrinsic coagulation pathway.[20] Fibrinogen adsorption kinetics onto polyethylene from $BaSO_4$-treated plasma and from normal plasma are shown in FIGURE 5. No significant differences between the curves are evident, suggesting that these clotting proteins do not influence fibrinogen adsorption from normal plasma onto polyethylene.

In a related experiment the adsorption kinetics of fibrinogen from refibrinogenated serum onto polyethylene were measured. FIGURE 5 shows that fibrinogen displacement occurred as readily from serum as from normal plasma. Since the formation of serum from blood results in the virtually complete activation and subsequent inhibition and/or degradation of many clotting proteins (factors V, VIII, IX, XIII, and prekallikrein), it at least appears that these factors do not play a major role in fibrinogen displacement from polyethylene. However, the differences between serum and plasma are complex so that it is difficult to interpret these data.

Adsorption from Kininogen-Deficient Plasma

Fibrinogen adsorbed to certain surfaces from plasma lacking HMWK is much more reactive to antifibrinogen[21] and the actual quantity adsorbed from undiluted plasma is much greater than from normal plasma.[11] To determine whether HMWK influences fibrinogen adsorption from plasma to other surfaces, a series of studies of fibrinogen adsorption from HMWK-deficient plasma were performed.

Fibrinogen adsorption to soda-lime glass from normal and kininogen-deficient human plasmas (after 2 hours at 37°C) is shown in FIGURE 6 (two lower curves). Fibrinogen adsorption reaches a maximum of 6–7 ng/cm^2 at a plasma concentration of 0.1% from both HMWK-deficient and normal plasmas, indicating that kininogen does not influence fibrinogen adsorption to glass under these conditions.

In one previous study of the effect of HMWK deficiency,[11] fibrinogen adsorption onto pyrex glass from normal and HMWK-deficient plasmas was measured at room temperature after five minutes, experimental conditions that differ significantly from those employed in the experiments described above. The effect of these differences was investigated by measuring fibrinogen adsorption onto glass from normal and kininogen-deficient plasmas after five minutes of incubation at 25°C. The results, shown in FIGURE 6 (upper two curves), indicate that fibrinogen adsorption from kininogen-deficient plasma was enhanced from highly diluted plasma relative to that observed from normal plasma, but no differences were evident at either 5% or 10% plasma concentration. In contrast, fibrinogen adsorption from 5% and 10% concentrations of HMWK-deficient plasma under these conditions was reported to be much greater than that from normal plasma.[11]

Fibrinogen adsorption from normal and kininogen-deficient plasmas onto both polyethylene and silicone rubber are shown in FIGURE 7. The adsorption from both normal and kininogen-deficient plasmas reached a maximum of 60–70 ng/cm^2 on

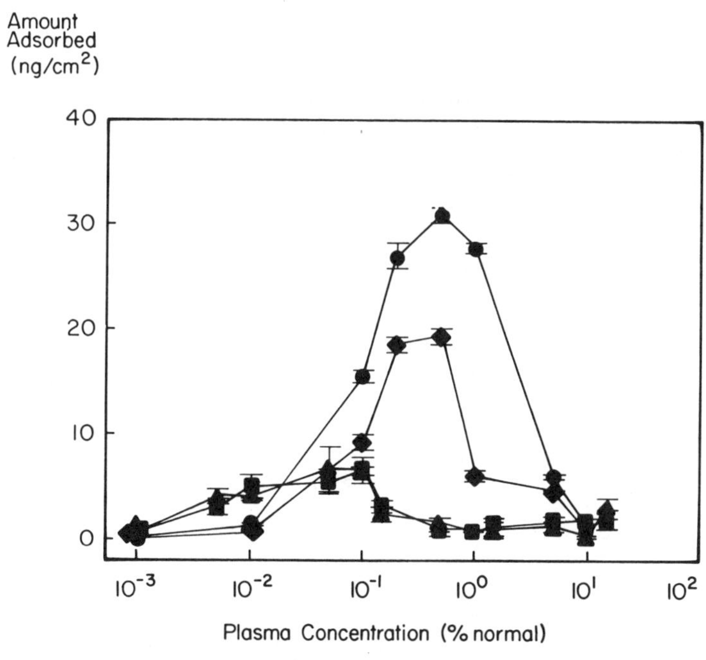

FIGURE 6. Fibrinogen adsorption to glass: effect of kininogen deficiency. Adsorption was measured from plasma after incubation for either 5 min at 25°C (*upper curves*) or for 2 h at 37°C (*lower curves*). Adsorption was measured after 5 min at 25°C for normal (*diamonds*) and deficient (*circles*) plasma and after 2 h at 37°C for normal (*triangles*) and deficient (*squares*) plasma.

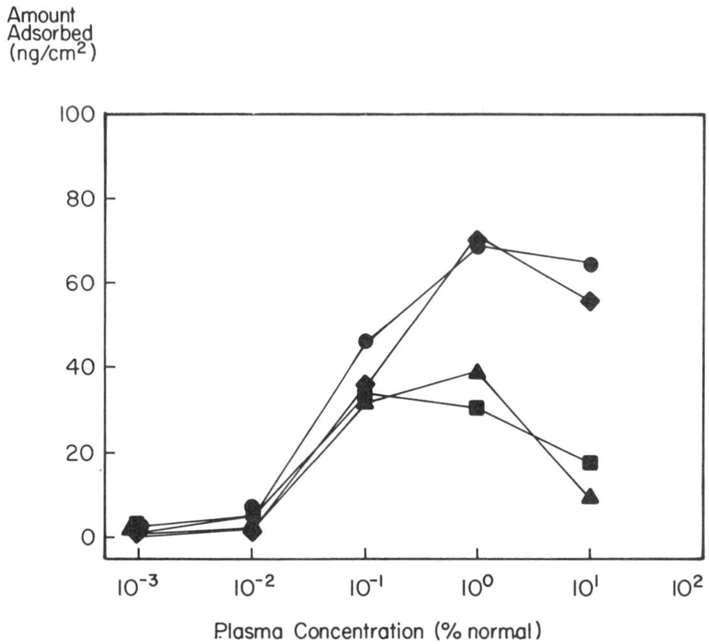

FIGURE 7. Fibrinogen adsorption to silicone rubber and polyethylene: effect of kininogen deficiency. Adsorption was measured to silicone rubber from normal (*triangles*) and deficient (*squares*) plasma and to polyethylene from normal (*diamonds*) and deficient (*circles*) plasma. The coefficient of variation averaged 19.9% and 22.5% for the data on silicone rubber from normal and deficient plasma, respectively, and 17.2% and 27.4% for the data on polyethylene from normal and deficient plasma, respectively.

polyethylene and 30–40 ng/cm^2 on silicone rubber. Thus, the absence of kininogen from plasma does not appear to affect fibrinogen adsorption onto these surfaces.

Finally, fibrinogen adsorption kinetics onto polyethylene from kininogen-deficient plasma are presented in FIGURE 5. Although adsorption from kininogen-deficient plasma seems to be enhanced relative to that measured from normal plasma, the effect is not large. The data do show that the characteristic decrease in adsorption as plasma contact time increases occurs at slightly later times compared to the kininogen-deficient plasma, *i.e.*, displacement is somewhat delayed. However, the total amount of fibrinogen that has been displaced, *i.e.*, maximal minus 2-hour adsorption, is essentially the same from both plasmas.

Adsorption from Prekallikrein-Deficient Plasma

In another study we have found that fibrinogen adsorption onto polyethylene from prekallikrein-deficient plasma is enhanced relative to that from normal plasma. Adsorption to polyethylene from prekallikrein-deficient plasma was nearly double that from normal plasma and did not pass through a maximum over the plasma concentration range studied.[22] Studies were therefore performed to see if prekallikrein could influence fibrinogen adsorption onto glass. The results of the experiment are shown in

FIGURE 8. Adsorption from prekallikrein-deficient plasma appears to be somewhat greater than that from normal plasma, but the effect is not as large as that observed with polyethylene in the previous study.[22] Maximum fibrinogen adsorption onto glass from both plasmas occurred at a plasma concentration of approximately 0.05%.

Adsorption from Kallikrein-inhibited Plasma

The higher adsorption of fibrinogen observed from plasmas deficient in either prekallikrein (FIG. 8) or kininogens (FIG. 6) suggested that contact activation may have occurred on glass from normal plasma despite the presence of citrate as an anticoagulant. Contact activation does not require Ca^{2+} and involves the formation of a more surface-active form of HMWK ($HMWK_a$, see DISCUSSION) that may be responsible for displacing fibrinogen. Since kallikrein is thought to be required to induce full activation of factors XI, XII, and HMWK,[24] contact activation was prevented by adding varying concentrations of Phe-Phe-Arg-CMK, an inhibitor of plasma kallikrein, to plasma. Phe-Phe-Arg-CMK reacts stoichiometrically with plasma kallikrein[23] and 100% inhibition represents a tetrapeptide concentration of 588 nM, the nominal concentration of prekallikrein in human plasma.[24] TABLE 2 shows that fibrinogen adsorption is invariant with inhibitor concentration at all plasma concentrations tested. Therefore, the activated forms of factors XI and XII, prekallikrein, and HMWK do not appear to be required for fibrinogen displacement from glass.

Although polyethylene and silicone rubber are not considered potent activators of the intrinsic pathway, it is possible that some contact activation occurs on these

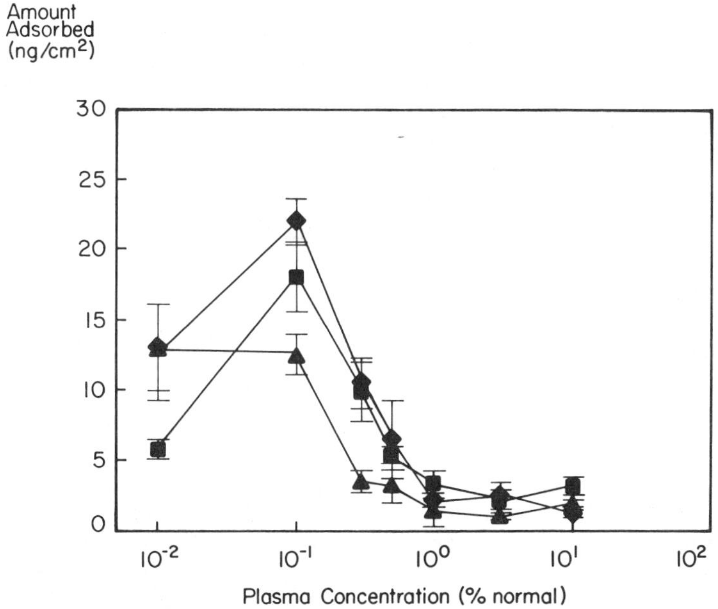

FIGURE 8. Fibrinogen adsorption to glass: effects of factor IX and prekallikrein deficiencies. Adsorption was measured from normal plasma (*triangles*) and plasma deficient in prekallikrein (*squares*) or factor IX (*diamonds*).

TABLE 2. Effect of Kallikrein Inhibitor on Fibrinogen Adsorption from Plasma to Glass[a]

Plasma Concentration (%)	% Inhibition[b]	Fibrinogen Adsorption (ng/cm²)
0.1	0	7.2 ± 2.7
	10	9.4 ± 1.0
	50	8.6 ± 1.9
	100	10.1 ± 1.2
0.2	0	17.8 ± 0.2
	10	15.3 ± 1.8
	50	18.2 ± 1.2
	100	15.7 ± 5.0
0.5	0	16.5 ± 1.5
	10	17.7 ± 0.4
	50	15.8 ± 1.4
	100	16.7 ± 0.8
1.0	0	5.8 ± 0.8
	10	7.0 ± 1.5
	50	5.6 ± 0.3
	100	5.8 ± 0.4

[a]Adsorption was done at 25°C for 5 minutes.

[b]One hundred percent inhibition corresponds to equal concentrations of inhibitor and prekallikrein in the plasma (588 nM). Smaller inhibitor concentrations were assumed to give proportionately less kallikrein inhibition. Data at four other plasma concentrations (not shown in the interest of space) were also taken. No differences in fibrinogen adsorption at any degree of inhibition were observed at those plasma concentrations either.

surfaces and causes displacement of fibrinogen. Therefore, 58.8 nM Phe-Phe-Arg-CMK (10% inhibition of kallikrein) was added to normal plasma and fibrinogen adsorption was measured after two hours at 37°C. Two hours was chosen to allow sufficient time for activation to occur in the uninhibited controls. FIGURE 9 shows that no significant differences between the isotherms were observed for either polyethylene or silicone rubber. Therefore, activation of coagulation factors by these surfaces does not appear to be involved in the observed displacement of fibrinogen.

Adsorption from Factor-IX-Deficient Plasma

Previous experiments have shown that fibrinogen adsorption to polyethylene is greater from factor-IX-deficient plasma than from normal plasma, similar to the effect of prekallikrein deficiency.[22] FIGURE 8 illustrates the fibrinogen adsorption isotherms onto glass from factor-IX-deficient and normal human plasmas. At a plasma concentration of 0.1%, almost double the amount of fibrinogen adsorbs to glass from factor-IX-deficient plasma compared to normal plasma but the adsorption values converge at larger plasma concentrations. Thus, the absence of factor IX from plasma does seem to influence fibrinogen adsorption onto glass but the effect is only observable from diluted plasma. The lack of any effect of prekallikrein deficiency at high plasma concentrations may perhaps explain why fibrinogen adsorption kinetics to polyethylene from undiluted plasma treated with $BaSO_4$ (which also removes factor IX) did not differ significantly from those measured from normal plasma (see FIGURE 5).

Behavior of Binary Protein Systems

The experiments with plasmas lacking the intrinsic coagulation factors HMWK, prekallikrein, and factor IX show that fibrinogen displacement still occurs on all surfaces examined in this study, although prekallikrein and factor IX seem to influence this effect to some extent. We then inquired whether fibrinogen displacement was a phenomenon unique to plasma. Fibrinogen adsorption isotherms were therefore measured from hemoglobin/fibrinogen and albumin/fibrinogen solutions onto glass (see FIGURE 10). Clearly, displacement of fibrinogen occurred from these simpler mixtures as well. Adsorption reached a maximum of 85 ng/cm^2 with hemoglobin as the competitor and 90 ng/cm^2 with albumin as the competitor. The smaller concentration of hemoglobin compared to albumin required to accomplish a similar reduction in fibrinogen adsorption is consistent with previous observations showing that hemoglobin is more surface active than albumin.[25] The kinetics of fibrinogen adsorption onto glass from a binary mixture of albumin and fibrinogen are shown in FIGURE 11. Displacement of fibrinogen adsorbed from this mixture clearly occurred. Thus, the effects of both dilution and contact time on fibrinogen adsorption from binary mixtures are similar to those observed from plasma.

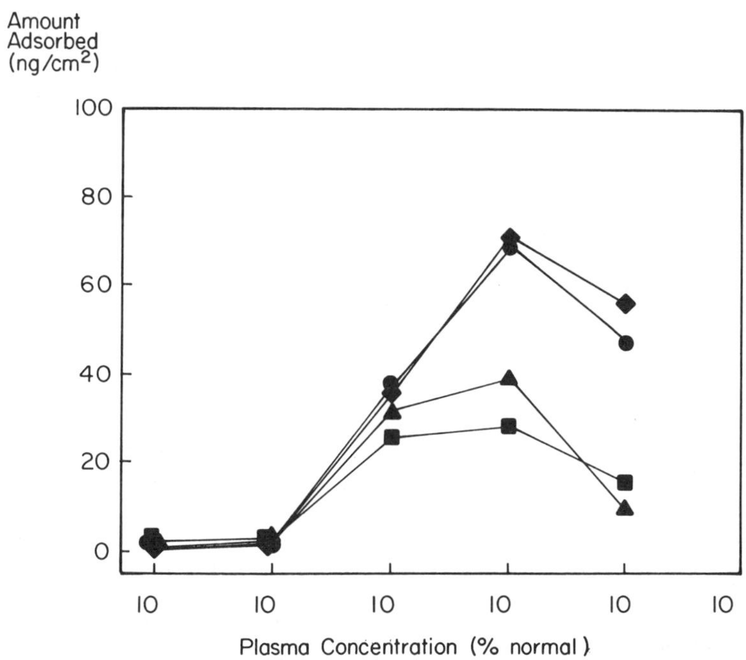

FIGURE 9. Fibrinogen adsorption to silicone rubber and polyethylene: effect of kallikrein inhibitor. Phe-Phe-Arg-CMK was added to plasma at a final concentration of 58.8 nM to inhibit 10% of the kallikrein. Adsorption was measured onto silicone rubber from normal (*triangles*) and inhibited (*squares*) plasma and onto polyethylene from normal (*diamonds*) and inhibited (*circles*) plasma. The coefficient of variation averaged 19.9% and 27.3% for the data on silicone rubber from normal and inhibited plasma, respectively, and 17.2% and 12.0% for the data on polyethylene from normal and inhibited plasma, respectively.

The effect of surface chemistry on competitive adsorption of fibrinogen in binary mixtures also parallels that observed in plasma adsorption studies. Fibrinogen adsorption from solutions containing both fibrinogen and hemoglobin onto poly(HEMA), poly(EMA), and a copolymer made from a 50/50 mixture of the two monomers (HEMA/EMA) is shown in FIGURE 12. Fibrinogen adsorption decreases as the ratio of hemoglobin to fibrinogen increases. Interestingly, a larger ratio of hemoglobin to fibrinogen was required to reduce adsorption to 50% of its maximum with the HEMA/EMA copolymer than was needed with either of the two homopolymers. These results are consistent with previous observations showing that fibrinogen

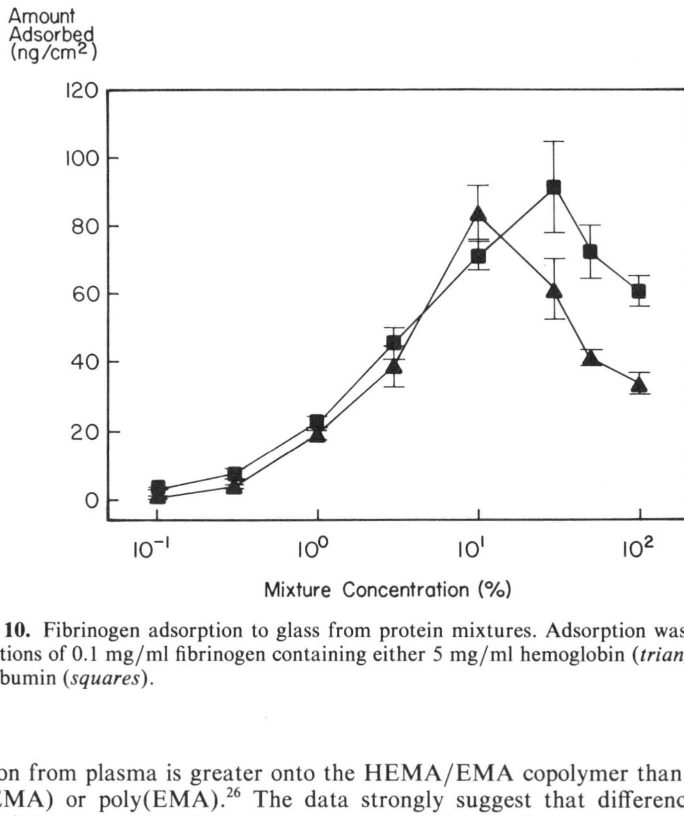

FIGURE 10. Fibrinogen adsorption to glass from protein mixtures. Adsorption was measured from solutions of 0.1 mg/ml fibrinogen containing either 5 mg/ml hemoglobin (*triangles*) or 10 mg/ml albumin (*squares*).

adsorption from plasma is greater onto the HEMA/EMA copolymer than on either poly(HEMA) or poly(EMA).[26] The data strongly suggest that differences in the affinity of fibrinogen for the substrate can exert large effects on the competitive effectiveness of proteins.

The effect of three different protein competitors on prothrombin adsorption to polyethylene is shown in FIGURE 13. A greater concentration of albumin than hemoglobin or fibrinogen was needed to reduce prothrombin adsorption by a similar amount. Therefore, fibrinogen and hemoglobin compete more effectively against prothrombin for adsorption sites than does albumin.

The data from these and other competitive adsorption experiments are summarized

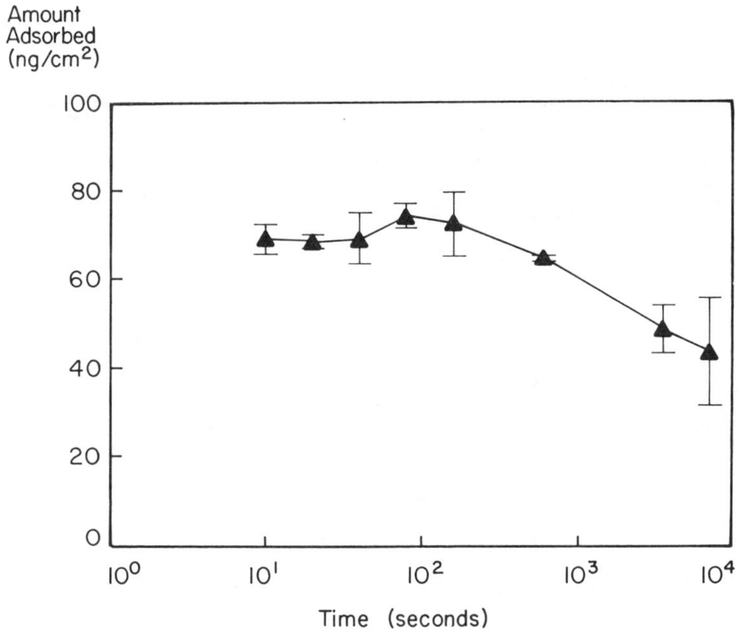

FIGURE 11. Kinetics of fibrinogen adsorption from an albumin solution to glass. Adsorption was measured from a solution containing both 0.1 mg/ml fibrinogen and 20 mg/ml albumin.

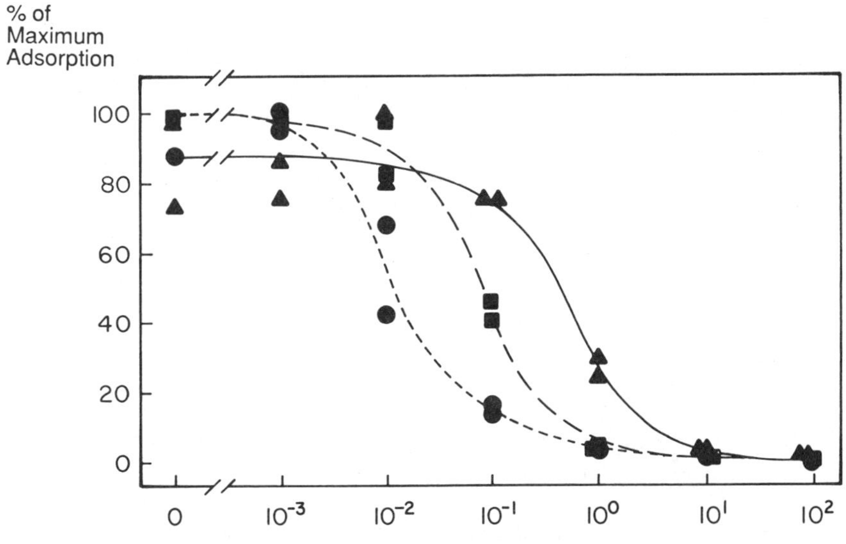

FIGURE 12. Fibrinogen adsorption from a hemoglobin solution: effect of surface. Adsorption was measured from a solution containing 0.1 mg/ml fibrinogen and varying concentrations of hemoglobin to HEMA (*triangles*), EMA (*squares*), and copolymer that was 50% HEMA and 50% EMA (*circles*). Individual measurements are plotted.

in TABLE 3. The parameter R^{50} is defined as the ratio of competing protein required to reduce the adsorption of the ^{125}I-labeled protein to 50% of what it would be from a pure solution. For example, at a prothrombin concentration of 0.01 mg/ml, albumin must be present at a concentration of 0.028 mg/ml in order to reduce the steady-state adsorption of prothrombin to half what it would be from a pure 0.01 mg/ml solution. Thus, R^{50} equals 0.028/0.01 or 2.8 in this case. Fibrinogen, on the other hand, need only be present at a concentration of 0.0016 mg/ml ($R^{50} = 0.16$) to accomplish the same feat, indicating that fibrinogen is a far superior competitor than albumin under these conditions.

In some binary protein experiments, the adsorption of the radiolabeled protein in the presence of a small amount of competing protein is greater by 10–30% than from a solution containing no competitor at all. In calculating the percentage of maximum adsorption, the greatest adsorption value recorded in the experiment was used. The maximum often occurred at a competing to radiolabeled protein ratio of 10^{-3} rather than zero. If the percentage of maximum adsorption is based instead on the adsorption from the protein solution lacking any competitor, the competition curves (like those in FIGURES 12 and 13) therefore sometimes change. The degree of change depends on the data set but is often negligible. Moreover, the relative change in R^{50} between experiments will not change at all. Thus, while the absolute magnitudes of R^{50} sometimes depend on how the maximum adsorption is defined, the comparisons of R^{50} we have made are still valid indicators of differences in competitive effectiveness.

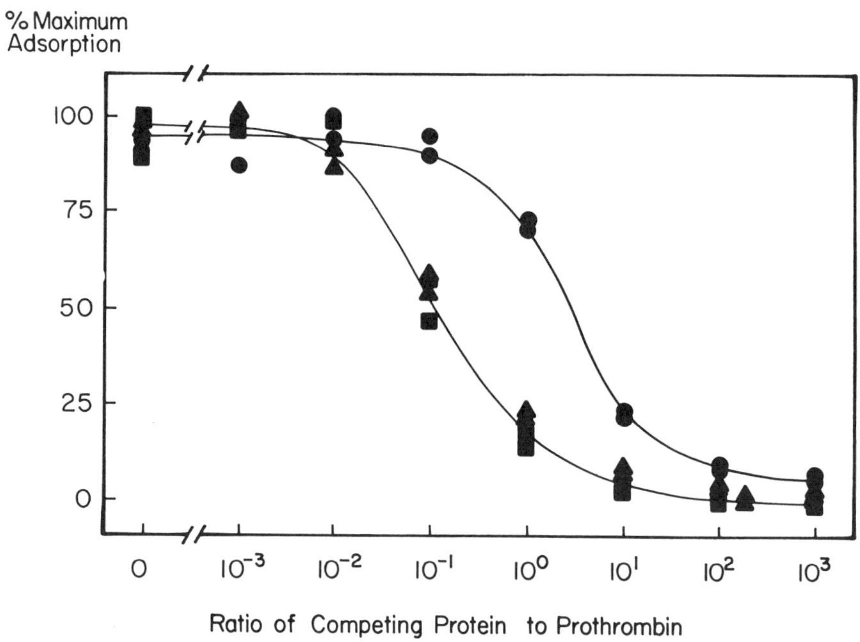

FIGURE 13. Prothrombin adsorption from binary protein mixtures. Adsorption was measured from solutions of 0.01 mg/ml prothrombin and varying concentrations of albumin (*circles*), fibrinogen (*triangles*), or hemoglobin (*squares*). Maximum absorption of prothrombin in the absence of competing proteins was 0.301 ± 0.014 $\mu g/cm^2$. Individual measurements are plotted.

TABLE 3. Summary of Binary Competitive Adsorption Data[a]

^{125}I-labeled Protein	Competitor	Surface	R^{50}
prothrombin	albumin	polyethylene	2.82
"	fibrinogen	"	0.16
"	hemoglobin	"	0.13
fibrinogen	hemoglobin	HEMA	0.02
"	"	EMA	0.08
"	"	HEMA/EMA	0.32
collagen	albumin	polyethylene	0.50
IgG	hemoglobin	HEMA	0.01
"	"	EMA	0.04
"	"	HEMA/EMA	0.08

[a]The ratio of competitor protein to ^{125}I-labeled protein required to reduce the latter's adsorption to 50% of its maximum is given by R^{50}. The ^{125}I-labeled protein concentration was kept constant in all experiments. The concentration was 0.01 mg/ml for prothrombin, but 0.1 mg/ml for the other ^{125}I-labeled proteins.

DISCUSSION

Fibrinogen adsorption from normal plasma onto every surface studied reached a maximum at an intermediate plasma concentration. Both the quantity of adsorbed fibrinogen and the plasma concentration at which maximum adsorption occurred varied with the type of substrate. Fibrinogen adsorption to glass and polyetherurethanes containing larger fractions of polyether (PPG and PTMG) was less than that on the more hydrophobic polymers. In addition, the plasma concentration at which maximum adsorption occurred was found to be greater for the hydrophobic substrates than for the hydrophilic ones. Fundamentally, these differences must arise from the fact that the affinity of a protein for a material depends strongly on the particular nature of the surface. However, the relationship between affinity and surface chemistry is poorly understood, although speculation on the importance of unfolding to allow interior hydrophobic residues to interact with apolar surfaces has been made.[27] We have shown, however, that fibrinogen adsorption from both plasma and a binary mixture of fibrinogen and hemoglobin is greater on the HEMA/EMA copolymer than on either the HEMA or EMA homopolymers, indicating that both hydrophilic and hydrophobic interactions are important in determining fibrinogen adsorption. The generally lower and weaker adsorption of proteins to hydrogels and to highly swollen, hydrophilic chromatography matrices noted in a recent review[28] agrees with our observations of lower adsorption to the more hydrophilic surfaces. However, a detailed explanation of these phenomena, in terms of which surface characteristics most strongly influence protein adsorption and how they exert their effects on proteins, cannot be given at this time.

The displacement of bound fibrinogen from polyethylene, as suggested by the decrease in adsorption with plasma contact time, is an unexpected result in the sense that protein adsorption to polymeric biomaterials has usually been considered to be irreversible. A recent study has demonstrated that some but not all adsorbed protein can be eluted from a surface using sodium dodecyl sulfate (SDS) or other, stronger detergents.[19] Yet adsorbed fibrinogen is removed from polyethylene quite effectively during continued exposure to plasma.

One explanation of fibrinogen displacment is that all plasma proteins possess varying degrees of surface activity and that collectively they can remove or displace adsorbed protein as efficiently as any detergent. In this model, displacement occurs as a result of the cumulative interaction of all proteins with the surfaces and each protein contributes to the process according to its intrinsic surface affinity and mass concentration. The coagulation factors would therefore not be expected to play an important role in displacement because of their typically very low concentrations in plasma. But they might still participate in displacement if they were very surface active, as they are believed to be. However, such a general explanation requires that displacement occur for other proteins as well and not just fibrinogen. On some polymers, at least, albumin adsorption from plasma has been found to pass through a maximum at early times.[4] Moreover, fibronectin adsorption passes through a maximum on both glass[29] and polystyrene[30] surfaces at intermediate serum concentrations. Finally, we have shown that fibrinogen adsorption onto glass from a binary mixture of fibrinogen and hemoglobin passes through a maximum, both as a function of time and mixture concentration. Thus, it appears that the mechanism(s) governing displacement reflect general properties of protein mixtures.

An alternative explanation, in which fibrinogen displacement is due to specific interactions of the clotting factors with surfaces, was suggested by previous studies of fibrinogen adsorption onto glass from HMWK-deficient plasma.[10,11] However, our attempts to extend this idea to other surfaces were not all successful. Thus, even though fibrinogen adsorption from normal plasma onto silicone rubber and polyethylene exhibited displacement, no differences were observed in either the adsorption kinetics or isotherms of fibrinogen from kininogen-deficient plasma onto those surfaces. In addition, the fibrinogen adsorption kinetics onto polyethylene from the $BaSO_4$-treated plasma and the refibrinogenated serum were similar to those seen with normal plasma, showing that displacement occurs whether or not all the coagulation factors are present in their proenzyme forms. On the other hand, we have seen that fibrinogen adsorption onto polyethylene is enhanced from prekallikrein- and factor-IX-deficient plasma relative to that measured from normal plasma.[22] The absence of these coagulation factors does seem to influence fibrinogen adsorption.

The idea that contact activation may have occurred on glass and caused displacement of fibrinogen was suggested by the higher adsorption of fibrinogen from HMWK- and prekallikrein-deficient plasmas to glass. During contact activation HMWK is cleaved by kallikrein to activated HMWK (HMWKa), a more surface-active form of the protein.[31] HMWK can also be cleaved by factor XIIa.[32] Since fibrinogen is unable to prevent HMWKa from adsorbing to kaolin,[31] HMWKa may be responsible for the displacement of fibrinogen from glass observed from normal plasma. When the reciprocal activation of prekallikrein and factor XII was prevented by adding Phe-Phe-Arg-CMK (a stoichiometric inhibitor of kallikrein) to plasma, there was no difference in the adsorption of fibrinogen to glass at any of the inhibitor concentrations. Therefore, HMWKa does not appear to be responsible for the displacement of fibrinogen. The possibility that HMWKa is present in plasma before the addition of inhibitor cannot be excluded. However, the observation that fibrinogen adsorption from factor-IX-deficient plasma, which contains all four of the contact activation factors, is greater than that from normal plasma shows that proteins other than HMWK or HMWKa influence the adsorption of fibrinogen to glass. HMWK may be responsible for displacement of fibrinogen at short incubation times (5 minutes, 25°C), but after 2 hours of adsorption other proteins become principally responsible for fibrinogen displacement since the amount of fibrinogen adsorbed after 2 hours from normal and HMWK-deficient plasmas is similar.

Collectively, these experiments suggest that fibrinogen adsorption and displacement from plasma depend on the affinities of all the proteins present in the mixture. Since displacement of fibrinogen by hemoglobin and albumin is not observed unless the ratio of competing protein is much higher than physiological ratios, this suggested explanation of fibrinogen displacement requires that all proteins in plasma act together to bring about displacement at the observed plasma concentrations. Certain clotting factors (prekallikrein and factor IX), despite existing in minute concentrations in plasma, can apparently influence fibrinogen adsorption, presumably because they possess large affinities for surfaces. The fact that fibrinogen displacement occurs from systems in which the progress of the intrinsic pathway has been stopped (*e.g.*, kallikrein-inhibited and $BaSO_4$-treated plasmas) and in which no clotting factors exist (mixtures of hemoglobin or albumin with fibrinogen) indicate that displacement is not solely a by-product of intrinsic pathway activation. Rather, displacement is the result of all plasma proteins expressing their innate affinity for adsorption sites. Depending on the nature of the surface, certain proteins will play a larger role in displacing bound fibrinogen but all plasma proteins probably contribute to the process.

Perhaps the most important realization to be made is that the adsorbed protein layer is in a dynamic equilibrium with the proteins in solution and thus the composition of the layer is constantly changing over time. This implies, then, that the responses of cells induced by the adsorbed proteins will depend on when the cells contact the adsorbed layer. If further experimentation can support this idea, then progress toward understanding the relationship between cellular responses involved in thrombosis and protein adsorption onto foreign materials will have been made.

SUMMARY

Fibrinogen adsorption from plasma exhibits an unusual displacement phenomenon (the Vroman effect) in that decreases in adsorption occur after longer contact time or as the plasma concentration increases. Fibrinogen adsorption and the displacement effect were found to depend markedly on the nature of the surface, the time and temperature of adsorption, and to a lesser extent on certain contact activation factors. Displacement still occurred from plasmas lacking kininogens, factor IX, and prekallikrein, and from plasma that had been treated with $BaSO_4$ to remove factors II, VII, IX, and X. Furthermore, displacement was also observed from fibrinogen solutions to which either albumin or hemoglobin had been added. In addition, competitive adsorption of binary protein mixtures was also shown to depend strongly on surface type. It therefore appears that fibrinogen adsorption from plasma is subject to similar if not identical competitive processes that occur in simpler protein mixtures. The final adsorption then reflects the influence of all the proteins in plasma, each competing for the limited number of adsorption sites according to the fundamental physical properties of surface activity and mass concentration.

ACKNOWLEDGMENTS

Technical assistance was provided by Winston Ciridon and Barbara Pederson and we are grateful to them for their efforts.

REFERENCES

1. Baier, R. E. & R. C. Dutton. 1969. Initial events in interactions of blood with a foreign surface. J. Biomed. Mater. Res. 3: 191–206.

2. PARK, K., D. F. MOSHER & S. L. COOPER. 1986. Acute surface-induced thrombosis in the canine ex vivo model: Importance of protein composition of the initial monolayer and platelet activation. J. Biomed. Mater. Res. **20:** 589–612.
3. PITT, W. G., K. PARK & S. L. COOPER. 1986. Sequential protein adsorption and thrombus deposition on polymeric biomaterials. J. Colloid Interface Sci. **111(2):** 343–362.
4. HORBETT, T. A. 1979. The kinetics of adsorption of plasma proteins to a series of hydrophilic-hydrophobic copolymers. Am. Chem. Soc. Div. Org. Coat. Plast. Chem. Pap. **40:** 642–646.
5. HORBETT, T. A., C. M. CHENG, B. D. RATNER, A. S. HOFFMAN & S. R. HANSON. 1986. The kinetics of baboon fibrinogen adsorption to polymers: In vitro and in vivo studies. J. Biomed. Mater. Res. **20:** 739–772.
6. HORBETT, T. A. 1984. Mass action effects on competitive adsorption of fibrinogen from hemoglobin solutions and from plasma. Thromb. Haemostas. **51(2):** 174–181.
7. VROMAN, L., A. L. ADAMS & G. C. FISCHER. 1982. Proteins, plasma, and blood in narrow spaces of clot-promoting surfaces. *In* Biomaterials: Interfacial Phenomena and Applications. Advances in Chemistry Series, Vol. 199. S. L. Cooper & N. A. Peppas, Eds.: 265–276. American Chemical Society. Washington, D. C.
8. BRASH, J. L. & P. TEN HOVE. 1984. Effect of plasma dilution on adsorption of fibrinogen to solid surfaces. Thromb. Haemostas. **51:** 326–330.
9. WOJCIECHOWSKI, P., P. TEN HOVE & J. BRASH. 1986. Phenomenology and mechanism of the transient adsorption of fibrinogen from plasma (Vroman effect). J. Colloid Interface Sci. **111:** 455–465.
10. VROMAN, L., A. L. ADAMS, G. C. FISCHER & P. C. MUNOZ. 1980. Interaction of high molecular weight kininogen, factor XII, and fibrinogen in plasma at interfaces. Blood **55(1):** 156–159.
11. BRASH, J. L., C. F. SCOTT, P. TEN HOVE & R. W. COLMAN. 1985. Desorption of plasma fibrinogen from glass: Role of high molecular weight kininogen (HMWK) and factor XI (abstract). Trans. Soc. Biomater. **11:** 105.
12. RATNOFF, O. D. & C. MENZIE. 1950. A new method for the determination of fibrinogen in small samples of plasma. J. Lab. Clin. Med. **37:** 316.
13. WEATHERSBY, P. K., T. A. HORBETT & A. S. HOFFMAN. 1977. Solution stability of bovine fibrinogen. Thromb. Res. **10:** 245–252.
14. HINSON, J. A. & T. L. MCMEEKIN. 1969. A rapid method for preparing crystalline human hemoglobin and the separation of crystalline hemoglobin A in quantity. Biochem. Biophys. Res. Commun. **35:** 94–101.
15. VAN ASSENDELFT, O. W. 1970. Spectrophotometry of Haemoglobin Derivatives. Charles C Thomas. Springfield, Ill.
16. HELMKAMP, R. W., R. L. GOODLAND, W. F. BALE, I. L. SPAR & L. E. MUTSCHLER. 1960. High specific activity iodination of gamma-globulin with iodine-131 monochloride. Cancer Res. **20:** 1495–1500.
17. YOON, S. C. & B. D. RATNER. 1986. Surface structure of segmented poly(ether urethanes) and poly(ether urethane ureas) with various perfluoro chain extenders. An x-ray photoelectron spectroscopic investigation. Macromolecules **19:** 1068–1079.
18. WEATHERSBY, P. K., T. A. HORBETT & A. S. HOFFMAN. 1977. Surface analysis of methacrylate graft copolymers varying in hydrophobicity. J. Bioeng. **1:** 381–394.
19. BOHNERT, J. L. & T. A. HORBETT. 1986. Changes in adsorbed fibrinogen and albumin interactions with polymers indicated by decreases in detergent elutability. J. Colloid Interface Sci. **111(2):** 363–377.
20. ZUCKER, M. B. & J. OWEN. 1982. Non-decalcified barium sulfate-adsorbed plasma, a potentially useful reagent for studying blood clotting, platelets or complement. Thromb. Haemostas. **47:** 182–184.
21. SCHMAIER, A. H., L. SILVER, A. L. ADAMS, G. C. FISCHER, P. C. MUNOZ, L. VROMAN & R. W. COLMAN. 1983. The effect of high molecular weight kininogen on surface-adsorbed fibrinogen. Thromb. Res. **33:** 51–67.
22. SLACK, S. & T. A. HORBETT. 1986. Physicochemical and biochemical aspects of fibrinogen adsorption from plasma and binary protein solutions onto polyethylene and glass. Submitted.

23. KETTNER, C. & E. SHAW. 1981. Inactivation of trypsin-like enzymes with peptides of arginine chloromethyl ketone. *In* Methods in Enzymology, Vol. 80. Proteolytic Enzymes. L. Lorand, Ed.: 826–842. Academic. New York.
24. GRIFFIN, J. H. & C. G. COCHRANE. 1979. Recent advances in the understanding of contact activation reactions. Semin. Thromb. Hemostas. **5(4):** 254–273.
25. HORBETT, T. A., P. K. WEATHERSBY & A. S. HOFFMAN. 1977. The preferential adsorption of hemoglobin to polyethylene. J. Bioeng. **1:** 61–78.
26. HORBETT, T. A. 1981. Adsorption of proteins from plasma to a series of hydrophilic-hydrophobic copolymers. 2. Compositional analysis with the prelabeled protein technique. J. Biomed. Mater. Res. **15:** 673–695.
27. HOFFMAN, A. S. 1974. Principles governing biomolecule interactions at foreign interfaces. J. Biomed. Mater. Res. Symp. **5**(Part 1): 77–83.
28. HORBETT, T. A. 1985. Protein adsorption to hydrogels. *In* Hydrogels in Medicine and Pharmacy, Vol. 1. N. L. Peppas, Ed.: 127–171. CRC Press. Boca Raton, Fla.
29. HORBETT, T. A. & M. SCHWAY. 1986. Correlations between mouse 3T3 cell spreading and serum fibronectin adsorption on glass and hydroxyethylmethacrylate-ethylmethacrylate copolymers. Submitted.
30. GRINNELL, F. & M. K. FELD. 1982. Fibronectin adsorption on hydrophobic and hydrophilic surfaces detected by antibody binding and analyzed during cell adhesion in serum containing medium. J. Biol. Chem. **257:** 4888–4893.
31. SCOTT, C. F., L. D. SILVER, M. SCHAPIRA & R. W. COLMAN. 1984. Cleavage of human high molecular weight kininogen markedly enhances its coagulant activity: Evidence that this molecule exists as a procofactor. J. Clin. Invest. **73:** 954–962.
32. WIGGINS, R. C. 1983. Kinin release from high molecular weight kininogen by the action of Hageman factor in the absence of kallikrein. J. Biol. Chem. **258(3):** 8963–8970.

Adsorption Kinetics of Protein Mixtures

A Tentative Explanation of the Vroman Effect

PETER A. CUYPERS,[a,b] GEORGE M. WILLEMS,[a]
H. COENRAAD HEMKER,[c] AND WIM TH. HERMENS[a]

[a]*Department of Biophysics*
[c]*Department of Biochemistry*
Biomedical Centre
University of Limburg
6200 MD Maastricht, The Netherlands

INTRODUCTION

When a surface is exposed to plasma, different proteins from the plasma will adsorb on the surface within several minutes. This adsorption from plasma or serum or protein mixtures depends on the concentration of the various proteins, the nature of the protein and surface, and the adsorption time. Despite numerous studies, the exact composition of the adsorbed protein layer from a multicomponent mixture such as plasma is not yet known.[1–3] Exposure of different surfaces to undiluted plasma results in a relatively limited adsorption of albumin, immunoglobulin, and fibrinogen compared with the adsorption of the same proteins from less concentrated solutions.[4] From experiments of Vroman[5] in which he used normal plasma and plasma lacking high molecular weight kininogen (HMWK), it was concluded that fibrinogen, initially adsorbed on hydrophilic surfaces exposed to normal plasma, is displaced by HMWK. These observations were confirmed by Brash.[3] Observations on the absorption of proteins from various dilutions of plasma showed that no fibrinogen is adsorbed from concentrated plasma, adsorption followed by desorption of fibrinogen occurs for moderately diluted plasma, and a stable adsorbed fibrinogen monolayer is formed for plasma dilutions of about 5% or less.[6–10] The observation that a protein, abundantly present in plasma, predominates initially in the adsorbed protein layer only to be replaced thereafter by a scarce component of the plasma proteins with a higher affinity for the adsorbing surface fits qualitatively into classical binding theory. The dilution effects, however, seem unexplainable in this framework.

In recent studies on the adsorption kinetics of three different proteins on a double layer of phospholipids it was found that the value of the intrinsic adsorption rate constant, k_{on}^{int}, is strongly dependent on the surface concentration of the adsorbed proteins. The experiments showed that k_{on}^{int} decays exponentially with increasing surface concentration Γ. The present study shows that this behavior results in an interaction parameter between the adsorbed proteins that may in principle cause such phenomena as the replacement of fibrinogen by HMWK, and, more importantly, also explains the different types of adsorption from different dilutions of plasma.

[b]Present address: DSM Research BV, P.O. Box 18, 6160 MD Geleen, The Netherlands.

MATERIALS AND METHODS

Materials

A double layer of 1,2-dioleoyl-*sn*-glycero-2-phosphoserine (DOPS) was stacked on a chromium slide as described in refs. 11 and 16. Bovine prothrombin and human fibrinogen were used. The proteins were either obtained commercially or prepared according to established procedures.[16]

Adsorption and desorption experiments were performed by ellipsometry as described in detail previously.[12–14] The surface concentration of proteins was calculated from the measured refractive index and thickness according to the modified Lorenz-Lorentz equation.[15] Sorption experiments were performed in Tris-HCl buffer, pH 7.5, containing 0.1 M NaCl and 1.5 mM $CaCl_2$.

Analysis of Sorption Kinetics

Introduction of Γ-dependent intrinsic adsorption and desorption rate constants, including the deviations from ideal Langmuir adsorption behavior, results in the following set of equations[16,17]

$$\frac{d}{dt}\Gamma(t) = k(\Gamma)_{\rm on}^{\rm app}(\Gamma_{\rm max} - \Gamma(t))c_{\rm b} - k(\Gamma)_{\rm off}^{\rm app}\Gamma(t) \qquad \textbf{(1a)}$$

with

$$k(\Gamma)_{\rm on}^{\rm app} = k(\Gamma)_{\rm on}^{\rm int}D/(D + \delta k(\Gamma)_{\rm on}^{\rm int}(\Gamma_{\rm max} - \Gamma)) \qquad \textbf{(1b)}$$

and

$$k(\Gamma)_{\rm off}^{\rm app} = k(\Gamma)_{\rm off}^{\rm int}D/(D + \delta k(\Gamma)_{\rm on}^{\rm int}(\Gamma_{\rm max} - \Gamma)), \qquad \textbf{(1c)}$$

where $\Gamma(t)$ = surface concentration ($\mu g/cm^2$) dependent on time t
$k(\Gamma)_{\rm on}$ = adsorption rate function ($cm^3/\mu g \cdot s$)
$k(\Gamma)_{\rm off}$ = desorption rate function (s^{-1})
$c_{\rm b}$ = protein concentration in the bulk ($\mu g/cm^3$)
D = diffusion constant of the protein (cm^2/s)
δ = thickness of the unstirred layer (cm)

The observed values of $k(\Gamma)_{\rm on}^{\rm app}$ and $k(\Gamma)_{\rm off}^{\rm app}$ can be approximated by exponential relations (see FIGURE 2):

$$k(\Gamma)_{\rm on}^{\rm int} = k_{+1}e^{-\alpha\Gamma}$$

and

$$k(\Gamma)_{\rm off}^{\rm int} = k_{-1}e^{+\beta\Gamma}, \qquad \textbf{(2)}$$

where α and β are respectively the interaction constants for the adsorption and desorption of this particular protein.[17]

From the preadsorption experiments (see RESULTS) it was concluded that the total amount of adsorbed protein has to be taken into account in these relations; for instance, for a mixture of two proteins

$$\Gamma = \Gamma_1 + \Gamma_2.$$

The equilibrium association constant K_a is defined by $K_a = k_{on}^{int}/k_{off}^{int}$. Using equations **1b, 1c,** and **2,** K_a can be written as:

$$K_a = k_{on}^{int}/k_{off}^{int} = k_{on}^{app}/k_{off}^{app} = Ke^{-\gamma\Gamma},$$

where $\gamma = \alpha + \beta$ and $K = k_+/k_-$ is the association constant in the limit of low surface coverage.

In equilibrium one has $d/dt\,\Gamma(t) = 0$ and it follows from equation **1a** that

$$\Gamma_{eq} = (k_{on}^{app}/k_{off}^{app})\,(\Gamma_{max} - \Gamma_{eq})c_b = Ke^{-\gamma\Gamma_{eq}}(\Gamma_{max} - \Gamma_{eq})c_b.$$

For two components one then obtains:

$$\Gamma_{eq} = \Gamma_{1eq} + \Gamma_{2eq} = (K_1e^{-\gamma_1\Gamma_{eq}}c_{1b} + K_2e^{-\gamma_2\Gamma_{eq}}c_{2b})(\Gamma_{max} - \Gamma_{eq}). \quad (3)$$

Knowing the parameters K_1, K_2, γ_1, γ_2, c_{1b}, c_{2b}, and Γ_{max}, this relation permits calculation of Γ_{eq}. Knowing Γ_{eq} one may then calculate Γ_{1eq} and Γ_{2eq}.

Instead of equation **3** one may also write:

$$\Gamma_{1eq}/\Gamma_{2eq} = [(K_1c_{1b})/(K_2c_{2b})]\,e^{-(\gamma_1 - \gamma_2)\Gamma_{eq}}. \quad (4)$$

This equation shows that the ratio of the adsorbed proteins is dependent on Γ_{eq}. If Γ_{eq} is

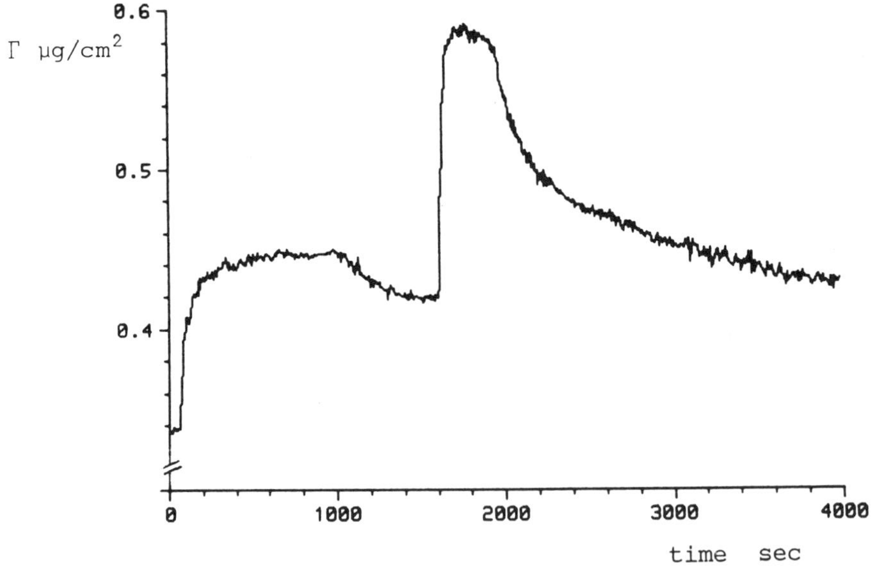

FIGURE 1. Measurement of adsorption and desorption of prothrombin, added 1600 s after preadsorption of fibrinogen (see text). The initial value of $\Gamma = 0.335\ \mu g/cm^2$ (at $t = 0$) was calculated for the DOPS double layer.

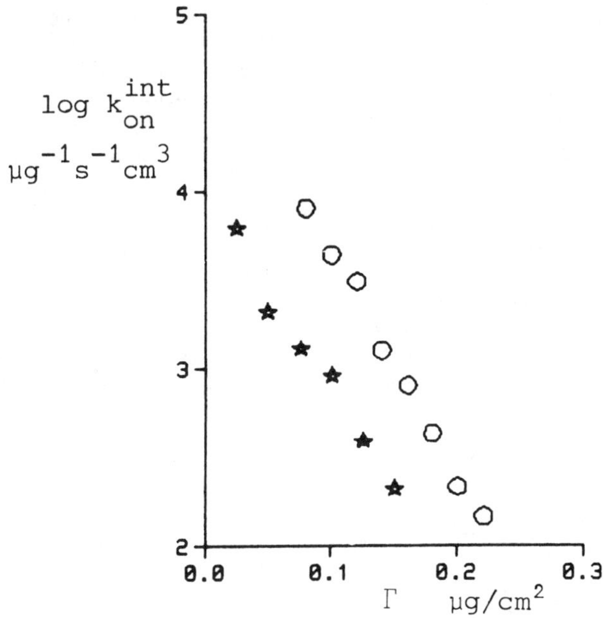

FIGURE 2. The effect of surface concentration Γ on the value of k_{on}^{int} (logarithmic plot); ○ = without preadsorption of fibrinogen; * = with preadsorption of 0.08 $\mu g/cm^2$ fibrinogen.

changed, for instance by changing the values of c_{1b} and c_{2b} by the same dilution factor, the ratio of the absorbed quantities of protein will also change.

RESULTS AND DISCUSSION

The Effect of Preadsorption of Fibrinogen on the Adsorption of Prothrombin

To investigate the effect of the presence of another absorbed protein on the absorption of prothrombin, a double layer of DOPS was stacked on a reflecting chromium surface and after 50 seconds 20 $\mu g/ml$ fibrinogen was added to the cuvette. The adsorption reaches a plateau value of 0.1 $\mu g/cm^2$ after 1000 s (FIGURE 1). The content of the cuvette was rinsed with buffer and a small desorption was observed. After 1600 s prothrombin adsorption was started by adding the protein to the cuvette (final concentration, 20 $\mu g/ml$). Within 100 seconds adsorption was completed at an adsorbed mass of 0.18 $\mu g/cm^2$. After 2000 seconds the desorption of prothrombin was measured by again rinsing the cuvette with buffer.

The results of 10 prothrombin adsorptions with and without preadsorption of fibrinogen are shown in FIGURE 2. The effect of a preadsorption of fibrinogen (0.08 $\mu g/cm^2$) on the adsorption of prothrombin is to lower the value of k_{on}^{int} by about a factor of ten and to cause a parallel shift to the left of about 0.06 $\mu g/cm^2$. Comparing these values, it is concluded that the adsorbing prothrombin molecules, in first approximation, do not discriminate between preadsorbed fibrinogen or prothrombin. Apparently the adsorption of one protein can be strongly influenced by the presence of another protein and in the case of a mixture of proteins the total adsorbed amount of proteins has to be taken into account. FIGURE 2 also shows the exponential relation between k_{on}^{int} and the surface concentration Γ, as has been observed before.[16,17]

Computer Simulations

In order to investigate the consequences of this model for the adsorption of a protein mixture, we performed some computer simulations. The choice of the parameter values of the model was guided by the following considerations.

From previous experiments with adsorptions of prothrombin and fibrinogen mixtures a value of $\Gamma_{max} = 0.3\ \mu g/cm^2$ was estimated and for Γ_{eq} a value of $0.25\ \mu g/cm^2$ was chosen arbitrarily. If the first protein must show preferential adsorption for a highly diluted mixture and be displaced by the second protein for an undiluted mixture, the following requirements must be satisfied (cf. equation **4**):

$$K_1 c_{b1} \gg K_2 c_{b2} \cong 1 \quad \text{and} \quad \frac{K_1 c_{b1}}{K_2 c_{b2}} e^{-(\gamma_1 - \gamma_2)0.25} \ll 1. \tag{5}$$

Therefore, the following numerical values were chosen:

$$K_1 c_{b1} = 10^4;\ K_2 c_{b2} = 10;\quad \frac{K_1 c_{b1}}{K_2 c_{b2}} e^{-(\gamma_1 - \gamma_2)0.25} = 10^{-2},$$

resulting in $\gamma_1 - \gamma_2 = 45\ (cm^2/\mu g)$.

For the dynamic simulations, values of $k_{+1} = k_{+2} = 1\ cm^3/\mu g \cdot s$ were chosen. For proteins with molecular weights of 100,000, this value corresponds to an association rate constant of approximately $10^8\ M^{-1}/s$. Thus a high, and identical, value of k_1 was chosen for both proteins, about one order of magnitude lower than the upper limit as predicted by Smoluchowsky theory. For the bulk concentrations protein values of $c_{b1} = 1000\ \mu g/cm^3$ and $c_{b2} = 10\ \mu g/cm^2$ were chosen, that is of the order of the plasma concentrations of fibrinogen and prothrombin, and the corresponding values of k_- thus became: $k_{-1} = 0.1\ s^{-1}$ and $k_{-2} = 1\ s^{-1}$. A value of $D/\delta = 10^{-3}$ cm/s was chosen in Equation **1**, in agreement with ref. 16.

It should be stressed, however, that the simulation results shown in FIGURES 3–5 are determined qualitatively by the conditions in equation **5** and do not depend critically on the other assumed parameter values. Also, the picture remains qualitatively unaltered if it is assumed that the effects of the absorbed quantities of both species are not strictly additive. This is suggested, for instance, by the finding that preadsorption of fibrinogen is slightly less effective in lowering k_{on} for prothrombin than preadsorption of prothrombin itself. Such effects could be expected for proteins having different values of γ and could be simply accounted for by assuming a relation of the type $\Gamma_{eq} = \Gamma_{1eq} + f\Gamma_{2eq}$, with f as a weight factor.

The above estimated value of γ, the interaction constant, of about $45\ cm^2/\mu g$ is in good agreement with the experimental values found. For the system tested until now γ values between $20\ cm^2/\mu g$ and $80\ cm^2/\mu g$ were found.[17]

The Ratio of the Adsorbed Proteins as a Function of Time and Dilution

FIGURE 3 shows the sequence and ratio of the adsorption of the two proteins. Initially the protein with the highest $K\,c_b$, value is adsorbed. At a surface concentration

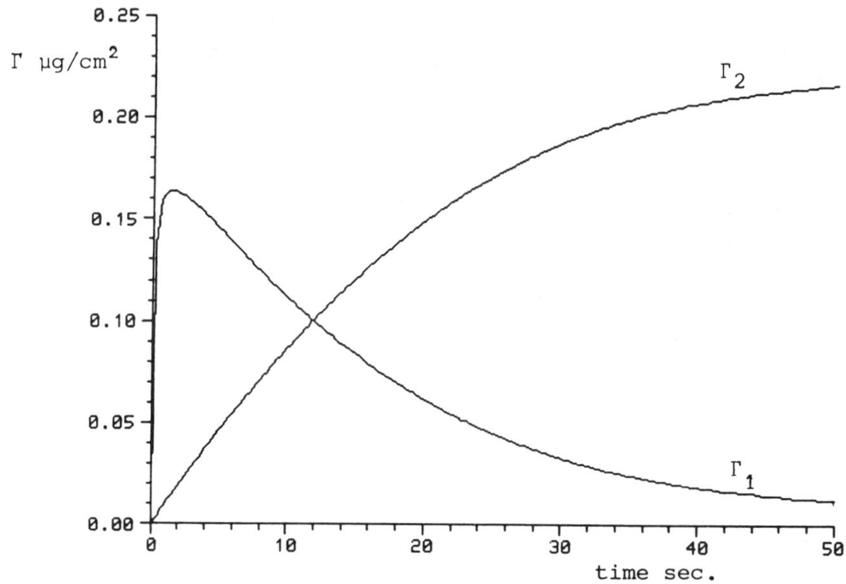

FIGURE 3. Sequential adsorption of proteins from a binary mixture. Parameter values are given in the text.

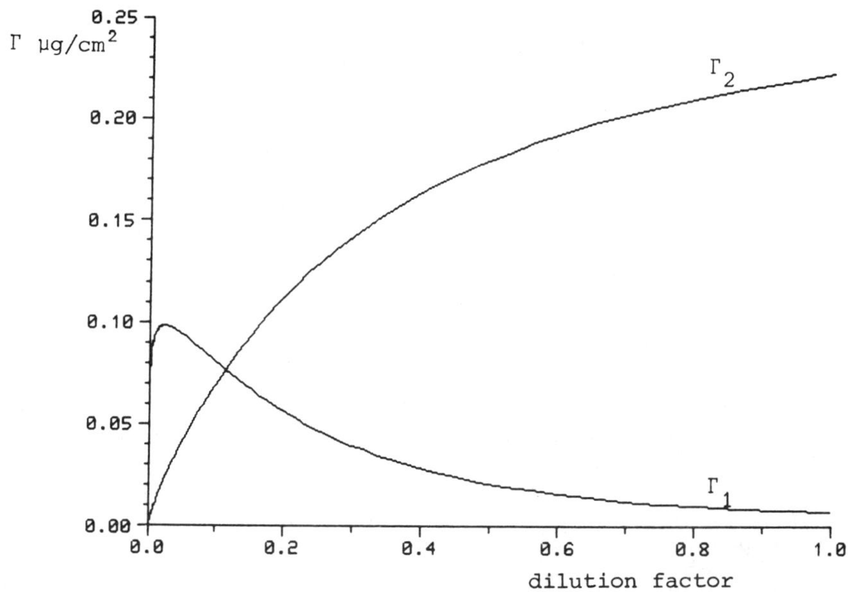

FIGURE 4. The effect of dilution on the final surface concentrations of the proteins from a binary mixture. Parameter values are as in FIGURE 3.

of about 0.16 $\mu g/cm^2$ the exponential interaction term already influences $\Gamma_{1eq}/\Gamma_{2eq}$ so strongly that the protein with the lower $K\,c_b$ value and a lower interaction constant γ can replace the first protein.

The concentrations of the adsorbed proteins as a function of dilution are presented in FIGURE 4. It is shown that, although the ratio of protein concentrations in the solution does not change upon dilution, there is a drastic change in the ratio of absorbed proteins. The effect of different values of the interaction constants is shown in FIGURE 5 for a range of values $\gamma_1 = 35$–$55\ cm^2/\mu g$.

The significance of an "interaction constant" between protein molecules needs some comment, as has been pointed out recently.[18] In a narrow sense it describes the situation where some real chemical or physical, either attractive or repulsive, forces

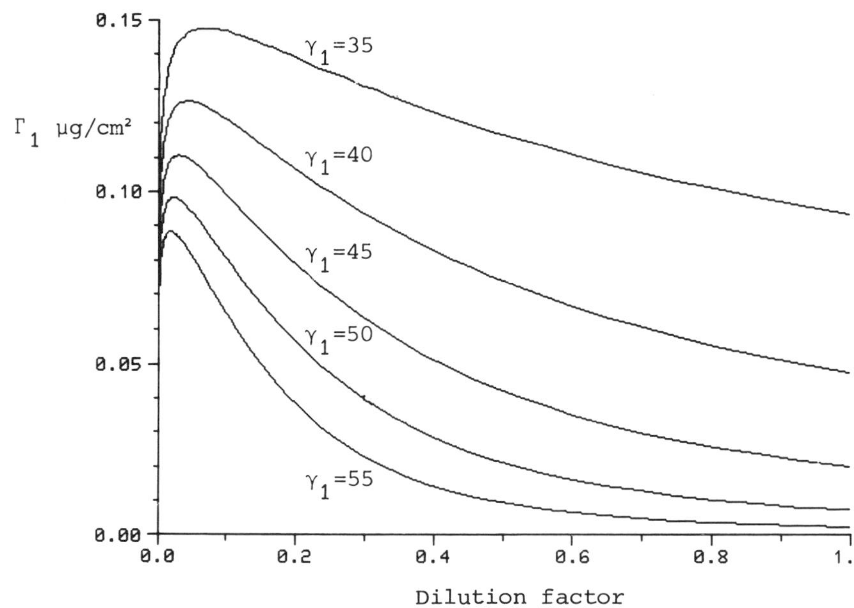

FIGURE 5. The effect of the interaction constant of protein *1* on the final adsorbed amount. Other parameter values are as in FIGURE 3.

exist between molecules that influence their distribution. The effect of pH and calcium ions on the interaction constant (e.g., for albumin, $\gamma = 76$ at pH $= 7.5$ and $\gamma = 23$ at pH $= 6.0$) strongly suggests the existence of such forces, particularly the presence of electrostatic interactions. However, the finite dimensions of the molecules could be sufficient to explain such effect. Their self-penetration is impossible and differences in molecular dimensions and orientations could largely influence the surface distribution of different proteins. It will be difficult to differentiate between various physicochemical forces and spacing effects, but their net effects seem to be reasonably well described by the exponential constants α and β in our model.

Fibrinogen displacement is not observed in HMWK-deficient plasma,[5,9,10] and this suggests some special property of the HMWK molecule resulting in a low value of the interaction constant γ at physiological pH. Indeed it is known that the light chain of

HMWK is responsible for the binding to negatively charged surfaces,[19] and this light chain has a rather unique amino acid composition with an average isoelectric point at pH 7.4. This implies that a large part of the molecule is uncharged at physiological pH, which could favor a low value of γ. It is tempting to speculate about such relations between the values of γ for different proteins and their amino acid composition and function. The same is true for a possible regulatory role of changes in the value of γ as a result of local triggers such as changes in pH or calcium concentrations. Such changes could cause altered compositions of a mixture of adsorbed proteins.

Sequential adsorption of proteins can be explained in a classical binding model by simply assuming that an abundant protein is displaced by a scarce protein with higher binding affinity. In such a model, however, dilution would not cause a qualitatively different behavior but would only make the process slower. A qualitative effect of dilution, as observed for fibrinogen, could still be explained in the framework of classical binding theory by assuming that, due to absorption, the highly diluted bulk phases becomes depleted of scarce proteins.[10] The model presented in the present study, however, may also explain such a qualitative effect of dilution in those cases[8] where depletion of protein from the bulk phase did not occur.

SUMMARY

A model for protein adsorption kinetics has been presented. This model includes diffusion-limited adsorption, adsorption and desorption rate constants k_{on} and k_{off}, which are dependent on the surface concentration, and an interaction term for the mutual influence of the adsorbed protein molecules. It has been shown that, in first approximation, values of k_{on} and k_{off} are exponential functions of the surface concentration. Assuming an adequate interaction term, it is possible to show with this model for a mixture of proteins that the ratio of the absorbed proteins is strongly dependent on the overall surface concentration even if the ratio of the bulk concentrations of these proteins is kept constant. Differences in interaction terms for the different proteins offer a possible explanation for the peculiar behavior of plasma protein adsorption on a surface at different dilutions of the plasma, the so-called Vroman effect.

ACKNOWLEDGMENT

We thank Dr. Thomas Horbett from the University of Washington, Seattle, and Dr. John Brash from the McMaster University, Hamilton, Ontario, for our stimulating discussions.

REFERENCES

1. VROMAN, L., A. ADAMS, M. KLINGS & G. FISCHER. 1975. Fibrinogen, globulins, albumin and plasma at interfaces. Adv. Chem. Ser. **145:** 255.
2. VROMAN, L. & A. ADAMS. 1969. Finding with the recording ellipsometer suggesting rapid exchange of specific plasma proteins at liquid/solid interfaces. Surf. Sci. **16:** 438–466.
3. BRASH, J. L., S. UNIYAL & B. M. C. CHAN. 1981. Interactions of proteins in plasma with various foreign surfaces. Artif. Organs **5**(Suppl.): 475–477.
4. VROMAN, L., A. ADAMS, M. KLINGS, G. FISHER, P. C. MUNOZ & R. P. SOLENSKY. 1977. Reactions of formed elements of blood with plasma proteins at interfaces. Ann. N.Y. Acad. Sci. **283:** 65–76.

5. VROMAN L., A. L. ADAMS, G. C. FISCHER & P. C. MUNOZ. 1980. Interaction of high molecular weight kininogen, factor XII and fibrinogen in plasma at interfaces. Blood **55:** 156–159.
6. BREEMHAAR, W., E. BRINKMAN, D. J. ELLENS, T. BEUGELING & A. BANTJES. 1984. Preferential adsorption of high density lipoprotein from blood plasma onto biomaterial surfaces. Biomaterials **5:** 269–274.
7. BRASH, J. L. & P. TEN HOVE. 1984. Effect of plasma dilution on adsorption of fibrinogen to solid surfaces. Thromb. Haemostas. **51**(3): 326–330.
8. HORBETT, T. A. 1984. Mass action effects on competitive adsorption of fibrinogen from hemoglobin solutions and from plasma. Thromb. Haemostas. **51**(2): 174–181.
9. WOJCIECHOWSKI, P., P. TEN HOVE & J. L. BRASH. 1986. Phenomenology and mechanism of the transient adsorption of fibrinogen from plasma (Vroman effect). J. Colloid Interface Sci. **111:** 455–465.
10. VROMAN, L. & A. L. ADAMS. 1986. Adsorption of proteins out of plasma and solutions in narrow spaces. J. Colloid Interface Sci. **111:** 391–402.
11. BLODGETT, C. 1935. Films built by depositing successive monolayers on a solid surface. J. Am. Chem. Soc. **57:** 1007–1022.
12. CUYPERS, P. A. 1976. Dynamic ellipsometry: Biochemical and biomedical applications. Ph.D. thesis. University of Limburg, Maastricht, the Netherlands.
13. CUYPERS, P. A., W. TH. HERMENS & H. C. HEMKER. 1977. Ellipsometric study of protein films on chromium. Ann. N.Y. Acad. Sci. **283:** 77–85.
14. KOP, M. J. M. M., P. A. CUYPERS, T. LINDHOUT, H. C. HEMKER & W. TH. HERMENS. 1984. The adsorption of prothrombin to phospholipid monolayers quantitated by ellipsometry. J. Biol. Chem. **259:** 13993–13998.
15. CUYPERS, P. A., J. W. CORSEL, M. P. JANSSEN, J. M. M. KOP, W. TH. HERMENS & H. C. HEMKER. 1983. The adsorption of prothrombin to phosphatidylserine multilayers quantitated by ellipsometry. J. Biol. Chem. **258:** 2426–2431.
16. CORSEL, J. W., G. M. WILLEMS, J. M. M. KOP, P. A. CUYPERS & W. TH. HERMENS. 1986. The role of intrinsic binding rate and transport rate in the adsorption of prothrombin. albumin and fibrinogen to phospholipid bilayers. J. Colloid Interface Sci. **11:** 544–553.
17. CUYPERS, P. A., G. M. WILLEMS, J. M. M. KOP, J. W. CORSEL, M. P. JANSSEN & W. TH. HERMENS. 1986. Kinetics of protein sorption on phospholipid membranes measured by ellipsometry. *In* Proteins at Interfaces. J. L. Brash & T. A. Horbett, Eds. American Chemical Society. Washington, D.C.
18. KAROLCZAK, M. 1984. The specification of the condition leading to interpretation of adsorption isotherms in the terms of excess electrochemical free energy of mixing and some implications of the interpretations. J. Colloid Interface Sci. **97:** 284–290.
19. KELLERMANN, J., F. LOTTSPEICH, A. HENSCHEN & W. MÜLLER-ESTERL. 1986. Completion of the primary structure of human high molecular mass kininogen. Eur. J. Biochem. **154:** 471–478.

Initiation of Blood Coagulation at Artificial Surfaces

ROBERT W. COLMAN, CHERYL F. SCOTT, ALVIN H. SCHMAIER, YANINA T. WACHTFOGEL, ROBIN A. PIXLEY, AND L. HENRY EDMUNDS, JR.[a]

Thrombosis Research Center
and
Department of Medicine
Temple University School of Medicine
Philadelphia, Pennsylvania 19122

[a]Department of Surgery
University of Pennsylvania
Philadelphia, Pennsylvania 19104

Over the past three decades a large body of information has been gathered by many investigators about the reactions of plasma proteins that initiate blood coagulation on artificial surfaces. The contact system comprises four proteins that exist in plasma in the zymogen or procofactor form, namely factor XII, (XII, Hageman factor), prekallikrein (PK, Fletcher factor), factor XI (XI, PTA) and high molecular weight kininogen (HMWK). Each of these proteins has been shown to be required to initiate, amplify, and propagate surface-mediated defense reactions.[1] Each of these proteins is converted to the corresponding active enzyme or cofactor during contact activation. The zymogens, XII (M_r 80,000), PK (M_r 88,000), and XI (M_r 160,000) are converted by limited proteolysis into the active serine proteases XIIa, kallikrein (K), and XIa. HMWK, a nonenzymatic procofactor, can be activated to a cofactor possessing increased coagulant activity (HMWKa) and then cleaved to an inactive cofactor form (HMWKi).

FIGURE 1 presents the current scheme for the initiation of the surface-mediated defense system. The activation of the contact system of plasma proteolysis is probably initiated by the binding of plasma XII to a negatively charged surface where autoactivation occurs: *i.e.,* the inert zymogen XII is converted to an active serine protease, XIIa, presumably by a trace amount of XIIa. In contrast, the substrates of XIIa, the zymogens PK and XI, cannot be activated on a surface in the absence of HMWK. PK and XI exist in bimolecular complexes[2–4] with the contact system procofactor, HMWK, which serves to place them on the surface for cleavage by factor XIIa. Thus, of the four proteins involved in the initiation of blood coagulation at artificial surfaces, only two interact directly with the surface.

To further delineate the interactions, we compared the adsorption of HMWK and factor XII to the artificial surface, kaolin, in normal plasma and plasma deficient in each of the contact factors.[5] Factor XII binds to kaolin independently of the presence of other proteins (FIG. 2B).[5] Although in normal plasma HMWK binds to negatively charged surfaces; significantly less binding occurs in plasma deficient in XII (FIG. 2A).[5] This observation suggests a means by which the adsorption of HMWK could be coordinated with the association of XII with the surface. The requirement for the presence of factor XII for adsorption of HMWK to the surface is indirect and is due to the need for cleavage of HMWK. Factor XIIa can directly cleave HMWK,[6] although this is minor when compared to the rate of HMWK cleavage by kallikrein.[5] This observation also explains the decreased binding of HMWK in plasma deficient in prekallikrein. These combined findings suggest that cleavage of HMW kininogen by either factor XIIa[6] or kallikrein[5] is required for adsorption of the cofactor to a negatively charged surface in a plasma environment.

Previous studies by Vroman[7] indicated that the ability to detect surface-adsorbed fibrinogen was affected by the presence of HMWK in plasma. These results were extended in a collaborative study between Vroman and our laboratory.[8] HMWK plays an important role in altering the association of plasma fibrinogen with surfaces. Plasma initially deposits fibrinogen onto most materials, but on hydrophilic (clot-promoting) surfaces, within 10 min, adsorbed plasma fibrinogen cannot be detected on the surface by antifibrinogen antisera. However, using HMWK-deficient and plasminogen-depleted plasma, fibrinogen remains immunologically identifiable. The interrelationship of adsorbed plasma fibrinogen with HMWK on hydrophilic surfaces (glass slides) has been delineated.[8] When plasma that is deficient in both low-molecular-weight kinonogen (LMWK) and HMWK was reconstituted with HMWK (0.40

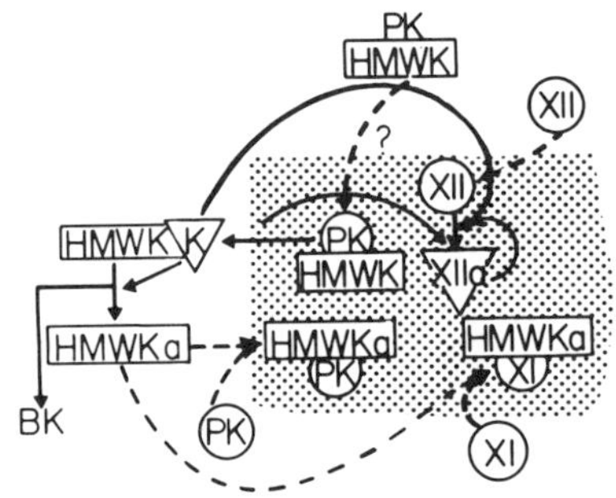

FIGURE 1. Initiation of the contact activation system. *Solid arrows* designate conversion; *dashed arrows,* translocation; *shaded area,* activating surface; *circles,* zymogen; *triangles,* enzyme; and *rectangles,* cofactor. Abbreviations are as in text. (From Colman.[1] Reprinted with permission from the *Journal of Clinical Investigation.*)

U/ml), fibrinogen was no longer detected on the surface by a monospecific antibody to that protein.[8] This behavior is specific for HMWK, since when the same plasma was reconstituted with LMWK (220 μg/ml) the amount of fibrinogen detected on the surface was unchanged (FIG. 3).[8] Further studies in an ellipsometer showed that HMWK increases the initial rate at which immunochemically reactive fibrinogen became undetectable.[8] This finding assumes more importance in view of the recent studies from Lindon *et al.,*[9] which indicated that the platelet adhesion to artificial surfaces increases with increasing surface coverage of adsorbed fibrinogen if the bound fibrinogen maintains a conformation such that its epitopes remain recognizable by antibody probes to fibrinogen.

Our observations suggested that in reciprocal fashion, fibrinogen might modulate the adsorption of HMWK to surfaces. We therefore compared the ability of intact, partially cleaved, and cleaved HMWK to adsorb to kaolin in the presence of plasma concentrations (3 mg/ml) of purified fibrinogen (FIG. 4).[5] The intact HMWK adsorbed to kaolin in the absence of fibrinogen to a limited extent. When HMWK was cleaved, the extent of adsorption at a given kaolin concentration increased. The

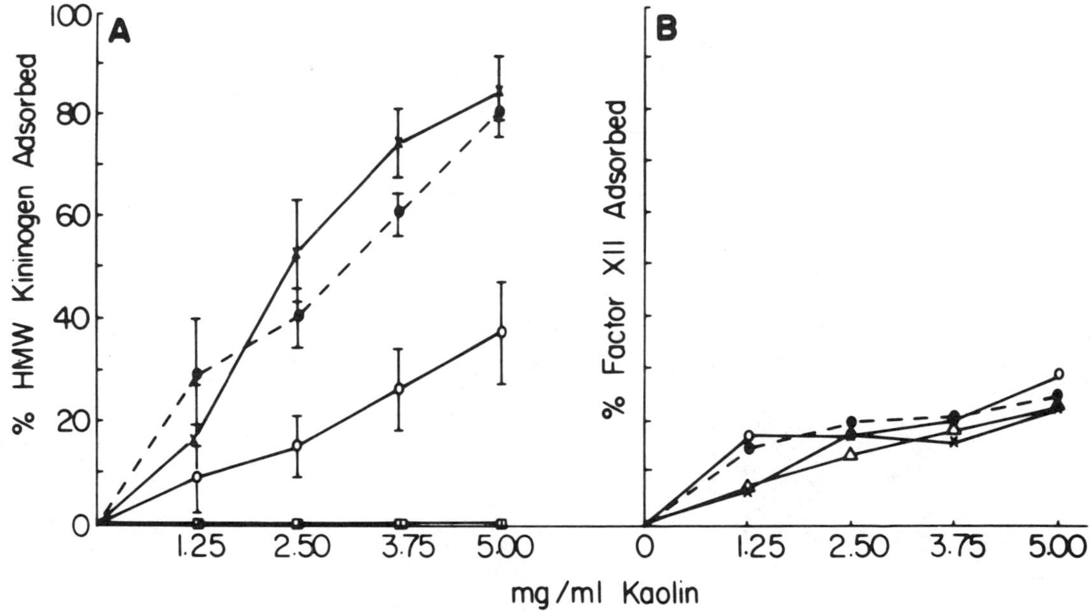

FIGURE 2. Effect of kaolin concentration on adsorption of (**A**) HMWK and (**B**) factor XII from deficient plasmas. Kaolin pellets, 0.125–0.5 mg, were prepared in 0.1 M sodium phosphate buffer containing 0.15 M NaCl. One hundred microliters of normal (●), factor-XII-deficient (□), factor-XI-deficient (×), prekallikrein-deficient (○), or HMWK-deficient (△) plasma was then suspended and incubated with the kaolin for 15 min at 23°C. The starting material and supernatants were assayed for HMWK and factor XII coagulant activity and the percentage adsorbed was calculated by difference. The data represent the mean ±SD of three to six experiments. (From Scott *et al.*[5] Reprinted with permission from the *Journal of Clinical Investigation.*)

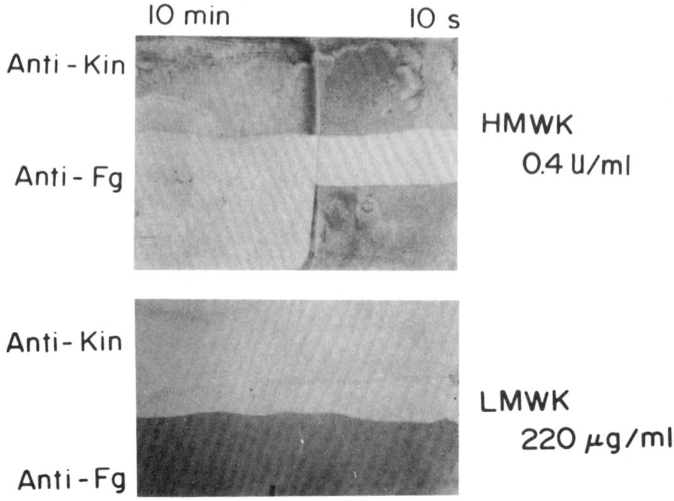

FIGURE 3. The effect of HMWK on surface-associated fibrinogen. Total kininogen-deficient plasma was reconstituted with HMWK (0.4 U/ml) or LMWK (220 μg/ml) and placed on glass slides. After incubation of the plasmas for 10 min or 10 s on the surface, the slides were rinsed and antikininogen (Anti-Kin) and antifibrinogen (Anti-Fg) antisera were overlaid on the slides. The dark shading was developed by Coomassie Brilliant Blue staining. The figure is one representative experiment of multiple determinations. (From Schmaier *et al.*[8] Reprinted with permission from *Thrombosis Research.*)

presence of fibrinogen, however, decreased the adsorption of intact and partially cleaved HMWK, but had no effect on fully cleaved HMWK. Thus, cleavage of HMWK enhanced its ability to adsorb to kaolin in the presence of a concentration of fibrinogen similar to that in plasma. Substitution of 30 mg/ml human serum albumin (HSA) for fibrinogen resulted in similar results to that with buffer alone. Therefore, fibrinogen regulates the ability of HMWK to associate with surfaces preventing uncleaved HMWK from adsorbing to kaolin.[5]

To ascertain which cleavage events were critical for the adsorption of HMWK to kaolin, radiolabeled HMWK and unlabeled HMWK were incubated for various times with plasma kallikrein (FIG. 5).[5] As cleavage progressed, increasing amounts of HMWK were found to adsorb to kaolin until maximal adsorption was observed between 3 and 4 hours of incubation. The maximal adsorption followed the maximal formation of the intermediate light chain ($M_r = 56{,}000$) and also paralleled bradykinin release. Thus, the first two cleavages of HMWK by kallikrein greatly enhances its ability to adsorb to kaolin in the presence of plasma concentrations of fibrinogen.[5]

To identify and quantify the actual species of HMWK that adsorbed to kaolin, various amounts of intact ^{125}I-labeled HMWK or cleaved ^{125}I-labeled HMWK were mixed with fibrinogen and incubated with kaolin in the presence and absence of a fivefold excess of unlabeled HMWK (FIG. 6).[5] There was no "specific" adsorption of the uncleaved HMWK. In contrast, the cleaved HMWK was associated with the kaolin and all but 12% was displaced by the excess, unlabeled cleaved HMWK. The kaolin-associated material was then eluted with SDS and subjected to SDS-PAGE electrophoresis. The SDS-extracted kaolin pellet contained 15% uncleaved HMWK

(M_r = 120,000), equivalent to the "nonspecific" adsorption observed after addition of a fivefold excess of unlabeled HMWK and 85% cleavage products (heavy and light chains). In contrast, the unadsorbed material contained 85% uncleaved HMWK and 15% cleavage products. This experiment reinforces the conclusion that cleavage of HMWK markedly amplifies its ability to adsorb to kaolin in the presence of fibrinogen and that uncleaved HMWK has little or no ability to adsorb to a negatively charged surface under such conditions.[5]

Recent studies have demonstrated that prekallikrein and factor XI are 60% homologous in amino acid sequence and indeed diverged only about 120 million years ago.[10] We tested the effect of factor XIa on the structure and function of HMWK and its ability to adsorb to surfaces.[11] Factor XIa cleaves HMWK, although the cleavage pattern differs from the one produced by kallikrein (FIG. 7). The initial cleavage by factor XIa yields a 75-kDa heavy chain and a 45-kDa light chain. The second and third cleavages by factor XIa release bradykinin from HMWK, albeit much more slowly than does kallikrein.[11]

More important than this difference in peptide bond cleavage is the ability of factor XIa to further proteolyze the 45-kDa light chain.[11] To investigate the effect of factor XIa cleavage of the 45-kDa light chain on HMWK coagulant activity, HMWK was incubated with factor XIa and/or kallikrein. Even at a molar ratio of kallikrein to HMWK of 1:33, no change in HMWK coagulant activity was detected. An increase in coagulant activity was not seen initially because during the coagulant assay cleavage of

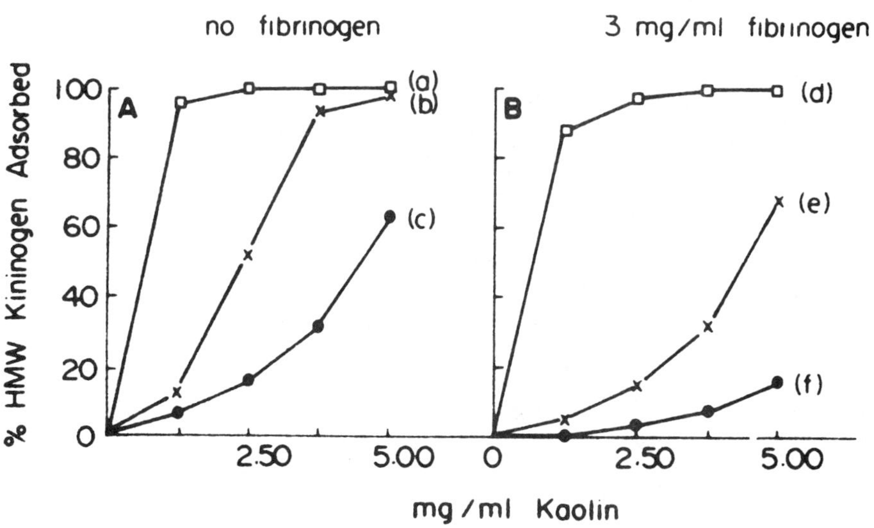

FIGURE 4. Effect of fibrinogen on adsorption of intact and cleaved HMWK. Three preparations of HMWK were used. The first preparation contained 90% of the M_r 120,000 band (*c* and *f*). A second preparation contained 65% of the M_r 120,000 band (*b* and *e*), and the third preparation was fully cleaved by kallikrein (*a* and *d*). One hundred microliters of each preparation, at 1 U/ml, was incubated in the (**A**) absence or (**B**) presence of 3 mg/ml purified plasminogen-free fibrinogen, with kaolin (0–5 mg/ml final concentration), for 10 min at 23°C. The starting material and supernatants from the kaolin pellets were assayed for HMWK coagulant activity. Each point is the average of duplicate determinations and the figure is representative of two to three similar experiments. (From Scott *et al.*[5] Reprinted with permission from the *Journal of Clinical Investigation.*)

HMWK occurs during the first stage of incubation. In contrast, increasing molar ratios (1:100 to 1:33) of factor XIa to HMWK progressively destroyed the activity of HMWK and simultaneously cleaved the light chain of HMWK. This same effect occurs in normal plasma, since on prolonged exposure of plasma to kaolin the coagulant activity decreases whereas in factor-XI-deficient plasma only a slight loss of HMWK coagulant activity occurs. Furthermore, there is an excellent correlation between the cleavage of the 45-kDa light chain of HMWK by factor XIa and the ability of HMWK to adsorb to kaolin (FIG. 8). When unlabeled and radiolabeled

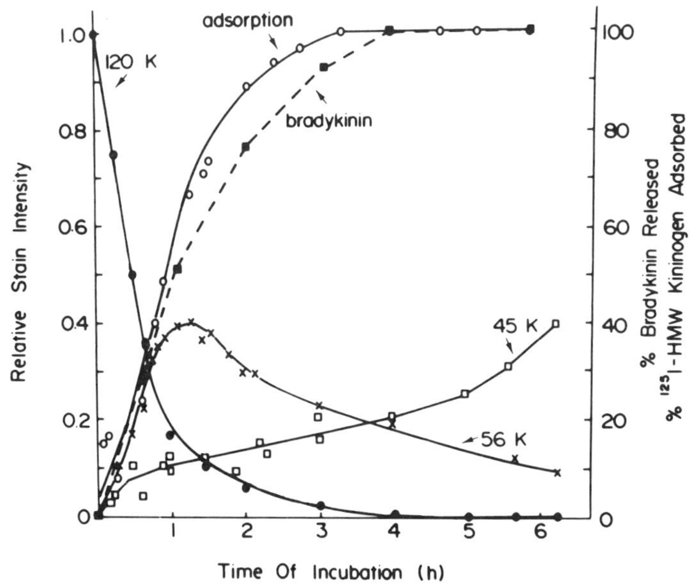

FIGURE 5. Kaolin adsorption of cleaved ^{125}I-labeled HMWK in a purified system containing fibrinogen. Aliquots of cleaved HMWK (3 μl) from a timed digest (25 μg kallikrein and 2500 μg HMWK in a final volume of 535 μl) were removed for bradykinin determination (■) after stopping the reaction with soybean trypsin inhibitor (40 μg). Additional 3-μl aliquots were incubated with 97 μl of fibrinogen (3 mg/ml) in buffer, and then 50 μl of each mixture was added to 0.125 mg prepared kaolin pellets for 6 min at 23°C. The starting material and supernatants were counted for γ radioactivity and the percentage of ^{125}I-labeled HMWK adsorbed to kaolin was calculated (O). After SDS-PAGE, the percentage of each M_r form—120,000 (●), 56,000 (×), 45,000 (□)—was calculated after densitometric scanning of the stained gel (see METHODS). (From Scott *et al.*[5] Reprinted with permission from the *Journal of Clinical Investigation.*)

HMWK is incubated with factor XIa, the coagulant activity closely parallels the concentration of the intact 45-kDa light chain.[11]

Contact-activated blood coagulation is regulated by a multifaceted control system of activators and inhibitors. Within this system, factor XI and prekallikrein are transported to the negatively charged surface via HMWK after it is activated (FIG. 1). However, the behavior of the two enzymes then sharply diverges. The enzyme, kallikrein, easily dissociates from the surface-bound HMWK.[12] However, factor XIa displays tightest binding to HMWK in a plasma environment,[13] and most factor XI remains surface bound. Therefore, the ability of factor XIa to destroy the light chain of

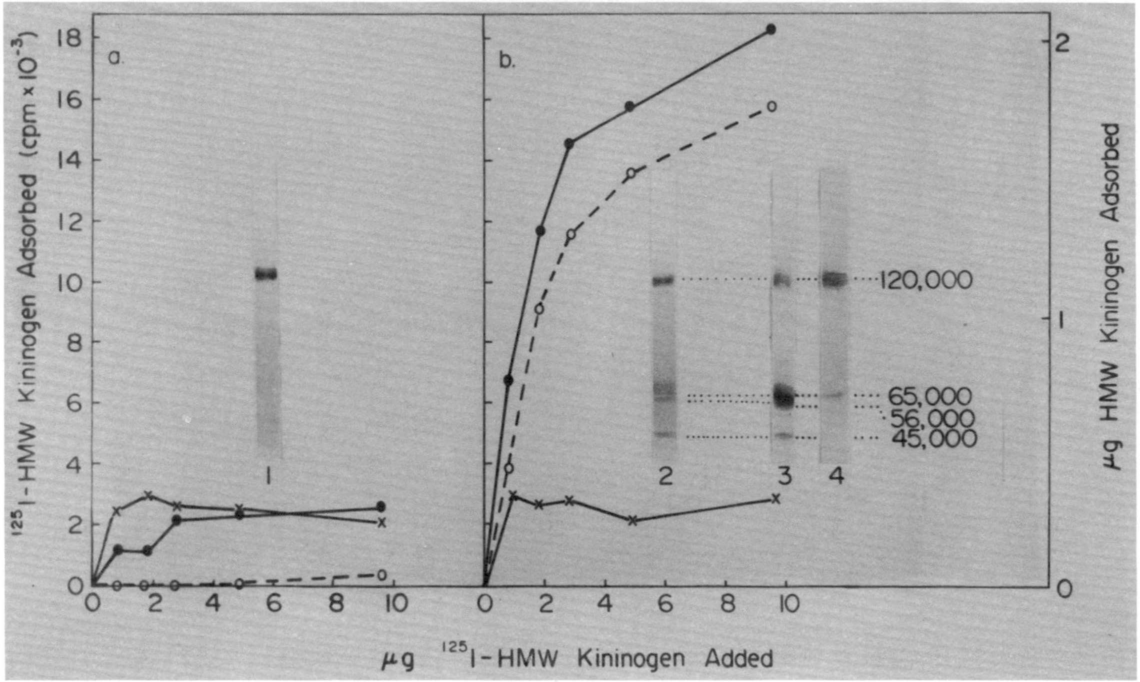

FIGURE 6. Effect of cleavage by kallikrein on the adsorption of ^{125}I-labeled HMWK to kaolin. Various amounts of ^{125}I-labeled HMWK starting material (**a**) were diluted with unlabeled HMWK 1 : 120 in order to reduce the specific radioactivity to 9800 cpm/μg. ^{125}I-labeled HMWK was incubated with kallikrein (1:48 wt/wt) for 2 h at 37°C (**b**) and with 218 μg of kaolin at 23°C for 6 min in the presence and absence of an additional fivefold excess of unlabeled HMWK. The samples were centrifuged at 12,000 ×g at 23°C for 1 min and the supernatants and pellets counted for radioactivity. The kaolin-associated radioactivity and amount of HMWK are plotted against the amount of HMWK incubated; ● = ^{125}I-labeled HMWK alone; × = ^{125}I-labeled HMW kininogen plus unlabeled HMWK with kaolin; ○ = specific adsorption (the difference between the above). *Inset:* The pellets obtained by incubation cleaved ^{125}I-labeled HMWK with kaolin were washed with 100 μl saline three times and this wash, containing <6% of the total radioactivity, was discarded. The pellets were then incubated for 10 min at 23°C with 1% SDS in Tris-Cl, pH 6.8. The soluble extracts as well as the unadsorbed material were run-reduced on a 10% SDS-PAGE, and an autoradiogram was performed at −70°C and percentage of total radioactivity was calculated as in METHODS. This photograph represents the 5 μg ^{125}I-labeled HMWK sample; *1,* uncleaved starting material; *2,* cleaved (partially) starting material; *3,* SDS-extracted pellet; *4,* supernatant. (From Scott *et al.*[5] Reprinted with permission from the *Journal of Clinical Investigation.*)

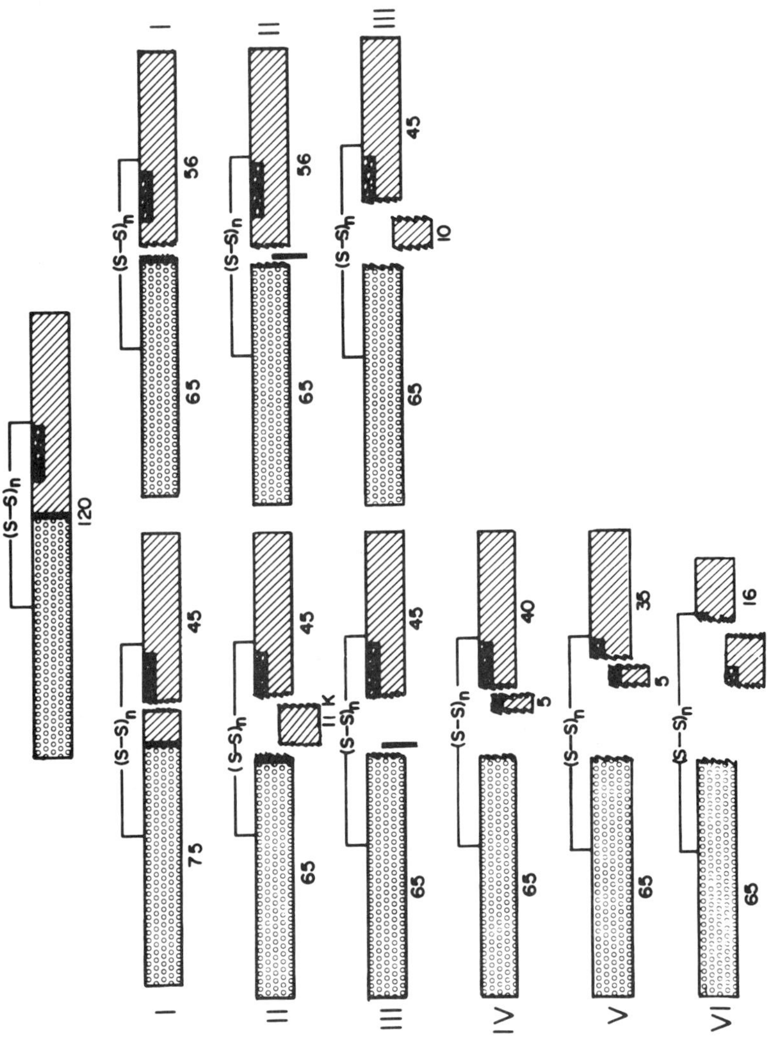

FIGURE 7. Model comparing HMWK patterns of cleavage by factor XIa (*left*) and kallikrein (*right*). (From Scott *et al.*[11] Reprinted with permission from the *Journal of Biological Chemistry*.)

HMWK provides a potential mechanism for allowing dissociation of the tightly bound factor XIa from its activating surface to be available to activate factor IX, which is associated with phospholipid micelles or platelets, thus propagating the hemostatic function of intrinsic blood coagulation. Furthermore, since the light chain is the portion of the HMWK molecule that adsorbs to a negatively charged surface[14] as well as binds to factor XI, factor XIa, prekallikrein, and kallikrein, destruction of the light chain could serve to curtail both the rate and extent of contact activation as well as to allow the inhibition of the active enzymes (kallikrein and factor XIa) by the plasma protease inhibitors.[13,15]

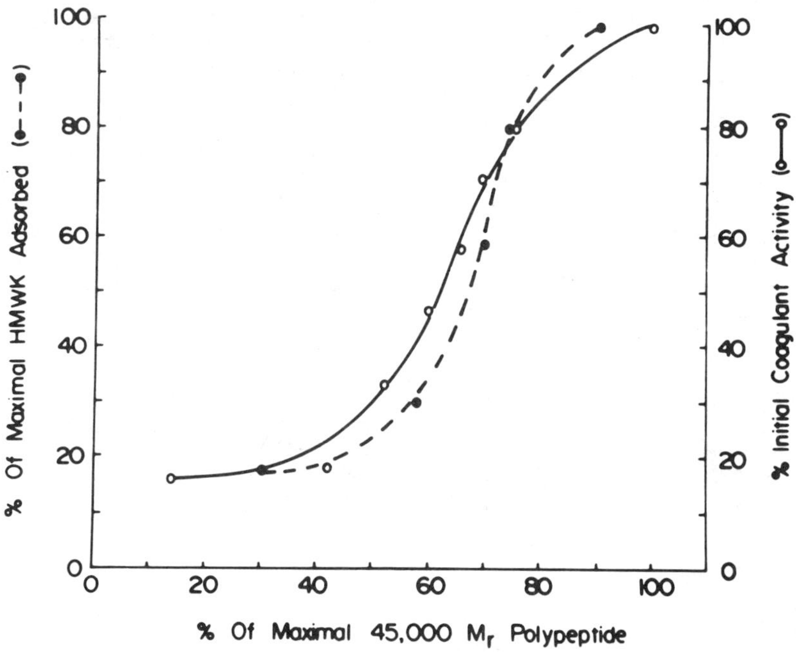

FIGURE 8. Correlation of HMWK coagulant activity with the ability of HMWK to adsorb to kaolin. The percentage of maximal HMWK which adsorbed to kaolin (●) was plotted as a function of the percent maximal ^{125}I-labeled 45-kDa polypeptide concentration in factor-XI-deficient plasma at each time point (see MATERIALS AND METHODS). The percentage of initial coagulant activity in purified HMWK samples after incubation with factor XIa (○) was plotted as a function of the maximal concentration of the 45-kDa light chain at each time point. (From Scott *et al.*[5] Reprinted with permission from the *Journal of Clinical Investigation*.)

The regulation of HMWK now appears to parallel the two other blood coagulation cofactors. Both factor V[16] and factor VIII:C[17] exist as procofactors whose coagulant activity is markedly augmented by thrombin. The potentiating effect produced by kallikrein on the degradation of HMWK by factor XIa is paralleled by the ability of activated protein C to degrade the activated cofactors factors Va[16] and VIIIa[17] more efficiently than their procofactors V and VIII. Finally, both kallikrein and factor XIIa can cleave HMWK to an active form, and both of these enzymes participate in production of factor XIa, the enzyme responsible for inactivating their cofactor. In a similar way, activated protein C, the enzyme which destroys the coagulant activity of thrombin-activated coagulation factors Va and VIIIa, depends on thrombin for its activation.

We have begun to probe the molecular basis of the binding of the light chain to surfaces. We hypothesized that the positively charged arginine residues might play an important role in binding to negatively charged surfaces. Modification with butanedione of four arginine residues prevented bradykinin release by preventing cleavage of HMWK.[18] This result was easily understood since arginine is the NH_2 terminal and the COOH terminal of bradykinin (Arg-Pro-Pro-Gly-Phe-Ser-Pro-Phe-Arg). In accordance with our construct that HMWK must be cleaved to exhibit coagulant activity, we observed a progressive loss of HMWK coagulant activity when up to 6.6 residues of arginine were modified.[18] The coagulant activity of cleaved HMWK is made up of two essential components: first, the ability of the cofactor to associate with the surface and second, the ability of HMWK to associate with prekallikrein and/or factor XI. We found that complex formation of HMWK with prekallikrein was unaffected by the modification of arginine residues by butanedione even though 90% of the coagulant activity was lost.[18] To account for the loss of coagulant activity, we therefore examined the ability of cleaved HMWK (active cofactor) to bind to an activating surface with and without modification by butanedione (FIG. 9).[18] HMWK was cleaved with plasma kallikrein prior to incubation with butanedione. ^{125}I-labeled HMWKa, with 15 residues of arginine modified, had less than 4% of the original coagulant activity. Although the modified labeled HMWK revealed the same saturation point as the unmodified HMWKa, ten times as much was required to achieve the same degree of

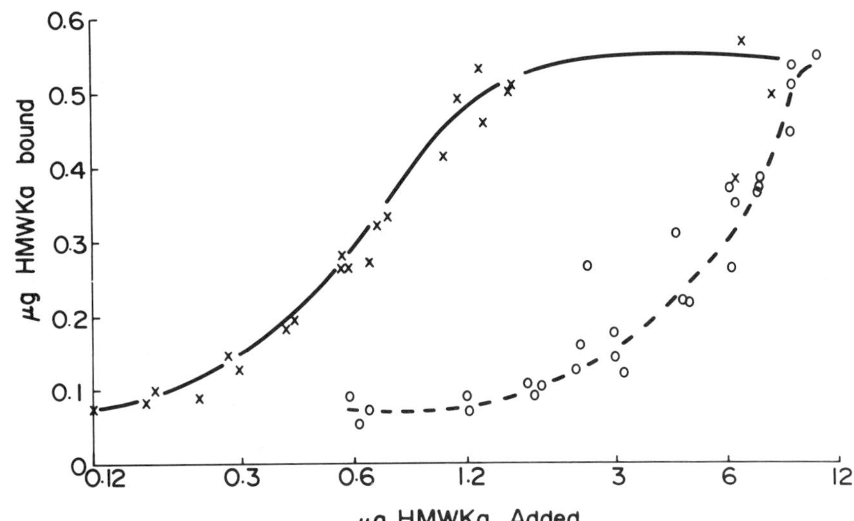

FIGURE 9. Effect of butanedione modification on the binding of ^{125}I-labeled HMWKa to kaolin. ^{125}I-labeled HMWKa was added to nonlabeled HMWKa. An aliquot was modified with butanedione. Various amounts of either the unmodified (×) or modified (O) HMWKa mixtures were added to microcentrifuge tubes containing 100 μg of kaolin, 300 μg of human serum albumin, and 300 μg of purified fibrinogen in a final volume of 100 μl. After 5 minutes at 25°C, the samples were centrifuged and the supernatants and pellets were counted for radioactivity. (From Chang *et al.*[18] Reprinted with permission from *Blood*.)

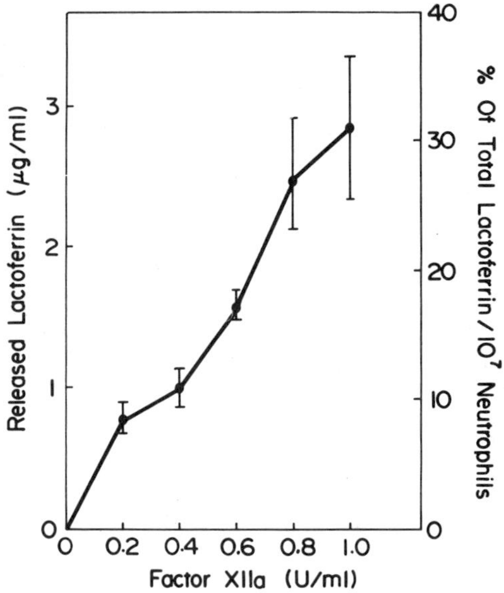

FIGURE 10. Lactoferrin release stimulated by factor XIIa. Neutrophils (1×10^7/ml) in HBSS containing 2 mmol/l $CaCl_2$ and 1.5 mmol/l $MgCl_2$ were incubated at 37°C for 20 minutes in the presence of increasing concentrations of factor XIIa. Samples were centrifuged at 13,000 ×g for 5 minutes at 23°C and lactoferrin was measured in these samples, using an indirect competitive ELISA for lactoferrin. Results are expressed as released lactoferrin (μg/ml), as well as the percentage of total lactoferrin per 10^7 neutrophils. These data represent the mean of two determinations. (From Wachtfogel *et al.*[24] Reprinted with permission from *Blood*.)

binding. This finding suggests that the arginine residues were essential for HMWKa association with the surface.

We must now ask what the significance is of this complex surface-activated proteolytic enzyme system. Although the title of this paper implies that the initiation of blood coagulation on artificial surfaces is the major role of this system, we believe that the contact system plays a more important role in body defenses. Furthermore, we are aware that deficiencies of HMWK, prekallikrein, or factor XI lead to *in vitro* coagulation impairment but not to an *in vivo* hemostatic disorder. The importance of the contact system may be in the ability of two of its constituent enzymes to stimulate neutrophils.

In 1972, Kaplan and associates[19] demonstrated that a partially purified preparation of human plasma kallikrein stimulated neutrophils to undergo chemotaxis in a Boyden chamber. In 1974, Goetzl and Austen[20] extended these observations to show that kallikrein also stimulates aerobic glucose metabolism and hexose monophosphate shunt activity of human neutrophils. Recently, our laboratory reinvestigated the effect of human plasma kallikrein on human neutrophils. Kallikrein has been found to aggregate neutrophils[21] and release the lysosomal enzyme elastase.[22] The active site of the kallikrein is required for aggregation and release of elastase, and furthermore, cleavage of the heavy chain of kallikrein prevents these processes.[23] The release of elastase by neutrophils also occurs in a normal plasma milieu, but plasma deficient in prekallikrein or factor XII promotes markedly decreased elastase release. C5 is not required for neutrophil stimulation and factor-XI-deficient plasma behaves like normal plasma.[23]

Another enzyme in the contact system, factor XIIa, is also an agonist for neutrophils.[24] Factor XIIa can aggregate neutrophils, release elastase from the azurophillic granules, and release lactoferrin from the specific granules (FIG. 10).[24] The active site of factor XIIa is required. The heavy chain of factor XIIa must also be present since factor XIIf, which corresponds closely to the light chain, is inactive in neutrophil stimulation.[24] The heavy chain has been shown to possess two domains homologous to growth factors and these may be the site for interaction with the neutrophil cell membrane.

The significance of the stimulation of neutrophils by enzymes activated by surface contact is well illustrated in clinical cardiopulmonary bypass.[25] During bypass, neutrophil counts fall as low as 67% by 45 min, but return to pre-bypass levels by 60 min (FIG. 11).[25] Lactoferrin levels rise throughout bypass and return to normal after 24 hours. A similar pattern is seen with elastase. In a simulated circuit, containing the pump and membrane oxygenator, lactoferrin rises dramatically. The lysosomal enzyme elastase is progressively released (FIG. 12).[25] The effect is inhibited by either PGE_1 or lidocaine, indicating that neutrophil activation by contact system enzymes is a direct effect on the cells. The relatively small decrease in neutrophil counts suggests that soluble agonists are involved.

To delineate which agonists might be involved, we have collaborated with Dr. Peter Harpel of Cornell University Medical Center.[26] We have investigated whether the

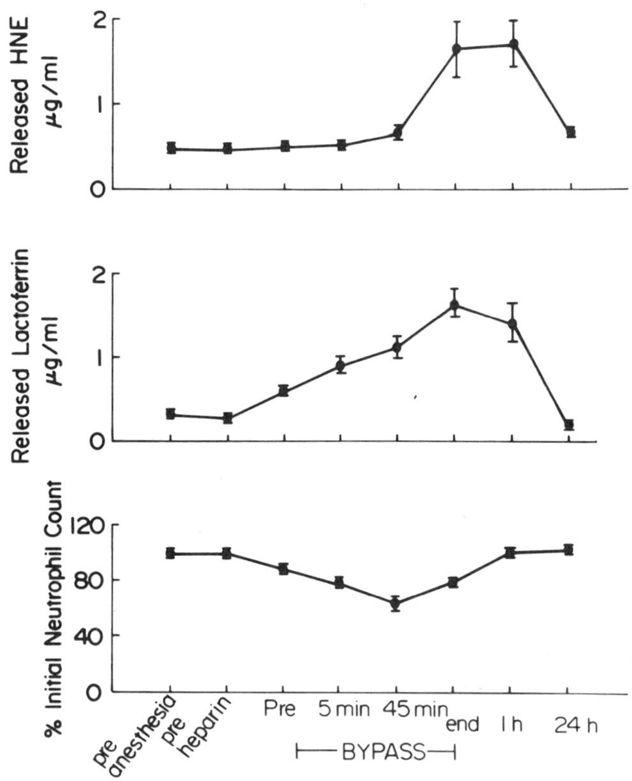

FIGURE 11. Neutrophil counts, plasma levels of neutrophil lactoferrin, and plasma levels of human neutrophil elastase (HNE) during clinical cardiopulmonary bypass (CCB). The percentage initial neutrophil count, released lactoferrin, and released HNE were determined before induction of anesthesia; after anesthesia, before heparin; after heparin, before CCB; 5 min after start of CCB; 45 min after start of CCB; just before CCB ended; 60 min after CCB; and 24 h after CCB. Each point represents the mean ±SEM of 10 patients. (From Wachtfogel *et al.*[24] Reprinted with permission from *Blood*.)

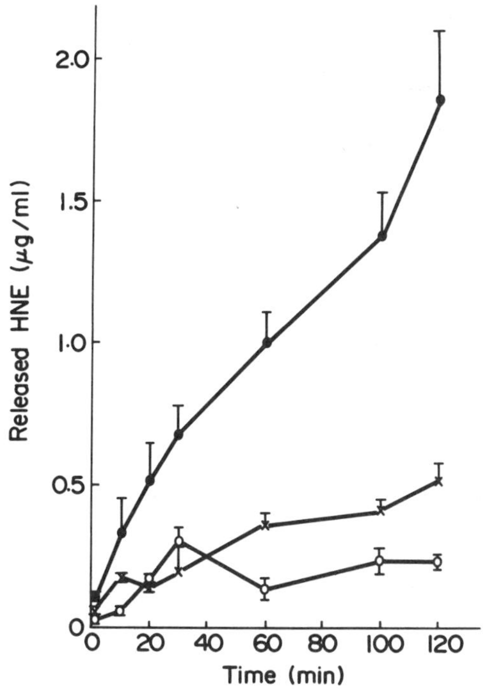

FIGURE 12. Plasma levels of human neutrophil elastase (HNE) in recirculated blood during simulated extracorporeal bypass (SECC). Released HNE is expressed as micrograms of HNE per ml of plasma. Values were obtained when heparin-anticoagulated blood was recirculated in the presence of PGE_1 (0.3 μM, ×), lidocaine (100 μM, ○), or absence of additional drug (●). Each point represents the mean ± SEM of 7 separate determinations. (From Wachtfogel *et al.*[24] Reprinted with permission from *Blood.*)

classical complement, contact, or plasmin pathways have been activated as potential sources of neutrophil agonists. Employing enzyme-linked immunosorbent "sandwich" assays specific for $C1_s$-$C\bar{1}$-inhibitor and kallikrein-$C\bar{1}$ inhibitor complexes respectively, we found that plasma levels of both of these formed complexes increases twofold after clinical cardiopulmonary bypass was completed and reverts to baseline within 24 hours postoperatively.[26] Since these complexes are cleared *in vivo,* we investigated their plasma levels during *in vitro* simulated extracorporeal circulation. Over a period of 2 hours, $C1_s$-$C\bar{1}$ inhibitor complexes rise tenfold and kallikrein-$C\bar{1}$ inhibitor complexes rise 12-fold.[26] However, there is no evidence of either *in vivo* or *in vitro* plasmin-α_2 plasmin inhibitor complex formation.[26] The occurrence of contact activation in the extracorporeal circulation despite the presence of up to 5 units per milliliter of heparin is consistent with our previous observations that the heparin-antithrombin III system has little if any effect on the inhibition of factor XIIa,[27] kallikrein,[28] or factor XIa.[29] These demonstrations of complexes containing $C\bar{1}$ and kallikrein indicate that activation of the classical pathway of complement and the contact system in plasma may be associated with neutrophil activation as seen during clinical cardiopulmonary bypass, presumably due to contact with hydrophillic surfaces.

The studies summarized in this paper indicate that the four contact proteins and their inhibitors represent an intricately regulated system that is responsible for the initiation of blood coagulation on artificial surfaces. Perhaps even more important is the fact that two of these enzymes can directly activate neutrophils, which may account for some of the poorly understood complications of prolonged cardiopulmonary bypass. The task ahead is to test whether the temporal association observed between activation of the contact system and neutrophil stimulation represents cause and effect.

REFERENCES

1. Colman, R. W. 1984. Surface mediated defense reactions. The plasma contact system. J. Clin. Invest. **73:** 1249–1253.
2. Mandle, R., Jr., R. W. Colman & A. K. Kaplan. 1976. Identification of prekallikrein and high molecular weight kininogen as a complex in human plasma. Proc. Natl. Acad. Sci. **73:** 4179–4183.
3. Scott, C. F. & R. W. Colman. 1980. Function and immunochemistry of prekallikrein high molecular kininogen complex in plasma. J. Clin. Invest. **65:** 413–422.
4. Thompson, R. E., R. Mandle, Jr. & A. P. Kaplan. 1977. Association of factor XI and high molecular weight kininogen in human plasma. J. Clin. Invest. **60:** 1376–1380.
5. Scott, C. F., L. D. Silver, M. Shapira & R. W. Colman. 1984. Cleavage of human molecular weight kininogen markedly enhances its coagulant activity: Evidence that this molecule exists as a procofactor. J. Clin. Invest. **73:** 954–962.
6. Wiggins, R. C. 1983. Kinin release from high molecular weight kininogen in the absence of kallikrein. J. Biol. Chem. **258:** 8963–8970.
7. Vroman, L., A. L. Adams, G. C. Fischer & P. C. Munoz. 1980. Interaction of high molecular weight kininogen, factor XII, and fibrinogen in plasma at interfaces. Blood **55:** 156–159.
8. Schmaier, A. H., L. Silver, A. L. Adams, G. C. Fischer, P. C. Munoz, L. Vroman & R. W. Colman. 1984. The effect of high molecular weight kininogen on surface-adsorbed fibrinogen. Thromb. Res. **33:** 51–64.
9. Lindon, J. N., G. McManama, L. Kushner, E. W. Merrill & E. W. Salzman. 1986. Does the confirmation of adsorbed fibrinogen dictate platelet interactions with artificial surfaces. Blood **68:** 355–362.
10. Veloso, D., J. Shilling, J. Shine, W. M. Fitch & R. W. Colman. 1986. Recent evolutionary divergence of plasma prekallikrein and factor X. Thromb. Res. **43:** 153–160.
11. Scott, C. F., L. D. Silver, A. D. Purdon & R. W. Colman. 1985. Cleavage of human high molecular weight kininogen by factor XIa *in vitro:* Effect on structure and function. J. Biol. Chem. **260:** 10856–10863.
12. Schapira, M., C. F. Scott & R. W. Colman. 1981. Protection of human plasma kallikrein from inactivation by C1 inhibitor and other protease inhibitors: The role of high molecular weight kininogen. Biochemistry **23:** 2738–2743.
13. Scott, C. F., M. Schapira, H. L. James, A. B. Cohen & R. W. Colman. 1982. The inactivation of factor XIa by plasma protease inhibitors. J. Clin. Invest. **69:** 844–852.
14. Silverberg, M., J. E. Nicoll & A. P. Kaplan. 1980. The mechanism by which the light chain of cleaved HMW-kininogen augments the activation of prekallikrein, factor XI and Hageman factor. Thromb. Res. **20:** 173–190.
15. Schapira, M., C. F. Scott, A. James, L. Silver, F. Kueppers, H. L. James & R. W. Colman. 1982. High molecular weight kininogen or its light chain protects human plasma kallikrein from inactivation by plasma protease inhibitors. Biochemistry **21:** 567–572.
16. Vehar, G. A. & E. W. Davie. 1980. Preparation and properties of bovine factor VIII (antihemophilic factor). Biochemistry **19:** 401–410.
17. Kisiel, W., W. M. Canfield, L. H. Ericsson & E. W. Davie. 1977. Anticoagulant properties of bovine plasma protein C following activation by thrombin. Biochemistry **16:** 5824–5831.

18. CHANG, J. J., C. F. SCOTT & R. W. COLMAN. 1986. Role of arginine residues in the coagulant activity of high molecular weight kininogen. Blood **67:** 805–810.
19. KAPLAN, A. P., A. B. KAY & K. F. AUSTEN. 1972. A prealbumin activator of prekallikrein. II. Appearance of chemotactic activity for human neutrophils by the conversion of human prekallikrein to kallikrein. J. Exp. Med. **135:** 81–97.
20. GOETZL, E. J. & K. F. AUSTEN. 1974. Stimulation of human neutrophil leukocyte aerobic glucose metabolism by purified chemotactic factors. J. Clin. Invest. **53:** 591–599.
21. SCHAPIRA, M., E. DESPLAND, C. F. SCOTT, L. A. BOXER & R. W. COLMAN. 1982. Purified human plasma kallikrein aggregates human neutrophils. J. Clin. Invest. **69:** 1199–1202.
22. WACHTFOGEL, Y. T., U. KUCICH, H. L. JAMES, C. F. SCOTT, M. SCHAPIRA, M. ZIMMERMAN, A. B. COHEN & R. W. COLMAN. 1983. Human plasma kallikrein releases neutrophil elastase during blood coagulation. J. Clin. Invest. **62:** 1672–1677.
23. COLMAN, R. W., Y. T. WACHTFOGEL, U. KUCICH, G. WEINBAUM, S. HAHN, R. A. PIXLEY, C. F. SCOTT, A. DEAGOSTINI, D. BURGER & M. SCHAPIRA. 1985. Effect of cleavage of the heavy chain of human plasma kallikrein and its functional properties. Blood **65:** 311–318.
24. WACHTFOGEL, Y. T., R. A. PIXLEY, U. KUCICH, W. ABRAMS, G. WEINBAUM, M. SCHAPIRA & R. W. COLMAN. 1986. Purified plasma Factor XIIa aggregates human neutrophils and causes degranulation. Blood **67:** 1731–1737.
25. WACHTFOGEL, Y. T., U. KUCICH, J. GREENPLATE, P. GLUSZKO, W. ABRAMS, G. WEINBAUM, R. K. WENGER, B. RUCINSKI, S. NIEWIAROWSKI, L. H. EDMUNDS & R. W. COLMAN. 1987. Human neutrophil degranulation during extracorporeal circulation. Blood. In press.
26. WACHTFOGEL, Y. T., P. HARPEL, L. H. EDMUNDS JR. & R. W. COLMAN. 1986. Formation of $C1_s$-$C\overline{1}$ inhibitor and kallikrein-$C\overline{1}$ inhibitor complexes during cardiopulmonary bypass (abstract). Blood. In press.
27. PIXLEY, R. A., M. SCHAPIRA & R. W. COLMAN. 1985. Effect of heparin on the inactivation rate of human activated factor XII by antithrombin III. Blood **66:** 198–203.
28. LAHIRI, B., A. BAGDASARIAN, B. MITCHELL, R. C. TALAMO, R. W. COLMAN & R. D. ROSENBERG. 1976. Antithrombin-heparin cofactor: An inhibitor of plasma kallikrein. Arch. Biochem. Biophys. **175:** 737–747.
29. SCOTT, C. F., M. SCHAPIRA & R. W. COLMAN. 1982. Effect of heparin on the inactivation rate of human XIa by antithrombin III. Blood **60:** 940–947.

The Activation of the Contact System of Human Plasma by Polysaccharide Sulfates

MICHAEL SILVERBERG AND SUSAN VEST DIEHL

Division of Allergy, Rheumatology, and Clinical Immunology
Department of Medicine
Health Sciences Center
State University of New York at Stony Brook
Stony Brook, New York 11794-8161

INTRODUCTION

Blood drawn into a clean glass tube will rapidly clot, yet if a plastic or siliconized tube is used, clotting is delayed. This phenomenon of "contact activation" is mediated by a group of plasma proteins, the contact system, whose interaction with a variety of negatively charged surfaces results in initiation of the intrinsic coagulation pathway.[1,2] These proteins also mediate the factor-XII-dependent pathways of kinin formation and fibrinolysis. The paradox of contact activation is that the congenital absence of any of the proteins of the contact system does not lead to overt clinical deficiencies, although the effect on the *in vitro* clotting assay is severe. However, there is increasing evidence that activation *in vivo* occurs in response to several situations including hereditary angioedema and gram negative sepsis. Also, blood or plasma in contact with non-physiological surfaces may generate significant quantities of bradykinin if contact activation occurs. Thus, the mechanism of the initiation of contact activation is a subject of considerable interest.

COMPONENT REACTIONS

The proteins involved in the initial reactions at the surface are factor XII (Hageman factor), prekallikrein, and high molecular weight kininogen. Both prekallikrein and factor XII circulate as zymogens but are converted to active proteases upon contact with a surface in the presence of high molecular weight kininogen.[3] Since the major activator of factor XII is kallikrein, and the major activator of prekallikrein is activated factor XII (FIG. 1), the contact system has the properties of positive feedback. As a result the events responsible for the initiation of the process become obscured and have been difficult to elucidate.

Earlier studies were conducted in whole plasma using relatively crude methods of assaying activation, but recently studies with purified components using kinetic assays have become feasible.[4–7] One of the outcomes of studies with synthetic substrates has been the realization that preparations of factor XII always have some enzymatic activity. This activity is inhibitable with protease inhibitors but it is very difficult to eliminate entirely. The explanation for this phenomenon appears to lie in the autoactivation of factor XII.[4] FIGURE 2 illustrates that factor XII incubated in a glass cuvette in the presence of substrate is able to evolve substantial enzymatic activity. The kinetics of this reaction are exponential, which is predicted by the simple model for autoactivation shown in FIGURE 3.

The autoactivation of human factor XII has been confirmed by a number of laboratories,[7–9] but bovine factor XII does not possess this property. Kinetically, the autoactivation of factor XII is much slower than the reactions between prekallikrein and factor XII shown in FIGURE 1. Nevertheless, factor XII autoactivation provides to us an extremely useful experimental tool with which to study the interaction between factor XII and the surface in the absence of other proteins, as will be illustrated below. When prekallikrein is added to the system, the positive feedback described in FIGURE 1 results in an extremely rapid acceleration of the rates of activation of either component. This is shown in FIGURE 4, which depicts an experiment similar to that shown in FIGURE 2 except that prekallikrein is also present. Using synthetic substrates specific for one enzyme or the other, we can see the very rapid generation of both enzymes compared with the rate of factor XIIa generation due to autoactivation.

The cuvette assay is a graphic demonstration of these reactions but is not readily amenable to the detailed kinetic analysis required for studies of the initiation of the contact reactions. Soluble dextran sulfate is a suitable activator of the system that can be used for such studies; using this material, we have demonstrated that activated

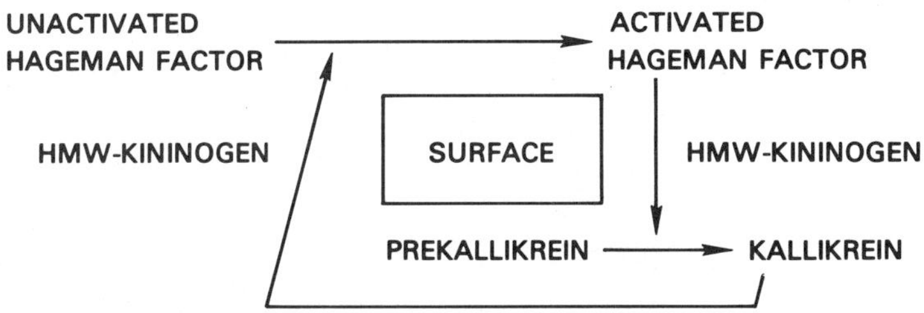

FIGURE 1. Diagram depicting the reciprocal activations of prekallikrein and factor XII in the presence of a surface and the cofactor high molecular weight kininogen.

factor XII is required for the activation of prekallikrein.[6] Tankersley and Finlayson[7] presented a detailed kinetic study of the rates of autoactivation of factor XII in the presence of dextran sulfate and the activation of prekallikrein by factor XIIa and of factor XII by kallikrein. The effects of the surface on these reactions are to increase the value of k_{cat}/K_m for prekallikrein activation by factor XIIa by 20-fold and to increase the reciprocal reaction by 10,000-fold. The rate of autoactivation is extremely low in the absence of the surface.

ROLE OF THE SURFACE

Although we talk about contact activation, it is not clear that the surface is actually able to induce activity that is not there in its absence. Thus the activations of prekallikrein by factor XIIa and of factor XII by kallikrein do proceed in the fluid phase. FIGURE 5 shows that the rate of prekallikrein activation seen when zymogen factor XII is added in the absence of surface increases with time until it reaches that obtained with activated factor XII, demonstrating that "contact activation" will also occur in the fluid phase, albeit slowly.

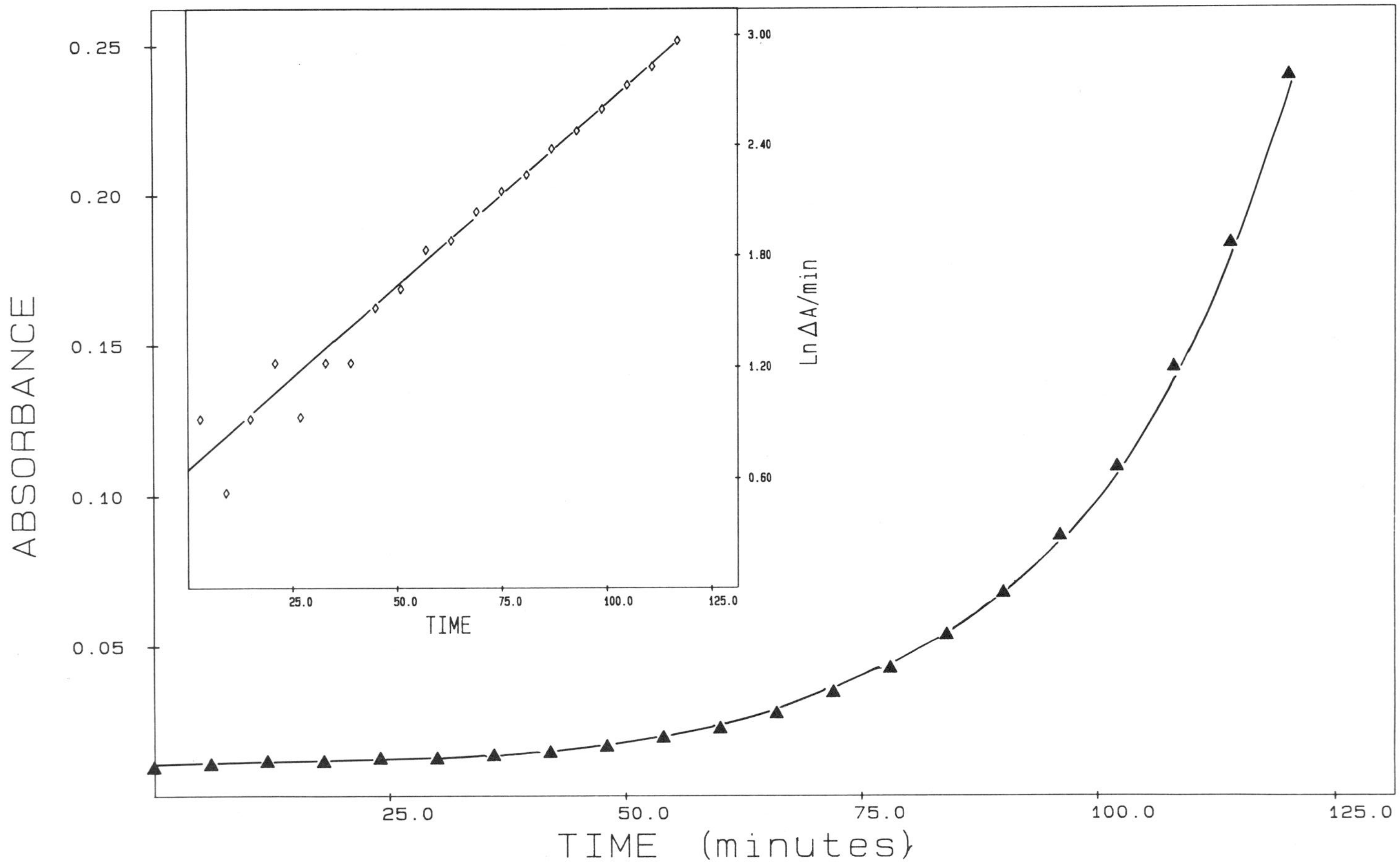

FIGURE 2. Factor XII (1.7 μg/ml) was incubated in a glass cuvette in 50 mM Tris HCl, pH 7.8, containing the substrate S2222 (500 μM). The logarithm of the rate of increase of absorbance was calculated at various times and plotted against the time (*inset*).

This notion is reinforced by studies of the effect of C1-INH on the autoactivation of factor XII in the presence or absence of activating surfaces.[10] The purpose of this study was to test the hypothesis that plasma inhibitors can prevent activation of factor XII. We found that, even in the absence of surface, factor XII became activated very slowly so that complexes of factor XIIa and C1-INH accumulated. By 48 hours of incubation, none of the original uncleaved factor XII is left. This lends support to the hypothesis that continued turnover of the system might be occurring *in vivo* with a very low level of active enzyme present at all times.

The surface, therefore, acts to accelerate reactions that are probably occurring slowly but continuously *in vivo*. TABLE 1 lists possible ways in which this might happen. The creation of a new enzyme from the zymogen by an induced conformational change was first proposed by Ratnoff and colleagues.[11] More recent studies, however, do not support this mechanism and there has been no unequivocal demonstration that zymogen ever possesses activity. The difficulties underlying such a potential demonstration are illustrated by the calculation of Tankersley and Finlayson[7] that at

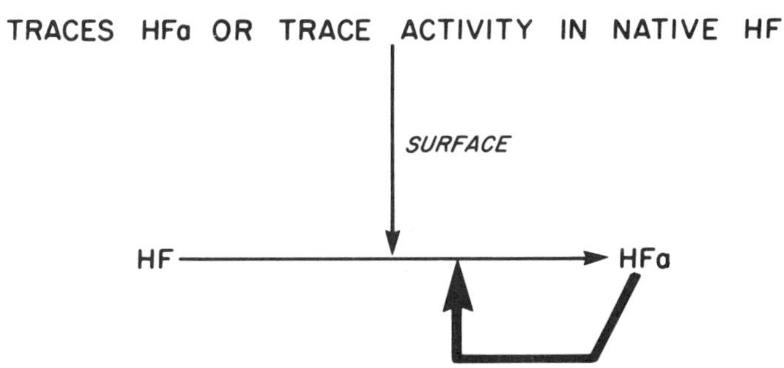

FIGURE 3. Scheme depicting the autoactivation of factor XII (*HF*). Whatever the initial stimulus, the rate of activation at any time is a function of the concentration of activated factor XII at that time, thus giving rise to the exponential kinetics seen in FIGURE 2.

physiological concentrations of factor XII and prekallikrein, the presence of one molecule of active enzyme of either species per milliliter would trigger reciprocal activation of both with a half-time of 13 seconds after the introduction of an activator such as dextran sulfate.

The induction of a new conformation of factor XII that is more readily cleaved to factor XIIa has been demonstrated by Griffin.[12] This effect was seen when different proteases were used as the activators and is probably a significant component of the catalytic effect of the surface.

The third possibility is that the reaction between surface and nonenzymatic cofactor is the important one. However, although high molecular weight kininogen appears to play an important role in plasma, the surface-catalyzed activations of purified factor XII and prekallikrein are clearly independent of any cofactor.

Finally, the factor that will be discussed in greater detail here is the localization of reactants to the surface. If proteins can reversibly bind to the surface there will be a zone of increased concentration local to the surface which will lead to increased rates of interaction. Some of these proteins will be molecules bound to the surface in

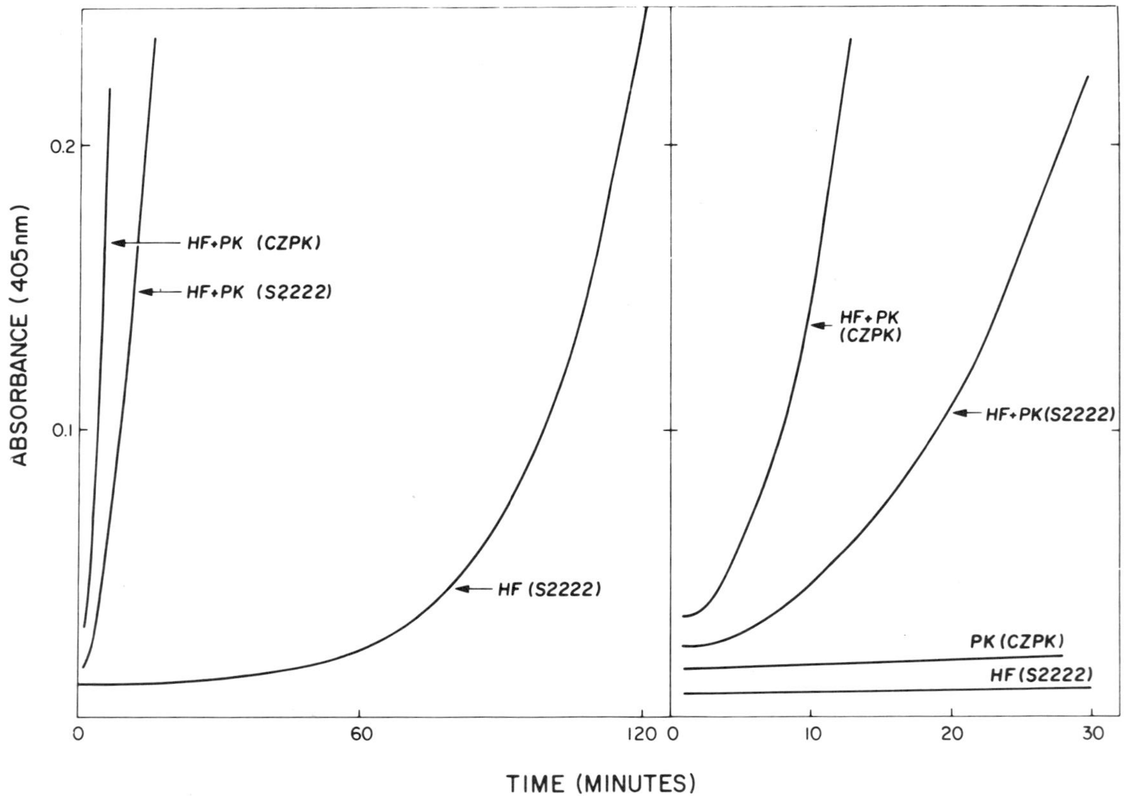

FIGURE 4. Factor XII (*HF*) was incubated in glass cuvettes with or without the addition of prekallikrein (*PK*) and 500 μM of either S2222, which is a substrate for activated factor XII but is not readily cleaved by kallikrein, or chromozym PK *(CZPK)*, which is a substrate for kallikrein but not for activated factor XII. *Right,* 1.35 μg/ml HF, 1.16 μg/ml PK; *Left,* 0.55 μg/ml HF, 0.47 μg/ml PK.

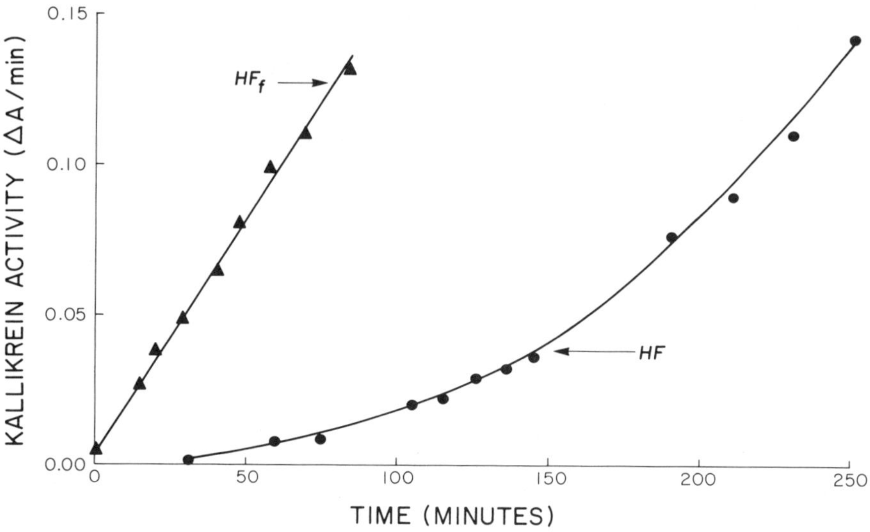

FIGURE 5. Activation of prekallikrein (36.3 μg/ml) by factor XII (*HF*, 8.27 ng/ml) or an equivalent molar concentration of factor XIIf (HF_f, 3.1 ng/ml) in the absence of a surface. At indicated times 5-μl aliquots were removed and assayed for kallikrein with chromozym-PK.

conformations more susceptible to activation, and so a many-fold increase in the activation rate is to be expected. The predictions of this model are shown in TABLE 2.

The possible identity of the putative physiological surface(s) required for contact activation and the nature of its interaction with the protein components of the system remain poorly understood. It has long been known that particulate materials bearing fixed negative charges, such as celite and kaolin, as well as glass, are active in promoting contact activation.[2] There were also early reports of various natural or synthetic sulfated polysaccharides that were identified that were able to support contact activation in plasma.[13–16] Of these, high molecular weight dextran sulfate is an efficient and reproducible activator,[16,17] though not a physiological compound. More recently, kinetic assays have been used to reexamine the activity of natural glycosaminoglycans, especially heparins,[18,19] which are the physiological substances most likely to be able to initiate contact activation. Our approach to the study of the interaction of contact proteins with surfaces has been to focus initially on the interaction of factor XII with defined fractions of dextran sulfate of varying size. In this manner we hope to be able to elucidate some of the features of the surface required for efficient activation.

TABLE 1. Possible Functions of the Surface

Hypothesis	Status
Create a new or better enzyme	unproved (and unlikely)
Create a new or better substrate	demonstrated (and important)
Create a new or better cofactor	unproved
Localize the reactants	probably important (see TABLE 2)

TABLE 2. Localization of Reactants

I. Effects
  A. Increase the local concentration of factor XII
    1. Increase local concentration of factor XIIa
  B. Increase ratios of reactant concentration to inhibitor concentrations
  C. Increase the susceptibility of unactivated factor XII to cleavage
II. Requirements
  A. Reversible binding of factor XII to activating surface
  B. Multiple binding sites clustered together
  C. Distinct binding anion binding sites on factor XII

STUDIES WITH DEXTRAN SULFATES

Sulfation of Dextrans

Since dextran sulfates are not available in a variety of molecular weight classes, we decided to sulfate commercially available preparations of dextran. Initially, the method of Nagasawa and Yoshidome[20] was used for the sulfation of dextrans. Quinolyl sulfate was synthesized from 8-hydroxyquinoline and chlorosulfonic acid in the presence of *N,N*-dimethylaniline in chloroform solution as described. The quinolyl sulfate was then used to sulfate dextran in dimethyl formamide in the presence of $CuCl_2$.

Soluble dextran of nominal molecular weight 200,000–275,000 sulfated with quinolyl sulfate did not support the autoactivation of factor XII when assayed by generation of amidolytic activity. Using the barium chloranilate assay for sulfate after a 6-hour hydrolysis at 100°C in 6N HCl, it appeared that the incorporation of sulfate into dextran from quinolyl sulfate was much lower than the sulfate content of the commercially obtained preparations. An alternative method is the direct sulfation of the dextran by chlorosulfonic acid in chloroform.[21] We prepared sulfated dextran of mw 200,000–275,000 by this method and compared the level of sulfate incorporation, using the barium chloranilate assay, of the three preparations of dextran sulfate (TABLE 3).

There was a clear correlation between incorporation of sulfate and the ability to support autoactivation. This was not in itself surprising but did demonstrate that the more rigorous sulfation reaction, using chlorosulfonic acid, was required. This reaction was therefore used to prepare a series of dextran sulfates and to sulfate Sephadex G50.

Relationship between the Autoactivation of Factor XII and the Molecular Size of Dextran Sulfate

Dextrans of nominal molecular weights from 200,000–275,000 down to 15,000–20,000 were sulfated and tested for their ability to support the autoactivation of factor

TABLE 3. Sulfation of Dextrans

Sulfation Reaction	SO_4 (% wt/wt)	Autoactivation
Commercial product	30	+++
Chlorosulfonic acid	25	++
Quinolyl sulfate	5	–

XII. We found that each of the sulfated dextrans was active and initially there appeared to be no clear correlation between activity in the assay and molecular weight, even down to a molecular weight of 5000. However, these preparations varied somewhat in sulfate content as well as molecular weight. We focused on three preparations that have similar high sulfate contents, those of 500,000, 15,000–20,000, and 5000 MW; we find a clear relationship between activity and molecular weight (TABLE 4).

The ability of dextran sulfate of molecular weight 5000 to support the autoactivation of factor XII was unexpected since only particulate or high molecular weight substances had ever been reported to function as "surfaces." It seemed possible that the dextran sulfates were forming complexes, perhaps with metal ions as described for ellagic acid.[22] Accordingly, dextran sulfate solutions were made up fresh in 10 mM EDTA or 5 mM *o*-phenanthroline and the incubation buffer for the autoactivation reactions was made 1 mM in EDTA. This did not diminish the anion-catalyzed activation, even by the 5000 MW dextran sulfate. Gel filtration on Sephadex G-50 in the presence of EDTA also did not abrogate the activity. Thus the ability of low molecular weight dextran sulfate to function as a surface was not due to the formation of higher molecular weight aggregates in the presence of metal ions.

To define further the effect of molecular weight of the dextran sulfate we chromatographed the 5000 MW preparation on columns of Sephadex G50 or G75,

TABLE 4. Properties of Dextran Sulfates

Nominal Molecular Weight	Sulfate (% by weight[a])	Apparent Rate Constant of Autoactivation (min^{-1})
500,000	48.2	0.435
15,000–20,000	50.9	0.294
5,000	50.2	0.089

Assays conducted at 53.2 μg/ml factor XII and 1.925 μg/ml dextran.
[a]Percent of total recovery of sulfate and dextran.

calibrated using a series of polystyrene sulfonates. Individual fractions of dextran sulfate were assayed for their ability to support the autoactivation of factor XII. When we determined the rate constants for autoactivation as a function of dextran concentration for each of five of the fractions eluted from G-75, we found that for each fraction the rate of activation rose to a peak and then declined with further increases in concentration. Significantly, the maximum rate of autoactivation obtained with different fractions, having molecular weights of 4800 and above, all occurred at about 3.0 μg/ml dextran sulfate. Thus, it appears that the maximum rate occurred at the same concentration of binding sites for each fraction, but that the value of that maximum increased as those sites were arranged into particles with a larger average number of binding sites per particle. The very smallest fraction examined, having a molecular weight of 3000, gave very low rates of autoactivation with an apparent peak in the region of 10 μg/ml. It is possible that this reflects the presence in this fraction of a small amount of material with higher molecular weight that is responsible for this activity and that between 3000 and 4000 MW the limit is reached below which no binding of factor XII can occur.

We extended these observations by fractionating the 15,000–20,000 MW dextran sulfate in the same fashion and assaying each fraction in the autoactivation reaction. We compared the rate constants with those obtained from the fractions derived from

5000 MW dextran sulfate at the same dextran concentration. The data from the two preparations appear to describe an identical relationship of autoactivation rate to molecular size of the dextran sulfate with a sharp increase occurring as a molecular weight of 10,000 is reached.

Following the discovery that low molecular weight dextran sulfate could support the autoactivation of factor XII, we extended the studies to include heparin. We found that the commercial preparations that we used did indeed support the autoactivation of factor XII. The rate of autoactivation with heparin was slower than with dextran sulfate, which may be a function of the lower sulfate content. Three different heparin preparations were used; USP heparin, a heparin fraction of 13,000–15,000 MW, and a fraction obtained by nitrous acid depolymerization and having a nominal molecular weight of 5000. When chromatographed on Sephadex G-75, these gave different elution profiles but the curves of autoactivation rate vs. elution position were superimposable. We confirmed that this was a true correlate of molecular size by taking two fractions from either end of one of the chromatograms and running over the same column. The fractions ran in the same positions as they had originally come from and supported autoactivation with the expected rate constants.

These results with two different preparations of dextran sulfate and three of heparin all showed similar variation of rate of autoactivation with elution from a gel-filtration column. In these experiments, protein and dextran concentrations were standardized so that the only variable was molecular size. The molecular weight range in which we found a strong effect of molecular size on activation rate is much lower than anticipated, and the implication is that only a small number of binding sites are required for activation. Calculations of the size of the smallest species that could support activation suggested that they should be able to bind one molecule of factor XII but not more, whereas species large enough to bind two molecules seemed to be able to support much more efficient activation. Other explanations are not yet ruled out, however, such as the possibility that a relatively large molecule of dextran sulfate is required to provide a binding site capable of inducing the required conformational change in the factor XII molecule.

Chromatography on Columns of Sulfated Dextran

We also sulfated sephadex beads to provide a particulate activator of more defined character than kaolin or similar materials. Sephadex G-50 was chosen for sulfation to eliminate the potential confusion of gel filtration effects and also to provide for direct comparison with SP-Sephadex; thus we wanted to be able to distinguish between a specific affinity reaction and simple ion exchange.

Sephadex G-50 was sulfated by the chlorosulfonic acid procedure and was shown by barium chloranilate assay to have incorporated 30.5% sulfate by weight. The beads were able to support the autoactivation of factor XII when incubated in the absence if inhibitors. Columns, 8 mm × 75 mm, were packed with Sephadex G-50, SP Sephadex C-50, and with the sulfated G-50. All were equilibrated with 50 mM Tris HCl, pH 7.5, containing 10 mM benzamidine, 0.15 M NaCl, and 0.001% Triton X-100. Under these conditions, factor XII is not bound or retarded by either the G-50 or the SP Sephadex but is bound tightly to the sulfated G-50. Washing with over 30 column volumes of equilibration buffer did not elute the factor XII, which was recovered by elution with gradients of sodium chloride or sodium sulfate. These data indicate that factor XII binds tightly to sulfated dextrans at physiological conditions, but the binding is reversible and thus is in agreement with the features expected (TABLE 2).

As a test of the prediction that factor XII must have discrete binding sites for negatively charged groups, we studied the ability of various anions to elute factor XII from the column. The basic method used was to elute the column with concentration gradients of the various compounds in equilibration buffer and to compare the conductivities at which the peak of eluted factor XII was found. The reference point is the conductivity of the equilibration buffer, which was 18.0 mS.

The column was eluted with a 0–0.2 M gradient of sodium sulfate; the factor XII was recovered at a conductivity of 33 mS, which represented a concentration much lower than that required with NaCl. This suggested that there might be some specificity to the interaction of factor XII with sulfate, or at least with divalent anions. We next tried a series of compounds containing either one negative group or two with different spacings. The results obtained with these are shown in TABLE 5.

These data seem to show a trend amongst the divalent compounds towards elution at lower concentration as the distance between the anionic groups increases. The anthraquinone compounds could not be dissolved at concentrations greater than 4 mM, but at this concentration the 2,6-disulfonate efficiently eluted factor XII from the

TABLE 5. Elution of Factor XII from Columns of Sulfated G-50

Compound	Conductivity of Elution (mS)
Monovalent	
Acetate	30
Phthalate	25,35 (two peaks)
Benzene sulfonate	25
Anthraquinone-2-sulfonate (4 mM)	no elution
Anthraquinone-2-carboxylate (4 mM)	no elution
Divalent	
Succinate	38
Fumarate	29–36
Malate	37
Benzene 1,4-disulfonate	27
Naphthalene 2,6-disulfonate	22
Anthraquinone 2,6-disulfonate (4 mM)	18.5

column. This effect was not due to the anthraquinone structure itself since neither of two mono-substituted anionic derivatives eluted the protein.

The results we have obtained so far seem to indicate that factor XII does indeed have at least two anionic binding sites and that compounds having anionic groups with suitable spacing may be able to bind preferentially. We looked to see if the most effective eluant, the anthraquinone 2,6-disulfonate, could block the autoactivation on factor XII with dextran sulfate, but in preliminary experiments we did not find inhibition.

CONCLUSIONS

Referring to TABLE 2 we find that the requirements have been met for a simple hypothesis of surface catalysis by localization of reactants. Thus factor XII binds reversibly to dextran sulfate and the rate of autoactivation is augmented when there is more than one binding site per "particle." The binding of factor XII to surfaces appears to be mediated through sites on factor XII that preferentially bind strong anionic groups such as sulfate. These factors, together with the enhancement of the rate of cleavage of surface-bound factor XII, are responsible for changing the balance between activation and inhibition during contact activation of human plasma.

REFERENCES

1. MARGOLIS, J. 1956. Glass surface and blood coagulation. Nature **178:** 805–806.
2. NOSSEL, H. L. 1964. The Contact Phase of Blood Coagulation. Blackwell Scientific Publications. Oxford.
3. KAPLAN, A. P. 1978. Initiation of the intrinsic coagulation and fibrinolytic pathways of man: The role of surfaces, Hageman factor, prekallikrein, high molecular weight kininogen and factor XI. Prog. Hemostas. Thromb. **4:** 127–175.
4. SILVERBERG, M., J. T. DUNN, L. GAREN & A. P. KAPLAN. 1980. Autoactivation of human Hageman factor: Demonstration utilizing a synthetic substrate. J. Biol. Chem. **255:** 7281–7286.
5. HOJIMA, Y., D. L. TANKERSLEY, M. MILLER-ANDERSSON, J. V. PIERCE & J. J. PISANO. 1980. Enzymatic properties of human Hageman factor fragment with plasma prekallikrein and synthetic substrates. Thromb. Res. **18:** 417–430.
6. SILVERBERG, M. & A. P. KAPLAN. 1982. Enzymatic activities of activated and zymogen forms of human Hageman factor (factor XII). Blood **60:** 64–70.
7. TANKERSLEY, D. L. & J. S. FINLAYSON. 1984. Kinetics of activation and autoactivation of human factor XII. Biochemistry **23:** 273–279.
8. TANS, G., J. ROSING & J. H. GRIFFIN. 1983. Sulfatide-dependent autoactivation of human blood coagulation factor XII (Hageman factor). J. Biol. Chem. **258:** 8215–8222.
9. GRIEP, M. A., K. FUJIKAWA & G. L. NELSESTUEN. 1985. Binding and activation properties of human factor XII, prekallikrein and derived peptides with acidic lipid vesicles. Biochemistry **24:** 4124–4130.
10. WEISS, R., M. SILVERBERG & A. P. KAPLAN. 1986. The effect of C1 inhibitor upon Hageman factor autoactivation. Blood **68:** 239–243.
11. MILLIN, C. R., H. SAITO, O. D. RATNOFF & A. G. WALTON. 1974. The secondary structure of human Hageman factor (factor XII) and its alteration by activating agents. J. Clin. Invest. **54:** 1312–1322.
12. GRIFFIN, J. H. 1978. Role of surface in surface-dependent activation of Hageman factor (blood coagulation factor XII). Proc. Natl. Acad. Sci. **75:** 1998–2002.
13. KELLERMEYER, W. F., JR. & R. W. KELLERMEYER. 1969. Hageman factor activation and kinin formation by cellulose sulfate solutions. Proc. Soc. Exp. Biol. Med. **130:** 1310–1314.
14. SCHWARTZ, H. J. & R. W. KELLERMEYER. 1969. Carrageenan and delayed hypersensitivity. II. Activation of Hageman factor by carrageenan and its possible significance. Proc. Soc. Exp. Biol. Med. **132:** 1021–1024.
15. MOSKOWITZ, R. W., H. J. SCHWARTZ, B. MICHEL, O. D. RATNOFF & T. ASTRUP. 1970. Generation of kinin-like agents by chondroitin sulfate, heparin, chitin sulfate, and human articular cartilage: Possible pathophysiologic implications. J. Lab. Clin. Med. **76:** 790–798.
16. KLUFT, C. 1977. Assay for prekallikrein levels and prekallikrein activation in human plasma using dextran sulfate as a soluble activator. Thromb. Hemostas. **38:** 220.
17. VAN DER GRAAF, F., F. J. A. KEUS, R. A. A. VLOOSWIJK & B. N. BOUMA. 1982. The contact activation mechanism in human plasma: Activation induced by dextran sulfate. Blood **59:** 1225–1233.
18. HOJIMA, Y., C. G. COCHRANE, R. C. WIGGINS, K. F. AUSTEN & R. L. STEVENS. 1984. In vitro activation of the contact (Hageman factor) system of plasma by heparin and chondroitin sulfate E. Blood **63:** 1453–1459.
19. SHIMADA, T., T. SUGO, H. KATO, K. YOSHIDA & S. IWANAGA. 1985. Activation of factor XII and prekallikrein with polysaccharide sulfates and sulfatides: Comparison with kaolin-mediated activation. J. Biochem. **97:** 429–439.

20. NAGASAWA, K. & H. YOSHIDOME. 1974. A metal catalysed reaction of 8-quinolyl sulphate and its application to the preparation of biochemically related sulphate esters. J. Org. Chem. **39:** 1681–1685.
21. RICKETTS, C. R. 1952. Dextran sulfate: A synthetic analogue of heparin. Biochem. J. **51:** 129–133.
22. BOCK, P. E., K. R. SRINIVASAN & J. D. SHORE. 1981. Activation of intrinsic blood coagulation by ellagic acid: Insoluble ellagic acid metal ion complexes are the activating species. Biochemistry **20:** 7258–7266.

Fibronectin Adsorption on Material Surfaces[a]

FREDERICK GRINNELL

Department of Cell Biology and Anatomy
University of Texas Health Science Center
Dallas, Texas 75235

INTRODUCTION

Some time ago, we reported that mammalian cells attach better to wettable surfaces.[1,2] For instance, studies on two different baby hamster kidney (BHK) cell lines showed that more cell attachment occurred on surfaces with air-water contact angles less than 60° than on surfaces with air-water contact angles greater than 70° (TABLE 1). The basis for such differences were unknown, but after fibronectin (FN) was identified as a serum component that promoted cell adhesion,[3-5] it seemed reasonable to suppose that the differences in cell adhesion on material surfaces might depend on differences in FN adsorption on the surfaces. In this paper, I will review briefly the results of our studies to test this hypothesis.[6-10]

FIBRONECTIN ADSORPTION ON SURFACES IN RELATION TO CELL ADHESION

We began our studies by measuring FN adsorption on surfaces in relation to BHK cell adhesion. Experiments were carried out using 35-mm diameter Falcon tissue culture (TC) dishes that have wettable surfaces and Falcon bacteriological culture (BACT) dishes that have nonwettable surfaces. Both types of dishes are made from polystyrene, but the former have been treated by the glow discharge technique.[11] Underwater contact angles on the dish surfaces were reported to be 88° and 31°, respectively.[12]

With solution concentrations less than 10 μg/ml, slightly more FN adsorption occurred on BACT dishes than on TC dishes (FIGURE 1). With solution concentrations of FN above 20 μg/ml, similar amounts of FN adsorption occurred on BACT dishes and TC dishes, *i.e.,* about 320 ng/cm^2. Significantly, however, FN adsorbed on TC dishes promoted cell spreading much more effectively than FN density of about 15 ng/cm^2, while complete cell spreading on BACT dishes required a FN density of 100 ng/cm^2.

EVIDENCE FOR DIFFERENT ORIENTATIONS OF ADSORBED FN

One explanation for the differences in biological activity between FN adsorbed on wettable surfaces and FN adsorbed on nonwettable surfaces was differences in the

[a]This research was supported by grant nos. CA14609 and HL24221 from the NIH.

TABLE 1. Attachment of BHK Cells to Surfaces Varying in Chemical Composition[a]

Surface	Air-Medium Contact Angle (Degrees)	% Cell Attachment	
		BHK-21-C13	BHK-21-13s
Glass	17 ± 2	56 ± 12	67 ± 1
TC polystyrene	28 ± 1	81 ± 2	81 ± 1
Stainless steel	45 ± 7	76 ± 1	84 ± 1
Aluminum	55 ± 5	79 ± 2	78 ± 2
Polycarbonate	59 ± 6	63 ± 7	76 ± 4
Polyethylene	71 ± 7	31 ± 3	33 ± 5
TPX	76 ± 5	28 ± 2	37 ± 2
Polypropylene	78 ± 9	30 ± 4	36 ± 12

[a]BHK cells in medium containing 5% fetal bovine serum were incubated for 60 min at 30°C on the surfaces indicated. At the end of the incubations the extent of cell attachment was measured. Contact angle measurements were made directly using a microscope equipped with rotatable crosshairs and a 360° reticle.

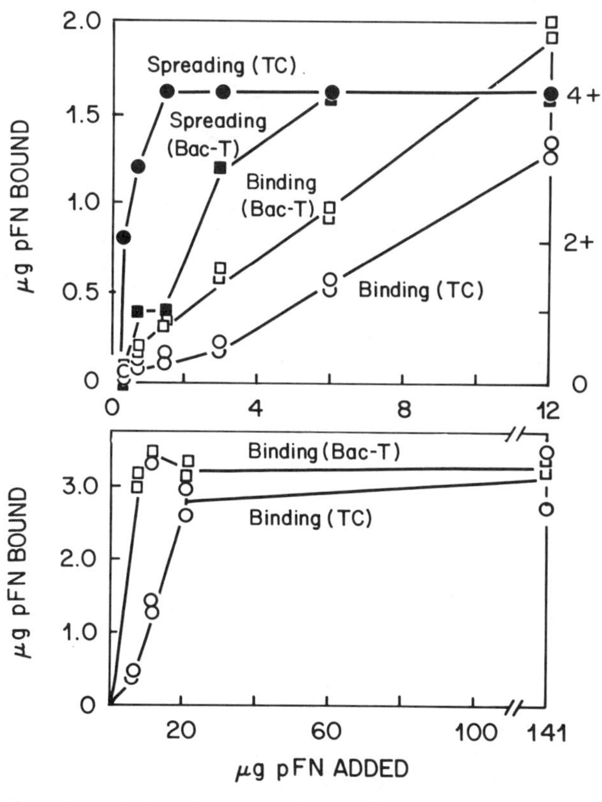

FIGURE 1. Adsorption of FN in relation to cell spreading. TC and BACT dishes were incubated for 10 min at 22°C with radiolabeled FN at the concentrations indicated. At the end of the incubations, the dishes were rinsed. Some samples were used to determine the amount of bound FN. Others were used to measure BHK cell spreading. (From Grinnell and Feld.[6])

orientation of FN molecules on the surfaces. Others have shown that there are chemical differences in protein bonding to wettable and nonwettable surfaces and emphasized the role of hydrophobic interactions in bonding to nonwettable surfaces.[13] Consistent with this view, we found that FN adsorbed on wettable surfaces was more easily extracted by NaOH or sodium doedecyl sulfate than was FN adsorbed on nonwettable surfaces. Moreover, FN adsorption on wettable surfaces was pH dependent, whereas FN adsorption on nonwettable surfaces was pH independent.[6]

To test directly possible differences in the orientation of FN adsorbed on wettable and nonwettable surfaces, we studied binding of polyclonal anti-FN antibodies to adsorbed FN (FIGURE 2). In these experiments, FN adsorption was measured directly using radiolabeled FN as in FIGURE 1 and indirectly based on the binding of anti-FN antibodies and radiolabeled anti-IgG.[7] Analyzed by the direct method, FN adsorption was slightly greater on BACT dishes than on TC dishes, as already mentioned.

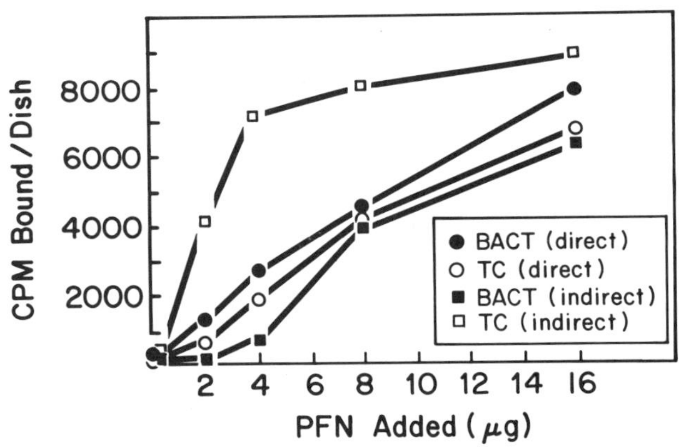

FIGURE 2. Adsorption of FN in the relation to antibody binding. TC and BACT dishes were incubated for 10 min at 22°C with radiolabled FN at the concentrations indicated. At the end of the incubations, the dishes were rinsed. Some samples were used to determine the amount of bound FN (direct). Others were incubated with anti-FN and radiolabeled anti-IgG to determine antibody binding (indirect). (From Grinnell and Feld.[7])

Analyzed by antibody binding, however, many more antigenic sites were exposed on FN bound to the wettable surfaces. For instance, after incubation with 4 μg/ml FN, about 70% as much FN adsorption occurred on wettable surfaces as on nonwettable surfaces, but 12 times more antibody molecules bound to the FN adsorbed on the wettable surfaces.

Studies in other laboratories are consistent with the observations described above. Antibody and lectin binding to FN adsorbed on wettable and nonwettable surfaces were shown to be different by ellipsometric measurements.[14] Also, analyses of adsorbed FN by contact angle measurements[15] and by total internal reflection fluorescence spectroscopy[16] indicated different conformations of adsorbed FN on wettable and nonwettable surfaces. Consequently, it seems reasonable to conclude that the orientation of adsorbed FN depends on the chemical features of the surfaces on which adsorption occurs, which is similar to what has been proposed for immunoglobulins.[17,18]

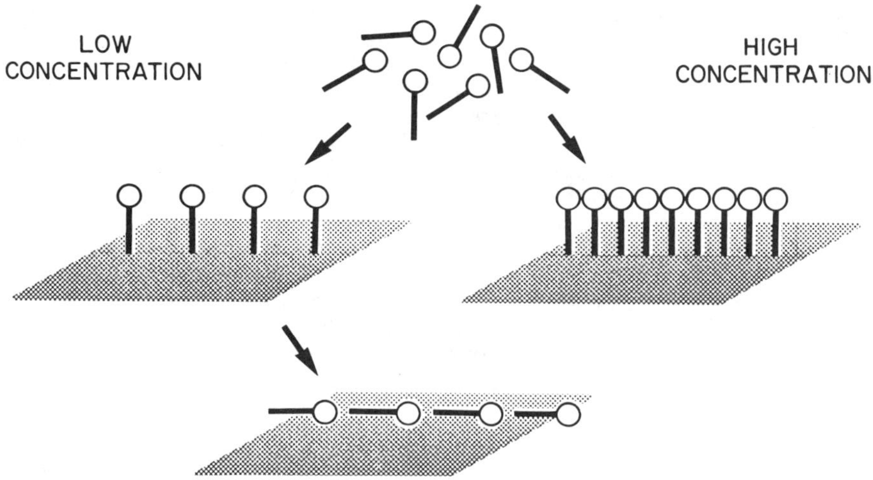

FIGURE 3. Theoretical model relating concentration dependence of protein adsorption to orientation of adsorbed proteins. See text for details.

MODULATION OF THE PACKING OF ADSORBED FN MOLECULES

As the concentration of FN was increased, differences in the reactivity of FN adsorbed on wettable and nonwettable surfaces were less evident (FIGURES 1 and 2). One possible explanation of the concentration dependence was that differences in the orientation of FN molecules adsorbed on the surfaces depended upon the initial FN concentration to which the surfaces were exposed. As shown by the theoretical model in FIGURE 3, molecules adsorbed on surfaces at low density have the space to orient differently from molecules adsorbed on surfaces at high density. It has been suggested that proteins adsorbed to surfaces will undergo conformation changes to maximize their binding energy if there is sufficient space on the surfaces for such changes to occur.[19,20]

Considered in the context of FIGURE 3, the results presented in FIGURES 1 and 2 suggested that FN adsorbed in a more biologically active orientation on surfaces exposed to high concentrations of FN. In addition, it seemed likely that FN adsorbed in

TABLE 2. Adsorption of FN on BACT Surfaces in the Presence and Absence of BSA[a]

Treatment	FN Adsorbed (ng/cm^2)	Cell Spreading
3.5 μg FN alone	43.5	none
3.5 μg/ml FN then 50 μg/ml BSA	45.5	none
3.5 μg/ml FN plus 50 μg/ml BSA	11.7	complete

[a]BACT dishes were incubated for 10 min at 22°C with radiolabeled FN, with radiolabeled FN followed by BSA, or with radiolabeled FN and BSA simultaneously. At the end of the incubations, the dishes were rinsed. Some samples were used to determine the amount of bound FN. Others were used to measure BHK cell spreading.

a more active orientation on wettable surfaces exposed to low FN concentrations. However, on nonwettable surfaces exposed to low FN concentrations FN adsorbed in a less active orientation. We predicted, therefore, that FN adsorbed on nonwettable surfaces would adsorb in the orientation with high biological activity if we altered the FN packing arrangement on the surfaces by adding another protein that could bind to the surfaces. This possibility was tested experimentally by incubating BACT dishes with low concentrations of FN in the presence of bovine serum albumin (BSA).[6] Representative data are shown in TABLE 2. On surfaces treated with FN alone or FN followed by BSA, similar amounts of FN were bound, and the adsorbed FN was unable to promote cell spreading. On surfaces incubated with FN in the presence of BSA, there was less FN bound, but the bound FN was much more active biologically. Dose-response studies showed that the effect on FN activity was maximal when the BSA level was at about 20 μg/ml.[7] Based on these studies, we concluded that BSA modified FN packing on the non-wettable surfaces, as a consequence of which a more biologically active orientation of adsorbed FN was obtained.

FN ADSORPTION ON SURFACES EXPOSED TO SERUM AND PLASMA

The experiments described above provided novel information about the orientation and packing of FN on surfaces. They did not clarify, however, why cells attach better on wettable surfaces than on nonwettable surfaces (TABLE 1), since cells attached similarly to both types of surfaces if the surfaces were coated with high concentrations of FN. Significantly, the studies summarized in TABLE 1 were carried out using medium that contained 10% fetal bovine serum (FBS). In related experiments, we found that diploid human fibroblasts in 10% serum-containing medium grow as well in FN-coated BACT dishes as in TC dishes, although they grow poorly in uncoated BACT dishes.[21] Consequently, we decided to change our focus from studying FN

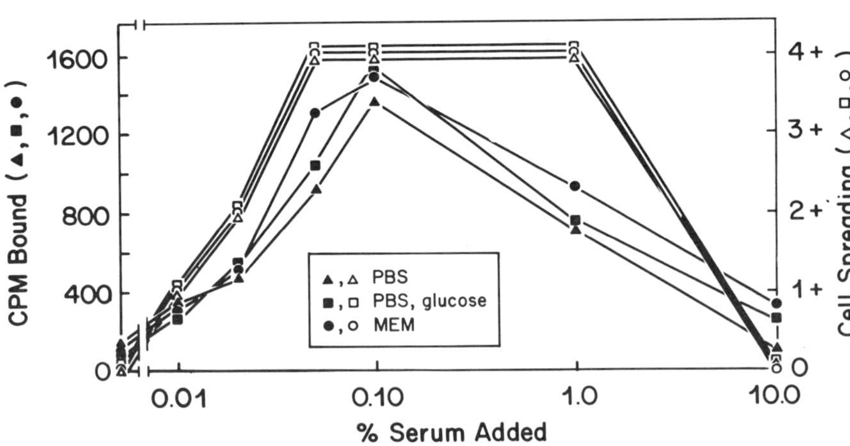

FIGURE 4. Adsorption of FN from serum solutions in relationship to cell spreading. TC dishes were incubated for 10 min at 22°C with human serum at the concentrations indicated prepared in the buffers shown. At the end of the incubations, the dishes were rinsed. Some samples were used to determine the amount of bound FN. Others were used to measure BHK cell spreading. (From Grinnell and Feld.[7])

TABLE 3. Desorption of FN Previously Adsorbed to Different Surfaces[a]

Test Surface	Desorption Buffer	% FN Desorbed
Glass	phosphate saline (PS)	15.7 ± 0.1
	PS + 10% FBS	70.0 ± 5.6
	PS + 7 mg/ml BSA	44.5 ± 2.1
	PS + 7 mg/ml ovalbumin	36.8 ± 4.5
TC polystyrene	PS	3.4 ± 0.6
	PS + 10% FBS	27.9 ± 0.4
BACT polystyrene	PS	0.8 ± 0.5
	PS + 10% FBS	9.4 ± 1.8

[a]Surfaces previously coated with radiolabeled FN were incubated for 1 h at 37°C with the buffers indicated. At the end of the incubations, the amounts of FN released into solution and remaining on the surfaces were measured.

adsorption on surfaces exposed to pure FN solutions to studying FN adsorption on surfaces exposed to serum.

Experiments were performed in which we incubated TC and BACT dishes with different concentrations of serum and then measured FN adsorption and BHK cell adhesion on the surfaces. As the serum concentration used to treat the surfaces was increased up to about 0.1%, the amount of FN adsorbed on the surfaces increased. At higher concentrations of serum, the amount of FN adsorbed on the surfaces decreased (FIGURE 4).[7] There was a corresponding increase in cell adhesion on surfaces treated with up to 0.1% serum and less cell adhesion on surfaces treated with higher serum concentrations. This bimodal pattern of adsorption was observed using TC and BACT dishes. Also, we measured FN adsorption and cell adhesion on surfaces treated with plasma, and the results were very similar to those observed with serum, at least under nonclotting conditions.[8,9]

The bimodal pattern of protein adsorption on surfaces exposed to serum or plasma solutions has been confirmed recently by laboratories studying other proteins including fibrinogen and immunoglobulin.[22–24] It seems likely that this pattern is a consequence of sequential, competitive adsorption-desorption of the different proteins of the complex mixtures.[22,25] Such a mechanism can explain the so-called "conversion" effect, which was observed when fibrinogen adsorption on surfaces was studied for short time periods.[26]

DESORPTION OF FN PREVIOUSLY ADSORBED TO SURFACES

The lack of FN adsorption on wettable or nonwettable surfaces exposed to 10% serum leads to the conclusion that TC or BACT dishes exposed to serum are coated primarily with nonadhesive proteins. As a result, cell adhesion requires replacement of the originally adsorbed nonadhesive protein layer with an adhesive protein layer, a modification process that can occur in fibronectin-depleted serum.[27,28] The results cannot be explained by the presence of another cell adhesion factor found in serum, *i.e.*, 70 kDa,[29] since the 70 kDa factor also has a bimodal adsorption pattern with a maximum on surfaces exposed to about 0.1% serum.[30] Therefore, the important difference between wettable and nonwettable surfaces may be the rate of nonadhesive protein replacement. Indeed, we have shown that after 4–6 h of cell culture in medium containing 10% serum, we can begin to detect a cell-dependent increase in the amount of FN on the surfaces of TC dishes that was not observed on the surfaces of BACT dishes.[7]

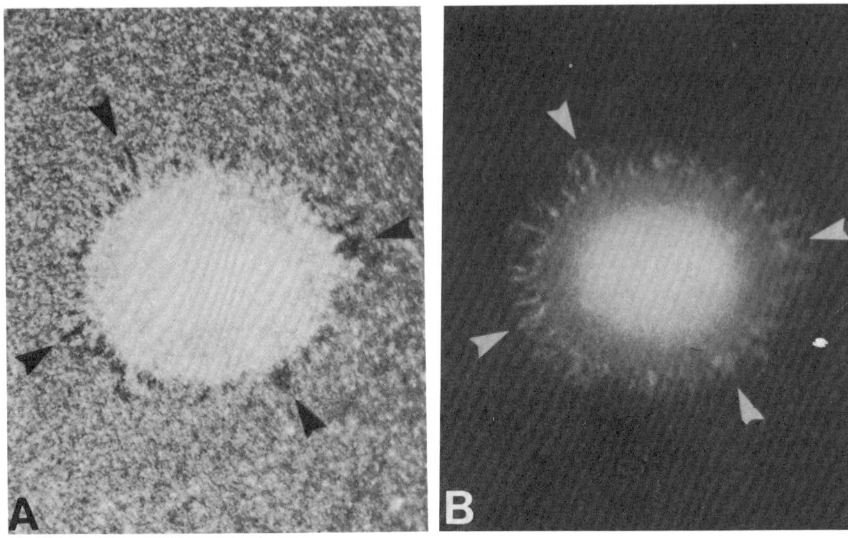

FIGURE 5. Removal of FN from glass surfaces at focal adhesion sites. Human fibroblasts were incubated for 30 min at 37°C on glass coverslips previously coated with fluorescein-conjugated FN. At the end of the incubations the cells were fixed and permeabilized and stained with antivinculin IgG and rhodamine-conjugated anti-IgG. Dark streaks in the bright fluorescein background (**A**, *arrows*) are sites where FN was removed from the glass surface. The same field viewed by rhodamine optics showed that the vinculin-containing focal adhesion sites (**B**, *arrows*) corresponded to the sites from which FN was removed. (From Grinnell.[10])

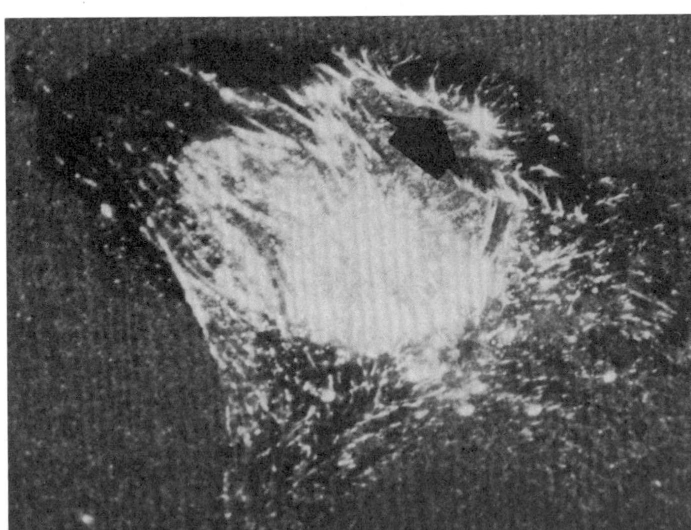

FIGURE 6. Removal of FN from beneath cells during adhesion. Same as FIGURE 5A except the incubation was carried out for 2 h. A large region of FN has been removed from the glass surface beneath the cells, and much of the removed FN is bound in fibrillar structures on the cell surface (*arrow*). (From Grinnell.[10])

In order to better understand how cells modify previously adsorbed protein layers, we have initiated studies on protein desorption. Others have reported that desorption is slower from nonwettable surfaces than from wettable surfaces[31] and can be promoted by the presence of protein in the medium[32]. Both of these features were observed with

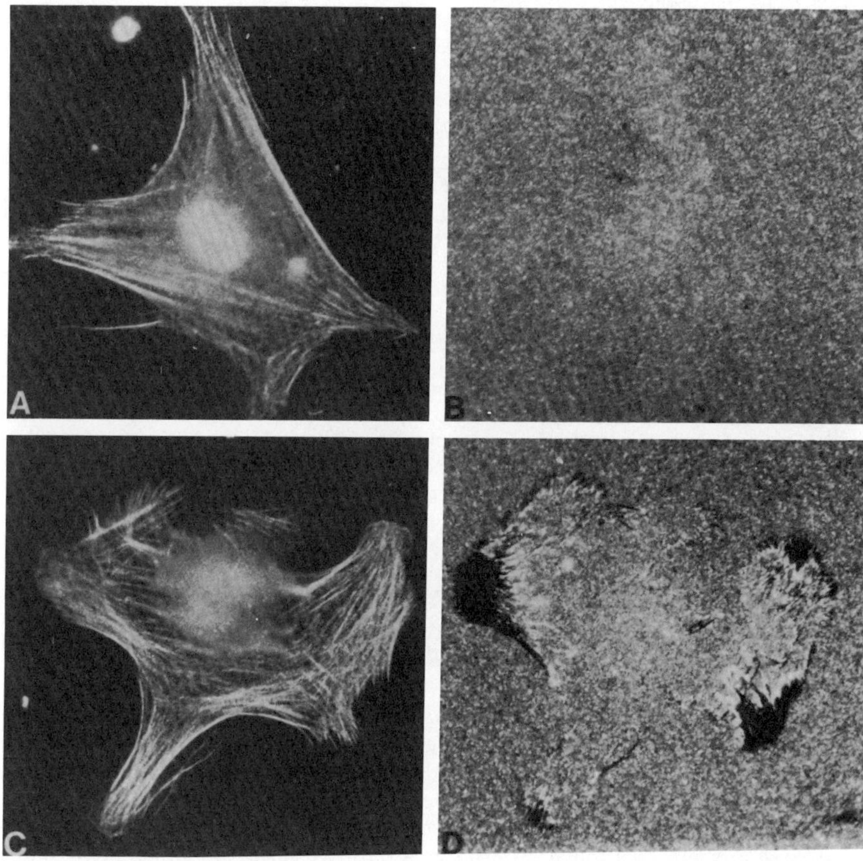

FIGURE 7. Removal of FN in serum-free medium. Human fibroblasts were incubated on fluorescein-conjugated FN-coated glass coverslips for 2 h at 37°C in (**A**,**B**) serum-free medium or in (**C**,**D**) serum-free medium containing 5 mg/ml BSA. At the end of the incubations the cells were fixed and permeabilized and stained with anti-actin IgG and rhodaminine-conjugated anti-IgG. Cells spread in serum-free medium and reorganized their actin cytoskeleton (**A**, rhodamine optics), but there was no removal of FN from the glass sufaces (**B**, fluorescein optics). In serum-free medium supplemented with BSA, cells spread (**C**), and FN was removed from the glass surfaces (**D**). (From Grinnell.[10])

FN (TABLE 3).[10] That is, when surfaces with adsorbed FN were incubated in buffer, FN desorption was greatest from glass and least from nonwettable polystyrene. Also, the presence of individual proteins or protein mixtures in the desorption buffer markedly increased the extent of desorption compared to protein-free buffer.

Cells in serum-containing medium also directly removed adsorbed FN from glass surfaces during adhesion[10] (and cf. ref. 33). The initial sites of removal were vinculin-staining focal adhesions (FIGURES 5A and 5B). These sites correspond to the tightest areas of cell adhesion, where the most stress would be applied by cells against the surfaces.[34,35] Eventually, large regions of FN were removed from the glass surfaces by the cells and organized into fibrillar structures on the cell surfaces (FIGURE 6). Significantly, removal of FN from surfaces did not occur in protein-free medium (FIGURES 7A and 7B), but was observed when the medium contained albumin (FIGURES 7C and 7D) or other proteins. The possible role of cells in reorganizing proteins previously adsorbed on surfaces is an important feature that has received little attention. Currently, we are studying the ability of cells to remove proteins other than FN from different surfaces.

CONCLUSIONS

The major findings of our studies can be summarized as follows:

1. FN adsorbs on different material surfaces in different molecular orientations that vary in biological activity. The orientation of FN adsorption depends not only on surface chemistry, but also on packing restraints imposed by the protein concentration.
2. On surfaces exposed to serum or plasma, FN exhibits a bimodal adsorption pattern. Maximum adsorption occurs on surfaces incubated with 0.1% serum or plasma, and lower FN adsorption occurs on surfaces incubated with higher serum or plasma concentrations. Such a bimodal adsorption pattern is consistent with the view that protein adsorption from complex protein mixtures occurs by a progressive adsorption-replacement mechanism.
3. FN desorption occurs more readily from wettable surfaces than from nonwettable surfaces. Desorption is promoted by the addition of other proteins to the incubation medium and by cellular shear forces generated at sites of cell adhesion.

Based on these findings, we favor the following hypothesis to explain the differences in cell adhesion dependent on surface chemistry that have been observed in studies using serum-containing medium. Surfaces exposed to medium containing 10% FBS are covered initially with nonadhesive proteins. Subsequently, cells replace the medium-derived nonadhesive proteins with cell-derived adhesion ligands. This replacement process occurs at a much faster rate on wettable surfaces than on nonwettable surfaces.

ACKNOWLEDGMENTS

I am indebted to Marian K. Feld and Trung V. Phan for their expert technical assistance in carrying out many of the studies described in this review.

REFERENCES

1. GRINNELL, F., M. MILAM & P. SRERE. 1972. Studies on cell adhesion. II. Adhesion of cells to surfaces of diverse chemical composition and inhibition of adhesion by sulfhydryl binding reagents. Arch. Biochem. Biophys. **153:** 193–198.

2. GRINNELL, F., M. MILAM & P. SRERE. 1973. Attachment of normal and transformed hamster kidney cells to substrata varying in chemical composition. Biochem. Med. **7:** 87–90.
3. KLEBE, R. 1974. Isolation of a collagen-dependent cell attachment factor. Nature **250:** 248–251.
4. PEARLSTEIN, E. 1976. Plasma membrane glycoprotein which mediates adhesion of fibroblasts to collagen. Nature **262:** 497–499.
5. GRINNELL, F., & D. HAYS. 1978. Cell adhesion and spreading factor: Similarity to cold insoluble globulin in human serum. Exp. Cell Res. **115:** 221–229.
6. GRINNELL, F. & M. FELD. 1981. Adsorption properties of fibronectin in relationship to biological activity. J. Biomed. Mater. Res. **15:** 363–381.
7. GRINNELL, F. & M. FELD. 1982. Fibronectin adsorption on hydrophilic and hydrophobic surfaces detected by antibody binding and analyzed during cell adhesion in serum-containing medium. J. Biol. Chem. **257:** 4888–4893.
8. GRINNELL, F. & T. V. PHAN. 1983. Deposition of fibronectin onto artificial material surfaces from human plasma and blood under clotting and non-clotting conditions. J. Cell. Phys. **116:** 289–296.
9. GRINNELL, F. & T. V. PHAN. 1985. Platelet attachment and spreading on polystyrene surfaces: Dependence on fibronectin and plasma concentration. Thromb. Res. **39:** 165–171.
10. GRINNELL, F. 1987. Focal adhesion sites and the removal of substratum-bound fibronectin. J. Cell Biol. In press.
11. GRINNELL, F. 1978. Cellular adhesiveness and extracellular substrata. Int. Rev. Cytol. **53:** 65–144.
12. SMITH, L. M. 1979. Cell adhesion as influenced by substrate surface properties. Ph.D. thesis, University of Utah, Salt Lake City, UT.
13. DILLMAN, W. J., JR. & J. F. MILLER. 1973. On the adsorption of serum proteins on polymer membrane surfaces. J. Colloid Interface Sci. **44:** 221–241.
14. JONSSON, U., B. IVARSSON, L. INGEMAR & L. BERGHEM. 1982. J. Colloid Interface Sci. **90:** 148–163.
15. STOKER, R. L. 1981. Adsorption of plasma fibronectin on quartz and glass substrates. M. S. thesis, University of Utah, Salt Lake City, UT.
16. IWAMOTO, G. K., L. C. WINTERTON, R. S. STOKER, R. A. VAN WAGENEN, J. D. ANDRADE & D. F. MOSHER. 1985. J. Colloid Interface Sci. **106:** 459–464.
17. KOCHWA, S., R. S. LITWAK, R. E. ROSENFIELD & E. F. LEONARD. 1977. Blood elements at foreign surfaces: A biochemical approach to the study of the adsorption of plasma proteins. Ann. N.Y. Acad. Sci. **283:** 37–49.
18. MORRISSEY, B. W. 1977. The adsorption and conformation of plasma proteins: A physical approach. Ann. N.Y. Acad. Sci. **283:** 50–64.
19. SODERQUIST, M. E. & A. G. WALTON. 1980. Structural changes in proteins adsorbed on polymer surfaces. J. Colloid Interface Sci. **75:** 386–397.
20. LUNDSTROM, I. 1985. Protein conformation at surfaces. *In* Oral Interactions. Reactions of Bone, Soft Tissue, and Saliva. P. O. Glantz, S. A. Leach & T. Ericson, Eds.: 9–23. IRL Press. Oxford.
21. GRINNELL, F. & J. MARSHALL. 1982. Coating bacteriological dishes with fibronectin permits spreading and growth of human diploid fibroblasts. Cell Biol. Int. Rep. **6:** 1012–1018.
22. HORBETT, T. A. 1984. Mass action effects on competitive adsorption of fibrinogen from hemoglobin solutions and from plasma. Thromb. Haemostas. **51:** 174–181.
23. BRASH, J. L. & P. TEN HOVE. 1984. Effect of plasma dilution on adsorption of fibrinogen to solid surfaces. Thromb. Haemostas. **51:** 326–330.
24. BREEMHAAR, W., E. BRINKMAN, D. J. ELLENS, T. BUEGELING & A. BANTJES. 1984. Preferential adsorption of high density lipoprotein from blood plasma onto material surfaces. Biomaterials **5:** 269–274.
25. VROMAN, L, A. L. ADAMS & G. C. FISHER, P. C. MUNOZ & M. STANFORD. 1982. Proteins, plasma, and blood in narrow spaces of clot-promoting surfaces. Adv. Chem. **199:** 265–276.

26. VROMAN, L. & A. L. ADAMS. 1969. Identification of rapid changes at plasma-solid interfaces. J. Biomed. Mater. Res. **3:** 43–67.
27. THOM, D., A. J. POWELL & D. A. REES. 1979. Mechanism of cellular adhesion. IV. Role of serum glycoproteins in fibroblast spreading on glass. J. Cell Sci. **35:** 281–305.
28. KNOX, P. & S. GRIFFITHS. 1980. The distribution of cell-spreading activities in sera: A quantitative approach. J. Cell Sci. **46:** 97–112.
29. KNOX, P. & S. GRIFFITHS. 1979. A cell spreading factor in human serum that is not cold insoluble globulin. Exp. Cell Res. **123:** 421–424.
30. BARNES, D. W., J. SILNUTZER, C. SEE & M. SHAFFER. 1983. Characterization of human serum spreading factor with monoclonal antibody. Proc. Natl. Acad. Sci. U.S.A. **80:** 1362–1366.
31. BRASH, J. L. 1977. Hydrophobic polymer surfaces and their interactions with blood. Ann. N.Y. Acad. Sci. **283:** 356–371.
32. BRASH, J. L., S. UNIYAL & Q. SAMAK. 1974. Exchange of albumin adsorbed on polymer surfaces. Trans. Am. Soc. Artif. Int. Organs **20:** 69–76.
33. AVNUR, A. & B. GEIGER. 1981. The removal of extracellular fibronectin from areas of cell-substrata contact. Cell **25:** 121–132.
34. MANGEAT, P. & K. BURRIDGE. 1984. Actin-membrane interaction in fibroblasts: What proteins are involved in this interaction? J. Cell Biol. **99:** 95s–103s.
35. BYERS, H. R., G. E. WHITE & K. FUJIWARA. 1984. Organization and function of stress fibers in cells in vitro and in situ: A review. Cell and Muscle Motility **5:** 83–137.

A Preliminary Comparison of the Thrombogenic Activity of Vitronectin and Other RGD-containing Proteins When Bound to Surfaces[a]

WILLIAM E. COLLINS,[b] DEANE F. MOSHER,[c,d]
BIANCA R. TOMASINI,[d] AND STUART L. COOPER[b]

[b]*Department of Chemical Engineering*
[c]*Department of Medicine*
[d]*Department of Physiological Chemistry*
University of Wisconsin
Madison, Wisconsin 53706

Recently several proteins that share no extensive homology with one another have been shown to interact with a set of homologous receptors on the surfaces of cells. The proteins, called "cell adhesion proteins," have two features in common: they each contain the sequence arginine-glycine-aspartic acid (RGD in the one-letter amino acid code) and the propensity to become deposited into the connective tissue matrix. The implication of this latter property is that the cell adhesion proteins are also structural proteins. Well-described examples of such proteins are found in blood plasma: fibronectin, vitronectin, von Willebrand factor, and fibrinogen. The cell surface receptors, called "integrins"[1] or "cytoadhesins,"[2] are heterodimers of α and β subunits. The α subunits are 130,000–170,000 daltons and are unique for each receptor, whereas β subunits are 90,000–110,000 daltons and apparently have the capacity to bind to several different α subunits; thus a given β subunit can be found in a variety of receptors.

The integrin-cell adhesion protein systems are thought to mediate the positioning and movement of cells. In support of this thesis, small tetra- or pentapeptides that contain the RGD sequence possess remarkable properties.[3] The peptides inhibit processes as diverse as gastrulation, neural crest migration, migration of prethymocytes into the embryonic thymus, platelet aggregation, cancer metastasis, and locomotion of slime mold. It is reasonable to conclude that the peptides work by binding to integrins and blocking the interaction of integrins with cognate cell adhesion proteins.

Over the past 7 years, we have used a canine *ex vivo* experimental model to characterize effects that various preadsorbed plasma proteins exert on thrombogenesis induced by candidate polymeric materials[4–6] and to assess the intrinsic acute thrombogenicity possessed by these materials.[7] Among the proteins that have been studied are fibronectin, von Willebrand factor, fibrinogen, and in recent preliminary investigations, vitronectin. In this paper the properties of vitronectin are briefly reviewed and the effects of vitronectin in the canine model described.

[a]This research was supported in part by the National Heart, Lung and Blood Institute of the National Institutes of Health through grant nos. HL-21001, HL-24046, and HL-29586.

CHARACTERISTICS OF VITRONECTIN

Several features of vitronectin structure-function have been determined. Vitronectin, like fibronectin, is a glycoprotein present at a concentration of 200–400 μg/ml in plasma[8] and in an insoluble form in tissues.[9] Vitronectin consists of 459 amino acid residues and, resembling plasma albumin and fibronectin, possesses at least one free sulfhydryl group and the propensity to multimerize.[10,11] Vitronectin has the same general structure as hemopexin and consists of 10 faintly homologous repeats.[12] The RGD sequence is found between the first and second of these repeats, and because small amounts of the first repeat circulate freely in plasma as somatomedin B, must be a physiologic cleavage site for some protease.[13] Vitronectin binds to and solubilizes the C5b-9 complex of complement, thus preventing cell lysis; in this guise the protein was isolated and characterized as "S-protein."[13-16] Vitronectin also binds strongly to the complex of thrombin and antithrombin III,[11,17-19] to heparin,[20] and to fibrillar collagen,[21] at least after it has been cycled through 8-M urea. An integrin found on osteosarcoma cells binds specifically to vitronectin and not to fibronectin.[22]

The principal source of plasma vitronectin is probably the liver.[23] The sources of tissue vitronectin are not known. There are many other questions that need to be answered about vitronectin before its physiologic and pathophysiologic roles in cell adhesion, the complement and blood coagulation systems, and connective tissue biology are understood. For anyone doing cell culture, however, vitronectin is an important protein. It binds extremely efficiently to glass[24] (hence the name of the protein) and polymer surfaces and competes with other plasma proteins for nonspecific binding sites on solid surfaces.[25] Accordingly vitronectin is the major adhesive protein when cells are cultured in medium containing greater than 5% serum.[26] Like other blood glycoproteins, such as prothrombin-thrombin[27] and fibrinogen,[28,29] the adsorption of vitronectin to solids affects its conformation and activity. For instance, one can diminish much of the cell-binding activity possessed by vitronectin using chromatography on an Ultrodex gel filtration column.[25]

RESULTS

Adsorption of Vitronectin to Polymers

We have determined the adsorption of vitronectin to five polymer surfaces (TABLE 1). These data represent the amount of ^{125}I-labeled vitronectin (purified as in ref. 10 and iodinated by the chloramine-T method) adsorbed to each selected polymer. Vitronectin adsorbed to the greatest extent on Teflon FEP, followed by, in order, polyethylene, silicone rubber, and Biomer, with the least affinity displayed toward oxidized polyethylene. Compared to adsorption data describing other globular blood proteins such as albumin[4,30-33] or fibronectin,[4,31,33-36] vitronectin adsorbs more avidly to polymers.

Diffusion and sedimentation characteristics of vitronectin were employed by calculating the dimensions of the prolate spheroid hydrodynamically equivalent to vitronectin. The hydrodynamic radius is 3.7 nm for vitronectin and its sedimentation coefficient is 4.6 S[11]; dimensions of 3.9 nm × 3.9 nm × 26.3 nm for the hydrodynamic analogue of vitronectin were calculated using these data.[37] By utilizing methods previously described, these dimensions were in turn used to obtain the value of absorbed vitronectin surface concentration corresponding to monolayer coverage of polymer surface. For randomly packed adsorbed vitronectin molecules, 0.09, 0.35, and

0.61 $\mu g/cm^2$ correspond to monolayers of vitronectin with its molecules in prevalently side-on, random, or end-on orientations, respectively. According to these data, the bulk concentration 0.01 mg/ml yielded surface concentrations squarely in the monolayer regime, and we chose this concentration for preadsorbing vitronectin for *ex vivo* characterization.

Effects of Adsorbed Vitronectin on Acute Thrombus Deposition and Embolization in a Canine ex Vivo *Model*

Ex vivo experiments (FIGURE 1) indicate that preadsorbed vitronectin stimulates thrombosis and related phenomena. TABLE 2 lists the peak platelet deposition obtained on five polymers that were either glycoprotein-preadsorbed or bare control.[4,6,38] Like vitronectin, human fibronectin, canine and human fibrinogen, and human fibronectin-antifibronectin complex were adsorbed for 120 minutes using bulk concentrations placing adsorption in the monolayer regime; native canine fibronectin was adsorbed for 30 minutes because our data (not shown) suggested that adsorbed fibronectin can show losses in its thrombotic activity at 120 minutes of adsorption. Five different vitronectin-preadsorbed materials were tested in a canine *ex vivo* model by using three replicates for each polymer type at each value of blood contact time t_c. Vitronectin was initially as thrombogenic as fibrinogen or fibronectin, and the data in TABLE 2 demonstrate that platelet deposition maxima obtained *ex vivo* on adsorbed vitronectin are comparable in magnitude to the maxima displayed by polymers pretreated with plasma proteins having established thrombogenicity. However, the maxima obtained on vitronectin-preadsorbed synthetics occur at much shorter blood contact times of 10 or 15 minutes compared to the 30 to 60 minute times of peak deposition for preadsorbed fibrinogen, fibronectin, or von Willebrand factor. Results for two more animals confirmed that maximum platelet and fibrinogen deposition occurred at t_c 10 or 15 minutes on vitronectin-preadsorbed polymers.

TABLE 1. Surface Concentrations of Human Vitronectin Adsorbed to Various Polymers

Material	Bulk Concentration of Vitronectin (mg/ml)	Γ and SD[a] ($\mu g/cm^2$)
Teflon FEP	0.0021	0.086 ± 0.0041
	0.0100	0.332 ± 0.030
silicone rubber	0.0021	0.077 ± 0.0052
	0.0100	0.263 ± 0.0097
polyethylene	0.0021	0.079 ± 0.0032
	0.0100	0.246 ± 0.058
Biomer	0.0021	0.072 ± 0.0038
	0.0100	0.228 ± 0.016
oxidized polyethylene	0.0021	0.056 ± 0.0031
	0.0100	0.248 ± 0.030

Adsorption was conducted at 22–24°C from vitronectin dissolved in PBS, pH 7.35, 0.02% NaN_3. Solutions of ^{125}I-labeled vitronectin were incubated with test polymers for 120 min and adsorbed radioactivity was quantified using an automated gamma counter.

[a]Standard deviation; $n = 3$.

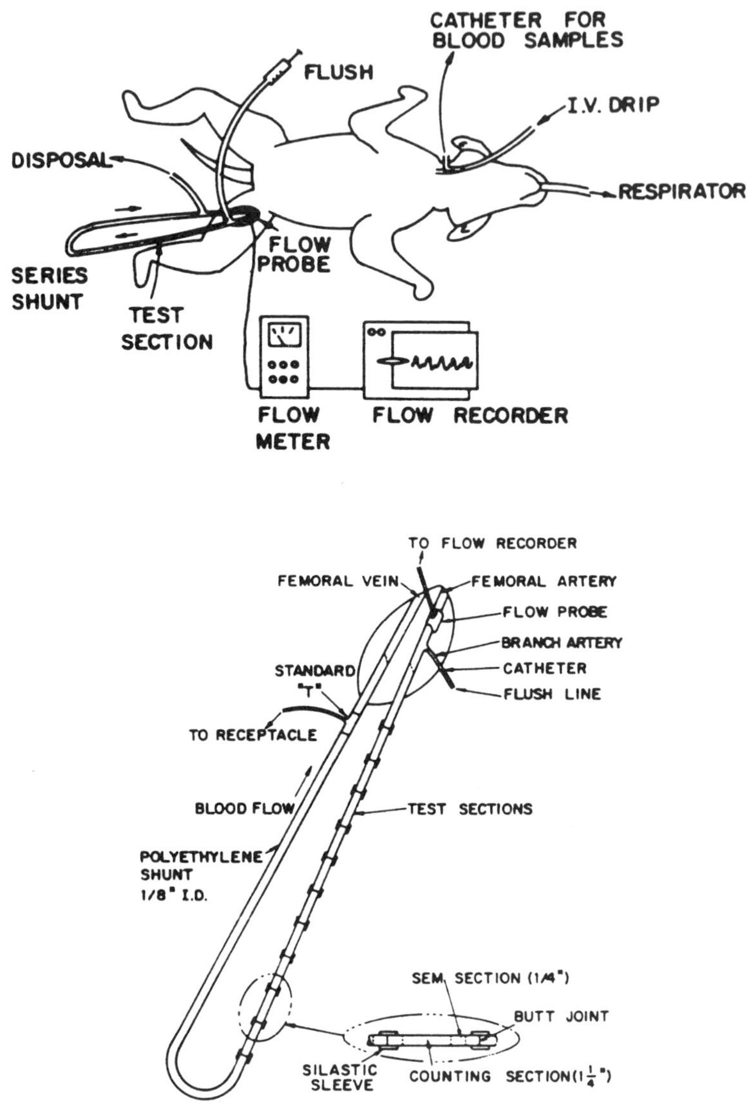

FIGURE 1. The canine *ex vivo* shunt experimental model measuring acute platelet and fibrinogen deposition on test polymers (see refs. 4 and 5 for further description of this experimental model).

Electron microscopy of preadsorbed samples at the time of peak platelet deposition revealed large mural thrombi and microscopy at later blood contact times revealed a carpet of minimally activated, dendritic platelets. These morphological trends were displayed on vitronectin-preadsorbed polyethylene (FIGURES 2A–C), Teflon FEP (FIGURES 3A and 3B), and silicone rubber (FIGURES 4A and 4B). To a less marked degree, the trends were also exhibited by oxidized polyethylene and biomer. Scanning electron microscopy at the time of maximal thrombus deposition revealed more fibrin (FIGURES 3A and 4A) than observed in previous studies.[4–6] The micrographs illustrate the substantial diversity in thrombus morphology evoked by different polymer types. For instance, at time of peak deposition, white blood cells were deposited on polyethylene, FEP, and silicone rubber, but were unequivocally spread on only polyethylene (FIGURE 2B) and silicone rubber (FIGURE 4B). At the deposition maxima, more deposited or entrapped erythrocytes were evinced by preadsorbed polyethylene than FEP (FIGURE 3A). Notably more fibrin deposited on silicone rubber (FIGURE 4A), greatly exceeding that deposited on the other polymers. These thrombi were lost, so that at 30 minutes a monolayer of isolated dendritic platelets prevailed with only occasional small thrombi (FIGURES 2C, 3B, and 4B).

DISCUSSION AND CONCLUSIONS

A number of the properties of vitronectin make this plasma protein a prime candidate to mediate the interaction of the formed elements of blood with artificial surfaces: its high concentration in plasma; its avidity for solid surfaces; its small size and high diffusivity; the presence of specific receptors on platelets and other cells; and the possibility of structural transformations upon binding to surfaces, to thrombin-antithrombin complexes, or to C5b-9 complexes and upon proteolytic cleavage. Our preliminary examination of vitronectin adsorption to polymers and activity when adsorbed lends support to this hypothesis. For example, vitronectin surface concentra-

TABLE 2. Effects of Polymer Surface Composition

		Maximum Platelet Deposition	
Material	Precoated Protein	Time (min)	Density (no. per 1000 μm^2)
SR	control	15	90 ± 40
	canine fibrinogen	45	600
	canine fibronectin	45	730 ± 610
	human fibronectin	30	1800 ± 900
	human FN-antifibronectin	30	900 ± 70
	human vitronectin	10	2020 ± 530
LDPE	control	15	370 ± 50
	canine fibrinogen	120	2000
	canine fibronectin	45	560 ± 330
	human vitronectin	10	2440 ± 170
Biomer	control	15	200 ± 2
	canine fibronectin	30	2080 ± 740
	human vitronectin	10	2200 ± 190
OXPE	control	20	3900 ± 400
	canine fibronectin	60	1230 ± 710
	human vitronectin	15	1380 ± 1020
FEP	human vitronectin	15	650 ± 120

Maximum platelet deposition on five protein-preadsorbed polymers appraised *ex vivo* using an acute canine experimental model. Proteins, except for canine fibronectin (30 min), were at room temperature preadsorbed to the polymer from Tyrode's solution for 120 min of incubation. The protein-preadsorbed polymer tubings were subsequently contacted with blood for a series of times ranging from 1 to 60 min (30 min maximum for vitronectin), and the adherent radioactivity from ^{51}Cr-labeled platelets was determined.

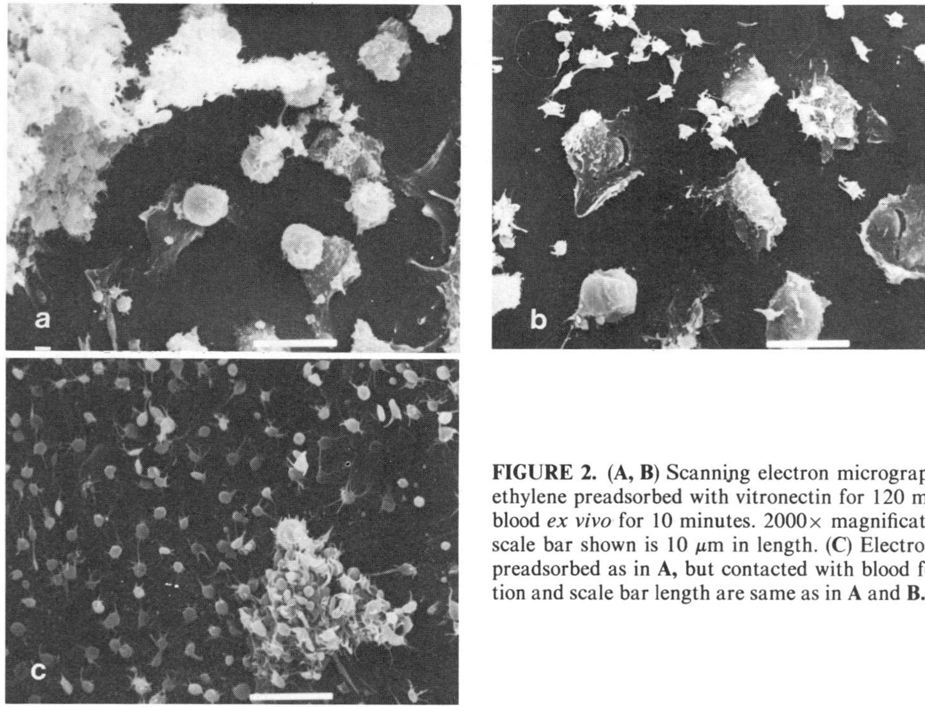

FIGURE 2. (**A, B**) Scanning electron micrographs of thrombosis on polyethylene preadsorbed with vitronectin for 120 minutes and contacted with blood *ex vivo* for 10 minutes. 2000× magnification was employed and the scale bar shown is 10 μm in length. (**C**) Electron micrograph of a sample preadsorbed as in **A,** but contacted with blood for 30 minutes. Magnification and scale bar length are same as in **A** and **B.**

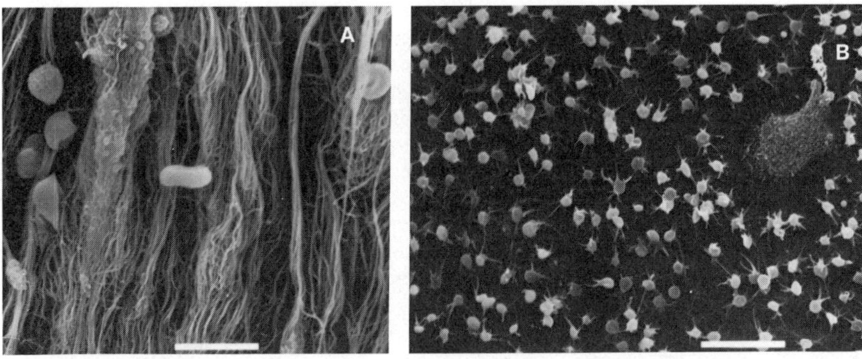

FIGURE 3. (**A**) Scanning electron micrographs of thrombosis on Teflon FEP preadsorbed with vitronectin. The conditions were the same as in FIGURE 2. The surface was contacted with blood for 15 minutes. (**B**) Micrograph of vitronectin-preadsorbed FEP for contact time 30 min. In both **A** and **B,** the magnification was 2000× and scale bar shown is 10 μm in length.

tions on five polymer adsorbents with widely dissimilar surface characteristics were quite high considering the low bulk concentrations employed in our experiments. Tested *ex vivo,* vitronectin-preadsorbed materials induced considerable peak platelet deposition, comparable to deposition obtained on glycoprotein adsorbates possessing established thrombogenicity.[4,5,38]

Some aspects of the platelet deposition on vitronectin-preadsorbed polymers appeared to be material-dependent and others did not. The magnitude of deposition maxima on vitronectin-preadsorbed surfaces depended on polymer type; the lowest maximum, 650 platelets/1000 μm^2, was observed on the fluorocarbon Teflon FEP, with oxidized polyethylene next and the remaining materials highest at 2020 to 2440 per 1000 μm^2. An instance of a response that seemed vitronectin-dependent was the rapid deposition and loss of large numbers of platelets; on each material investigated, the peak in the number of adherent platelets occurred at relatively short times of 10 to

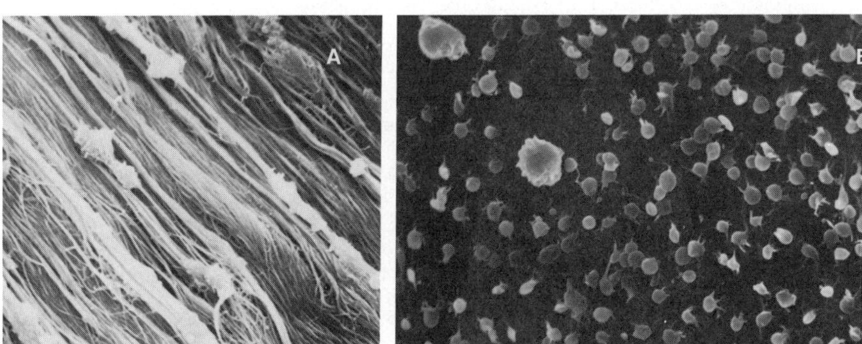

FIGURE 4. (**A**) Scanning electron micrograph of silicone rubber preadsorbed using vitronectin and blood contacted for 10 minutes. (**B**) Micrograph of vitronectin-preadsorbed silicone rubber contacted with blood for 30 minutes. Magnification was 2000× and scale bar shown is 10 μm in length.

15 minutes. The propensity for substantially attenuated deposition at the longer blood contact time of 30 minutes also "depended" upon the presence of adsorbed vitronectin. At this time point, each material displayed markedly decreased deposition, perhaps through embolization. Though other thrombogenic glycoproteins that were adsorbed to polymers invoke maximum platelet and fibrin deposition at longer contact times (typically 30 minutes), it is too early to interpret the significance of the disparate temporal behavior *ex vivo* of these glycoproteins and vitronectin. It is believed that polymer properties affect the thrombogenicity of glycoproteins such as fibrinogen[4,6] and fibronectin[4,38]; scanning electron micrographs of thrombi formed on vitronectin adsorbed to different polymers also indicate that surface properties affect thrombus morphology and perhaps also influence the thrombotic activity of advitronectin.

REFERENCES

1. HYNES, R. O. 1987. Integrins: A family of cell surface receptors. Cell **48:** 549–554.
2. PLOW, E. F., J. C. LOFTUS, E. G. LEVIN, D. S. FAIR, D. DIXON, J. FORSYTH & M. H. GINSBERG. 1986. Immunologic relationship between platelet membrane glycoprotein GP IIb/IIIa and cell surface molecules expressed by a variety of cells. Proc. Natl. Acad. Sci. U.S.A. **83:** 6002–6006.
3. RUOSLAHTI, E. & M. D. PIERSCHBACHER. 1986. Arg-Gly-Asp: A versatile cell recognition signal. Cell **44:** 517–518.
4. YOUNG, B. R., L. K. LAMBRECHT, S. L. COOPER & D. F. MOSHER. 1982. Plasma proteins: Their role in initiating platelet and fibrin deposition on biomaterials. Adv. Chem. Ser. **199:** 317–350.
5. LAMBRECHT, L. K., B. R. YOUNG, R. E. STAFFORD, K. PARK, R. M. ALBRECHT, D. F. MOSHER & S. L. COOPER. 1985. The influence of preadsorbed canine von Willebrand factor, fibronectin and fibrinogen on *ex vivo* artificial-surface-induced thrombosis. Thromb. Res. **41:** 99–117.
6. PARK, K., D. F. MOSHER & S. L. COOPER. 1986. Acute surface-induced thrombosis in the canine *ex vivo* model: Importance of protein composition of the initial monolayer and platelet activation. J. Biomed. Mater. Res. **20:** 589–612.
7. LELAH, M. D., L. K. LAMBRECHT & S. L. COOPER. 1984. A canine *ex vivo* series shunt for evaluating thrombus deposition on polymer surfaces. J. Biomed. Mater. Res. **18(5):** 475–496.
8. SHAFFER, M. C., T. P. FOLEY & D. W. BARNES. 1984. Quantitation of spreading factor in human biologic fluids. J. Lab. Clin. Med. **103:** 783–791.
9. HAYMAN, E. G., M. D. PIERSCHBACHER, Y. ÖHGREN & E. RUOSLAHTI. 1983. Serum spreading factor (vitronectin) is present at the cell surface and in tissues. Proc. Natl. Acad. Sci. U.S.A. **80:** 4003–4009.
10. DAHLBÄCK, B. & E. R. PODACK. 1985. Characterization of human S-protein, an inhibitor of the membrane attack complex of complement. Demonstration of a free reactive thiol group. Biochemistry **24:** 2368–2374.
11. PREISSNER, K. T., R. WASSMUTH & G. MÜLLER-BERGHAUS. 1985. Physiochemical characterization of human S-protein and its function in blood coagulation system. Biochem. J. **231:** 349–355.
12. STANLEY, K. K. 1986. Homology with hemopexin suggests a possible scavenging function for S-protein/vitronectin. FEBS Lett. **199:** 249–253.
13. JENNE, D. & K. K. STANLEY. 1985. Molecular cloning of S-protein, a link between complement, coagulation and cell-substrate adhesion. EMBO J. **4:** 3153–3157.
14. PODACK, E. R. & H. J. MÜLLER-EBERHARD. 1979. Isolation of human S-protein, an inhibitor of the membrane attack complex of complement. J. Biol. Chem. **254:** 9907–9914.
15. PREISSNER, L. T., N. HEIMBURGER, E. ANDERS & G. MÜLLER-BERGHAUS. 1986. Physiochemical, immunochemical and functional comparison of human S-protein and vitronectin. Biochem. Biophys. Res. Comm. **134:** 951–956.

16. TOMASINI, B. R. & D. F. MOSHER. 1986. On the identity of vitronectin and S-protein: Immunological crossreactivity and functional studies. Blood **68:** 737–742.
17. JENNE, D., H. FERDINAND & S. BHAKDI. 1985. Interaction of complement S-protein with thrombin-antithrombin complexes: A role for the S-protein in hemostasis. Thromb. Res. **38:** 401–412.
18. PODACK, E. R., B. DAHLBÄCH & J. H. GRIFFIN. 1986. Interaction of S-protein of complement with thrombin and antithrombin III during coagulation. J. Biol. Chem. **261:** 7387–7392.
19. ILL, C. R. & E. RUOSLAHTI. 1985. Association of thrombin-antithrombin III complex with vitronectin in serum. J. Biol. Chem. **260:** 15610–15615.
20. BARNES, D. W., J. E. REINZ & B. AMOS. 1985. Heparin-binding properties of human serum spreading factor. J. Biol. Chem. **260:** 9117–9122.
21. GEBB, C., E. G. HAYMAN, E. ENGVALL & E. RUOSLAHTI. 1986. Interaction of vitronectin with collagen. J. Biol. Chem. **261:** 16698–16703.
22. PYTELA, R., M. PIERSCHBACHER & E. RUOSLAHTI. 1985. A 125/115 kDa cell surface receptor specific for vitronectin interacts with the arginine-glycine-aspartic acid adhesion sequence derived from fibronectin. Proc. Natl. Acad. Sci. U.S.A. **82:** 5766–5770.
23. BARNES, D. W. & J. REING. 1985. Human spreading factor: Synthesis and response by HepG2 hepatoma cells in culture. J Cell Physiol. **125:** 207–214.
24. BARNES, D. W., L. MOUSETIS, B. AMOS & J. SILNUTZER. 1984. Glass-bead affinity chromatography of cell attachment factors of human serum. Anal. Biochem. **137:** 196–204.
25. KNOX, P. J. 1984. Kinetics of cell spreading in the presence of different concentrations of serum or fibronectin-depleted serum. J. Cell Sci. **71:** 51–59.
26. HAYMAN, E. G., M. D. PIERSCHBACHER, S. SUZUKI & E. RUOSLAHTI. 1985. Vitronectin, a major cell attachment-promoting protein in fetal bovine serum. Exp. Cell Res. **160:** 245–258.
27. CHUANG, H. Y. & S. P. MITRA. 1984. Adsorption and reactivity of human prothrombin to artificial surfaces. J. Biomed. Mater. Res. **18:** 695–705.
28. CHAN, B. M. C. & J. L. BRASH. 1981. Conformational change in fibrinogen desorbed from glass. J. Colloid Interface Sci. **84:** 263–265.
29. CHUANG, H. Y. K. 1984. *In situ* immunoradiometric assay of fibrinogen adsorbed to artificial surfaces. J. Biomed. Mater. Res. **18:** 547–559.
30. BRASH, J. L. & Q. M. SAMAK. 1978. Dynamics of interactions between human albumin and polyethylene surface. J. Colloid Interface Sci. **65:** 495–504.
31. KOLTISKO, R. & A. WALTON. 1985. Chromatographic analysis of protein adsorption. *In* Surface and Interfacial Aspects of Biomedical Polymers, Vol. 2. J. D. Andrade, Ed.: 217–239. Plenum. New York.
32. SHIRAHAMA, H. & T. SUZAWA. 1985. Adsorption of BSA onto styrene/2-hydroxyethyl methacrylate copolymer latex. J. Colloid Interface Sci. **104:** 416–421.
33. WINTERTON, L. C., J. D. ANDRADE, J. FEIJEN & S. W. KIM. 1986. Heparin interaction with protein adsorbed surfaces. J. Colloid Interface Sci. **111:** 314–342.
34. GRINNELL, F. & H. K. FELD. 1981. The adsorption characteristics of plasma fibronectin in relationship to biological activity. J. Biomed. Mater. Res. **15:** 363–381.
35. JÖNSSON, U., B. VARSSON, I. LUNDSTRÖM & L. BERGHEM. 1982. Adsorption behavior of fibronectin on well-characterized silica surfaces. J. Colloid Interface Sci. **90:** 148–163.
36. IWAMOTO, G. K., L. C. WINTERTON, R. S. STOKER, R. A. VAN WAGEREN, J. D. ANDRADE & D. F. MOSHER. 1985. Fibronectin adsorption detected by interfacial fluorescence. J. Colloid Interface Sci. **106:** 459–464.
37. VAN HOLDE, K. 1971. Physical Biochemistry. 2d edit. Prentice-Hall. Englewood Cliffs, NJ. pp. 141–157.
38. COLLINS, W. E., D. F. MOSHER, A. R. DIWAN, K. D. MURTHY, S. R. SIMMONS, R. M. ALBRECHT & S. L. COOPER. 1987. *Ex vivo* platelet deposition on fibronectin-preadsorbed surfaces. Scanning Microsc. In press.

Methods of Investigating Protein Interactions on Artificial and Natural Surfaces

LEO VROMAN

Interface Laboratory
Veterans Administration Medical Center
Brooklyn, New York 11209

INTRODUCTION

The following line of reasoning has led biomaterial sciences to the study of protein adsorption: (1) Normal endothelium does not cause thrombosis. (2) Tubes of most materials do cause thrombosis. (3) This thrombus formation is preceded by deposition of plasma proteins on the tube surface. (4) Endothelium therefore either does not adsorb proteins out of plasma or does so in such a way that no thrombosis results. (5) We must find materials whose surfaces handle plasma the way endothelium does. (6) The question of primary importance is, therefore: How does the endothelium handle plasma? (7) To answer this question, we should separate blood from blood vessel wall, and then reunite them in a controlled way (*e.g.*, after adding purified labeled protein to the plasma).

This narrow path of logic leads to several inspiring pitfalls. The first three points assume that thrombus formation can be traced back to initial protein adsorption in a linear way, while in reality each event along that way can have multiple consequences. Points 4 to 7 assume that the relationship between endothelium and blood can be traced back to a point in the developing organism when this differentiation did not yet exist, and that this point can be recreated by interrupting the present context. I doubt that we can "rerun" the first meeting between blood and vessel this way. Our plasma proteins as well as our blood cells evolved together with the endothelial and other surfaces that formed and maintain them. Each protein species developed its own properties allowing it (1) to survive, (2) to function in a singular way at a singular place and time within its submolecularly structured yet mobile world, and (3) to die for the survival of that world.

The mere size of our efforts to dissect a live system is enough to yield measurable and therefore unnatural data. When some blood is captured and taken from its live environment into an artificial container (or when this live environment is invaded by an artificial device), an event is begun of a magnitude for which the blood has not prepared itself. The syringe, test tube, or device offers such a large virginal field to the blood that it will cover itself with a carpet of uniform and synchronized molecular events—a carpet so large that we can observe and time its formation or notice its effect on its host.

The separation of blood components such as proteins also requires manipulations on a relatively gigantic scale. Consequently, a sample of purified protein is as informative as the display of an object dug up by an archaeologist: it will not easily betray its original use and will completely hide its individual history.

With the advent of successful endothelial cell culture came the possibility of creating a "bloodless blood vessel wall." We can now observe how this surface handles plasma proteins, but in trying to fit these observations into the normal blood-vessel relationship we will be led again into a trap. The fact that a certain protein will be adsorbed by cultured cells will suggest that *in vivo* the blood vessel wall will also adsorb this protein, or must have adsorbed it, but the question as to when this occurs remains. Did it take place while its cells were being formed? The event may be traced with purified protein injected into recipients congenitally deficient in this protein, but then the patient's endothelium, having been deprived of whatever information the protein lacking would have carried, cannot be considered normal.

It appears that the more complex substrates will yield more complex and indirect answers. At the same time, with increased complexity and increased resemblance to living surfaces, these indirect answers, such as evidence of the physiological activity rather than the quantity of specific adsorbed proteins, may become more biologically rather than physically meaningful.

ARTIFICIAL SURFACES

Immobile Substrates

On unnaturally large and immobile surfaces, blood will generate measurably large images of an otherwise natural event. Such images can be regarded as a mean or mode of protein adsorption on a uniform surface. However, in reviewing the various methods of observation, we must remember that the time schedule of adsorption and interactions among proteins in whole plasma is affected by physical material surface properties (*e.g.*, roughness with a mode of gap size, local critical surface tension, or flow) as well as by chemical ones. This time schedule will intersect with that of platelet and white cell arrivals and departures.

Methods of measuring protein adsorption on artificial surfaces rely in part on those used for studying the surface itself,[1] while others are being developed more specifically to study protein adsorption; these have been reviewed and tabulated thoroughly.[2] Fourier transform infrared spectroscopy using attenuated total reflection (FT-IR/ATR),[3] and improved ellipsometry[4] combined with X-ray photoelectron spectroscopy[5] are now allowing measurement during adsorption under various flow conditions. These methods provide data and permit some conclusions about sites of protein attachment, thickness, density, and perhaps orientation of the adsorbates. All require very flat surfaces to yield observably large numbers of very small but numerous and simultaneous submolecular or molecular events.

In extreme contrast to the perfectly flat surface, a suspension of particles made of the identical material has lost its uniformity but has gained a large total surface area[6]; this allows measurement of supernatant depletion and of radiolabeled protein adsorption and release. Direct observation using partial gold decoration with electron microscopy indicates that protein distribution even on rather uniform surfaces is not uniform[7] or at least does not remain uniform when exposed to the hardships of preparation for observation, especially on rough surfaces where narrow gaps generate complex interactions during and after protein adsorption.[8]

Our own observations have relied for a long time on detection of adsorbed proteins by matching antibodies, with or without the use of ellipsometry. We found that on clot-promoting surfaces, plasma deposits fibrinogen and then removes it,[9] mostly by replacing it with high molecular weight kininogen (HMWK).[10] Similar results were obtained by measuring adsorption and release of ^{125}I-labeled fibrinogen in plasma flowing through narrow glass tubing.[11] The graded narrow spaces between a flat surface and a convex lens resting belly-down on it cause undiluted plasma to leave fibrinogen in spaces of 10 to 20 μm, and HMWK in wider spaces[12]; a set of concentric rings of various proteins is left by diluted plasma.[13]

Intriguing as these phenomena are, they are only meaningful to a biologist if the adsorbed proteins can be shown to have some biological activity. Since specific proteins at interfaces are already known to have specific effects (or "functions"), we can use these as a more physiological expression of surface protein concentration. We can then combine this value with the degree of antigenicity shown by the adsorbate in contact with various monoclonal antibodies as a measure of orientation, and with more physical data (film thickness and density using ellipsometry; FTR; intrinsic fluorescence at the interface; electron microscopy). Much information is gained where these data are not parallel. For example, steric limitations will distort immunological quantification when with increasingly dense packing, space among adsorbed fibronectin molecules becomes smaller than the size of an antibody molecule. On the other hand, increased packing of fibronectin on a hydrophilic substrate enhances its antigenicity, probably by forcing orientation that favors exposure of the antigenic site.[14] One biological activity of fibrinogen on a surface, namely its ability to cause deposition of platelets, is paralleled by its immunological rather than by its radiolabel quantification, indicating that, rather than overall density, specific interindividual distances of the adsorbed fibrinogen are most biologically significant.[15]

Mobile Substrates

Spacing and interaction among adsorbed protein molecules can be observed on a mobile substrate such as the air-liquid interface. Langmuir noted half a century ago that these interactions vary in effect among various protein species.[16] Modifications of his surface film balance[17] allow sensitive measurement of film pressure and viscosity, and of their modification when the film is penetrated by other molecules.[18] Compressed and decompressed films can be transferred to solid substrates for study by all of the techniques used for proteins adsorbed out of bulk described above.

Mobility of the substrate as well as its chemical composition and topology must be considered if we want to approach physiological (*e.g.*, cell surface) conditions. For example, ellipsometry of proteins onto phospholipid layers that in turn are kept immobilized on a reflecting substate[4] is only a first step toward studying the same proteins interacting with phospholipid micelles or near-liquid cell membranes.

A phospholipid bilayer formed at a liquid-liquid interface would provide a more sophisticated model. A protein could be introduced into the aqueous phase, to be followed by some form of physical quantification of adsorption as well as of immunological and functional (*e.g.*, clot and cell adhesion promoting) evaluation. Even then, the closer we come to the endothelial surface we try to imitate, the more obvious it will be that our artificial systems are true models only of diseases that have not yet been invented.

THE NATURAL SURFACE

In addition to the rather philosophical problems we face when trying to study adsorption of proteins on endothelium, there are some practical and obvious ones: it will be difficult to distinguish between effects caused by proteins formed and transmitted by the endothelium and those caused by proteins added experimentally.

Nevertheless, endothelial cell surfaces and cultures can now be induced to change and thereby show how they handle proteins[19] or how a protein handles them.[20] Chances

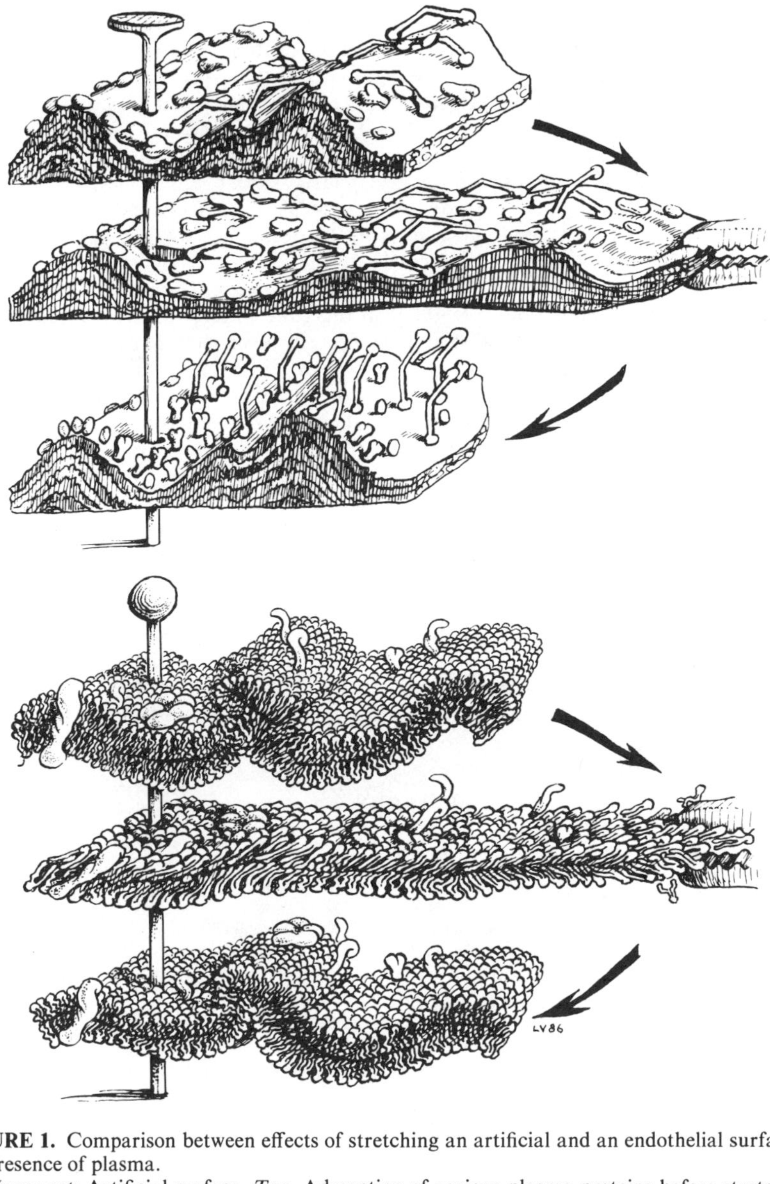

FIGURE 1. Comparison between effects of stretching an artificial and an endothelial surface in the presence of plasma.

Upper set: Artificial surface. *Top,* Adsorption of various plasma proteins before stretching. *Middle,* Further adsorption on new substrate sites exposed by stretching. *Lower,* Reorientation of adsorbed molecules upon return to original substrate shape.

Lower set: Endothelial surface. *Top,* Little adsorption of plasma proteins on the protein-studded phospholipid bilayer. *Middle,* Rearrangement of the membrane proteins in the bilayer as it adjusts to being stretched. *Lower,* Upon relaxation, the overall shape of the endothelium is regained, but on the molecular scale the plasma-endothelial interface has become rearranged.

are increasing that we will discover invisible structures in the endothelium by their interactions with added purified proteins, and that we will begin to understand pathological conditions by creating them in the laboratory accidentally. Even then it will be difficult to trace the protein's fate and to determine whether it ever was "truly" physically adsorbed, or rather physically embraced and emulsified or actively and very specifically held and transported.

While all of these interactions would involve substrate mobility on a molecular scale, others may be provoked by the relatively large-scale changes induced by flexing or stretching and relaxing of the substrate. I have tried to envision and compare events occurring on an artificial and on a natural (endothelial) surface that are being stretched and then being allowed to recover, all in presence of blood plasma (FIGURE 1). Upon contact with the artificial surfaces (upper drawing of upper set) proteins are adsorbed and replace each other. Stretched at this time (middle drawing of upper set), the substrate will have new sites available for protein adsorption. When the material is now allowed to recover (third drawing of upper set), adsorbed protein molecules will lose part of their multiple footholds and may stand up. As a result, even in a single cycle of stretching, the material itself may regain its original configuration but its protein adsorbate will not. Further cycles should produce further complications.

In contrast, the endothelial structure is so mobile that it will adapt to charge and apolar residue configuration of any approaching plasma protein molecule and no firm "irreversible" adsorption of that molecule will result (see lower set of drawings, FIGURE 1). Little may change in surface properties by stretching to a limited degree, but when allowed to regain its overall structure, the endothelium surface—being mobile and nearly liquid—will not regain exactly the molecular configuration it had. Further cycles should not lead to further complications.

Thus, the apparent simplicity of the interaction of plasma and endothelial surface is maintained by the complexity of the substrate. The complexity of the interaction of plasma and polymer surface is caused by the simplicity of the substrate.

REFERENCES

1. RATNER, B. D. 1982. Adv. Chem. Ser. **199:** 9–23.
2. ANDRADE, J. D., Ed. 1985. Surface and Interfacial Aspects of Biomedical Polymers, Vols. 1 and 2. Plenum. New York.
3. CHITTUR, K. K., D. J. FINK, R. I. LEININGER & T. B. HUTSON. 1986. Fourier transform infrared spectroscopy/attenuated total reflection studies of protein adsorption in flowing systems: Approaches for bulk correction and compositional analysis of adsorbed and bulk proteins in mixtures. J. Colloid Interface Sci. **111:** 419–433.
4. CORSEL, J. W., G. M. WILLEMS, J. M. M. KOP, P. A. CUYPERS & W. TH. HERMENS. 1986. The role of intrinsic binding rate and transport rate in the adsorption of prothrombin, albumin, and fibrinogen in phospholipid bilayers. J. Colloid Interface Sci. **111:** 544–554.
5. SUNDGREN, J.-E., P. BODO, B. IVARSSON & I. LUNDSTROM. 1986. Adsorption of fibrinogen on titanium and gold surfaces studied by ESCA and ellipsometry. J. Colloid Interface Sci. **113:** 530–543.
6. BRASH, J. L. & J. A. THIBODEAU. 1986. Identification of proteins adsorbed from human plasma to glass bead columns: Plasmin-induced degradation of adsorbed fibrinogen. J. Biomed. Mater. Res. **20:** 1263–1275.
7. EBERHART, R. C., M. E. LYNCH, F. H. BILGE, J. F. WISSINGER, M. S. MUNRO, S. R. ELLSWORTH & A. J. QUATRONE. 1982. Protein adsorption on polymers. Visualization, study of fluid shear and roughness effects, and methods to enhance albumin binding. Adv. Chem. Ser. **199:** 293–315.
8. KLEIN, J. 1986. Surface interactions with adsorbed macromolecules. J. Colloid Interface Sci. **111:** 305–313.

9. VROMAN, L. & A. L. ADAMS. 1969. Identification of rapid changes at plasma-solid interfaces. J. Biomed. Mater. Res. **3:** 43–67.
10. VROMAN, L. & A. L. ADAMS. 1980. Interaction of high molecular weight kininogen, factor XII, and fibrinogen in plasma at interfaces. Blood **55:** 156–159.
11. WOJCIECHOWSKI, P., P. TEN HOVE & J. L. BRASH. 1986. Phenomenology and mechanism of the transient adsorption of fibrinogen from plasma (Vroman effect). J. Colloid Interface Sci. **111:** 455–465.
12. ADAMS, A. L., G. C. FISCHER, P. C. MUNOZ & L. VROMAN. 1984. Convex-lens-on-slide: a simple system for the study of human plasma and blood in narrow spaces. J. Biomed. Mater. Res. **18:** 643–654.
13. VROMAN, L. & A. L. ADAMS. 1986. Adsorption of proteins out of plasma and solutions in narrow spaces. J. Colloid Interface Sci. **111:** 391–402.
14. GRINNELL, F. & M. FELD. 1982. Fibronectin adsorption on hydrophilic and hydrophobic surfaces detected by antibody binding and analyzed during cell adhesion in serum-containing medium. J. Biol. Chem. **257:** 4888–4893.
15. SALZMAN, E. W., J. LINDON, G. MCMANAMA & J. A. WARE. 1987. Role of fibrinogen in activation of platelets by artificial surfaces. This volume.
16. LANGMUIR, I. 1938. Protein monolayers. Cold Spring Harbor Symp. **6:** 171–189.
17. VROMAN, L., S. KANOR & A. L. ADAMS. 1968. Surface film pressure recording system. Rev. Sci. Instrum. **39:** 278–279.
18. VROMAN, L. & A. L. ADAMS. 1969. Effect of heparin on reactions at aminated polymer-blood interfaces. J. Colloid Interface Sci. **31:** 188–195.
19. FRIEDMAN, M., U. S. RYAN, W. C. DAVENPORT, E. L. CHANEY, D. L. STRICKLAND & L. KWOCK. 1986. Reversible alterations in cultured pulmonary artery endothelial cell monolayer morphology and albumin permeability induced by ionizing radiation. J. Cell. Physiol. **129:** 237–249.
20. MALIK, A. B. 1986. Thrombin-induced endothelial injury. Sem. Thromb. Hemostas. **12:** 184–196.

Complement Activation in Extracorporeal Circuits

DENNIS E. CHENOWETH

Travenol Laboratories, Round Lake, Illinois 60073

INTRODUCTION

Complement activation reactions normally make an important contribution to host defense mechanisms by promoting localized generation of acute inflammatory mediators. However, it is now apparent that blood contact with many types of biomaterials initiates complement activation and, in the case of extracorporeal medical devices, fosters systemic production of bioactive molecules that can provoke specific types of clinical sequelae. Consequently, biomaterial scientists have begun to emphasize delineation of the complement-activating potential of blood-contacting materials employed in the manufacture of medical devices. For example, our previous investigations have centered on both laboratory and clinical evaluation of hemodialyzers and cardiopulmonary bypass oxygenators.[1] In particular, studies aimed at characterizing the complement-activating potential of hemodialyzers have been extremely useful for defining the membrane or material characteristics that regulate clinical exposure to the human anaphylatoxins as well as for delineating the pathophysiologic responses that result from systemic complement activation.[2-4] Before discussing and interpreting these specific findings, it will be helpful to summarize briefly our current understanding of the mechanisms of complement activation and the biological properties of the human anaphylatoxins.

COMPLEMENT ACTIVATION

Alternative Pathway Mechanisms

It is generally accepted that the complement activation observed during hemodialysis proceeds by alternative pathway mechanisms. The proteins and biochemical events that compose the alternative pathway have previously been described in detail[5] and may be briefly summarized as follows.

Activation of the alternative pathway involves four distinct phases: initiation, deposition of C3b, recognition, and amplification. The first phase, initiation, begins in plasma and involves spontaneous formation of a short-lived intermediate termed metastable C3b. The active site of this reactive species consists of an activated thiolester that can undergo nucleophilic attack (FIGURE 1). Consequently, this reactive form of C3 can deposit on and become covalently attached to biomaterials or other surfaces that possess nucleophilic characteristics. The second step, recognition, involves discrimination between materials that serve as activators or nonactivators. This process of discrimination occurs very soon after C3b becomes attached to the surface and essentially results from regulation of the binding of the inhibitory protein factor H to the surface-bound C3b. For example, materials that behave as activators of the alternative pathway tend to limit binding of factor H to C3b and favor assembly of the positive regulatory components, factors B, D, and P. When this occurs, C3b in the presence of factors B and D and Mg^{2+} forms a C3 convertase capable of generating many molecules of C3b that are identical to the original C3b that was initially deposited on the surface. In this way, amplification of the signal through a positive-feedback mechanism takes place and rapid assembly of the C3 and C5 convertase enzymes is achieved. By contrast, some materials behave as nonactivators of the alternative pathway. In these cases, factor H binding to surface-bound C3b is greatly enhanced when compared to that of factor B. Thus, nonactivating surfaces are characterized by the fact that they promote catabolic inactivation of C3b and termination of the amplification feedback mechanism.

The biochemical characteristics that impart either activating or nonactivating properties to a material have not been completely described. However, current evidence supports the hypothesis that surface nucleophiles contribute importantly to the activating potential of a foreign material (FIG. 1). By constrast, negatively charged surface constituents facilitate factor H binding to C3b, thus causing a material to

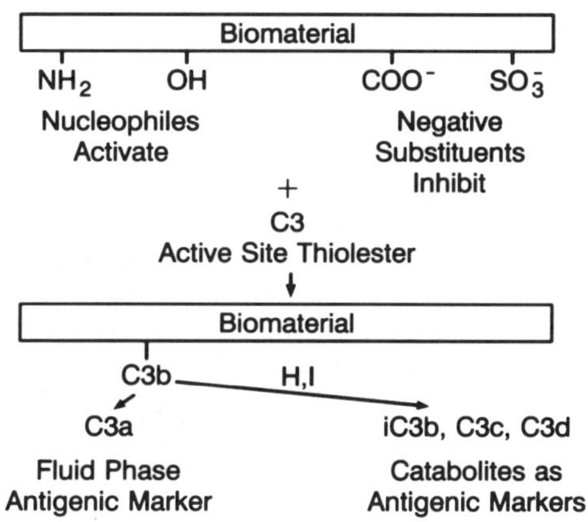

FIGURE 1. Schematic diagram summarizing the molecular mechanisms of the complement alternative pathway activation.

behave as a nonactivator. For example, the presence of sialic acid has been shown to promote high-affinity association between particle-bound C3b and factor H without influencing the affinity of C3b for factor B.[6] Additionally, chemical modification studies have clearly demonstrated that substitution of dextran with either carboxylic or benzylamine sulphonated groups conferred the capacity to inhibit formation of the amplification C3 convertase.[7] Finally, studies performed with particle-bound heparin provide an interesting example of the ability of anionic materials to act as inhibitors of the alternative pathway activation events.[8]

It is also important to note that factors H and I function as inhibitors of the alternative pathway because they are enzymes that cleave surface-bound C3b to yield the inactive catabolite iC3b (FIG. 1). Subsequently, other plasma enzymes such as plasmin kallikrein or elastase cleave iC3b to liberate the C3c fragment into the fluid phase while leaving the active site containing C3d fragment covalently attached to the surface. The final step in the breakdown and catabolism of C3 is hydrolysis of the ester or amide bond that covalently links the C3d fragment to the surface and resultant liberation of this fragment from the material into the fluid phase. It should also be recognized that these same catabolic events take place when C3b becomes attached to an activating surface, although at a greatly diminished rate. Thus, activating biomaterials would be expected to display both surface-bound C3b and/or iC3b as well as measurable levels of C3c- and C3d-related antigens in the fluid phase after a reasonable period of incubation.

In summary, although both complement-activating and nonactivating materials may have surface nucleophiles, activating substances provide an environment that favors binding of factor B to C3b, thus facilitating feedback amplification of C3 convertase formation. As a result, an activating surface rapidly becomes saturated with C3b molecules and significant quantities of the C3a cleavage product are released into the fluid phase. By contrast, nonactivating materials frequently have negatively charged groups on their surface and are characterized by the fact that they promote binding of factor H to C3b. Consequently, nonactivating surfaces display a few bound iC3b molecules and levels of fluid-phase C3a antigen remain essentially unchanged. Subsequent catabolism of surface-bound C3b results in the time-dependent liberation of C3c, C3d, and other C3-derived fragments from the material surface into solution.

The Human Anaphylatoxins

The anaphylatoxins C3a and C5a are bioactive polypeptides that are produced during complement activation.[9] Human C3a is cleaved from C3 by the C3 convertase (C3b, Bb) that is formed during the amplification phase of the alternative pathway activation events. The C5 convertase C3b(n), Bb, formed by deposition of additional C3b molecules on the C3 convertase, acts to cleave C5 and liberate C5a into the fluid phase. Generation of these anaphylatoxin molecules by alternative pathway enzymes may be detected by employing specific radioimmunoassay (RIA) procedures.[10]

Additionally, RIA quantitation of both C3a and C5a antigens permits calculation of a constant designated the "coupling efficiency." This constant permits an assessment of the activating or nonactivating character of a material.[11,12] For example, potent activators of the alternative pathway, such as zymosan, behave as they do because they prohibit binding of factors H and I to C3b. Consequently, both the C3 and C5 convertases are readily formed on the particle surface and essentially equimolar (mole fraction) concentrations of C3a and C5a antigen are liberated into the fluid phase, *i.e,* the "coupling efficiency" of zymosan approaches 100%.[11] By contrast, factors H and I associate more readily with C3b when solution-phase activators, such as bacterial lipopolysaccharide, are employed as stimuli. Therefore, fewer C5 and C3 converting enzymes are established and the mole fraction of liberated C5a is less than that of C3a, *i.e,* the "coupling efficiency" of these weak activators is 25% or less.[11]

The anaphylatoxins that are produced when blood contacts a biomaterial are particularly important for at least two reasons. As depicted in FIGURE 2, the C3a antigen serves as a reliable plasma marker of complement activation because the [des-Arg-77] C3a ($C3a_{des\ Arg}$) polypeptide is biologically inert and accumulates readily in blood.[9] More importantly, the C5a and/or [des-Arg-74] C5a ($C5a_{des\ Arg}$) that is formed as a result of blood-material contact is a potent bioactive molecule that may provoke a variety of pathophysiologic responses.[9]

Extracorporeal production of C5a anaphylatoxin results in clinical manifestations that are directly related to the quantity of C5a produced at the blood-material interface. Generation of even modest amounts of this potent biological effector provides sufficient C5a to bind to the C5a receptor of peripheral blood granulocytes passing through the extracorporeal circuit.[13] When this happens, the C5a-activated neutrophils and monocytes are returned to the patient, where they may become sequestered in the microvasculature. These biological events account for the granulocytopenia commonly observed during hemodialysis performed with complement-activating membranes. In addition to these acute phenomena, it has been suggested that C5a-stimulated neutrophil may initiate local tissue injury while it is in contact with the pulmonary endothelial cell and the C5a-activated monocyte might elaborate interleukin-1 (IL-1), which in turn could produce systemic manifestations of inflammation.[14]

It is also now apparent that C5a can have direct effects on the pulmonary vasculature. For example, both our published studies performed with swine[15] and our more recent unpublished investigations employing a sheep model demonstrate that intravenous infusion of either porcine or human C5a provokes a significant increase in the pulmonary artery pressure (PAP) and the systemic arterial pressure (SAP) while causing a dimunition in the cardiac output (CO) and hypoxemia. Interestingly,

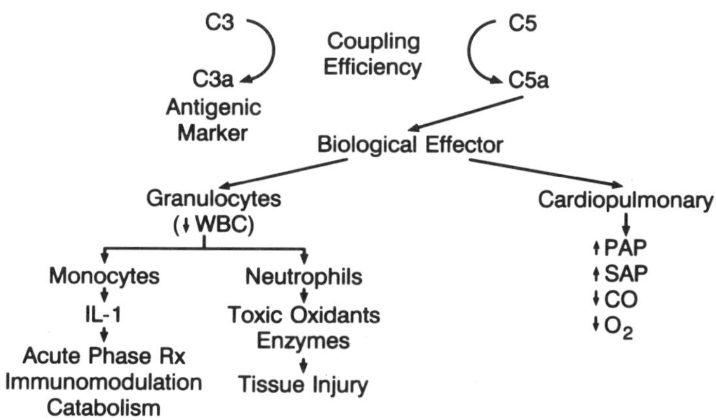

FIGURE 2. Schematic diagram depicting the biological consequences of anaphylatoxin production in extracorporeal circuits.

C5a-induced pulmonary hypertension is consistently detected prior to the onset of C5a-induced granulocytopenia, thus demonstrating the direct actions of the anaphylatoxin on the pulmonary vasculature.

COMPLEMENT ACTIVATION DURING HEMODIALYSIS

Observations

Initially, Craddock and his coworkers provided the first evidence of complement activation in extracorporeal circuits when they employed bioassays to demonstrate that C5a (des-Arg) resulted when blood contacted cellulosic hemodialyzer membranes. Subsequently, development of specific anaphylatoxin radioimmunoassays (RIAs) permitted extension of these observations to include evaluation of cardiopulmonary bypass circuitry and other types of hemodialyzers.[1] Currently, the greatest amount of

TABLE 1. Complement Activation and Granulocytopenia Produced by Various Dialyzers (in Normalized Percentage Values)

Dialyzer Type	Plasma C3a	Leukopenia
Cuprophan	100	100
Cellulose acetate	67	43
Hemophan	60	62
Polycarbonate	40	53
Polysulfone	24	12
Reused cuprophan	15	38
Polyacrylonitrile sodium methallylsulfonate (Hospal AN-69)	5	0

basic and clinical information has been obtained from studies of hemodialyzers. For this reason, it is worthwhile to review this data base and to attempt to correlate this information with what is known about the human complement system and the human anaphylatoxins.

The complement-activating potential of various types of dialyzer membrane materials can be clinically defined in two ways. First, the maximal amount of C3a antigen produced during the initial phases of hemodialysis can be quantitated by RIA methods. Second, the magnitude of the leukopenic response induced by hemodialysis with a particular type of dialyzer can be readily measured. As shown in TABLE 1, when the complement-activating potential of several different types of dialyzers is defined in this way, Cuprophan hollow fiber devices made with unmodified cellulosic membrane consistently produce the greatest amount of C3a generation and the greatest degree of leukopenia. Modification of the cellulosic material, either by acetylation (cellulose acetate) or introduction of tertiary amino groups (Hemophan), results in a 30–40% reduction in the maximum amount of plasma C3a detected during the first 15 minutes of dialysis. The leukopenic response provoked by these modified cellulosic dialyzers is also corresponding reduced. Perhaps the most "biocompatible" form of modified Cuprophan is that unique membrane which results from use and formalin storage of new dialyzers. Clinical studies performed with these reused Cuprophan dialyzers demonstreate that they produce only about 15% of the C3a formation induced by new dialyzers.[3]

Synthetic membranes consistently exhibit a lower complement-activating potential than cellulosic membranes. As shown in TABLE 2, both polycarbonate and polysulfone membrane dialyzers provoke only moderate C3a formation when evaluated clinically. The most interesting synthetic membrane appears to be a polyacrylonitrile-sodium methallylsulfonate copolymer, the Hospal AN-69 membrane. Dialyzers manufactured with this synthetic material produce only small quantities of C3a antigen that can be

TABLE 2. Classification of Hemodialyzers

	Biological Consequences	
Complement-activating Capacity	Granulocytopenia	Pulmonary Hypertension
high	yes	yes
moderate	yes	no
low	no	no

detected in the efferent (outlet) line of the dialyzer and fail to induce granulocytopenia in the dialyzed patient.[2]

In addition to direct quantitation of C3a antigen and determination of peripheral blood leukocyte counts, the complement-activating potential of dialyzers may be defined by physiologic measurements. For example, as mentioned previously, purified porcine C5a produces a significant increase in the pulmonary artery pressure when injected intravenously into swine.[4] Similar results have been observed when sheep were employed as the test animal (unpublished observation). Thus, measurements of PAP during dialysis performed on swine or sheep have been exploited to estimate the amount of C5a produced during the procedure. These types of studies have demonstrated that unmodified cellulosic membranes produce a two-to-threefold elevation of the mean PAP within 5 minutes after the onset of dialysis. By contrast, the newer modified cellulosic membranes (Hemophan), although they still activate complement with 60% of the activity of Cuprophan, do not provoke this physiologic response. Similarly, the synthetic membranes that display reduced complement-activating potential, such as polysulfone and AN-69, also fail to produce a significant increase in PAP during dialysis.

TABLE 3. Factors Governing Patient Exposure to C5a Anaphylatoxin during Extracorporeal Circulation

- I. Factors effecting complement activation
  - A. Number of reactive groups
  - B. Reactivity of surface groups
  - C. Nature and number of surface regulatory constituents
- II. Factors effecting anaphylaxtoxin distribution
  - A. Transport through materials (membrane)
  - B. Binding to materials
  - C. Interaction with blood cells in the extracorporeal circuit

In summary, detailed clinical and laboratory studies suggest that hemodialyzer membrane materials tend to fall into one of three different categories (TABLE 2). The first category is exemplified by unmodified cellulosic membranes. These display a great capacity to activate complement and are characterized by the fact that they provoke both granulocytopenia and pulmonary hypertension. The second group consists of a large number of modified cellulosic and synthetic membranes that display about half the complement-activating potential of Cuprophan. These membranes are distinctly different from unmodified cellulosic ones because, although they do induce pulmonary vascular leukosequestration, they fail to promote pulmonary hypertension. The Hospal An-69 membrane is most typical of the final category. Dialyzers containing this synthetic copolymer display low complement-activating potential and fail to induce either granulocytopenia or pulmonary hypertension.

Hypotheses

Results of studies performed to date suggest that there is one central issue to resolve when considering complement activation in extracorporeal circuits. That is to identify the factors that govern the quantity of the bioactive C5a molecule is delivered from the extracorporeal circuit to the patient during the therapeutic procedure.

Knoweldge of the mechanisms of complement activation, the biological properties of human C5a anaphylatoxin, and the observed performance of different hemodialysis membrane materials permits a hypothetical delineation of these critical factors and provides a conceptual framework for understanding biomaterial-complement interactions.

The author speculates that the factors that account for patient exposure to C5a anaphylatoxin during extracorporeal circulation can be divided into two broad categories. First, it is postulated that certain membrane characteristics will effect the complement activation process directly (TABLE 3). For example, experimental evidence supports the contention that both the relative number and chemical reactivity of surface nucleophiles contributes significantly in this regard.[15]

Additionally, it is now appreciated that other membrane surface groups may play a critical role in regulating surface activation events. Particular emphasis is being placed on those that are negatively charged. These regulatory phenomena may be experimentally manifested as a reduction in the "coupling efficiency."

Second, factors that effect anaphylatoxin distribution would also be expected to modify patient exposure to C5a that is produced within the extracorporeal circuit. In this case, emphasis has been placed on the fact that the low molecular weight cationic C5a molecule may either by transported through certain porous membranes or bound tightly to other anionic membranes. For example, the apparent "biocompatibility" of the AN-69 membrane appears to result from the fact that it binds both C3a and C5a after they are produced.[16] Finally, basic investigations have demonstrated that C5a is irreversibly bound to granulocytes under physiologic conditions. Thus it is likely that binding of this anaphylatoxin to the cellular elements of blood in the extracorporeal circuit induces cellular activation while reducing the plasma levels of the glycopolypeptide. As a consequence, patients may exhibit granulocytopenia but be spared from exposure to the freely circulating bioactive C5a.

SUMMARY

Clinical studies performed with various types of hemodialyzers provide a data base and conceptual framework for understanding blood-material interactions that result in complement activation. Current findings suggest that the complement-activating potential of biomaterials may be defined by quantitating either fluid-phase C3a antigen or measurement of surface-bound C3 fragments. Furthermore, systematic studies can reveal material properties that regulate both the production and distribution of the human anaphylatoxins. Assessing the fate of the C5a anaphylatoxin is particularly important because it is likely that generation of this bioactive molecule in extracorporeal circuits initially triggers granulocyte responses and may produce cardiopulmonary manifestations if the C5a is formed in sufficient quantities. It seems likely that detailed knowledge of these varied phenomena will permit rational design of newer "biocompatible" materials and membranes.

REFERENCES

1. CHENOWETH, D. E. 1986. Anaphylatoxin formation in extracorporeal circuits. Complement **3:** 152–165.
2. CHENOWETH, D. E., A. K. CHEUNG & L. W. HENDERSON. Anaphylatoxin formation during hemodialysis: Effects of different dialyzer membranes. Kid. Int. **24:** 764–769.
3. CHENOWETH, D. E., A. K. CHEUNG, D. M. WARD & L. W. HENDERSON. 1983. Anaphyla-

toxin formation during hemodialysis: Comparison of new and reused dialyzers. Kid. Int. **24:** 770–774.

4. CHEUNG, A. K., M. LEWINTER, D. E. CHENOWETH, W. Y. W. LEW & L. W. HENDERSON. 1986. Cardiopulmonary effects of Cuprophane-activated plasma in the swine: Role of complement products. Kid. Int. **29:** 799–806.
5. PANGBURN, M. K. 1986. The alternative pathway. *In* Immunobiology of the Complement System. G. D. Ross, Ed.: 45–62. Academic Press. Orlando, FL.
6. KAZATCHKINE, M. D., D. T. FEARON & K. F. AUSTEN. 1979. Human alternative complement pathway: Membrane associated sialic acid regulates the competition between B and beta-1-H for cell bound C3b. J. Immunol. **122:** 75–79.
7. MAUZAC, M., F. MAILLET, J. JOZEFONVICZ & M. D. KAZATCHKINE. 1985. Anticomplementary activity of dextran derivatives. Biomaterials **6:** 61–63.
8. KAZATCHKINE, M. D., D. T. FEARON, D. D. METCALFE, R. D. ROSENBERG & K. F. AUSTEN. 1981. Structural determinants of the capacity of heparin to inhibit the formation of the human amplification C3 convertase. J. Clin. Invest. **67:** 223–228.
9. CHENOWETH, D. E. 1986. Complement mediators of inflammation. *In* Immunobiology of the Complement System. G. D. Ross, Ed.: 63–86. Academic Press. New York.
10. CHENOWETH, D. E. 1984. Biocompatibility of hemodialysis membranes. Evaluation with C3a anaphylatoxin radioimmunoassays. Asaio J. **7:** 44–49.
11. CHENOWETH, D. E. 1986. Complement activation produced by biomaterials. Trans. Am. Soc. Artif. Intern. Organs. **32:** 226–232.
12. CHENOWETH, D. E. & L. W. HENDERSON. 1987. Complement activation during hemodialysis: Laboratory evaluation of hemodialyzers. Artif. Organs **11:** 155–162.
13. CHENOWETH, D. E. & T. E. HUGLI. 1978. Demonstration of a specific C5a receptor on intact human polymorphonuclear leukocytes. Proc. Natl. Acad. Sci. U.S.A. **75:** 3943–3947.
14. GOODMAN, M. G., D. E. CHENOWETH & W. O. WEIGLE. 1982. Induction of interleukine-1 secretion and enhancement of humoral immunity by binding of human C5a to macrophage surface C5a receptors. J. Exp. Med. **156:** 912–917.
15. CHENOWETH, D. E. 1984. Complement activation during hemodialysis: Clinical observations, proposed mechanisms and theoretical implications. Artif. Organs **8:** 281–287.
16. CHEUNG, A. K., D. E. CHENOWETH, D. OTSUKA & L. W. HENDERSON. 1986. Compartment distribution of complement activation products in artificial kidneys. Kid. Int. **30:** 74–80.

Summary

Plasma Systems

PAUL DIDISHEIM

National Institutes of Health
Bethesda, Maryland 20892

This session has dealt with the adsorption of certain specific plasma proteins onto artificial surfaces and their activation resulting from contact with those surfaces. John Brash reviewed some of his findings on the Vroman effect, in which fibrinogen is rapidly adsorbed onto surfaces initially and is subsequently displaced by factors of the contact phase of coagulation including high molecular weight kininogen (HMWK) and factor XII. The fraction of fibrinogen remaining on the surface appears to have been degraded by plasmin, suggesting surface-induced activation of plasminogen. Thomas Horbett showed how the Vroman effect varies in magnitude and plasma concentration depending upon the nature of the surface. It appears that displacement is a general phenomenon of all protein mixtures rather than being limited to contact activation factors. Peter Cuypers presented evidence that sequential adsorption and the Vroman effect can be explained by the surface concentration of the adsorbed proteins. Robert Colman showed how the contact factors need to be cleaved and thus changed into their active form before they can be adsorbed onto a surface. Michael Silverberg demonstrated activation of contact factors by soluble "surfaces" such as dextran sulfate and heparin; these molecules must be large enough to possess multiple binding sites for the contact proteins.

Dennis Chenoweth presented evidence that blood contact with extracorporeal devices is associated with complement activation by the alternative pathway resulting in the production of C3a and C5a. Plasma C3a levels are readily measured but C5a is not, owing to its binding to leukocytes and their subsequent removal from the circulation. Measurement of these activities may be useful in evaluating biomaterials for their compatibility with blood. Frederick Grinnell presented data suggesting that fibronectin adsorbs on surfaces in different orientations depending on protein concentration and surface chemistry, and that fibronectin desorption occurs selectively beneath cells adherent to the surface. Deane Mosher reviewed the structure, homology, and functions of four proteins that are adhesive for platelets: fibrinogen, fibronectin, von Willebrand factor, and vitronectin, discussed the properties of the GPIIb-GPIIIa complex on the platelet membrane, which is the receptor that recognizes these proteins, and compared their role in platelet adhesion to surfaces. Leo Vroman reviewed the phenomenon he identified, which others have named the "Vroman effect." He also described a simple, rapid, inexpensive method for measuring proteins adsorbed to surfaces based on the color reaction between proteins and the different oxides bound to specific antibody.

Summarizing these reports, it is evident that protein adsorption onto surfaces is a highly dynamic event, varying with time, surface, and the structure, functions, and concentration of the proteins being examined. The dynamic nature of these events complicates their interpretation with the regard to the "compatibility" of surfaces with blood. The extent to which these rapidly changing events are related to the clinical problems observed with cardiopulmonary bypass, hemodialysis, catheters, vascular grafts, or total artificial hearts is not yet clear. It seems likely, however, that the adsorption and activation of certain of these plasma proteins play key roles in the subsequent cellular and molecular events that are critical to the function of these devices, at least in the short term. Whether these early events have any bearing on the long-term *in vivo* responses of implanted devices, including thromboembolism, excessive tissue proliferation, and calcification, is unknown at present. This is an important question, and it is my hope that it will be specifically addressed in future investigations.

Surface Abnormalities and Conduit Characteristics as a Cause of Blood Trauma in Artificial Internal Organs

The Interaction of Fluid-Dynamic, Physicochemical and Cell Biological Reactions in Thrombus Formation

L. J. WURZINGER AND H. SCHMID-SCHÖNBEIN

Departments of Anatomy and Physiology
Technical University Aachen
D-5100 Aachen, Federal Republic of Germany

INTRODUCTION

From the very beginning of their use, both the functional behavior and the tolerance of artificial blood-perfused organs by patients were jeopardized by hemolysis on one hand, and thrombosis and paradoxic bleeding on the other hand, *i.e.,* symptoms related to "blood trauma" in a foreign environment. According to scientific concepts of the sixties and early seventies, hemolysis was related to "turbulent flow,"[1] and thrombosis and bleeding to the exposure of blood to a "foreign" surface.[2] The ability of nonendothelial surfaces to trigger the activation of a pivotal coagulation enzyme (factor XII) and subsequently the intrinsic cascade of coagulation with the final polymerization of fibrinogen was imagined to produce thrombi in regions of "blood stasis." Soon, however, it became evident that high flow forces in an environment with nonendothelial lining produced an activation of platelets, the cellular components of the hemostatic system.[3] Furthermore, consideration of the scope of effects of activated factor XII as a multifunctional trigger revealed the intricate interrelations between the enzyme activation cascades of coagulation, fibrinolysis, the complement system, and the kinin system.[4] In an early comprehensive biological interpretation of "blood trauma" in artificial organs, we interpreted this process as an activation of the "unspecific defense system" (UDS) of the organism.[5] In these terms the "hematological response" of the body to an artificial blood-perfused organ was considered as a manifestation of a fundamental physiological function, *i.e.,* that of the "old" humoral and cellular defense to any kind of noxious events or agents. This basic response has its corollary in the activation of the phylogenetically "new" specific immune system by xenotransplanted internal organs. In essence, the unspecific defense reaction consists of an activation of networks of enzymatic processes escaping physiological control.

Recent developments in the biochemistry of cellular functions, catalytic reactions, and membranes have profoundly changed our concepts concerning the UDS in general, and that of the hemostatic system in particular. On one hand, the once pivotal role of contact-activated factor XII in hemostasis has been supplemented by a concept of "altered cell membranes," providing catalytic sites for the proteolytic activation of plasmatic proenzymes.[6] On the other hand, considerable knowledge has accumulated about molecular details of proenzyme networks and enzyme inactivators in blood. The widespread underlying common mechanism appears to be that of "limited proteolysis," which converts zymogens into active serine proteases by conformational changes.[7] Thus the molecular basis of the detection of "noxious signals" and the amplification by enzyme cascades, initially discovered for the plasmatic coagulation system, is now being appreciated as a general principle in the triggering of the complement system, the kinin system, and the renin angiotensin system. The self-amplification of the serine protease network has its counterpart in a positive feedback of tissue hormone-mediated cell biological activation processes, involving cells of the blood, the vessel wall, and the interstitial space.[8] Positively fed back, biochemically mediated cell-cell interactions occur between members of any subclass as well as among members of different cell types. There also exist reactions connecting the various systems of serine proteases with themselves, and cell activation processes.

The host of reactions unveiled during the last two decades is bewildering. At the moment it appears difficult to estimate their respective biological significance. Their prominence in the scientific literature reflects the availability and sensitivity of methods of their study rather than proven validity. From a cybernetic standpoint, however, one problem stands out: How can positively fed back systems be stable? From a biochemist's point of view this question leads to the deciphering of an equally complex system of inhibitory proteins and the postulation of reaction equilibria. Looked at from this perspective, a thrombus is the result of a local disbalance between "coagulation" and "fibrinolysis." From a rheologist's point of view, however, a much simpler answer can be offered: the equilibrium between activation and inhibition largely depends on "supply and removal." The unactivated state is primarily maintained by undisturbed laminar blood flow. We would like to postulate that the "powder barrel" of cells, mediators, and enzymes is kept from "exploding" simply by the fundamental physics of Poiseuille flow. The mutual sliding of fluid lamellae, with speed increasing towards the vessel center, automatically provides dilution in flowing blood. This means that repetitive collisions of substrates with enzymes and cofactors or cells with mediators are extremely rare. No matter how high the gain of positively fed back hemostatic reactions may be in closed systems, as in reaction tubes, wash out in vessels in less than 0.1 s, as estimated from the ratio of segment volume and flow rate, attenuates turnover.

It should not be ignored, however, that fluid dynamic factors are most certainly involved in the triggering and promotion of hemostatic reactions. First, uninterrupted blood flow provides transport of proenzymes and cellular components, mainly platelets, to the "site of need." Second, during the last two decades evidence has accumulated for a stimulating effect of fluid dynamic forces on platelets.[9]

Starting from this premise, the biochemical aspects of which were dealt with in detail in two meetings sponsored by the Concerted Action on Extracorporeal Oxygenation of the Commission of European Communities, our group has since focused on several aspects of the rheology, fluid dynamics, cell biology, and enzyme biochemistry of the UDS, with special interest focused on the boundary conditions prevailing during its activation in artificial organs.

SHORT-TIME EXPOSURE OF PLATELETS TO LAMINAR SHEAR STRESS

The effects of high shear forces on blood cells have been investigated over the last two decades. The most significant work has been conducted by the groups in St. Louis and at Rice University in Houston with the aid of rotational viscometers, permitting "defined" shear exposure of blood cells. Defined shear exposure is characterized by the shear stress, calculated as the product of the shear rate and the apparent viscosity of the suspension, and the time it acts upon blood cells. However, most of the published studies with conventional viscometers extend single shear stress exposures over 5 minutes. In artificial organs, *e.g.*, heart valve prostheses, blood cells are expected to pass through regions of high shear within times considerably shorter than a second, probably in a few milliseconds (ms).[10] For the short-time shearing of blood cells, we used a modified Couette viscometer[11] (FIG. 1). By applying a continuous sample flow in axial direction through the gap between the two cylinders of the Couette system, the time the blood cells spend within the gap can be varied between 7 and 700 ms. Rotation of the inner cylinder generates shear rates up to 214,000/s in the Couette slit, equalling a shear stress of 255 N/m^2 (2550 $dynes/cm^2$) at an average viscosity of 1.2 mPa.s of platelet-rich plasma (PRP).

It is well known that platelets are extremely prone to undergo fast secondary reactions.[12] This notwithstanding, all studies published so far lack precise information about the time passing between the end of shear exposure and the inhibition of secondary reactions. In papers published before 1980 hardly any information about inhibitory measures can be found. Care was therefore taken to block these reactions within 30 s after passage of the shearing gap. This was done by pipetting the sheared

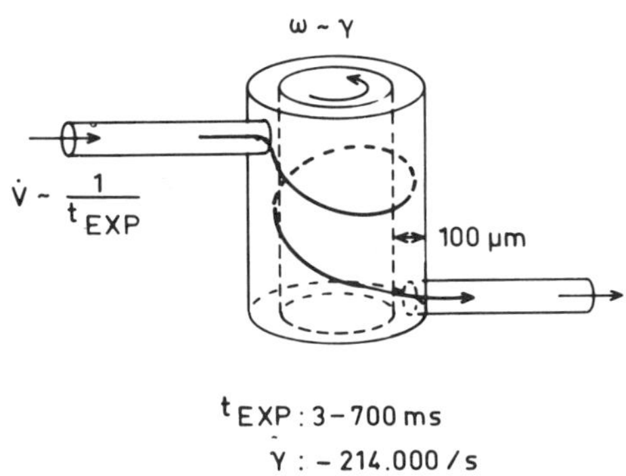

FIGURE 1. Schematic drawing illustrating the pathway of a suspended particle through the axial flow through Couette viscometer employed for short-time shearing of blood cells.[11]

PRP onto an inhibitory mixture of EDTA, theophylline, and PGE_1 at 0–4°C before platelets were spun down for determination of intraplatelet marker substances in the supernatant.[13]

Basic insight into the mechanism of "shear-induced" platelet activation was gained from exposure of platelets to shear stresses between 57 N/m^2 and 255 N/m^2 for times ranging from 7 to 700 ms.[14] Unspecific lytic damage of the platelet plasma membrane as a consequence of the impact of fluid mechanical forces is usually detected by the extracellular appearance of cytoplasmic marker substances like lactic dehydrogenase (LDH). On the other hand, β-thromboglobulin (β-TG) represents a platelet protein stored in alpha granules and is actively released in response to stimuli, without affecting the platelets' structural integrity. It is, however, a plain but frequently neglected fact that β-TG leaks out from damaged platelets too and is by no means specific for platelet activation.

We were able to confirm the damaging and β-TG-releasing properties of shear forces mentioned in previous studies. A contradiction of the literature,[15–17] where a lower threshold of shear stress is reported for the induction of the release of granule proteins than for LDH, was that neither differences of shear stress threshold levels for

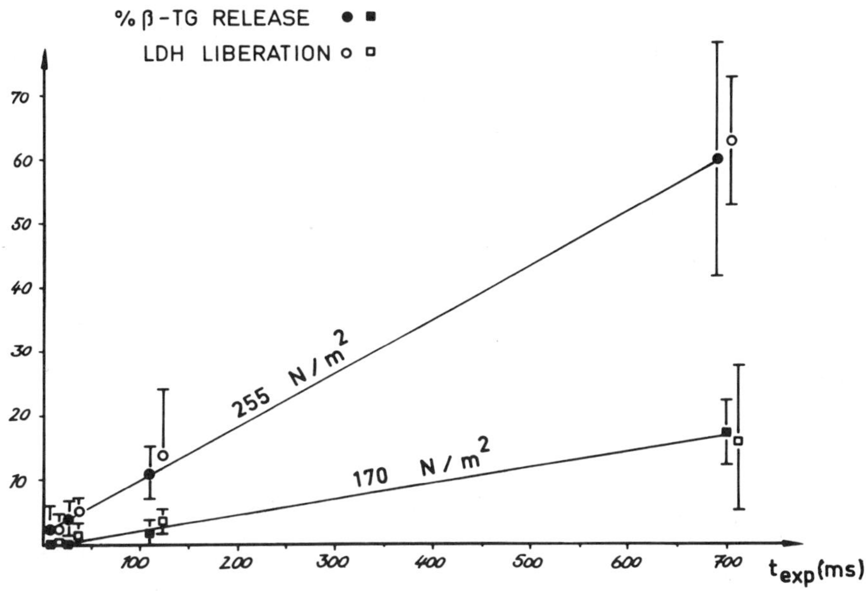

FIGURE 2. Diagram showing the linear increase of β-TG and LDH in the supernatant of sheared platelet-rich plasma with increasing exposure time.

their liberation, nor any significant difference in the amount of both marker proteins could be found[14] (FIG. 2).

On the other hand Stypventime, as a parameter for platelet factor 3 (PF 3) availability, proved to be more sensitive to the impact of shear stress than the leakage of LDH or β-TG from damaged platelets (TABLE 1). In the presence of activated clotting factors X and V and calcium ions, the proteolytic conversion of prothrombin to thrombin and thus fibrin formation depends critically upon the presence of phosphatidylserine (PS) in the outer leaflet of the phospholipid bilayer of the platelet membrane. In resting platelets PS is located almost exclusively in the inner half of the lipid bilayer. Strong stimulation of platelets with thrombin and collagen causes a translocation of PS from the inner to the outer leaflet within the intact platelet membrane,[18] thereby eliciting the described catalytic properties. The molecular events underlying the

TABLE 1. Threshold Shear Stress Levels (N/m^2) Necessary to Induce Platelet Alterations Depending on Time of Shear Exposure

Platelet Parameter	Exposure Time (ms) 700	113	27	7
Platelet factor 3	<57	57	108	170
Reduction of platelet count	<57	108	57	>255
Liberation of β-TG	57	170	255	255
Liberation of LDH	57	170	170	255
Inhibition of ADP-induced aggregation	108	255	>255	>255

The figures give the shear stress levels in N/m^2 leading to a significant change ($p < 0.05$) of a parameter for a given exposure time. (Data taken from Wurzinger *et al.*[14])

extreme sensitivity of Stypven time and PF 3 availability to lytic damage of platelets are a matter of conjecture at present. Leakage of 1% of total platelet LDH content is reported to cause a 40% reduction of Stypven time.[18] Accordingly, a 36% reduction of Stypven time following at 27 ms lasting exposure to 170 N/m^2 is most likely a consequence of an LDH-monitored lysis rate of roughly 1%.[14]

Obviously the assay of marker proteins or the determination of catalytic properties of the platelet surface fails to provide decisive clues to cell biological effects of shear forces on platelets, although the linear dependence of β-TG liberation from the exposure time is an argument against the notion of a direct release-stimulating effect of shear stress (FIG. 2).

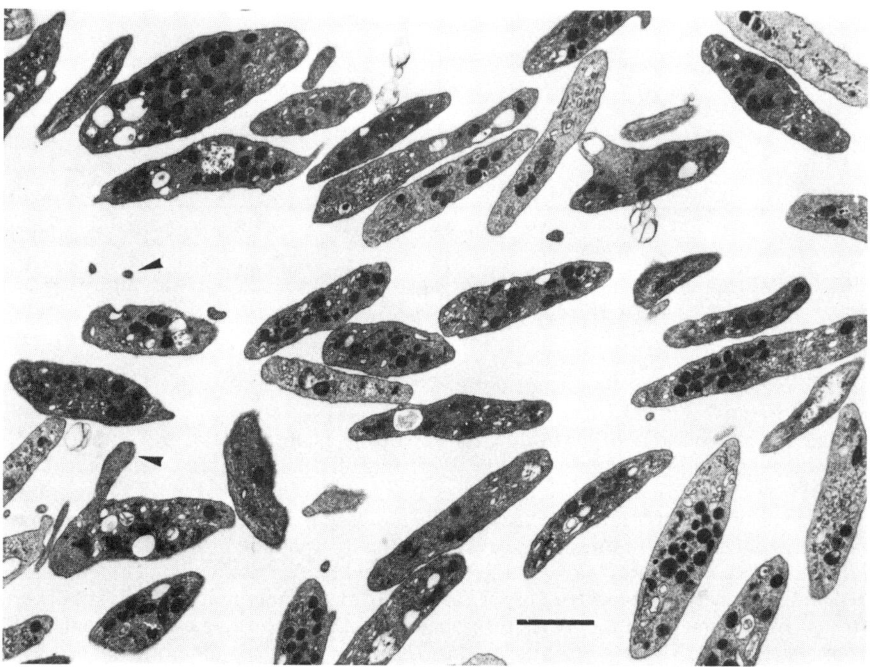

FIGURE 3. TEM micrograph of control platelets that have passed the viscometer without high shear exposure. Note discoid forms with few protrusions (*arrowheads*). *Bar*: 1 μm.

Transmission electron micrographs of PRP fixed within 20 to 30 s after shear exposure contain almost exclusively activated platelets, which compared to "inactive smooth disks" (FIG. 3) show a round shape, numerous cytoplasmic protrusions, and centralized organelles. Depending on the length and level of shear exposure, a varying proportion of platelets becomes "lytic." Lytic platelets are characterized by ballooning degeneration as a consequence of influx of extracellular fluid through a leaky plasma membrane. Their cytoplasmic density appears reduced and their internal architecture irreversibly broken down (FIG. 4). In some instances membrane material and free granules, probably from completely destroyed platelets, can also be found. The appearance of the material in FIGURE 5 renders the discussion about the mechanism by

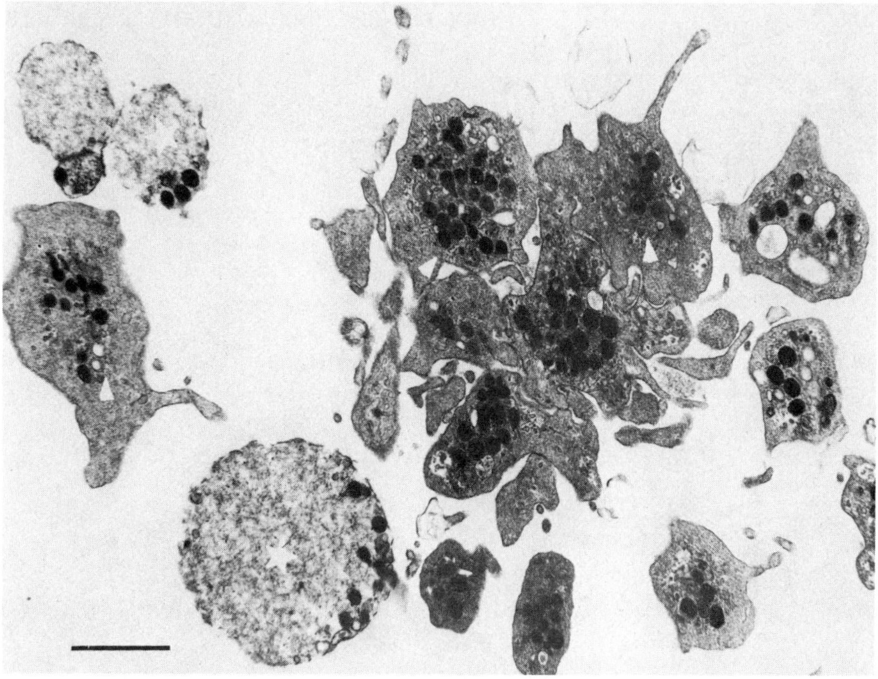

FIGURE 4. TEM micrograph showing platelets after exposure to 170 N/m^2 for 113 ms. Platelets are rounded and a small aggregate has formed. *White arrowheads* mark centralized granules; *white asterisks* mark irreversibly ballooned, "lytic" platelets. *Bar*: 1 μm.

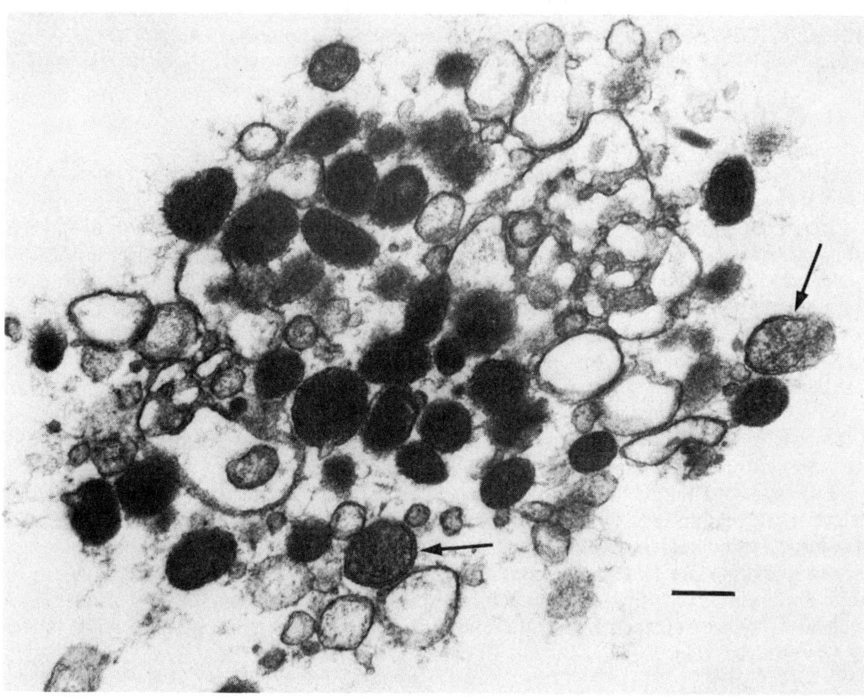

FIGURE 5. TEM micrograph containing loose organelles (*arrows* indicate mitochondria) and membrane vesicles of completely destroyed platelet. *Bar*: 0.2 μm.

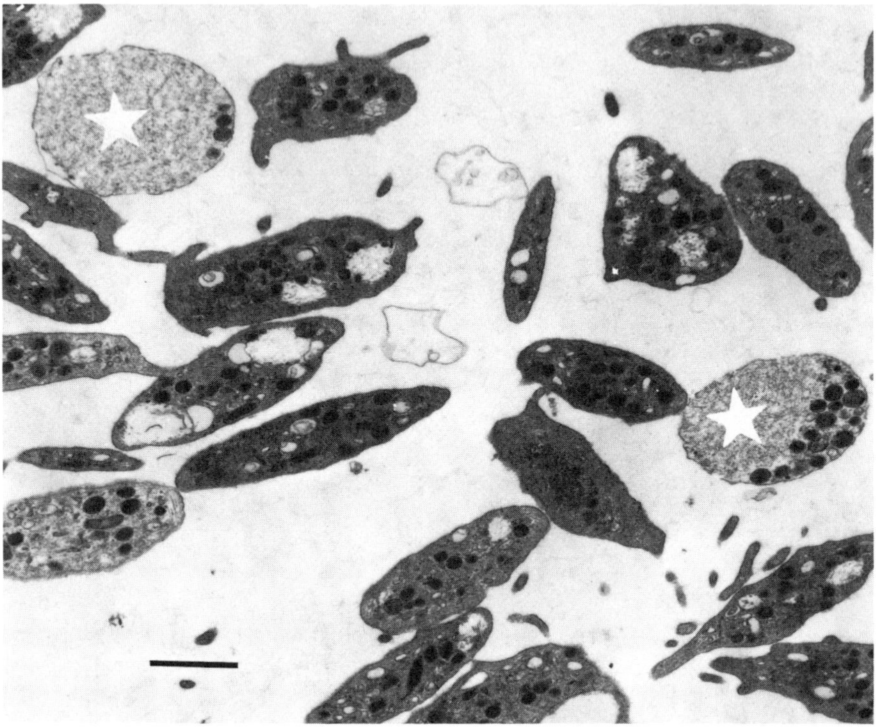

FIGURE 6. TEM micrograph with platelets having undergone same shear stress (170 N/m^2; 113 ms) as the platelets in FIGURE 4, but in presence of "ADP scavengers." Note discoid, resting platelets. *Asterisks* mark irreversibly damaged platelets. *Bar*: 1 μm.

which fluid mechanical forces might cause PS to switch to the outer leaflet of the platelet membrane a rather academic one.

Irreversibly damaged platelets are readily recognized and cannot be confused with intact platelets in any state of activation. The latter can be determined precisely by means of morphometric techniques, *e.g.*, measuring the flatness of the shape of platelets or the centralizarion of organelles.[19] Therefore ultrastructural morphometry appears to be superior to biochemical techniques when it comes to the question of activation or trauma of a platelet population. An increasing proportion of damaged platelets before a background of activated platelets correlates with increasing shear stress and/or exposure time. However, when PRP is sheared in the presence of ADP-scavenging enzyme-substrate systems, the platelet-activating effect of fluid mechanical forces vanishes, without affecting its damaging effect (FIG. 6).

Exposure of PRP to shear forces mimicking both in magnitude and time course the situation during passage of artificial organs *in vivo* leads *in vitro* to the following chain of events. High shear stress damages a proportion of platelets, with their cytoplasmic contents leaking out. The latter contain ADP and ATP, rapidly degraded to ADP, in such amounts[20] that shape change is completed within a few seconds after shear exposure. Active release of granule contents, however, takes minutes if ADP is the triggering agent.[21] The sole result of fluid mechanical stress upon platelets under *in vivo* conditions appears to be "thrombocytorrhexis."

SHORT-TIME EXPOSURE OF RED CELLS TO LAMINAR SHEAR STRESS

Suspensions of washed RBC with a hematocrit of 40% and a viscosity in the range of 2.0 to 2.8 mPa.s were subjected to high shear stresses in the same flow-through viscometer, observing a protocol analogous to the platelet experiments.[22] The lysis of RBC subjected to high shear forces is correlated in a linear fashion to the duration of shear exposure, as was the lysis rate of platelets. In spite of their greater diameter, red blood cells appear to tolerate shear stresses acting for $10^{-2} - 1$ s significantly better than do platelets (FIG. 7).

This is reflected in an increase of hemoglobin-monitored lysis rate with the square of the shear stress, whereas LDH-monitored lysis of sheared platelets rises proportionally to the third or fourth power of shear stress. Considering the ultrastructural features of both cell types, this substantial difference in "shear pliability" becomes quite conceivable. Whereas RBCs are basically membrane-coated droplets of a highly viscous but nevertheless fluid hemoglobin solution, platelets are stuffed with organelles

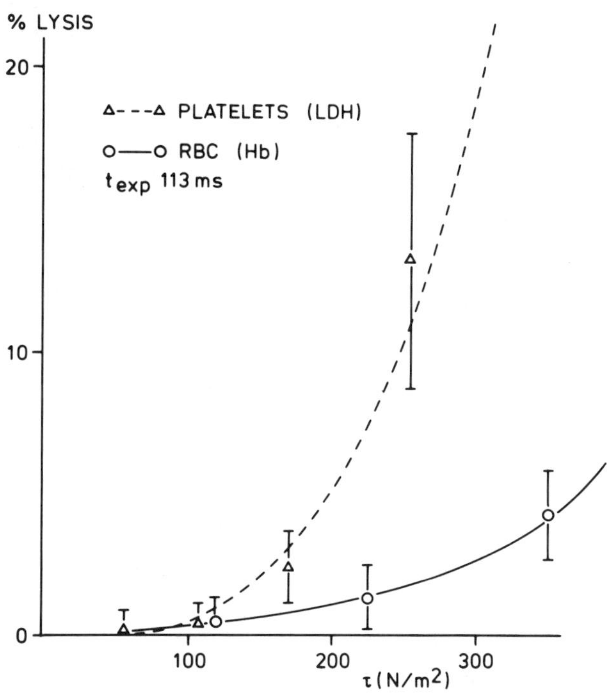

FIGURE 7. Comparative illustration of shear-induced lysis of platelets and red cells as a function of shear stress. Lysis of RBC is determined by assaying hemoglobin in the supernatant of washed RBC (hematocrit = 0.40).

and above all contain a stiffening ring of microtubules. Depolymerization of this microtubular cytoskeleton results indeed in a higher deformability and a lower lysis rate when exposed to fluid mechanical forces.[23,24]

In contrast to former results obtained in RBC suspended in high viscosity media (>40 mPa.s), no changes in shape of the "surviving" RBC or microspheres were detected upon interference contrast microscopical examination of sheared suspensions.[25] It thus far remains uncertain whether this discrepancy is due to the unphysiological ratio of the viscosity of the intracellular to the extracellular fluid in the quoted studies or to the extreme suddenness of shear exposure (up to 200,000 N/m^2 per s) to which cells are subjected upon passage through the Heuser-Opitz flow-through viscometer.

The liberation of small K^+ ions at shear stress levels definitely too low to cause leakage of the large hemoglobin molecules, which prompted the notion of the opening of membrane "pores" at sublytic shear stress,[26] could not be reproduced in the described experimental setup either.[22]

INTERACTIONS BETWEEN RED CELLS AND PLATELETS IN HIGH SHEAR FIELDS

Convincing evidence has been put forward in the past that a variety of relevant platelet reactions in various test systems are enhanced in the presence of RBC. Platelet adherence to subendothelium is correlated with the hematocrit,[27] whereas *in vitro* hemostasis fails in the absence of RBC.[28] The mechanism whereby RBC should exert

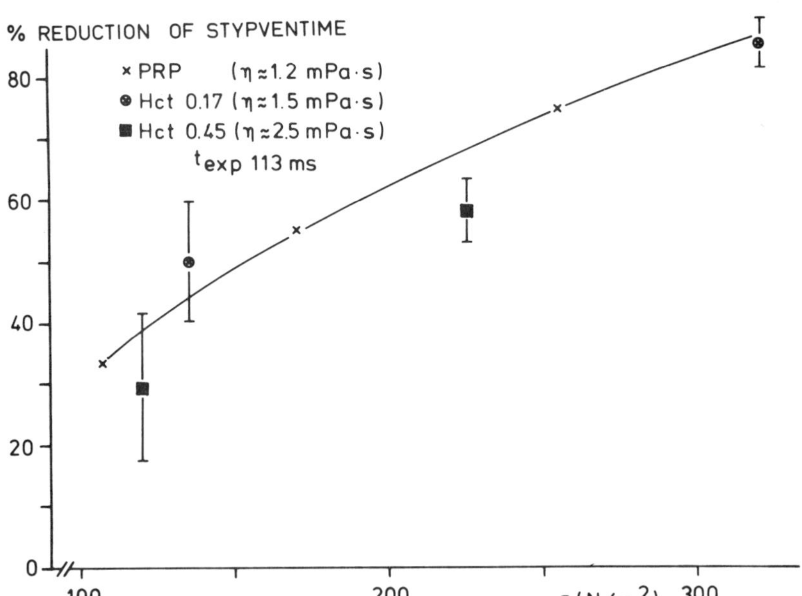

FIGURE 8. The line indicates the reduction of Stypven time in PRP for PF 3 activity, following exposure to shear stress for 113 ms. Measurements with RBC added are indicated by round or square symbols ($\bar{x}$ + SD).

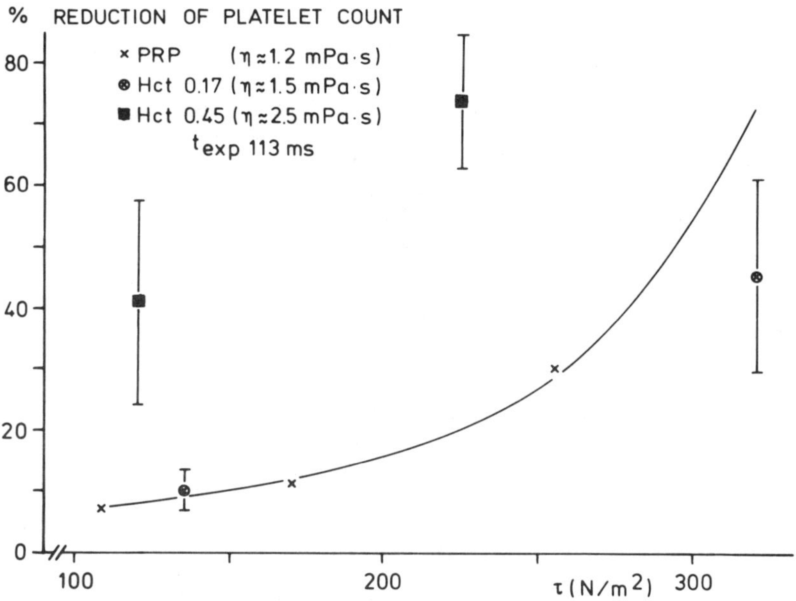

FIGURE 9. The drawn line indicates the loss of single platelets, mainly by aggregation, following exposure to shear stress for 113 ms. Addition of RBC is denoted by the same symbols as in FIGURE 8. Only RBC in whole-blood concentration induce significantly higher platelet losses under shear.

this effect so obviously important for the basic hemostatic function of platelets was investigated extensively. In a recent study Reimers and colleagues were able to show that red cells promoted platelet aggregation during 300 s exposure to 5 N/m^2 by two mechanisms.[29] First, adenine nucleotides escaping from sheared red cells provide proaggregatory biochemical stimulation. Second, an ADP-independent biophysical effect, probably "shear-enhanced diffusion," seems to play a significant role too.

By subjecting PRP supplemented with packed RBC to a hematocrit of 0.17 or 0.45 for 113 ms to high shear fields ($48–214 \times 10^3$/s), we found:

1. A significant increase of lysis-dependent parameters like PF 3 availability and β-TG liberation is observed with an increasing proportion of RBC present. The shear-induced fall in single platelet count, going far beyond the degree of possibly shear-destroyed platelets, and being a consequence of extensive aggregation already in PRP, is accordingly aggravated by addition of red cells. Addition of RBC, however, increases viscosity and consequently the actual shear force acting upon suspended cells. Extrapolating data from the literature,[30] viscosities of 1.5 mPa.s for a hematocrit of 0.17 and 2.5 mPa.s for whole blood diluted 1:10 with anticoagulant were considered conservative estimates.
2. Following correction for the hematocrit-dependent increase in shear stress, the presence of RBC does not significantly alter the increase in PF 3 availability in response to shear exposure (FIG. 8), nor does it change β-TG liberation.
3. However, taking the reduction of platelet count as a measure for platelet aggregation, it becomes evident that RBC at a hematocrit of 0.45 drastically enhance platelet aggregation following shear exposure on the order of 10^{-1}

seconds. At a hematocrit of 0.17 no increase in single platelet loss as compared to plain PRP occurs (FIG. 9).

During millisecond exposure to shear stress a biophysical effect of red cells in the sense of "shear-enhanced diffusivity" appears to dominate the influence of RBC on platelets. Based on microscopic observation in tube flow we prefer the term "microconvection " and suspect that a gross increase in platelet collisions plays a role in the enhancement of "shear-induced" platelet aggregation.[31] This interpretation does not preclude the possibility of a biochemical proaggregatory effect of ADP, becoming operational during the sampling time of our experiments.

LOCALIZED VORTEX FORMATION IN NONCYLINDRICAL BLOOD CONDUITS AS "BIOCHEMICAL FLOW REACTOR"

Acting for realistic time intervals shear forces beyond 100 N/m^2 primarily exert biophysical effects on blood cells. Besides increasing contact among themselves, lytic damage by tearing the plasma membrane appears to predominate. The extent of the subsequent activation of platelets and the coagulation system, leading to a "prethrombotic state" in the blood, appears to be largely a matter of experimental boundary conditions. They must, therefore, undoubtedly be considered secondary events.

In straight undisturbed tube flow, be it in artificial or natural blood conduits, the fluid dynamic boundary conditions do not foster the complicated interactions between mediators and cells and enzymes and proenzymes that constitute the early steps of thrombogenesis. As outlined in the INTRODUCTION undisturbed laminar flow in cylindrical conduits constitutes a truly "open" system, which differs profoundly from "closed" systems typically encountered in laboratory equipment, *e.g.*, aggregometers and coagulometers.

The localization of thrombi at segments deviating from cylindrical shape assigns a paramount role to fluid dynamic boundary conditions in the initiation and propagation of thrombosis. Typical examples would be valve prostheses (FIG. 10), entry ports with sudden expansion or constriction of conduit diameter, branchings, and bends.[32] Contemporary fluid dynamic analysis of the details of flow-through noncylindrical conduit segments has uncovered details of what is known as "separated flow." Application of microrheological techniques[33] and high-resolution laser Doppler anemometry[34] revealed more details of secondary flow that can be put into a functional perspective. The aforementioned examples of noncylindrical conduits are characterized by the occurrence of closed vortices ("eddies"), the contents of which are largely precluded from convective exchange with the "main stream." A vortex following a marked constriction preferentially receives blood flowing near the wall (FIG. 10), which in a constricted conduit segment has experienced peak shear stresses. For artificial heart valves shear forces certainly transgress the level critical for lysis of blood cells.[35] We therefore feel justified in introducing the term "traumatizing streamline," the blood elements traveling on which become, at least temporarily, trapped and thoroughly mixed in the recirculating poststenotic vortex. The feeding by the traumatizing streamline as well as its fluid dynamic seclusion render poststenotic vortices a "sieve" for damaged blood cells. They provide the closed environment wherein mediators from shear-destroyed platelets and red cells, mainly adenine nucleotides, can exert their platelet-activating effect. The abundance of procoagulant phospholipids facilitates the activation of thrombin, further activating platelets via a positive feedback loop. As far as macroscopic dimensions of vortices are concerned, convective mixing of its contents, molecules as well as cells, appears important for the propagation of the activation of the hemostatic system through repeated collisions of activated enzymes with their cofactor and substrate molecules, as well as contacts of mediators with their target cells.

The question of whether the lifetime of poststenotic vortices in pulsatile flow suffice to develop a prethrombotic state in blood must be left open to further elucidation. TEM micrographs suggest that during a lifetime of 0.5 s, platelet shape change reaction has proceeded to a notable extent (FIG. 11). Moreover pulsatile flow does not automatically mean a complete wash out of the vortex within each cardiac cycle.[36] With a residual volume of the vortex persisting throughout diastole, it becomes a permanent source of activated platelets and coagulation enzymes.

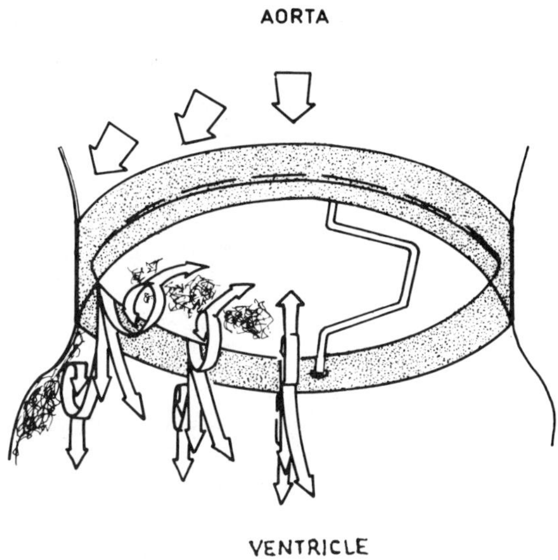

FIGURE 10. Schematic drawing of a Björk-Shiley valve prosthesis in aortic position from beneath. The streamlines of the jet flowing during diastole through the leak around the nonoccluding disk of the closed valve are shown on the left. Shear stresses well over 250 N/m^2 have been measured to act in the diastolic backflow jet, giving rise to mechanical blood trauma and thrombus formation on the ventricular side of the disk and the ventricle wall, where stagnation point flow occurs.

THE REATTACHMENT POINT AS THE SITE OF CONVECTIVE TRANSPORT OF ACTIVATED HEMOSTATIC COMPONENTS TO THE WALL

From the point where a sudden increase in conduit diameter causes the "main stream" to separate from the wall, vortices extend downstream until the main stream reattaches to the wall, and surface parallel laminar flow is reestablished. There streamlines inclined towards the wall provide convection onto the conduit lining. As the position of the reattachment point depends on the flow rate, it is bound to oscillate back and forth in pulsatile flow. The diastolic decrease in flow rate is inevitably associated with an involution of vortices, irrespective of their location. This means that "activated" blood is released into the circulation from the faltering vortex in diastole.

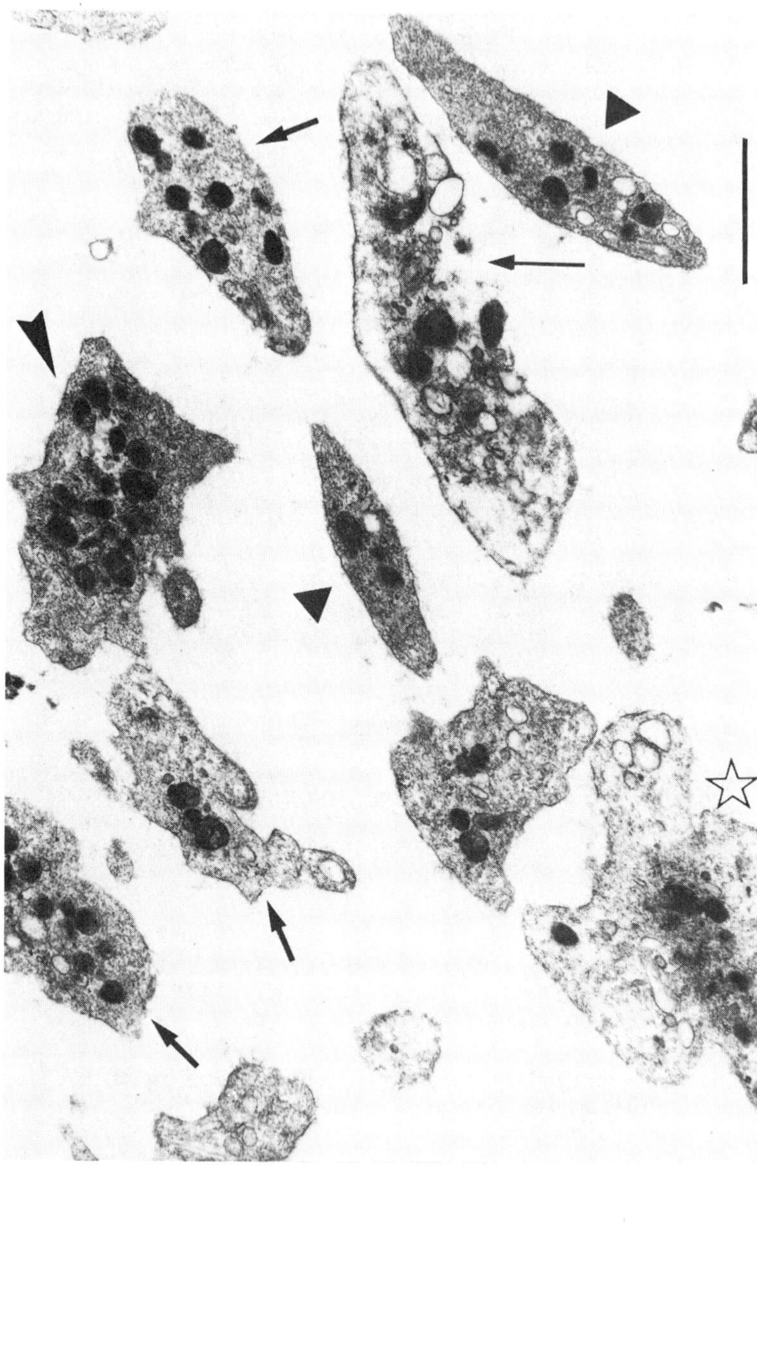

FIGURE 11. PRP fixed within 2 s after 113 ms exposure to 255 N/m^2. Platelets in various stages of activation and damage can be seen. *Triangles* show resting disks; *short arrows* show platelets early in shape change; the *arrowhead* marks a rounded platelet with pseudopods and centralized granules; the *long arrow* shows a discoid but leaky platelet, the *asterisk* a platelet almost ballooned. *Bar:* 1 μm.

Activated molecular and cellular components of the hemostatic system leave the vortex via streamlines at the border to the mainstream, which convey them to the reattachment points. This results in a strictly localized "showering" of the wall by the receding stagnation point, a mechanism we have suggested be named "Naumann vortex transport," in honor of the late A. Naumann.[37]

It is little wonder that reattachment points are sites where thrombosis takes place in natural and artificial vessels when two peculiarities of Naumann vortex transport are borne in mind: (1) convective transport of platelets to the wall by stagnation point

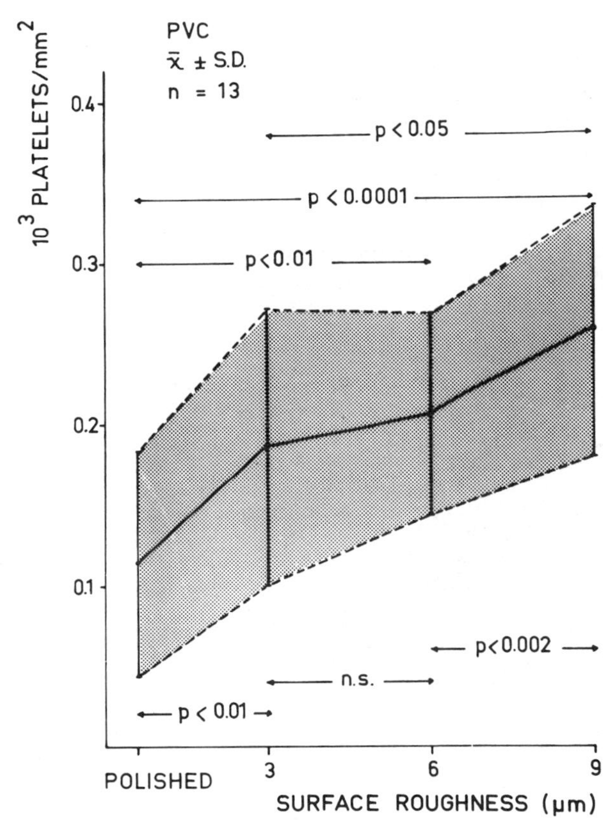

FIGURE 12. Platelet adhesion on a PVC polymer film as a function of surface irregularity.

flow is more effective by at least 2 orders of magnitude than RBC-mediated "microconvection" in surface parallel flow;[32] (2) compared to resting platelets, vortex-activated platelets have a greatly enhanced ability to form permanent thrombotic deposits.[38]

Using a technique that mimics the flow situation at the reattachment point[39] we could demonstrate the adhesion-enhancing effect of platelets stimulated with ADP, as well as the inhibitory effect of PGI_2. When testing polymer surfaces with defined roughness, we found that surface irregularities of the dimensions of single platelets ($\approx$3 μm) did in fact increase platelet deposition onto that surface by a factor of 1.5 (FIG. 12). In our view this underlines the importance of irregularities of conduit geometry, even on the micrometer level, for convective transport of blood cells to the wall and thrombogenesis in artificial blood conduits.

CONCLUSION AND SUMMARY

The activation of the complex network of enzyme cascades and cellular functions that make up the hemostatic system in particular and the unspecific defense system (UDS) in general requires a "closed" environment as provided by reaction tubes under *in vitro* conditions. *In vivo,* when blood is flowing rapidly through artificial conduits, comparatively simple fluid dynamic peculiarities regularly encountered at sites with noncylindrical conduit configuration are responsible for the activation of the hemostatic system with the adverse formation of thrombi. Three steps of pathogenetic significance can be delineated: (1) A localized increase in shear forces may inflict unspecific damage on blood cells. (2) The action of mediators from leaky cells, with intact platelets in fluid dynamically secluded vortices, allows simple damage to proceed to activation of platelets and enzymes. The self-amplificating properties of the system are only limited by the lifetime of the vortex. (3) Diastolic devolution of the vortex causes the spillage of activated "hemostatic components" onto the conduit lining at the reattachment point, thereby denoting the site of manifestation of a thrombogenic stimulus.

REFERENCES

1. GEHRMANN, G. & F. LOOGEN. 1964. Mechanische hämolytische Anämie nach Implantation künstlicher Aortenklappen. Dt. Med. Wschr. **89:** 625–630.
2. FORBES, C. D. & C. R. M. PRENTICE. 1978. Thrombus formation and artificial surfaces. Br. Med. Bull. **34:** 822–830.
3. BROWN, C. H., L. B. LEVERETT, C. W. LEWIS, C. P. ALFREY, JR. & J. D. HELLUMS. 1975. Morphological, biochemical, and functional changes in human platelets subjected to shear stress. J. Lab. Clin. Med. **86:** 462–472.
4. MÜLLER-ESTERL, W. 1985. The kinin-forming pathway and its role in blood-contact activation. *In* Enzyme Activation in Blood-Perfused Artificial Organs. H. Schmid-Schönbein, L. J. Wurzinger & R. E. Zimmermann, Eds.: 33–50. Martinus Nijhoff. Boston.
5. SCHMID-SCHÖNBEIN, H. 1979. Biological analysis of blood trauma: The response of the unspecific defense system to foreign technical apparatus. *In* Basic Aspects of Blood Trauma. H. Schmid-Schönbein & P. Teitel, Eds.: 1–22. Martinus Nijhoff. Boston.
6. ZWAAL, R. F. A., P. COMFURIUS & L. L. M. VAN DEENEN. 1977. Membrane asymmetry and blood coagulation. Nature **268:** 358–360.
7. ZIMMERMANN, R. E. 1985. Interactions of proteolytic systems in the plasma. *In* Enzyme Activation in Blood-Perfused Artificial Organs. H. Schmid-Schönbein, L. J. Wurzinger & R. E. Zimmermann, Eds.: 1–8. Martinus Nijhoff. Boston.
8. VARGAFTIG, B. B., M. CHIGNARD, J. LEFORT & J. BENVENISTE. 1980. Platelet-tissue interaction: Role of platelet-activating factor (PAF-acether). Agents Actions **10:** 502–506.
9. HELLUMS, J. D. & R. A. HARDWICK. 1981. Response of platetels to shear stress: A review. *In* Rheology of Biological Systems. D. R. Gross & N. H. C. Hwang, Eds.: 160–183. Sijthoff & Noordhoff. Alphen a. d. Rijn.
10. TILLMANN, W., H. REUL, M. HEROLD, K.-H. BRUSS & J. VAN GILSE. 1984. In-vitro wall shear measurements at aortic valve prostheses. J. Biomech. **17:** 263–279.

11. HEUSER, G. & R. OPITZ. 1980. A Couette viscometer for short time shearing of blood. Biorheology **17:** 17–24.
12. WÜTHRICH, C., D. A. DERANLEAU, D. DUBLER & E. F. LÜSCHER. 1984. Human blood platelet secretion: Optical multichannel analyser measurement using acriflavine as a release indicator. Biochemistry **23:** 1224–1229.
13. LUDLAM, C. A., S. MOORE, A. E. BOLTON, D. S. PEPPER & J. D. CASH. 1975. The release of a human platelet specific protein measured by a radioimmunoassay. Thromb. Res. **6:** 543–551.
14. WURZINGER, L. J., R. OPITZ, P. BLASBERG & H. SCHMID-SCHÖNBEIN. 1985. Platelet and coagulation parameters following millisecond exposure to laminar shear stress. Thromb. Haemostas. **54:** 382–386.
15. ANDERSON, G. H., J. D. HELLUMS, J. L. MOAKE & C. P. ALFREY. 1978. Platelet response to shear stress: Changes in serotonin uptake, serotonin release, and ADP induced aggregation. Thromb. Res. **13:** 1039–1047.
16. ANDERSON, G. H., J. D. HELLUMS, J. L. MOAKE & C. P. ALFREY. 1978. Platelet lysis and aggregation in shear fields. Blood Cells **4:** 499–507.
17. STEVENS, D. E., J. H. JOIST & S. P. SUTERA. 1980. Role of platelet prostaglandin synthesis in shear-induced platelet alterations. Blood **56:** 753–758.
18. ZWAAL, R. F. A., J. ROSING, G. TANS, E. M. BEVERS & H. C. HEMKER. 1980. Topological and kinetic aspects of phospholipids in blood coagulation. *In* The Regulation of Coagulation. K. G. Mann & F. B. Taylor Eds.: 95–115. Elsevier. Amsterdam.
19. WURZINGER, L. J., R. OPITZ, M. WOLF & H. SCHMID-SCHÖNBEIN. 1987. Ultrastructural investigations on the question of mechanical activation of blood platelets. Blut **54:** 97–107.
20. UGURBIL, K., H. HOLMSEN & R. G. SHULMAN. 1979. Adenine nucleotide storage and secretion in platelets as studied by ^{32}P nuclear magnetic resonance. Proc. Natl. Acad. Sci. U.S.A. **76:** 2227–2231.
21. CHARO, I. F., R. D. FEIMMAN & T. C. DETWILER. 1977. Interrelations of platelet aggregation and secretion. J. Clin. Invest. **60:** 866–873.
22. WURZINGER, L. J., R. OPITZ & H. ECKSTEIN. 1986. Mechanical bloodtrauma: An overview. Angeiologie **38:** 81–97.
23. WHITE, J. G., S. M. BURRIS, D. TUKEY, C. SMITH & C. C. CLAWSON. 1984. Micropipette aspiration of human platelets: Influence of microtubules and actin filaments on deformability. Blood **64:** 210–2144.
24. WURZINGER, L. J., R. OPITZ, M. WOLF & H. SCHMID-SCHÖNBEIN. 1986. Pharmacological interference with platelet damage by high shearing forces. *In* Recent Advances and New Developments in Hemostaseology. H. K. Breddin, N. Bender & R. E. Scharf, Eds.: 19–20. Karger, Basel.
25. LAMBERT, J. 1979. Mechanical red cell disruption. *In* Basic Aspects of Blood Trauma. H. Schmid-Schönbein & P. Teitel, Eds.: 300–311. Martinus Nijhoff. Boston.
26. BLACKSHEAR, P. L., JR. 1972. Mechanical hemolysis in flowing blood. *In* Biomechanics: Its Foundations and Objectives. Y. C. Fung, Ed.: 501–528. Prentice-Hall. Englewood Cliffs, NJ.
27. TURITTO, V. T. & H. R. BAUMGARTNER. 1975. Platelet interaction with subendothelium in a perfusion system: Physical role of red cells. Microvasc. Res. **9:** 335–344.
28. BERGQVIST, D. & K. E. ARFORS. 1980. Hemostatic plug formation in the isolated rabbit mesenteric preparation: An analysis of red blood cell participation. Thromb. Hemostas. **44:** 6–11.
29. REIMERS, R. C., S. P. SUTERA & J. H. JOIST. 1984. Potentiation by red blood cells of shear-induced platelet aggregation: Relative importance of chemical and physical mechanisms. Blood **64:** 1200–1206.
30. SCHMID-SCHÖNBEIN, H. 1977. Microrheology of erythrocytes and thrombocytes, blood viscosity and the distribution of blood flow in the microcirculation. *In* Handbuch der allgemeinen Pathologie, Vol. III (7). Mikrozirkulation. H. Meessen, Ed. Springer. Berlin.
31. BLASBERG, P., L. J. WURZINGER & H. SCHMID-SCHÖNBEIN. 1983. Microrheology of thrombocyte deposition: Effect of stimulation, flow direction, and red cells. *In* Fluid

Dynamics as a Localizing Factor for Atherosclerosis. G. Schettler, R. M. Nerem, H. Schmid-Schönbein, H. Mörl & C. Diehm, Eds.: 60–70. Springer. Heidelberg.

32. Murphy, E. A., H. L. Rowsell, H. G. Downie, G. A. Robinson & J. F. Mustard. 1962. Encrustation and atherosclerosis: The analogy between early in vivo lesions and deposits which occur in extracorporeal circulations. Can. Med. Ass. J. **87:** 259–274.
33. Goldsmith, H. L. 1972. The flow of model particles and blood cells and its relation to thrombogenesis. Prog. Hemostas. Thromb. **1:** 97–110.
34. Liepsch, D. & S. Moravec. 1984. Pulsatile flow of non-Newtonian fluids in distensible models of arteries. Biorheology **21:** 571–587.
35. Yoganathan, A. P., Y. R. Woo & H. W. Sung. 1986. Turbulent shear stress measurements in the vicinity of aortic heart value prostheses. J. Biomech. **19:** 433–442.
36. Hugh, A. E. & A. Fox. 1970. The precise localization of atheroma and its association with stasis at the origin of the internal carotid artery: A radiographic investigation, Br. J. Radiol. **43:** 377–384.
37. Schmid-Schönbein, H. & L. J. Wurzinger. 1986. Transport phenomena in pulsating post-stenotic vortex flow. An interactive concept of fluid-dynamic, hemorheological and biochemical processes in white thrombus formation. Nouv. Rev. Fr. Hematol. **28:** 257–267.
38. Wurzinger, L. J., P. Blasberg, M. van de Loecht, W. Suwelack & H. Schmid-Schönbein. 1984. Model experiments on platelet adhesion in stagnation point flow. Biorheology **22:** 399–413.
39. Wurzinger, L. J., P. Blasberg, F. Horii & H. Schmid-Schönbein. 1986. A stagnation point flow technique to measure platelet adhesion onto polymer films from native blood: A technical report. Thromb. Res. **44:** 401–406.

Rheology of Leukocytes[a]

SHU CHIEN,[b] KUO-LI PAUL SUNG,[b]
GEERT W. SCHMID-SCHÖNBEIN,[d] RICHARD SKALAK,[c]
EMILY A. SCHMALZER,[b] AND SHUNICHI USAMI[b]

[b]*Department of Physiology and Cellular Biophysics*
Columbia University
New York, New York 10032

[c]*Department of Civil Engineering and Engineering Mechanics*
and the Bioengineering Institute
Columbia University
New York, New York 10027

[d]*Department of Applied Mechanics and Engineering Sciences*
University of California, San Diego
La Jolla, California 92093

The rheological properties of blood cells constitute a significant factor in controlling flow dynamics in the microcirculation.[1] Because white blood cells (WBCs) have a larger volume and lower deformability[2,3] than the red blood cells (RBCs), they can play a significant role in affecting microcirculatory flow[4] despite their much lower volume concentration.

White blood cells are essentially spherical when observed in the living microcirculation. They may be passively deformed by hemodynamic stresses when traversing narrow capillaries, but they normally do not undergo active deformation during flow in the circulation.[5,6] Spontaneous active deformation of WBCs with protopod formation occurs *in vivo* during emigration across the endothelium,[7] migration in a chemotactic gradient,[8] and phagocytosis.[9] When human WBCs are kept *in vitro* in the presence of free Ca^{2+} ions they undergo spontaneous deformation and generate protopods. Such spontaneous active deformation is suppressed and the WBCs can maintain an essentially spherical shape if they are suspended in a Ca^{2+}-free medium with the presence of a chelator, *e.g.*, ethylenediamine tetraacetate (EDTA).[10]

Analysis of the rheological behavior of WBCs requires quantitative knowledge about their morphological characteristics, including the volume and surface area of the cell and of its nucleus. Although the WBCs are spherical in outline, the presence of membrane foldings provides an excess membrane area that allows cell deformation without area expansion. These morphological parameters together with the mechanical properties of the cell components determine the WBC deformability, especially during large deformations such as those involved in their release from the bone marrow or extravasation into the interstitium.

This paper represents a summary of several studies performed in our laboratory related to WBC rheology.[10–18] The mechanical properties of human WBCs in both the passive state (in the presence of EDTA) and the active state (in the presence of Ca^{2+}) have been studied by measuring the small deformation of these cells in response to a low aspiration pressure applied via a micropipette with a diameter considerably

[a]This work was supported by research grants from the National Heart, Lung and Blood Institute (nos. P01–HL–16851 and T32–HL–07114) and the Cystic Fibrosis Foundation.

smaller than that of the WBC. The analysis of the experimental results with the aid of a theoretical model has allowed the determination of the intrinsic rheological properties without significant contributions of the geometric factors. Large deformations of WBCs were also investigated by studying their filterability through polycarbonate sieves with 5 μm pores; the results of these tests are affected by both the geometric and intrinsic rheological properties of the cell.

METHODS

These studies were performed on fresh blood samples obtained from healthy human subjects using EDTA as anticoagulant unless otherwise noted.

Studies on WBC Morphology

White blood cells in freshly drawn blood samples were fixed in a buffered 2% glutaraldehyde solution (pH = 7.4). The cells were then washed in buffered 0.9% NaCl solution, postfixed with 1% OsO_4 for 1 h, and washed in cacodylate buffer and in distilled water. These postfixed cells were then processed for examination in a Zeiss (EM9 S2) transmission electron microscope. The three-dimensional geometry of the WBCs was calculated with the aid of stereological technique[19] from thin sections at random radial positions of the cells.

Micropipette Tests

The RBCs were allowed to sediment at room temperature for 25–40 min. The supernatant plasma containing WBCs, platelets, and a few RBCs, was collected with a Pasteur pipette. This WBC-rich plasma was diluted with a prefiltered, buffered saline-albumin solution to a concentration of approximately 50 WBCs/mm^3. The solution contained 0.9 g/dl NaCl, 0.1 g/dl EDTA, 0.25 g/dl bovine serum albumin, and 12 mM Tris, with pH adjusted to 7.4 by the dropwise addition of 1 N HCl. The osmolality as measured by means of the freezing point depression method was 300–310 milliosmoles (mOsm) per kg H_2O.

The experimental setup and procedure for the micropipette aspiration studies have been described elsewhere.[10,20] About 0.5–1 ml of the cell suspension was loaded in a small round chamber located on the stage of an inverted microscope. Individual WBCs were viewed with an 100× objective (NA 1.25, oil immersion) and a 20× eyepiece, and the viewing field was monitored through a video camera connected to the eyepiece for the display and recording of the video image.

Micropipettes with inner radii of 1.1–1.7 μm were filled with the buffered saline-albumin solution and mounted on a hydraulic micromanipulator. The wide end of the micropipette was connected to a pressure regulation system. The pressure level was monitored with the use of a Statham transducer connected to a recorder.

To analyze the time course of deformation of the neutrophils, sequential photographs were taken from the video images during single-frame replay on the video monitor. The data on the displacement of the cell into the pipette were entered into a PDP 11/10 minicomputer and analyzed by using a theoretical model,[10,16] in which the neutrophil is treated as a standard solid consisting of an elastic element K_1 in parallel with a Maxwell element (an elastic element K_2 in series with a viscous element μ).

Filtration Tests

Suspensions of RBCs and WBCs in various proportions were prepared from fresh human blood samples using a Tris-buffered Ringer solution (pH 7.4, containing 0.5 g/dl serum albumin) as the suspending medium. The suspension was pumped at a constant flow rate of 1.6 ml/min through polycarbonate sieves (Nuclepore Corp., Pleasanton, CA) with a mean pore diameter of 4.79 ± 0.19 (SD) μ, a pore density of $3.6 \times 10^5/\text{cm}^2$, and an effective filtration area of 0.79 cm^2. The filtration pressure (P) was recorded as a function of time (t) with the use of a Statham pressure transducer and a Grass recorder. Filtration pressure (P_o) was also determined for the Ringer solution. In some of the experiments the filter was removed at the end of the test and processed for electron microscopic examinations.

RESULTS AND DISCUSSION

WBC Morphology

All WBCs freshly fixed were spherical in their overall outline and had no protopods. Numerous cell membrane foldings are seen in an isotonic medium (300 mOsm) and also in hypertonic solution; they disappear in hypotonic solution (*e.g.*, 105 mOsm) and the cell shape becomes almost that of a smooth sphere.

TABLE 1. Geometric Characteristics of Human Erythrocytes and Leukocytes

	Whole Cell				Nucleus		
	Volume (μm^3)	Surface Area μm^2	Surface Area % Excess	D min[a] (μm)	Volume (μm^3)	Surface Area μm^2	Surface Area % Excess
Erythrocytes	90	140	44	2.7	—	—	—
Neutrophils	190	300	88	2.6	35	102	97
Eosinophils	206	324	92	2.6	37	99	84
Lymphocytes	120	270	130	1.8	50	90	40
Monocytes	230	430	137	2.2	52	108	62

[a]Minimum diameter the cell can achieve at constant area and volume for a cylindrical shape with hemispherical caps; the influence of nucleus on D_{min} is ignored in the calculation. (Data from Chien *et al.*[15])

The average volumes and membrane areas of various types of WBCs and their nuclei in isotonic medium are given in TABLE 1. The percentage of excess membrane area (σ) was calculated from the difference between the average cell membrane area (A_c) and the area (A_s) needed to cover a smooth sphere with the same volume as the cell:

$$\sigma = 100(A_c - A_s)/A_s. \quad (1)$$

The WBCs in physiological tonicity, because of the presence of membrane foldings, have more excess membrane area than the discoid RBCs. The value of σ varies among the various types of WBCs studied, averaging approximately 100%. The nuclei of the WBCs also have excess membrane areas. When suspended in hypotonic media the cell and the nucleus increase their volumes, while their membrane areas remain essentially constant and the values of σ decrease.

Passive Small Deformation of WBCs

These studies were performed on WBCs in EDTA and Ca^{2+}-free medium. The time course of deformation of a neutrophil in saline-albumin solution (pH 7.4, 300 mOsm, 21–23°C) in response to an aspiration pressure (ΔP = 3 mm H_2O) applied via a

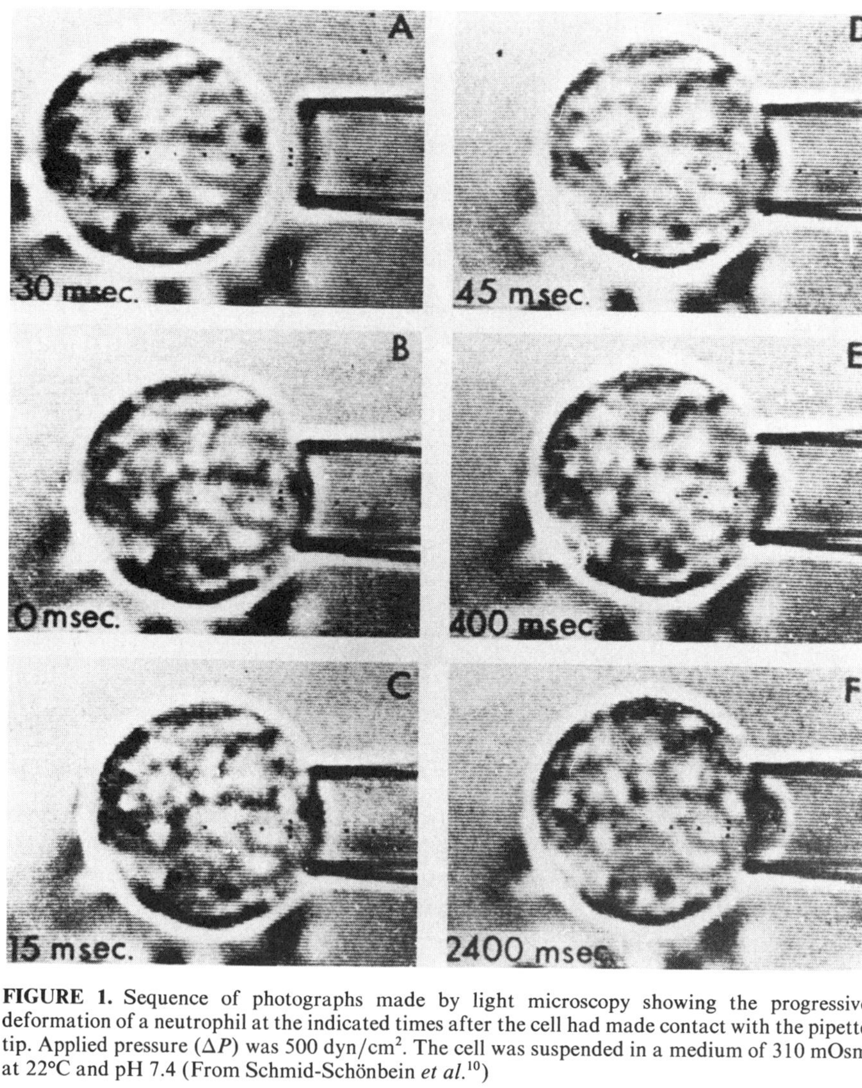

FIGURE 1. Sequence of photographs made by light microscopy showing the progressive deformation of a neutrophil at the indicated times after the cell had made contact with the pipette tip. Applied pressure (ΔP) was 500 dyn/cm^2. The cell was suspended in a medium of 310 mOsm at 22°C and pH 7.4 (From Schmid-Schönbein *et al.*[10])

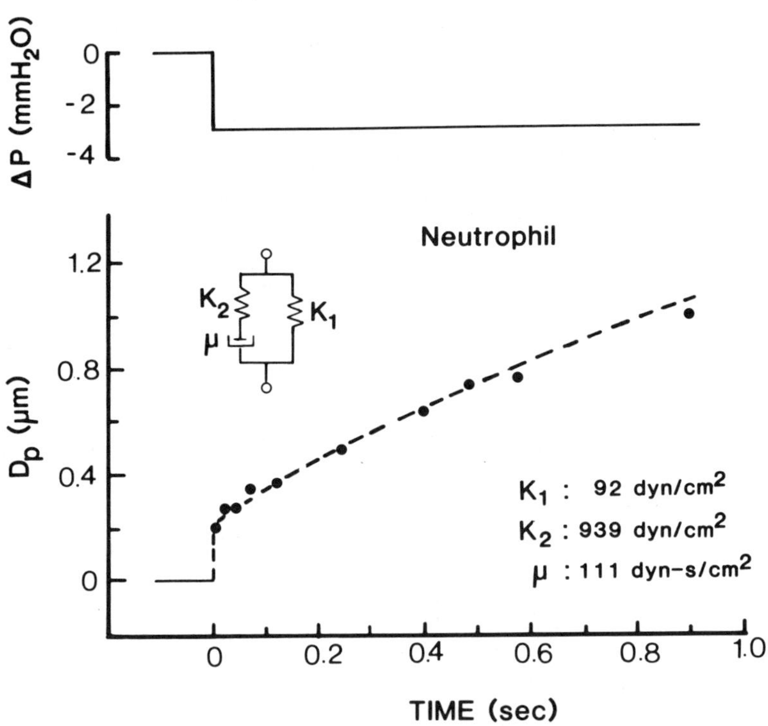

FIGURE 2. Time courses of deformation, $d(t)$, of a human neutrophil in response to a step aspiration pressure, $\Delta P(t)$. The data points were fitted with the theoretical model (*dashed line*) by the use of the K_1, K_2, and μ values tabulated in the figure. (From Chien *et al.*[15])

micropipette (radius = 1.7μm) is illustrated by the example in FIGURE 1. The WBC moves rapidly toward the pipette tip and seals it within 1 or 2 television frames (16–32 ms). At the time the WBC makes contact with the pipette tip (zero time), it already shows an elastic deformation essentially synchronous with the applied pressure. As shown in FIGURE 2, the initial rapid response is followed by a slow creep displacement; the dashed line for $d(t)$ represents the best fit of the standard solid model[10] to the experimental data, and the coefficients K_1, K_2 and μ are listed in the figure. Thus, at the beginning of neutrophil deformation, the cell behaves like an elastic body with a shear modulus of $(K_1 + K_2)/2$. The initial slope of the deformation curve at the end of the initial deformation is proportional to $K_1K_2/[(K_1^2 + K_2^2)\mu]$, and the maximum

TABLE 2. Viscoelastic Coefficients of Leukocytes in Small Passive Deformation[a]

Coefficients	Neutrophils	B Lymphocytes	T Lymphocytes
K_1 (dyn/cm^2)	275 ± 14	221	451
K_2 (dyn/cm^2)	737 ± 40	502	819
μ (dyn/sec · cm^2)	130 ± 6	145	206

[a]The leukocytes were suspended in isotonic saline-albumin-EDTA solution (pH 7.4, 310 mOsm, 21–23°C). Values given for neutrophils (n = 75) are mean ± SEM (Data from Chien *et al.*[15])

displacement after long times is proportional to $1/K_1$. The values obtained for K_1, K_2, and μ are shown in TABLE 2. The results are similar for neutrophils and peripheral B lymphocytes; the peripheral T lymphocytes tend to have higher viscoelastic coefficients.

The standard solid model gives the average properties of the cell, including the stress contributions by all cytoplasmic structures and the membrane. In an isotonic medium, when there exists a large excess membrane area, the contribution of the cell geometry to the viscoelastic behavior during small deformations is probably negligible.[10] The response is dominated by the cell interior, including the cortical cytoskeletal network subjacent to the cell membrane.

The viscoelastic behaviors of WBCs can be compared with those of RBCs. In order to effect a comparable steady-state deformation into micropipettes with an inner radius (R_p) $\simeq 0.5$ μm, the value of the stress parameter $(\Delta P)R_p$ needed for neutrophils is approximately four times that for RBCs. The time constant (τ) of the neutrophil

TABLE 3. Comparison of Rheological and Geometric Properties of Human Erythrocytes and Neutrophils

	Erythrocytes	Neutrophils
Cell volume (μm^3)	90	190
Surface area (μm^2)		
Measured	140	300
Calculated for sphere with same volume	97	160
Excess surface area (μm^2)	43(44%)	140 (88%)
Minimum cylindrical diameter (μm)	2.7	2.6
Deforming stress needed for $D_{pm}/R_p = 3$ (dyn/cm)[a]	0.025	0.10
Time constant for small deformation (ms)	20–120[a,b]	650
Cellular viscosity (poise)	0.7	130

[a] D_{pm} is the steady-state deformation and R_p is the pipette radius. The value for erythrocytes reflects membrane behavior.

[b] Time constant for initial, rapid deformation phase; this value reflects membrane behavior of erythrocytes.

deformation can be calculated as

$$\tau = \mu[(1/K_1) + (1/K_2)]. \tag{2}$$

The τ value of approximately 650 ms is nearly an order of magnitude larger than that of the RBC membrane.[20] The viscosity of the neutrophil interior is approximately 130 P, which is more than four orders of magnitude higher than the value of $0.07P$ for the viscosity of the normal RBC interior.[21] The rheological and geometric properties of human neutrophils and RBCs are compared in TABLE 3.

Effects of Physicochemical Factors on Neutrophil Deformability

The effects of variations in osmolality (52 to 664 mOsm) have been studied in neutrophils.[13] The values of K_1, K_2, and μ rise nearly exponentially with increasing osmolality of the suspension medium from 200 mOsm to 660 mOsm (FIGURE 3); this reflects the effect of an increase of intracellular solid concentration. With a reduction of osmolality from 200 to 150 mOsm, K_2 increases slightly, but K_1 and μ are not significantly changed. This relative constancy of the viscoelastic coefficients probably

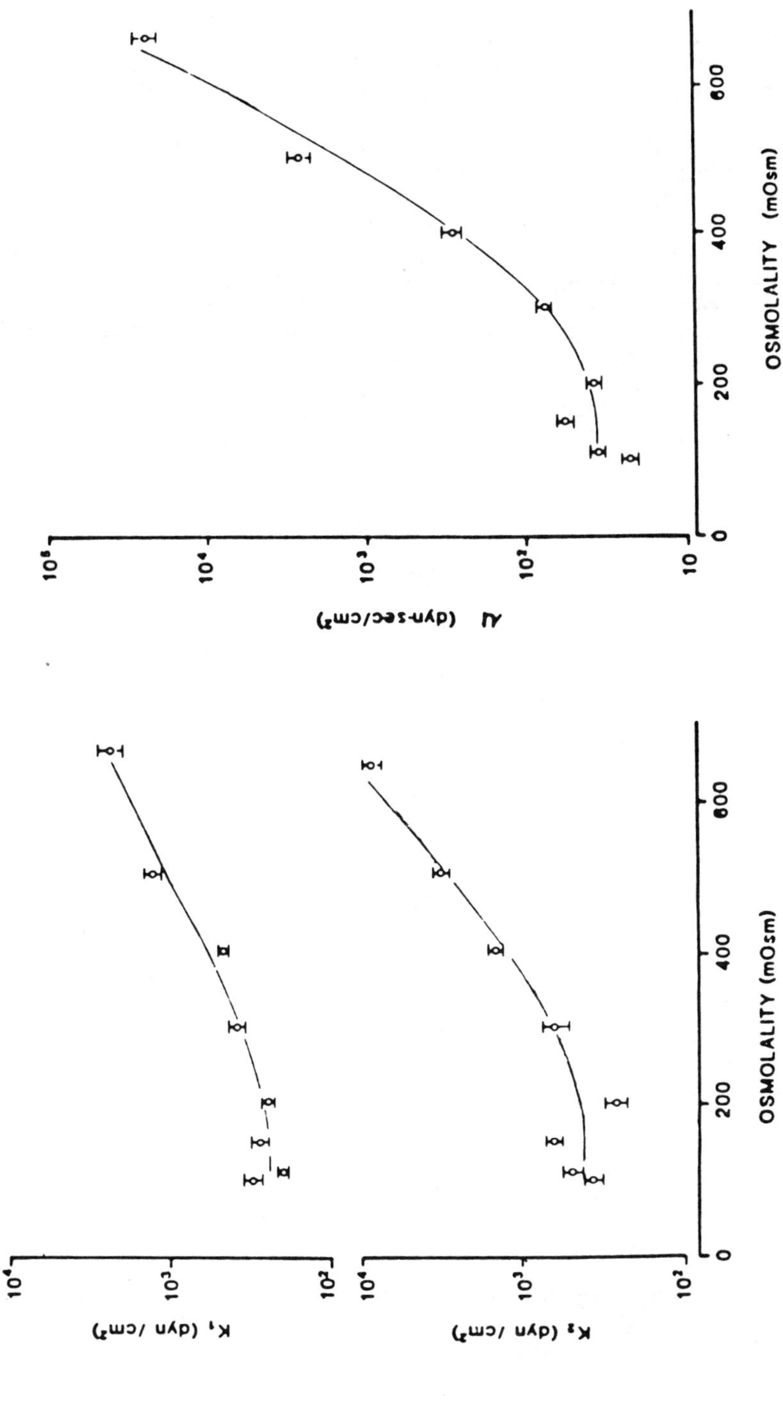

FIGURE 3. The viscoelastic coefficients K_1, K_2, and μ as a function of osmolality of the suspension media at room temperature at pH 7.4. *Vertical bars* represent SEM. (From Sung *et al.*[13])

represents a balance between the decrease in solid concentration and the increase in cell sphericity. In suspending media with an osmolality ≤100 mOsm, the neutrophil, if not yet lysed, does not deform in response to aspiration pressure as the cell becomes swollen to approach a smooth sphere. At these very low osmolalities, the smoothly spherical cell is essentially nondeformable despite the marked dilution of the cell interior.

Incubation of neutrophils with colchicine causes the disruption of microtubules. The mechanical properties of WBCs in EDTA treated with colchicine have been compared with untreated controls run at the same time (FIGURE 4).[17] Colchicine treatment does not alter the value of K_1, but it results in significant decreases of both K_2 (to 61% of control) and μ (to 15% of control). Incubation of neutrophils with cytochalasin B, an agent causing the disruption of microfilaments, results in a decrease of all three elements (K_1 to 40% of control, K_2 to 50%, and μ to 12%). These findings suggest that both the microfilaments and microtubules play significant roles in governing the passive rheological properties of the neutrophils; their disruption leads to a decrease in the viscoelastic coefficients of the cell. Furthermore, the results indicate that the microfilaments and the microtubules have different roles in the control of the cellular rheological properties. The microtubules apparently are not important in determining K_1, whereas the disruption of microfilaments has an influence on all three elements.

Viscoelastic Properties of Neutrophils in the Active State

These studies were performed on neutrophils obtained from fresh heparinized blood samples and suspended in a Ringer-albumin solution (Ca^{2+} concentration = 2 mM) without EDTA.[12] These WBCs deform spontaneously to develop irregular cell shapes with protopod projections, as described by Lichtman *et al.*[22]

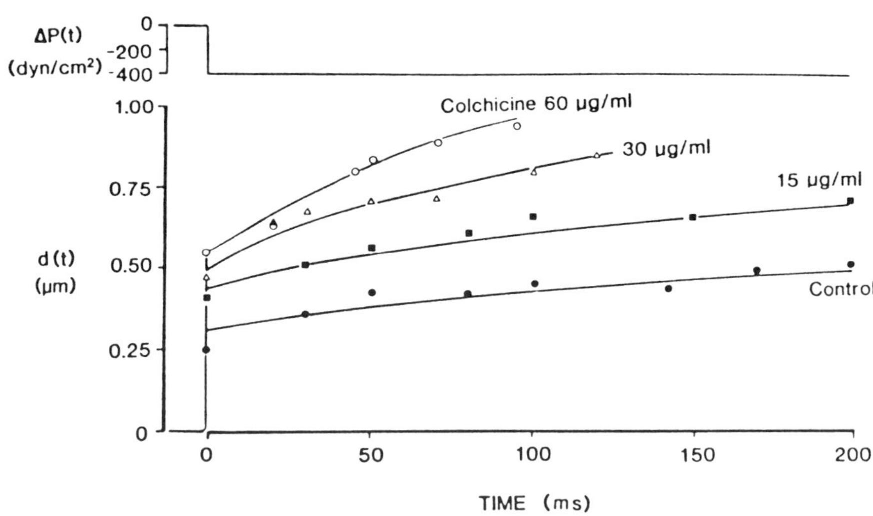

FIGURE 4. Micropipette aspiration pressure, $\Delta P(t)$, and deformation, $d(t)$, for neutrophils treated for 30 min with 15, 30, and 60 μg/ml colchicine and for control neutrophils. (From Chien and Sung.[17])

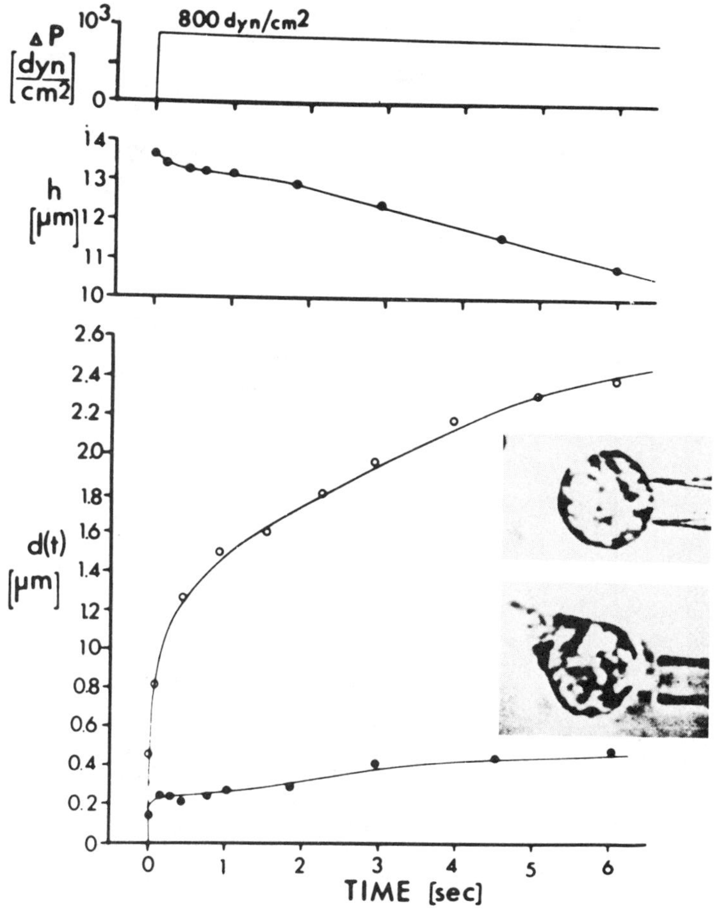

FIGURE 5. Micropipette aspiration pressure, $\Delta P(t)$, and deformation, $d(t)$, for a cell aspirated at the main cell body (*open circles*) and at a small protopod (*closed circles*). (From Schmid-Schönbein *et al.*[12])

In those neutrophils with protopod formation, the rheological properties of the main cell body and the protopod have been compared by measuring their deformation responses to the same micropipette aspiration pressure. Following the application of an aspiration pressure ΔP of 800 dyn/cm^2, the resulting deformation $d(t)$ at the main cell body shows the typical slow creep, as in the passive state (FIGURE 5). In response to the same ΔP of 800 dyn/cm^2, the deformation in the region of the protopod is significantly smaller and shows very little creep. When an aspirated protopod rejoins the main body of the cell, a prominent nonlinear creep develops during the maintenance of a steady aspiration pressure.

Actin-like and myosin-like proteins, as well as other proteins which interact to control their polymerization, are present in WBCs.[23–25] Gelation of these proteins probably generates the protopods and changes the mechanical properties of the cell. The granules, mitochondria, and nucleus, which together account for 37% of the cell volume, are excluded from the protopod.[12] Local changes in Ca^{2+} concentration probably play a significant role. A theoretical analysis describing the mechanical phenomena of active deformation has been made.[16]

Filterability of WBCs through Polycarbonate Sieves

To study the passage of whole WBCs through narrow channels, the filterability of WBC suspensions across polycarbonate sieves has been measured by the constant flow

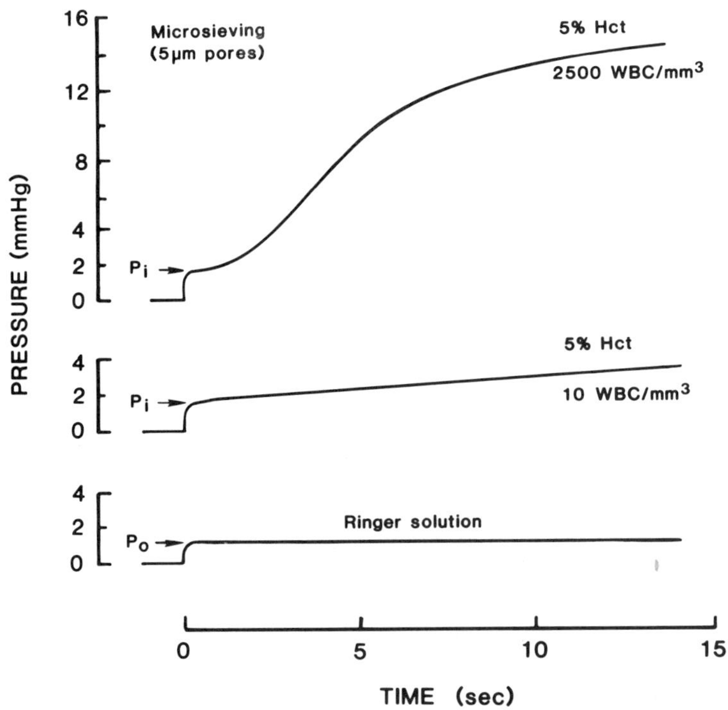

FIGURE 6. Pressure-time curves of (from bottom to top) a cell-free Ringer solution, a cell suspension containing 5% hematocrit and 10 WBCs/mm^3, and a cell suspension containing 5% hematocrit and 2500 WBC/mm^3, filtered through 5 μm polycarbonate sieves at a constant flow rate. (From Chien *et al.*[15])

technique.[26,27] When a cell-free Ringer-albumin solution is pumped through a polycarbonate sieve at a constant flow rate, the filtration pressure P_o rises to attain a constant level in 1 second or less (FIGURE 6). The filtration pressure time curve for a suspension of RBCs at a hematocrit of 5% (containing very few WBCs), pumped through the same sieve at the same flow rate, shows an initial rise in filtration pressure to attain a quasi-steady pressure reading P_i in less than 2 seconds, and this is followed by a gradual subsequent pressure rise with continued filtration at a constant flow rate. The value of P_i varies linearly with hematocrit up to 25%, or a red cell concentration,

[RBC], of $\simeq 3.3 \times 10^6/\text{mm}^3$. At a given [RBC], *e.g.*, $6 \times 10^5/\text{mm}^3$, P_i is not significantly affected by WBC concentration, [WBC], up to $0.12 \times 10^5/\text{mm}^3$. An increase in [WBC], however, causes a significant acceleration in the pressure rise after the attainment of P_i. In order to obtain a comparable slope of this pressure rise, the [RBC] needed is approximately 700-fold higher than [WBC]. That is, each WBC is equivalent to about 700 RBCs in causing this pressure rise. This result is in keeping with the finding that the cellular viscosity of WBCs is three orders of magnitude higher than the viscosity of the RBC content (TABLE 3). Another interesting point to be noted is that the normal [RBC] of $5 \times 10^6/\text{mm}^3$ is approximately 700 times the normal [WBC] of $7 \times 10^3/\text{mm}^3$.

The geometric relationship between the cell volume and membrane area of WBCs is such that they should be able to deform to pass through as narrow a channel (2.7 μm or less) as the RBCs (TABLE 3). The relative inability of WBCs to traverse 5 μm channels, as compared to RBCs, is mainly attributed to the difference in their viscoelastic properties. As mentioned above, although the steady-state deformation behavior of WBCs is only four times stiffer than that of RBCs, the cellular viscosity of WBCs is more than 1000 times higher than that of RBCs (TABLE 3). Another factor that would impede WBC passage through 5 μm channels is the presence of the nucleus, which is less deformable than the cell cytoplasm.

The filtration data indicate that the P_i represents an average behavior of the overall cell population studied, with each cell having essentially equal weighting; the slope of the subsequent pressure rise, however, is dominated by the less deformable cells, even though they may be present only in a very low proportion. This comes about because the less deformable cells traverse the narrow pores very slowly or not at all, thus progressively reducing the number of pores available for filtration as the constant flow delivery of cells proceeds with time. These results illustrate the potential importance of increased [WBC] in causing microvascular obstruction. The obstruction of the filter pores by WBCs can be shown by scanning and transmission electron microscopy.[15]

Treatment of WBCs with 10 mM pentoxifylline causes a reduction in filtration resistance through 5 μm polycarbonate sieves; studies of fractionated WBC populations indicate that the effect is exerted on monocytes and polymorphonuclear leukocytes, but not lymphocytes.[29] The increase in WBC filterability following pentoxifylline can be correlated with a concurrent inhibition of protopod formation.[29]

Physiological and Pathophysiological Implications of WBC Rheology

The results of these morphometric and rheological investigations have considerable implications concerning the functional roles of WBCs in health and disease. The low deformability and slow transit of WBCs through narrow vessels influence the flow dynamics in a microcirculatory network.[30] In a divergent bifurcation, the entry of a WBC into one branch will raise the flow resistance and reduce the flow rate in that branch (FIGURE 7A). As a result, the RBCs arriving subsequently at the branch point will be diverted into the other branch until the attainment of a new balance of resistances and flow rates.[28] In a convergent branch, *e.g.*, postcapillary venules, the interaction between a WBC and RBCs arriving from the two feeding capillaries may displace the WBC toward the venular endothelium (FIGURE 4B) and force them to roll along the wall.[6,30] Therefore, the WBCs tend to occupy a strategic position for the perception of chemotactic signals from the extravascular space and the ready emigration across the vessel wall when needed. The migration of WBCs toward the vessel wall is further enhanced when there is RBC aggregation.[31,32]

The strong influence of [WBC] on filter plugging indicates that an abnormal

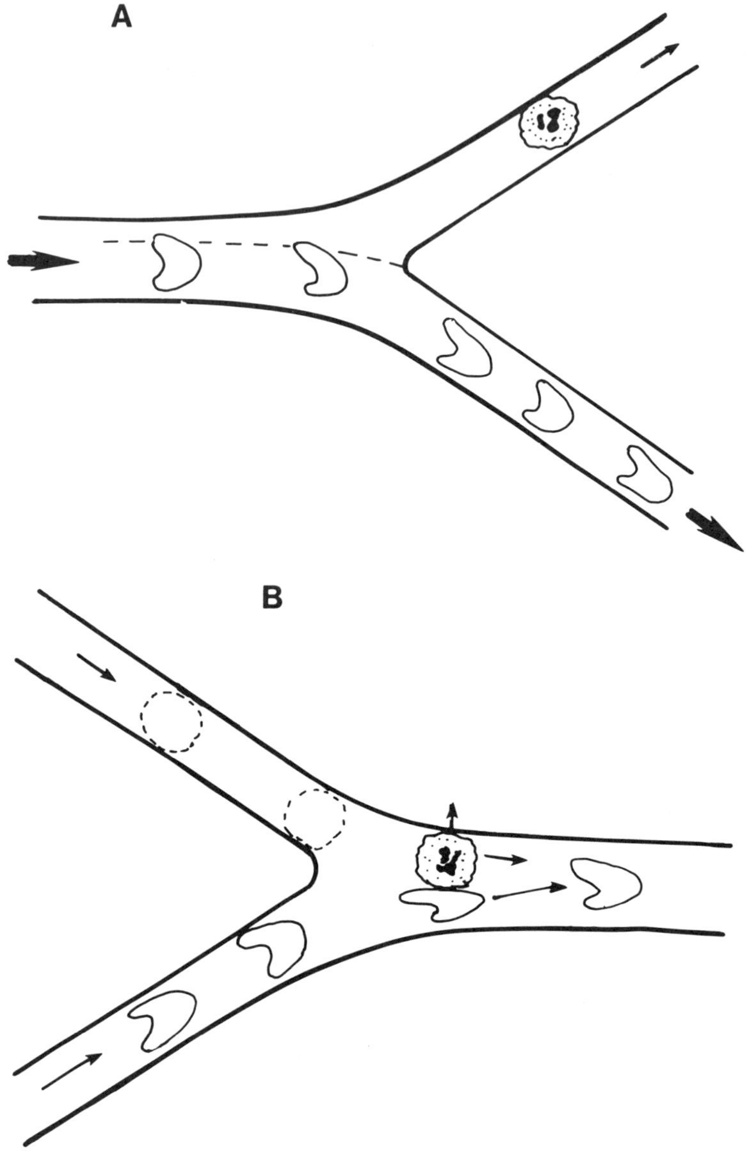

FIGURE 7. (**A**) Schematic drawing of a divergent capillary bifurcation showing the influence of the entry of a WBC into one branch on the flow rates (indicated by the relative sizes of the *arrows*), the partitioning of the streamlines in the parent vessel (indicated by the *dashed line*), and the preferential entry of the subsequently arriving RBCs into the other branch. (**B**) Schematic drawing of a convergent microvascular branch point showing the influence of RBCs on the WBC, causing the WBC to remain in a flow stream very close to the endothelium. (From Chien *et al.*[15])

elevation of [WBC] may lead to microvascular obstruction.[33] In addition to total [WBC], other important factors to be considered are the relative proportion of the various types of leukocytes, their rheological properties, and their adhesiveness to the walls of the flowing channel. The deformability and adhesiveness of the WBCs may be adversely affected in various low flow states, including cerebral ischemia, thus enhancing the probability of microvascular obstruction by WBCs and aggravating the flow disturbance.[4,34] On the other hand, compensatory vasodilation may improve the passage of WBCs, and this may be the mechanism by which leukemic patients can survive very high concentrations of circulating leukocytes. Therefore, the pathophysiological role of WBCs in affecting the microcirculation must be considered in concert with other parameters and functions, *e.g.*, vessel geometry, flow dynamics, and interactions between WBCs and other cells.

SUMMARY

The rheological properties of human leukocytes (WBCs) have been studied by micropipette aspiration and filtration tests. A small aspiration pressure applied via a micropipette (diameter $\simeq$3 μm) causes the WBC to undergo a rapid elastic deformation followed by a slow creep. The data can be analyzed with a viscoelastic model: an elastic element K_1 in parallel with a Maxwell element (elastic element K_2 in series with viscous element μ). Neutrophils and B lymphocytes are similar in K_1, K_2, and μ, but these values are higher for T lymphocytes. Treatment of neutrophils with colchicine decreases K_2 and μ without changing K_1, whereas cytochalasin B decreases all three coefficients; these results indicate the importance of cytoskeletal microtubules and microfilaments in WBC rheology. In the presence of Ca^{2+}, WBCs form protopods which have increased viscoelastic coefficients. Inhibition of protopod formation with pentoxifylline is associated with an increase in WBC deformability. The ruffled surface of the apparently round WBC provides an area about twice that needed to enclose a smooth sphere of the same volume; this geometric feature plays an important role in whole WBC deformability tested through 4–5 μm filter pores or micropipettes. Because of its larger volume and higher cellular viscosity, each WBC is equivalent to approximately 700 erythrocytes in its tendency to block 5-μm channels. The rheology of WBCs has significant implications in their functional behavior, including flow through the microcirculation and interaction with endothelial cells.

REFERENCES

1. Chien, S. 1982. Rheology in the microcirculation in normal and low flow states. Adv. Shock Res. **8:** 71–90.
2. Lichtman, M. A. 1973. Rheology of leukocytes, leukocyte suspensions and blood in leukemia. J. Clin. Invest. **52:** 350–358.
3. Miller, M. E. & K. A. Myers. 1975. Cellular deformability of the human peripheral blood polymorphonuclear leukocyte: Method of study, normal variation, and effects of physical and chemical alterations. J. Reticuloendothel. Soc. **18:** 337–345.
4. Braide, M., B. Amundsson, S. Chien & U. Bagge. 1984. Quantitative studies on the influence of leukocytes on the vascular resistance in a skeletal muscle preparation. Microvasc. Res. **27:** 331–352.
5. Bagge, U. & P. I. Branemark. 1977. White blood cell rheology: An intravital study in man. Adv. Microcirc. **7:** 1–17.
6. Schmid-Schönbein, G. W., S. Usami, R. Skalak & S. Chien. 1980. The interaction of

leukocytes and erythrocytes in capillary and postcapillary vessels. Microvasc. Res. **19:** 45–70.
7. MARCHESI, V. T. & H. W. FLOREY. 1960. Electron micrographic observations on the emigration of leukocytes. Q. J. Exp. Physiol. **45:** 343–347.
8. GALLIN, J. I. & P. C. QUIE, Eds. 1978. Leukocyte Chemotaxis: Methods, Physiology and Clinical Implications. Raven Press. New York.
9. ELSBACH, P. 1974. Phagocytosis. *In* The Inflammatory Process, Chap. 1. 2d edit. B. W. Zweifach, L. Grant, R. T. McCluskey, Eds: 363–410. Academic. New York.
10. SCHMID-SCHÖNBEIN, G. W., K. L. P. SUNG, H. TÖZEREN, R. SKALAK & S. CHIEN. 1981. Passive mechanical properties of human leukocytes. Biophys. J. **36:** 243–256.
11. SCHMID-SCHÖNBEIN, G. W., Y. Y. SHIH & S. CHIEN. 1980. Morphometry of human leukocytes. Blood **56:** 866–875.
12. SCHMID-SCHÖNBEIN, G. W., R. SKALAK, K. L. P. SUNG & S. CHIEN. 1982. Human leukocytes in the active state. *In* White Blood Cells: Morphology and Rheology as Related to Function. U. Bagge, G. V. Born, P. Gaehtgens, Eds. Martinus Nijhoff. The Hague.
13. SUNG, P., G. W. SCHMID-SCHÖNBEIN, R. SKALAK, G. B. SCHUESSLER, S. USAMI & S. CHIEN. 1982. Influence of physicochemical factors on rheology of human neutrophil. Biophys. J. **39:** 101–106.
14. CHIEN, S., E. A. SCHMALZER, M. M. L. LEE, T. IMPULLUSO & R. SKALAK. 1983. Role of white blood cells in filtration of blood cell suspensions. Biorheology **20:** 11–27.
15. CHIEN, S., G. W. SCHMID-SCHÖNBEIN, K. L. P. SUNG, E. A. SCHMALZER & R. SKALAK. 1984. Viscoelastic properties of leukocytes. *In* White Cell Mechanics: Basic Science and Clinical Aspects. H. I. Meiselman, M. A. Lichtman, P. L. LaCelle, Eds: 19–51. Alan R. Liss. New York.
16. SKALAK, R., S. CHIEN & G. W. SCHMID-SCHÖNBEIN. 1984. Viscoelastic deformation of WBC: Theory and analysis. *In* White Cell Mechanics: Basic Science and Clinical Aspects. H. J. Meiselman, M. A. Lichtman & P. L. LaCelle, Eds: 1–18. Alan R. Liss. New York.
17. CHIEN, S. & K. L. P. SUNG. 1984. Effect of colchicine on viscoelastic properties of neutrophils. Biophys. J. **46:** 383–386.
18. CHIEN, S. 1985. Influence of inflammation on white cell rheology. *In* Cellular Aspects of Inflammation: Potentials for Drugs. G. A. Marcel, Ed.: 11–18. Lab. Roussel. Paris.
19. UNDERWOOD, E. 1970. Quantitative Stereology. Addison-Wesley. Reading, MA.
20. CHIEN, S., K. L. P. SUNG, R. SKALAK, S. USAMI & A. TÖZEREN. 1978. Theoretical and experimental studies on viscoelastic properties of erythrocyte membrane. Biophys. J. **24:** 463–487.
21. COKELET, G. R. & H. J. MEISELMAN. 1968. Rheological comparison of hemoglobin solutions and erythrocyte suspensions. Science **162:** 275–277.
22. LICHTMAN, M. A., P. A. SANTILLO, E. A. KEARNEY, G. W. ROBERTS & R. I. WEED. 1976. The shape and surface morphology of human leukocytes in vitro: Effect of temperature, metabolic inhibitors and agents that influence membrane structure. Blood Cells **2:** 507–531.
23. HARTWIG, J. H. & T. P. STOSSEL. 1975. Isolation and properties of actin, myosin, and a new actin binding protein in rabbit alveolar macrophages. J. Biol. Chem. **250:** 5696–5705.
24. SHIBATA, N., T. TAKUBO & N. SENDA 1979. Ca^{2+}-sensitive contractile protein from leucocytes. *In* Cell Motility: Molecules and Organelle. S. Hatano, H. Ishikawa, H. Sato, Eds: 13–31. University Park Press. Baltimore.
25. STOSSEL, T. P. & T. D. POLLARD. 1973. Myosin in polymorphonuclear leukocytes. J. Biol. Chem. **248:** 8288–8294.
26. SCHMALZER, E. A., R. SKALAK, S. USAMI, M. VAYO & S. CHIEN. 1983. Influence of red cell concentration on filtration of blood cell suspensions. Biorheology **20:** 29–40.
27. USAMI, S., S. CHIEN & J. F. BERTLES. 1975. Deformability of sickle cells as studied by microsieving. J. Lab. Cliln. Med. **86:** 274–279.
28. SCHMID-SCHÖNBEIN, G. W., S. USAMI, R. SKALAK & S. CHIEN. 1980. Cell distribution in capillary networks. Microvasc. Res. **19:** 18–44.
29. SCHMALZER, E. A. & S. CHIEN. 1984. Filterability of supopulations of leukocytes: Effect of pentoxifylline. Blood **2:** 542–546.

30. BAGGE, U. & R. KARLSSON. 1980. Maintenance of white blood cell margination at the passage through small venular junctions. Microvasc. Res. **20:** 92–95.
31. CHIEN, S., S. USAMI & R. SKALAK. 1984. Blood flow in small tubes. *In* Handbook of Physiology: Microcirculation, Vol. 1. E. M. Renkin & C. Michel, Eds: 217–249. American Physiological Society. Washington, D.C.
32. NOBIS, U. & P. GAEHTGENS. 1981. Rheology of white blood cells during blood flow through narrow tubes. Bibliotheca Anat. **20:** 211–214.
33. PRESTON, F. E., R. J. SOKOL, J. S. LILEYMAN, D. A. WINFIELD & E. K. BLACKBURN. 1978. Cellular hyperviscosity as a cause of neurological symptoms in leukemia. Br. Med. J. **1:** 476–8.
34. BAGGE, U., B. AMUNDSON & C. LAURITZEN. 1980. White blood cell deformability and plugging of skeletal muscle capillaries in hemorrhagic shock. Acta Physiol. Scand. **108:** 159–163.

The Interaction between Leukocytes and Endothelium *in Vivo*[a]

GEERT W. SCHMID-SCHÖNBEIN,[b] RICHARD SKALAK,[c] SCOTT I. SIMON,[b] AND ROBERT L. ENGLER[d]

[b]*Department of Applied Mechanics and Engineering Sciences-Bioengineering*
University of California, San Diego
La Jolla, California 92093

[c]*Department of Civil Engineering and Engineering Mechanics*
Bioengineering Institute
Columbia University
New York, New York 10027

[d]*Department of Medicine*
Cardiology Division and Research Service
Veterans Administration Medical Center
La Jolla, California 92093

INTRODUCTION

The significance of leukocyte-endothelium interaction as part of the inflammatory process has long been recognized.[1] Recent evidence suggests that the adhesion to endothelium plays a key role during the obstruction of capillaries and in the no-reflow phenomenon.[2] Adhesion between granulocytes and endothelium requires close contact between membranes (in the nanometer range) so that molecular interaction becomes possible. A multitude of naturally occurring and synthetic agents appear to be able to modulate the adhesion. It is an essential part of the action of the specific and unspecific immune cells.

Traditional methods to estimate the strength of adhesion between leukocytes and endothelium membranes have relied largely on indirect measurements of adhesion, such as the number of cells per area of endothelium. They have led to the discovery of a number of agents and chemicals which modulate the adhesion *in vivo* (TABLE 1). Numerous other factors have been discovered by means of *in vitro* tests of adhesion to tissue cultures or artificial surfaces.[19] There is evidence that adhesion is modulated in some circulatory circumstances by plasma factors and membrane proteins, by their synthesis and transport in the cell, and by their motility in the membrane. In several cases of cell interaction, adhesion is associated with pseudopod projection and this adhesion is of fundamental importance to determine cell traffic in organs during normal conditions and infections, chronic disease, aging, and death. The need to understand the details of adhesion and its modulation is apparent.

Dembo and Bell[20] have provided a theoretical framework for the molecular

[a]This work was supported in part by USPHS grant no. HL-10881, by a grant from Dr. Karl Thomae, GmbH, Federal Republic of Germany, and the Academic Senate of the University of California, San Diego.

interaction during adhesion in terms of specific receptor sites and nonspecific repulsion between membranes. The receptors are assumed to be laterally mobile in the membrane and capable of making reversible bonds with an appropriate substrate. The limiting cell shapes during attachment and with surface-volume ratios were derived. Such a formulation is attractive but cannot be exploited currently because of a lack of quantitative experimental observations.

In order to obtain specific information on the leukocyte-endothelium membrane adhesion, measurements of the adhesion energy are needed. Since a number of natural substances appear to be involved, it is desirable to obtain the measurement *in vivo*. In this report the natural rolling of granulocytes on the endothelium of postcapillary venules will be used as basis for estimation of the adhesion energy in this *in vivo* situation.

TABLE 1. Some Factors Affecting Granulocyte Adhesion to Vascular Endothelium *in Vivo*

Trauma (heat, shear, compression, etc.)	Clark and Clark[3] Zweifach[4]
Saline wash	Giddon and Lindke[5] Görög and Born[6]
Lysosomal proteins	Janoff and Zweifach[7]
Ca^{2+}	Allison and Lancaster[8] Atherton and Born[9]
Glucocorticoid	Ebert and Barclay[10]
Lidocaine	Giddon and Lindke[5]
Casein, *E. coli* culture filtrate	Atherton and Born[9]
fMLP peptides	Fehr and Jacob[11]
Leukotriene B_4	Dahlén *et al.*[12]
Prostaglandin inhibitors (sulfinpyrazone, aspirin, indomethacin)	Tuma[13]
Complement	Hammerschmidt *et al.*[14]
Viral infection of endothelial cells	MacGregor *et al.*[15]
PAF-ester	Benveniste *et al.*[16]
Neuraminidase treatment of endothelial cells	Görög and Born[6]
Adenosine (*in vitro*)	Cronstein *et al.*[17]
Basic membrane glycoprotein (lactoferrin)	Boxer *et al.*[18]

ANALYSIS

The Adhesion Energy

In the undeformed state, granulocytes have a spherical shape with numerous membrane surface folds. During attachment to the endothelium the cell membrane unfolds and forms a contact area. Separation of the membranes requires energy, namely the adhesion energy E_a, to break the bonds. E_a is associated with a fracture stress, γ, such that

$$\gamma = \frac{dE_a}{dA_c}, \tag{1}$$

where A_c is the area of contact being debonded during the separation process. E_a is the resultant of all energies involved in the membrane interaction due to osmotic forces, electrostatic forces, van der Waal forces, molecular bridging, etc.; γ has the dimension of a tension (dyn/cm) and serves as a measure for the strength of the adhesion. The objective of our experiments and analysis is to obtain an estimate of γ.

Leukocyte Rolling on the Endothelium

Since the leukocyte cytoplasm has viscoelastic properties,[22] the energy provided by the bloodstream during rolling of the cells on vascular endothelium is dissipated predominantly into two parts. There is energy loss due to deformation of the cell, E_d, and there is a energy loss to overcome the adhesion, E_a. The cell also gains some energy, E_a^*, due to contact formation at its leading edge. Since the cell is small the kinetic energy may be neglected. If we also neglect active pseudopod formation and the associated energy gain from biochemical sources, then the rate of work done on the cell is equal to the sum of the dissipation rates:

$$\frac{dE}{dt} = \frac{dE_a}{dt} - \frac{dE_a^*}{dt} + \frac{dE_d}{dt}.$$

For a viscoelastic material, such as the leukocyte protoplasm, E_d consists of an elastic part that is recoverable and a viscous part that is dissipated. During the typical rolling to be considered below, however, the net rate of energy gain, $-dE_a^*/dt$, is small due to dissipation during extrusion of the plasma fluid film and stretching of the membrane; then

$$\frac{dE}{dt} = \frac{dE_a}{dt} + \frac{dE_{-d}}{dt}. \tag{2}$$

On the other hand, if the cell is adhered to the wall of a vessel without flow, $dE/dt = 0$, and there is only attachment without detachment, so $dE_a/dt = 0$. Then, from equation **1**:

$$\frac{dE_a^*}{dt} = -\frac{dE_d}{dt}.$$

This is the case of passive cell spreading. The energy gained due to formation of attachment bonds is transformed into the energy needed for the elastic deformation of the cell plus the viscous dissipation. The degree of spreading is limited by the available membrane area and possibly by the receptor density.[20]

To find the work done on the cell rolling on the wall without slip, we note that the velocity of the cell is approximated by a rigid body motion (using the index notation of Fung[21]):

$$v_i = e_{ijk}\,\omega_j\,r_k^P + v_i^P, \tag{3}$$

where v_i^P is the velocity at the cell centroid P and r_k^P the radius vector from P, ω_j is the cell rotational velocity, and e_{ijk} is the permutation symbol as usually defined in index notation; double indices indicate a summation over spatial directions from 1 to 3.

The surface traction, T_i, on the plasma membrane of the cell due to the plasma fluid stress σ_{ij} is

$$T_i = \sigma_{ij}\,\nu_j, \tag{4}$$

where ν_j is the outer normal unit vector from the surface of the cell. The rate of work done by the blood flow is

$$\frac{dE}{dt} = \iint_{S_f} T_i v_i \, dS, \tag{5}$$

where S_f is the part of the cell surface exposed to the plasma flow. Substitution of equations **3** and **4** into **5** gives

$$\frac{dE}{dt} = \iint_{S_f} \sigma_{ij}\nu_j v_i^P \, dS + \iint_{S_f} \sigma_{ij}\nu_j e_{imk}\omega_m r_k^P \, dS \tag{6}$$

$$= v_i^P \iint_{S_f} \sigma_{ij}\nu_j \, dS + \omega_m \iint_{S_f} \sigma_{ij}\nu_j e_{imk} r_k^P \, dS \tag{7}$$

$$= v_i^P F_i + \omega_m M_m, \tag{8a}$$

where F_i is the resultant force on the cell, and M_i the resultant moment taken about point P. In a unidirectional rolling motion with centroid velocity v_W and rotational velocity ω_W, equation **8a** reduces to

$$\frac{dE}{dt} = v_W F + \omega_W M. \tag{8b}$$

To find the work done by the internal stresses, σ_{ij}, in deforming the cell cytoplasma, note that the rate of work done by the cell surface traction T_i and by the body force X_i is

$$\frac{dE_d}{dt} = \int_S T_i v_i \, dS + \int_V X_i v_i \, dV.$$

With equation **4** and using the Gauss theorem we obtain

$$\frac{dE_d}{dt} = \int_V \frac{\partial}{\partial x_j}(\sigma_{ij} v_i) + X_i v_i \, dV$$

which in equilibrium reduces to

$$\frac{dE_d}{dt} = \int_V \sigma_{ij} \dot{V}_{ij} \, dV, \tag{9}$$

where V_{ij} is the rate of deformation tensor,

$$\dot{V}_{ij} = \frac{1}{2}\left(\frac{\partial v_i}{\partial x_j} + \frac{\partial v_j}{\partial x_i}\right), \tag{10}$$

S the cell surface, and V is the cell volume. Equation **9** applies irrespective of the cell material properties. In the passive state the cell cytoplasm for small strains can be approximated by a standard solid viscoelastic model[22]:

$$\sigma'_{ij} + \frac{\mu}{k_2}\dot{\sigma}'_{ij} = e'_{ij} k_1 + \dot{e}'_{ij}\mu\left(1 + \frac{k_1}{k_2}\right), \tag{11}$$

where σ'_{ij} is the stress deviator such that

$$\sigma'_{ij} = \sigma_{ij} - \tfrac{1}{3}\,\sigma_{kk}\,\delta_{ij} \tag{12}$$

and $\dot{\sigma}'_{ij} = d\sigma'_{ij}/dt$ is the material time derivative; δ_{ij} is the Kronecker symbol and e'_{ij} the strain deviator

$$\begin{aligned} e'_{ij} &= e_{ij} - \tfrac{1}{3}\,e_{kk}\,\delta_{ij} \\ &= e_{ij}, \end{aligned} \tag{13}$$

since the cytoplasma in the absence of fluid escape is incompressible and we assume $e_{kk} = 0$. For small strains $\dot{e}_{ij} = \dot{V}_{ij}$. This completes the general formulation of the leukocyte rolling. The process is assumed to be driven by fluid stresses only without involvement of pseudopod formation. This is in agreement with the observation that the leukocyte rolling motion ceases instantaneously if the surrounding fluid flow is stopped. The motion produced by pseudopods is significantly slower and essentially independent of plasma flow.

Next we present a dimensional analysis of the variables involved in the experimental measurement of the fracture stress and thereafter we estimate its value. In the absence of a complete solution of the problem we shall make an estimate of the fracture stress using an idealized case.

Dimensional Analysis

Since the Reynolds number of the flow field around the leukocyte on postcapillary endothelium is small ($10^{-2} - 10^{-3}$), the resultant force and moment acting on the cell are in first approximation proportional to the midstream red cell velocity, v_R, and white cell velocity v_W according to $v_R - \alpha v_W$ and $v_R - \beta v_W$, respectively. ω is proportional to v_W, so that according to equation **8**

$$\frac{dE}{dt} = C_1\,v_W\,v_R - C_2\,v_W^2 \tag{14}$$

where v_W is the axial velocity component of the leukocyte centroid parallel to the wall. The rate of work done by the internal stresses (equation **9**) for small cytoplasmic deformation is proportional to v_W^2, so that in linear approximation

$$\frac{dE_d}{dt} = C_3\,v_W^2, \tag{15}$$

where C_1, C_2, C_3, α and β are two constants whose value depends on the shape of the cell, its material properties, the plasma viscosity, and the diameter. During the rolling motion with a continuous peeling of membrane along the trailing edge

$$\frac{dE_a}{dt} = \gamma\,\frac{dA_c}{dt} = \gamma h v_W, \tag{16}$$

according to equation **1**; h is the width of the contact area normal to the rolling direction. Combining equations **14** to **16** with **2** yields

$$\gamma = \frac{v_R}{h}\left(C_1 - (C_2 + C_3)\,\frac{v_W}{v_R}\right). \tag{17}$$

This equation shows that for modest degrees of deformation and constant v_R and geometry the fracture stress is a function of the ratio of leukocyte and centerline velocity. The lower the velocity ratio the higher the fracture stress. Thus, measurements of this velocity ratio together with the vessel and cell geometry serve as a basis for estimation of the fracture stress. Furthermore, measurement of the velocity ratio can serve as a measure of the fracture stress if the effects of different drugs or agents on adhesion are to be investigated. This is the rationale for the experiments to be reported below.

The Magnitude of the Fracture Stress

In the absence of a complete analysis to find γ we shall make an order of magnitude estimate with some idealizations. According to equations **1** and **2**,

$$\gamma = \left(\frac{\mathrm{d}A_c}{\mathrm{d}t}\right)^{-1} \left(\frac{\mathrm{d}E}{\mathrm{d}t} - \frac{\mathrm{d}E_d}{\mathrm{d}t}\right). \tag{18}$$

To estimate the work done by the blood ($\mathrm{d}E/\mathrm{d}t$) according to equation **8b** we note that the resultant shear force F and moment M on such a cell at rest and in contact with the wall is[23]

$$F = \tilde{C}_1\, 6\pi\mu_{PL} \left(\frac{d_c}{2}\right)^2 \dot{V} \tag{19a}$$

and

$$M = \tilde{C}_2\, 4\pi\mu_{PL} \left(\frac{d_c}{2}\right)^3 \dot{V} \tag{19b}$$

$\tilde{C}_1 = 1.7005$ and $\tilde{C}_2 = 0.944$ are constants, μ_{PL} is the plasma viscosity, d_c the cell diameter, and $\dot{V}$ the shear rate at the wall in the absence of the cell. In Poisseuille flow $\dot{V} = v_R\, 4/d$, where v_R is the centerline velocity and d the vessel diameter. Since a rolling cell with overall spherical shape has a rotational velocity $\omega_W = v_W/(d_c/2)$ then after substitution of equations **19** into equation **8b**

$$\frac{\mathrm{d}E}{\mathrm{d}t} = v_W\, v_R \frac{4\pi\mu_{PL}}{d} \left(\frac{d_c}{2}\right)^2 (6\,\tilde{C}_1 + 4\,\tilde{C}_2). \tag{20}$$

When a white blood cell forms contact with the endothelium the largest deformation occurs adjacent to the contact area. To estimate the work done by the internal stresses we shall neglect such detailed features and consider a modest compression of the cell such as is often seen in such vessels. We assume that the cell is compressed into an obloid spheroid with wall contact and with axis $a_1 = (1 + \epsilon)(d_c/2)$ parallel to the wall and $a_2 = (1 - \epsilon)\,(d_c/2)$ normal to the wall; ϵ is a small strain such that $\epsilon > 0$ and $\epsilon \ll 1$. This is a case similar to the tank treading motion discussed by Keller and Skalak.[24] The motion is assumed to be in a plane which is parallel to the vessel axis and perpendicular to the vessel wall. Following a material point around its elliptical path, the displacement components relative to axes rotating with the particle angular velocity ω are

$$u = (x \cos 2\omega t + y \sin 2\omega t)\,\epsilon \tag{21a}$$

$$v = (x \sin 2\omega t = y \cos 2\omega t)\,\epsilon \tag{21b}$$

$$\omega = 0,$$

x, y, and z being coordinates with origin in the center of the ellipsoidal cell and ω the angular velocity of rotation, which is related to the cell centroid velocity v_W and axis $a_1 = (1 - \epsilon)(d_c/2)$ as

$$\omega = 2\pi\, v_W / a_1. \tag{22}$$

The strains for small deformation theory are

$$e_{ij} = \frac{1}{2}\left(\frac{\partial u_i}{\partial x_j} + \frac{\partial u_j}{\partial x_i}\right),$$

so that in this case the only nonvanishing strain components are

$$e_{11} = \epsilon \cos 2\omega t \tag{23a}$$

$$e_{22} = -\epsilon \cos 2\omega t \tag{23b}$$

$$e_{12} = \epsilon \sin 2\omega t. \tag{23c}$$

The nonzero components of the small strain rate are

$$\dot{e}_{11} = -2\omega\epsilon \sin 2\omega t \tag{24a}$$

$$\dot{e}_{22} = 2\omega\epsilon \sin 2\omega t \tag{24b}$$

$$\dot{e}_{12} = 2\omega\epsilon \cos 2\omega t \tag{24c}$$

which in this case are equal to the rate of deformation tensor $\dot{V}_{ij}$

$$\dot{e}_{ij} = \frac{\partial e_{ij}}{\partial t} = \dot{V}_{ij}. \tag{25}$$

Since the cell cytoplasm is incompressible the strain and strain rate deviator are $e_{ij} = e'_{ij}$ and $\dot{e}_{ij} = \dot{e}'_{ij} = \dot{V}'_{ij}$, respectively. The associated deviatoric stress components can be derived from the constitutive equation **11** for the cell cytoplasm as

$$\sigma'_{11} = A \cos 2\omega t + B \sin 2\omega t \tag{26a}$$

$$\sigma'_{22} = -A \cos 2\omega t - B \sin 2\omega t \tag{26b}$$

$$\sigma'_{12} = -B \cos 2\omega t + A \sin 2\omega t \tag{26c}$$

where

$$A = \left(\tau_0 - 2\omega \frac{\mu}{k_2}\tau_1\right) \bigg/ \left[1 + \left(2\omega \frac{\mu}{k_2}\right)^2\right]$$

$$B = \left(\tau_1 - 2\omega \frac{\mu}{k_2}\tau_0\right) \bigg/ \left[1 + \left(2\omega \frac{\mu}{k_2}\right)^2\right]$$

with $\tau_0 = \epsilon k_1$ and $\tau_1 = -\epsilon 2\omega\mu(1 + k_1/k_2)$.

Using equations **24**, **25**, and **26**, we can now compute the energy dissipation by the cytoplasmic stresses according to equation **9** to find an average value after a full cell rotation of

$$\frac{\overline{dE_d}}{dt} = \frac{\epsilon^2 \omega V}{1 + \left(2\omega \frac{\mu}{k_2}\right)^2} \left[\omega\mu\left(1 + \frac{1}{k_2}\right) - k_1\right], \quad \textbf{(27)}$$

where V is the cell volume. In order to obtain a numerical value for the fracture stress γ according to equation **18**, we note from previous measurements[22] that on average for neutrophils $\mu = 130$ dyn sec/cm^2, $k_1 = 275$ dyn/cm^2, and $k_2 = 737$ dyn/cm^2. The normal compression is typically $\epsilon = 0.1$ for cells rolling with $v_W = 0.01022$ cm/s at a centerline velocity $v_R = 0.2$ cm/sec in a vessel with diameter $d = 22$ μm (see EXPERIMENTAL RESULTS). To estimate the break of contact area at the trailing edge of the cell we assume for a uniform membrane attachment

$$\frac{dA_c}{dt} = v_W \ell, \quad \textbf{(28)}$$

where ℓ is the width of the contact which for a neutrophil with diameter $d_c = 8$ μm is of the order of $\ell = 6$ μm. Assuming a plasma viscosity $\mu_{PL} = 0.014$ dyn sec/cm^2 we can find the fracture stress from equations **18**, **20**, and **27** as

$$\gamma = 3.4 \times 10^{-3} \text{ dyn/cm}.$$

In this case the energy dissipated in the cell protoplasm is about 22% of the total energy provided by the bloodstream. The majority (78%) is dissipated by the peeling process. If the cell should become subject to a large deformation, for example during elongation into a teardrop shape, the internal dissipation may increase in magnitude, particularly during rapid rolling.

EXPERIMENTAL METHODS

Sprague-Dawley rats 15–20 weeks of age were given general anesthesia with Alfathesin, 10 mg/kg i.p. followed by 10 mg/(kg · h) continuous femoral intravenous infusion (Glaxovet, Baronia, Australia). The mesentery was exposed through an abdominal midline incision and draped loosely over a transparent pedestal for microscope transillumination. The intestine was covered with a plastic sheet and the mesentery was suffused with a balanced Krebs electrolyte solution saturated in the reservoir with 95% N_2 and 5% CO_2 gas mixture at pH = 7.7 and 36°C. The animal was covered and kept at 37°C body temperature with a heating pad.

Individual postcapillary venules in the mesentery were observed through an intravital microscope (Leitz, Wetzlar, FRG) with a 25× salt water immersion lens (NA = 0.8) and 10× ocular lens (FIGURE 1). The vessel was viewed with bright field illumination and fluorescence illumination (Ploempak, Leitz, West Germany) after intravital staining of leukocytes with acridin orange (2% solution in saline, continuous i.v. infusion at about ½ ml/h). The image of the cells and vessels was recorded with a silicone-intensified target TV camera (Model 4400 COHU, San Diego) displayed on a monitor and stored on a videocassette recorder for replay.

In each venule the following measurements were obtained: (1) the red cell centerline velocity v_R by means of the dual split photometric velocimeter by Tompkins *et al.*[25] with the calibration of Lee *et al.*,[26] and (2) the centroid axial velocity of individual white cells v_W during single frame replay of the video record. The position of

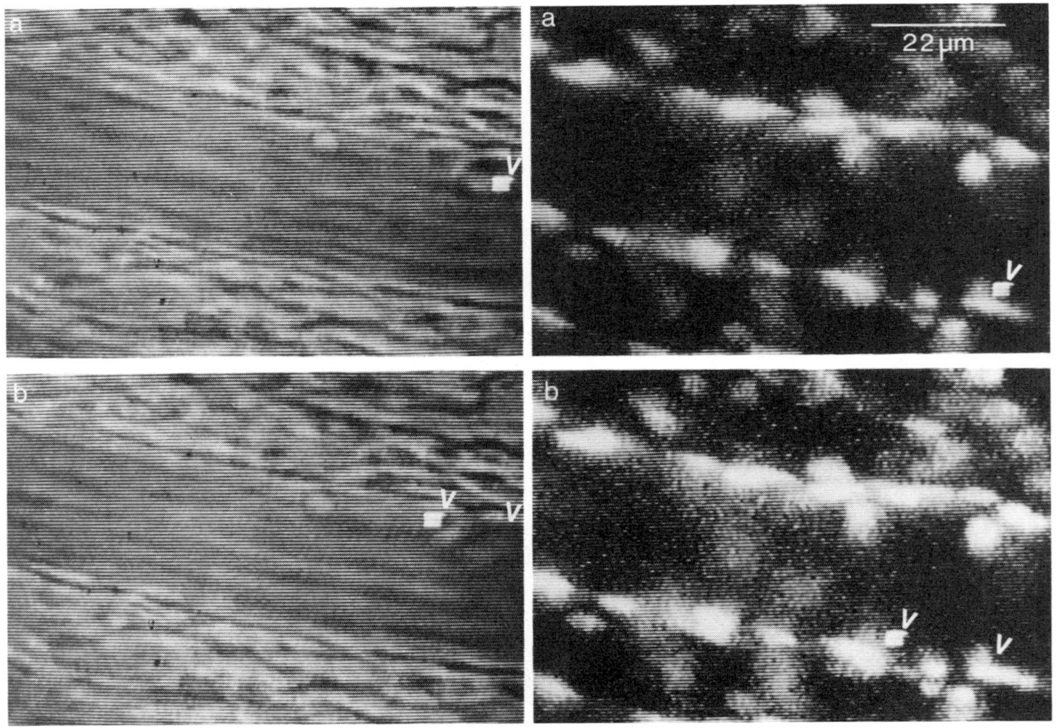

FIGURE 1. Micrograph of a postcapillary venule in the rat mesentery under bright field illumination (*left panels*) and fluorescence illumination (*right panels*). For fluorescence microscopy the cells were stained intravitally with a fluorochrome (acridin orange). The micrographs were taken directly from the television screen. Two TV frames are shown in each case, about 100 ms apart from each other. The flow direction in the venule is from the right to the left and white square marker (indicated by the *arrow*) shows the position of the rolling white blood cells. In panels **b** the initial and final positions are marked.

the white cells was marked on each TV frame by placement of a videomarker controlled through a joystick (Model 204A, Videophotoanalyzer, IPM, San Diego) and whose position is recorded through an analog-digital converter in a laboratory computer. From these white cell positions the cell velocity v_W was computed with appropriate length and time calibration.

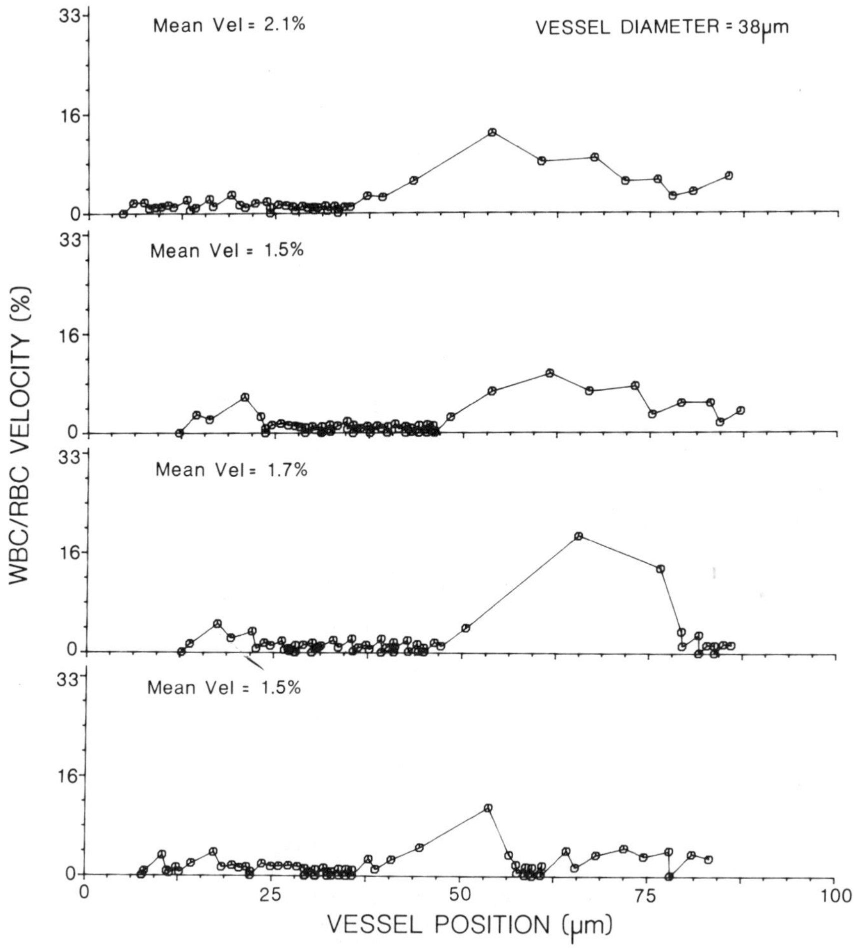

FIGURE 2. The ratio of white cell rolling velocity and center line red cell velocity v_W/v_R as a function of vessel position for a set of four randomly selected granulocytes on the endothelium of a venule with diameter of about 38 μm. The mean velocity ratios were computed as temporal averages. The center line velocity v_R was essentially unchanged over the observation period.

EXPERIMENTAL RESULTS

FIGURE 2 shows the experimental records of the velocity ratio v_W/v_R of four different neutrophils passing the same local segment of a postcapillary venule. The vessel position is the same in all four cases, showing that there is a region (up to about 40–50 μm) where granulocytes are rolling slower than in the more distal wall region (between 50 and 75 μm in FIGURE 2). Such endothelial locations with slow rolling cells are common in the vessels and have been found in all animals investigated so far. FIGURE 3 shows the velocity ratio, v_W/v_R, as a function of position averaged over 20 cells. The averages for the 20 cells were computed at selected locations in intervals of 5 μm along the length of the vessel segment under observation (shown by the open

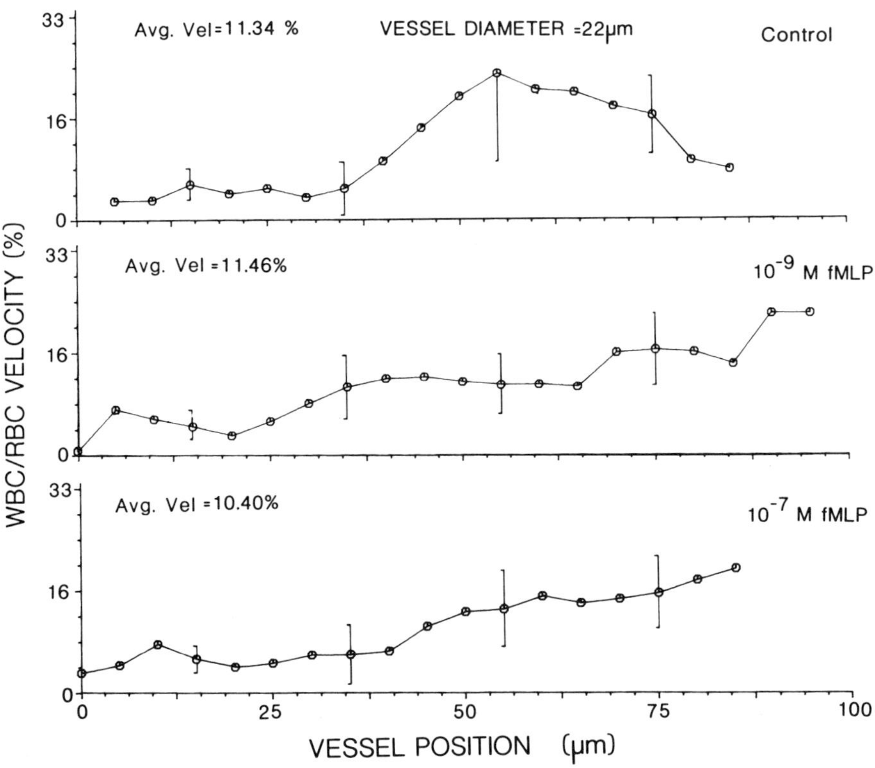

FIGURE 3. The velocity ratio, v_W/v_R, as a function of vessel position. The velocity ratio was averaged over 20 granulocytes at selected locations along the endothelium (vessel position). Only granulocytes that are still rolling are included in this data set. Three cases are shown: a control period, and during 10^{-9} M and during 10^{-7} M fMLP topical application for about 10–15 minutes.

symbols in FIG. 3). Three cases are shown: a control period within about 30 minutes after exposure, and two periods during which 10^{-9} M and 10^{-7} M *n*-formyl-methionyl-leucyl-phenylalanine (fMLP) were applied to the mesentery in the superfusion solution. The velocity ratio was derived only for those cells that continue to roll along the endothelium. Regions that initially show slow rolling, so-called sticky spots (between about 0 and 30 μm in FIGURE 3) do not show a significant reduction of rolling velocity, whereas regions with higher rolling velocities show considerably slower rolling in the presence of fMLP. It should be noted that in addition to a reduced rolling velocity the subpopulation of permanently adhering cells in the presence of fMLP is increased considerably. Thus for many cells the fracture stress is increased to the point where detachment from the endothelium is impossible under the resultant force and moment exerted by the bloodstream. If the temporal average velocity ratio is computed by inclusion of such stationary granulocytes (FIGURE 3) it is 6.5% and 2.1% in the presence of 10^{-9} M and 10^{-7} M fMLP, respectively.

DISCUSSION

One of the limitations of an *in vivo* test of adhesion is the range over which the fracture stress can be estimated. Since the applied force and moment on the cell is generated by the bloodstream the cell cannot be detached when there is strong adhesion to the endothelium. An example would be the attachment in the presence of high concentrations of fMLP ($>10^{-6}$ M). In such a situation all cells adhere to the endothelium without rolling motion, they project pseudopods and spread, and the fluid forces are too small to detach the cells. The adhesion energy cannot be directly measured *in vivo*. This situation is also common for virtually all *in vitro* adhesion tests, such as perfusions over a tissue culture or artificial surface, nylon fiber, or glass bead extractions. It can be overcome, however, with the double micropipette technique.[27,28] In spite of this limitation the current *in vivo* test shows the adhesion over a range that is of interest for blood flow and transport of these cells in the microcirculation. It can be utilized to test the effect of different agents, it serves to unravel heterogeneities of the local endothelium and their underlying mechanisms, and it can be applied to several different organs.

There exist a wide range of natural and synthetic agents that modulate the adhesion between granulocytes and endothelium.[29] Agents that reduce the adhesion improve microvascular perfusion in general.[2] The discovery that specific membrane-associated adhesion proteins and their partial blockade by monoclonal antibodies[30] have a direct effect on adhesion *in vivo* has opened the way for a molecular understanding of the adhesion process and its modulation by short chain proteins and protein fragments such as fMLP and others.

The measurements of rolling velocity reported previously fall into the same order of magnitude as found in this study.[31–34] It is on the order of 10% or less of the center line red cell velocity. It should be noted that due to the laminar flow in such small postcapillary vessels, rolling on the endothelium may occur even if the fracture stress were zero. In such a situation the cell will become detached if there is a local protrusion of endothelial cells (wall roughness) and if there are hydrodynamic interactions with red cells. Random interactions with other cells rolling on the endothelium and detachments occur so that the individual cell behaviors are not exactly the same. Averages are quite stable, but the fluctuations are large. If the adhesion energy is reduced to zero, such as after application of a Ca^{2+} chelating agent, all granulocytes detach from the endothelium.

ACKNOWLEDGMENTS

The authors wish to thank Ms. Dawn Newcom, Mr. Frank De Lano, and Mr. William Bloomer, Jr. for assistance with the experiments, and Karen Kosakowski for typing the manuscript.

REFERENCES

1. GRANT, L. 1973. The sticking and emigration of white blood cells in inflammation. *In* The Inflammatory Process, Vol. II. 2d edit. B. W. Zweifach, L. Grant & R. T. McCluskey, Eds.: 205–250. Academic Press. New York.
2. SCHMID-SCHÖNBEIN, G. W. & R. L. ENGLER. 1986. Granulocytes as active participants in acute myocardial ischemia and infarction. Am. J. Cardiovasc. Pathol. **1:** 15–30.
3. CLARK, E. R. & E. L. CLARK. 1935. Observation on polymorphonuclear leukocytes in living animal. Am. J. Anat. **57:** 385–438.
4. ZWEIFACH, B. W. 1954. The exchange of materials between blood vessels and lymph compartments. Transactions of the Fifth Conference on Connective Tissues. Josiah Macy Jr. Foundation. New York. pp. 38–77.
5. GIDDON, D. B. & J. LINDKE. 1972. In-vivo quantitation of local anesthetic suppression of leukocyte adherence. Am. J. Pathol. **68:** 327–334.
6. GÖRÖG, P. & G. V. R. BORN. 1982. Increased adhesiveness of granulocytes in rabbit ear-chamber blood vessels perfused with neuraminidase. Microvasc. Res. **23:** 380–384.
7. JANOFF, A. & B. W. ZWEIFACH. 1964. Adhesion and emigration of leukocytes produced by cationic proteins of lysosomes. Science **144:** 1456–1458.
8. ALLISON, F. & M. G. LANCASTER. 1960. Studies on the pathogenesis of acute inflammation. II. The relationship of fibrinogen and fibrin to the leucocytic sticking reaction in ear chambers of rabbits injured by heat. J. Exp. Med. **111:** 45–64.
9. ATHERTON, A. & G. V. R. BORN. 1972. Quantitative investigations of the adhesiveness of circulating polymorphonuclear leucocytes to blood vessel walls. J. Physiol. (London) **222:** 447–474.
10. EBERT, R. H. & W. R. BARCLAY. 1952. Changes in connective tissue reaction induced by cortisone. Ann. Intern. Med. **37:** 506–518.
11. FEHR, J. & H. S. JACOB. 1977. In vitro granulocyte adherence and in-vivo margination: Two associated complement dependent functions. J. Exp. Med. **146:** 641–652.
12. DAHLÉN, S.-E., J. BJÖRK, P. HEDQVIST, K.-E. ARFORS, S. HAMMARSTRÖM, J.-A. LINDGREN & B. SAMUELSSON. 1981. Leukotrienes promote plasma leakage and leukocyte adhesion in postcapillary venules: In vivo effects with relevance to the acute inflammatory response. Proc. Natl. Acad. Sci. **78:** 3887–3891.
13. TUMA, R. F. 1985. White cell adherence in microvessels. Prog. Appl. Microcirc. **7:** 31–42.
14. HAMMERSCHMIDT, D. E., P. D. HARRIS, J. H. WAYLAND, P. R. CRADDOCK & H. S. JACOB. 1981. Complement-induced granulocyte aggregation in-vivo. Am. J. Pathol. **102:** 146–150.
15. MACGREGOR, R., H. FRIEDMAN, E. MECARAK & N. KEFALIDES. 1980. Virus infection of endothelial cells increases granulocyte adherence. J. Clin. Invest. **65:** 1469–1477.
16. BENVENISTE, J. & E. COËFFIER. 1985. Leukocyte-platelet interaction in inflammation. Prog. Appl. Microcirc. **7:** 68–77.
17. CRONSTEIN, B. N., R. I. LEVIN, J. BELANOFF, G. WEISSMANN & R. HIRSCHHORN. 1986. Adenosine: An endogenous inhibitor of neutrophil-mediated injury to endothelial cells. J. Clin. Invest. **78:** 760–770.
18. BOXER, L., B. BJORKSTEN, J. BJORK, H. YANG, J. ALLEN & R. BAEHNER. 1982. Neutropenia induced by systemic infusion of lactoferrin. J. Lab. Clin. Med. **99:** 866–872.
19. MACGREGOR, R. R. 1980. Granulocyte adherence. *In* The Cell Biology of Inflammation, chap 9. G. Weissman, Ed: 267–298. Elsevier/North-Holland Biomedical Press. Amsterdam.
20. DEMBO, M. & G. I. BELL. 1987. The thermodynamics of cell adhesion. Curr. Top. Membr. Transp. **29:** 71–89.
21. FUNG, Y. C. 1977. A First Course in Continuum Mechanics. 2d edit. Prentice-Hall. Englewood Cliffs, NJ.
22. SCHMID-SCHÖNBEIN, G. W., K.-L.P. SUNG, H. TÖZEREN, S. CHIEN & R. SKALAK. 1981. Passive mechanical properties of human leukocytes. Biophys. J. **36:** 243–256.
23. TÖZEREN, A. & R. SKALAK. 1977. Stress in a suspension near rigid boundaries. J. Fluid Mech. **82:** 289–307.

24. KELLER, S. R. & R. SKALAK. 1982. Motion of a tank-treading ellipsoidal particle in a shear flow. J. Fluid Mech. **120:** 27–47.
25. TOMPKINS, W. R., R. MONTI & M. INTAGLIETTA. 1974. Velocity measurements by self tracking correlator. Rev. Sci. Instrum. **45:** 647–649.
26. LEE, T. Q., G. W. SCHMID-SCHÖNBEIN & B. W. ZWEIFACH. 1983. The application of an unproved dual-slit photometric analyzer for volumetric flow rate measurements in microvessels. Microvasc. Res. **26:** 351–361.
27. EVANS, E. A. & K. BUXBAUM. 1981. Affinity of red blood cell membrane for particle surfaces measured by the extent of particle encapsulation. Biophys. J. **34:** 1–12.
28. SUNG, P. K.-L., L. A. SUNG, M. CRIMMINGS, S. J. BURAKOFF & S. CHIEN. 1986. Determination of junction avidity of cytolytic T cell and target cell. Science **234:** 1405–1408.
29. HARLAN, J. M. 1985. Leukocyte-endothelial interactions. Blood **65:** 513–525.
30. LINDBOM, L., C. LUNDBERG, K. LUNDBERG, J. HARLAN & K.-E. ARFORS. 1986. Prevention of experimentally induced neutrophil accumulation in vivo (abstract). Int. J. Microcirc.: Clin. Exp. **5:** 232.
31. ATHERTON, A. & G. V. R. BORN. 1973. Relationship between the velocity of rolling granulocytes and that of blood flow in venules. J. Physiol. (London) **233:** 157–165.
32. MAYROVITZ, H. N. 1982. The relationship between leukocyte and erythrocyte velocity in arterioles. *In* White Blood Cells: Morphology and Rheology Related to Function. U. Bagge, G. V. R. Born & P. Gaethgens, Eds.: 82–87. Martinus Nijhoff. The Hague.
33. GAEHTGENS, P., K. LEY, A. R. PRIES & R. MÜLLER. 1985. Mutual interaction between leukocytes and microvascular blood flow. Prog. Appl. Microcirc. **7:** 15–28.
34. MAYROVITZ, H. N., M. WIEDEMANN & R. F. TUMA. 1977. Factors influencing leukocyte adherence in microvessels. Thromb. Haemostas. **38:** 823–830.

Blood Elements at Surfaces: Platelets[a]

BARRY S. COLLER

Division of Hematology
State University of New York at Stony Brook
Stony Brook, New York 11794

The behavior of blood platelets at surfaces is a complex phenomenon in which the rheology controls the kinetic interactions, and several biochemical and cellular factors determine the outcome of the interactions. These latter factors can be organized into four broad categories: (1) the nature of the surface; (2) the integrity of the platelets with regard to their surface receptors, activating mechanisms, and content of self-activating agents; (3) the presence and integrity of plasma proteins that act as platelet cofactors; and (4) the presence of fluid-phase activators and inhibitors of platelet function (TABLE 1). This paper is designed to present an overview of each of these categories, emphasizing recent advances in our understanding of the basic mechanisms involved and potential therapeutic interventions.

THE NATURE OF THE SURFACE

Damage to a blood vessel *in vivo* results in the loss of the integrity of the endothelial cell lining, a surface to which platelets do not normally adhere; superficial damage will expose the subendothelial matrix whereas more severe damage may expose deeper structures in the vessel wall.[1] The composition of the subendothelial matrix and these deeper structures are still poorly defined, but since platelets readily adhere to these surfaces, they clearly contain potent platelet-reactive elements. The best characterized of these is collagen, which has been extensively studied for its ability to induce platelet aggregation in platelet-rich plasma. Considerable evidence indicates that collagen must be in a fibrillar form in order to bind to, and activate, platelets; the underlying collagen chain composition appears to be less important than this architectural feature.[1] Although considerable insight has developed on the interaction of platelets with purified collagen species both in fluid phase and when immobilized on a variety of surfaces,[2] much less is known about the structure of collagen in the damaged vessel wall as "seen" by a circulating platelet. Based on qualitative morphologic studies, it has been stated that minor blood vessel damage probably does not expose collagen, whereas deeper injury probably does; quantitation of the amount of exposure is difficult, however, and extrapolations from experimental injury to natural injury must be made with caution. Moreover, since there is no way to inactivate the interaction between platelets and collagen selectively, it is not clear to what extent, if at all, the platelet-collagen interaction actually contributes to platelet adhesion. One possible insight into this issue can be derived from the clinical history of a patient with a long bleeding time whose platelets could not be aggregated by collagen and were deficient in glycoprotein Ia[3,4] (see below). The patient had a history of easy bruising (especially with significant trauma) and heavy menses, but she did not bleed excessively from cuts,

[a]This work was supported by grant no. 19278 from the National Heart, Lung and Blood Institute.

TABLE 1. Major Determinants of Platelet Behavior at Surfaces

- I. Flow
  - A. Rate
  - B. Geometry
  - C. Shear
  - D. Turbulence
  - E. Effect of other cellular elements
- II. The reactive surface
  - A. Natural
    - 1. Blood vessel location
    - 2. Nature of injury
    - 3. Exposed mediator(s)
      - a) Collagen
      - b) Immobilized von Willebrand factor
      - c) Noncollagenous microfibrils
      - d) Fibronectin
      - e) Thrombospondin
  - B. Artificial
    - 1. Fibrinogen deposition
    - 2. Fibrinogen transformation
- III. The platelets
  - A. Receptors
    - 1. For fluid-phase agonists
    - 2. For inhibitors
    - 3. For glycoproteins (GPIa, GPIb, GPIIb-IIIa, GPIV)
  - B. Metabolic pathways
    - 1. Arachidonic acid (cyclooxygenase, thromboxane synthetase, lipoxygenase)
    - 2. Phospholipase C/diglyceride lipase: diacyglycerol/inositol trisphosphate/protein kinase C
    - 3. Cyclic AMP generation
    - 4. Calcium metabolism
  - C. Effector pathways
    - 1. Contractile mechanism
    - 2. Release reaction
    - 3. Procoagulant activity
  - D. Content of adhesion- and aggregation-augmenting agents
    - 1. Dense bodies (ADP, epinephrine, serotonin)
    - 2. α-Granules (fibrinogen, fibronectin, thrombospondin, von Willebrand factor)
- IV. Soluble protein cofactors
  - A. Fibrinogen
  - B. Von Willebrand factor
- V. Activators
  - A. Fluid phase
    - 1. Singly
      - a) ADP
      - b) Thrombin
      - c) Epinephrine
      - d) Serotonin
      - e) TXA_2 (PGG_2, PGH_2)
      - f) Platelet-activating factor
    - 2. In combination
  - B. Solid phase
    - 1. Collagen
    - 2. Immobilized von Willebrand factor
    - 3. Immobilized fibrinogen
    - 4. Immobilized fibronectin
    - 5. Immobilized thrombospondin
- VI. Inhibitors
  - A. PGI_2
  - B. PGE_1
  - C. Adenosine

did not have excessive nosebleeds or gum bleeding, and she withstood multiple surgical procedures and tooth extractions without incident. If this patient's platelets are truly incapable of interacting with collagen *in vivo*, it is likely that such interaction plays an important role in the blood vessels in the skin, but a considerably lesser role in blood vessels in other tissues. This emphasizes the likely heterogeneity of blood vessesls in different tissues, as well as the heterogeneity that is likely to result from different types of injuries (gentle endothelial denudation of capillaries at the one extreme and complete severing of arteries at the other).

Von Willebrand factor (vWF) is also present on the subendothelial surfaces of blood vessels, and there is considerable evidence that platelets will adhere to immobilized von Willebrand factor via glycoprotein Ib.[1,5-8] This is of especial interest since platelets do not appear to interact with fluid-phase von Willebrand factor unless one of several nonphysiologic agents (ristocetin, botrocetin, polybrene, or polylysine) is also present.[5,9] Thus, immobilizing von Willebrand factor must result in some change—in its conformation, concentration, or microenvironment—that results in this alteration in behavior.[5] There are two potential sources of the immobilized von Willebrand factor, namely that which is deposited abluminally by endothelial cells and is always present on the subendothelial surface, and that which binds to blood vessel surfaces from the pool of plasma von Willebrand factor after the blood vessel has been damaged.[5,8,10] The relative contributions of each source in attaining hemostasis is still not fully understood, but both appear necessary for optimal interaction between platelet and vessel wall. It is presumed that von Willebrand factor binds to one or more elements in the subendothelium and in evolving thrombi; based on *in vitro* studies, several candidate proteins have been identified (collagen, noncollagenuous microfibrils, fibrin),[1,5,11] but evidence also exists for specific binding of von Willebrand factor to sulfated glycolipids.[12] The physiologic significance of each of these interactions, however, remains uncertain.

Fibronectin has also been proposed as a subendothelial protein to which platelets adhere.[1,6,13] This protein, like von Willebrand factor, exists both in plasma and as an immobilized protein deposited on the abluminal side of endothelial cells. Platelets activated with certain agonists such as thrombin can bind fluid-phase fibronectin,[14] and there is considerable *in vitro* evidence that fibronectin contributes to platelet adhesion to, and/or spreading on, collagen surfaces;[2,15,16] *ex vivo* evidence also points to a role in platelet adhesion to, and/or spreading on, subendothelial surfaces.[6,13] Complicating the interpretation of these data is the ability of collagen, fibrin, and acidic mucopolysaccharides to bind directly to fibronectin, making it difficult to be certain that the fibronectin is actually involved directly in the binding to platelets.[17]

Thrombospondin is another adhesive glycoprotein synthesized by endothelial cells and deposited on the subendothelial surfaces.[18] Unlike von Willebrand factor and fibronectin, however, its plasma concentration is very low. It too can interact with a large number of proteins, including fibrinogen, and will bind to platelets that are stimulated with several different agonists in a way that stabilizes aggregates that are formed.[19,20] A putative receptor has been identified (glycoprotein IV),[21] although the amount of binding that occurs to this glycoprotein as opposed to binding to platelet-bound fibrinogen under physiologic circumstances is unknown. Thrombospondin's role in platelet adhesion remains to be defined, especially since at least one preliminary report suggests that platelets do not adhere to surfaces coated with it.[22]

Platelet deposition on artificial surfaces appears to be controlled by the adsorption of fluid-phase proteins onto the artificial surface. In particular, the adsorption of fibrinogen appears to augment platelet adhesion dramatically.[23-25] Since unactivated platelets do not bind appreciable amounts of fibrinogen whereas apparently unactivated platelets bind readily to fibrinogen-coated surfaces, these phenomena parallel the dilemma posed before concerning immobilized von Willebrand factor. Although still unresolved, two studies bear on this point: (1) coupling fibrinogen at high density to solid beads by a relatively gentle chemical reaction resulted in interaction of the beads with apparently unactivated platelets, suggesting that the high concentration rather than an adsorption-dependent conformational change may be important,[26] and (2) the ability of artificial surfaces to bind platelets was found to be directly related to the amount of adsorbed fibrinogen that maintained the ability to interact with an antifibrinogen antibody, suggesting that major conformational changes in adsorbed fibrinogen results in decreased rather than increased platelet reactivity.[25]

THE PLATELET

The platelet's capacity to interact normally with surfaces and with other platelets depends upon the integrity of its surface membrane receptors, its metabolic pathways, its effector mechanisms, and its content of adhesion- and aggregation-augmenting agents.

Receptors

The platelet membrane has receptors for agonists that stimulate platelets, inhibitors that prevent platelet activation, and plasma glycoproteins that mediate both the interactions between platelets and surfaces and between platelets and other platelets.

The fluid-phase activators of platelets that may play a role *in vivo* include both small, nonprotein molecules (ADP, epinephrine, serotonin, thromboxane A_2, platelet-activating factor) thought to interact with specific receptors on platelets in a reversible manner characteristic of many agonist-receptor mechanisms, and a proteolytic enzyme (thrombin) that requires its proteolytic activity for platelet activation and induces activation according to a complex kinetic mechanism.[27] A specific platelet glycoprotein (GPV) has been shown to be cleaved by thrombin, but there is controversy about whether GPV functions as the thrombin receptor.[28] The receptors for all of the fluid phase agonists may not be platelet-specific since these agents are known to have effects on other cells. Although these platelet receptors have been well characterized with regard to agonist structure-activity relationships, they have not been well characterized at the biochemical level. Thus, it is not known if significant differences exist between the platelet receptors and the receptors on other cells. From a strategic point of view, therefore, these receptors may not be attractive targets for platelet inhibitors because if the platelet receptor is similar or identical to the receptors in other cells, such inhibitors may have untoward effects in other tissues. Moreover, there are very few data concerning which of these agonists, alone or in combination, participate in normal hemostastic processes and in the various pathological phenomena.

Fluid-phase inhibitors of platelet aggregation, including PGI_2, adenosine, and perhaps PGE_1 may also regulate platelet function under normal and/or pathological conditions.[27,29,30] Although early speculation suggested that PGI_2 may circulate in concentrations high enough to provide a tonic level of platelet inhibition, measurements of circulating PGI_2 levels indicate that they are probably too low to perform this function.[31] They may, however, reach effective levels at the sites of vascular injury, especially if platelets are activated and provide prostaglandin intermediates to the endothelial cells.[31,32] The *in vivo* role of PGE_1, if any, is even less well defined. Competitive binding studies suggest that PGI_2 and PGE_1 share the same receptor.[29] Adenosine can inhibit platelet function and it has been suggested that the antiplatelet drug, dipyridamole, enhances adenosine's inhibitory effect by preventing the uptake of adenosine by erythrocytes.[30] Adenosine's interaction with the platelet membrane is complex, and may involve more than one receptor.

Glycoprotein Ib (GPIb) and the glycoprotein IIb-IIIa complex (GPIIb-IIIa) are the two best defined receptors for adhesive glycoproteins and so they will be reviewed in some detail. Glycoprotein Ia and glycoprotein IV have recently been proposed as receptors for collagen and thrombospondin, respectively, and they will only briefly be mentioned.

GPIb

Biochemical analysis of this protein indicates that it is composed of a larger α-chain (M_r 145,000) and a smaller β-chain (M_r 22,000) held together by one or more disulfide bonds.[33,34] The α-chain is readily cleaved near its insertion into the membrane by a variety of proteases, including the calcium-activated protease(s) present in platelets and many other cells; the large external fragment (M_r 130,000) so produced has been termed glycocalicin.[35] Glycocalicin is very rich in *O*-linked carbohydrate, with approximately 90 sialic acid residues per molecule, making it highly negatively charged.[33] The β-chain also contains carbohydrate and extends out from the surface of the platelet.[33] The β-chain extends through the membrane and has a free sulfhydryl group and a phosphorylation site on its endofacial portion.[34,36,37] Glycoprotein Ib appears to have a noncovalent association with another glycoprotein, GPIX (M_r 17–20,000), since both of these glycoproteins are immunopurified with monoclonal antibodies directed against either protein.[38,39] In addition the platelets in patients cogenitally deficient in GPIb also lack GPIX.[39,40]

Convincing evidence from studies using monoclonal antibodies, protease-digested platelets, and platelets congenitally deficient in GPIb indicates that GPIb acts as a binding site for von Willebrand factor when platelets are treated with ristocetin.[5,34,38] The binding site for von Willebrand factor has been localized to the glycocalicin portion of the molecule, most likely in the outermost portion of the molecule containing the disulfide loop.[41] Studies assessing the *ex vivo* adhesion and aggregation of platelets to segments of blood vessels denuded of endothelium indicate the GPIb probably mediates the interaction between platelets and subendothelial von Willebrand factor,[5,7] although the GPIIb-IIIa receptor has recently been shown to be able to mediate at least some of the vWF-dependent adhesion to collagen.[42] Whether the interaction between platelets and von Willebrand factor that is responsible for some of the platelet-platelet interactions in the *ex vivo* vessel wall model[8] is also mediated by GPIb remains to be determined.

As part of our studies on GPIb, we postulated that as platelets undergo cytolysis after attaching to surfaces, they might release some of the calcium-activated protease from their cytoplasm into the plasma, where the millimolar calcium concentration would activate the enzyme.[43] The enzyme could then cleave GPIbα molecules, leading either to platelet emobilization (if it cleaved GPIbα molecules that were involved in the adhesion of platelets to a surface), or to release of glycocalicin into the circulation (if it cleaved GPIbα molecules that were not involved in adhesion). Using our monoclonal antibody to GPIb that also reacts with glycocalicin, we were, in fact, able to detect an average of several micrograms of glycocalicin per ml of normal plasma.[43] Patients with aplastic anemia and no bone marrow megakaryocytes had very low levels of glycocalicin, indicating that platelets and megakaryocytes are probably the sole sources of plasma glycocalicin.[43] This is of interest because recent reports indicate that a GPIb-like molecule may be present on endothelial cells as well as platelets.[44] At present we believe that the plasma glycocalicin level is a complex function of platelet count, platelet turnover, platelet mass, and megakaryocyte mass. As such it appears to be able to distinguish whether the low platelet counts found in some patients are due to a decrease in the production of platelets or to an increase in their destruction.[45] It remains to be determined whether plasma glycocalicin will also reflect thrombotic or prethrombotic states.

GPIIb-IIIa

Glycoprotein IIb (a two-chain molecule composed of a larger α-chain of M_r 120,00) and a small β-chain of (M_r 23,000) held together by one or more disulfide bonds) and glycoprotein IIIa (a one-chain molecule of M_r 110,000 when reduced and M_r 90,000 when nonreduced) exist as a calcium-dependent complex on both resting and activated platelets.[33,34,46–49] The proteins appear to be made from different mRNAs,[50] but there is conflicting evidence as to whether they are homologous.[51–53] This matter should be resolved by cloning the two glycoproteins, a feat that is underway in several laboratories. As arranged on the surface of platelets, GPIIb-IIIa complexes are present in very high concentration (~40,000 sites per platelet), estimated to represent nearly 50% of the platelet surface.[54]

Although early studies suggested that GPIIb and GPIIIa are specific for platelets, recent data indicate that there are immunologically similar molecules in endothelial cells and perhaps monocytes.[55-57] Moreover, evidence points to homology between GPIIb-IIIa and a family of glycoprotein receptors present on granulocytes, monocytes, and lymphocytes (LFA-1; Mac-1; p150,95), the cellular receptors for vitronectin and fibronectin, and a neural cellular adhesion molecule (N-CAM).[58-63] GPIIb-IIIa functions as the receptor for fibrinogen when platelets are stimulated with any of the agonists thought to operate *in vivo*, whereas little or no binding occurs to platelets that are unstimulated.[63,64] GPIIb-IIIa is also responsible for the binding of platelets to fibrinogen-coated surfaces such as glass.[65] When fibrinogen is not present in the surrounding medium, both von Willebrand factor and fibronectin can bind to GPIIb-IIIa after platelet activation with thrombin,[20,66,67] indicating a more general ability of the complex to bind adhesive glycoproteins. The details of the binding mechanisms are discussed below, but all three molecules contain the RGD (arginine-glycine-aspartic acid) amino acid sequence and the RGD peptide can inhibit the binding of all three molecules.[68] Evidence for the physiological significance of fibrinogen binding to the receptor is well established since patients with afibrinogenemia have prolonged bleeding times and abnormalities in platelet aggregation *in vitro*,[26] but the physiological significance of the binding of von Willebrand factor and fibronectin to this receptor needs to be better defined, especially since fibrinogen, which is present in plasma at much greater concentration than von Willebrand factor, competes for binding to GPIIb-IIIa.[67]

The mechanism by which agonists activate platelets so that fibrinogen binds to the GPIIb-IIIa receptor has been studied in our own and other laboratories.[16] It is established that the receptor is always present on the surface of platelets and so activation must result in a change in the conformation of the receptor of the receptor itself or its microenvironment. Using fragments and cross-linked aggregates of a monoclonal antibody that binds preferentially or exclusively to the activated form of the receptor,[69] I was able to show that activation alters the receptor so as to allow larger molecules access to the binding site on the complex.[70] An IgM monoclonal to GPIIb-IIIa, which is larger than the IgG antibody used in my studies, has been reported to show even greater selectivity for the activated form of the receptor.[71] The hypothesis that activation affects size-dependent access to the binding site on the receptor is also supported by the observation that the RGD peptide and a small peptide containing the fibrinogen γ-chain binding site (see below) bind equally well to unactivated and activated platelets.[72,73]

There are two points that are worth emphasizing with regard to the GPIIb-IIIa receptor (1) *In vitro* studies of platelets from patients with no GPIIb-IIIa receptors and normal platelets on which the GPIIb-IIIa receptors have been blocked with monoclonal antibodies indicate that all platelet aggregation induced by the agonists thought to operate *in vivo* depends upon this receptor.[27,34] Thus, blockade of this receptor can theoretically block platelet aggregation *in vivo* completely. (2) Although the arachidonic acid pathway can augment activation of the GPIIb-IIIa receptor by the production of thromboxane A_2 and release of ADP and epinephrine, agonists such as ADP, collagen, and thrombin can activate platelets so as to "expose" the GPIIb-IIIa receptor even if arachidonic acid metabolism is completely blocked by aspirin's inhibition of cyclooxygenase.[27]

The potency of the anti-GPIIb-IIIa monoclonal antibodies in blocking platelet aggregation *in vitro* encouraged us to explore the possibility that they might be useful therapeutic agents in disorders characterized by vaso-occlusion or thromboemboli. We chose to use $F(ab')_2$ fragments rather than intact antibody for fear that platelets coated with intact antibody would be very rapidly cleared in the spleen by macrophages bearing receptors for the Fc portion of immunoglobulin. After establishing that an intravenous dose of 0.8 mg per kg of antibody 7E3 could almost completely inhibit *ex vivo* platelet aggregation and block ~85% of the GPIIb-IIIa sites on platelets without causing spontaneous bleeding or other obvious ill effects,[74] we went on to show that such treatment had a profound antithrombotic effect in a model developed by Dr. John Folts involving partially stenosed coronary arteries in dogs and carotid arteries in monkeys.[75] In fact, the antibody was the most potent agent studied in this system. In collaboration with investigators at Massachusetts General Hospital, we have also found preliminary evidence that the antibody is effective in preventing reocclusion of severely stenosed coronary arteries in dogs after reperfusion of an upstream thrombus by recombinant tissue plasminogen activator.[76] These studies encourage us to pursue further the therapeutic potential of such antibodies. Another antibody to the GPIIb-IIIa receptor has more recently been reported to inhibit vascular graft closure in a baboon model using a dose of 10 mg/kg.[77]

GPIa and GPIV

Based on the selective absence of collagen-induced platelet aggregation in a patient with a severe deficiency of GPIa, this glycoprotein of M_r 167,000 (reduced) has been proposed as the receptor for collagen.[3,4] Other proteins have previously been proposed to function as the collagen receptor and so this issue remains unsettled.[27] GPIV has been suggested to act as the platelet receptor for thrombospondin because a monoclonal antibody that reacts with GPIV blocks the binding of thrombospondin to activated platelets.[21] The functional consequences of this interaction are now being explored.

Metabolic Pathways

In addition to biochemical pathways that generate energy, platelets have several metabolic pathways that are more directly involved in platelet activation: arachidonic acid metabolism, the phospholipase-C–diglyceride lipase pathway, cAMP generation, and calcium metabolism.

Arachidonic acid can be released from membrane phospholipid by several different mechanisms and the resulting free arachidonate can be further metabolised by either lipoxygenase or cyclooxygenase.[78] The latter pathway, which can be blocked by acetylsalicylic acid, generates a series of protaglandin intermediates and the potent platelet aggregating agent thromboxane A_2.[78] The thromboxane produced by the platelet appears to activate platelets by interacting with a receptor on the surface of platelets, and so it must exit from the platelet and then bind to the same or a neighboring platelet. The lipoxygenase pathway leads to other intermediates and, in cells with the appropriate enzymes (*e.g.*, granulocytes), the final products are the chemotactic and spasmogenic leukotrienes.[79] Recent data indicate that the metabolism in these pathways can be dramatically affected by cooperative effects between platelets and other cells (endothelial cells, granulocytes) that have different enzymatic capabilities.[79] Although the arachidonic acid pathway generates powerful platelet activating agents, it is important to emphasize that it is not absolutely required for either platelet aggregation or the platelet release reaction. Thus, aspirin-treated platelets cannot generate thromboxane A_2, but they can aggregate in response to ADP and undergo the release reaction in response to thrombin.

The phospholipase-C–diglyceride lipase pathway generates two important mediators of platelet activation: diacylglycerol and inositol trisphosphate.[80] The former decreases the calcium concentration needed to activate protein kinase C[81], an enzyme that phosphorylates target proteins thought to be involved in both platelet activation and the release reaction via mechanisms that are still not clearly defined. Inositol trisphosphate can increase the intracellular concentration of calcium by interacting with receptors on the closed membrane system that sequesters calcium in platelets (dense tubular system) so as to cause release of the calcium.[82,83] Recent studies indicate that other phosphorylated forms of inositol may also act as mediators.[84] At present it is not clear whether the activation of this pathway is a prerequisite for platelet aggregation and release of granule contents by all of the different agonists.

Platelets contain the enzyme adenylate cyclase and can generate cAMP in response to PGI_2 and other stimuli.[30] Elevation in cAMP inhibits platelet function at multiple levels, including inhibition of calcium release, inhibition of arachidonic acid metabolism, inhibition of actin phosphorylation (with diminution in the contractile mechanism), and a direct effect on the platelet membrane, apparently mediated through cytoskeletal elements, that alters the aggregability of platelets by von Willebrand factor.[85]

Calcium metabolism is considered crucial to platelet function because many, if not all, of the agonists that activate platelets also increase cytosolic calcium concentrations, and calcium may thus function as the final common messenger for all of these phenomena.[86,87] Overall calcium homeostasis is a complicated function of external calcium, calcium-binding proteins (including the GPIIb-IIIa complex), a plasma membrane calcium pump, and the dense tubular system, which sequesters and releases calcium in response to different stimuli. Mitochondrial calcium and calcium contained within dense granules are probably not involved in the calcium fluxes that regulate platelet function.

Effector Pathways

In order to translate the activation signal into a response that affects neighboring platelets and the evolving fibrin thrombus, platelets can contract, release the contents of their granules, and help to promote the formation of fibrin.[27] The contractile mechanisms includes actin, myosin and a variety of ancillary proteins (actin-binding protein, talin, vinculin, α-actinin, gelsolin, profilin, spectrin, tropomyosin, etc.) that coordinate the contractile response. Control of contraction is thought to be primarily exercised by phosphorylation of the myosin light chain, which, in turn, is controlled by a calcium- and calmodulin-dependent kinase.[88] This contractile capacity is responsible *in vitro* for clot retraction and so it is presumed to result in consolidation of thrombi *in vivo*. The contractile mechanism may also play a role in granule extrusion (released reaction), but most of the data bearing on this issue are circumstantial. The release reaction can enhance the platelet response in several ways, including making more platelet agonists (ADP, epinephrine, serotonin) available at the site of initial platelet activation, thus recruiting more platelets into the platelet aggregate (thrombus); increasing the local concentration of the adhesive glycoproteins contained with α-granules (fibrinogen, thrombospondin, fibronectin, and von Willebrand factor); and exposing receptors for activated clotting factors (and perhaps activating α-granule factor V) so as to facilitate thrombin generation, which, in turn, further activates platelets.[27] The biochemical and biophysical events that actually mediate platelet granule exocytosis remain mysterious, but they must in some final way promote the fusion of granule membranes with either the plasma membrane or the membranes of the open canalicular system.

Platelet coagulant activity is a generic term that accounts for more rapid generation of thrombin by coagulation factors in the presence of platelets than in their absence.[89] In fact, a variety of different activities probably help to mediate this phenomenon, including, but not limited to, the interaction of factor XI with the platelet membrane and its subsequent activation; the availability of platelet phospholipids to act as a matrix for the coagulation reactions; the exposure of activated factor V, which can serve as a receptor for factor Xa; and the binding of thrombin. Platelet activation and/or lysis is required for full expression of these effects, depending upon the agonist used and the particular mechanism being investigated. The accelerated generation of thrombin on or near the platelet surface can facilitate fibrin deposition, induce further platelet activation, and/or activate factor XIII, which can cross-link fibrin and stabilize a thrombus against plasmin, the fibrinolytic enzyme.

Content of Adhesion- and Aggregation-augmenting Agents

Deficiencies of the contents of dense bodies (ADP, epinephrine, serotonin) or α-granules (fibrinogen, von Willebrand factor, fibronectin, thrombospondin) as occur in some congenital and acquired disorders[27] can compromise the positive feedback phenomena that serve to augment the platelet response.

SOLUBLE PROTEIN COFACTORS

Fibrinogen

In order for platelet aggregation to proceed normally, there must be an adequate concentration of fibrinogen. *In vitro* experiments indicate that as little as 20 mg/dl is sufficient.[63,64] Since the normal range of plasma fibrinogen concentrations is 200–400 mg/dl, quantitative abnormalities are rarely a serious clinical problem except in patients with cogenital hypo- or afibrinogenemia, or patients with profound difibrination syndromes. Structural studies indicate that fibrinogen binds to platelets via segments of both the Aα- and γ-chains, fibrinogen being a dimer of three nonidentical chains (Aα, Bβ, and γ).[63,64] The γ-chain segment that is important in platelet binding has been localized to the 10–12 amino acids at the carboxy terminus of the molecule, and since the dimers are joined at the amino termini, this places the fibrinogen binding regions at the outer ends of the molecule. This arrangement gives the fibrinogen molecule the potential of spanning receptors of two different platelets that are as much as 475 Å apart, the full molecular diameter of the fibrinogen molecule. In fact, for any molecule to function as a bridge between cells, it must be multivalent (so that it can interact with two different cells simultaneously) and be of sufficient molecular diameter to span the gap between the cells. The location of the Aα-chain binding sites has been tentatively localized to a tripeptide of arginine-glycine-aspartic acid (RGD) near the carboxy-terminal end of the molecule, although another RGD sequence occurs in the Aα-chain in the tightly coiled region joining the amino-terminal and carboxy-terminal regions. The binding of both Aα- and γ-chains to platelets permits one to construct another model by which fibrinogen spans between platelets, namely a sideways orientation in which the γ- and Aα-chains on one side of the molecule bind to two different platelets with a similar arrangement on the other side of the molecule; in this case, the platelets will be closer together than in the first case.[90] Such a model may not, however, be easily reconciled with the behavior of fibrinogen molecules lacking the carboxy-terminal regions of the Aα-chain.[63]

The RGD tripeptide appears to be of general importance in cell adhesion phenomena since (1) fibrinogen, fibronectin, and von Willebrand factor all contain at least one RGD sequence and RGD-containing peptides can inhibit the binding of all three molecules to the platelet glycoprotein IIb-IIIa receptor,[68,91] (2) RGD-containing peptides can inhibit the binding of fibronectin to other receptors of mammalian cells,[92] (3) another extracellular matrix protein involved in cell spreading, vitronectin (serum spreading factor, S-protein) contains an RGD sequence,[97] as does the *E. coli* phage receptor and the Sindbis virus coat protein,[93] and (4) RGD-containing peptides can inhibit metastasis formation in an animal model.[94] The relationship, if any, between the γ-chain peptide (which contains an AGD sequence but no RGD sequence) and RGD remains obscure since conflicting data have been presented on whether RGD and the γ-chain peptide bind to the same site.[95–97] Moreover, the mechanism by which RGD inhibits binding of fibrinogen needs more precise definition with regard to potential noncompetitive conformational changes.

Qualitative changes in fibrinogen could also theoretically affect its platelet-binding activity, and congenital and acquired fibrinogens with both increased and decreased platelet cofactor activity have been reported.[98,99] Plasmin degradation products of fibrinogen vary in both their content of the different chains and the basic dimeric structure and so might potentially compete with normal fibrinogen for binding to platelets; careful kinetic analyses suggest that such molecules do not, in fact, have a high binding affinity for platelets, but they can cause inhibition of normal fibrinogen binding by interacting with fibrinogen itself.[63]

Von Willebrand Factor

Von Willebrand factor meets the minimal criteria for a bridging molecule, being made up of multiple, essentially identical subunits (each of M_r 200,000 with the basic unit consisting of a disulfide-linked dimer of M_r 400,000, and the plasma forms being disulfide-linked multimers containing somewhere between 1 and 40 of these basic units).[5] *In vitro,* von Willebrand factor can mediate platelet aggregation, presumably by spanning between platelets, either by binding to platelet GPIb in the presence of the antibiotic ristocetin, or by binding to platelet GPIIb-IIIa in the presence of thrombin or ADP.[5] In fact, studies employing monoclonal antibodies or selective proteolysis of von Willebrand factor have identified two different binding domains on the von Willebrand molecule, one for GPIb and the other for GPIIb-IIIa.[100,101] The physiologic role for fluid-phase binding of von Willebrand factor to each of these receptors needs to be better defined since (1) no fluid phase analogue of ristocetin has been identified, (2) fibrinogen competes effectively with von Willebrand factor for binding to GPIIb-IIIa when both are present at their usual plasma concentrations (~3 mg/ml vs. ~10 μg/ml),[67,102] and (3) the aggregation that is mediated by von Willebrand factor binding to GPIIb-IIIa may only occur at calcium concentrations well below that found *in vivo*.[103]

At present, the most convincing evidence points to fluid-phase von Willebrand factor being able to bind to subendothelial surfaces so as to augment platelet adhesion mediated by GPIb. *Ex vivo* data also suggest that von Willebrand factor may mediate platelet-platelet interactions,[8] but it is not clear whether this is mediated by GPIb or GPIIb-IIIa. Most recently, von Willebrand factor associated with fibrin has been reported to bind to platelets via GPIb, providing one possible "physiologic" ristocetin.[11] Such a mechanism cannot, however, explain the adhesion of platelets to blood vessel walls that is thought to precede fibrin formation.

An astonishing array of both qualitative and quantitative disorders of von Willebrand factor has been described, giving rise to the von Willebrand syndromes, which are characterized by variably severe bleeding diatheses.[104]

ACTIVATORS

Fluid Phase

A variety of fluid-phase agents have been identified that might potentially exist at sites of vascular injury and activate platelets. When analyzed according to the full range of platelet responses (shape change, "exposure" of the GPIIb-IIIa receptor, "exposure" of the GPIb receptor, release of arachidonic acid, initiation of the phospholipase C system, induction of the release reaction), these activators show characteristic differences.[27] Thus, for example, ADP, a relatively "weak" agonist, produces little release of platelet granule contents unless platelet aggregation occurs, whereas thrombin can induce release even in the absence of aggregation.

Several considerations bear emphasizing as one tries to extrapolate from the *in vitro* studies to *in vivo* phenomena: (1) Few direct data are available on which agonists are actually present at the site of vessel injury *in vivo*. Moreover, it is quite likely that different forms of injury may result in the presence of different mediators. For example, injuries that include damage to erythrocytes are likely to result in high local concentrations of ADP, whereas injuries that involve tissues rich in tissue factor production are likely to contain significant amounts of thrombin. Rheologic consideration, affecting the rate of removal of the agonists, may also have a profound effect on the final result. (2) It is likely that all *in vivo* injuries result in the presence of several different activators working in concert rather than as single activators. One observation that probably reflects this phenomenon is that individuals taking aspirin and patients with hemophilia have normal or modestly increased bleeding times, whereas hemophiliacs taking aspirin or other nonsteroidal anti-inflammatory medications have markedly prolonged bleeding times.[105] This suggests that thrombin formation and thromboxane production both contribute to arrest of bleeding in this setting and that their effects are synergistic. Thus, in addition to the separate patterns of activation produced by individual agonists, it is crucial to understand the effects of combinations of agonists. Interesting results are emerging from such studies, for example, the discovery that subaggregating doses of epinephrine can sensitize platelets to other agonists and can even overcome the inhibition of platelet aggregation caused by aspirin and PGI_2, both *in vivo* and *ex vivo*.[75,106–108] This phenomenon may help to explain aspirin's disappointing performance as an antiplatelet agent and offers a potential link between platelet function and events that affect catecholamine levels such as "stress" and cigarette smoking.[75] (3) Despite the great insights that have been derived from analyzing *in vitro* data obtained in the aggregometer, it must be remembered that such studies are conducted on anticoagulated blood from which platelet-rich plasma has been prepared. Thus, platelets are isolated from the other formed elements of the blood and studied in an unphysiologically low calcium concentration; both of these "artifacts" have been shown to affect platelet behavior.[109,110] Aggregometer studies are also carried out with an empirically determined stirring mechanism that cannot reflect the range of shear rates and geometries encountered *in vivo*. These limitations are leading investigators into new approaches that will better simulate the conditions that exist *in vivo* (different anticoagulants, whole blood aggregometry, better-defined and adjustable shear-rate conditions), but each new technique introduces its own new artifacts. One particularly interesting approach involves native blood exposed to rabbit aortic segments that have been de-endothelized, in which platelet and fibrin deposition is assessed at a variety of shear rates. Such studies have found that very few platelets are required for fibrin deposition, and that, paradoxically, increasing the shear rate increases platelet deposition and decreases fibrin deposition.[111]

Solid Phase

Since collagen requires a fibrillar form in order to activate platelets, that is, to induce the release reaction and/or produce thromboxane A_2, it is probably best to consider it a solid-phase activator. Von Willebrand factor and fibrinogen, which act as plasma cofactors when in solution, appear to be able to activate platelets under some circumstances when platelets adhere to surfaces on which the proteins have been previously adsorbed; in fact even soluble fibrinogen polymers that have been cross-linked with antibodies are able to activate gel-filtered platelets.[112] This may not be universally the case, however, since platelets do not undergo measurable release when they interact with beads to which fibrinogen has been covalently attached.[26] Less is known about the activation, if any, of platelets that bind to immobilized fibronectin or thrombospondin.

INHIBITORS

The response of platelets at a surface will also be affected by the presence of inhibitors. PGI_2 is an extremely potent inhibitor *in vitro,* but even its inhibitory effects on platelet aggregation can be overcome with subaggregating concentrations of epinephrine.[106] At present it is impossible to measure the concentration of PGI_2 or the other inhibitors that may function *in vivo,* PGE_1 and adenosine, at the site of injury and so discussions of their contribution remain speculative.

SUMMARY

This brief review is designed to highlight the limitations of our knowledge given the difficulties in simulating the *in vivo* condition in models established *in vitro* and *ex vivo.* Despite this uncertainty, mounting evidence indicates that the GPIIb-IIIa receptor mediates crucial platelet functions and that control over its interactions may offer the potential for altering platelet behavior *in vivo.* Since this receptor appears to be part of a generalized family of adhesive protein receptors that utilize the tripeptide RGD as a recognition signal, insights derived from platelet function may have broad biological implications.

ACKNOWLEDGMENTS

I would like to thank Lesley Scudder for outstanding technical assistance and Shirley Murray for outstanding secretarial assistance.

REFERENCES

1. PACKHAM, M. A. & J. F. MUSTARD. 1984. Platelet adhesion. Prog. Hemostas. Thromb. **7:** 211–288.
2. HOUDIJK, W. P. M., K. S. SAKARIASSEN, P. F. E. M. NIEVELSTEIN & J. J. SIXMA. 1985. Role of factor VIII-von Willebrand factor and fibronectin in the interaction of platelets in flowing blood with monomeric and fibrillar human collagen types I and III. J. Clin. Invest. **75:** 531–540.
3. NIEUWENHUIS, H. K., J. W. N. AKKERMAN, W. P. M. HOUDIJK & J. J. SIXMA. 1985. Human blood platelets with a defect of response to collagen fail to express surface glycoprotein Ia. Nature **318:** 470–472.
4. NIEUWENHUIS, H. K., K. S. SAKARIASSEN, W. P. M. HOUDIJK, P. F. E. M. NIEVELSTEIN & J. J. SIXMA. 1986. Deficiency of platelet membrane glycoprotein Ia associated with a decreased platelet adhesion to subendothelium: A defect in platelet spreading. Blood **68:** 692–695.
5. COLLER, B. S. 1985. Platelet-von Willebrand factor interactions. *In* Platelet Membrane Glycoproteins. J. N. George, A. T. Nurden & D. R. Phillips, Eds.: 215–244. Plenum. New York.
6. BOOYSE, F. M. S., S. FEDER & A. J. QUARFOOT. 1982. Culture-produced subendothelium. II. Effect of plasma, FVIII R:WF and fibronectin on interaction of normal platelets with normal and von Willebrand porcine aortic subendothelium. Thromb. Res. **28:** 299–311.
7. SAKARIASSEN, K. S., P. F. E. M. NIEVELSTEIN, B. S. COLLER & J. J. SIXMA. 1986. The role of platelet membrane glycoproteins Ib and IIb-IIIa in platelet adherence to human artery subendothelium. Br. J. Haematol. **63:** 681–691.
8. TURITTO, V. T., J. H. WEISS & H. R. BAUMGARTNER. 1984. Platelet interaction with rabbit subendothelium in von Willebrand's disease: Altered thrombus formation distinct from defective platelet adhesion. J. Clin. Invest. **74:** 1730–1741.
9. COLLER, B. S. 1983. Biochemical and electrostatic considerations in primary platelet aggregation. Ann. N.Y. Acad. Sci. **416:** 693–708.
10. STEL, H. V., K. S. SAKARIASSEN, PH.G. DE GROOT, J. A. VAN MOURIK & J. J. SIXMA. 1985. Von Willebrand factor in the vessel wall mediates platelet adherence. Blood **65:** 85–90.
11. LOSCALZO, J., A. INBAL & R. I. HANDIN. 1986. Von Willebrand protein facilitates platelet incorporation in polymerizing fibrin. J. Clin. Invest. **78:** 1112–1119.
12. ROBERTS, D. D., S. B. WILLIAMS, H. R. GRALNICK & V. GINSBURG. 1986. Von Willebrand factor binds specifically to sulfated glycolipids. J. Biol. Chem. **261:** 3306–3309.

13. HOUDIJK, W. P. M. & J. J. SIXMA. 1985. Fibronectin in artery subendothelium is important for platelet adhesion. Blood **65:** 598–605.
14. PLOW, E. F. & M. H. GINSBERG. 1981. Specific saturable binding of plasma fibronectin to thrombin-stimulated platelets. J. Biol. Chem. **256:** 9477–9482.
15. CHAZOV, E. I., A. V. ALEXEEV, A. S. ANTONOV, V. E. KOTELIANSKY, V. L. LEYTIN, E. V. LYUBIMOVA, V. S. REPIN, D. D. SVIRIDOV, V. P. TORCHILIN & V. N. SMIRNOV. 1981. Endothelial cell culture of fibrillar collagen: Model to study platelet adhesion and liposome targeting to intercellular collagen matrix. Proc. Natl. Acad. Sci. U.S.A. **78:** 5603–5607.
16. LAHAV, J., M. A. ALEXANDER & R. O. HYNES. 1982. Analysis of platelet adhesion with a radioactive chemical cross-linking reagent: Interaction of thrombospondin with fibronectin and collagen. Cell **31:** 253–262.
17. HYNES, R. A. 1986. Fibronectins. Sci. Am. **254(6):** 42–51.
18. SILVERSTEIN, R. L., L. L. K. LEUNG & R. L. NACHMAN. 1986. Thrombospondin: A versatile multifunctional glycoprotein. Arteriosclerosis **6:** 245–253.
19. LEUNG, L. L. K. 1984. Role of thrombospondin in platelet aggregation. J. Clin. Invest. **74:** 1764–1772.
20. PLOW, E. F., R. P. MCEVER, B. S. COLLER, V. L. WOODS, JR., G. MARGUERIE & M. H. GINSBERG. 1985. Related binding mechanisms for fibrinogen, fibronectin, von Willebrand factor and thrombospondin on thrombin-stimulated platelets. Blood **66:** 724–727.
21. ASCH, A. S., J. BARNWELL, R. L. SILVERSTEIN & R. L. NACHMAN, 1986. Glycoprotein IV is the thrombospondin membrane receptor. Clin. Res. **34:** 450A
22. LAHAV, J. 1986. Platelet thrombospondin is non-thrombogenic. Thromb. Res. Suppl. **VI:** 56.
23. ZUCKER, M. B. & L. VROMAN. 1969. Platelet adhesion induced by fibrinogen adsorbed on glass. Proc. Soc. Exp. Biol. Med. **131:** 318–320.
24. MUSTARD, J. F. & M. A. PACKHAM. 1970. Factors influencing platelet function: Adhesion, release, and aggregation. Pharmacol. Rev. **22:** 97–187.
25. LINDON, J. N., G. MCMANAMA, L. KUSHNER, E. W. MERRILL & E. W. SALZMAN. 1986. Does the conformation of absorbed fibrinogen dictate platelet interactions with artificial surfaces. Blood **68:** 355–362.
26. COLLER, B. S. 1980. Interaction of normal, thrombasthenic, and Bernard-Soulier platelets with immobilized fibrinogen. Defective platelet-fibrinogen interactions in thrombasthenia. Blood **55:** 169–178.
27. COLLER, B. S. 1984. Disorders of platelets. *In* Disorders of Hemostasis. O. Ratnoff & C. D. Forbes, Eds.: 73–176. Plenum. New York.
28. SOLUM, N. A. 1986. Platelet membrane proteins. Semin. Hematol. **22:** 289–302.
29. WEKSLER, B. B. 1982. Prostacyclin. Prog. Hemostas. Thromb. **6:** 113–138.
30. WEISS, H. J. 1982. Platelets: Pathophysiology and Antiplatelet Drug Therapy. Alan R. Liss. New York.
31. CHESTERMAN, C. N., R. OWE-YOUNG, J. MACPHERSON & S. A. KRILIS. 1986. Substrate for endothelial prostacyclin production in the presence of platelets exposed to collagen is derived from the platelets rather than the endothelium. Blood **67:** 1744–1750.
32. MARCUS, A. J., B. B. WEKSLER, E. A. JAFFE & M. J. BROCKMAN. 1980. Synthesis of prostacyclin from platelet-derived endoperoxides by cultured human endothelial cells. J. Clin. Invest. **66:** 979–989.
33. CLEMETSON, K. J. 1985. Glycoproteins of the platelet plasma membrane. *In* Platelet Membrane Glycoproteins. J. N. George, A. T. Nurden & D. R. Phillips, Eds.: 51–85. Plenum. New York.
34. COLLER, B. S., L. E. SCUDDER, E. I. PEERSCHKE, E. L. KALOMIRIS, & M. STEINBERG. 1986. Platelet physiology and platelet membrane glycoproteins. *In* Biology and Pathology of Platelet-Vessel Wall Interactions. A. T. Nurden & Y. Legrand, Eds.: 181–199. Academic. New York.
35. HAGEN, I. & N. O. SOLUM. 1985. Structure and function of platelet membrane glycoproteins as studied by crossed immunoelectrophoresis. *In* Platelet Membrane Glycoproteins. J. N. George, A. T. Nurden & D. R. Phillips, Eds.: 105–127. Plenum. New York.

36. Wyler, B., D. Bienz, K. J. Clemetson & E. F. Luscher. 1986. Glycoprotein Ib-beta is the only phosphorylated major membrane glycoprotein of human platelets. Biochem. J **234:** 373–378.
37. Kalomiris, E. L. & B. S. Coller. 1985. Thiol-specific probes indicate that the beta-chain of platelet glycoprotein Ib is a transmembrane protein with a reactive endofacial sulfydryl group. Biochemistry **24:** 5430–5436.
38. Coller, B. S., E. I. Peerschke, L. E. Scudder & C. A. Sullivan. 1983. Studies with a murine monoclonal antibody that abolishes ristocetin-induced binding of von Willebrand factor to platelets: Additional evidence in support of GPIb as a platelet receptor for von Willebrand factor. Blood **61:** 99–110.
39. Berndt, M. C., C. Gregory, B. H. Chong, H. Zola & P. A. Castaldi. 1983. Additional glycoprotein defects in Bernard-Soulier's syndrome: Confirmation of genetic basis by parental analysis. Blood **62:** 800–807.
40. Clemetson, K. J., J. L. McGregor, E. James, N. Dechavane & E. F. Luscher. 1982. Characterization of the platelet membrane glycoprotein abnormalities in Bernard-Soulier syndrome and comparison with normal by surface-labeling techniques and high resolution two-dimensional gel electrophoresis. J. Clin. Invest. **70:** 304–311.
41. Handu, M., K. Titani, L. Z. Holland, J. R. Roberts, T. S. Zimmerman & Z. M. Ruggeri. 1986. The von Willebrand factor binding domain of glycoprotein Ib. Characterization by monoclonal antibodies and partial amino acid sequence analysis of proteolytic fragments. Circulation **74** (Suppl. II): 238.
42. Fressinand, E., K. S. Sakariassen, J. P. Girma, D. Meyer & H. R. Baumgartner. 1986. Role of GPIIb/IIIa as well as GPIb in von Willebrand factor-mediated platelet adhesion to collagen. Thromb. Res. Suppl. **VI:** 138.
43. Coller, B. S., E. Kalomiris, M. Steinberg & L. E. Scudder. 1984. Evidence that glycocalicin circulates in normal plasma. J. Clin. Invest. **73:** 794–799.
44. Asch, A. S., M. Fujimoto, B. Adelman & R. L. Nachman. 1986. An endothelial cell GPIb like molecule mediates von Willebrand factor binding. Circulation **74** (Suppl. II): II–232.
45. Steinberg, M. H., J. G. Kelton & B. S. Coller. 1986. Plasma glycocalicin differentiates thrombocytopenia due to decreased production from thrombocytopenia due to increased destruction. Circulation **74** (Suppl. II): II–235.
46. Coller, B. S. 1986. Mechanism(s) of exposure of the GPIIb/IIIa complex receptor for adhesive glycoproteins. *In* Monoclonal Antibodies and Human Blood Platelets. INSERM Symposium No. 27. J. L. McGregor, Ed.: 93–102. Elsevier. Amsterdam.
47. Kunicki, T. J. 1985. Organization of glycoproteins within the platelet plasma membrane. *In* Platelet Membrane Glycoproteins. J. N. George, A. T. Nurden & D. R. Phillips, Eds.: 87–103. Plenum. New York.
48. Shattil, S. J., L. F. Brass, J. S. Bennett & P. Pandhi. 1985. Biochemical and functional consequences of dissociation of the platelet membrane glycoprotein IIb-IIIa complex. Blood **66:** 92–98.
49. Fitzgerald, L. A. & D. R. Phillips. 1985. Calcium regulation of the platelet membrane glycoprotein IIb-IIIa complex. J. Biol. Chem. **260:** 11366–11374.
50. Bray, P. F., J. P. Rosa, V. R. Lingapa, Y. W. Kan, R. P. McEver & M. A. Shuman. 1986. Biogenesis of the platelet receptor for fibrinogen: Evidence for separate precursors for glycoprotein IIb and IIIa. Proc. Natl. Acad. Sci. U.S.A. **83:** 1480–1484.
51. Leung, L. L. K., T. Kinoshita & R. L. Nachman. 1981. Isolation, purification and partial characterization of platelet membrane glycoprotein IIb and IIIa. J. Biol. Chem. **256:** 1994–1997.
52. McEver, R. P., J. U. Baenziger & P. W. Majerus. 1982. Isolation and structural characterization of the polypeptide subunits of membrane glycoprotein IIb-IIIa from human platelets. Blood **59:** 80–85.
53. Newman, P. J. & R. A. Kahn. 1983. Structural relationship of human platelet membrane glycoproteins IIb (GPIIb) and IIIa (GPIIIa). Blood **62:** 264a.
54. Mosher, D. F., D. M. Pesciotta, J. C. Loftus & R. M. Albrecht. 1985. Secreted alpha granule proteins: The race for receptors. *In* Platelet Membrane Glycoproteins. J. N. George, A. T. Nurden & D. R. Phillips, Eds.: 171–191. Plenum. New York.

55. FITZGERALD, L. A., I. F. CHARO & D. R. PHILLIPS. 1985. Human and bovine endothelial cells synthesize membrane proteins similar to human platelet glycoproteins IIb and IIIa. J. Biol. Chem. **260:** 10893–10896.
56. NEWMAN, P. J., Y. KAWAI, R. R. MONTGOMERY & T. J. KUNICKI. 1986. Synthesis by cultured human umbilical vein endothelial cells of two proteins structurally and immunlogically related to platelet membrane glycoproteins IIb and IIIa. J. Cell Biol. **103:** 81–86.
57. ALTIERI, D. C., P. M. MANNUCCI & A. M. CAPITANIO. 1986. Binding of fibrinogen to human monocytes. J. Clin. Invest. **78:** 968–976.
58. PYTELA, R, M. D. PIERSCHBACHER, M. H. GINSBERG, E. F. PLOW & E. RUOSLAHTI. 1986. Platelet membrane glycoprotein IIb/IIIa. Member of a family of Arg-Gly-Asp-specific adhesion receptors. Science **231:** 1559–1562.
59. BURNS, G. F., L. COSGROVE, T. TRIGLIA, J. A. BEALL, A. F. LOPEZ, J. A. WERKMEISTER, C. G. BEGLEY, A. P. HADDAD, J. F. D'APICE, M. A. VADAS & J. C. CAWLEY. 1986. The IIb-IIIa glycoprotein complex that mediates platelet aggregation is directly implicated in leukocyte adhesion. Cell **45:** 269–280.
60. LOFTUS, J., E. F. PLOW, R. PYTELA, M. PIERSCHBAKER, J. J. RYCKWAERT, E. RUOSLAHTI & M. GINSBERG. 1986. Immunochemical and structural comparison of GPIIb-IIIa and the vitronectin receptor. Circulation (Suppl. II): II–63.
61. PLOW, E. F., J. C. LOFTUS, E. G. LEVIN, D. S. FAIR, D. DIXON, J. FORSYTH & M. H. GINSBERG. 1986. Immunologic relationship between platelet membrane glycoprotein GPIIb/IIIa and cell surface molecules expressed by a variety of cells. Proc. Natl. Acad. Sci. U.S.A. **83:** 6002–6006.
62. CHARO, I., L. A. FITZGERALD, B. STEINER, S. C. RAWL, L. F. BEKAERT & D. R. PHILLIPS. 1986. Platelet glycoproteins IIb and IIIa: Evidence for a family of immunologically and structurally related glycoproteins in mammalian cells. Proc. Natl. Acad. Sci. U.S.A. **83:** 8351–8356.
63. PEERSCHKE, E. I. B. 1985. The platelet fibrinogen receptor. Semin. Hematol. **22:** 241–259.
64. BENNETT, J. S. 1985. The platelet-fibrinogen interaction. *In* Platelet Membrane Glycoproteins. J. N. George, A. T. Nurden & D. R. Phillips. Eds.: 193–214. Plenum. New York.
65. COLLER, B. S., E. I. PEERSCHKE, L. E. SCUDDER & C. A. SULLIVAN. 1983. A murine monoclonal antibody that completely blocks the binding of fibrinogen to platelets produces a thrombasthenic-like state in normal platelets and binds to glycoproteins IIb and/or IIIa. J. Clin. Invest. **72:** 325–338.
66. RUGGERI, Z. M., L. DE MARCO, L. GATTI, R. BADER & R. R. MONTGOMERY. 1983. Platelets have more than one binding site for von Willebrand factor. J. Clin. Invest. **72:** 1–12.
67. GRALNICK, H. R., S. B. WILLIAMS & B. S. COLLER. 1984. Fibrinogen competes with von Willebrand factor for binding to the glycoprotein IIb/IIIa complex when platelets are stimulated with thrombin. Blood **64:** 797–800.
68. PLOW, E. F., M. PIERSCHBACHER, E. RUOSLAHTI, G. A. MARGUERIE & M. H. GINSBERG. 1985. The effect of Arg-Gly-Asp containing peptides on fibrinogen and von Willebrand factor binding to platelets. Proc. Natl. Acad. Sci. U.S.A. **82:** 8057–8061.
69. COLLER, B. S. 1985. A new murine monoclonal antibody reports an activation-dependent change in the conformation and/or microenvironment of the platelet GPIIb/GPIIIa complex. J. Clin. Invest. **76:** 101–108.
70. COLLER, B. S. 1986. Activation affects access to the platelet receptor for adhesive glycoproteins. J. Cell Biol. **103:** 451–456.
71. SHATTIL, S. J., J. A. HOXIE, M. CUNNINGHAM & L. F. BRASS. 1985. Changes in the platelet membrane glycoprotein IIb-IIIa complex during activation. J. Biol. Chem. **260:** 11107–11114.
72. LAM, S. C-T., J. FORSYTH, M. D. PIERSCHBACHER, E. RUOSLAHTI, E. F. PLOW & M. H. GINSBERG. 1985. A synthetic peptide containing a fibronectin cell attachment sequence inhibits platelet aggregation and binds specifically and saturably to platelets. Fed. Proc. **44:** 1994.

73. KLOCZEWIAK, M. A., S. D. TIMMONS, T. J. LUKAS & J. J HAWIGER. 1984. Structural attributes of synthetic peptides inhibiting and promoting aggregation of human platelets. Circulation 70 (Suppl. II): II–358.
74. COLLER, B. S. & L. E. SCUDDER. 1985. Inhibition of dog platelet function by in vivo infusion of $F(ab')_2$ fragment of a monoclonal antibody to the platelet GPIIb/GPIIIa receptor. Blood **66:** 1456–1459.
75. COLLER, B. S., J. D. FOLTS, L. E. SCUDDER & R. S. SMITH. 1986. Antithrombotic effect of a monoclonal antibody to the platelet glycoprotein IIb/IIIa receptor in an experimental animal model. Blood **68:** 783–786.
76. YASUDA, T., H. K. GOLD, R. G. LEINBACH, M. KANKE, J. FALLON, L. E. SCUDDER & B. S. COLLER. 1986. A monoclonal anti-platelet antibody prevents acute coronary reocclusion following thrombolysis in dogs despite residual high-grade stenosis. Clin. Res. **34:** 634.
77. HANSON, S., L. HARKER, Z. Ruggeri & T. ZIMMERMAN. 1986. Antiplatelet GPIIb/IIIa antibody (LJ-CP8) prevents thrombus formation and occlusion of small caliber vascular grafts. Circulation (Suppl. II): II-236.
78. MARCUS, A. J. 1984. The eicosanoids in biology and medicine. J. Lipid Res. **25:** 1511–1516.
79. MARCUS, A. J. 1986. Transcellular metabolism of eicosanoids. Prog. Hemostas Thromb. **8:** 127–142.
80. HOLMSEN, H. 1985. Platelet metabolism and activation. Semin Hematol. **22:** 219–240.
81. NOMURA, H., H. NAKANISHI, K. ASE, U. KIKKAWA & Y. NISHIZUKA. 1986. Phosphoinositide metabolism in signal transduction. Prog. Hemostas. Thromb. **8:** 143–158.
82. AUTHI, K. S., B. J. EVENDEN & N. CRAWFORD. 1986. Metabolic and functional consequences of introducing inositol 1,4,5-triphosphate into saponin-permeabilized human platelets. Biochem. J. **233:** 709–718.
83. BRASS, L. & S. JOSEPH. 1986. A role for inositol triphosphate in intracellular calcium mobilization and granule secretion in platelets. J. Biol. Chem. **260:** 15172–15179.
85. COLLER, B. S. 1981. Inhibition of von Willebrand factor-dependent platelet function by increased platelet cyclic AMP and its prevention by cytoskeleton-disrupting agents. Blood **57:** 846-855.
86. MURER, E. H. 1985. The role of platelet calcium. Semin Hematol. **22:** 313–323.
87. BRASS, L. F. 1984. Ca^{2+} homeostasis in unstimulated platelets. J. Biol. Chem. **259:** 12563–12570.
88. FOX, J. E. B. 1985. The organization of platelet contractile proteins. *In* Platelet Membrane Glycoproteins. J. N. George, A. T. Nurden & D. R. Phillips, Eds.: 273–298. Plenum. New York.
89. WALSH, P. N. 1985. Platelet-mediated coagulant protein interactions in hemostasis. Semin. Hematol. **22:** 178–186.
90. HAWIGER, J. Personal communication.
91. GARTNER, T. K. & J. S. BENNETT. 1985. The tetrapeptide analogue of the cell attachment site of fibronectin inhibits platelet aggregation and fibrinogen binding to activated platelets. J. Biol. Chem. **260:** 11891–11894.
92. PIERSCHBACHER, M. D. & E. RUOSLAHTI. 1984. Variants of the cell recognition site of fibronectin that retain attachment-promoting activity. Proc. Natl. Acad. Sci. U.S.A. **81:** 5985–5988.
93. TOMASINI, B. R. & D. F. MOSHER. 1986. On the identity of vitronectin and S-protein: Immunologic crossreactivity and functional studies. Blood **68:** 737–742.
94. HUMPHRIES, M. J., K. OLDEN & K. M. YAMADA. 1986. A synthetic peptide from fibronectin inhibits experimental metastasis of murine melanoma cells. Science **233:** 467–470.
95. HUGGERI, Z. M., R. HOUGHTEN, S. RUSSEL & T. S. ZIMMERMAN. 1986. Inhibition of platelet function with synthetic peptides designed to be high affinity antagonists of fibrinogen binding to platelets. Proc. Natl. Acad. Sci. U.S.A. **83:** 5708–5712.
96. GARTNER, T. K., J. W. POWER, E. H. BEACHEY, J. S. BENNETT & S. J. SHATTIL. 1985. The tetrapeptide analogue of the alpha chain and decapeptide analogue of the gamma chain of fibrinogen bind to different sites on the platelet fibrinogen receptor. Blood **66**(Suppl. 1): 1104.
97. LAM, S., M. SMITH, E. PLOW, A. ANDRIEUS, J. RYCKWAERT, G. MARGUERIE & M.

GINSBERG. 1986. Evidence that Arg-Gly-Asp and fibrinogen gamma peptides share a common binding site on platelets. Circulation (Suppl. II): II–62.

98. THORSEN, L. I., F. BROSSTAD, N. O. SOLUM & H. STORMORKEN. 1986. Increased binding to ADP-stimulated platelets and aggregation effect of the dysfibrinogenemia Oslo I as compared with normal fibrinogen. Scand. J. Hematol. **36:** 203–210.

99. PEERSCHKE, E. I. B. & D. K. GALANAKIS. 1985. Binding of fibrinogen to ADP-treated platelets: Importance of the A-alpha chain. *In* Fibrinogen-Structural Variants and Interactions. A. Henschen, B. Hessel, J. McDonagh & T. Saldeen, Eds.: 369–377. Walter de Gruyter. Berlin.

100. GIRMA, J. P., M. KALAFATIS, G. PIETU, J. M. LAVERGNE, M. W. CHOPEK, T. S. EDINGTON & D. MEYER. 1986. Mapping of distinct von Willebrand factor domains interacting with platelet GPIb and GPIIb/IIIa and with collagen using monoclonal antibodies. Blood **67:** 1356–1366.

101. HOUDIJK, W. P. M., M. E. SCHIPHORST & J. J. SIXMA. 1986. Identification of functional domains on von Willebrand factor by binding of tryptic fragments to collagen and to platelets in the presence of ristocetin. Blood **67:** 1498–1503.

102. SCHULLEK, J., J. JORDAN & R. R. MONTGOMERY. 1984. Interaction of von Willebrand factor with human platelets in the plasma milieu. J. Clin. Invest. **73:** 421–428.

103. PACKHAM, M. A., E. J. HARFENIST, R. L. KINLOUGH-RATHBONE, M. CATTANEO & J. F. MUSTARD. 1986. Effect of [Ca^{2+}] in the suspending medium on the ability of von Willebrand factor and fibrinogen to support ADP-induced aggregation of human platelets. Thromb. Res. Suppl. **VI:** 121.

104. COLLER, B. S. 1987. Von Willebrand disease. *In* Hemostasis and Thrombosis: Basic Principles and Clinical Practice. R. W. Colman *et al.,* Eds: 60–96. J. B. Lippincott. Philadelphia.

105. EYSTER, M. E., R. A. GORDON & J. O. BALLARD. 1981. The bleeding time is longer than normal in hemophilia. Blood **58:** 719–723.

106. RAO, G. H. R., G. ESCOLAR & J. G. WHITE. 1986. Epinephrine reverses the inhibitory influence of aspirin on platelet-vessel wall interactions. Thromb. Res. **44:** 65–74.

107. BUTTRICK, P. M., C. A. FORSCHER, I. I. SUSSMAN & H. S. MUELLER. 1982. Subaggregatory doses of catecholamines prevent prostacyclin-induced inhibition of platelet aggregation. Am. Heart J. **109:** 1258–1263.

108. BERTHA, B. G. & J. D. FOLTS. 1984. Inhibition of epinephrine-exacerbated coronary thrombus formation by prostacyclin in the dog. J. Lab. Clin. Med. **103:** 204–214.

109. REIMERS, R. C., S. P. SUTERA & J. H. JOIST. 1984. Potentiation by red blood cells of shear-induced platelet aggregation: Relative importance of chemical and physical mechanisms. Blood **64:** 1200–1206.

110. MUSTARD, J. F., D. W. PERRY, R. L. KINLOUGH-RATHBONE & M. L. PACKHAM. 1975. Factors responsible for ADP-induced release reaction of human platelets. Am. J. Physiol. **228:** 1757.

111. WEISS, H. J., V. T. TURITTO & H. R. BAUMGARTNER. 1986. Role of shear rate and platelets in promoting fibrin formation on rabbit subendothelium. Studies utilizing patients with quantitative and qualitative platelet defects. J. Clin. Invest. **78:** 1072–1082.

112. MCMANAMA, G., J. N. LINDON, M. KLOCZEWIAK, M. A. SMITH, J. A. WARE, J. HAWIGER, E. W. MERRILL & E. W. SALZMAN. 1986. Platelet aggregation by fibrinogen polymers crosslinked across the E domain. Blood **68:** 363–371.

Regulation of Platelet-Fibrin Thrombi on Subendothelium[a]

HARVEY J. WEISS,[b] HANS R. BAUMGARTNER,[c] AND VINCENT T. TURITTO[d]

[b]*Department of Medicine*
The St. Luke's-Roosevelt Hospital Center
New York, New York 10019
and
College of Physicians and Surgeons
Columbia University
New York, New York 10032

[c]*Department of Experimental Medicine*
F. Hoffmann-La Roche & Co.
Basel, Switzerland

[d]*Department of Medicine*
Division of Cardiology
Mt. Sinai Medical School
New York, New York 10029

INTRODUCTION

Both normal hemostasis and pathological thrombosis are due, in part, to the formation of platelet-fibrin thrombi at sites of blood vessel injury. We have studied this process utilizing a technique developed by Baumgartner[1] for exposing de-endothelialized segments of rabbit aorta to human blood under controlled flow conditions. Initially our studies focused on factors that influence the deposition of platelets on the subendothelium. More recently, we have utilized this technique for studying fibrin deposition. The results of these studies have demonstrated that platelet and fibrin deposition on the subendothelium are strongly influenced by plasma and cellular factors, by properties of the vessel wall, and by flow.

MATERIALS AND METHODS

The perfusion chamber is an annular device on whose central core is mounted an everted segment of rabbit aorta previously denuded of endothelium by means of a balloon catheter.[1–4] Blood entering the chamber passes through the annular space formed by the subendothelial surface and the outer cylinder wall, thereby permitting platelets to interact with the exposed subendothelial surface. The flow parameters, dimensions, and temperature (37°C) control for the chamber have been previously described.[3–5]

[a]This work was supported in part by U.S. Public Health Service grant nos. HL27346, 37444, and 35103, and a grant from the Charles Slaughter Foundation.

Everted vessel segments were exposed at varying shear rates and exposure times to citrated or nonanticoagulated blood. Citrated blood, adjusted for the hematocrit value to a final plasma concentration of 19.7 mmol/l sodium citrate, was circulated through the chamber in a closed system using a peristaltic pump to maintain the desired blood flow.[1-5] For studies using nonanticoagulated blood, blood from the anticubital vein was drawn directly through an infusion set into the chamber and was not recirculated.[6-8] The flow rate was controlled by the pump and was accurately determined after each run by measuring the actual amount of blood perfused.[3] The wall shear rate for each flow rate used was determined as previously described.[3,5]

After perfusion, vessel segments were embedded in an oriented manner, and cross sections 0.8 μm in thickness were stained and evaluated morphormetrically by light microscopy[2-9] (FIGURE 1). Platelet interaction with the subendothelium was evaluated by two microscopical techniques that were performed on the same cross-sectional area of a vessel segment. For determining platelet adhesion, the presence of platelets was evaluated at 10 μm intervals, and platelet-subendothelial interaction was evaluated as either C (platelets attached but not spread on the surface) or S (platelets spread on the surface), and may, in addition, have superimposed aggregates of platelets (thrombi) extending for varying distances into the lumen (FIGURE 1). Platelet adhesion is defined as $C + S$, expressed as a percentage of the total number evaluated (~1000) per vessel segment. To evaluate more precisely the dimensions of the platelet thrombi, vessel segments were projected onto the recording plate of a manual picture analysis system (MOP/AMOI, Kontron AG, Zurich, Switzerland).[6-10] The thrombus volume per unit surface area is calculated from the total cross-sectional area of all platelet aggregates in a section normalized by the cross-sectional length of the subendothelial surface.[10] The maximum thrombus height is the average peak-to-base distance for the three tallest thrombi in a section. Further details of the MOP technique have been previously published.[10,11]

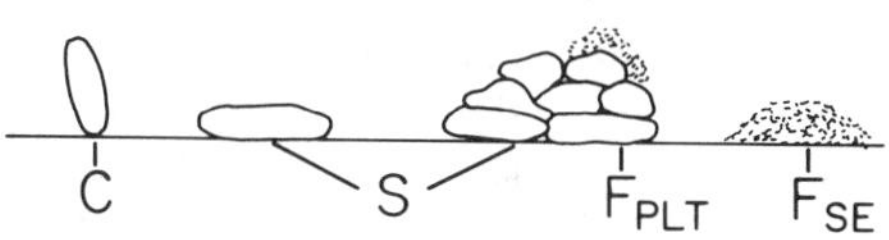

FIGURE 1. Morphometric evaluation of platelet and fibrin deposition on subendothelium. Schematic representation of platelet and fibrin deposition. Platelet adhesion is defined as the sum of contact (C) and spread (S) platelets (see METHODS). Total fibrin (F_T) is the sum of fibrin on subendothelium (F_{SE}) and fibrin on platelets (F_{PLT}).

Fibrin (presence or absence) on the subendothelium (F_{SE}) and on platelets (F_{PLT}) was evaluated systematically at 10 μm intervals (~1000 intersections) and total fibrin ($F_T = F_{SE} + F_{PLT}$) expressed as a percentage of the total number of evaluations.[6-8,10] Calculation of total surface coverage with fibrin (F_T) takes into account fibrin that is deposited directly on the subendothelial surface (F_{SE}) as well as fibrin that is observed on platelets that are attached to the surface (F_{PLT}). In order to account for the different levels of surface coverage with platelets observed in various patient groups, we calculated, for each subject, a parameter $F_{PLT}/(C + S)$, and designated this normalized value as platelet-bound fibrin.

In addition to the morphometric evaluation described above, we also measured, by radioimmunoassay, fibrinopeptide A (FPA) levels in blood exiting the chamber.[6,8]

Studies were performed on normal subjects (ages 21–50) and patients with congenital disorders of platelet function or deficiencies of plasma coagulation factors.

FACTORS DETERMINING DEPOSITION OF PLATELETS ON THE SUBENDOTHELIUM

General Considerations

The fluid dynamic and reaction rate parameters determining platelet deposition on the subendothelium in the annular perfusion system has been extensively analyzed using classical boundary layer theory to describe the overall convective-diffusive transport situation.[5,12–15] This well-established theoretical approach makes it possible to distinguish events related to purely flow effects from those more humoral in nature. Such an analysis places on a solid theoretical foundation, supported by experimental measurements,[3,16–18] the relevance of conditions under which proposed biochemical mechanisms should be tested (and additionally conditions at which they should not be tested) to the events of platelet adhesion and thrombus formation. Analysis by classic mass-transport theory predicted an adhesion of platelets to subendothelium that was highly dependent on the wall shear rate.[5,14] This analysis indicated that platelet attachment to subendothelium was determined predominantly by physical factors controlling the rate of platelet transport to the subendothelium at low shear rates ($<800\ s^{-1}$). In contrast, the influence of platelet surface reactivity became more evident at higher shear rates.[5] Platelet adhesion in native blood was also found to be highly dependent on shear rate, although at each shear rate where comparisons were made, adhesion was less in native than in citrated blood.[3]

In addition, platelet deposition was found to be highly dependent on the concentration of red cells, an effect attributed in part to the fact that red cells, by increasing the radial movement of platelets,[19] enhance their diffusivity several orders of magnitude compared to that theoretically predicted and experimentally measured in platelet-rich plasma.[16,20,21]

Role of von Willebrand Factor and Glycoprotein Ib in Platelet Adhesion

Utilizing these techniques, we described, in 1973 and subsequently, a shear-rate-dependent decrease in platelet adhesion in both von Willebrand's disease (vWD)[2,3,13,22] and the Bernard-Soulier syndrome,[3,4] thereby providing evidence for the complementary role of plasma von Willebrand factor (vWF) and its platelet receptor glycoprotein Ib (deficient in Bernard-Soulier platelets[23]) in mediating platelet-vessel wall attachment. More recently, we have shown that von Willebrand factor may also mediate platelet-to-platelet, as well as platelet-to-surface, attachment on subendothelium.[11] These findings were similar to previous ones demonstrating a role of von Willebrand factor in promoting platelet aggregation in packed bead columns.[24]

The shear rate dependence of the platelet adhesion defect in both congenital[3] and antibody-induced[25] von Willebrand's disease is consistent with theoretical predictions that assumed reduced platelet attachment kinetics of von Willebrand platelets.[14] Hence, in von Willebrand's disease (even at low shear rates) platelet adhesion is influenced by both attachment kinetics and transport (unlike normal blood where transport factors predominate). As shear rate is increased, kinetic factors become increasingly dominant, which accounts for the shear rate dependence of the platelet adhesion defect in von Willebrand's disease. Recent studies indicate that shear rates as high as $16{,}000\ s^{-1}$ may exist in the microvasculature.[26] Thus, the adhesion defects we have demonstrated in von Willebrand's disease have been obtained at shear rates that might exist in blood vessels involved in hemostasis. That these findings are physiologically relevant is further supported by the Sakariassen *et al.*, who found, utilizing a modification of the original Baumgartner technique, that the correction of the bleeding time after administration of desamino-D-arginine vasopressin (DDAVP) in patients with von Willebrand's disease correlates well with enhanced platelet adhesion to subendothelium.[27] It is interesting to note that the adhesion rate of von Willebrand platelets, both in native and citrated blood, actually decreases with shear rate, whereas in normal platelets the adhesion rate increases.[3] This shear-rate-dependent decrease of adhesion is, to a large extent, responsible for the shear-rate-dependent adhesion defect in von Willebrand's disease. Because classic theory, in which attachment kinetics are independent of fluid dynamic conditions, predicts in the limit an adhesion rate that is independent of shear rate, the experimentally observed decrease in adhesion with shear rate in von Willebrand's disease suggests a direct influence of flow in reducing reaction kinetics. The mechanisms that may account for this effect are considered elsewhere.[10]

Mechanisms Involved in vWF-mediated Adhesion

Studies by Sakariassen *et al.* have shown that plasma vWF mediates platelet adhesion by first binding to subendothelium.[28] In addition, platelet adhesion may also be mediated, in part, by von Willebrand factor that is already present in the subendothelium.[29,30] The major role of von Willebrand factor is to mediate the initial contact of platelets with the subendothelium,[9,31] although a secondary role in promoting spreading cannot be ruled out.[32] The molecular basis for the properties of vWF which mediate adhesion are currently under investigation. Studies utilizing monoclonal antibodies have identified a domain on the von Willebrand factor molecule that is associated with both ristocetin-induced platelet aggregation and platelet adhesion,[33] although the molecular loci involved in these two biological functions of the protein may not be identical.[34] Functional domains of von Willebrand factor that bind to glycoprotein Ib (GPIb) and promote platelet adhesion have been identified on a 116 kDa fragment obtained after proteolytic cleavage with trypsin[35] and on a 320 kDa fragment obtained after cleavage with *S. aureus* V-8 protease.[36] Further studies have shown the ligand for the GPIb receptor that is involved in platelet adhesion resides on a small (28–33 kDa) segment of the amino terminal port of the von Willebrand factor molecule.[37] The role of the multimer structure of von Willebrand factor in promoting adhesion is not clear, but adhesion may not require the full complement of multimers.[38]

Role of Glycoprotein IIb-IIIa

GPIIb-IIIa has been identified as the membrane receptor protein on platelets that can bind a group of adhesive proteins (including fibrinogen, von Willebrand factor, and fibronectin[39]) after platelet stimulation by agonists such as thrombin and ADP, but not ristocetin.[40–42] The domain on von Willebrand factor that binds to GPIIb-IIIa has been localized to a fragment, obtained after proteolytic cleavage, which is distinct from that containing the GpIb binding site.[37] In the absence of GPIIb-IIIa (as in Glanzmann's thrombasthenia) the platelets do not aggregate in response to ADP, owing to impaired binding of fibrinogen.[23] In addition, a possible role for von Willebrand factor in promoting GPIIb-IIIa–mediated aggregation in some circumstances has been suggested.[43]

Utilizing the perfusion chamber, we have studied the role of GPIIb-IIIa in mediating platelet deposition on subendothelium. In patients with thrombasthenia the platelets deposit as a monolayer on the subendothelium, further demonstrating the requirement of GPIIb-IIIa in mediating platelet-to-platelet interaction.[7,44] Although initial studies did not disclose a defect in platelet adhesion,[44] our more recent studies utilizing different experimental conditions demonstrated a defect in platelet adhesion both in patients with thrombasthenia and in normal blood that was treated with a monoclonal antibody to GPIIb-IIIa.[7] Further analysis suggested that GPIIb-IIIa is involved in the spreading of platelets on the subendothelium,[7] in contrast to GPIb, which is required principally in the initial attachment of platelets to the surface.[9,31] Similar conclusions concerning GPIIb-IIIa have been reached by Sakariassen *et al.*[45] The specific adhesive protein involved in GPIIb-IIIa–mediated platelet adhesion remains to be determined. Studies in a patient with congenital afibrinogenemia suggest that it is not fibrinogen.[3,6,11]

Other Factors Mediating Interaction of Platelet and Vessel Wall

We have recently studied platelet factors other than GPIb and GPIIb-IIIa that may be involved in the interaction of platelets with the vessel wall. We observed decreased thrombus formation in patients with storage pool deficiency (SPD) selectively deficient in platelet dense granules (δ-SPD), and the degree of abnormality was in proportion to the magnitude of the dense granule defect.[7] These findings strongly suggest that dense-granule-bound substances, in all likelihood ADP, either influence the growth of thrombi on subendothelium or help to maintain thrombus stability in growing thrombi subjected to the high shear stresses (650 to 2600 s^{-1}) utilized in these studies,[7] comparable to those encountered physiologically. The even smaller thrombi observed in patients with combined deficiencies of α-granules and dense granules ($\alpha\delta$-SPD)[7] further suggest an additional role of substances, including von Willebrand factor, which are stored in α-granules.

We also observed decreased platelet adhesion in some patients with δ-SPD, similar to previous observations on storage-pool-deficient (Fawn-hooded) rats[46] and consistent with the recent conclusions of Timmons *et al.* that platelet adhesion may be influenced, in part, by ADP released from platelets.[47] However, platelet adhesion in δ-SPD was strongly influenced (at a shear rate of 2600 s^{-1}) by the hematocrit value.[7] These findings suggest a possible role for red cells that could compensate for the platelet defect at higher shear rates, consistent with previous observations.[18] This possibility is currently under investigation.

Proteins present in the subendothelium may also influence adhesion. In addition to subendothelial von Willebrand factor,[48] which has been shown to influence adhesion,[29,30] a role for fibronectin has also been reported.[49,50,51] Some of the mechanisms involved in platelet adhesion on subendothelium are shown in FIGURE 2. Finally, another platelet glycoprotein, Ia, has been recently shown to play a role in mediating platelet adhesion.[31]

FACTORS AFFECTING FIBRIN DEPOSITION ON SUBENDOTHELIUM

We have recently turned our attention to studying plasma and platelet factors that influence the deposition of fibrin on the subendothelium. These studies were initiated in order to examine mechanisms involved in fibrin deposition on a vascular surface exposed to blood under a range of flow conditions found in various parts of the circulatory system.

General Observations

Studies were performed on nonanticoagulated blood from normal subjects and from patients with a variety of coagulation and platelet defects. The everted vessel segments were exposed to blood at shear rates ranging from 50 to 2600 s^{-1} and for perfusion times of 5 and 10 min. In normal subjects, we observed an inverse relationship between platelet and fibrin deposition.[8] Platelet deposition reached a minimum (adhesion = 5%) at a shear rate of 50 s^{-1} and increased progressively with increasing shear rate, consistent with behavior predicted by classical mass transfer theory, as discussed above. In contrast, fibrin deposition on subendothelium reached a

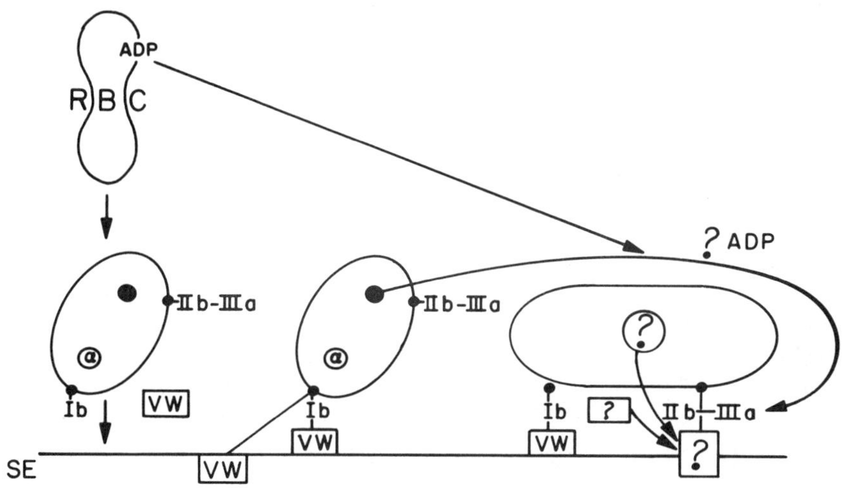

FIGURE 2. Mechanisms involved in the adhesion of platelets on the subendothelium. The initial attachment of platelets to subendothelium (*SE*) requires the binding of von Willebrand factor (*VW*) present in blood or subendothelium to glycoprotein Ib. Glycoprotein IIb-IIIa is involved in the subsequent spreading of platelets on the surface through one or more adhesive proteins (currently being studied) present in either blood, platelet α-granules, or subendothelium. In addition, adhesion requires glycoprotein Ia, a substance present in platelet dense granules (possibly ADP), and fibronectin present in subendothelium. Adhesion is also strongly influenced by red blood cells (*RBC*), which greatly enhance platelet diffusivity and could also increase platelet reactivity.

maximum at 50 s^{-1} and decreased with increasing shear rate.[8] This observation is discussed in more detail below.

Role of Plasma Coagulation Factors

Detailed studies on the coagulation mechanism have demonstrated that the contact of blood with negatively charged surfaces resulted in the sequential activation of factors XII (requiring kallikrein and high molecular weight kininogen), XI, IX, X (requiring factor VIII and platelets), prothrombin (requiring factor V and platelets),

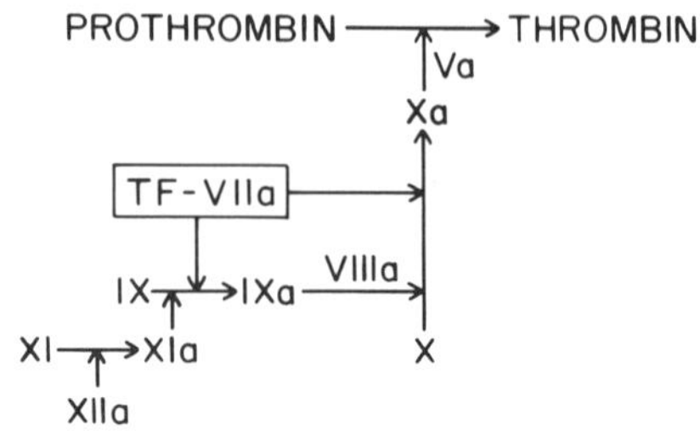

FIGURE 3. Tissue-factor-mediated coagulation pathways. Tissue factor (TF) bound to factor VIIa can activate factor IX (as well as factor X), thereby producing a mechanism for activating factor IX that does not require either factor XIIa or factor XIa.

and fibrinogen.[52,53] This sequence, however, does not explain the absence of bleeding symptoms in patients with factor XII deficiency[52] (and some patients with factor XI deficiency[54,55]), in contrast to the severe bleeding characteristically seen in patients deficient in factors VIII and IX. A possible explanation of these findings is suggested by recent observations that tissue factor-VIIa complex can (in addition to directly activating factor X) also activate factor IX,[56–59] thereby providing an alternative mechanism for the activation of factor IX that "bypasses"' the requirement for factor XI (FIGURE 3).

To determine which plasma coagulation factors are required for the deposition of fibrin on subendothelium, we studied patients with congenital deficiencies of factors XII, XI, IX, and VIII.[6] As seen in FIGURE 4, the standard partial thromboplastin time (PTT) performed in glass tubes was markedly prolonged in all four groups of patients, the most severe defect occurring in patients with factor XII deficiency. In contrast, the

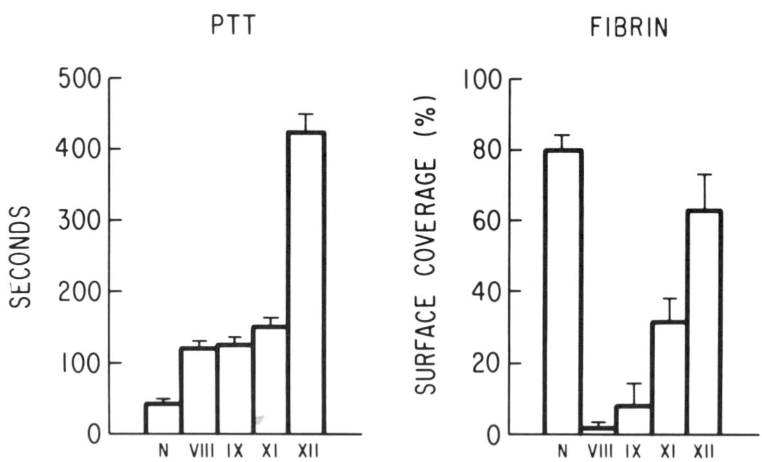

FIGURE 4. Plasma coagulation studies and subendothelial fibrin deposition in patients with coagulation disorders. The plasma partial thromboplastin time (*PTT*) was prolonged in all patients and was most abnormal in factor XII deficiency (*left*). In contrast (*right*), significantly more fibrin deposition on subendothelium (studied at a shear rate of 650 s^{-1}) was observed in patients with factor XII and factor XI deficiency than in those deficient in factors VIII and IX. *Bars* represent the SEM. (Data from Weiss *et al.*[6]).

deposition of fibrin on subendothelium at a shear rate of 650 s^{-1} was greater in patients with factor XII and XI deficiency than in those deficient in factors VIII and IX (FIGURE 4). Comparable results were obtained for FPA levels in blood exiting the chamber.[6] In addition, we observed (FIGURE 5) smaller platelet thrombi in hemophilia (but not afibrinogenemia), suggesting that thrombin was a major factor in determining the formation of platelet thrombi under these shear conditions. Thus, the results obtained for fibrin deposition, FPA, and platelet thrombus dimensions appeared to

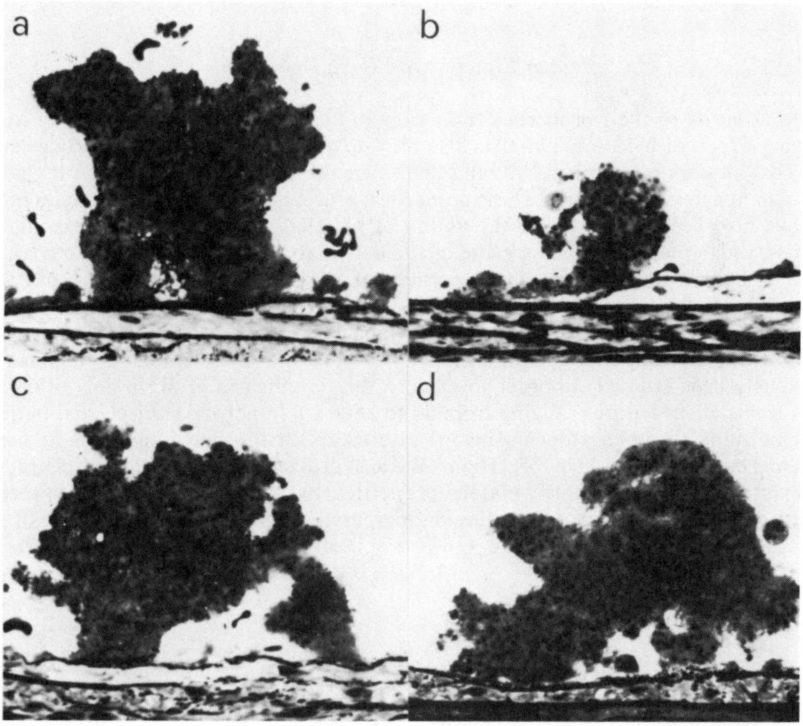

FIGURE 5. Platelet thrombi on subendothelium in patients with coagulation defects. Representative light micrographs of cross sections of rabbit aorta exposed to native human blood flowing at 10 ml/min (650 s^{-1} wall shear rate) for 5 min in an annular chamber. The thrombi shown correspond in their height approximately to the average heights of the three tallest thrombi observed. (**a**) Control subject. (**b**) Patient with hemophilia (factor VIII deficiency). (**c**) Patient with factor XII deficiency. (**d**) Patient with fibrinogen deficiency. Magnification: 750×. (For complete details, see Weiss *et al.*[6])

correlate better with the severity of clinical bleeding than those obtained by more standard coagulation tests.

The above findings suggest that tissue factor-VIIa activation of factor IX could be a critical step in mediating fibrin deposition on subendothelium, provided it can be shown that the subendothelium possesses tissue factor activity. In our initial studies we reported normal values for fibrin deposition and FPA levels in two patients with factor VII deficiency,[6] a finding that is inconsistent with the above hypothesis. We utilized an exposure time of 5 min, similar to the conditions used for studying the other coagulation-deficient patients. We have recently utilized a shorter perfusion period and observed, in factor-VII-deficient patients, both decreased fibrin deposition and FPA levels after 2 min (but not 5 min, see FIGURE 6). These findings demonstrate the presence of tissue factor activity in the subendothelium and suggest that direct activation of factor IX by tissue factor-VIIa could play a critical role in mediating fibrin deposition on subendothelium and account for the results shown in FIGURE 4. Direct experimental verification of this hypothesis will require more extensive studies on the kinetics governing the activation of coagulation factors on the subendothelium.

Role of Platelets in Fibrin Deposition

In addition to their properties (adhesion and aggregation) that contribute to the primary arrest of bleeding, platelets also provide a surface that can greatly accelerate the coagulation mechanism,[60–62] and hence could play an important role in the permanent arrest of bleeding. These properties, previously referred to as platelet factor 3, have now been attributed to the ability of platelets to bind activated coagulation factors, thus greatly enhancing some of the enzymatic activities involved in coagulation.[60–62] Besides playing a role in the permanent arrest of bleeding, these procoagulant properties of platelets could also contribute to the formation of the fibrin component of intravascular thrombi, but the extent to which the coagulant properties of platelets may be influenced by flow conditions in various parts of the circulatory system has not previously been studied. In order to explore this, we measured fibrin deposition and FPA levels at shear rates ranging from 50 to 2600 s^{-1} in normal subjects and patients with immune thrombocytopenia in order to establish the flow conditions at which platelets contribute to fibrin formation.[8] We also utilized patients with well-characterized platelet defects to identify platelet properties that may contribute to this process.

In normal subjects, platelet adhesion increased progressively from a value of 5 ± 1% at a shear rate of 50 s^{-1} to 52 ± 6% at a shear rate of 2600 s^{-1} and the average

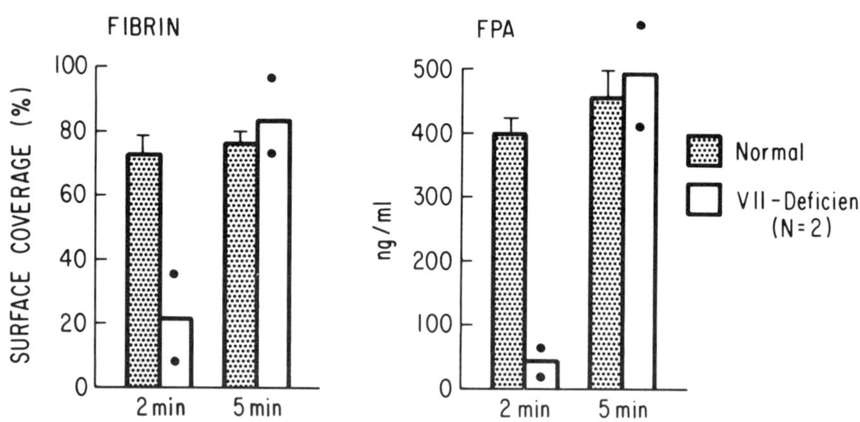

FIGURE 6. Fibrin deposition and FPA levels in factor VII deficiency. Fibrin deposition on subendothelium and FPA levels of blood exiting the chamber were determined in two patients with congenital factor VII deficiency (factor VII levels 1–2%). Subendothelium was exposed to nonanticoagulated blood for either 2 or 5 min at a shear rate of 650 s^{-1}. *Bars* are the SEM.

TABLE 1. Characteristics of Scott Syndrome[8,63–65]

- Normal platelet aggregation and secretion
- Decreased platelet factor 3
- Impaired prothrombin consumption (whole blood)
- Decreased binding of factor Xa to platelets
- Impaired platelet catalytic activity in converting (1) prothrombin to thrombin (in presence of FXa and FVa); and (2) factor X to Xa (in presence of FVIII and FIXa)
- Impaired agonist-induced exposure of acidic phospholipids

maximum thrombus height increased from 368 μm to 130 ± 22 μm.[8] Thus, the effect of increasing shear rate was to enhance both the attachment ($C + S$) of platelets to the surface as well as to increase the size of the platelet thrombi that formed over adherent platelets. The opposite was true for fibrin deposition on the subendothelium, which reached maximum at 50 s^{-1}, and decreased sharply at shear rates greater than 650 s^{-1}.[8] The latter was also the case for blood FPA levels. From the above findings, a shear rate of 650 s^{-1} seemed appropriate for examining a possible role of platelets and platelet properties in fibrin deposition. At this shear rate, we found (utilizing patients with thrombocytopenia) that platelets were required for fibrin deposition; little or no fibrin was deposited on the subendothelium when platelet adhesion was less than 4%, corresponding to blood platelet counts less than 5000 per μl.[8] Studies performed in patients with functional platelet disorders provided additional information on the specific properties of platelets that contribute to fibrin deposition at this shear rate. Decreased fibrin deposition was observed in a patient with Scott syndrome[8] who has a specific defect in platelet procoagulant activity.[63] This disorder is characterized by an impaired capacity of the platelets to catalyze the conversion of factor X to factor Xa (in the presence of factors IXa and VIII[64]) and prothrombin to thrombin (in the presence of factor V[64,65]), the latter owing to a decreased factor-Xa-binding capacity of the platelets[65] (TABLE 1). These abnormalities may be due to reduced exposure of membrane phospholipids after agonist-induced stimulation of the platelets.[64] In contrast to the findings in Scott syndrome, both fibrin deposition and FPA values were completely normal (and possibly increased) in thrombasthenia (GPIIb-IIIa deficiency).[8] The findings obtained in Scott syndrome and thrombasthenia are shown in FIGURE 7. They demonstrate the marked deficiency in fibrin deposition in Scott syndrome despite normal, and perhaps even enhanced, platelet adhesion. In addition, the platelet thrombi were reduced in volume, as occurs in hemophilia (FIGURE 5), again illustrating the important role of thrombin in promoting platelet-to-platelet interaction under these shear conditions. The normal (and perhaps even increased) fibrin deposition observed in patients with thrombasthenia (FIGURE 7) indicate that a monolayer of platelets (including those deficient in GPIIb-IIIa) is completely active in promoting fibrin deposition on subendothelium. These findings suggest that a drug which can induce a platelet defect similar to that observed in Scott syndrome (in contrast to thrombasthenia) might prevent platelet-fibrin thrombi at shear rates (200–800 s^{-1}) comparable to those in the coronary circulation.[66]

We also studied two patients deficient in GPIb (Bernard-Soulier syndrome) and compared the results with moderately thrombocytopenic patients having comparably decreased platelet adhesion values.[8] As seen in FIGURE 8, total fibrin deposition was somewhat decreased in the Bernard-Soulier patients, but was normal in the patients with thrombocytopenia (as noted above, fibrin deposition is decreased in patients with *marked* thrombocytopenia). As indicated in MATERIALS AND METHODS, measurement of total fibrin takes into account the deposition of fibrin both on the subendothelium (F_{SE}) and on platelets (F_{PLT}). The abnormal fibrin deposition in the Bernard-Soulier

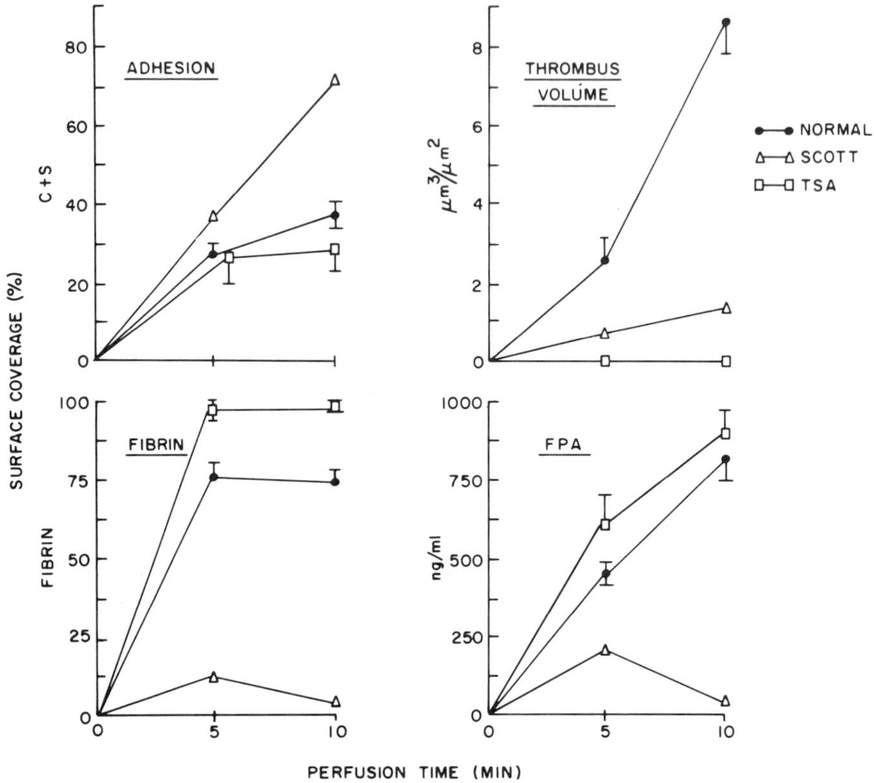

FIGURE 7. Fibrin and platelet deposition on subendothelium. Scott syndrome and thrombasthenia. Subendothelium was exposed to nonanticoagulated blood for 5 or 10 min at a shear rate of 650 s^{-1}. Parameters for platelet deposition (adhesion and thrombus volume, *above*) and coagulation (fibrin deposition and FPA levels, *below*) are shown for normal subjects, patients with thrombasthenia ($n = 3$), and a patient with Scott syndrome. *Bars* represent the SEM. (Data from Weiss *et al.*[8])

syndrome appears to be due primarily to a decreased deposition of fibrin on platelets (FIGURE 8). As seen further in FIGURE 9, the decreased amount of platelet-bound fibrin in these patients was particularly striking when expressed as the normalized value $F_{PLT}/C + S$, particularly for the 10 min perfusion period, and is in marked contrast with the normal values obtained in patients with thrombocytopenia at comparable levels of platelet adhesion. This reduction in platelet-bound fibrin observed in patients with GpIb deficiency may be related to the recent findings of Loscalzo *et al.* that von Willebrand protein and GpIb facilitate the incorporation of polymerizing fibrin onto platelets.[67]

Effect of Shear Rate

The above studies indicate that platelets, and the platelet properties specifically impaired in Scott syndrome, are required for fibrin deposition at a shear rate of 650

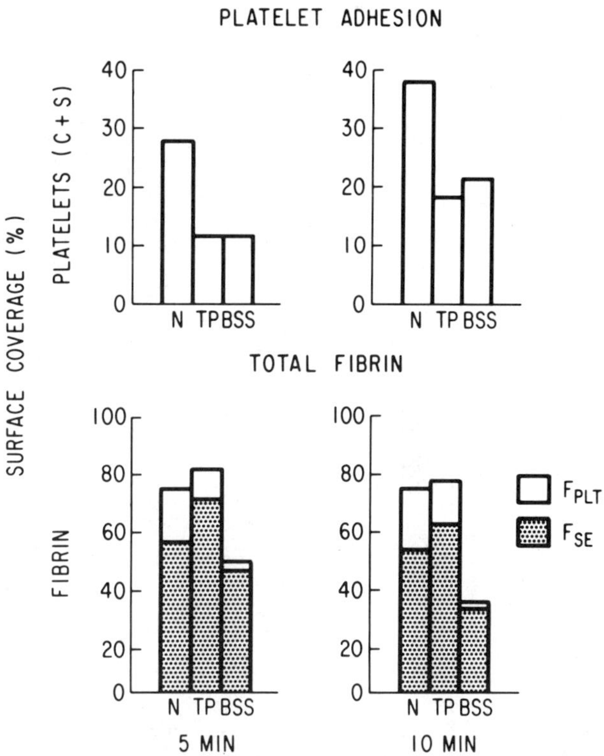

FIGURE 8. Platelet and fibrin deposition in thrombocytopenia and the Bernard-Soulier syndrome. Platelet adhesion and fibrin deposition were determined after exposure of subendothelium to nonanticoagulated blood for 5 min at a shear rate of 650 s^{-1}. The average values shown are for normal subjects ($n = 24$), two patients with the Bernard-Soulier syndrome (*BSS*), and six patients with immune thrombocytopenia (*TP*) whose values for platelet adhesion were comparable to those of the Bernard-Soulier patients. The total fibrin deposition on the surface reflects fibrin deposited directly on the subendothelium (F_{SE}) as well as fibrin that is associated with platelets (F_{PLT}). (Data from Weiss *et al.*[8])

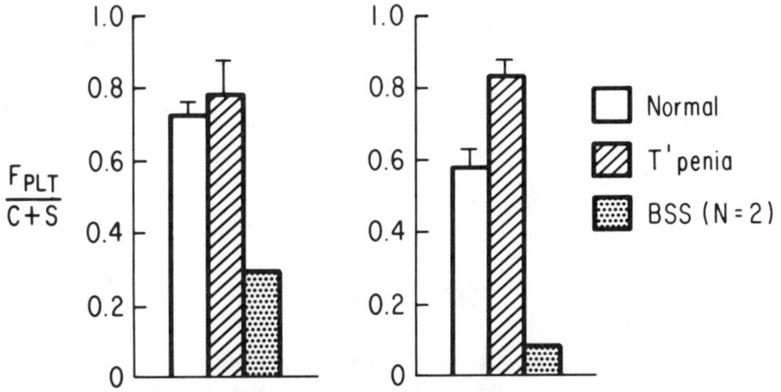

FIGURE 9. Platelet-bound fibrin in thrombocytopenia and the Bernard-Soulier syndrome. Conditions were the same as in FIGURE 8, and the results are shown for perfusion times of 5 and 10 min. The parameter $F_{PLT}/C + S$ (platelet-bound fibrin) normalizes the deposition of fibrin on platelets for variations in platelet adhesion. *Bars* represent the SEM. (Data from Weiss *et al.*[8])

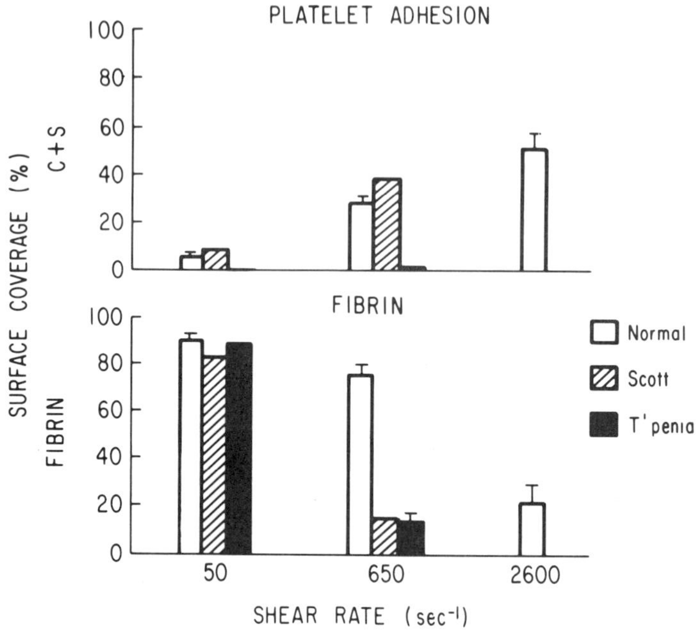

FIGURE 10. Shear-rate dependence of platelet adhesion and fibrin deposition in Scott syndrome and thrombocytopenia. Values for platelet adhesion and total fibrin deposition obtained at shear rates of 50, 650, and 2600 s^{-1} are shown for normal subjects, a patient with Scott syndrome, and four patients with immune thrombocytopenia (T'penia) in whom platelet adhesion values at the shear rate of 650 s^{-1} were markedly reduced (less than 4%). Note that at a shear rate of 50 s^{-1} fibrin deposition was relatively independent of platelets in all groups, whereas at 2600 s^{-1} fibrin deposition in the normal subjects is decreased despite increasing values for platelet adhesion. *Bars* represent the SEM.

s^{-1}. Studies were performed to examine the platelet requirements at other shear rates. As seen in FIGURE 10, fibrin deposition values of 82–90% were observed in normal subjects (despite low values of platelet adhesion), in Scott syndrome, and in a patient with thrombocytopenia whose adhesion value was 0%. These findings indicate that platelets are not required for fibrin deposition at a shear rate (50 s^{-1}) observed in large veins and are consistent with clinical observations that thrombocytopenia does not appear to confer any absolute or relative protection against developing a venous thrombus. As may also be seen in FIGURE 10, fibrin deposition in normal subjects decreases at a shear rate of 2600 s^{-1}, despite increasing platelet deposition (adhesion) on the surface, as discussed earlier.

CONCLUSIONS

The results of our studies demonstrate the complex role of various plasma coagulation factors, specific platelet properties, and the procoagulant properties (tissue factor) of the vessel in mediating fibrin deposition on both subendothelium and on adherent platelets. Further, they demonstrate the strong, and inverse, relationship of fibrin deposition with shear rate, the relative lack of a platelet requirement at low shear rates (where fibrin deposition can occur despite little or no platelet deposition), the progressive decrease in fibrin deposition at shear rates greater than 650 s^{-1} (despite increasing platelet deposition), and specific abnormalities in patients with various types of platelet disorders. Thus, a satisfactory explanation must account for not only the well-studied mechanisms for activation of the coagulation mechanism, but also for the rheological factors that determine the concentrations of activated coagulation proteins either in the boundary layer or those immobilized by surface binding to platelets on the subendothelial surface. As discussed by Leonard,[68] the concentration of proteins activated, but not bound, at the surface through the coagulation mechanism will be strongly influenced by flow factors, and the net concentration will be determined both by the biochemical reactions producing activated coagulation factors and by convective-diffusive factors that serve to moderate the concentrations of unactivated and activated coagulation proteins.

In general, because the boundary layer for activated species (products) is diluted as wall shear rate increases, it follows that the effective concentration of activated coagulation factors in the boundary layer will also decrease. This might explain the inverse relationship between fibrin deposition and shear rate observed with normal blood.[8] Since platelets have been shown to bind activated coagulation factors such as factors Xa,[69,70] Va,[71,72] and IXa[73] to their surface, the presence of adherent platelets on the subendothelium could, with increasing shear rates, serve to maintain activated coagulation proteins in the boundary layer at a concentration that would otherwise be reduced through convective diffusion in their absence (see FIGURE 11). Thus, at low shear rates (50 s^{-1}), the concentration of activated coagulation factors in the boundary layer might be sufficient to support fibrin deposition despite the absence of platelets, whereas at very high shear rates (2600 s^{-1} and above), even the presence of platelets is insufficient to maintain the required concentration. The shear-dependent defect of

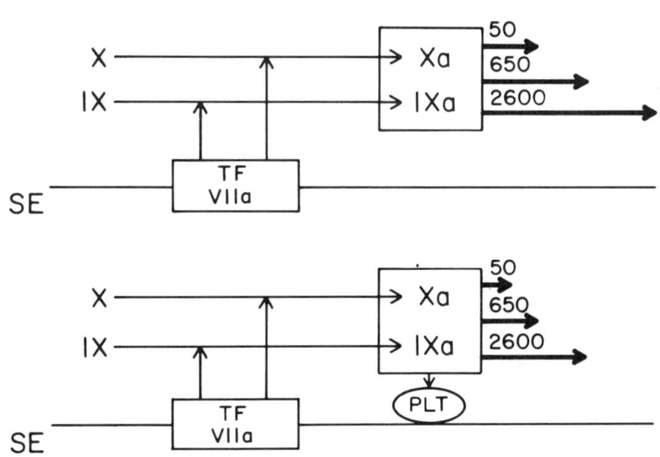

FIGURE 11. Possible effect of shear rate and platelets on fibrin deposition on subendothelium. The removal (*heavy arrows*) of activated coagulation factors such as factors IXa and Xa (generated, in part, from their precursors by subendothelial TF-VIIa) from the vicinity of the vessel is strongly influenced by blood flow and the capacity of the platelets to bind them at their surface. Platelets, though binding these factors, may serve to counteract the effect of flow. Thus, at a shear rate of 50 s^{-1} (but not 650 s^{-1} and above), the factors may be adequate even without platelets (*above*), whereas platelets may be necessary (*below*) at higher shear rates (650 s^{-1}). At even higher shear rates (2600 s^{-1}) flow effects may predominate.

fibrin formation in a patient with Scott syndrome,[8] a disorder in which impaired binding of factor Xa has been previously demonstrated,[65] is consistent with such a theory.

The findings in the present study emphasize the importance of considering flow in evaluating both the requirement for platelets in accelerating fibrin formation as well as the specific platelet properties that are involved in this process. For one, they provide evidence that platelets play a relatively minor role in accelerating fibrin formation at low shear rates even when they are observed to be present in small numbers. These observations do not lend any support to the possibility that inhibiting the procoagulant activities of platelets would be particularly useful in preventing thrombosis at low shear conditions, such as those observed in large veins. Our studies, however, do provide strong evidence that inhibiting the procoagulant properties of platelets, such as those which are abnormal in Scott syndrome, might by potentially useful in inhibiting fibrin formation in large arteries, such as the coronaries, where shear rates of 200 to 800 s^{-1} are characteristically observed.[66] This could be particularly relevant in view of recent evidence from clinical studies with fibrinolytic agents that fibrin is a major component of the thrombotic material in major epicardial vessels during the early stages of an evolving transmural myocardial infarction.[74] In addition, by inhibiting thrombin formation, the size of the platelet thrombi that form over the adherent platelets would also be decreased (FIGURES 4B and 7), thereby preventing the type of mixed platelet-fibrin thrombi that may initiate episodes of cerebral and cardiac ischemia.

REFERENCES

1. BAUMGARTNER, H. R. 1973. The role of blood flow in platelet adhesion, fibrin deposition and formation of mural thrombi. Microvasc. Res. **5:** 167–179.
2. TSCHOPP, T., H. J. WEISS & H. R. BAUMGARTNER. 1974. Decreased adhesion of platelets to subendothelium in von Willebrand's disease. J. Lab. Clin. Med. **83:** 296–300.
3. WEISS, H. J., V. T. TURITTO & H. R. BAUMGARTNER. 1978. Effect of shear rate on platelet interaction with subendothelium in citrated and native blood. Shear-rate dependent decrease of adhesion in von Willebrand's disease and the Bernard-Soulier syndrome. J. Lab. Clin. Med. **92:** 750–764.
4. WEISS, H. J., T. B. TSCHOPP, H. R. BAUMGARTNER, I. I. SUSSMAN, M. M. JOHNSON & J. J. EGAN. 1974. Decreased adhesion of giant (Bernard-Soulier) platelets to subendothelium. Further implications on the role of the von Willebrand factor in hemostasis. Am. J. Med. **57:** 920–925.
5. TURITTO, V. T. & H. R. BAUMGARTNER. 1979. Platelet interaction with subendothelium in flowing rabbit blood: Effect of blood shear rate. Microvasc. Res. **17:** 38–54.
6. WEISS, H. J., V. T. TURITTO, W. J. VICIC & H. R. BAUMGARTNER. 1984. Fibrin formation, fibrinopeptide A release, and platelet thrombus dimensions on subendothelium exposed to flowing native blood: Greater in factor XII and XI than in factor VIII and IX deficiency. Blood **63:** 1004–1014.
7. WEISS, H. J., V. T. TURITTO & H. R. BAUMGARTNER. 1986. Platelet adhesion and thrombus formation on subendothelium in platelets deficient in glycoproteins IIb-IIIa, Ib, and storage granules. Blood **67:** 322–330.
8. WEISS, H. J., V. T. TURITTO & H. R. BAUMGARTNER. 1986. Role of shear rate and platelets in promoting fibrin formation on rabbit subendothelium. Studies utilizing patients with quantitative and qualitative platelet defects. J. Clin. Invest. **78:** 1072–1082.
9. TURITTO, V. T., H. J. WEISS & H. R. BAUMGARTNER. 1983. Decreased platelet adhesion on vessel segments in von Willebrand's disease: A defect in initial platelet attachment. J. Lab. Clin. Med. **102:** 551–564.
10. BAUMGARTNER, H. R., V. T. TURITTO & H. J. WEISS. 1980. Effect of shear rate on platelet interaction with subendothelium in citrated and native blood. II. Relationships among platelet adhesion, thrombus dimensions and fibrin formation. J. Lab. Clin. Med. **95:** 208–221.

11. TURITTO, V. T., H. J. WEISS & H. R. BAUMGARTNER. 1984. Platelet interaction with rabbit subendothelium in von Willebrand's disease: Altered thrombus formation distinct from defective platelet adhesion. J. Clin. Invest. **74:** 1730–1741.
12. TURITTO, V. T., H. J. WEISS & H. R. BAUMGARTNER. 1980. The effect of shear rate on platelet interaction with subendothelium exposed to citrated human blood. Microvasc. Res. **19:** 352–365.
13. WEISS, H. J., H. R. BAUMGARTNER, T. B. TSCHOPP & V. T. TURITTO. 1977. Interaction of platelets with subendothelium: A new method for identifying and classifying abnormalities of platelet function. Ann. N.Y. Acad. Sci. **283:** 293–309.
14. TURITTO, V. T. & H. R. BAUMGARTNER. 1975. Platelet deposition on subendothelium exposed to flowing blood: Mathematical analysis of physical parameters. Trans. Am. Soc. Artif. Intern. Organs **21:** 593–601.
15. TURITTO, V. T., H. J. WEISS & H. R. BAUMGARTNER. 1979. Rheological factors influencing platelet interaction with vessel surfaces. J. Rheol. **23:** 735–749.
16. TURITTO, V. T. & H. R. BAUMGARTNER. 1975. Platelet interaction with subendothelium in a perfusion system: Physical role of red blood cells. Microvasc. Res. **9:** 335–344.
17. TURITTO, V. T. & H. J. WEISS. 1983. Platelet and red cell involvement in mural thrombogenesis. Ann. N.Y. Acad. Sci. **416:** 363–374.
18. TURITTO, V. T. & H. J. WEISS. 1980. Red cells: Their dual role in thrombus formation. Science **207:** 541–543.
19. GOLDSMITH, H. L. & T. KARINO. 1977. Microscopic considerations: The motions of individual particles. Ann. N.Y. Acad. Sci. **283:** 241–255.
20. TURITTO, V. T., A. M. BENIS & E. F. LEONARD. 1972. Platelet diffusion in flowing blood. Ind. Eng. Chem. Fund **11:** 216–223.
21. GRABOWSKI, E. F., L. I. FRIEDMAN & E. F. LEONARD. 1972. Effects of shear rate on the diffusion and adhesion of blood platelets to a foreign surface. Ind. Eng. Chem. Fund **11:** 224–232.
22. WEISS, H. J., H. R. BAUMGARTNER, T. B. TSCHOPP, V. T. TURITTO & D. COHEN. 1978. Correction by factor VIII of the impaired platelet adhesion to subendothelium in von Willebrand's disease. Blood **51:** 267–279.
23. GEORGE, J. N., A. T. NURDEN & D. R. PHILLIPS. 1984. Molecular defects in interactions of platelets with the vessel wall. N. Engl. J. Med. **311:** 1084–1098.
24. MCPHERSON, J. & M. B. ZUCKER. 1976. Platelet retention in glass bead columns: Adhesion to glass and subsequent platelet-platelet interaction. Blood **47:** 55–67.
25. BAUMGARTNER, H. R., T. B. TSCHOPP & D. MEYER. 1980. Shear rate dependent inhibition of platelet adhesion and aggregation on collagenous surfaces by antibodies to human factor VIII/von Willebrand factor. Br. J. Haematol. **44:** 127–139.
26. SCHMID-SCHÖNBEIN, G. W. & B. W. ZWEIFACH. 1975. RBC velocity profiles in arterioles and venules of the rabbit omentum. Microvasc. Res. **10:** 153–164.
27. SAKARIASSEN, K. S., M. CATTANEO, A. VAN DER BERG, Z. M. RUGGERI, P. M. MANNUCCI & J. J. SIXMA. 1984. DDAVP enhances platelet adherence and platelet aggregate growth on human artery subendothelium. Blood **64:** 229–236.
28. SAKARIASSEN, K. S., P. A. BOLHUIS & J. J. SIXMA. 1979. Human blood platelet adhesion to artery subendothelium is mediated by factor VIII: vWF bound to the subendothelium. Nature **279:** 636–638.
29. TURITTO, V. T., H. J. WEISS, T. S. ZIMMERMAN & I. I. SUSSMAN. 1985. Factor VIII/von Willebrand factor and subendothelium mediates platelet adhesion. Blood **65:** 823–831.
30. STEL, H. V., K. S. SAKARIASSEN, P. G. DE GROOT, J. A. VAN MOURIK & J. J. SIXMA. 1985. Von Willebrand factor in the vessel wall mediates platelet adherence. Blood **65:** 85–90.
31. NIEUWENHUIS, H. K., K. S. SAKARIASSEN, W. P. M. HOUDIJK, P. F. E. M. NIEVELSTEIN & J. J. SIXMA. 1986. Deficiency of platelet membrane glycoprotein Ia associated with a decreased platelet adhesion to subendothelium: A defect in platelet spreading. Blood **68:** 692–695.
32. BOLHUIS, P. A., K. S. SAKARIASSEN, H. J. SANDER, B. N. BOUMA & J. J. SIXMA. 1981. Binding of factor VIII-von Willebrand factor to human arterial subendothelium precedes increased platelet adhesion and enhances platelet spreading. J. Lab. Clin. Med. **97:** 568–576.
33. STEL, H. V., K. S. SAKARIASSEN, B. J. SCHOLTE, E. C. I. VEERMAN, T. H. KWAST, P. G. DE

GROOT, J. J. SIXMA & J. A. VAN MOURIK. 1984. Characterization of 25 monoclonal antibodies to factor VIII-von Willebrand factor: Relationship between ristocetin-induced platelet aggregation and platelet adherence to subendothelium. Blood **63:** 1408–1415.

34. MEYER, D., H. R. BAUMGARTNER & T. S. EDGINGTON. 1984. Hybridoma antibodies to human von Willebrand factor. II. Relative role of intramolecular loci in mediation of platelet adhesion to the subendothelium. Br. J. Haematol. **57:** 609–620.
35. SIXMA, J. J., K. S. SAKARIASSEN, H. V. STEL, W. P. M. HOUDIJK, D. W. IN DER MAUR, R. J. HAMER, P. G. DE GROOT & J. A. VAN MOURIK. 1984. Functional domains on von Willebrand factor: Recognition of discrete tryptic fragments by monoclonal antibodies that inhibit interaction of von Willebrand factor with platelets and with collagen. J. Clin. Invest. **74:** 736–744.
36. SAKARIASSEN, K. S., E. FRESSINAUD, J. P. GIRMA, H. R. BAUMGARTNER & D. MEYER. 1986. Mediation of platelet adhesion to fibrillar collagen in flowing blood by a proteolytic fragment of human von Willebrand factor. Blood **67:** 1515–1518.
37. GIRMA, J.-P., M. KALAFATIS, G. PIETU, J.-M. LAVERGNE, M. W. CHOPEK, T. S. EDGINGTON & D. MEYER. 1986. Mapping of distinct von Willebrand factor domains interacting with platelet GPIb and GPIIb/IIIa and with collagen using monoclonal antibodies. Blood **67:** 1356–1366.
38. SIXMA, J. J., K. S. SAKARIASSEN, N. H. BEESER-VISSER, M. OTTENHOF-ROVERS & P. A. BOLHUIS. 1984. Adhesion of platelets to human artery subendothelium: Effect of factor VIII-von Willebrand factor of various multimeric compositions. Blood **63:** 128–139.
39. PYTELA, R., M. D. PIERSCHBACHER, M. H. GINSBERG, E. F. PLOW & E. RUOSLAHTI. 1986. Platelet membrane glycoprotein IIb/IIIa: Member of a family of Arg-Gly-Asp-specific adhesion receptors. Science **231:** 1559–1562.
40. RUGGERI, Z. M., L. DEMARCO, L. GATTI, R. BADER & R. R. MONTGOMERY. 1983. Platelets have more than one binding site for von Willebrand factor. J. Clin. Invest. **72:** 1–12.
41. RUGGERI, Z. M., R. BADER & L. DEMARCO. 1982. Glanzmann's thrombasthenia: Deficient binding of von Willebrand factor to thrombin-stimulated platelets. Proc. Natl. Acad. Sci. U.S.A. **79:** 6038–6041.
42. FUJIMOTO, T. & J. HAWIGER. 1982. Adenosine diphosphate induces binding of von Willebrand factor to human platelets. Nature **297:** 154–157.
43. DEMARCO, L., A. GIROLAMI, T. S. ZIMMERMAN & Z. RUGGERI. 1986. Von Willebrand factor interaction with the glycoprotein IIb/IIIa complex: Its role in platelet function as demonstrated in patients with congenital afibrinogenemia. J. Clin. Invest. **77:** 1272–1277.
44. TSCHOPP, T. B., H. J. WEISS & H. R. BAUMGARTNER. 1975. Interaction of platelets with subendothelium in thrombasthenia: Normal adhesion, impaired cohesion. Experientia **31:** 113–116.
45. SAKARIASSEN, K. S., P. F. E. M. NIEVELSTEIN, B. S. COLLER & J. J. SIXMA. 1986. The role of platelet membrane glycoproteins Ib and IIb-IIIa in platelet adherence to human artery subendothelium. Br. J. Haematol. **63:** 681–691.
46. TSCHOPP, T. B. & H. R. BAUMGARTNER. 1977. Defective platelet adhesion and aggregation on subendothelium exposed in vivo or in vitro to flowing blood of fawn-hooded rats with storage pool disease. Thromb. Haemostas. **38:** 620–629.
47. TIMMONS, S., M. KLOCZEWIAK & H. HAWIGER. 1984. ADP-dependent common receptor mechanism for binding of von Willebrand factor and fibrinogen to human platelets. Proc. Natl. Acad. Sci. U.S.A. **81:** 4935–4939.
48. RAND, J. H., I. I. SUSSMAN, R. E. GORDON, S. V. CHU & V. SOLOMON. 1980. Localization of factor-VIII-related antigen in human vascular subendothelium. Blood **55:** 752–756.
49. HOUDIJK, W. P. M., P. G. DE GROOT, P. F. E. M. NIEVELSTEIN, K. S. SAKARIASSEN & J. J. SIXMA. 1986. Subendothelial proteins and platelet adhesion: von Willebrand factor and fibronectin, not thrombospondin, are involved in platelet adhesion to extracellular matrix of human vascular endothelial cells. Arteriosclerosis **6:** 24–33.
50. HOUDIJK, W. P. M & J. J. SIXMA. 1985. Fibronectin in artery subendothelium is important for platelet adhesion. Blood **65:** 598–604.
51. BOOYSE, F. M., S. FEDER & A. J. QUARFOOT. 1982. Culture-produced subendothelium. II. Effect of plasma, F.VIIIr:WF and fibronectin on interaction of normal platelets with normal and von Willebrand porcine aortic subendothelium. Thromb. Res. **28:** 299–311.

52. RATNOFF, O. D. 1977. Blood clotting mechanism: An overview. *In* Haemostasis: Biochemistry, Physiology, and Pathology. D. Ogston & B. Bennett, Eds.: 1–21. John Wiley & Sons. New York.
53. SAITO, H. 1984. Normal hemostatic mechanisms. *In* Disorders of Hemostasis. O. D. Ratnoff & C. D. Forbes, Eds.: 23–42. Grune and Stratton. New York.
54. EDSON, J. R., J. G. WHITE & W. KRIVIT. 1967. The enigma of severe factor XI deficiency without hemorrhagic symptoms. Distinction from Hageman factor and "Fletcher factor" deficiency. Thromb. Diath. Haemorrh. **18:** 342–348.
55. RIMON, A., S. SCHIFFMAN, D. I. FEINSTEIN & S. I. RAPAPORT. 1976. Factor XI activity and factor XI antigen in homozygous and heterozygous factor XI deficiency. Blood **48:** 165–174.
56. OSTERUD, B. & S. I. RAPAPORT. 1977. Activation of factor XI by the reaction product of tissue factor and factor VII: Additional pathway for initiating blood coagulation. Proc. Natl. Acad. Sci. U.S.A. **74:** 5260–5264.
57. ZUR, M. & Y. NEMERSON. 1980. Kinetics of factor IX activation via the extrinsic pathway. Dependence of K_m on tissue factor. J. Biol. Chem. **255:** 5703–5707.
58. JESTY, J. & S. A. SILVERBERG. 1979. Kinetics of tissue factor-dependent activation of coagulation factors IX and X and in a bovine plasma system. J. Biol. Chem. **254:** 12337–12345.
59. MARLAR, R. A., A. J. KLIESS & J. H. GRIFFIN. 1982. An alternative extrinsic pathway of human blood coagulation. Blood **60:** 1353–1358.
60. WALSH, P. N. & A. H. SCHMAIER. 1985. Platelet-coagulation protein interactions. *In* Hemostasis and Thrombosis. R. W. Colman, J. Hirsh, J. Marder & E. W. Salzman, Eds.: 689–709. J. B. Lippincott. Philadelphia.
61. HEMEKER, H. C., J. L. M. L. VAN RIJN, J. ROSING, G. VAN DIEIJEN, E. M. BEVERS & R. F. A. ZWAAL. 1983. Platelet membrane involvement in blood coagulation. Blood Cells **9:** 303–317.
62. MAJERUS, P. W., J. P. MILETICH, W. H. KANE, S. L. HOFMAN, N. STANFORD & C. M. JACKSON. 1980. The formation of thrombin on the platelet surface. *In* The Regulation of Coagulation. K. G. Mann & F. B. Taylor, Eds.: 215–222. Elsevier. New York.
63. WEISS, H. J., W. J. VICIC, B. A. LAGES & J. ROGERS. 1979. Isolated deficiency of platelet procoagulant activity. Am. J. Med. **67:** 206–213.
64. ROSING, J., E. M. BEVERS, P. COMFURIUS, H. C. HEMKER, G. VAN DIEIJEN, H. J. WEISS & R. F. A. ZWAAL. 1985. Impaired factor X and prothrombin activation associated with decreased phospholipid exposure in platelets from a patient with a bleeding disorder. Blood **65:** 1557–1561.
65. MILETICH, J. P., W. H. KANE, S. L. HOFMANN, N. STANFORD & P. W. MAJERUS. 1979. Deficiency of factor Xa-factor Va binding sites on the platelets of a patient with a bleeding disorder. Blood **54:** 1015–1022.
66. TURITTO, V. T. & H. R. BAUMGARTNER. 1985. Platelet-surface interactions. *In* Hemostasis and Thrombosis. R. W. Colman, J. Hirsh, V. J. Marder & E. W. Salzman, Eds.: 555–571. J. B. Lippincott. Philadelphia.
67. LOSCALZO, J., A. INBAL & R. I. HANDIN. 1986. Von Willebrand protein facilitates platelet incorporation in polymerizing fibrin. J. Clin. Invest. **78:** 1112–1119.
68. LEONARD, E. F. 1982. Rheology of thrombosis. *In* Hemostasis and Thrombosis. R. W. Coleman, J. Hirsh, V. J. Marder & E. W. Salzman, Eds.: 755–765. J. B. Lippincott. Philadelphia.
69. MILETICH, J. P., C. M. JACKSON & P. W. MAJERUS. 1978. Properties of the factor Xa binding site on human platelets. J. Biol. Chem. **253:** 6908–6916.
70. KANE, W. H., M. J. LINDHOUT, C. M. JACKSON & P. W. MAJERUS. 1980. Factor Va-dependent binding of factor Xa to human platelets. J. Biol. Chem. **255:** 1170–1174.
71. TRACY, P. B., M. E. NESHEIM & K. G. MANN. 1981. Coordinate binding of factor Va and factor Xa to the unstimulated platelet. J. Biol. Chem. **256:** 743–751.
72. KANE, W. H. & P. W. MAJERUS. 1982. The interaction of human coagulation factor Va with platelets. J. Biol. Chem. **257:** 3963–3969.
73. HEEB, M. J., J. GREENGARD & C. P. NOVA. 1985. Binding of human factors IX and IXa to washed platelets (abstract). Thromb. Haemostas. **54:** 131.
74. LAFFEL, E. L. & E. BRAUNWALD. 1984. Thrombolytic therapy: A new strategy for the treatment of acute myocardial infarction. N. Eng. J. Med. **311:** 710–717.

Insights into the Mechanism of Platelet Retention in Glass Bead Columns[a]

MARJORIE B. ZUCKER,[b] SANDRA BROWNLEA,[c] AND JEAN McPHERSON[c]

[b]*Department of Pathology*
New York University Medical Center
New York, New York 10016

[c]*Faculty of Medicine*
University of Newcastle
Newcastle, New South Wales, Australia

Von Willebrand's disease (vWD) is a hereditary (autosomal) hemorrhagic disorder characterized by reduced and/or abnormal von Willebrand factor (vWF or VIII-related antigen, VIII:RAg) in plasma, and reduced plasma levels of factor VIII (VIII:C or antihemophilic factor). The primary deficiency is that of vWF.[1]

The prolonged bleeding time in patients with vWD is characteristic of a platelet disorder. Microscopic examination of bleeding time puncture wounds reveals masses of platelets that do not adhere to the cut blood vessels, and thus are ineffective for hemostasis.[2] *In vitro* tests in which blood is perfused past de-endothelialized everted arterial rings have established the importance of vWF in platelet adhesion to the vascular subendothelium.[3,4] Standard *in vitro* tests of platelet aggregation and secretion are normal. Platelet agglutination with ristocetin is reduced in severe vWD and can be corrected by addition of vWF. This agglutination does not require platelet activation. It does require the presence of glycoprotein Ib (GPIb) on the platelet membrane and is absent in patients with the Bernard-Soulier syndrome, whose platelets lack this glycoprotein.[1]

The platelet retention test is the only measurement of *in vitro* platelet function that is abnormal in blood from patients with vWD and that does not require vascular tissue or ristocetin. Although the test was first described in 1960 by Hellem,[5] shown to be abnormal in vWD in 1963,[6,7] and discussed in two earlier New York Academy of Sciences conferences,[8,9] it is still poorly understood.

To perform the test, 5 ml of native or heparinized blood is pumped rapidly through a column of glass beads. Each milliliter emerging from the column is collected separately with EDTA and platelet counts performed. For each milliliter, the retention is the difference between the postcolumn count and the precolumn count expressed as a percentage of the precolumn count. In normal blood, the number of platelets retained in the column is low for the first milliliter but increases progressively in subsequent milliliters. FIGURE 1A illustrates a typical test in a normal subject and the reduced retention in a patient whose plasma contained no measurable vWF. The shear rate is very important; if blood is pumped through the bead column slowly, retention is normal even in severe vWD.[10] Similarly, the requirement for vWF in platelet adhesion to the subendothelium is demonstrable only when the shear rate is high.[11]

We developed a two-stage test (FIGURE 1B) in an attempt to clarify the

[a]This study was supported in part by grant no. HL–27752 from the National Institutes of Health.

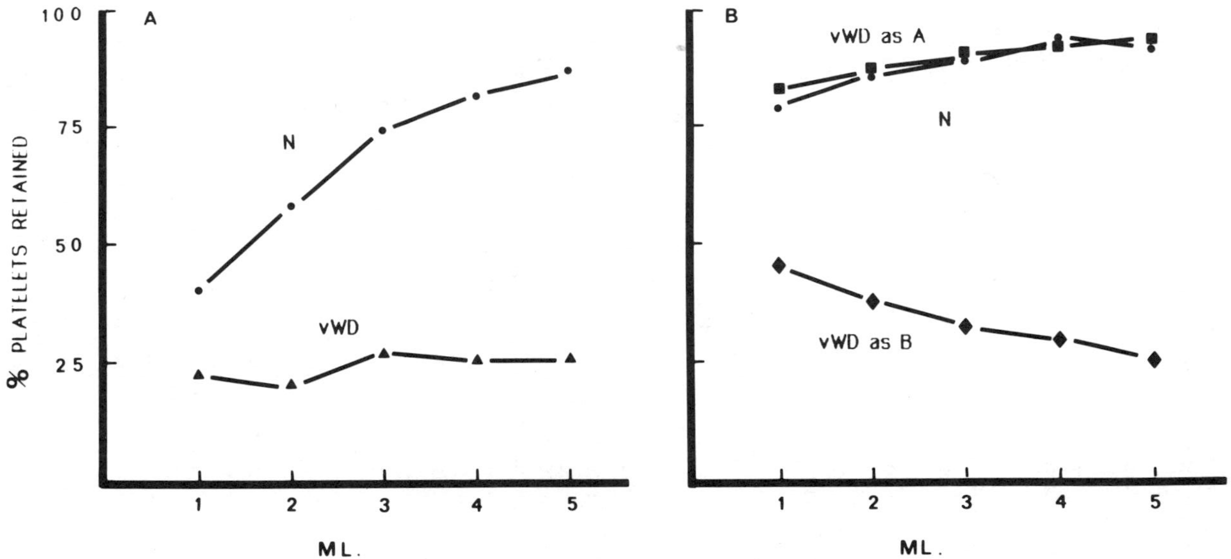

FIGURE 1. (**A**) One-stage tests of platelet retention in normal blood (*N*) and blood from a patient with severe von Willebrand's disease (*vWD*). Ten ml of blood that had been drawn into a syringe containing 4 U heparin per ml blood were pumped through a column containing 2 g of glass beads at a speed of 5.7 ml per min. Each ml of blood was collected into concentrated EDTA and the number of platelets counted. (**B**) Two-stage tests of platelet retention. One ml of heparinized blood (blood *A*) was passed through a column of glass beads followed by 5 ml of isotonic saline and then 5 ml of blood (blood *B*). Platelet counts were carried out on each ml of emerging blood B. *N*, Blood A and blood B were normal; *vWD-A*, blood A was from a vWD patient and blood B was normal; *vWD-B*, blood A was normal and blood B was from a vWD patient.

mechanisms of platelet retention.[12] One milliliter of blood, called blood A, was pumped through the column of glass beads. The column was rinsed with buffer or plasma, then 5 ml of blood, designated B, was passed through the column and the platelets were counted in each milliliter emerging from the column. If blood A was normal, retention was high even in the first milliliter of blood B. The constituents of blood A that were necessary to enhance retention in the first milliliters of blood B were fibrinogen, divalent cations, and platelets that were able to bind to fibrinogen (*i.e.,* not thrombasthenic platelets, which lack GPIIb-IIIa). Neither von Willebrand factor nor ADP were required in this stage. Platelets adhere to fibrinogen-coated areas. Vroman and his colleagues[13] have shown that fibrinogen is rapidly adsorbed when plasma is exposed to glass, but is replaced within seconds by high molecular weight kininogen. A layer of blood up to about 20 μm thick does not contain enough high molecular weight kininogen to replace the fibrinogen. The contact zones between the beads in a glass bead column provide such narrow blood-filled spaces, probably explaining why platelets can adhere.

When blood containing a low level of vWF was used as blood B, retention was slightly enhanced in the first milliliter, but then fell to and remained at very low levels. Thus, while vWF is not required for the adhesion of platelets to glass beads in the first stage, it is necessary for the subsequent progressive formation of platelet aggregates in the column.[12] Since the test measures more than platelet adhesion to glass, it should not be called the platelet adhesiveness test. Turitto *et al.*[14] suggested recently that vWF plays a part in the formation of the platelet aggregates that attach to platelets adherent to the subendothelium of perfused vascular rings.

Two observations indicate that platelet GPIb is involved in mediating the effect of vWF: (1) platelet retention is diminished in blood from patients with the Bernard-Soulier syndrome, whose platelets lack GPIb (summarized in ref. 15); and (2) platelet retention is impaired by a monoclonal antibody (mAb), 6D1, which is directed against GPIb and inhibits ristocetin-induced binding of vWF to platelets.[15]

The second stage of platelet retention also requires platelet GPIIb-IIIa, since retention was low in all 5 ml when blood from patients with thrombasthenia was used as blood B following normal blood as A.[12] These glycoproteins become "exposed" on normal platelets that have interacted with ADP or thrombin and form the receptor for fibrinogen. The bound dimeric fibrinogen molecule then forms the bond that holds the platelets together in an aggregate.[16] The requirement for GPIIb-IIIa in the first stage of retention is in accord with their role in the adhesion of platelets to fibrinogen.[17] Are these glycoproteins necessary in the second stage because fibrinogen binds together the platelet aggregates in the glass bead column? The finding that blood from a patient with afibrinogenemia was indistinguishable from normal when it was used as blood B[12] suggested that fibrinogen was not essential. In fact, heparinized (but not citrated) platelet-rich plasma from this afibrinogenemic patient aggregated well with ADP.[18] Thus either the trace concentration of fibrinogen in the patient's plasma was adequate to support retention and aggregation, or fibrinogen was not needed.

Purified vWF can bind to GPIIb-IIIa on washed platelets that have been activated with ADP or thrombin.[19,20] In normal plasma, vWF does not bind appreciably to stimulated platelets because the concentration of fibrinogen is 250 times higher than that of vWF.[21] Ruggeri's laboratory has carried out studies with two monoclonal antibodies against GPIIb-IIIa. Fab′ fragments of MAb LJ-P9 inhibited binding of fibrinogen, fibronectin, and vWF to stimulated platelets and inhibited ADP-induced aggregation.[22] Fab′ fragments of the other MAb, LJ-P5, did not affect binding of fibrinogen to stimulated platelets, but inhibited the vWF binding that occurs in the absence of physiologic concentrations of fibrinogen.[22,23] This antibody did not inhibit ADP-induced aggregation of platelets in normal plasma, which presumably depends on fibringen binding, but did inhibit aggregation in plasma of patients with afibrinogenemia. Thus it appears that vWF binding to GPIIb-IIIa is not significant in ADP-induced aggregation of platelets in normal plasma, mediated by fibrinogen binding, but that it can support ADP-induced aggregation when fibrinogen is virtually absent.[23]

In order to determine whether these findings are relevant to responses in a glass bead column, we tested the effect of two of Dr. Ruggeri's antibodies on platelet retention (TABLE 1). Fab′ fragments of LJ-CP8 (which like LJ-P9 inhibits fibrinogen and vWF binding to GPIIb-IIIa; personal communication from Dr. Ruggeri) markedly inhibited retention when used in a one-stage test, or when added to either blood A or blood B in a two-stage test. These results support our earlier conclusion that fibrinogen must be present in blood A and suggest that binding of fibrinogen to GPIIb-IIIa normally occurs in blood B during retention. In contrast, Fab′ fragments of LJ-P5 failed to affect platelet retention, supporting the conclusion of Ruggeri's group that vWF binding to GPIIb-IIIa does not occur in the presence of physiologic concentrations of fibrinogen. Surprisingly, however, a recent study[24] showed that this antibody only slightly inhibited the second stage of retention in blood of a subject with severe afibrinogenemia. This finding supports the observation of Cattaneo *et al.*[25] that there is a component of ADP-induced platelet aggregation that is not dependent on plasma proteins but is dependent on glycoprotein IIb-IIIa.[25]

TABLE 1. Effect of Monoclonal Antibodies (Fab′) to GPIIb-IIIa on Platelet Retention in Glass Bead Columns

		Effect on Retention		
			Two Stage	
Material Added	Concentration (μg/ml Plasma)	One Stage	First Stage	Second Stage
Ruggeri LJ-P5	172	none	none	none
Ruggeri LJ-CP8	44	inhibition	inhibition	inhibition

If vWF binding to GPIIb-IIIa is not responsible for the second stage of platelet retention in a glass bead column, what is the role of vWF? Investigators in several laboratories have shown that vWF from patients with type IIB vWD,[26,27] or vWF from which sialic acid has been removed,[28] can induce platelet aggregation. The altered vWF binds to GPIb (without added ristocetin), causing "exposure" of GPIIb-IIIa. These glycoproteins then bind fibrinogen, resulting in platelet aggregation. These observations suggest the interesting possibility that rapid passage of blood through a glass bead column causes changes in the vWF molecule that permit it to bind to GPIb, resulting ultimately in retention of platelets within the column.

In addition to vWF, ADP must be present for normal platelet retention. This is clear because conversion of ADP to ATP by addition of creatine kinase and creatine phosphate (CK-CP) markedly reduced retention. In the two-stage retention test adding CK-CP or prostaglandin E_1 to blood A did not inhibit retention in blood B, but adding them to the saline or plasma used to flush the column between blood A and blood B or to blood B itself prevented the enhancement of retention seen when blood B followed normal blood as A.[12] Furthermore, passage of blood through the glass bead column was associated with release of ADP. ATP was released as well, and the ATP:ADP ratio of the released nucleotides was 1.6. Platelets seem a likely source for these nucleotides, since released hemoglobin was not detected, erythrocytes have a

TABLE 2. *In Vitro* Effects of Monoclonal Antibodies against vWF

Antibody			vWF-Dependent Function Affected									
			Platelet Agglutination with Ristocetin		Platelet Adhesion to Subendothelium		vWF Adhesion to Collagen		vWF Binding to Thrombin-stimulated Platelets		Retention in Glass Bead Column	
Designation	Source	Ref.	Conc. (μg/ml)	Inhib. (%)	Conc. (μg/ml)	Inhib. (%)	Conc. (μg/ml)	Inhib. (%)	Conc. (μg/ml)	Inhib. (%)	Conc. (μg/ml)	Inhib. (%)
RAg 35	Netherlands	4, 36, 37	1	100	1	100	24	0	not reported		1.0	100
RAg 38	Netherlands	36	500	50	500	54	—	—	not reported		3.2	100
											1.0	50
RAg 201	Netherlands	36, 37	500	0	500	33	7	100	not reported		3.2	100
											1.0	50
RAg Asc[a]	Netherlands	—	500	0	500	0	500	0	not reported		3.2	100
											1.0	50
vWF 9[b]	France	38–40	100	10	20	95	—	—	5	100	5.0	100
											2.5	50

Antibody concentrations represent plasma concentration assuming 50% hematocrit. Antibody was incubated with blood for 20 min before measuring retention (shown in last two columns).

[a]This antibody binds to vWF but does not affect its function (personal communication from Dr. J. Sixma).

[b]Fab and $F(ab')_2$ fragments were equally inhibitory.

much higher ratio of nucleotides, and less adenine nucleotide was liberated from blood with low retention (in vWD, thrombasthenia, or thrombocytopenia).[8,29,30] More recent studies by Joist's group on citrated blood subjected to shear stress suggested, however, that erythrocytes may contribute ADP without hemolysis.[31] Nucleotides from platelets are usually secreted from the dense granules, a pool that is not in equilibrium with the cytoplasmic metabolic nucleotides and in which the ratio of ATP:ADP is between 0.6 and 1.1. Joist's group showed that platelets in sheared blood aggregated and released [^{14}C]serotonin and β-thromboglobulin. Aspirin did not affect aggregation, and reduced release of [^{14}C]serotonin and β-thromboglobulin by only 50% although it prevented malondialdehyde formation.[32,33] In our studies, release of nucleotides during the platelet retention test, and platelet retention itself, were not inhibited by aspirin (which prevents thromboxane A_2 formation), nor was the release of nucleotide accompanied by the release of [^{14}C]serotonin, as it would be in the usual secretory response.[27,28] Thus, although platelets seem to be the source of most of the released adenine nucleotides in blood subjected to shear or passed through a glass bead column, thromboxane A_2 formation does not play a major role and the mechanism of release is obscure.

Although ADP is necessary for normal retention, it can also inhibit retention. Retention is much reduced when blood is disturbed by passing it rapidly between syringes,[32] or even by slow centrifugation and remixing. This inhibition can be mimicked by adding a very low concentration of ADP (in rabbit blood as well[33]), and is partially alleviated by removing ADP enzymatically.[29,30,34] The inhibition caused by disturbance of blood suggests that many studies of platelet adhesion and aggregation are being carried out with inhibited platelets.

Investigators have recently prepared MAb against vWF and studied their effects on various functions of vWF. TABLE 2 summarizes the effect of some of these antibodies on retention and other platelet functions. We tested four of the antibodies prepared by van Mourik and studied by Sixma's group. All of them inhibited the one-stage platelet retention test, as well as the second (vWF-requiring) stage of the two-stage test, but had no effect on the first stage, *i.e.*, when added to blood A. RAg 35 was the most active, causing complete inhibition when added to blood at a plasma concentration of 1.2 μg/ml. RAg 38, RAg 201, and RAg Asc caused only partial inhibition at this concentration, but complete inhibition at 4 μg/ml. Meyer provided us with antibody vWF 9 against the IIb-IIIa binding site on vWF. This antibody also inhibited retention strongly when used in the one-stage assay, or as blood B in the two-stage test (TABLE 2).

This lack of specificity suggested that inhibition of retention might occur because a complex of vWF with any of the antibodies became bound to the platelet Fc receptor, which is thought to be closely associated with GPIb.[41] Three pieces of evidence argue against this interpretation. First, a polyclonal antibody to factor IX, a protein present in plasma in about the same concentration as vWF, failed to affect platelet retention at plasma concentrations up to 200 μg per ml. Second, Fab and $F(ab')_2$ fragments to Meyer's antibody, prepared by us, were just as effective in inhibiting retention as the whole antibody. Third, heat-aggregated IgG, which stimulates platelets by binding to the Fc receptor, at least in the absence of plasma,[42] did not affect platelet retention even at plasma concentrations as high as 50 μg/ml.

In summary, binding of fibrinogen to GPIIb-IIIa appears necessary for platelet retention in normal blood. Binding of vWF to GPIIb-IIIa is not important in retention in normal blood but may contribute to the normal second stage of retention reported previously in afibrinogenemic blood. Studies of MAbs to vWF did not indicate that any domain of the vWF molecule is particularly important for platelet retention. Rather, since binding of any one of five MAbs rendered the vWF molecule ineffective in supporting platelet retention, we conclude that the conformation of the entire molecule is critical to this measure of platelet function. It is possible that attachment of any MAb to the molecule prevents the conformational change in vWF that we suggest may take place during rapid passage of blood through a glass bead column.

ACKNOWLEDGMENT

We are very grateful to Drs. J. A. van Mourik (Netherlands Red Cross Blood Transfusion Service, Amsterdam), J. J. Sixma (University Hospital, Utrecht), D. Meyer (Hôpital Bicêtre, Paris), and Z. M. Ruggeri (Scripps Clinic, San Diego, CA) for generously providing us with the antibodies for these studies.

REFERENCES

1. Weiss, H. J. 1983. Von Willebrand's disease. *In* Hematology, Chap. 155. W. F. Williams, E. Beutler, A. J. Erslev & M. A. Lichtman, Eds.: 1413–1420. McGraw-Hill. New York.
2. Sawada, Y., D. N. Fass, J. A. Katzmann, R. C. Bahn & E. J. W. Bowie. 1986. Hemostatic plug formation in normal and von Willebrand pigs: The effect of the administration of cryoprecipitate and a monoclonal antibody to Willebrand factor. Blood **67:** 1229–1239.
3. Tschopp, T., H. J. Weiss & H. Baumgartner. 1974. Decreased adhesion of platelets to subendothelium in von Willebrand's disease. J. Lab. Clin. Med. **83:** 296–300.
4. Stel, H. V., K. S. Sakariassen, P. G. de Groot, J. A. van Mourik & J. J. Sixma. 1985. Von Willebrand factor in the vessel wall mediates platelet adherence. Blood **65:** 85–90.
5. Hellem, A. J. 1960. The adhesiveness of human blood platelets in vitro. Scand. J. Clin. Lab. Invest. **12**(Suppl. 51).
6. Zucker, M. B. 1963. In vitro abnormality of the blood in von Willebrand's disease correctable by normal plasma. Nature **197:** 601–602.
7. Salzman, E. W. 1963. Measurement of platelet adhesiveness: A simple in vitro technique demonstrating an abnormality in von Willebrand's disease. J. Lab. Clin. Med. **62:** 724–735.
8. Zucker, M. B., P. L. Rifkin, N. M. Friedberg & B. S. Coller. 1972. Mechanisms of platelet function as revealed by the retention of platelets in glass bead columns. Ann. N.Y. Acad. Sci. **201:** 138–144.
9. Zucker, M. B. & J. McPherson. 1977. Reactions of platelets near surfaces *in vitro:* Lessons from the platelet retention test. Ann. N.Y. Acad. Sci. **283:** 128–137.
10. O'Brien, J. R. & J. B. Heywood. 1967. Some interactions between human platelets and glass: von Willebrand's disease compared with normals. J. Clin. Pathol. **20:** 56–64.
11. Weiss, H. J., V. T. Turitto & H. R. Baumgartner. 1978. Effect of shear rate on platelet interaction with subendothelium in citrated and native blood. I. Shear dependent decrease of adhesion in von Willebrand's disease and Bernard-Soulier syndrome. J. Lab. Clin Med. **92:** 750–764.
12. McPherson, J. & M. B. Zucker. 1976. Platelet retention in glass bead columns: Adhesion to glass and subsequent platelet-platelet interactions. Blood **47:** 55–67.
13. Adams, A. L., G. C. Fischer, P. C. Munoz & L. Vroman. 1984. Convex-lens-on-slide: A simple system for the study of human plasma and blood in narrow spaces. J. Biomed. Mater. Res. **18:** 643–654.
14. Turitto, V. T., H. J. Weiss & H. R. Baumgartner. 1984. Platelet interaction with rabbit subendothelium in von Willebrand's disease: Altered thrombus formation distinct from defective platelet adhesion. J. Clin. Invest. **74:** 1730–1741.
15. Coller, B. S., E. I. Peerschke, L. E. Scudder & C. A. Sullivan. 1983. Studies with a murine monoclonal antibody that abolishes ristocetin-induced binding of von Willebrand factor to platelets: Additional evidence in support of GP Ib as a platelet receptor for von Willebrand factor. Blood **61:** 99–110.

16. PEERSCHKE, E. I. 1985. The platelet fibrinogen receptor. Semin. Hematol. **22:** 241–259.
17. COLLER, B. S. 1980. Interaction of normal, thrombasthenic, and Bernard-Soulier platelets with immobilized fibrinogen: Defective platelet-fibrinogen interaction in thrombasthenia. Blood **55:** 169–178.
18. WEISS, H. J. & J. ROGERS. 1971. Fibrinogen and platelets in the primary arrest of bleeding. Studies in two patients with congenital afibrinogenemia. N. Engl. J. Med. **283:** 369–374.
19. FUJIMOTO, T. & J. HAWIGER. 1982. Adenosine diphosphate induces binding of von Willebrand factor to human platelets. Nature **297:** 154–156.
20. RUGGERI, Z. M., L. DE MARCO, L. GATTI, R. BADER & R. R. MONTGOMERY. 1983. Platelets have more than one binding site for von Willebrand factor. J. Clin. Invest. **72:** 1–12.
21. GRALNICK, H. R., S. B. WILLIAMS & B. S. COLLER. 1984. Fibrinogen competes with von Willebrand factor for binding to glycoprotein IIb/IIIa complex when platelets are stimulated with thrombin. Blood **64:** 797–800.
22. LOMBARDO, V. T., E. HODSON, J. R. ROBERTS, T. J. KUNICKI, T. S. ZIMMERMAN & Z. M. RUGGERI. 1985. Independent modulation of von Willebrand factor and fibrinogen binding to the platelet membrane glycoprotein IIb/IIIa complex as demonstrated by monoclonal antibody. J. Clin. Invest. **76:** 1950–1958.
23. DE MARCO, L., A. GIROLAMI, T. S. ZIMMERMAN & Z. M. RUGGERI. 1986. Von Willebrand factor interaction with the glycoprotein IIb/IIIa complex. Its role in platelet function as demonstrated in patients with congenital afibrinogenemia. J. Clin. Invest. **77:** 1272–1277.
24. MCPHERSON, J, S. BROWNLEA & M. B. ZUCKER. 1987. Effect of monoclonal antibodies against von Willebrand factor and platelet glycoproteins IIb/IIIa on the platelet retention test. Blood **70:** 546–550.
25. CATTANEO, M., R. L. KINLOUGH-RATHBONE, A. LECCHI, C. BEVILACQUA, M. A. PACKHAM & J. F. MUSTARD. 1987. Fibrinogen-independent aggregation and deaggregation of human platelets: Studies in two afibrinogenemic patients. Blood **70:** 221–226.
26. HOLMBERG, L., A. C. KRISTOFFERSSON, S. LAMME, I. M. NILSSON, A. AWIDI & N. O. SOLUM. 1985. Platelet-von Willebrand factor interactions in Type IIB von Willebrand's disease. Scand. J. Haematol. **35:** 305–314.
27. DE MARCO, L., A. GIROLAMI, T. S. ZIMMERMAN & Z. M. RUGGERI. 1985. Interaction of purified type IIB von Willebrand factor with the platelet membrane glycoprotein Ib induces fibrinogen binding to the glycoprotein IIb/IIIa complex and initiates aggregation. Proc. Natl. Acad. Sci. U.S.A. **82:** 7424–7428.
28. GRALNICK, H. R., S. B. WILLIAMS & B. S. COLLER. 1985. Asialo von Willebrand factor interactions with platelets. Interdependence of glycoproteins Ib and IIb/IIIa for binding and aggregation. J. Clin. Invest. **75:** 19–25.
29. FRIEDBERG, N. M. & M. B. ZUCKER. 1972. ADP as the cause of reversible inhibition of platelet retention in glass bead columns. J. Lab. Clin. Med. **80:** 603–612.
30. MCPHERSON, V. J., M. B. ZUCKER, N. M. FRIEDBERG & P. L. RIFKIN. 1974. Platelet retention in glass bead columns: Further evidence for the importance of ADP. Blood **44:** 411–425.
31. REIMERS, R. C., S. P. SUTERA & J. H. JOIST. 1984. Potentiation by red blood cells of shear-induced platelet aggregation: Relative importance of chemical and physical mechanisms. Blood. **64:** 1200–1206.
32. STEVENS, D. E., J. H. JOIST & S. P. SUTERA. 1980. Role of platelet-prostaglandin synthesis in shear-induced platelet alterations. Blood **56:** 753–758.
33. MORITZ, M. W., R. C. REIMERS, R. K. BAKER, S. P. SUTERA & J. H. JOIST. 1983. Role of cytoplasmic and releasable ADP in platelet aggregation induced by laminar shear stress. J. Lab. Clin. Med. **101:** 537–544.
34. COLLER, B. S. & M. B. ZUCKER. 1971. Reversible decrease in platelet retention by glass bead columns (adhesiveness) induced by disturbing the blood. Proc. Soc. Exp. Biol. Med. **136:** 769–771.
35. DODDS, W. J., J. M. DINOVO & J. A. BERGERON. 1981. A native whole blood assay for blood materials interaction. Thromb. Haemostas. **45:** 12–17.
36. STEL, H. V., K. S. SAKARIASSEN, B. J. SCHOLTE, E. C. I. VEERMAN, T. H. VAN DER KWAST,

P. G. de Groot, J. J. Sixma & J. A. van Mourik. 1984. Characterization of 25 monoclonal antibodies to factor VIII-von Willebrand factor: Relationship between ristocetin-induced platelet aggregation and platelet adherence to subendothelium. Blood **63:** 1408–1415.

37. Sixma, J. J., K. S. Sakariassen, H. V. Stel, W. P. M. Houdjik, D. W. In der Maur, R. J. Hamer, P. G. de Groot & J. A. van Mourik. 1984. Functional domains on von Willebrand factor. Recognition of discrete tryptic fragments by monoclonal antibodies that inhibit interaction of von Willebrand factor with platelets and with collagen. J. Clin. Invest. **74:** 736–744.

38. Nokes, T. J. C., N. A. Mahmoud, G. F. Savidge, A. H. Goodall, D. Meyer, T. S. Edgington & R. M. Hardisty. 1984. Von Willebrand factor has more than one binding site for platelets. Thromb. Res. **34:** 361–366.

39. Meyer, D., H. R. Baumgartner & T. S. Edgington. 1984. Hybridoma antibodies to human von Willebrand factor. II. Relative role of intramolecular loci in mediation of platelet adhesion to the subendothelium. Br. J. Haematol. **57:** 609–620.

40. Girma, J-P., M. Kalafatis, G. Pietu, J.-M. Lavergne, M. W. Chopek, T. S. Edgington & D. Meyer. 1986. Mapping of distinct von Willebrand factor domains interacting with platelet GPIb and GPIIb/IIIa and with collagen using monoclonal antibodies. Blood **67:** 1356–1366.

41. Moore, A., G. D. Ross & R. L. Nachman. 1978. Interaction of platelet membrane receptors with von Willebrand factor, ristocetin and the Fc region of immunoglobulin G. J. Clin. Invest. **62:** 1053–1060.

42. Pfueller, S. L., S. Weber & E. F. Lüscher. 1977. Studies of the mechanism of the human platelet release reaction induced by immunologic stimuli. III. Relationship between the binding of soluble IgG aggregates to the Fc receptor and cell response in the presence and absence of plasma. J. Immunol. **118:** 514–524.

Cell-Cell Interactions in the Eicosanoid Pathway[a]

A. J. MARCUS, L. B. SAFIER, H. L. ULLMAN, N. ISLAM, M. J. BROEKMAN, J. R. FALCK, S. FISCHER, AND C. v. SCHACKY

Divisions of Hematology-Oncology
Departments of Medicine
New York Veterans Administration Medical Center
Cornell University Medical College
New York, New York 10010

INTRODUCTION

Eicosanoids are oxygenated metabolites derived from free arachidonic acid. Formation of these autacoids in stimulated cells and tissues is rather ubiquitous, but their precise physiologic or pathophysiologic role has not been defined.[1] It appears likely that the biological effects of eicosanoids are exerted in the microenvironment.

Eicosanoid research has focused mainly on single cell types and on reactions of the cyclooxygenase pathway. Formation of cyclooxygenase products is inhibited by nonsteroidal anti-inflammatory drugs and more is known about functional parameters of eicosanoids such as prostacyclin (PGI_2) and thromboxane A_2 (TXA_2).[2] Research on products of the lipoxygenase pathway is relatively more recent, and is assuming increasing importance because lipoxygenase products may play a role in inflammatory and allergic reactions, as well as host defense mechanisms in general.[3] Furthermore, production of lipoxygenase metabolites is not inhibited, and may be enhanced, during administration of nonsteroidal anti-inflammatory agents. Our recent research strategy has evolved from the hypothesis that hemostasis, thrombosis, and host defense mechanisms are multicellular events simultaneously involving both the cyclooxygenase and lipoxygenase eicosanoid pathways.

ARACHIDONIC ACID METABOLISM IN INDIVIDUAL CELL TYPES

Studies of arachidonate metabolism in specific cells should be initiated by ascertaining the pattern of eicosanoid production upon exposure to various agonists. Such basic information allows for identification of a new eicosanoid(s) when the cell is interacted with another cell type. This approach also provides information as to whether different cells can biochemically modify each others' precursors, intermediates, and end products. Examples of eicosanoid patterns in individual cells are shown

[a]This work was supported by grants from the Veterans Administration, the National Institutes of Health (grant nos. HL-18828-12 SCOR to AJM, MJB, and CvS, HL-29034 to MJB, GM 31278 to JRF), the Edward Gruenstein Fund, the Sallie Wichman Fund, the S. M. Louis Fund (to AJM), and the Deutsche Forschungsgemeinschaft (to SF and CvS). MJB is an established investigator of the American Heart Association.

TABLE 1. Arachidonate Metabolites from Thrombin-stimulated Platelets

Product	dpm	%[a]
$PGF_2\alpha$	603	1.6
TXB_2	12,909	34.1
PGE_2	500	1.3
PGD_2	449	1.2
HHT	13,863	36.6
12-HETE	7,568	20.0
Free 20:4	1,189	3.1

[a]Percentage of total dpm (minus phospholipid and neutral lipid) recovered from thin-layer chromatography plate.

in TABLES 1 and 2. When 1×10^8 arachidonate-labeled platelets were stimulated with 5 U/ml thrombin, the profile shown in TABLE 1, as analyzed by thin-layer radiochromatography, was obtained. The major cyclooxygenase products were TXB_2 and 12-hydroxyheptadecatrienoic acid (HHT), which occurred in approximately equal amounts. Small quantities of $PGF_{2\alpha}$, PGE_2, and PGD_2 were produced as well. 12-HETE is the major lipoxygenase product in stimulated platelets.

Since human endothelial cells respond to thrombin, ^{3}H-labeled arachidonic acid was added to 5.5×10^6 endothelial cells, followed by thrombin (5 U/ml).[4] The major metabolite was 6-keto-$PGF_{1\alpha}$, the end product of prostacyclin formation (TABLE 2). $PGF_{2\alpha}$ was also prominent and PGE_2, PGD_2, and hydroxy acids were minor components. Knowledge of these profiles permitted studies of direct interactions between platelets and endothelial cells. It could be shown that platelet-derived prostaglandin endoperoxides were metabolized by endothelial cells in close contact to form PGI_2.[4] This meant that platelets could directly enhance the inherent synthetic capability of endothelial cells to produce PGI_2.[5]

The most commonly used stimulus for studies of the eicosanoid profile in human neutrophils is ionophore A23187. In our experience, purified neutrophil preparations only produce lipoxygenase products. These include leukotriene B_4 (LTB_4), 5-HETE, and trihydroxy acids (THETE).[6]

PLATELET-NEUTROPHIL INTERACTIONS

We have recently been studying platelet-neutrophil interactions involving the platelet lipoxygenase product 12-HETE. Stimulated platelets synthesize 12-HETE in

TABLE 2. Arachidonate Metabolites from Thrombin-stimulated Endothelial Cells

Product	cpm	%[a]
6-keto-$PGF_1\alpha$	116,008	65.5
$PGF_2\alpha$	30,484	17.2
PGE_2	6,060	3.4
PGD_2	2,119	1.2
Hydroxy acids	6,559	3.7
Free 20:4	3,220	1.8

[a]Percentage of counts minus phospholipid and solvent front recovered from thin-layer chromatography plate.[4]

abundance *in vitro.* If platelets are pretreated with aspirin, 12-HETE production is increased. In experiments with combined suspensions of stimulated platelets and unstimulated neutrophils, we identified a new eicosanoid, 12,20-dihydroxyeicosatetraenoic acid (12,20-DiHETE), which neither cell alone could produce.[7,8] This compound was produced from platelet 12-HETE by the unstimulated neutrophil via an ω-hydroxylation of the cytochrome P-450 type. Evidence that this was indeed a cytochrome P-450 mechanism can be summarized as follows: (1) Formation of 12,20-DiHETE from 12-HETE by neutrophils was inhibited by classical cytochrome P-450 antagonists. (2) Exposure of neutrophils to carbon monoxide inhibited 12,20-DiHETE formation by 94%, an effect which was totally reversible upon reoxygenation.[9] (3) As is characteristic of other cytochrome P-450 enzyme systems, NADPH was a required cofactor and the enzyme system was localized in the microsomal subcellular compartment of the neutrophil. The ω-hydroxylase under study was particularly susceptible to proteolysis as induced by cell disruption. It was necessary to pretreat intact cells with diisopropylfluorophosphate (DFP) prior to fractionation procedures.

Since the major eicosanoid produced by stimulated neutrophils is LTB_4, we studied the effect of LTB_4 addition on 12,20-DiHETE production. LTB_4 was added to a neutrophil suspension 15 seconds prior to 12-HETE. Progressive inhibition of 12-HETE ω-hydroxylation was observed. At a concentration of 0.22 μM, 12-HETE ω-hydroxylation was blocked by 21% and when equal amounts of 12-HETE and LTB_4 were present (4.4 μM), 93% inhibition of 12-HETE omega-hydroxylation was observed. It is therefore plausible that the neutrophil LTB_4 ω-hydroxylase and the 12-HETE ω-hydroxylase may be similar or identical enzymes.[9]

In an extension of the above research, we have observed time-dependent formation of a new compound by unstimulated neutrophils exposed to 12-HETE.[10] The compound is more polar than 12,20-DiHETE, as determined by reversed-phase high performance liquid chromatography. We ascertained that the parent compound of the new eicosanoid was 12,20-DiHETE by incubation of purified 12,20-DiHETE with neutrophils. There was a progressive decrease in 12,20-DiHETE as formation of the polar metabolite increased. Additional preliminary data indicate that the new metabolite of 12,20-DiHETE is 12-hydroxyeicosatetraen-1,20-dioic acid (12-HETE-1,20-dioic acid). UV spectral studies indicated that 12-HETE-1,20-dioic acid had an identical maximum at 236 nm to that of 12-HETE and 12,20-DiHETE. When equimolar concentrations of 20-hydroxy-LTB_4 and 12,20-DiHETE (2.8 μM) were added to neutrophils, formation of 12-HETE-1,20-dioic acid was inhibited by 28%. This inhibition increased to 49% when 8μM 20-hydroxy-LTB_4 was added.

It therefore appears that unstimulated neutrophils possess a finely regulated metabolic system for processing platelet-derived 12-HETE. These metabolites may exert physiological effects yet to be described or they may represent disposal mechanisms for biologically active 12-HETE.

CLASSIFICATION OF CELL-CELL INTERACTIONS

As already mentioned, multiple cell types participating in the hemostatic, thrombotic, and inflammatory processes are brought into close proximity. This increases the probability of metabolic interactions between these cells as described above.[5] Experimental results in our own and several other laboratories have indicated that these cell interactions can be classified in an orderly manner.[5]

Type I: Different Cells Share a Common Precursor

Type IA

A stimulated cell synthesizes its own precursor, but it is also capable of obtaining the same precursor from a neighboring cell. This results in production of more endogenous end product. An example would be utilization of platelet-derived endoperoxides by endothelial cells for prostacyclin production.[4,11]

Type IB

A cell cannot produce a precursor endogenously, but inherently possesses biochemical mechanisms for further transforming a precursor obtainable from another stimulated cell in proximity. McGee and Fitzpatrick[12] demonstrated that human erythrocytes were capable of producing LTB_4 from LTA_4 released from stimulated neutrophils. In addition neutrophil leukotriene A_4 can be transferred to endothelial cells for synthesis of leukotriene C_4.[13]

Type II: A Cell Can Transform an Eicosanoid of Another Into a New Compound That Neither Cell Can Synthesize Alone

Type IIA

Both cells are activated. One example would be utilization of 12-HETE from stimulated platelets by activated neutrophils to produce 5,12-DiHETE.[6] In this instance 12-HETE released by platelets was processed by the activated neutrophil 5-lipoxygenase. Interestingly, 5-HETE can be processed to 5,12-DiHETE by the activated platelet 12-lipoxygenase.

Type IIB

One cell in the system is activated and the other is not. As discussed in detail above, 12-HETE from activated platelets can be converted to 12,20-DiHETE by resting neutrophils.[7,8] There is a sharp contrast between the totally stimulated system (type IIA) and that described here (type IIB) wherein only one cell is in the activated state.

Type III: An Eicosanoid or Intermediate Synthesized by One Cell Can Act as an Agonist or Inhibitor of Eicosanoid Production in Another Cell

The biological effects attributable to the action of cyclooxygenase products can be induced in the lung by stimulation with leukotrienes C_4, D_4, and E_4.[14] Thus, active eicosanoids derived from one cell type can stimulate production of eicosanoid mediators with different biological properties from other cell types.

SUMMARY

In vitro experiments carried out in several laboratories indicate that cell components of hemostatic plugs, thrombi, and inflammatory lesions are capable of sharing precursors and intermediates of both the lipoxygenase and cyclooxygenase systems. These cells produce new eicosanoids in a stimulus-specific manner. It is therefore important to further elucidate mechanisms by which eicosanoids are formed during cell-cell interactions and the functional implications thereof.

REFERENCES

1. MARCUS, A. J. 1984. J. Lipid Res. **25:** 1511–1516.
2. MARCUS, A. J. 1978. J. Lipid Res. **19:** 793–826.
3. SAMUELSSON, B. 1983. Science **220:** 568–575.
4. MARCUS, A. J., B. B. WEKSLER, E. A. JAFFE & M. J. BROEKMAN. 1980. J. Clin. Invest. **66:** 979–986.
5. MARCUS, A. J. 1986. Prog. Hemostas. Thromb. **8:** 127–142.
6. MARCUS, A. J., M. J. BROEKMAN, L. B. SAFIER, H. L. ULLMAN, N. ISLAM, C. N. SERHAN, L. E. RUTHERFORD, H. M. KORCHAK & G. WEISSMANN. 1982. Biochem. Biophys. Res. Commun. **109:** 130–137.
7. MARCUS, A. J., L. B. SAFIER, H. L. ULLMAN, M. J. BROEKMAN, N. ISLAM, T. D. OGLESBY & R. R. GORMAN. 1984. Proc. Natl. Acad. Sci. U.S.A. **81:** 903–907.
8. WONG, P. Y.-K., P. WESTLUND, M. HAMBERG, E. GRANSTRÖM, P. H.-W. CHAO & B. SAMUELSSON. 1984. J. Biol. Chem. **259:** 2683–2686.
9. MARCUS, A. J., L. B. SAFIER, H. L. ULLMAN, N. ISLAM, M. J. BROEKMAN & C. VON SCHACKY. 1987. J. Clin. Invest. **79:** 179–187.
10. MARCUS, A. J., L. B. SAFIER, H. L. ULLMAN, N. ISLAM, M. J. BROEKMAN & C. VON SCHACKY. 1987. Clin. Res. **35:** 601A (abstract).
11. SCHAFER, A. I., D. D. CRAWFORD & M. A. GIMBRONE, JR. 1984. J. Clin. Invest. **73:** 1105–1112.
12. MCGEE, J. E. & F. A. FITZPATRICK. 1986. Proc. Natl. Acad. Sci. U.S.A. **83:** 1349–1353.
13. FEINMARK, S. J. & P. J. CANNON. 1986. J. Biol. Chem. **261:** 16466–16472.
14. PIPER, P. J. 1983. Br. Med. Bull. **39:** 255–259.

Endothelial Cell Perturbation and Low-Density Lipoprotein

Quantitative Autoradiography[a]

ERIC M. MORREL,[b] JAMES A. HOLLAND,[c]
KIRKWOOD A. PRITCHARD,[c] CLARK K. COLTON,[b]
AND MICHAEL B. STEMERMAN[c]

[b]*Department of Chemical Engineering*
Massachusetts Institute of Technology
Cambridge, Massachusetts 02139

[c]*Department of Medicine*
New York Medical College
Valhalla, New York 10595

INTRODUCTION

The mechanism of the initiation and formation of the atherosclerotic plaque remains unclear. The response to injury hypothesis[1–3] suggests that endothelial cell loss induces intimal thickening and lipid accumulation, which are early steps in plaque formation. Many studies have confirmed that experimental de-endothelialization can induce an atherogenic response.[1,4–11] A number of recent studies with experimental hypercholesterolemic animals,[12–17] however, have observed more subtle morphological changes in the early stages of atherogenesis without the overt loss of endothelial cells. Apparent evidence of endothelial loss was not seen until plaque development was notable.[14,15] Moreover, only a limited number of studies[18–22] have demonstrated nonmechanically induced endothelial cell desquamation with exposure of the subendothelium. Furthermore, dead endothelial cells may remain a part of the intact monolayer until they are sloughed without exposing the underlying subendothelium.[23,24] The infrequency of naturally occurring de-endothelialization suggests that endothelial cell loss may not be a common cause for initiation of the atherogenic process. Instead of cell denudation, endothelial dysfunction without cell loss could be the first event in atherogenesis.[25]

The endothelium is a barrier to macromolecular transport into the arterial wall.[26–28] Loss of this barrier function represents one form of endothelial dysfunction. Regions of enhanced permeability to the protein binding azo-dye Evans blue are seen in normal pigs[29–33] and rabbits.[31,32] Areas of increased Evans blue permeability are correlated with elevated uptake of ^{131}I-labeled albumin,[29–32] ^{131}I-labeled fibrinogen,[32] and ^{3}H-labeled cholesterol.[30] Endothelial cell morphology is slightly altered in these regions,[33] but there is no evidence of de-endothelialization.

[a]This work was supported by grant nos. HL21429, HL33742 and A483439 from the NIH-NHLBI and by a Herman Tarnower Research Award from the Westchester-Putnam Chapter of the American Heart Association.

FOCI OF ENHANCED ENDOTHELIAL PERMEABILITY

Utilizing horseradish peroxidase (HRP) as a macroscopic marker of enhanced permeability, Stemerman noted numerous spots of intense brown color scattered over the surface of the aorta of normocholesterolemic rabbits.[17] These regions are found to be focal sites of enhanced permeability to HRP.[17] Feeding rabbits a lipid-enriched diet increased the area covered by HRP foci by fivefold while raising the total cholesterol from 50 to 400 mg/dl. Others[34–36] have also observed variability in vessel wall permeability to HRP at the electron microscope level. The regions studied by Stemerman and coworkers[17,37,38] are scattered over the rabbit aortic luminal surface, appearing as foci (on average 200 μm in diameter, range 150–650 μm) of brown HRP reaction product. HRP-stained regions are most prevalent in the arch and upper abdominal aorta. The number of spots per square centimeter range from about 150 in the arch to 50 in the upper abdominal aorta and 15 HRP sites per square centimeter in the descending thoracic aorta. The corresponding fractional area coverage is roughly 3.0% in the arch, 1.5% in the thoracic aorta, and 0.5% in the descending thoracic aorta. Staining is more common proximal and distal rather than lateral to aortic ostia.[38]

Stemerman *et al.*[37] measured the uptake of ^{125}I-labeled LDL within sites of low and high HRP permeability. Following 10 min of ^{125}I-labeled LDL circulation and 1 min of HRP circulation, animals were sacrificed, perfusion fixed with glutaraldehyde, and sites of low and high HRP permeability were excised from the descending thoracic aorta. Samples of the high permeability foci included both the intima and the underlying media from each site and were roughly 0.1 mm^2 in luminal surface area. Intimal-medial samples from low permeability regions were typically 15 mm^2 in luminal surface area. ^{125}I-labeled LDL concentrations were up to 50 times greater in foci of enhanced HRP permeability when compared with low permeability zones.

QUANTITATIVE AUTORADIOGRAPHY

A method of absolute quantitative autoradiography,[39] which permits the measurement of ^{125}I-labeled LDL concentrations within 1 μm cross sections of tissue, has now been incorporated into the study of foci of enhanced HRP/LDL permeability. The use of 1-μm cross sections as samples permits high-resolution studies of radiolabeled tracer uptake into small areas. Additionally, with autoradiography, the distribution of a radiolabeled tracer within a sample can be observed directly. Arterial wall tissue samples are excised from rabbits in which ^{125}I-labeled LDL is injected 30 min and HRP 1 min prior to sacrifice. Samples of HRP high and low permeability sites are embedded in epoxy resin for ultramicrotomy. One micron sections are cut and autoradiographed along with gelatin standards of known ^{125}I-labeled LDL radioactivity concentation. The autoradiographic grain densities measured over the tissue samples are translated into ^{125}I-labeled LDL concentrations by comparison with a calibration curve calculated from the gelatin standards. In this way, the concentration of ^{125}I-labeled LDL across the arterial wall within a one micron section is measured. Autoradiography reveals ^{125}I-labeled LDL concentrations one to two orders of magnitude higher in HRP foci than in low permeability regions. The highest concentrations are localized directly beneath the endothelium and are an order of magnitude greater than measured previously with whole sample counting.[37] The region of elevated ^{125}I-labeled LDL concentration, after 30 min tracer circulation, measured about 100 μm in diameter and penetrated about 30 μm into the media. The endothelium in these unstained autoradiograms appeared unaltered.

In two animals, in addition to an injection of HRP and ^{125}I-labeled LDL as described above, the lower third of the descending thoracic aorta was de-endothelialized and Evans blue dye was injected 35 min prior to sacrifice. The grain density pattern in de-endothelialized regions is strikingly different from either the white (low permeability) or brown HRP (enhanced permeability) sites. There is a high grain density over nearly half the media with a slow decrease toward the luminal adventitial border. Grain density measurements translated into ^{125}I-labeled LDL concentration profiles reveal markedly increased concentrations in brown HRP regions and blue de-endothelialized regions when compared to white areas. The magnitude and shapes of the brown and blue profiles, however, are different, suggesting that different uptake mechanisms are operative. With the endothelium removed, the concentration near the lumen averages about 7% of the plasma value, and decreases continuously moving away from the lumen into the underlying media. By contrast, the concentration near the lumen in the brown regions approaches 25% of the plasma value and drops rapidly in the inner 20% of the media. The shape of the profile in the HRP foci is consistent with predominantly diffusive transport in the media, whereas the profile shape suggests that convection may dominate when the endothelium is removed. The high concentration near the lumen in the brown foci suggests that (1) the rate of transendothelial transport is extremely high compared to normal, and (2) LDL is sequestered in the subjacent media to a greater extent than usual, perhaps by binding to tissue components or smooth muscle cell receptors with subsequent internalization.

ENDOTHELIAL CELL TURNOVER

The increased presence of IgG permeable cells[23,24] and elevated uptake of Evans blue *in vivo*[40] have been correlated with increased cell proliferation. Evidence for foci of endothelial growth activity has been described.[41–43] Any of these findings contribute in part to understanding the observation of foci of enhanced HRP-LDL permeability. Preliminary tritiated thymidine uptake studies were performed in HRP injected animals to determine if HRP brown staining correlated with endothelial growth activity.

Twelve animals were injected with ^{3}H-labeled thymidine 17, 9, and 1 hour prior to sacrifice. Samples for en face autoradiography were dissected from the aorta and stripped of adventitial and medial tissue without damaging the intima. The autoradiograms from these studies revealed no consistent association between HRP uptake and tritiated thymidine uptake. These results indicate that only a subset of all replicating endothelial cells permit subsequently enhanced transport of macromolecules the size of HRP. A second possible interpretation is that the period within the cell cycle during which the region around a replicating cell is permeable occurs long before or after DNA synthesis.

ENDOTHELIAL CELL PERTURBATION IN CULTURE

Study of the mechanism(s) of focal endothelial cell dysfunction is difficult *in vivo*. We have recently investigated the feasibility of studying the response of the endothelium to protracted exposure of high low-density lipoprotein concentrations.[44] We have used an all-human system to culture endothelium in the presence of atherogenic levels of LDL for up to one month. These experiments, thus far, show no direct overt cytotoxicity associated with such treatment. There was a notable steady change in eicosanoid generation as measured by release of increased prostacycline, determined by measures of 6-keto $PGF_1\ \alpha$ from these cells as compared with controls. Thus LDL imparts a disturbance to normal EC function *in vitro* without induction of overt cytotoxicity.

SUMMARY

The focal entry and accumulation of LDL within the arterial wall of the normal animal may represent an early stage in the development of the atherosclerotic plaque. Concentrations of LDL 10 to 100 times normal medial concentrations might be difficult to clear from the arterial wall, permitting accumulation of lipid. Elevated LDL concentrations, in proximity to smooth muscle cells, appear to stimulate SMC proliferation.[2,5] High LDL concentrations might also enhance mononuclear cell adhesion to endothelium.[45] Since LDL has a high affinity for heparin and heparin for growth factors, LDL accumulation may be a mechanism for the concentration of such materials in the intima. The observation of markedly enhanced macromolecular permeability foci could be related to several potential mechanisms of initiation of atherosclerosis. This observation is of particular note when the focal occurrence of atherosclerosis is considered. Although atherosclerosis is seen as a generalized thickening of the intima, it is the focal narrowing of the lumen that is often responsible for the stenosis which produces symptoms such as angina or myocardial infarction.

ACKNOWLEDGMENTS

The authors wish to thank Tracey Holden and Nancy Rogers for their technical assistance and Sue Murphy for help with the preparation of this manuscript.

REFERENCES

1. Stemerman M. B. & R. Ross. 1972. Experimental arteriosclerosis. 1. Fibrous plaque formation in primates, an electron microscopic study. J. Exp. Med. **136:** 769–789.
2. Ross, R. & J. A. Glomset. 1976. The pathogenesis of atherosclerosis I. N. Engl. J. Med. **295:** 369–377.
3. Ross, R. & J. A. Glomset. 1976. The pathogenesis of atherosclerosis II. N. Engl. J. Med. **295:** 420–425.
4. Spaet, T. H., C. Rhee & C. Geiger. 1978. Delayed consequences of endothelial removal from rabbit aorta. Adv. Exp. Med. Biol. **102:** 165–173.
5. Minick, C. R., M. B. Stemerman & W. Insull, Jr. 1977. Effect of regenerated endothelium on lipid accumulation in the arterial wall. Proc. Natl. Acad. Sci. U.S.A. **74:** 1724–1728.
6. Ross, R. & L. Harker. 1976. Hyperlipidemia and atherosclerosis. Chronic hyperlipidemia initiates and maintains lesions by endothelial cell desquamation and lipid accumulation. Science **193:** 1094–1100.
7. Nam, S. C., W. M. Lee, J. Jarmolych, K. T. Lee & W. A. Thomas. 1973. Rapid production of advanced atherosclerosis in swine by a combination of endothelial injury and cholesterol feeding. Exp. Mol. Pathol. **18:** 369–379.
8. Stemerman, M. B. 1973. Thrombogenesis of the rabbit arterial plaque. An electron microscope study. Am. J. Pathol. **73:** 7–26.
9. Bjorkerud, S. 1969. Atherosclerosis initiated by mechanical trauma in normolipidemic rabbits. J. Atheroscler. Res. **9:** 209–213.

10. BJORKERUD, S. & G. BONDJERS. 1971. Arterial repair and atherosclerosis after mechanical injury. I. Permeability and light microscope characteristics of endothelium in non-atherosclerotic and atherosclerotic lesions. Atheroslcerosis **13:** 355–363.
11. BJORKERUD, S. & G. BONDJERS. 1973. Arterial repair and atherosclerosis after mechanical injury, Part 5: Tissue response after induction of large superficial transverse injury. Atherosclerosis **18:** 235–255.
12. DAVIES, P. F., M. A. REIDY, T. N. GOODE & D. E. BOWYE. 1976. Scanning electron microscopy in the evaluation of endothelial integrity of the fatty lesion in atherosclerosis. Atherosclerosis **25:** 125–130.
13. GOODE, T. B., P. E. DAVIES, M. A. REIDY & D. E. BOWYER. 1977. Aortic endothelial cell morphology observed in situ by scanning electron microscope during atherogenesis in the rabbit. Atherosclerosis **27:** 235–251.
14. FAGGIOTTO, A & K. ROSS. 1984. Studies of hypercholesterolemia in the non-human primate. II. Fatty streak conversion to fibrous plaque. Arterisoclerosis **4:** 341–356.
15. FAGGIOTTO, A., R. ROSS & L. HARKER. 1984. Studies of hypercholesterolemia in the non-human primate. I. Changes that lead to fatty streak formation. Arteriosclerosis **4:** 323–340.
16. SCHWARTZ, S. M., M. A. REIDY & G. K. HANSSON. 1983. Injury at the vascular surface. *In* Fluid Dynamics as a Localizing Factor for Atherosclerosis. G. Schettler *et al.,* Eds.: 188–199. Springer-Verlag. Berlin, Heidelberg.
17. STEMERMAN, M. B. 1981. Effects of moderate hypercholesterolemia on rabbit endothelium. Atherosclerosis **1:** 25–32.
18. GUTSTEIN, W. H., G. A. FARRELL & C. ARMELLINI. 1973. Blood flow disturbance and endothelial cell injury in preatherosclerotic swine. Lab. Invest. **29:** 134–149.
19. FRY, D. L. 1976. Hemodynamic forces in atherosclerosis. *In* Cerebrovascular Diseases. P. Scheinberg, Ed.: 77–95. Raven. New York.
20. LEWIS J. C. & B. A. KOTTKE. 1977. Endothelial damage and thrombocyte adhesion in pigeon atherosclerosis. Science **196:** 1007–1009.
21. OSBORNE-PELLEGRIN, M. J. 1979. "Spontaneous" lesions of the intima in the rat caudal artery. Principal morphologic characteristics and occurrence as a function of age and sex. Lab. Invest. **40:** 668–677.
22. OSBORNE-PELLEGRIN, M. J. & D. WEILL. 1983. "Spontaneous" endothelial injury in the rat caudal artery. Exp. Mol. Pathol. **39:** 61–79.
23. HANSSON, G. K., G. A. STARKEBAUM, E. P. BENDITT & S. M. SCHWARTZ. 1984. Fc-mediated binding of IgG to vimentin-type intermediate filaments in vascular endothelial cells. Proc. Natl. Acad. Sci. U.S.A. **81:** 3103–3107.
24. HANSSON G. K. & S. M. SCHWARTZ. 1983. Evidence for cell death in the vascular endothelium in vivo and in vitro. Am. J. Pathol. **112:** 278–286.
25. STEMERMAN, M. B., C. K. COLTON & E. M. MORREL. 1984. Perturbation of the endothelium. *In* Progress in Hemostasis and Thrombosis, Vol. 7. T. H. Spaet, Ed. Grune and Stratton. New York
26. BRATZLER, R. L., G. M. CHISOLM, C. K. COLTON, K. A. SMITH, D. B. ZILVERSMIT & R. S. LEES. 1977. The distribution of labeled albumin across the rabbit thoracic aorta in vivo. Circ. Res. **40:** 182–190.
27. BRATZLER, R. L., G. M. CHISOLM, C. K. COLTON, K. A. SMITH & R. S. LEES. 1977. The distribution of labeled low-density lipoproteins across the rabbit thoracic aorta in vivo. Atherosclerosis **28:** 289–307.
28. RAMIREZ, C. A., C. K. COLTON, K. A. SMITH, M. B. STEMERMAN & R. S. LEES. 1984. Transport of ^{125}I-albumin across normal and deendothelialized rabbit thoracic aorta in vivo. Arteriosclerosis **4:** 283–291.
29. PACKHAM M. A., H. G. ROSWELL, I. JORGENSEN & J. F. MUSTARD. 1967. Localized protein accumulation in the wall of the aorta. Exp. Mol. Pathol. **7:** 214–232.
30. SOMER, J. B. & S. M. SCHWARTZ. 1971. Focal ^{3}H-cholesterol uptake in pig aorta. Atherosclerosis **13:** 293–304.
31. BELL, E. P., I. L. ADAMSON & C. J. SCHWARTZ. 1974. Aortic endothelial permeability to albumin: Focal and regional patterns of uptake and transmural distribution of ^{125}I-albumin in the young pig. Exp. Mol. Pathol. **20:** 281–292.
32. BELL, F. P. & A. S. GALLUS & C. J. SCHWARTZ. 1974. Focal and regional patterns of

uptake and the transmural distribution of ^{131}I-fibrinogen in the pig aorta, in vivo. Exp. Mol. Pathol. **20:** 281–292.

33. CAPLAN, B. A., R. G. GERRITY & C. J. SCHWARTZ. 1974. Endothelial cell morphology in focal areas of in vivo Evans blue uptake in the young pig aorta. I. Quantitative light microscopic findings. Exp. Mol. Pathol. **21:** 102–117.
34. WEBSTER, W. S., S. P. BISHOP & J. C. GEER. 1974. Experimental aortic intimal thickening. II. Endothelialization and permeability. Am. J. Pathol. **76:** 265–284.
35. SCHWARTZ, S. M. & E. P. BENDITT. 1972. Studies on aortic intima. I. Structure and permeability of rat thoracic aortic intima. Am. J. Pathol. **66:** 241–252.
36. HUTTNER, I., M. BOUTET & R. H. MORE. 1973. Studies on protein passage through arterial endothelium. II. Regional differences in permeability to find structural protein tracers in arterial endothelium of normotensive rat. Lab. Invest. **28:** 678–685.
37. STEMERMAN, M. B., E. M. MORREL, K. R. BURKE, C. K. COLTON, K. A. SMITH & R. L. LEES. 1986. Local variation in arterial wall permeability to low density lipoprotein in normal rabbit aorta. Arteriosclerosis, **6:** 64–69.
38. UHTHOFF, P. A. F. M. S. thesis, Massachusetts Institute of Technology. In preparation.
39. SCHNITZER, J. J., E. M. MORREL, C. K. COLTON, K. A. SMITH & M. B. STEMERMAN. Absolute quantitative autoradiography of ^{125}I-labeled proteins incorporating automated grain density analysis. J. Histochem. Cytyochem. In press.
40. CAPLAN, B. A. & C. J. SCHWARTZ. 1973. Increased endothelial cell turnover in areas of in vivo Evans blue uptake in the pig aorta. Atherosclerosis **17:** 401–417.
41. GERRITY, R. G., M. RICHARDSON, B. A. CAPLAN, J. F. CADE, J. HIRSCH & C. J. SCHWARTZ. 1976. Endotoxin injury, enface morophology, ^{3}H-thymidine uptake and circulating endothelial cells in the dog. Exp. Mol. Pathol. **24:** 59–69.
42. SCHWARTZ, S. M. & E. P. BENDITT. 1973. Cell replication in the aortic endothelium: A new method for study of the problem. Lab. Invest. **28:** 699–707.
43. SCHWARTZ, S. M. & E. P. BENDITT. 1976. Clustering of replicating cells in aortic endothelium. Proc. Natl. Acad. Sci. U.S.A. **73:** 651–653.
44. HOLLAND, J. A. 1988. Sustained endothelial culture with atherogenic levels of low density lipoprotein. In preparation.
45. ALDERSON, L. M., G. ENDEMANN, S. LINDSEY, A. PONCZUK, R. L. HOOVER & K. C. HAYES. 1986. LDL enhances monocyte adhesion to endothelial cells in vitro. Am. J. Pathol. **123:** 334–342.

Endothelial Cell Modulation of Primary Platelet Hemostasis[a]

ERIC F. GRABOWSKI

Division of Pediatric Hematology/Oncology
New York Hospital-Cornell Medical Center
New York, New York 10021

OVERVIEW

The adhesion-aggregation of platelets to a site of vessel wall injury is a quintessential blood flow phenomenon. First, platelets are driven to the vicinity of the vessel wall by a form of convective diffusion in which red cells both mechanically augment the effective platelet diffusivity[1,2] and enhance the near-wall platelet concentration.[3] Secondly, red cells subjected to physiologic shear forces release sufficient adenine nucleotides to induce primary platelet aggregation.[4] This "humoral" effect of erythrocytes is likely to contribute to primary hemostasis in a shear-stress-dependent manner. Thirdly, endothelial cells are able to modulate platelet aggregation at a site of vessel injury by producing prostacyclin (and perhaps other antithrombotic substances) in a manner that increases with vessel shear rate[5]; production for a large range of arterial shear rates appears to be limited by plasma-borne substrate (arachidonate). This manner of production ensures a concentration of prostacyclin in the near-wall region that remains relatively independent of shear rate.

IMAGING PRIMARY HEMOSTASIS

In our work, epifluorescence videomicroscopy has allowed real-time imaging of platelet adhesion-aggregation to a simulated vessel wall injury.[6] The injury model is an endothelial cell monolayer (ECM) across which, prior to ECM exposure to flowing blood, a 6-0 sterile suture is drawn in a direction transverse to flow. Microinjuries measuring 70 ± 15 μm (mean ± SD) in width (FIG. 1) result. The fluorescent label is the TAB murine monoclonal antibody (courtesy of Dr. R. P. McEver) directed against human platelet GpIIb, together with a fluorescein-conjugated goat $F(ab')_2$ against murine immunoglobulin. The injured ECMs, grown to confluence on rectangular cover glasses precoated with microfibrillar collagen, constitute one wall of a flow chamber mounted on a vertical microscope stage. On microinjury sites and at shear rates of 100 to 700 s^{-1}, computer-enhanced video images show adherence, remodeling, and growth of chains of platelet aggregates (FIG. 2). Aligned with the flow direction, these chains have a spacing of approximately 30 μm, a length similar to the average endothelial cell diameter. One may speculate that such chains provide a scaffold for wound healing insofar as they are likely to be rich in agents chemotactic for leukocytes and in platelet-derived growth factor.

Computer enhancement of video images consists of real-time image digitalization

[a]This work was supported by grant no. HL 33095 from the National Institutes of Health, and by the Children's Blood Foundation.

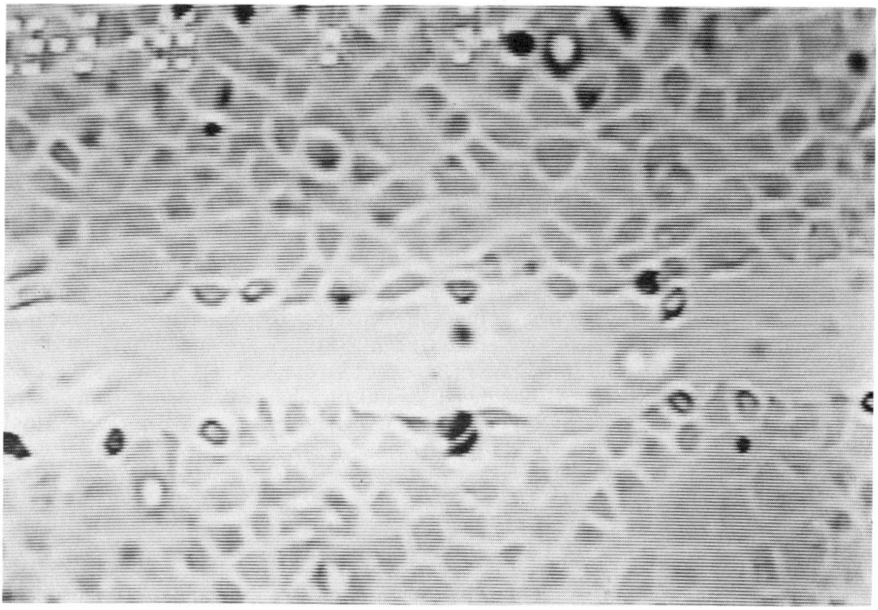

FIGURE 1. Microinjury site on otherwise confluent monolayer of bovine aortic endothelial cells. Injury width is 80 μm.

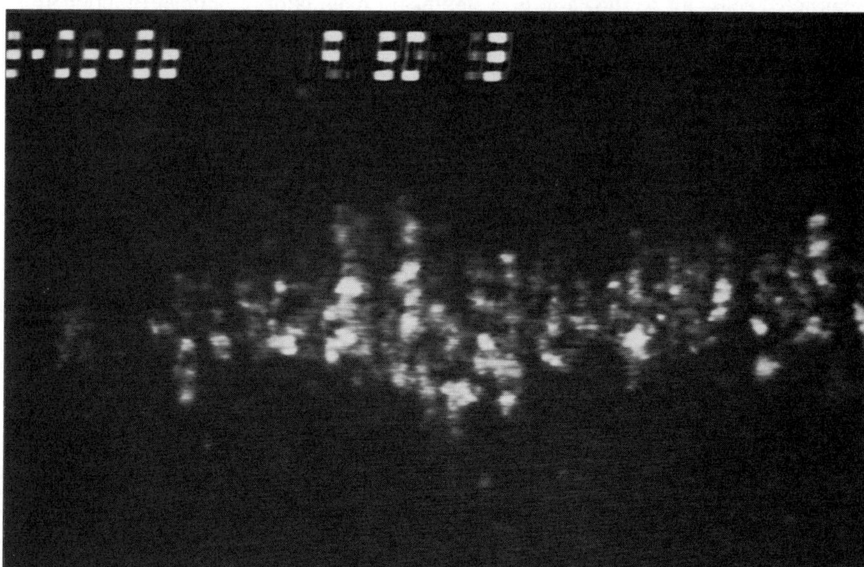

FIGURE 2. Platelet adhesion-aggregation at microinjury site in whole blood after 5 minutes at a surface shear rate of 270 s^{-1}. Because of camera inversion and reversal of image, blood flow is from top to bottom. Image corresponds to an area 435 μm $\times$ 580 μm.

and background subtraction, digital amplification, and image "running" summation. Off-line measurements of total thrombus volume, the dimensions of individual platelet thrombi, and the degree of coverage of the injury area by platelet adhesion-aggregation are performed. The first assumes that local aggregate height is proportional to local fluorescence intensity.

MODULATORY ROLE OF ENDOTHELIUM

When the ECMs are pretreated with 1.0 mM FC lysine acetylsalicylate, the mean aggregate height increases ($2p < 0.05$) to 260 ± 64% (mean ± SE, $n = 6$) of control, the percent surface area of the injury site covered by platelets is augmented ($2p < 0.05$) from 14.8 ± 4.3 to 49.2 ± 5.2 (mean ± SE, $n = 6$), and outflow levels by RIA of serum thromboxane B_2 increase ($2p < 0.01$) from 5.08 ± 1.61 to 9.35 ± 2.65 ng/ml (mean ± SE, $n = 6$). Although no significant changes are seen in levels of prostacyclin by RIA for 6-keto-$PGF_1\ \alpha$, these levels did decrease in five of seven paired experiments.

SUMMARY

Rheology has profound effects on the rate, structure, and modulation of primary hemostasis. Many of these effects can be studied via real-time, epifluorescence videomicroscopy of platelet adhesion-aggregation to a site of injury to an endothelial cell monolayer exposed to flowing blood. In particular, with the model described, endothelial cells can be shown to be a significant modulator of platelet function at an injury site.

REFERENCES

1. Turitto, V. T., A. M. Benis & E. F. Leonard. 1972. Ind. Eng. Chem. Fund. **11:** 216–223.
2. Grabowski, E. F., L. I. Friedman & E. F. Leonard. Ind. Eng. Chem. Fund. **11:** 224–232.
3. Tillies, A. W. & E. C. Eckstein. 1987. Microvasc. Res. In press.
4. Reimers, R., S. P. Sutera & J. H. Joist. 1984. Blood. **64:** 1200–1206.
5. Grabowski, E. F. *et al.* 1983. Blood. **62:** 301a.
6. Grabowski, E. F. 1987. Blood. In press.

Summary

Cellular Systems

ERIC F. GRABOWSKI

Division of Pediatric Hematology/Oncology
New York Hospital-Cornell Medical Center
New York, New York 10021

The microenvironment of flowing blood in contact with natural and artificial surfaces is one rich in continuous communication among different cell types. In our own work (see preceding paper), for example, endothelial cells can be shown to modulate platelet aggregation at a site of vessel injury perfused with whole blood at arterial shear rates. The modulating agents are endothelial cell products inhibitable by aspirin.

In this session, Dr. Holger Schmid-Schönbein presented a block diagram overview of the flow factors, physicochemical concepts, and cell reactions important in thrombosis at a surface. This set the stage for Drs. Shu Chien and Geert Schmid-Schönbein, who shed light on the specific rheology of the leukocyte. Dr. Chien identified elastic and viscous parameters using a micropipette approach. These parameters reflect the structure of cytoskeletal microtubules and microfilaments, and likely change with cell activation. Dr. Schmid-Schönbein considered leukocytes in rolling contact with endothelium. He found that the degree to which leukocyte net motion lags behind the vessel's centerline flow velocity is proportional to the energy required to separate leukocyte and endothelial membranes.

Platelet function at surfaces was discussed by Drs. Barry Coller, Harvey Weiss, and Marjorie Zucker. Dr. Coller summarized our knowledge of platelet activation at surfaces: factors include plasma fibrinogen, von Willebrand factor, the integrity of platelet glycoprotein receptors, and the diacylglycerol inositol trisphosphate and prostaglandin-thromboxane A_2 pathways. Dr. Weiss showed that a tissue-factor-like property of platelets (as well as of subendothelium) is important to fibrin deposition on subendothelium at arterial shear rates. Dr. Zucker employed a variety of monoclonal antibodies to clarify the factor or factors behind platelet retention in a glass bead column. She found a possible role for von Willebrand factor binding to platelet glycoprotein Ib.

The study of cell-cell communication on a biochemical level was well illustrated by Dr. Aaron Marcus, whose studies of platelet-neutrophil interaction are fundamental. Stimulated platelets, for instance, synthesize 12-HETE, the proinflammatory monohydroxy lipoxygenase product of arachidonic acid. Unstimulated neutrophils may modulate platelet 12-HETE levels *in vivo* by their ability to metabolize 12-HETE to 12,20-DiHETE.

Lastly, Dr. Michael Stemerman described the penetration of low-density lipoprotein into vessel walls at discrete locations. These locations are characterized not by endothelial cell loss, but rather by locally increased permeability to horseradish peroxidase. In other words, an endothelium that appears morphologically intact need not be functionally intact.

Flow Patterns in Vessels of Simple and Complex Geometries[a]

TAKESHI KARINO, HARRY L. GOLDSMITH, MINEO MOTOMIYA, SHOJI MABUCHI, AND YASUNORI SOHARA

McGill University Medical Clinic
Montreal General Hospital
Montreal, Quebec H3G 1A4, Canada

INTRODUCTION

Disturbed flows associated with the particular geometry of vessels are considered not only to play an important role in the focal deposition of platelets and white cells on artificial surfaces and the localization of thrombosis and atherosclerosis *in vivo,* but also to exert some detrimental effects on both the circulating blood cells and the vessel wall, resulting in hemolysis of red cells, activation and aggregation of platelets and white cells, and formation of aneurysms and dilatation of the vessel wall in regions of disturbed flow. Ideally, therefore, it is desirable to avoid creating any flow disturbance, but if this is inevitable, to minimize the size and intensity of the disturbed flows that may form in living vessels as the result of vascular surgery or in channels of artificial organs and vascular prostheses. Except for the case of very high flow rates (or high Reynolds numbers well over 2000), turbulent flow either in the straight parts of arteries *in vivo,* or in any artificial conduit having a circular cross section, is not likely to be seen. Therefore, in the context of the present paper, we will limit our description and discussion only to the phenomena that occur at Reynolds numbers smaller than 2000 and in steady flow.

During the past 10 years or so we have been carrying on a series of investigations on the role of fluid mechanical factors in the localization of thrombosis and atherosclerosis in man, and studying the flow patterns in various vessels of simple and complex geometries by means of flow visualization and cinemicrographic techniques. In this paper we will summarize our findings on the detailed three-dimensional structures of disturbed flows formed in glass models of stenoses and T-junctions, compare them with those observed in isolated transparent natural arteries and veins prepared from dogs and humans postmortem, and then identify the differences in geometrical structures and flow patterns between the artificial vessels and the natural blood vessels in order to find out the optimum conditions to eliminate or minimize the region of disturbed flow that may form *in vivo* as well as in any channel of artificial vessels.

[a]This work was supported by Medical Research Council of Canada grant nos. MT 1835 and MT 7084, grant no. HL 29502 from the National Heart, Lung and Blood Institute, USPHS, and the Quebec Heart Foundation.

METHODS

A sudden tubular expansion, serving as an idealized model of an axisymmetric stenosis, was constructed by tightly and concentrically fitting a 150-μm inner diameter thick-walled glass tube into a 500-μm inner diameter thin-walled outer glass tube. Glass model T-junctions having various branching angles and tube diameter ratios were constructed either by fitting and gluing together two pieces of thin walled glass tubing having inner diameters of 1.05, 2.0, and 3.0 mm at desired angles from 30° to 90°, or by glass blowing. Transparent natural arteries and veins were prepared from dogs and humans postmortem by fixing the vessels under the physiological transmural pressures, dehydrating them with ethanol and suspending or immersing them in oil of wintergreen containing 5% ethanol.[1] Flow was visualized by taking 16-mm cine films of the motions of tracer polystyrene microspheres in dilute suspensions undergoing steady flow at various flow rates. The developed films were subsequently projected on a drafting table and analyzed frame by frame.

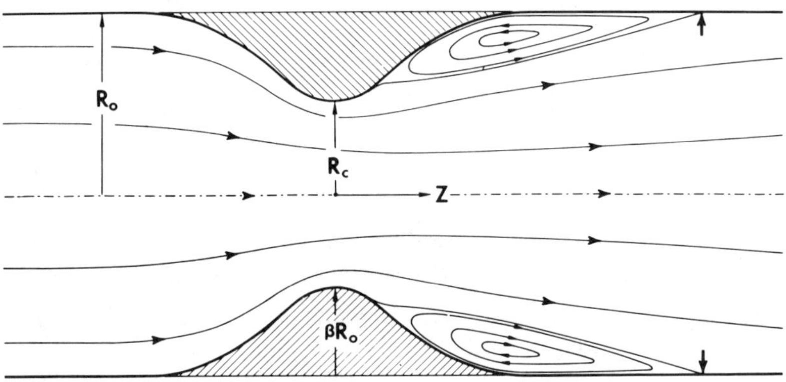

FIGURE 1. Schematic representation of flow through a bell-shaped axisymmetric constriction (median plane). An annular vortex is formed downstream of the narrowest point of the vessel lumen. The *arrows* indicate the reattachment points of the separated flow on the vessel wall. (From Goldsmith and Karino.[3])

RESULTS

Flow through Channels of Nonuniform Diameter

As demonstrated by Reynolds over a hundred years ago,[2] flow in a circular vessel will remain laminar and undisturbed until the Reynolds number, a dimensionless parameter defined as $Re = D\overline{U}\rho/\mu$ (with D the tube diameter, $\overline{U}$ the mean fluid velocity, ρ and μ the fluid density and viscosity, respectively) exceeds the critical value of ~2300. However, once an irregularity is produced in the vessel diameter, a number of problems arise even at much lower Re. FIGURE 1 illustrates the flow through a bell-shaped axisymmetric stenosis. When a fluid is subjected to steady flow through the tube at a constant driving pressure in the axial Z direction, it is suddenly accelerated as it passes by the stenosis and then is immediately decelerated. As a result, there occurs a positive, adverse static pressure gradient distal to the stenosis. In the mainstream, the kinetic energy of the fluid is sufficient to overcome this pressure gradient. However, the fluid adjacent to the wall consumes its much smaller kinetic energy before having moved very far, and it is eventually forced to a standstill and caused to flow backward by the adverse pressure gradient existing near the vessel wall distal to the stenosis. Fresh fluid arrives and experiences the same retardation, and as the decelerated portion of the stream rapidly increases in volume, the mainstream is pushed away from the boundary, forcing the separation of streamlines from the vessel wall slightly downstream of the constriction. In this way, flow separation occurs. The fluid in the reverse flow regions coils itself up and a vortex (an annular ring vortex) is formed between the forward-flowing mainstream and the vessel wall distal to the stenosis. The point of separation of the streamline from the vessel wall and the point of reattachment of the once separated streamline on the vessel wall beyond the vortex are called, respectively, the separation and reattachment points. This is one way by which flow disturbances are created within flowing blood. Flow separation usually occurs near the downstream edge of the constriction, and the critical Re for the formation of the vortex is largely affected by the amplitude and sharpness of the stenosis.[3] As a result of flow separation and vortex formation, which consume extra energy due to the internal friction of the viscous fluid circulating in the vortex, a sudden decrease in driving pressure downstream of the stenosis occurs. In the circulation, this may lead to a drop in flow rate and a poorer supply of blood and hence oxygen, resulting in the development of local ischemia and thrombosis. If Re is high enough, the vortex may oscillate and even exhibit shedding in turbulent flow, especially in the arterial circulation where the effect of pulsation is more marked and causes vibration of the vessel wall around the reattachment point. Such mechanical vibration has been found to induce weakening of the vessel wall, especially of the elastin in the intima, resulting in the development of a poststenotic dilatation in the region of disturbed flow.[4] Shedding of the vortices has been held responsible for the generation of poststenotic murmurs.[5]

It has also been demonstrated that such undesirable flow patterns have some detrimental effects on blood cells with respect to their interactions with each other and with the vessel wall. It has been shown that in dogs partial occlusion of the coronary arteries[6] and implantation of an orifice ring into the inferior vena cava[7] resulted in the formation of a thrombus at the site of vessel constriction. The factor responsible for thrombus formation at such sites was attributed to the turbulence of the flow generated by the stenosis.[8]

To investigate the exact mechanisms of thrombus formation at such sites, we have previously carried out a series of microrheological investigations on the flow behavior and interactions of red cells and platelets with each other and with the vessel wall in the region of disturbed flow distal to a sudden tubular expansion, which served as an idealized model of a stenosis. FIGURE 2 shows the flow patterns observed in the region of disturbed flow formed downstream of an expansion of a 150-μm into 500-μm glass tube. As predicted by fluid mechanical theory,[9] a triangular-shaped captive annular ring vortex formed distal to the expansion. As a result of detailed investigations, we discovered the following three important characteristics of the vortex:

1. The vortex is a region of stagnant flow in which single cells and small aggregates of cells migrate out after long residence times while circulating in its orbits, resulting in the establishment of lowered hematocrits in the region of separated flow, whereas large aggregates of cells are trapped indefinitely in both steady and pulsatile flow.[10]
2. The vortex is a region of shear flow in which collisions between platelets

circulating in its orbits for long periods of time result in the spontaneous formation of aggregates that increase in size without the addition of any activating agents.[11]

3. The vortex is a region of disturbed flow in which the collision of blood cells with the vessel wall is significantly enhanced through their convective transport along the radially directed streamlines of the flow around the reattachment (stagnation) point, resulting in the localized adhesion of platelets on both sides of the reattachment point.[12]

It is not likely that such a perfectly axisymmetric stenosis exists in the circulation even under pathological conditions. However, it is not rare to find sudden axisymmetric

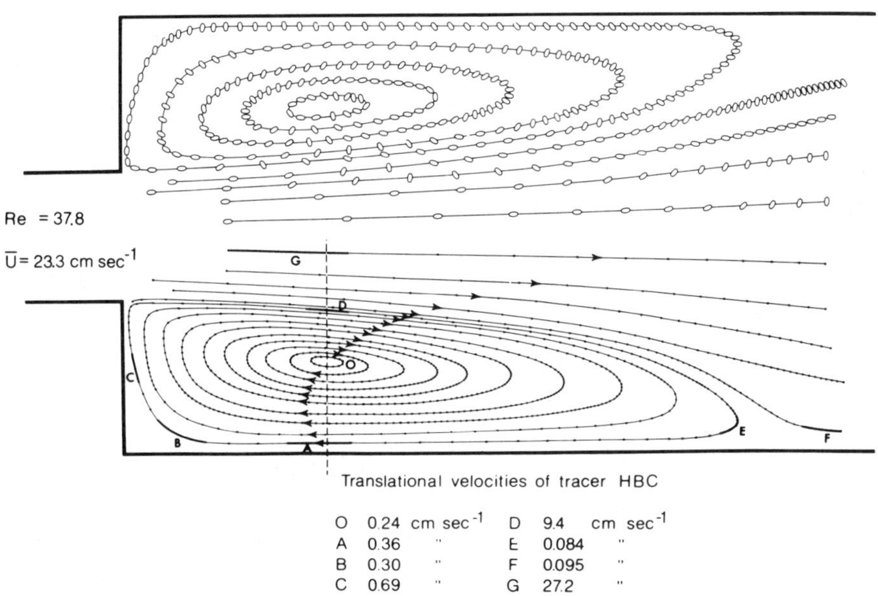

FIGURE 2. Flow patterns in the median plane of an annular vortex formed downstream of a sudden expansion of a 150-μm into a 500-μm glass tube at Re = 37.8. The orientations of red cells are drawn on the orbits in the upper portion of the diagram. The *arrows* indicate the velocity distribution in the vortex and adjacent mainstream. The letters *A* to *G* and *O* indicate the positions at which particle velocities listed were measured; *HBC*, hardened blood cells. (From Karino and Goldsmith.[10] Reprinted with permission from the *Philosophical Transactions of the Royal Society of London.*)

changes in vessel diameter in channels of some artificial organs and prosthetic devices, where the phenomena described above may have some implications for thrombogenesis in regions of disturbed flow. In the circulation, one may find similar flow patterns downstream of the aortic valve, arterial stenoses caused by the development of atherosclerotic plaques, and the venous valves. Here we present an example of disturbed flows observed in the venous circulation.

FIGURE 3 illustrates the detailed flow patterns observed along the common median plane of a 2-mm diameter dog saphenous vein containing a bileaflet valve. As shown in the figure, flow separation at the edge of the valve leaflet resulted in the formation of large paired vortices located symmetrically on both sides of the bisector plane of the valve leaflets in each valve pocket under physiological flow conditions. Particles continually entered the valve pockets from the mainstream, spending long periods of time describing a series of spiral orbits of decreasing diameter while moving away from the bisector plane, and eventually left the vortex. With concentrated suspensions of hardened red cells it was found that another smaller counter-rotating secondary vortex, driven by the large primary vortex, existed deep in each valve pocket (blank area of FIGURE 3) where venous thrombi are believed to originate.[13] Furthermore, with a suspension of 25% hematocrit hardened red cells, it was found that the hematocrit in this secondary vortex remained appreciably lower than that in the primary vortex. In

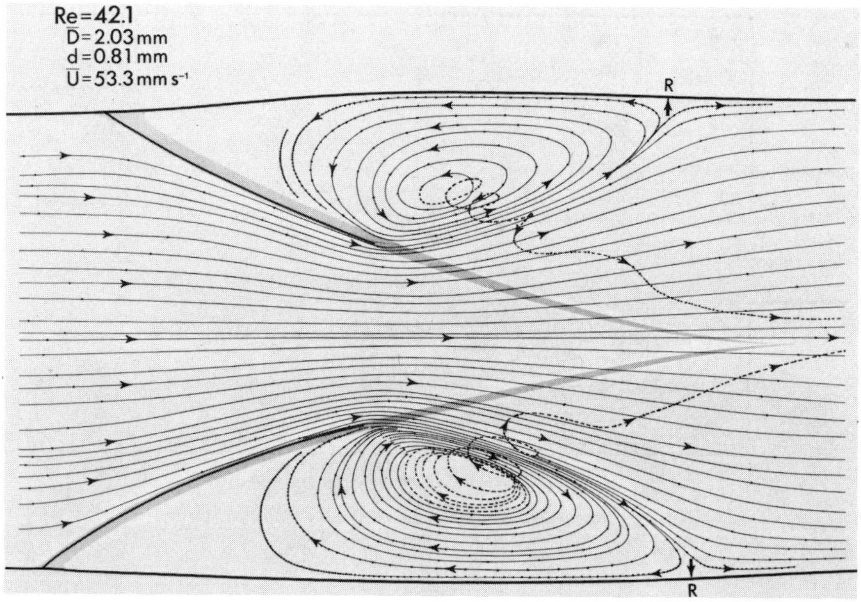

FIGURE 3. Detailed flow patterns in the common bisector plane of the valve leaflets in a 2-mm diameter dog saphenous vein containing a bileaflet valve, showing the formation of a recirculation zone in each valve pocket. In fact, these consist of a pair of vortices located symmetrically on both sides of the bisector plane. The *solid lines* are the paths of particles located in or close to, and the *dashed lines* those located far away from, the bisector plane (the projection of the particle paths on the bisector plane). The arrows at *R* indicate the location of the reattachment point. (From Karino and Motomiya.[25] Reprinted by permission from *Thrombosis Research.*)

such stagnant regions, fluid circulated with extremely low velocities, thus creating a very low shear field that allowed the hardened red cells to form aggregates. It is, therefore, possible that in some pathological states red cells and platelets form much larger aggregates which could be trapped in this secondary vortex, as was previously found in an annular vortex formed in a model of a stenosis,[10-12] or sediment toward the deepest portion of the valve pocket. Furthermore, since these regions are isolated from the mainstream by the primary vortices, transport of materials including oxygen and carbon dioxide to and from the blood in the mainstream would be inhibited, resulting in a lowered concentration of oxygen in the valve pockets, as has been demonstrated by

Hamer *et al.* in dogs and humans.[14] The results suggest a possible mechanism of thrombus formation in the valve pockets through severe hypoxemia, which causes endothelial damage, leading to the adhesion and aggregation of fresh normal platelets and leukocytes, taken into the valve pocket by sudden disturbances of the flow, onto the injured vessel wall, leading to the eventual formation of fibrin clots as nidi for thrombus formation.

Flow through Simple Branching Vessels

Formation of vortices (eddies) at the site of flow division is a common phenomenon in both open channels such as rivers and canals (two-dimensional channels) and closed channels such as water conduits and blood vessels (three-dimensional channels). However, the nature of the eddies and the detailed flow patterns are quite different. In two-dimensional bifurcations with rectangular cross sections all the fluid elements move parallel to the common median plane of the parent and daughter channels, and no secondary flow (flow in the direction normal to the mainstream) is created at the flow divider. The recirculation flow which forms at the hips of the bifurcation bears the typical characteristics of a vortex with closed orbits.[15] However, in three-dimensional (tubular) bifurcations with circular cross-sections, the flow is much more complex and quite different from that formed in the two-dimensional case.

To investigate the exact nature of the disturbed flow formed at the junction of three-dimensional bifurcations, we have studied the detailed flow patterns in various glass models of branching vessels having circular cross sections.[16-17]

Right Angle T-Junctions

FIGURE 4 shows an example of flow patterns, traced out from the motions of tracer microspheres, in the common median plane of 3-mm diameter right angled square (top) and rounded (bottom) T-junctions at the same inflow Reynolds number, Re_o, when the main branch was partially occluded so that 80% of the flow left through the side branch. Under these conditions ($Q_1/Q_o = 0.2$), a large recirculation zone was formed in the main tube in both T-junctions, and a small secondary one in the side branch in only the square T-junction. The formation and the sizes of these recirculation zones were found to be largely dependent on the flow ratio Q_1/Q_o as well as on Re_o. When observed along the common median plane it was found that the recirculation zones in both main and side tubes consisted of a pair of spiral secondary flows located symmetrically on both sides of the common median plane of the T-junction. Particles in the mainstream were deflected at the flow divider and traveled laterally and very slowly along the wall above and below the common median plane, and encircled the mainstream. Some of them entered the core of the main recirculation zone in the straight main branch and described complicated multiple orbits, others changed direction and moved backward along the outer wall of the main branch. They then changed direction again and crossed the mainflow encircling above or below it in the junction region far out of the common median plane (indicated by the dashed path lines in FIGURE 4) and entered the side tube and side recirculation zone downstream of which a counter-rotating double helicoidal flow developed. All the particles entering the smaller recirculation zone at the entrance of the side branch originated from the larger main recirculation zone in the main tube. When the degree of occlusion of the main tube was gradually reduced, the larger recirculation zone in the main tube

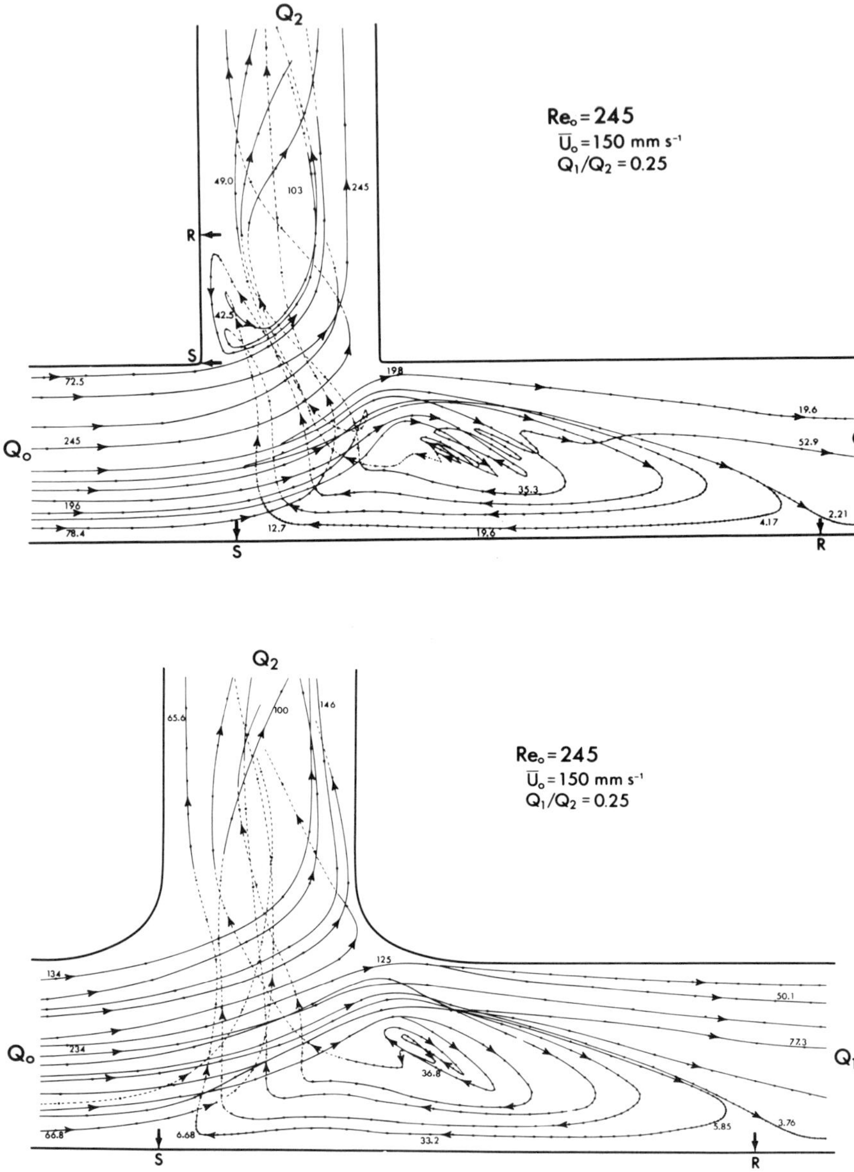

FIGURE 4. Flow patterns in a 3-mm uniform diameter 90° square (*top*) and rounded (*bottom*) T-junctions showing the formation of main and side (only in the top) recirculation zones in the main and side tubes, respectively. The arrows at *S* and *R* indicate the respective separation and stagnation points of the flow, and the numbers on the paths indicate the particle linear velocities in mm · s^{-1}. (From Karino *et al.*[16] Reprinted with permission from *Biorheology*.)

became smaller and eventually disappeared as the flow ratio was reversed (Q_1/Q_o = 0.8), while the recirculation zone in the side branch grew in size.

With respect to the effects of curvature of the wall at the junction, there were significant differences between the square and rounded T-junctions as demonstrated in FIGURE 4. At a given flow ratio, Q_1/Q_o, the side recirculation zone was formed at much lower Re_0 in the square than in the rounded T-junction. In the rounded T-junction, it existed over a much narrower range of Q_1/Q_o and disappeared altogether at $Q_1/Q_o <$ 0.35. In the square T-junction, the two recirculation zones coexisted even at $Q_1/Q_o \sim 0$, provided $Re_0 > 60$. By contrast, the main recirculation zone first appeared at somewhat lower Re_0 in the rounded than in the square T-junction. Thus, at a given Re_0 and Q_1/Q_o, a much larger main recirculation zone with more rapidly circulating fluid existed in the rounded than in the square T-junction, though the side recirculation zone may not form at all as in the case depicted in FIGURE 4. These data show that formation of the side recirculation zone is largely affected by the curvature of the wall at the bend opposite to the flow divider, while that of the main recirculation zone is affected by the curvature at the flow divider, indicating that the side recirculation zone has its origin in flow separation at the bend while the main recirculation zone is created as a result of flow deflection and resultant formation of strong secondary flows at the flow divider.

Formation of such recirculation flows was observed also in actual arterial T-junctions in the dog abdominal aorta.[1] The general flow patterns at each branching site of the celiac, cranial-mesenteric, and right and left renal arteries were similar to those observed in various glass models. FIGURE 5 illustrates the detailed flow patterns observed at the aorto-celiac artery junction at its geometrical flow ratio (flow rate ratio calculated by assuming that the flow in the parent tube is distributed into the two daughter tubes proportionally to their cross-sectional area evaluated at the apex of the flow divider). As shown in the figure, paired spiral secondary flows, symmetrical about the common median plane of the aorta and branch, were formed adjacent to the vessel wall at $Re_0 \sim 300$, grew bigger with increasing Re_0, and reached a fully disturbed flow at $Re_0 \sim 900$ (the largest orbit then reached the opposite wall and the paired spiral secondary flow completely encircled the undisturbed mainflow). With further increasing Re_0, the recirculation zone grew in length and the eddies increased in intensity and then, at $Re_0 \sim 1200$, there was a sudden transition from disturbed to turbulent flow. Here an interesting observation was made on the geometrical structure of the natural vessel. Close examination of the wall at each junction revealed that curvature of the wall at the flow divider was very sharp ($< 90°$), with a sudden stepwise decrease in aortic diameter distal to the branch, whereas that at the opposite corner was gently rounded. From the results obtained in the glass model T-junctions described earlier, this represents the optimum condition for minimizing the size of both main and side recirculation zones which may form in the aortic T-junction. In fact, it was found that under physiological conditions $Re_0 > 700$, and at a geometrical flow ratio there was no side recirculation zone (in the side branch) and the main recirculation zone (in the main branch) was small and confined to a thin layer close to the vessel wall surrounding the mainstream. Hence, in the circulation, conditions at arterial branches appear to be optimal for minimizing the formation of recirculation zones.

Acute Angle T-Junctions

The effects of branching angle, θ, and tube diameter ratio, d/D, on the formation of disturbed flow at sites of flow division were studied by measuring the critical Reynolds number, Re_c, for the onset of the main and side recirculation flow which formed in various glass model square T-junctions. It was found that Re_c for the main recircula-

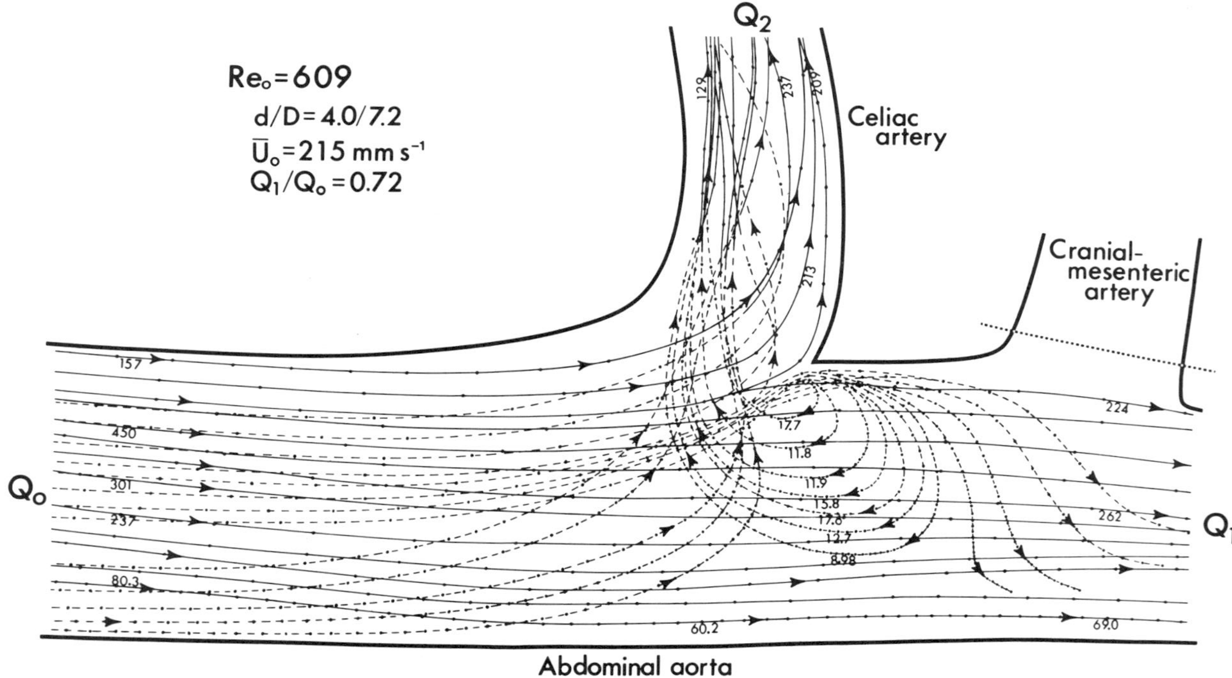

FIGURE 5. Detailed flow patterns at the aorto-celiac artery junction of a dog abdominal aorta, showing the formation of paired thin-layered spiral secondary flows on both sides of the common median plane of the main and side branches, adjacent to the vessel wall surrounding the undisturbed mainstream. The *solid lines* are the paths of particles in or close to the common median plane, and the *dashed lines* the paths far away from the common median plane (projection of the particle paths on the common median plane). The *numbers* on the streamlines indicate the particle velocities in $mm \cdot s^{-1}$. (From Karino and Motomiya.[1] Reprinted with permission from *Biorheology*.)

tion zone was the lowest at 90° for all Q_1/Q_o, whereas for the side recirculation zone it decreased as the branching angle increased from 45° to 135° (recirculation zone became bigger with increasing branching angle). Thus, as shown in FIGURE 6 for a 30° T-junction with 2-mm side tube, the main recirculation zone (paired spiral secondary flows) became much smaller than that observed in uniform diameter right angle T-junctions (c.f. FIGURE 4) and was confined to a thin layer adjacent to the tube wall, wrapped around the predominant undisturbed mainflow. No side recirculation zone was formed at the geometrical flow ratio. With decreasing tube diameter ratio, d/D (side to main), Re_c for both the main and side recirculation zones increased drastically. Thus, for 90° T-junctions with $d/D < 0.5$, no main recirculation zone was formed at the geometrical flow ratio. The Re_c for the side recirculation zone appeared to be a maximum around the geometrical flow ratio, indicating that this is the optimum condition for minimizing the size of the recirculation zone and thus the region of disturbed flow which forms in branching vessels.

Acute angle T-junctions and bifurcations as shown in FIGURE 6 will be found at many sites along the arterial tree. One of the best examples of disturbed flow in such vessels is that of the human carotid artery bifurcation.[18] It was found that a standing recirculation zone, consisting of a pair of complex spiral secondary flows located symmetrically on both sides of the common median plane of the bifurcation, was formed in the carotid sinus over wide ranges of Re_o and flow ratios Q_1/Q_o (internal/common carotid). As shown in FIGURE 7, particles were deflected at the flow divider, and traveled laterally along the vessel wall on both sides of the common median plane, almost at right angles to and encircling the mainstream. They then changed direction, moving back along the outer wall of the internal carotid artery at the site of the sinus, describing spiral orbits near the outer wall of the bifurcation, and rejoined the mainstream. Downstream from the stagnation point (R), a strong counter-rotating double helicoidal flow developed. At the geometrical flow ratio ($Q_1/Q_o \sim 0.65$), recirculation flows were formed only in the internal carotid artery at $Re_o \sim 170$, grew in size with increasing Re_o, but were always confined within the carotid sinus. The recirculation zone increased in length from about 4 mm at $Re_o = 300$ to a maximum of about 9 mm at $Re_o > 800$. The fact that a standing recirculation zone was formed in the carotid sinus at $Re_o \sim 170$, which is well below the physiological values of 500–600,[19-20] makes it plausible that such a standing recirculation flow exists in the carotid sinus even in normal subjects under physiological flow conditions. In this case, disturbed flow was created as a result of the combined effect of flow separation at the leading edge of the carotid sinus indicated by a letter S, and development of strong secondary flow due to the sudden deflection of flow at the flow divider of the bifurcation. Since the flow patterns in the carotid sinus resemble that of the annular vortex described earlier, it is likely that interactions of blood cells with the vessel wall and mass transfer are much enhanced by the disturbed flow, leading to high incidences of thrombosis and atherosclerosis in this region.[21-22]

Obtuse Angle T-Junctions

With increasing branching angle over 90°, the portion of the flow deflected at the flow divider increased, resulting in the formation of strong secondary flows in each daughter tube. FIGURE 8 shows the detailed flow patterns observed in a 135° glass model T-junction when the flow entered the side tube. As shown in the figure, particles located close to the common median plane of the T-junction in the parent tube were deflected symmetrically on both sides of the common median plane as they approached the vessel wall (flow divider) at almost right angles. They then encountered each other

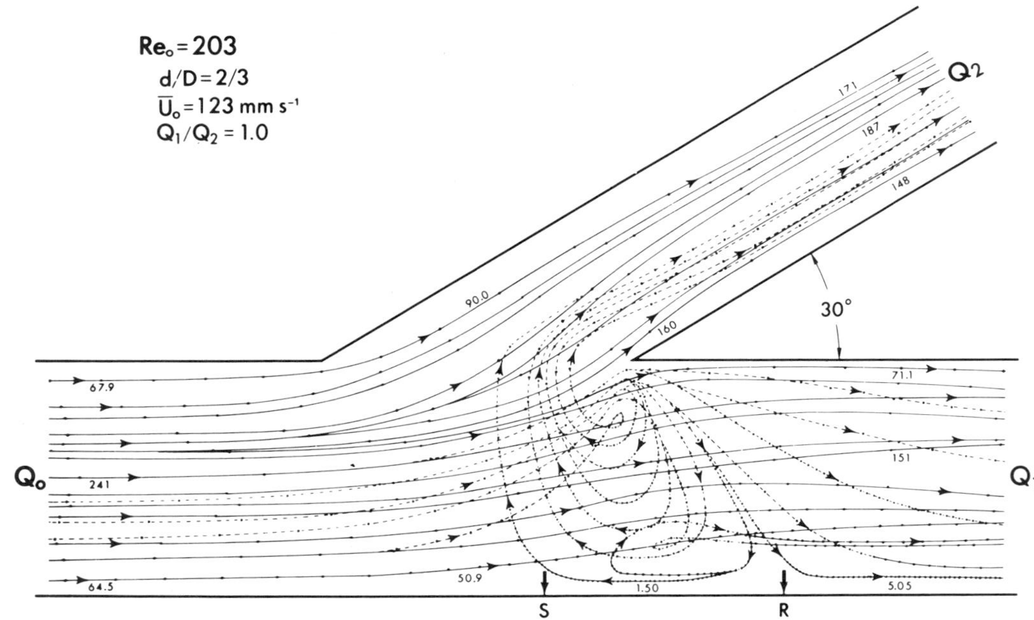

FIGURE 6. Flow patterns in a 30° nonuniform diameter T-junction showing the formation of paired, thin-layered spiral secondary flows on both sides of the common median plane of the T-junction. The arrows at S and R indicate the respective separation and stagnation points, and the numbers on the streamlines indicate the particle linear velocities in $mm \cdot s^{-1}$. (From Karino and Goldsmith.[17] Reprinted with permission from *Biorheology*.)

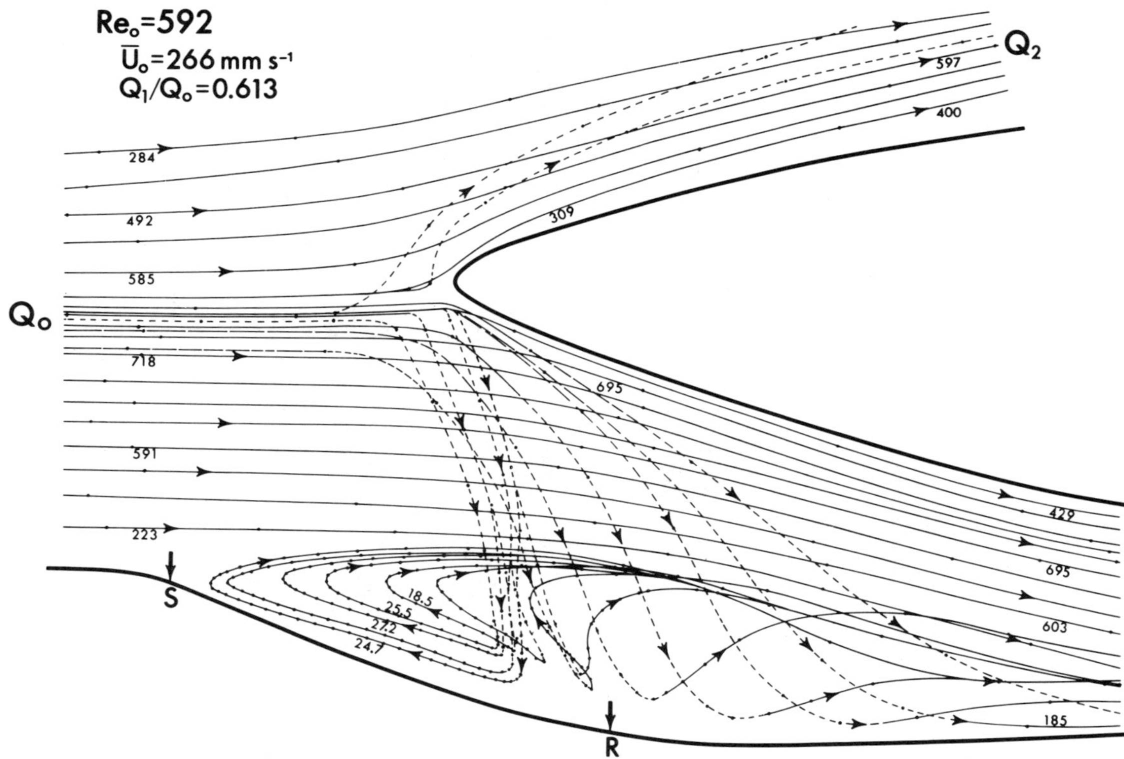

FIGURE 7. Detailed flow patterns in the human carotid artery bifurcation in steady flow, showing the formation of a recirculation zone (paired spiral secondary flows) and a counter-rotating double helicoidal flow, both located symmetrically on either side of the common median plane in the internal carotid artery. The *solid lines* are the paths of particles in or close to, and the *dashed lines* paths far away from, the common median plane (the projection of the particle paths on the common median plane). The arrows at *S* and *R* denote the respective locations of the separation and stagnation points. The numbers on the streamlines (particle paths) indicate the particle translational velocities in mm · s^{-1}. (From Motomiya and Karino.[18] Reprinted with permission from *Stroke*.[1])

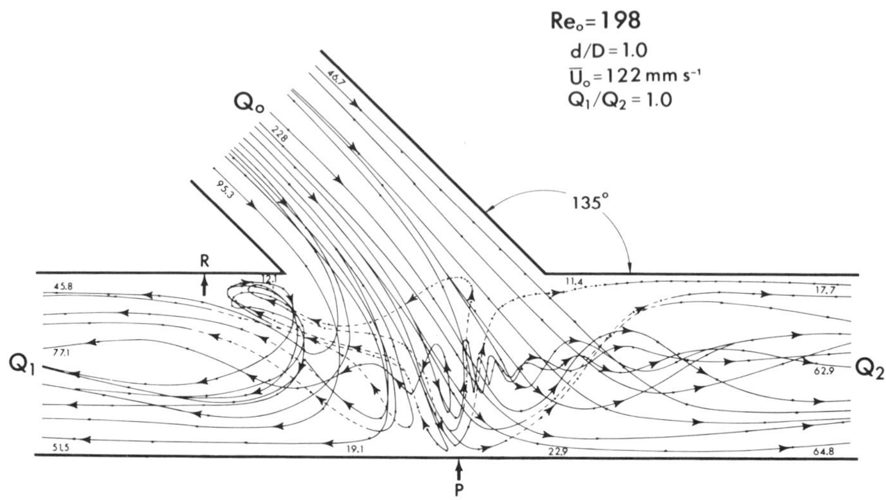

FIGURE 8. Flow patterns in a 135° T-junction with flow entering the side tube showing the formation of double helicoidal flows in each daughter tube. The arrows at *P* and *R* indicate the stagnation points. The numbers on the streamlines indicate the particle velocities in mm · s^{-1}. (From Karino and Goldsmith.[17] Reprinted with permission from *Biorheology*.[1])

on the common median plane on the other side of the flow divider after describing semicircles and rejoined the mainstream near the common median plane and repeated the same deflection. Thus a strong counter-rotating double helicoidal flow was created in one or both daughter tubes. Furthermore, due to the sudden change in flow direction, flow separation occurred at the edge of each bend, where part of the deflected flow entered and formed a recirculation zone as shown in the figure. The size and intensity of the double helicoidal flow increased with increasing Re_o and the portion of the flow in a particular branch. Such a flow pattern was found also in some regions of human cerebral arteries. FIGURE 9 illustrates the detailed flow patterns observed at the internal carotid-posterior communicating artery junction. As shown in the figure, fluid elements in the mainflow in the internal carotid artery having high velocity directly impinged onto the vessel wall around the flow divider and were deflected on both sides of the common median plane of the bifurcation almost at right angles to the vessel wall, entered one of the daugher vessels, and described spiral orbits of gradually decreasing diameter similar to those observed in glass model T-junctions (c.f. FIGURE 8). Such flow patterns, especially the strong impingement of fluid elements onto the vessel wall, may be responsible for the observed high frequency of aneurysm formation around the flow divider of this particular junction.[23]

Symmetric Bifurcations

These can be found at many sites in the circulation. The largest one is the common iliac artery bifurcation. Here we present the one encountered in human cerebral arteries as an example. FIGURE 10 illustrates the detailed flow patterns observed in one of the middle cerebral artery bifurcations having an almost perfectly symmetrical structure and spatial arrangement of the daughter vessels. As shown in the figure, a standing recirculation zone, very similar to that observed in the carotid artery bifurcation, was formed along the outer wall of one or both daughter vessels (depending on Re_0 and the flow ratios in the two daughter vessels).

It was also found that atherosclerotic thickening of the vessel wall was localized at the exact locations where recirculation zones were formed. Furthermore, as is evident from the figure, even when the flow in the parent vessel was distributed equally to the two daughter vessels, the region of disturbed flow (formed along the outer walls of the bifurcation) was much longer in the right side branch where the region of atherosclerotic wall thickening was also longer than that in the left side branch where the wall thickening was confined to only a narrow area, suggesting a strong correlation between the longitudinal length of the regions of disturbed flow and that of the atherosclerotic wall thickening.

Flow through Complex Branching Vessels

So far we have described the detailed flow patterns observed in vessels of simple geometry having a plane of symmetry (whether it is the tube axis or the common median plane). In such vessels we found that the flow patterns were also symmetric

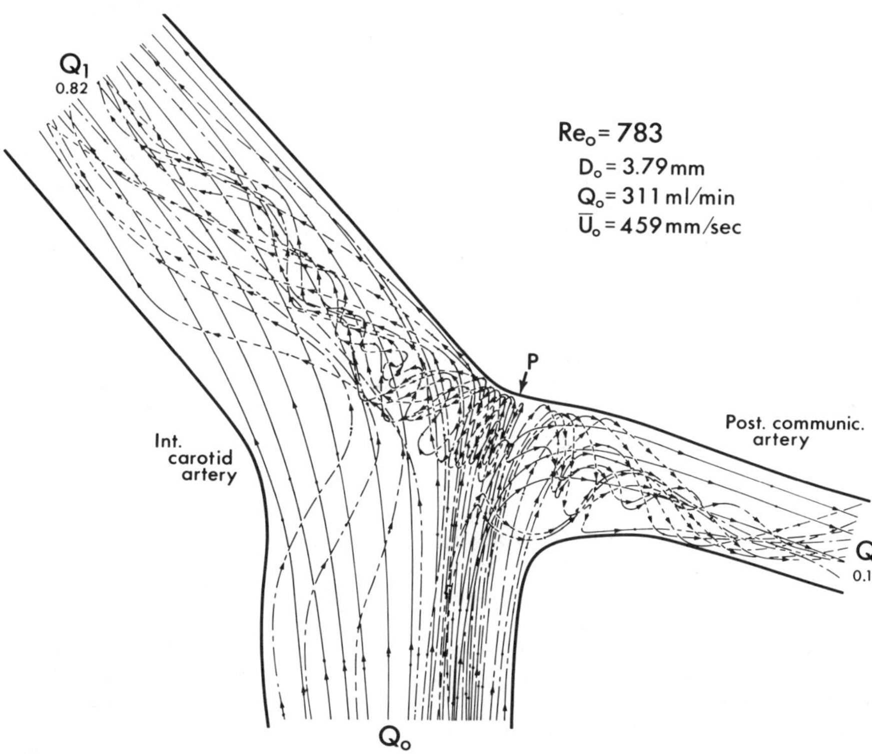

FIGURE 9. Detailed flow patterns observed at the human internal carotid-posterior communicating artery junction showing the formation of strong helicoidal flows in each daughter vessel. The arrow at *P* indicates the stagnation point.

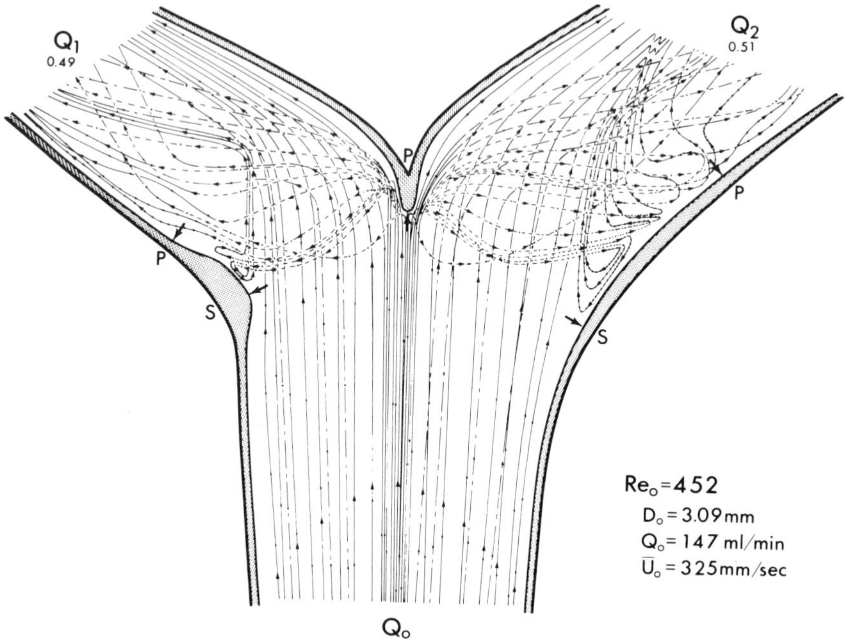

FIGURE 10. Detailed flow patterns at the human middle cerebral artery bifurcation showing the formation of secondary flows and recirculation zones along the outer walls of the bifurcation in steady flow. Note that the exact locations and the longitudinal lengths of the formed recirculation zones closely match those of the atherosclerotic wall thickening. The *solid lines* are the paths of particles in or close to the common median plane, and the *dashed lines* the paths far away from the common median plane. The arrows at *S* and *P* denote the respective locations of the separation and stagnation points.

about the plane of geometrical symmetry. However, there are many cases in the circulation where symmetry of flow is not assured. Here we present two examples of highly asymmetric flow observed in isolated transparent natural arteries.

Aortic Arch

FIGURE 11 illustrates detailed flow patterns observed in the aortic arch of a young dog in steady flow when the flow rate in each daughter vessel was adjusted to its geometrical flow ratio.[24] As shown in the figure, it was found that the flow in the aortic arch consists of three major components: quasi-parallel undisturbed flow located close to the common median plane of the ascending aorta and the two daughter branches, spiral secondary flows located near the ventral periphery of the aorta and the side branches, and the mainflow to the side branches. Flow separation does occur at the inner (lower) wall of the aortic arch. However, no recirculation zone was formed downstream of the separation point. Instead, the region of separated flow was filled with the peripheral spiral secondary flows. Thus, looking down the aorta, the flow in the aortic arch appeared as a single helicoidal flow revolving in a clockwise direction, rather than the two that had been anticipated. When the flow rates in the side branches were reduced from the control values, a recirculation zone was formed in each branch adjacent to the vessel wall opposite to the flow divider. Particles in the mainstream were deflected sideways at the flow divider and traveled laterally. Some entered the side branches, while others traveled backward along the vessel wall, and after describing multiple spiral orbits, rejoined the mainflow in the descending aorta or the side branches. Formation of the asymmetric flow is considered to be largely due to the facts that the axes of the side branches are located not exactly on the median plane of the ascending aorta and the two side branches, but off-center toward the dorsal wall of the aorta, and that the aortic arch itself is bent slightly dorsally distal to the branching point of the left subclavian artery.

Basilar Artery Bifurcation

At the basilar artery Y-bifurcation, the flow was disturbed and formation of complex secondary flows was demonstrated over wide ranges of Re_o and flow ratios. FIGURE 12 illustrates an example of the flow patterns observed in a basilar artery bifurcation having approximately equal diameter daughter vessels. As shown in the figure for the case of $Q_1 \approx Q_2$, particles in the mainstream were deflected sideways at the flow divider, traveled backward along the vessel wall, and entered one of the right or left superior cerebellar arteries. With increasing Re_o, the deflected particles started

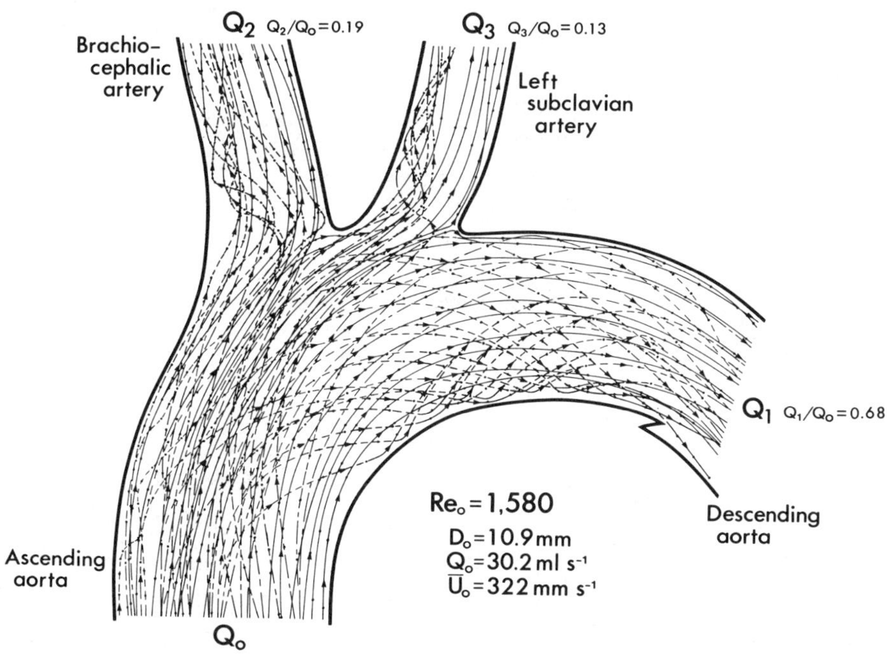

FIGURE 11. Detailed flow patterns in the dog aortic arch showing the existence of the parallel undisturbed mainflow, single clockwise spiral helicoidal flow in the aorta, and the secondary flows generated at the flow divider of the side branches. (From Sohara & Karino.[24] Reprinted with permission from Pergamon Press.)

to describe multiple spiral orbits, creating a region of highly disturbed flow over the entire lumen of the basilar artery between the right and left superior cerebellar arteries and the flow divider of the bifurcation. The degree of flow disturbance increased with increasing proportion of flow in the superior cerebellar arteries. Formation of such an asymmetric disturbed flow appears to be caused by the particular asymmetric arrangement of the side branches and mismatch of the flow rate entering each daughter vessel.

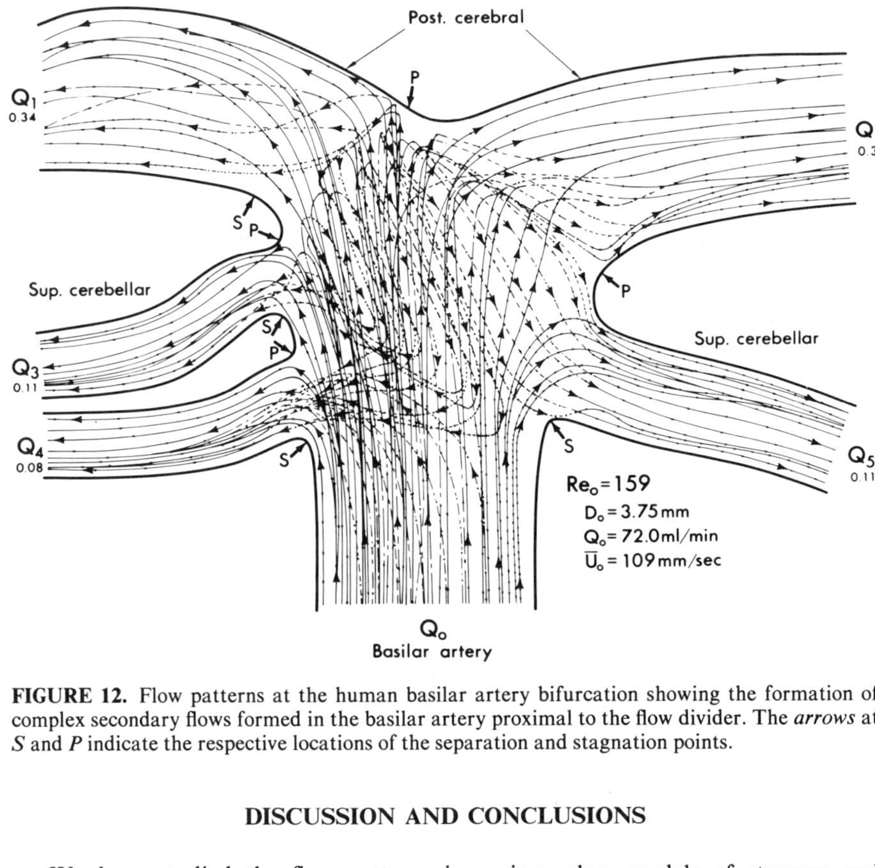

FIGURE 12. Flow patterns at the human basilar artery bifurcation showing the formation of complex secondary flows formed in the basilar artery proximal to the flow divider. The *arrows* at *S* and *P* indicate the respective locations of the separation and stagnation points.

DISCUSSION AND CONCLUSIONS

We have studied the flow patterns in various glass models of stenoses and branching vessels as well as in isolated transparent natural blood vessels, and described the three-dimensional structure of disturbed flows formed in each vessel. It was made clear at this point that disturbed flows are formed within the flowing blood by at least one or a combination of the following three mechanisms: (i) through a flow separation caused by the irregularity of the vessel wall, (ii) through a development of strong secondary flows (as a result of flow deflection) caused by sudden changes in the direction of flow as it occurs at bends, T-junctions, and bifurcations, and (iii) through mismatching of flow rate entering each daughter vessel at the branching sites of T-junctions and bifurcations that force the backflow of the excess fluid entering a particular branch due to the inertia of the fluid. Thus, in an axisymmetric stenosis, an annular ring vortex with closed orbits was formed downstream of the constriction as a result of a flow separation. A similar flow pattern was also observed in natural vessels in the pocket of venous valves. The exact flow patterns were, however, somewhat different from those of the annular ring vortex formed downstream of an axisymmetric stenosis. In the annular vortex, theory predicts closed streamlines[15] and there could be no flow of blood cells from the mainstream into the vortex unless there were frequent and vigorous particle interactions between the crowded cells in flowing blood. By contrast, in the valve-pocket recirculation zone, the streamlines were not closed and there was continuous inflow of fluid and cells from the mainstream, thereby assuring the exchange of material between the recirculation zone in the valve pocket and the mainstream. In this sense, venous valves are well designed to minimize stagnation of the circulating blood, though there still are some potential problems, as discussed elsewhere.[25]

In T-junctions and bifurcations having circular cross-sections, it was found that in both glass models and natural blood vessels, complex spiral secondary flows and recirculation zones were formed in the junction region by a combination of the three mechanisms discussed earlier. Formation of such disturbed flow was largely affected by the inflow Reynolds number, the flow ratios in the daughter vessels, the curvature of the walls at the flow divider and the bend opposite to it, and the branching angle. Except for the case of very complex branching vessels as seen in the aortic arch and the basilar artery junction, disturbed flows were always formed in a paired structure in both the main and side daughter vessels, but were never in the form of a closed vortex as predicted for two-dimensional branching vessels.

The results demonstrated convincingly that the flow separation and formation of paired spiral secondary flows and standing recirculation zones, observed in various models of stenoses[10-12] and branching vessels,[16-17] do occur also in natural blood vessels at Reynolds numbers much lower than those prevailing *in vivo,* making it plausible that such disturbed flows do exist also *in vivo* in many parts of the human circulation under normal physiological conditions. It should be noted, however, that in many natural vessels the formation of spiral secondary flows and recirculation zones was observed at much higher Reynolds number than in corresponding glass model stenoses and branching vessels, suggesting that valves and branching vessels *in vivo* are designed much better than those of artificial organs and prosthetic devices. In this sense, it is necessary to study further the detailed geometric structure of natural blood vessels.

Our work was originally aimed at elucidating the possible connection between flow and localization of the vascular diseases, thrombosis, atherosclerosis, and aneurysms in the human circulation. The knowledge acquired from these investigations may help not only to understand the fluid dynamics of the human circulation in connection with the localization of the vascular diseases, but also to interpret the results of some angiological tests. It will also provide certain guidelines for the optimal design of flow channels in artificial organs and prosthetic devices which suffer from the common problem of thrombus formation, as well as for surgical procedures in coronary bypass operations and other vascular reconstructions which, due to the altered flow patterns in some cases, expose the patient to a risk of postoperative thrombosis.

If we attempt to draw some guidelines for the optimal design of flow channels on the basis of our own findings, they could be summarized as follows:

1. Never create sudden and axisymmetric changes of vessel diameter.
2. In bifurcations and T-junctions, the curvature of the wall should be as sharp as possible at the flow divider and as gentle as possible at the bend opposite to it.

3. In any branching vessel, the branching angle should be kept as small as possible.
4. In any simple and complex T-junction, it is desirable that the diameter of the side tubes be smaller than half of the parent tube, and the flow rate in the side branches should not exceed that based on their geometrical flow ratios.
5. In bifurcations, the flow rate in each daughter vessel should be equal to its geometrical flow ratio.

ACKNOWLEDGMENTS

We thank C. Artigas, S. Spain and E. de Heuvel for their excellent technical assistance, and D. Besso and P. Lilley for typing the manuscript.

REFERENCES

1. Karino, T. & M. Motomiya. 1985. Flow visualization in isolated transparent natural blood vessels. Biorheology **20:** 119–127.
2. Reynolds, O. 1883. An experimental investigation of the circumstances which determine whether the motion of water shall be direct or sinus and of the law of resistance in parallel channels. Trans. R. Soc. Lond. **A174:** 935–982.
3. Goldsmith, H. L. & T. Karino. 1978. Mechanically induced thromboemboli. *In* Quantitative Cardiovascular Studies: Clinical and Research Applications of Engineering Principles. N.H.C. Hwang, D. R. Gross & D. J. Patel, Eds.: 289–351. University Park Press. Baltimore.
4. Sinclair, A. S. & M. R. Roach. 1975. Effect of vibration on isolated dog bronchi. J. Appl. Physiol. **38:** 780–785.
5. Bruns, D. L. 1959. A general theory of the causes of murmurs in the cardiovascular system. Am. J. Med. **27:** 360–374.
6. Folts, J. D., E. B. Crowell & G. G. Rowe. 1976. Platelet aggregation in partially obstructed vessels and its elimination with aspirin. Circulation **54:** 365–370.
7. Foster, E. D. & A. R. C. Dobell. 1971. Evaluation of rigid prosthetic rings as in vivo intravascular thrombogenic models. J. Surg. Res. **11:** 550–558.
8. Stein, P. D. & H. N. Sabbah. 1974. Measured turbulence and its effect on thrombus formation. Circ. Res. **35:** 608–614.
9. Macagno, E. O. & T. K. Hung. 1967. Computational and experimental study of a captive annular eddy. J. Fluid Mech. **28:** 43–64.
10. Karino, T. & H. L. Goldsmith. 1977. Flow behaviour of blood cells and rigid spheres in an annular vortex. Phil. Trans. R. Soc. **B279:** 413–445.
11. Karino, T. & H. L. Goldsmith. 1979. Aggregation of human platelets in an annular vortex distal to a tubular expansion. Microvasc. Res. **17:** 217–237.
12. Karino, T. & H. L. Goldsmith. 1979. Adhesion of human platelets to collagen on the wall distal to a tubular expansion. Microvasc. Res. **17:** 238–262.
13. Sevitt, S. 1978. Pathology and pathogenesis of deep vein thrombi. *In* Venous Problem. J. J. Bergan & J. S. T. Yao, Eds.: 257–279. Year Book Medical Publishers. Chicago.
14. Hamer, J. D., P. C. Malone & I. A. Silver. 1981. The pO_2 in venous valve pockets: Its possible bearing on thrombogenesis. Br. J. Surg. **68:** 166–170.
15. Hung, T. K. & S. A. Naff. 1969. A mathematical model of systolic blood flow through a bifurcation. Proceedings of Eighth International Conference on Medicine and Biological Engineering.
16. Karino, T., H. M. Kwong & H. L. Goldsmith. 1979. Particle flow behavior in models of branching vessels. I. Vortices in 90° T-junctions. Biorheology **16:** 231–248.
17. Karino, T. & H. L. Goldsmith. 1983. Particle flow behavior in models of branching

vessels. II. Effects of branching angle and diameter ratio on flow patterns. Biorheology **22:** 87–102.

18. MOTOMIYA, M. & T. KARINO. 1984. Flow patterns in the human carotid artery bifurcation. Stroke **15:** 50–56.
19. KRISTIANSEN, K. & J. KROG. 1962. Electromagnetic studies on the blood flow through the carotid system in man. Neurology **12:** 20–22.
20. UEMATSU, S., A. YANG, T. J. PREZIOSI, R. KOUBA & T. J. K. TOUNG. 1983. Measurement of carotid blood flow in man and its clinical application. Stroke **14:** 256–266.
21. SAMUEL, K. C. 1956. Atherosclerosis and occlusion of the internal carotid artery. J. Path. Bact. **LXXI:** 391–401.
22. IMPARATO, A. M., T. S. RILES & F. GORSTEIN. 1979. The carotid bifurcation plaque: Pathologic findings associated with cerebral ischemia. Stroke **10:** 238–244.
23. RHOTON, A. L., JR. 1980. Anatomy of saccular aneurysms. Surg. Neurol. **14:** 59–66.
24. SOHARA, Y. & T. KARINO. 1985. Secondary flow in the dog aortic arch. *In* Fluid Control and Measurement. M. Harada, Ed.: 143–147. Pergamon. Oxford.
25. KARINO, T. & M. MOTOMIYA. 1984. Flow through a venous valve and its implication in thrombogenesis. Thromb. Res. **36:** 245–257.

Transport of Platelets in Flowing Blood[a]

EUGENE C. ECKSTEIN, DAVID L. BILSKER,
CHRISTOPHER M. WATERS, J. SHANE KIPPENHAN,
AND ARNO W. TILLES

Department of Biomedical Engineering
University of Miami
Coral Gables, Florida 33124

INTRODUCTION

Flow causes deformations and interactions of blood cells that, among other things, augment platelet transport greatly beyond that attributable to Brownian motion.[1–7] Effective dispersion coefficients are typically one or two orders of magnitude greater than the values for Brownian diffusion. Such transport can be envisioned as a dispersive process that results from a random walk of designated platelets or platelet analogues. The changes of direction of the "walking" particle are the result of interactions ("collisions") with the red cells and other platelets. Modeling platelet motions in blood flow with such random walks envisages a directionally unbiased outcome of the interactions of platelets with the suspended cells. When considering such models of platelet transport, one should remember that available measurements of augmented platelet diffusion coefficients were made in flows with low or moderate shear rates and invoked only traditional equations of diffusive transport. Microrheological events that may produce bias in the cellular collisions are considered below, along with a more comprehensive random walk model that includes the effects of biased collisions.

The comprehensive random walk model adds an important feature: a convective style of transport. The lateral platelet movement that results from many collisions, some or all of which are biased, includes an effective directed motion, a velocity, in addition to a diffusive motion. In a complete model other blood components, i.e., plasma and red cells, will also have effective lateral motions caused by these collisions. All effective velocities (those for red cells, platelets, and plasma) are interrelated by an equation for mass (or volume) conservation. This paper examines blood flows far from the entrance of a tube where the average arrangement of red cells and plasma is well set. For this reason, the effective velocities of red cells and plasma are ignored. As platelets move through the entry region, they assume an average distribution across the flow as a result of their interactions with other cells. Any subsequent rearrangement of platelets is unlikely to be associated with a significant volume flow rate. Extension from this situation to an undeveloped entrance region may be straightforward. This judgment is based upon the facts that the platelets have a small effective velocity and that they form a small volume fraction of the blood; accordingly, the changes in red cell and plasma distributions required by mass conservation will be insignificant.

The second part of the paper reviews experimental evidence related to descriptions of platelet transport that include a flow-induced effective lateral velocity. It describes experimental methods used to study the distribution of platelet analogues during blood

[a]This work was supported by NIH grant no. HL–33100.

flow. Each distribution of nonreactive platelet analogues reflects, in a simple situation, the outcomes of many individual random walks associated with flow-augmented platelet transport. Portions of the observed distributions are consistent with the predictions of a model that balances effective lateral convection and augmented diffusion. The model provides a means to estimate the effective wall-directed platelet velocity.

PRIOR WORK AND THEORETICAL MODELS

Transport phenomena are divided into convective and diffusive events according to differences in temporal behavior, as illustrated by the characteristic mathematical dependence upon t and $t^{1/2}$, respectively. The wealth of mathematical solutions for convective and diffusive transport problems is a good reason to maintain this conventional dichotomy in the description of platelet transport. Since blood is a concentrated cellular suspension, convective and diffusive models should be applied only after close examination of the behavior of the flowing suspension. The text below examines platelet transport in situations that do not have significant reactivity of the blood components, *i.e.,* coagulation, platelet activation, and deposition are prevented by drugs or experimental design or are not considered in the theory. This restriction simplifies the consideration of random walks and diffusive motions, but it does not prohibit extension of the concepts to reactive situations, since methods exist to extend random walk models to include reaction.[8]

The convective motion of blood is usually taken to be the same as that of a liquid of appropriate viscosity.[1] Methods exist to handle situations at low shear rates where the modeling of blood viscosity by a single simple coefficient is inappropriate. Other methods treat blood flow in small tubes where the distribution of red cells across the stream is sufficiently nonuniform to affect the accuracy of the overall model. Even with such complications, the convective concept can be used to describe relatively commonplace situations. One example is steady flow through a conduit of significant size, where streamlines can be identified and where the nominal displacement can be obtained from the integral of the velocity along the path provided by the streamline.

Transport of suspended material perpendicular to the streamlines of a steady flow is due to flow-induced lateral forces and to the diffusive motion of the material. (Diffusive transport can also occur along the direction of the streamlines, but it is usually unimportant in blood flow since it is much less than the convective motion.) The motions of particles in tube flows have been quantitatively described and reviewed.[2] The lateral motions of individual particles in dilute suspensions depend upon the particle Reynolds number, the ratio of particle and tube diameters, and the deformability of the particle. Rigid particles in dilute suspensions show little or no net motion across streamlines, while deformable particles in dilute suspensions are associated with relatively large directed lateral motions.[3] As suspensions become more concentrated, the lateral motions no longer result in direct relocation of particles to special positions because the large number of particles prevents long directed migrations. One viewpoint, particularly appropriate for moderate and high concentrations, is that the flow-induced collisions of suspended particles in the central region of the flow produce an outward motion (force) that counteracts the inwardly directed migration caused by wall-originated fluid forces.[1] Description of such situations should include the particle concentration as a dimensionless parameter; among other things, it will aid in depicting events that restrict lateral motions in nondilute suspensions.

The flow-induced collisions that restrict motions of individual particles near the wall also give rise to lateral motions in the bulk of the fluid. The path followed by an individual particle has an erratic form that suggests modeling with a random walk.[3] Like self-diffusion of dyed fluid elements in a Newtonian fluid, these motions result in lateral dispersion of material to other streamlines. Such lateral motion is small for laminar flows of Newtonian liquids, but is much larger for turbulent flows. These motions, which can be observed without a physical concentration gradient when a label is artificially imposed on selected material, are the basis for diffusion (dispersion) of material down concentration gradients. Goldsmith and coworkers have shown that both normal red cells and latex-bead platelet analogues have significant lateral diffusive motion in concentrated ghost cell suspensions.[3,5,6] Employing the relationships that relate simple random walks and diffusion, they calculated effective lateral diffusion coefficients from direct observations of the path of tracer particles. To enable the tracking of individual particles, these experiments were done at shear rates of 30 s^{-1} or less.

Turitto *et al.* used the method developed by G. I. Taylor to obtain values of the diffusion coefficient of platelets in blood flow.[7] Their experiments used wall shear rates ranging from 40 to 440 s^{-1}. The upper value of shear rate is below that in much of the circulation and in many prosthetic devices. While dispersion coefficients were directly obtained from their data at low wall shear rates, coefficients for wall shear rates over 200 s^{-1} were determined after allowing for a nonuniform radial distribution of platelets. The Taylor method uses conventional principles of convective-diffusive transport and hence implicitly invokes the same random walk concepts that Goldsmith applied to the cellular interactions in flowing blood. It does not account for any bias in the collisions that augment the lateral motion.

Values of platelet dispersion coefficients obtained by Turitto *et al.* are in reasonable agreement with those obtained by Goldsmith. These values have been used to estimate the amount of thrombus deposited onto reactive surfaces in flowing blood (for a discussion, see ref. 1). The inverse process, *i.e.*, the use of experimental studies of platelet deposition to determine dispersion coefficients for flowing blood, is inappropriate as the reactions and circumstances that produce thrombotic deposits are only crudely modeled. Such studies may not account for the local concentrations or the fluxes that deliver material to surfaces. (Support for this viewpoint is provided by several profiles of platelet analogues that are shown below.) An experimentally proven, general picture of platelet transport for high shear rates and significant hematocrits has yet to be assembled.

Random Walks and Dispersion

A single mathematical equation governs both simple random walks and the processes of diffusion or dispersion.[8,9] For example, the distribution of a number of objects undergoing one-dimensional random walks that start at the origin and the distribution of mass diffusing from an infinitely thin planar source at the origin have the same methematical form. Both are described by a Gaussian curve that is centered at the origin whose width at the half-height varies with the square root of time. Each situation is described by what is commonly referred to as the diffusion equation. For random walks described by the diffusion equation, it is assumed that each step is independent of the previous one and that there is no preferred direction for the steps. This model is reasonable for collisions among equal particles. Work reviewed above shows that this model can adequately describe platelet transport in flowing blood despite differences of size, shape, and flexibility for red cells and platelets. It should be noted that it did not work perfectly at moderate wall shear rates,[7] and thus should be considered proven only for describing platelet motion due to cellular interactions in flows of low shear rate or in regions of flow with low shear rates.

If the random walk model is used to describe the flow-induced interactions among platelets (or latex beads) and red cells at higher shear rates (shear stresses), then it is useful to consider walks where the probability of outcome is not equal in all directions. Random walks with external forces, those occurring in anisotropic media, or those with persistence of motion from the last collision result in a diffusion equation that includes terms with a convective form.[10] To describe the effect of these outside factors, the probabilities describing the turns of the random walk (due to collisions of particles in the flow) are altered so that the outcomes for motion are not the same in all directions. The major effect of using random walks biased to account for nonuniform interactions among the platelets and red cells is that the characteristic lateral platelet motion is no longer purely diffusive. The resulting motion also has a convective nature, and as implied by the data shown below, this motion moves platelets toward the wall even in nonreactive blood flow through impermeable tubes. The occurrence of a convective velocity as a result of a collision process is not surprising since there is a similar outcome in the kinetic theory of gases.

Prior microrheological studies suggest that collisions between platelets and red cells are appropriately modeled with biased probabilities, especially when the wall shear rate is moderate or high or when the region of interest is within a few cell diameters of the wall. Red cells and platelets differ in rigidity. Shear-dependent transitions of red cell orientation in dilute suspensions may be especially relevant to modeling the collisions of platelets and red cells. At low shear rates, the red cells tumble and assume orbits of the same nature as rigid particles.[4,11] In dilute suspensions, the red cell is known to deform and become aligned with the flow at higher shear rates.[4] In particular, a large fraction of the red cells are known to assume orbits with $C = 0$ at moderate shear rates[4,11] (C is discussed in ref. 11). In this orbit the cell becomes aligned with the flow and will exhibit cellular elongation with application of additional shear stress. Similar orientation and elongation of a fraction of the red cells appears to occur in concentrated blood suspensions.[12] Since the region of interest for the more comprehensive model is near the wall, it should also be remembered that isolated deformable bodies, such as red cells, exhibit larger and different shear-induced lateral motions than rigid bodies.[1,2] In contrast to these shear-induced changes of red cell shape and behavior, the platelet exhibits the rotational characteristics of a rigid disk for all shear rates of interest.[13] Thus, it is reasonable to expect that there are unequal probabilities that describe the inward or outward motion for the individual steps of a random walk of a rigid body (the platelet) that sustains "collisions" with bodies of different rheological character. In essence, there is a loss of the random outcome for interactions of platelets with red cells at moderate or higher shear rates because a significant fraction of the red cells are aligned with the flow. At lower shear rates the red cells have a more random orientation, and as indicated by the successful application of dispersion coefficients measured for low shear rates,[1] the outcome of interactions is apparently equal for inward and outward steps. The use of unequal probabilities may be particularly applicable when the collisions take place in the near-wall flow field, which exerts different forces on the particles undergoing collisions. During any collision process, the larger and more flexible red cells would have a greater tendency to be displaced toward the center, while the smaller, more rigid platelets would experience a lesser force and thus tend to be displaced toward the wall.

The nonuniform distribution of red cells in the near-wall region may also be a source of bias. To visualize this possibility, it is useful to consider the net outcome of some small number of interactions among a platelet and the nearby red cells. The near-wall region includes a peripheral plasma layer, which has no red cells, and a much larger region that is relatively depleted of red cells. The average time between collisions would be greater for locations nearer to the wall because of the lack of particles. The time required for a "unit collision" would be longer near the wall than at locations near the center. Such events, caused by environmental anisotropy, would bias the probabilistic description of each platelet's random walk.

The above random walks concepts can be applied to predict the distribution of platelets or platelet-sized latex beads during steady blood flow through a tube. In regions of the flow where the microrheological events produce "collisions" between platelets and red cells that are unbiased, the usual picture of dispersion in a limited space will be observed: the local distribution of platelets will be uniform. Consider, however, a flow with a radial zone where the probabilities describing individual steps are biased for some reason, *e.g.*, larger, longer or more frequent displacements in some direction. This zone is likely to be near the wall of the tube. The more comprehensive random walk model predicts a convective type of platelet motion that attempts to build an excess of material. The excess will be limited by conventional dispersion, which remains a major part of the random walk model and always acts to reduce concentration gradients. Consideration of the biasing modes discussed above suggests that in flows of moderate to high shear rate, the collision events are more likely to move the platelets toward the wall than away from it. This directed motion is the convective velocity that would build an excess near the impermeable wall. The excess should be a short distance from the wall because wall-repulsive forces will prevent the convective motion of platelets directly to the wall.

EXPERIMENTAL EVIDENCE

The experimental results described below act as illustrations that biased random walks are useful models of platelet transport for blood flows in small tubes. For experimental purposes, whole blood was modeled by suspensions of washed red blood cells and fluorescent latex beads (2½ microns in diameter); the suspending fluid was an iso-osmotic solution of dextrose with approximately ½ wt% albumin to maintain cell shape. The use of platelet analogues ensured that no significant wall reaction or adhesion occurred. Concentration distributions were obtained by observations of bead positions through the use of fluorescence microscopy.

Our first studies used stroboscopic epifluorescence photomicroscopy to determine local populations of platelet analogues in a glass channel. Photographs were taken at different distances from the channel wall by using the fine focus adjustment to select planes of focus (aligned parallel to the wall) within the channel. The numbers of focused beads in several pictures of one location were averaged, and the averages from several locations were assembled to form histograms representing the concentration profiles. Experimental trials for each set of rheological parameters were repeated three times. The height of each cell of the raw histogram was normalized with respect to the maximum of the average counts for that trial. This normalization of raw data avoided differences due to small variations of the bead concentration in the reservoir blood and facilitated comparisons of different histograms. Each histogram presented here will thus represent wall distances vs. normalized bead concentrations. More details of the procedure appear elsewhere.[14]

These studies demonstrated several important facts, the first of which was that the distributions of the platelet-sized latex beads were often nonuniform. The excess near the wall was consistent with the above arguments for an effective lateral velocity that is the result of a biased random walk. The near-wall excess of beads only occurred for significant levels of hematocrit. While a slight effect was seen for 7%, a significant effect appeared for 15%. This dependence on hematocrit was consistent with the random walk view of platelet transport in flowing blood, where the "collisions" of platelets with red cells were the major source of the enhanced dispersion. The level of near-wall excess was quite large for the suspension with 30% red cells (see FIGURE 1).

A second important fact demonstrated by these experiments was that large near-wall excesses occurred only for an elevated wall shear rate. Histograms for 210 and 430 s^{-1} with 15% hematocrit in the 50 micron channel, shown in FIGURE 2, illustrate this point. Examination of histograms for other wall shear rates indicated

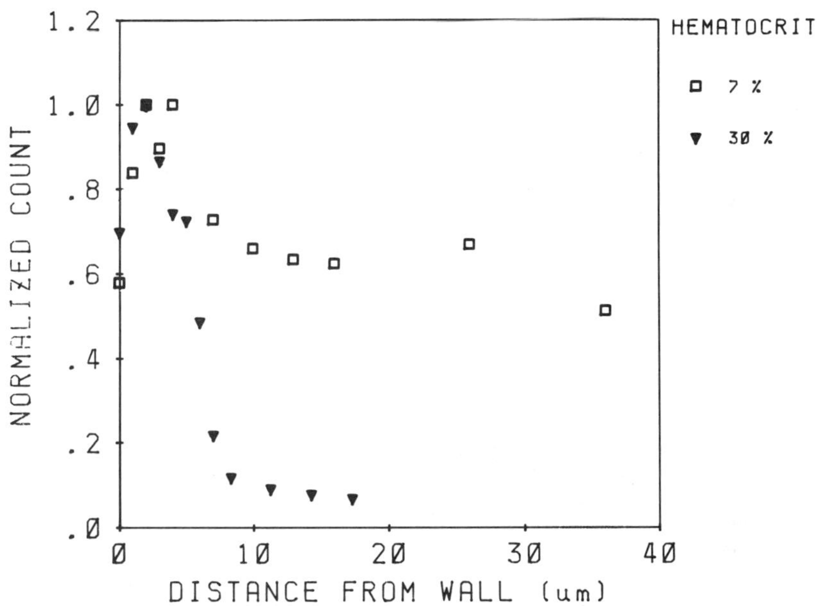

FIGURE 1. Graph of normalized bead count versus distance for suspensions with 7% and 30% hematocrit. The wall shear rate was 1630 s^{-1} and bead diameter was 2.38 μm. Experiments were done in channels 50 μm high and 1 mm wide; observations of the profiles were made 5 cm from the channel entrance.

that the shear rate dependence was essentially that of a step function. Values of wall shear rate of 430 s^{-1} and above were associated with larger near-wall excesses.

The experiments also demonstrated that flow-induced deformation of the red cells influences the distributions of platelet-sized particles. Concentration profiles for 15% suspensions of hardened red cells flowing through 50-micron channels had a small near-wall excess for both low and high wall shear rates.[15] In particular, they did not have the large excess that was seen with suspension flow of normal cells at wall shear rates of 430 s^{-1} or above. Since both suspended species were rigid, neither of them could be significantly deformed, and thus the smaller near-wall excess was probably due only to geometric aspects of the suspension flow that caused biased collisions in the near-wall region.

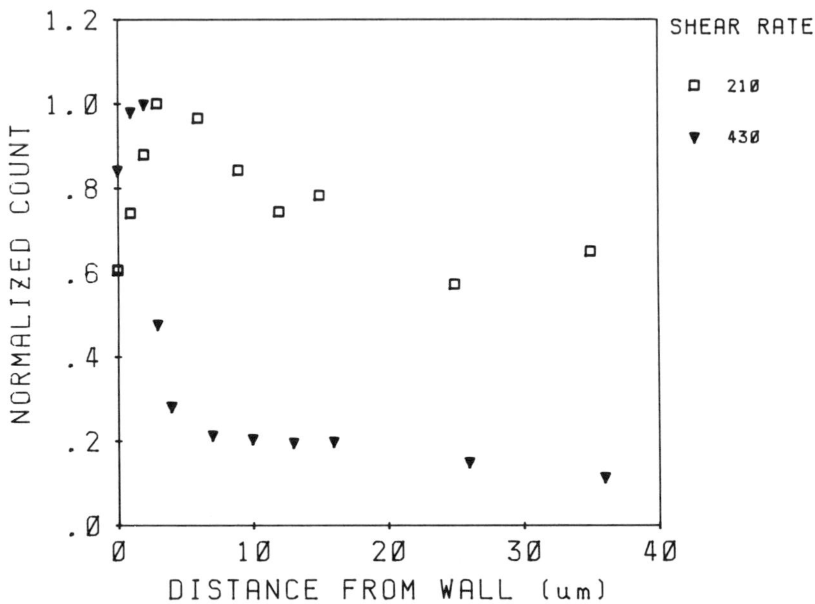

FIGURE 2. Graph of normalized bead count versus distance for wall shear rates of 210 and 430 s^{-1}. The hematocrit of the suspensions was 15% in both cases; bead and channel parameters were the same as in FIGURE 1.

The shear rate dependence found with normal cells could be altered by changing the viscosity of the suspending fluid. Experiments with flows of 15% hematocrit suspensions through 50-micron channels showed that when the viscosity of the suspending fluid was increased by inclusion of dextran 40 to 3.1 times that of the usual suspending fluid, a large near-wall excess occurred for a wall shear rate of 210 s^{-1}. Dextran 40 was chosen because it causes by itself no significant changes in the rheological behavior of red cells; it simply alters the viscosity of the suspending fluid.[16] In these experiments, the elevated viscosity resulted in more stress on the red cell membrane for a given wall shear rate. The increase in shear stress under these conditions was large enough to change the percentage of oriented and elongated cells,[4,12] and presumably cause biased collisions that result in a nonuniform bead distribution.

A recently developed experimental method allows work at higher hematocrits and in larger channels.[17] Briefly, this method involves stopping the flow of a suspension through a tube by rapidly freezing it with liquid nitrogen. Early work has used thin-walled polyethylene tubes with an inner diameter of 200 μm and a flow rate that produced a wall shear rate of approximately 500 s^{-1}. Segments of the tube are collected and cross-sectioned without allowing the blood to thaw. Images of the sections are collected on videotape and replayed in order to digitize the positions of the fluorescent latex beads. Distances from the wall are then calculated by computer. These distances are assembled into histograms representing the concentration profiles of beads. Data from these experiments also show near-wall excesses, as can be seen for a 30% suspension in FIGURE 3. These observations indicate that the height of the near-wall excess is smaller in the larger tube, but that the elevated concentration extends further from the wall. The 200-micron size is sometimes cited as the smallest size for which effects due to the finite size of the red cells in the vessel (Fahraeus-style events) are unimportant.[7] If this is applicable here, then the extent of the nonuniform concentration is an indication of events in much larger tubes.

A logarithmic plot of the percentage of observations versus the radial location is shown in FIGURE 4. This plot shows a relatively linear distribution of points in the histogram in the region between 5 and 35 microns from the wall. Recalling the model and assumptions discussed previously, *i.e.*, that a uniform radial convection of particles will be balanced by diffusion along a concentration gradient, one can write the equation

$$vC = -D\frac{dC}{dx},$$

in which v is an average convective velocity, C is the local concentration, D represents an effective diffusion coefficient, and x is a distance coordinate. Solution of this equation provides a concentration profile of the form $C_0 \exp(-vx/D)$, where C_0 is an integration constant. This relationship, the slope of the log plot, and values of D from experiments at relatively low wall shear rates[1,3,5,7] provide a way to estimate the convective velocity v. Using a value for D of 10^{-7} cm^2/s, v is 0.4 μm/s. This velocity represents the average or effective lateral motion of platelets in the near-wall region where the estimate was made. The experimental value of this velocity is not surprising

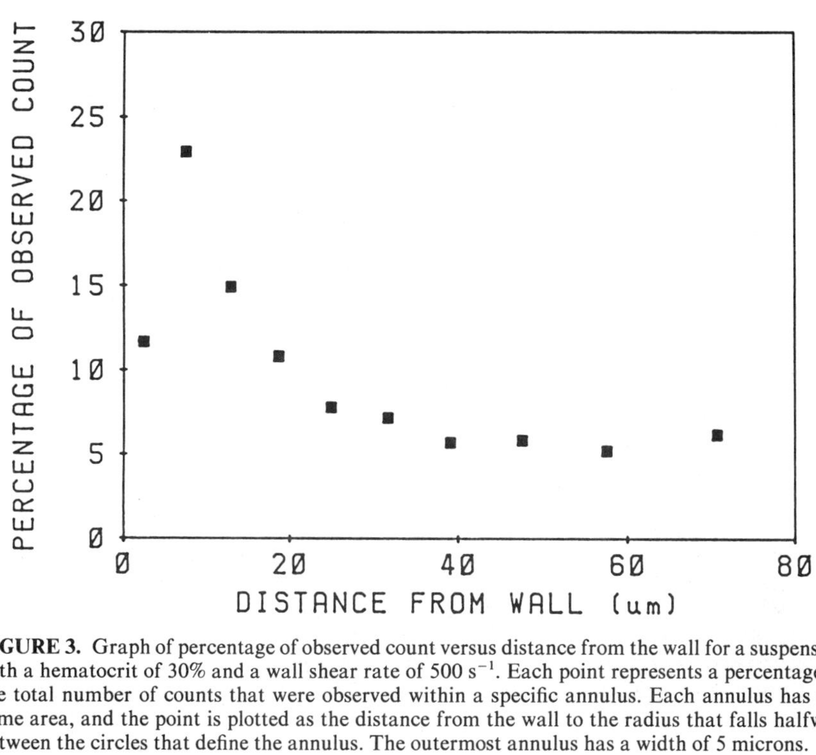

FIGURE 3. Graph of percentage of observed count versus distance from the wall for a suspension with a hematocrit of 30% and a wall shear rate of 500 s^{-1}. Each point represents a percentage of the total number of counts that were observed within a specific annulus. Each annulus has the same area, and the point is plotted as the distance from the wall to the radius that falls halfway between the circles that define the annulus. The outermost annulus has a width of 5 microns.

if one considers the scale of lateral motion shown by individual particles. (See, *e.g.*, Figure 2b of Goldsmith and Karino.[5])

The equation that balances dispersion and convective motion indicates that the effective convective velocity must be zero in some regions. Two regions of particular interest are the central region of the flow and the peak of the distribution, located near the wall. For the slope of the distribution profile to be zero, the velocity must be zero (unless the concentration itself goes to zero). There will be no lateral convective motion on the centerline, because symmetry implies the lack of a preferred direction. This condition may exist for some distance from the center because that region is one of low shear stress, and hence lesser percentages of the red cells there will be oriented or elongated. Accordingly, the amount of bias in the collisions will probably also be lower

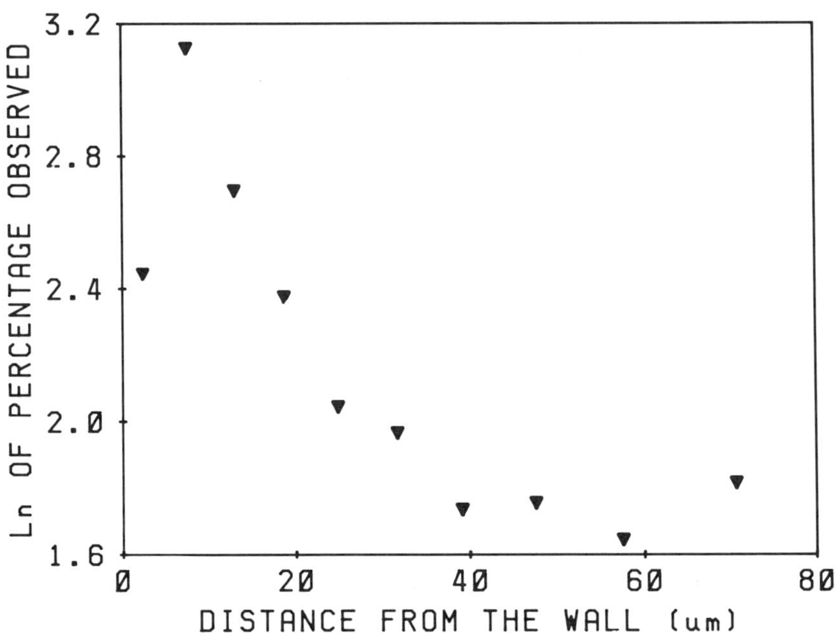

FIGURE 4. Graph of the natural logarithm of the percentage of observed count versus distance from the wall for a suspension with a hematocrit of 30%. Percentages are defined as described in the legend to FIGURE 3.

here. It seems likely that the effective convective motion in the lateral direction changes smoothly between regions where it is zero and those where it is finite.

The occurrence of a zero value of net lateral convective motion near the wall is reasonable, since there is a wall-induced force acting on each particle. The force, which in dilute suspension would cause migration of individual particles away from the wall, acts against the biased collision events that would move a platelet toward the wall. The decreased concentrations near the walls are illustrations of this balance. Altering this force balance, as occurs in ultrafiltering devices, could greatly change the shape of the bead distribution and perhaps control the rate of ultrafiltration. When the ultrafiltration velocity exceeded the equivalent velocity caused by the wall repulsion, the effective lateral convective motion in the zone farther from the wall could deliver platelets to the wall. This delivery of platelets to the wall could occur without red cells because they are larger and more flexible, and thus are more strongly repelled by the wall. This scenario is consistent with the work by Blackshear *et al.*, who demonstrated that the presence of red cells leads to enhanced levels of bead deposition into ultrafiltering dialysis membranes.[18]

Future work will include collection of other experimental data illustrating the near-wall excess and a more detailed exploration of the random walk model that has been discussed here.

SUMMARY

Distribution and transport of platelets in flowing blood were studied experimentally using suspensions of washed red cells and fluorescent latex beads as platelet analogues. Distributions of the platelet analogues were obtained from stroboscopic epifluorescence photomicrographs of flow in 50-μm channels and from images of the cut cross sections of cryogenically frozen thin-walled 200-μm tubes. Concentration profiles of platelet analogues had a substantial near-wall excess for situations with a substantial hematocrit (>10%) and a substantial wall shear rate (>400 s^{-1}). The viscosity of the suspending fluid was found to affect the size of the near-wall excess and its shear-dependent onset. Additionally, the shear-rate dependence of the near-wall excess did not occur with suspensions of hardened red cells. The excess extended a substantial distance from the wall in the 200-μm tubes and a portion of the profile could be fitted to an exponential curve. The random walk model that is used to describe enhanced platelet diffusion is envisioned as a walk (lateral platelet motion) caused by shear-induced collisions with red cells. A more comprehensive random walk model that includes biased collisions produces an effective lateral motion of convective nature in addition to a diffusional motion; it is used to explain the observed nonuniform distributions of platelet analogues.

REFERENCES

1. GOLDSMITH, H. L. & V. T. TURITTO. 1986. Rheological aspects of thrombosis and haemostasis: Basic principles and applications. Thromb. Haemostas. **55:** 415–435.
2. GOLDSMITH, H. L. & S. G. MASON. 1967. The microrheology of dispersions. *In* Rheology: Theory and Application, Vol. 4. F. R. Eirich, Ed: 85–250. Academic. New York.
3. GOLDSMITH, H. L. 1971. Red cell motions and wall interactions in tube flow. Fed. Proc. **30:** 1578–1588.
4. GOLDSMITH, H. L. & J. MARLOW. 1972. Flow behavior of erythrocytes. I. Rotation and deformation in dilute suspensions. Proc. R. Soc. Lond. Ser. B. **182:** 351–384.
5. GOLDSMITH, H. L. & T. KARINO. 1977. Microscopic considerations: The motions of individual particles. Ann. N.Y. Acad. Sci. **283:** 241–255.
6. GOLDSMITH, H. L. & J. MARLOW. 1979. Flow behavior of erythrocytes. II. Particle motions in concentrated suspensions of ghost cells. J. Colloid Interface Sci. **71:** 383–407
7. TURITTO, V. T., A. M. BENIS & E. F. LEONARD. 1972. Platelet diffusion in flowing blood. Ind. Eng. Chem. Fundam. **11:** 216–223.
8. CHANDRASEKHAR, S. 1954. Stochastic problems in physics and astronomy. *In* Selected Papers on Noise and Stochastic Processes. N. Wax, Ed.: 3–91. Dover. New York.
9. LAVENDA, B. H. 1985. Brownian motion. Sci. Am. **252**(2): 70–85.
10. PATLAK, C. S. 1953. Random walk with persistence and external bias. Bull. Math. Biophys. **15:** 311–338.
11. BITBOL, M. 1986. Red blood cell orientation in orbit C = 0. Biophys J. **49:** 1055–1068

12. Bitbol, M., F. Leterrier, J. Dufaux & D. Quemada. 1985. Measurement of erythrocyte orientation in flow by spin labeling. III. Erythrocyte orientation and rheological conditions. Biorheology **22:** 43–53.
13. Teirlinck, H. C., G. J. Tangelder, D. W. Slaaf, A. M. M. Muijtjens, T. Arts & R. S. Reneman. 1984. Orientation and diameter distribution of rabbit blood platelets flowing in small arteries. Biorheology **21:** 317–331.
14. Tilles, A. W. & E. C. Eckstein. 1987. The near-wall excess of platelet-sized particles in blood flow: Its dependence on hematocrit and wall shear rate. Microvasc. Res. **33:** 211–223.
15. Tilles, A. W. & E. C. Eckstein. 1986. Blood models: RBC deformability and platelet distributions. Presented at the 39th Annual Conference on Engineering in Medicine and Biology. Baltimore, MD.
16. Tran-Son-Tay, R., G. B. Nash & H. J. Meiselman. 1985. Effects of dextran and membrane shear rate on red cell membrane viscosity. Biorheology **22:** 335–340.
17. Bilsker, D. L., J. S. Kippenhan & E. C. Eckstein. A freeze-capture method for the study of platelet distributions. Submitted.
18. Blackshear, P. L., K. W. Bartelt & R. J. Forstrom. 1977. Fluid dynamic factors affecting particle capture and retention. Ann. N.Y. Acad. Sci. **283:** 270–279.

Cells and Aggregates at Surfaces[a]

VINCENT T. TURITTO,[b] HARVEY J. WEISS,[c]
HANS R. BAUMGARTNER,[d] LINA BADIMON,[b] AND
VALENTIN FUSTER[b]

[b]*Department of Medicine*
Mount Sinai Medical Center
New York, New York 10029

[c]*Department of Medicine*
St. Lukes-Roosevelt Hospital
New York, New York 10019

[d]*Department of Pharmaceutical Research*
F. Hoffmann-La Roche & Co.
4002 Basel, Switzerland

During the past 10 years, considerable progress has been achieved concerning the physical and chemical events that govern the interaction of cells with surfaces. The attachment of cellular material to a foreign surface and the subsequent growth of the cellular deposit is a fundamental biological phenomenon that underlies numerous homeostatic functions in living organisms and in addition forms the bases for pathological processes ranging from metastases of tumor cells and thrombosis to the evolution of the atherosclerotic process. In this article we shall be concerned primarily with the interaction of blood platelets and damaged vascular material as a model for the cellular events important in thrombosis. The first microscopically visible step in the interaction of platelets with a vascular or prosthetic surface is adhesion of the cell to the surface, which under the appropriate conditions is rapidly followed by the subsequent cohesion of platelets to each other. We will consider primarily the latter event, the growth and stabilization of platelet aggregates on surfaces, with the understanding that aggregate growth is essentially dependent on prior and continuing adhesion of cells to the substrate. The adhesion of cells, especially platelets, directly to the surface is an event that has been considerably advanced from both a theoretical and experimental viewpoint since the proceedings of the previous New York Academy of Sciences conference on this subject ten years ago[1]; however, this event is covered in several chapters in the present volume and the subject of platelet adhesion has been recently reviewed.[2]

PHYSICAL EFFECTS OF FLOW ON CELL-SURFACE INTERACTIONS

Blood flow classically determines both the arrival and removal of cells and other elements from the surface (FIGURE 1). The strength of binding of cells to the surface and of cells to other cells relative to the shear forces imposed on the cells at the surface essentially determines whether arrival or removal will predominate for a given surface (or cell). The various possibilities are depicted in FIGURE 1. Typically, platelets

[a]This work supported in part by grants from the U.S. Public Health Service (HL 35103, HL27346, and HL17430) and funds contributed by Boehringer-Ingelheim.

exposed to a subendothelial surface form the aggregate type (FIGURE 1C) shown in FIGURE 2, whereas, under the same conditions, red cell deposition on the same surface or most other surfaces would be represented by FIGURE 1A. Platelets attaching to various artificial substrates have been generally characterized by FIGURES 1A or 1B, at least in anticoagulated blood systems.

As flow or more precisely the local shear rate is increased, the behavior of cell deposition could theoretically undergo a transition from an aggregate pattern, such as in FIGURE 1C, to that shown in either FIGURE 1A or 1B due to the increased shear forces imposed by the flow on the cells; such changes would necessarily depend on the relative cell-surface and cell-cell bonding strengths. However experimentally, when platelets are exposed to subendothelium for a range of wall shear rates, a quite different pattern is observed (FIGURE 3). Deposition, as measured by thrombus height,

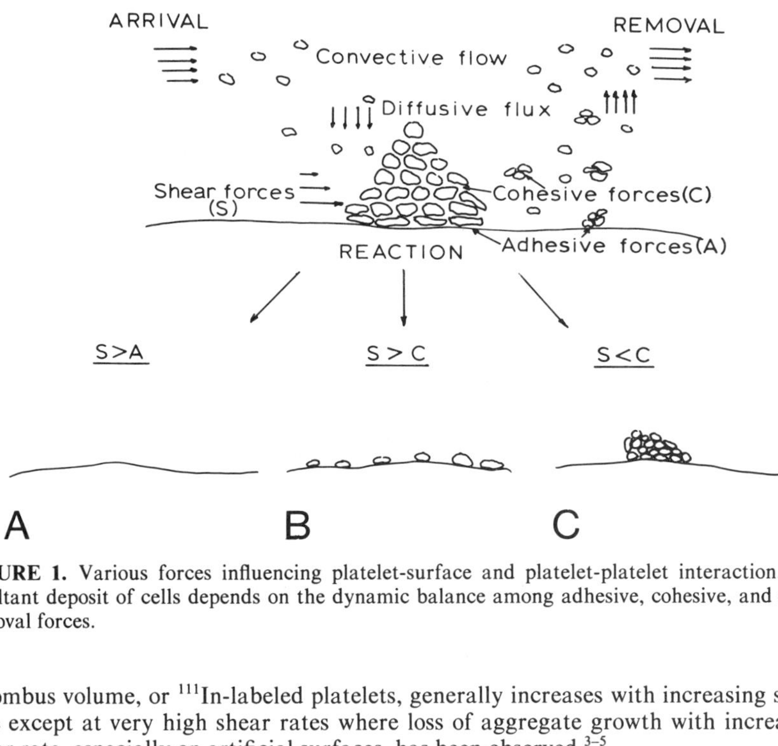

FIGURE 1. Various forces influencing platelet-surface and platelet-platelet interaction. The resultant deposit of cells depends on the dynamic balance among adhesive, cohesive, and shear removal forces.

thrombus volume, or ^{111}In-labeled platelets, generally increases with increasing shear rate except at very high shear rates where loss of aggregate growth with increasing shear rate, especially on artificial surfaces, has been observed.[3–5]

The increase in thrombus growth with local shear rate reflects one of two possibilities. The classical explanation is that the increase is due to the enhanced arrival and cohesion of platelets in the vicinity of the surface. Boundary layer analysis, which has been developed primarily for the direct attachment of cells to the subendothelial surface,[6–8] suggests that the maximum increase in arrival rate should be a fractional power of the wall shear rate. The magnitude of the fractional power could vary from one-third in the case of molecular deposits to approximately two-thirds, as determined experimentally for red-cell-enhanced adhesion of blood platelets.[6] In fact, when the initial slope is determined from a double logarithmic plot of platelet deposition (^{111}In-labeled platelets) versus shear rate, the value is considerably

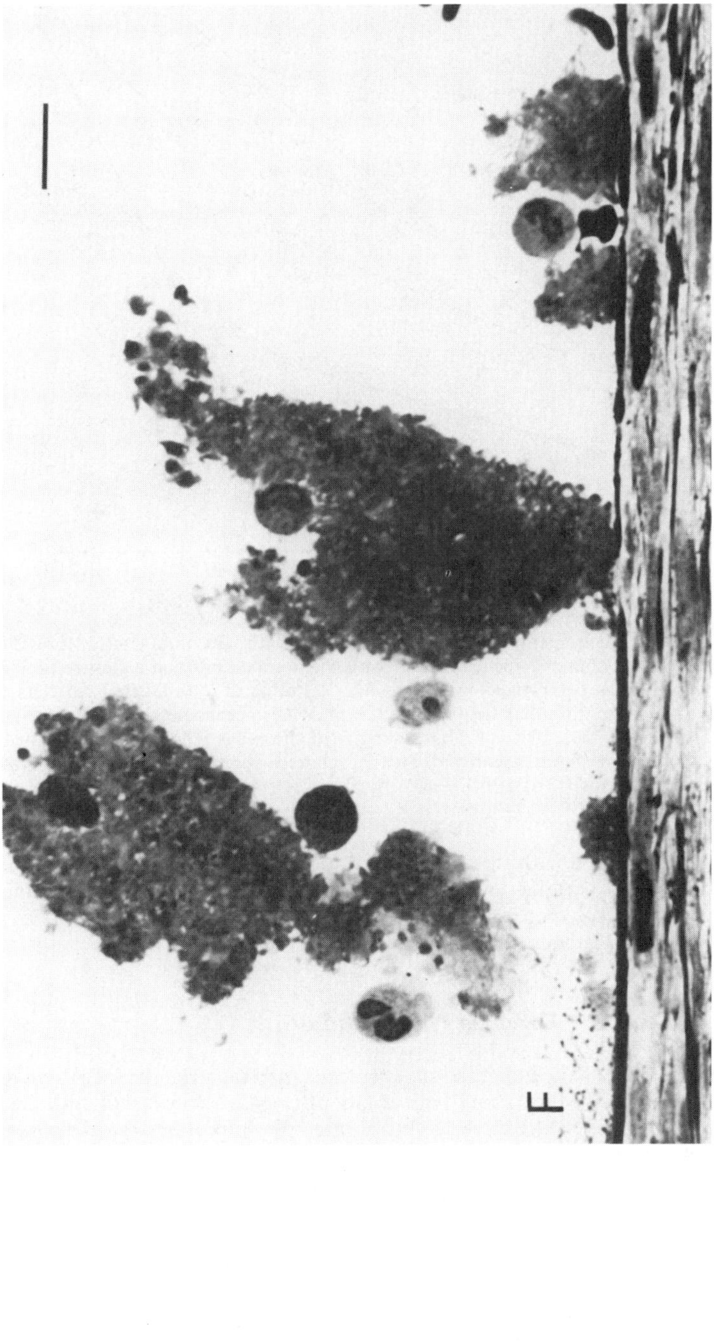

FIGURE 2. Interaction of human blood with de-endothelialized rabbit aorta. Nonanticoagulated blood is exposed at a flow rate of 20 ml/min (wall shear rate of 1300 s^{-1}) for 5 min. Growth of platelet aggregates is nonsymmetrical and appears highly resistant to fluid shear forces. Flow is perpendicular to plane of figure. Fibrin deposition is indicated by *F*. *Bar* represents 10 μm. (From Turitto *et al.*[53])

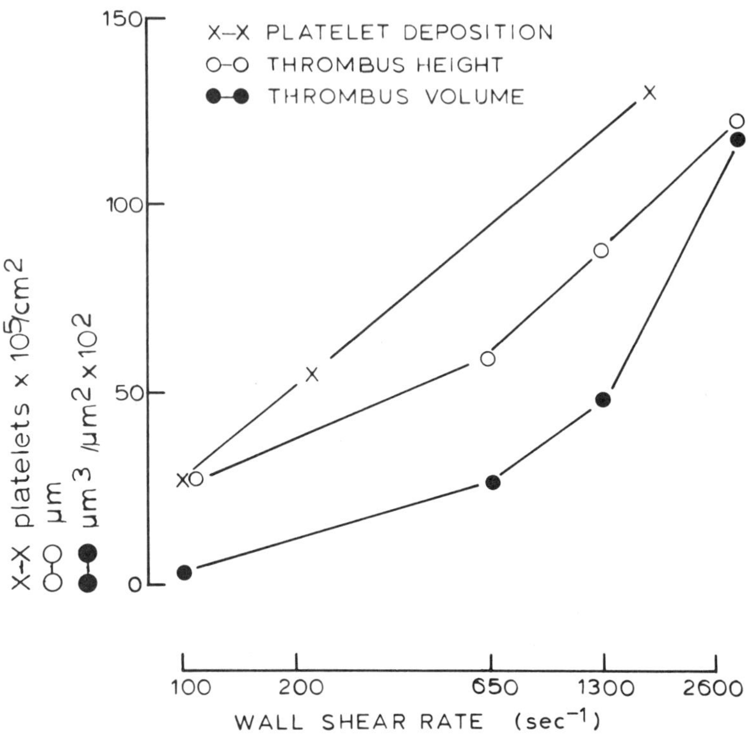

FIGURE 3. Various measurements of platelet interaction with subendothelium representing platelet-platelet cohesion obtained for a range of wall shear conditions and exposure time of 5 min: platelet deposition as determined by radiometric counting of ^{111}In-labeled platelets (pig blood, pig vessel); average thrombus height as determined by morphometric evaluation of the three highest thrombi (human blood, rabbit vessel); and thrombus volume as determined by morphometric planimetry of cross-sectional area of platelet thrombi (human blood, rabbit vessels). (For details, see refs. 23 and 70.)

enhanced (1.41) compared with that determined for platelet adhesion (0.6–0.7).[9] The enhanced deposition of platelets over that predicted from classical considerations is related to several possible mechanisms by which the local arrival of platelets at the growing thrombus may be increased.

Enhanced Platelet Diffusivity

A number of studies have indicated that red cells may increase the local arrival of platelets at surfaces.[10–13] In fact, studies in our laboratory have shown that both the red cell concentration and the local wall shear rate are important for determining thrombus growth on subendothelium. As seen in FIGURE 4 at low values of hematocrit, thrombi will not form regardless of the wall shear rate. This minimum shear rate necessary for inducing thrombus formation on subendothelium decreases with increasing hematocrit, as shown in FIGURE 4.

We and others[14,15] have suggested from direct measurement of platelet diffusivity in flowing blood that the enhanced movement of platelets induced by colliding red cells will increase the deposition rate several orders of magnitude over that predicted by Brownian motion alone. Moreover, since the collision frequency of red cells with each other and with platelets is dependent on the local shear conditions, the platelet diffusivity will be dependent on the local shear rate, with the resultant deposition rate exceeding the classical (one-third power) dependency on wall shear rate, in accord with experimental observations of platelet adhesion.[6,7]

The dependency of thrombus formation on flow has not been analyzed previously with respect to the influence of hematocrit. The studies depicted in FIGURE 3 are performed at normal levels of hematocrit, 30–45%. Detailed studies of total thrombus deposition at various levels of hematocrit have not as yet been performed using ^{111}In-labeled platelets as marker. However, the studies shown in FIGURE 4 suggest a marked dependency of thrombus formation (platelet aggregates greater than 5 μm in height) on hematocrit at high shear rates. In this figure the rate of thrombus formation increases with hematocrit as wall shear rate is increased from 800 to 2600 s^{-1}. At the hematocrits of 50% and 60% the increase is approximately 11- and 24-fold, respectively, with only a 4-fold increase in wall shear rate. This increase indicates a very strong power-low dependence, considering that the morphometric technique fails to reflect quantitatively the contribution of platelets which deposit on thrombi once the 5 μm height is exceeded. As discussed in previous publications, the factors influencing platelet deposition at these high shear rates and hematocrits may be both physical and biochemical in nature.[10,12,13] The biochemical nature of the effect of red cells on thrombus formation is currently being investigated by several groups and will be discussed in a later section. In addition to platelet diffusivity, several other physical

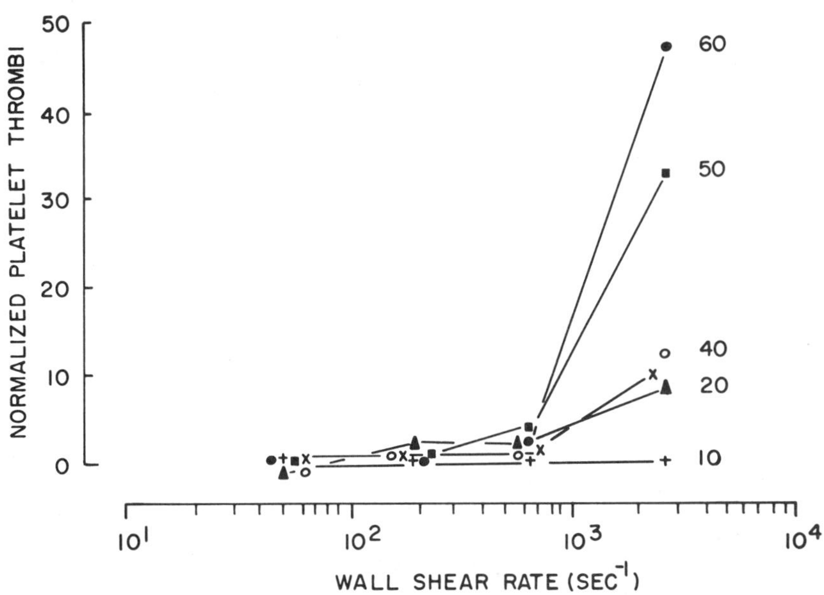

FIGURE 4. Thrombus deposit normalized by the exposure time on subendothelium exposed for various shear conditions to blood adjusted to hematocrits of 10, 20, 30, 40, 50 and 60%. (From Turitto and Weiss.[10])

factors must be considered to contribute to the influence of hematocrit and shear rate in platelet deposition.

Altered Concentration Profiles

The interchange of cells with a surface depends on the local cell concentration gradient in the direction perpendicular to the surface. Classically, this gradient is determined from a balance between reaction (deposition) at the surface and resupply of cells by convective flow and diffusive motion. For example, a high rate of resupply relative to reaction leads to a kinetic controlled reaction rate with a corresponding zero gradient (cell concentration at wall equals bulk concentration). Conversely, a low resupply relative to reaction leads to a diffusion-rate-limiting reaction rate with a maximal gradient (cell concentration equals zero at the surface). The cell concentration gradient which is formed due to the balance between net supply and reaction defines the mass transfer boundary layer, which for fluids is well within the fluid dynamical boundary layer (its dimensions for cellular species are between one and two orders of magnitude less than the distance over which changes in fluid motion occurs).

Recent experimental evidence indicates that radial concentration profiles near surfaces may not be uniform even in the absence of cellular reaction. That is, the effect of flow on the cells is to alter the local concentration gradient of red cells and platelets by an as yet undefined mechanism. Early studies[15,16] suggested that in long narrow tubes (L/D of approximately 10^4) platelets suspended in plasma migrated away from the tube wall, so that a local depletion was observed near the surface. Conversely, when red cells were added to the suspension, the platelets migrated radially outward, such that an excess of platelets at the surface was observed. More precise measurements of this directed (nonrandom) migration supporting the concept that both red cells and flow factors can alter local concentration profiles have been recently performed.[17–19] (For a more extensive discussion of this topic, see the paper in this volume by Eckstein.[73]) Basically, concentration profiles for platelet-like particles that result in a maximum in platelet concentration within tens of microns from the wall can be expected. It is clear that such changes can certainly influence the overall deposition of cellular material on surfaces. What is not clear at present is the relative magnitude of this effect compared with the diffusional effect discussed previously. An important consideration is the rapidity with which such nonuniform gradients can be formed; since the forces on such particles are not expected to be strong, the entrance length for formation may be considerably longer than most vascular surfaces or test devices, and thus the effect would be relatively insignificant.

Impaction and Interception of Cells at Surfaces

Minor modifications of classical transport theory have been successful in describing the initial deposition of platelets to both vascular and artifical surfaces. However, when the deposition becomes multilayer there are major difficulties in describing experimental observations with theoretical predictions. For example, the growth of platelet aggregates occurs at discrete locations rather than uniformly as would be expected from continuum theory (FIGURE 2). While such nonhomogeneous growth could be attributable to surface nonhomogeneities, a more likely explanation is that initial deposition of particles with finite dimensions creates a "shadow effect" as well as a local nidus of increased surface availability. This is a well-known effect in filtration science[20,21] and is illustrated in FIGURE 5. As a cell attaches to the surface, its physical dimensions prevent newly arriving cells from reaching the surface immediately downstream (area 2). The dimensions of this sheltered zone will depend on the particle dimensions and flow conditions; that is, the extent to which the deposit alters the local fluid flow. For example, if one assumed that flow remained identical to the conditions prior to attachment (which is a physical impossibility since the flow in the immediate vicinity of the cell must be altered), then only particles that did not collide with the attached cells (whose centers must be on streamlines a minimum of 1.5 times the cell diameter from the wall surface) would be able to bypass the adherent cell and have the opportunity of attaching downstream by diffusing the distance of the cell from the wall. Since diffusion is a slow process, relative to convection, the sheltered area would be maximal under such conditions. Conversely, for fluid flow that follows exactly the contour of the attached cell (Stokes flow), streamlines less than a cell radius from the attached cell surface will be displaced and return to a similar distance from the wall after passing the adherent cell; cells located on such streamlines will have a much shorter diffusional distance to the wall and the sheltered area will be significantly reduced compared to the former conditions. While such flow conditions are more realistic, especially with cellular dimensions, as the aggregate grows, alterations in the local streamlines must occur, collisional impacts with growing

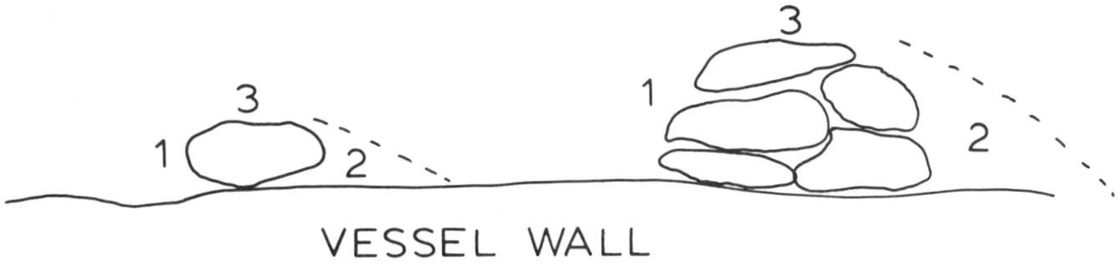

FIGURE 5. Sketch of physical changes in surface availability that can occur due to the deposition of cells with finite dimensions. The surface undergoes a transition from homogeneous availability to a state where discrete growth can occur. *1,* Active sites extending into lumen. *2,* Sheltered areas. *3,* Enhanced shear.

thrombi increase due to their intrusion into the blood flow, and the dimensions of the sheltered area grow with time. Analysis of the mass exchange under such conditions becomes exceedingly complex, but may be quite important for a better understanding of the stabilization of thrombus masses that eventually occlude the lumen. In this region what essentially become created on a microscopic scale are areas of high and low shear flow regimes (the peaks and sheltered valleys of the growth process, respectively). As indicated by Weiss *et al.,*[22] in another paper in this volume, very different mechanisms are favored at high and low shear conditions. Platelets are rapidly deposited and secrete their granule contents at high shear rates, whereas activation of the coagulation pathway with the local deposition of fibrin is observed predominantly at low shear rates. Given the requirement of platelets for fibrin to deposit on subendothelium[23] and the well-established effects of thrombin on platelet function,[24–26] having such events in close proximity may tend to maximize both pathways.

BIOCHEMICAL FACTORS INFLUENCING THROMBUS GROWTH

Thrombus formation is a dynamic process, that is, the precipitation of cellular and proteinaceous elements from the blood onto vascular or other surfaces occurs in the presence of flow. The past 10 years have seen the gradual recognition that blood flow not only influences the development of thrombi both quantitatively and qualitatively; that is, the specific role of certain proteins, such as von Willebrand factor, is determined by the flow conditions. As such, a number of systems designed to expose surfaces to controlled flow conditions have evolved, stemming from devices introduced in the early 1970s by Friedman *et al.* for prosthetic surfaces[27] and by Baumgartner for vascular material.[28] The various biochemical factors that will be discussed in this article will consider primarily those important for thrombus growth on arterial subendothelium, an area in which our understanding has progressed much more rapidly than in the field of biomaterials in general.

TABLE 1 lists a number of the factors that have been described as important (or surprisingly unimportant) in the development of thrombus formation on subendothelium; the factors to be considered will be those that influence thrombus formation independently of platelet adhesion. As previously discussed, most of these factors have been studied at high shear rates ($>650\ s^{-1}$) since extensive platelet-platelet interaction does not occur at lower shear rates. These components will be briefly discussed in the following sections.

TABLE 1. Influence of Various Components on Thrombus Formation

	Degree of Influence	Ref.
Plasma Components		
Platelet count	++++	29,30
Hematocrit	++++	10,13,31,32
Ca^{++} ion	++++	6,34,35
PGI_2 (PGE_1)	++++	38,39
Heparin	+	29,34
Aspirin	++	34,37
Von Willebrand factor	+++	53,54
Fibrinogen	±	53
Procoagulant factors	++++	29,34,53,54
Vessel Wall Components		
Collagen	++++	67,71
Von Willebrand factor	?	64
Other adhesive proteins (fibrinogen, fibronectin)	?	—
Tissue factor	?	—
Platelet-related Components		
GPIb	?	45,46
GPIIb-IIIa	++++	23,59
Dense granules	+++	44,59
α Granules	?	44,59

Plasma Components

Cells

The cellular components of blood can influence thrombus formation through both physical and chemical mechanisms. Platelets are obviously necessary physically to produce the typical white thrombus found in arteries, whereas red cells, generally entrapped in fibrin, are often the main constituent of the red thrombus characteristic of veins or the "tail" of the platelet thrombus. The dependence of thrombus deposition on platelet concentration, as occurs naturally[29] or as produced artificially in the laboratory,[30] has been described on subendothelial surfaces. More recently, platelets have been found to be necessary for the deposition of fibrin on subendothelial surfaces; thus, the physical dimensions of the thrombus can be influenced by the physical presence of platelets through various mechanisms.[22,23]

As previously discussed red cells contribute to the physical movement of platelets in flowing blood. Their ability to induce such movement is largely determined by their concentration (hematocrit), although red cell size[31] and deformability[32] have also been shown to contribute to platelet-surface interactions. Presumably these factors influence platelet-platelet cohesion and thus thrombus formation, but the latter has not been demonstrated. Red cells also contribute a biochemical factor that induces thrombus growth at high hematocrits and shear rates.[10,13] The obvious candidate for such an effect is the extensive quantity of ADP which is contained in the red cell and which may be released as a result of stress-related lysis.[33] Platelets themselves contain numerous moieties, either on their membrane or within certain cellular compartments, which contribute actively to thrombus formation; these will be considered below.

Nonproteinaceous Substances

The formation of platelet thrombi on de-endothelialized surfaces is quite sensitive to the concentration of calcium, much more so than the platelet-surface attachment.[6,34] Thrombus formation is generally reduced when blood is collected into a calcium-chelating anticoagulant compared to native (nonanticoagulated) blood or heparinized blood.[29,34] In general, heparin has been found to have little significant effect on thrombus formation compared with native blood, although various values of thrombus dimensions may be slightly reduced in the presence of heparin, a finding that is likely related to the inhibition of procoagulant factors (ref. 34, and unpublished results in human blood). The inhibitory effect of reduced calcium may be magnified by the use of increased concentration of sodium citrate[6] or 1% EDTA,[35] whereas little effect is seen on platelets for heparin levels varying from 2.5 to 10 U/ml (unpublished results).

Various drugs have been investigated for their effect on thrombus formation. Aspirin has a pronounced effect on reducing thrombus formation on subendothelium when blood is anticoagulated with sodium citrate[36]; this inhibition is comparable to that seen in platelet aggregation studies. However, when *nonanticoagulated* blood is drawn directly from either human[37] or rabbit[34] sources and exposed to subendothelium, the effect of aspirin on thrombus formation is much reduced, and aspirin in such situations appears to be only a mild inhibitor of platelet-platelet interaction. Under similar conditions, both dipyridamole and sulfinpyrazone were found not to inhibit platelet-platelet interaction, as measured by the thrombus height or thrombus volume, at concentrations of 100/μmol/kg given orally to rabbits.[34] Identical findings with dipyridamole given to humans over a week's time were also observed.[37]

The most potent inhibitors of thrombus formation on subendothelium are the prostaglandins PGE_1 and PGI_2,[38,39] the latter of which virtually abolishes platelet-platelet interactions at nanomolar concentrations in citrated[39] and native blood (unpublished results).

Plasma Proteins

During the past 10 years, much work has been directed at elucidating the platelet and protein mechanisms involved in thrombosis. The foundation supporting much of this work has been the classification of various bleeding disorders with respect to specific platelet and plasma defects. Work on the specific classification, utilizing well-defined perfusion systems, was begun in the mid-seventies. By the time of the last conference[40] defects in the attachment of platelets to subendothelium in von Willebrand disease[41] and Bernard-Soulier syndrome[42] and in the development of platelet-platelet interactions (mural thrombus formation) in thrombasthenia[43] and storage-pool disease[44] had been described. Thus, a plasma protein, vWF, and a platelet membrane protein were thought to be necessary for normal platelet adhesion to subendothelium; a deficient or defective membrane component and the reduced granular content of platelets were believed to be primarily responsible for the inhibited aggregate growth. Considerable investigation over the past 10 years has helped delineate (1) the platelet glycoproteins GPIb and GPIIb-IIIa, deficient in Bernard-Soulier syndrome and thrombasthenia,[45,46] respectively, (2) the characteristics of the vWF and its role in adhesion,[47–50] and (3) the proteinaceous and biochemical constituents of the platelet granules and their involvement in platelet-vessel wall interaction.[51,52]

The platelet proteins, both membrane and intracelluar, involved in platelet-platelet interaction will be discussed below. A plasma protein recently demonstrated to be involved in platelet-platelet deposition on subendothelium is von Willebrand factor, a high molecular weight multimer absent in severe von Willebrand's disease.[53,54] The defect in thrombus formation due to the absence of vWF has been shown with both human and pig blood to occur at lower shear conditions ($<1300\ s^{-1}$ in native blood) than necessary to produce a defect in platelet-subendothelial interaction.[53] Thus, platelet-platelet interactions appear more sensitive to the effect of shear rate (stress) than platelet-surface interactions on subendothelium. Interestingly, fibrinogen, which is thought to be necessary for platelet aggregation from *in vitro* studies of platelet aggregation, appears not to be involved significantly in thrombus formation, as indicated by the normal values of thrombus dimensions on subendothelium in afibrinogenemia.[53] The latter observation may be related to the ability of vWF to substitute for fibrinogen in binding to the platelet membrane.[55–57] A major question to be answered has to do with the relative roles of vWF and fibrinogen in thrombosis in normal subjects. The adhesive protein most recently implicated in thrombus formation (associated with platelet-platelet interaction) is fibronectin.[58] The mechanisms by which these proteins interact (presumably with GPIIb-IIIa on platelets) and the extent to which such proteins may substitute for each other are areas of intense research at present.

Platelet-related Substances

Two sources of platelet material are available to participate in thrombus formation: (1) those present on the surface membrane, and (2) those normally contained within the platelet granules that are secreted upon stimulation.

Two glycoproteins on the surface that are associated with thrombus formation have been identified. The glycoprotein complex GPIIb-IIIa, which, as discussed previously, upon stimulation of the platelet with exogenous ADP or thrombin binds von Willebrand factor, fibronectin, and fibrinogen, is considered essential for thrombus formation. Patients who lack this receptor bleed. This bleeding is associated with a failure to develop platelet-platelet aggregates on subendothelium in either native or citrated blood.[59] The glycoprotein Ib is the receptor site for von Willebrand factor and is deficient in Bernard-Soulier syndrome.[45,46] The site has been most directly associated with platelet-subendothelial interaction (adhesion); however, whether it may also be involved in the platelet-platelet defect in von Willebrand's disease[53,60] is not clear at present, since vWF binds to both glycoproteins Ib and IIb-IIIa.

However, deficiency of GPIb, as in Bernard-Soulier syndrome[61] results in a partial inhibition of platelet-platelet interaction on subendothelium, unlike the absent cohesion produced by GPIIb-IIIa deficiency.[23] Thus, if GPIb plays a significant role in thrombus formation, it apparently will do so only in concert with GPIIb-IIIa.

The release of platelet granular material has been associated with the ability to form platelet aggregates on subendothelium. Decreased levels of dense body substances, such as ADP, ATP, and serotonin, lead to strikingly reduced levels of thrombus dimensions on subendothelium exposed to native blood in patients with δ-storage pool disease.[59] This observation has been attributed mainly to ADP; the degree of abnormality is related to the level of dense granular content. Even smaller thrombus dimensions were observed in patients with combined deficiencies of dense and α-granules, suggesting that α-granule substances may also contribute to the ability of thrombi to grow in the presence of flowing blood. The protein responsible for platelet-platelet interactions in the α-granules of platelets is not known at present. (vWF, fibrinogen, fibronectin, and thrombospondin are among the potential candidates). However, it has been reported that transplantation of normal bone marrow into pigs with severe von Willebrand disease partially corrected the bleeding time in these animals,[74] suggesting that platelet vWF is one factor involved in hemostatic plug formation.

Components of the Vessel Wall

Various plasma and/or platelet proteins that have been described as mediating platelet-platelet interaction have also been localized in the vessel wall.[62,63] The role of vascular proteins, such as vWF, fibrinogen, fibronectin, etc., on platelet-platelet interaction has never been demonstrated; it is more likely that such immobilized proteins might contribute primarily to platelet-vessel wall interactions (and thereby to thrombus deposits), and such behavior has been described.[64–66]

The vascular protein that might play an important role in the development of platelet thrombus formation is collagen. Fibrillar collagen either from Achilles tendon (type I), as exposed by digestion of subendothelium (type I and III) or as purified from various sources and coated onto surfaces, develops extensive masses of platelets when exposed to flowing blood.[67–71] Collagen acts presumably through its ability to stimulate platelet secretion or directly alter the platelet membrane. Aggregates not only grow extensively into the lumen but also appear resistant to embolysis over prolonged periods of time compared to subendothelium. A major consideration is the availability of the various collagens to blood elements. The more reactive fibrillar collagens, types I and III, are not normally exposed in the intimal layers, although they are abundant in the deeper vessel layers and may be exposed upon deep vascular injury or plaque rupture. Types IV and V, which do not generally interact strongly with platelets,[72] are more common in the basement membrane area. Thus, it is possible that collagen is not greatly involved in a mild type injury in which only basement membrane components are exposed, but acquires more importance in deeper vascular injury.

A final observation concerns the generation of procoagulant moieties by the vessel wall. Recent findings indicate the presence of tissue factor in vascular subendothelium (unpublished result, this laboratory). The generation of activated clotting factors in the blood has been shown to enhance greatly the growth and/or stability of platelet aggregates in subendothelium. Thus, by modulating the production of factors such as thrombin, tissue factor may indirectly mediate the extent of platelet-platelet interaction. The pathways by which vascular surfaces communicate with platelets in the presence of an active coagulation system are only beginning to be explored. It is clear that a better understanding of thrombosis on surfaces requires recognition of

Virchow's century-old triad: the thrombotic event is highly dynamic in nature and involves both chemical and physical considerations of fluid dynamic, blood, and vascular factors acting in concert.

REFERENCES

1. Vroman, L. & E. F. Leonard, Eds. 1977. Ann. N.Y. Acad. Sci. **283:** 1–560.
2. Turitto, V. T. & H. R. Baumgartner. 1987. Platelet-surface interactions. *In* Hemostasis and Thrombosis: Basic Principles and Clinical Practice. 2d edit. R. Coleman, J. Hirsh, V. Marder & E. Salzman, Eds. J. P. Lippincott. New York. pp. 555–571.
3. Sauvage, L. R., M. W. Walker, K. Berger, S. B. Robel, M. M. Lischko, S. G. Yates & G. A. Logan. 1979. Current arterial prosthesis: Experimental evaluation by implantation in the carotid and circumflex coronary arteries of the dog. Arch. Surg. **114:** 687–691.
4. Christenson, J. T., J. Mergerman, K. C. Hanel, G. J. L'Italien, H. W. Strauss & W. M. Abbott. 1981. The effect of blood flow rates on platelet deposition in PTFE arterial bypass grafts. Trans. Am. Soc. Artif. Intern. Organs **27:** 188–91.
5. Lelah, M. D., L. K. Lamrecht & S. L. Cooper. 1984. A canine ex vivo series shunt for evaluating thrombus deposition on polymer surfaces. J. Biomed. Mater. Res. **18:** 475–496.
6. Turitto, V. T., H. J. Weiss & H. R. Baumgartner. 1980. The effect of shear rate on platelet interaction with subendothelium exposed to citrated human blood. Microvasc. Res. **19:** 352–365.
7. Turitto, V. T. & H. R. Baumgartner. 1979. Platelet interaction with subendothelium in flowing rabbit blood: Effect of blood shear rate. Microvasc. Res. **17:** 38–54.
8. Turitto, V. T. & H. R. Baumgartner. 1975. Platelet deposition on subendothelium exposed to flowing blood: Mathematical analyses of physical parameters. Trans. Am. Soc. Artif. Intern. Organs **21:** 593–600.
9. Badimon, L., V. Turrito, J. A. Rosemark, J. J. Badimon & V. Fuster. Characterization of a tubular flow chamber for studying platelet interaction with biological and prosthetic materials: Deposition of ^{111}In-labelled platelets on collagen, subendothelium and Gore-Tex®. J. Lab. Clin. Med. In press.
10. Turitto, V. T. & H. J. Weiss. 1983. Platelet and red cell involvement in mural thrombogenesis. Ann. N.Y. Acad. Sci. **416:** 363–376.
11. Brash, J. L., J. M. Brophy & I. A. Feuerstein. 1976. Adhesion of platelets to artificial surfaces. Effect of red cells. J. Biomed. Res. **10:** 429–443.
12. Turitto, V. T. & H. R. Baumgartner. 1975. Platelet interaction with subendothelium in a perfusion system: Physical role of red blood cells. Microvasc. Res. **9:** 335–344.
13. Turitto, V. T. & H. J. Weiss. 1980. Red blood cells: Their dual role in thrombus formation. Science **207:** 541–543.
14. Goldsmith, H. L. & J. Marlow. 1979. Flow behavior of erythrocytes. II. Particle motions in concentrated suspensions of ghost cells. J. Colloid Interface Sci. **71:** 383–407.
15. Turitto, V. T., A. M. Benis & E. F. Leonard. 1972. Platelet diffusion in flowing blood. Ind. Eng. Chem. Fund. **11:** 216–223.
16. Turitto, V. T. 1972. The Measurement of Platelet Kinetics in Flowing Blood. Ph.D. dissertation, Columbia University, New York.
17. Bock, M. R. & E. C. Eckstein. 1980. Preliminary report on platelet concentration in capillary tube flow of whole blood. Biorheology **17:** 455.
18. Eckstein, E. C. 1982. Rheophoresis: A broader concept of platelet dispersivity. Biorheology **19:** 717.
19. Blasberg, P., L. J. Wurzinger & H. Schmid-Schönbein. 1983. Microrheology of thrombocyte deposition: Effect of stimulation, flow direction and red cells. *In* Fluid Dynamics as a Localizing Factor for Atherosclerosis. G. Schettler, R. M. Nerem, H. Schmid-Schönbein, H. Morl & C. Diehm, Eds.: 103–115. Springer-Verlag. Berlin.
20. Wang, C., M. Beizaie & C. Tien. 1977. Deposition of solid particles on a collector: Formulation of a new theory. AIChE J. **23:** 879–890.

21. TIEN, C., C. WANG & D. T. BAROT. Chainlike formation of particle deposits in fluid-particle separation. 1977. Science **196:** 983–85.
22. WEISS, H. J., H. R. BAUMGARTNER & V. T. TURITTO. 1987. Regulation of platelet-fibrin thrombi on subendothelium. This volume.
23. WEISS, H. J., V. T. TURITTO & H. R. BAUMGARTNER. 1986. Role of shear rate and platelets in promoting fibrin formation on rabbit subendothelium: Studies utilizing patients with quantitative and qualitative platelet defects. J. Clin. Invest. **78:** 1072–1082.
24. MAJERUS, P. W. & J. P. MILETICH. 1978. Relationship between platelets and coagulation factors in hemostasis. Ann. Rev. Med. **29:** 41–49.
25. JAMIESON, G. A. & T. ORUMURA. 1978. Reduced thrombin binding and aggregation in Bernard-Soulier platelets. J. Clin. Invest. **61:** 861–864.
26. MCGOWAN, E. B., A. DING & T. C. DETWILER. 1983. Correlation of thrombin-induced glycoprotein V hydrolysis and platelet activation. J. Biol. Chem. **258:** 11243–11248.
27. GRABOWSKI, E. F., L. I. FRIEDMAN & E. F. LEONARD. 1972. Effects of shear rate on the diffusion and adhesion of blood platelet to a foreign surface. Ind. Eng. Chem. Fund. **11:** 224–232.
28. BAUMGARTNER, H. R. 1973. The role of blood flow in platelet adhesion, fibrin deposition and formation of mural thrombi. Microvasc. Res. **5:** 167–179.
29. BAUMGARTNER, H. R., V. T. TURITTO & H. J. WEISS. 1980. Effects of shear rate on platelet interaction with subendothelium in citrated and native blood. II. Relationships among platelet adhesion, thrombus dimensions and fibrin formation. J. Lab. Clin Med. **95:** 208–221.
30. TURITTO, V. T. & H. R. BAUMGARTNER. 1974. Effect of temperature on platelet interaction with subendothelium exposed to flowing blood. Hemostasis **3:** 224–236.
31. AARTS, P. A. M. M., P. A. BOLHUIS, K. S. SAKARIASSEN, B. M. HEETHAAR & J. J. SIXMA. 1983. Red blood cell size is important for adherence of blood platelets to artery subendothelium. Blood **62:** 214.
32. AARTS, P. A. M. M., R. M. HEETHAAR & J. J. SIXMA. 1984. Red blood cell deformability influences platelet-vessel wall interaction in flowing blood. Blood **64:** 1228–1233.
33. REIMERS, R., S. P. SUTERA & J. H. JOIST. 1984. Potentiation by red blood cells of shear-induced platelet aggregation: Relative importance of chemical and physical mechanisms. Blood **64:** 1200–1206.
34. BAUMGARTNER, H. R. 1979. Effects of acetylsalicyclic acid, sulfinpyrazone and dipyridamole on platelet adhesion and aggregation in flowing native and anticoagulated blood. Haemostasis **8:** 340–352.
35. TURITTO, V. T., H. J. WEISS & H. R. BAUMGARTNER. 1983. Decreased platelet adhesion on vessel segments in von Willebrand disease: A defect in initial platelet attachment. J. Lab. Clin. Med. **102:** 551–564.
36. WEISS, H. J., T. B. TSCHOPP & H. R. BAUMGARTNER. 1985. Impaired interaction (adhesion-aggregation) of platelets with the subendothelium in storage-pool disease and after aspirin ingestion: A comparison with von Willebrand's disease. N. Engl. J. Med. **293:** 619–623.
37. WEISS, H. J., V. T. TURITTO, W. J. VICIC & H. R. BAUMGARTNER. 1981. Effect of aspirin and dipyridamole on the interaction of human platelets with subendothelium: Studies using citrated and native blood. Thromb. Haemostas. **45:** 136–141.
38. BAUMGARTNER, H. R., R. MUGGLI, T. B. TSCHOPP & V. T. TURITTO. 1976. Platelet adhesion, release and aggregation in flowing blood: Effects of surface properties and platelet function. Thromb. Haemostas. **35:** 124–138.
39. WEISS, H. J. & V. T. TURITTO. 1979. Prostacyclin (prostaglandin I_2, PGI_2) inhibits platelet adhesion and thrombus formation on subendothelium. Blood **53:** 244–250.
40. WEISS, H. J., H. R. BAUMGARTNER, T. B. TSCHOPP & V. T. TURITTO. 1977. Interaction of platelets with subendothelium: A new method for identifying and classifying abnormalities of platelet function. Ann. N. Y. Acad. Sci. **283:** 293–309.
41. TSCHOPP, T. B., H. J. WEISS & H. R. BAUMGARTNER. 1974. Decreased adhesion of platelets to subendothelium in von Willebrand's disease. J. Lab. Clin. Med. **83:** 296–300.
42. WEISS, H. J., T. B. TSCHOPP, H. R. BAUMGARTNER, I. I. SUSSMAN, M. M. JOHNSON & J. J. EGAN. 1974. Decreased adhesion of giant (Bernard-Soulier) platelets to subendothelium:

Further implications on the role of the von Willebrand factor in hemostasis. Am. J. Med. **57:** 920–925.

43. TSCHOPP, T. B., H. J. WEISS & H. R. BAUMGARTNER. 1975. Interaction of thrombasthenic platelets with subendothelium: Normal adhesion, absent aggregation. Experientia **31:** 113–116.
44. WEISS, H. J., T. B. TSCHOPP & H. R. BAUMGARTNER. 1975. Impaired interaction (adhesion-aggregation) of platelets with the subendothelium in storage-pool disease and after aspirin ingestion: A comparison with von Willebrand's disease. N. Engl. J. Med. **293:** 619–623.
45. JENKINS, C. S. P., D. R. PHILLIPS, K. J. CLEMETSON, D. MEYER, M. J. LARRIEU & E. F. LUSCHER. 1976. Platelet membrane glycoproteins implicated in ristocetin-induced aggregation: Studies of the proteins on platelets from patients with Bernard-Soulier syndrome and von Willebrand's disease. J. Clin. Invest. **57:** 112.
46. JAMIESON, G. A., T. OKUMURA, B. FISHBACK, M. M. JOHNSON, J. J. EGAN & H. J. WEISS. 1979. Platelet membrane glycoproteins in thrombasthenia, Bernard-Soulier syndrome and storage-pool disease. J. Lab. Clin. Med. **93:** 652.
47. WEISS, H. J., V. T. TURITTO & H. R. BAUMGARTNER. 1978. Effect of shear rate on platelet interaction with subendothelium in citrated and native blood. J. Lab. Clin. Med. **92:** 750–764.
48. SAKARIASSEN, K. S., P. A. BOLHUIS & J. J. SIXMA. 1979. Human blood platelet adhesion to artery subendothelium is mediated by factor VIII-von Willebrand factor bound to the subendothelium. Nature **279:** 636.
49. WEISS, H. J., H. R. BAUMGARTNER, T. B. TSCHOPP, V. T. TURITTO & D. COHEN. 1978. Correction by factor VIII of the impaired platelet adhesion to subendothelium in von Willebrand disease. Blood **51:** 267–279.
50. TURITTO, V. T., H. J. WEISS & H. R. BAUMGARTNER. 1983. Decreased platelet adhesion on vessel segments in von Willebrand's disease. A defect in initial platelet attachment. J. Lab. Clin. Med. **102:** 551–564.
51. HOLMSEN, H. 1987. Platelet secretion. *In* Hemostasis and Thrombosis: Basic Principles and Clinical Practice. R. W. Colman, J. Hirsh, V. J. Marder, E. W. Salzman, Eds. J. B. Lippincott Co. Philadelphia. pp. 606–617.
52. KAPLAN, K. L. 1981. Platelet granule proteins: Localization and secretion. *In* Platelets in Biology and Pathology 2. J. L. Gordon, Ed. Elsevier/North Holland. Amsterdam. pp. 77–90.
53. TURITTO, V. T., H. J. WEISS & H. R. BAUMGARTNER. 1984. Platelet interaction with rabbit subendothelium in von Willebrand's disease: Altered thrombus formation distinct from defective platelet adhesion. J. Clin. Invest. **74:** 1730–1741.
54. BADIMON, L. J. J. BADIMON, J. RAND, V. T. TURITTO & V. FUSTER. Platelet deposition on von Willebrand deficient vessels: Extracorporeal perfusion studies in von Willebrand's disease swine utilizing native and heparinized blood. J. Lab. Clin. Med. In press.
55. RUGGERI, Z. M., L. DEMARCO, L. GATTI, R. BADER & R. R. MONTGOMERY. 1983. Platelets have more than one binding site for von Willebrand factor. J. Clin. Invest. **72:** 1.
56. GRALNICK, H. R., S. B. WILLIAMS & B. S. COLLER. 1984. Fibrinogen competes with von Willebrand factor for binding to the glycoprotein IIIb-IIIa complex when platelets are stimulated with thrombin. Blood **64:** 797.
57. PLOW, E. F., A. SROUJI, D. MEYER, G. MARGUERIE & M. H. GINSBERG. 1984. Evidence that three adhesive proteins interact with a common recognition site on activated platelets. J. Biol. Chem. **259:** 5388.
58. BASTIDA, E., G. ESCOLAR, R. CASTILLO, A. ORDINAS & J. J. SIXMA. 1987. Fibronectin is required for platelet adhesion and for thrombus formation on subendothelium and collagen surfaces. Thromb. Haemostas. **58:** 705.
59. WEISS, H. J., V. T. TURITTO & H. R. BAUMGARTNER. 1986. Platelet adhesion and thrombus formation on subendothelium in platelets deficient in glycoprotein IIb-IIIa, Ib and storage granules. Blood **67:** 322–330.
60. SAWADA, Y., D. N. FASS, J. A. KATZMANN, R. C. BAHN & E. J. W. BOWIE. 1986. Hemostatic plug formation in normal and von Willebrand pigs: The effect of the

administration of cryoprecipitate and a monoclonal antibody to Willebrand factor. Blood **67:** 1229–1239.

61. JAMIESON, G. A., T. OKUMARA, B. FISHBACK, M. JOHNSON & H. J. WEISS. 1979. Platelet membrane glycoproteins in thrombasthenia, Bernard-Soulier syndrome, and storage pool disease. J. Lab. Clin. Med. **93:** 652–660.
62. RAND, J. H., I. I. SUSSMAN, R. E. GORDON, S. V. CHU & V. SOLOMON. 1980. Localization of factor VIII-related antigen in human vascular subendothelium. Blood **55:** 752–756.
63. RAND, J. H., L. BADIMON, R. E. GORDON & V. FUSTER. The distribution of von Willebrand factor in porcine intima varies with blood vessel type and location. Arteriosclerosis. **7:** 287–291.
64. TURITTO, V. T., H. J. WEISS, T. S. ZIMMERMAN & I. I. SUSSMAN. 1985. Factor VIII/von Willebrand factor in subendothelium mediates platelet adhesion. Blood **65:** 823–831.
65. HOUDIJK, W. P. M., P. G. DE GROOT, P. F. E. M. NIEVELSTEIN, K. S. SAKARIASSEN & J. J. SIXMA. 1985. Subendothelial proteins and platelet adhesion: Von Willebrand factor and fibronectin, not thrombospondin, are involved in platelet adhesion to extracellular matrix of human vascular endothelial cells. Arteriosclerosis **6:** 24–33.
66. STEL, H. V., K. S. SAKARIASSEN, P. G. DE GROOT, J. A. VAN MOURIK & J. J. SIXMA. 1985. The von Willebrand factor in the vessel wall mediates platelet adherence. Blood **65:** 85–90.
67. BAUMGARTNER, H. R. 1977. Platelet interaction with collagen fibrils in flowing blood. I. Reaction of human platelets with α-chymotrypsin-digested subendothelium. Thromb. Haemostas. **37:** 1–17.
68. MUGGLI, R. & H. R. BAUMGARTNER. 1978. Platelet interactions with collagenous substrates in the presence of flowing blood. *In* Collagen-Platelet Interaction. H. Gastpar, Ed: 289–298. Schattauer Verlag. New York.
69. BADIMON, L., J. J. BADIMON, A. GALVEZ, J. H. CHESEBRO & V. FUSTER. 1986. Influence of arterial damage and wall shear rate on platelet deposition: Ex vivo study in a swine model. Arteriosclerosis **6:** 312–320.
70. BADIMON, L., J. J. BADIMON, V. T. TURITTO & V. FUSTER. 1987. Thrombosis: Studies under flow conditions. This volume.
71. BADIMON, L., J. J. BADIMON, V. T. TURITTO, S. VALLABHAJOSULA & V. FUSTER. Platelet thrombus formation on collagen type I under blood shear rate conditions typical of stenotic and normal vessels: Effect of blood coagulation and circulating von Willebrand factor. Submitted.
72. HOUDIJK, W. P. M., K. S. SAKARIASSEN, M. OTTENHOF-ROVERS, J. J. SIXMA & J. RAUTERBERG. 1983. Platelet interaction with interstitial and basement membrane collagen. Thromb. Haemostas. **50:** 190.
73. ECKSTEIN, E. E., D. L. BILSKER, C. M. WATERS, J. S. KIPPENHAN & A. W. TILLES. 1987. Transport of platelets in flowing blood. This volume.
74. BOWIE, E. J. W., L. A. SOLBERG, JR., D. N. FASS, C. M. JOHNSON, G. J. KNUTSON, M. L. STEWART & L. J. ZOECKLEIN. 1986. Transplantation of normal bone marrow into a pig with severe von Willebrand's disease. J. Clin. Invest. **78:** 26–30.

Interactions of Human Blood Cells with the Vascular Endothelium[a]

HARRY L. GOLDSMITH AND TAKESHI KARINO

McGill University Medical Clinic
Montreal General Hospital
Montreal, Quebec H3G 1A4, Canada

INTRODUCTION

To a large extent, the interaction of the formed elements with the blood vessel wall are governed by fluid mechanical factors. Local flow patterns and fluid mechanical stress, as well as the balance between inwardly directed hydrodynamic and outwardly directed dispersive forces, determine the flux of cells toward the vessel wall, and thus play a decisive role in the maintenance of vascular homeostasis and in the genesis of vascular diseases such as thrombosis and atherosclerosis.

The purpose of this paper is to summarize our knowledge of the fluid dynamics of cell-wall interactions in support of the thesis that, in the circulation, wall encounters can occur by two different mechanisms: dispersion within the blood and convective transport to the wall.

Dispersion within the Blood

Cell-wall encounters arise from the continual shear-induced collisions between red cells that lead to lateral displacements of their paths as well as those of white cells and platelets. Thus, cells flowing in the periphery of vessels are frequently displaced to the wall.

Convective Transport to the Wall

Corpuscles are carried toward the wall along curved streamlines having pronounced radial velocity components. Such flow patterns are found in regions of disturbed flow that exist downstream of aortic and venous valves, mural thrombi and stenoses, and at bifurcations of major arteries.

Evidence for the above two mechanisms comes from our own *in vitro* studies of the microrheology of human blood cells in straight tubes less than 200 μm in diameter,[1–3] in models of stenoses[4–6] and T-junctions,[7,8] as well as in transparent segments of human and dog arterial T-junctions[9,10] and bifurcations,[11] and in dog venous valves.[12] In these various investigations, cellular and fluid motions in the interior of the suspensions were observed and photographed through a microscope and quantitated by analysis of 16-mm cine films.[5,13]

[a]This work was supported by Medical Research Council of Canada grant nos. MT 1835 and MT 7084, grant no. HL 29502 from the National Heart, Lung and Blood Institute, USPHS, and the Quebec Heart Foundation.

The dispersion mechanism for cell-wall interactions has been strongly supported by the studies of other investigators on, for example, the increase in platelet diffusivity in flowing blood[14] and the effect of red cells on platelet adhesion to subendothelium[15,16] and other surfaces.[17,18] The convective transport mechanism is supported by evidence that some of the regions of disturbed flow found in the model studies, for example, at flow dividers of aortic T-junctions and the outer wall of the carotid sinus, are generally the preferred sites of thrombosis and atherosclerosis.[19–21]

DISPERSION IN FLOWING BLOOD

Dilute Suspensions of Cells

In the absence of cell-cell interactions, the transport of corpuscles in tube flow occurs by convection due to bulk flow and by diffusion due to Brownian motion. Providing cell : tube diameter ratios $\ll 1$,[22] cells are carried by the plasma in convective transport at velocities equal to those of the fluid, *i.e.*, at mean velocities $\overline{U}$ from ~300 mm · s^{-1} in a major artery of ~6 mm diameter, down to ~50 mm · s^{-1} in small arteries of ~0.3 mm diameter and ~0.5 mm · s^{-1} in capillaries.[23,24] Assuming for the moment a parabolic Poiseuille velocity distribution, the velocity, $u(r)$, of a cell in the axial direction at a radial distance r from the tube axis is

$$u(r) = 2\overline{U}\left(1 - \frac{r^2}{R^2}\right), \tag{1}$$

R being the tube radius. Thus a platelet, whose center of rotation is located only 4 μm from the vessel wall would, in 1 second, travel 1600 and 5300 μm parallel to the wall in the major and small artery, respectively.

By contrast, the distance the platelet would be carried in diffusive transport in a direction normal to the wall, characterized by the translational Brownian diffusion constant, D_t, is much smaller[25]:

$$D_t = \frac{\overline{\Delta x^2}}{2\Delta t} = \frac{kT_K}{K_t\eta}. \tag{2}$$

Here $\overline{\Delta x^2}$ is the mean square distance traveled by the cell in time Δt, k the Boltzmann constant, T_K the absolute temperature, η the suspending fluid viscosity, and K_t the translational resistance coefficient. Values of the latter for motion along, and tranverse to, the axis of revolution of an oblate spheroid such as a red cell or a platelet have been given.[3,26] The mean value of K_t for a platelet, whose mean axis of revolution is 0.46 μm and whose mean equivalent ellipsoidal axis ratio $\bar{r}_e$ is 0.36,[27] is 3.19×10^{-2} mm. Thus, D_t for platelets in plasma at 37°C, with η 1.2 mPa s is 1.12×10^{-7} mm^2 · s^{-1}, and the root mean square distance traveled in 1 second, $(\overline{\Delta x^2})^{1/2}$ is 0.47 μm. Actual collisions with the wall due to Brownian diffusion are highly improbable since the hydrodynamic resistance increases sharply as the particle center of rotation approaches within one particle diameter of the interface.[28] However, if the particle interacts chemically (*e.g.*, activated platelet and a collagen surface) or physically (*e.g.*, opposite charges between particle and surface), it can be drawn to the wall and adhere while still a small distance from the interface.

Levich[29] has given a solution for the convective-diffusive transport of solute molecules in a liquid undergoing Poiseuille flow which has been applied by Leonard, Turitto, *et al.* to small particles such as platelets in plasma.[30,31] If it is assumed that the particle axial velocity at a radial distance y from the tube wall is equal to that of the undisturbed fluid, and that curvature of the shear field can be neglected, the steady-state flux, J, to the surface is then

$$J = D_t \left(\frac{\partial n}{\partial y}\right) y = 0$$

$$= 0.67 n_0 \left(\frac{G(R) D_t^2}{2z}\right)^{1/3}, \quad \textbf{(3)}$$

where n and n_0 are the respective local and bulk number concentration of cells, z the axial distance along the tube, and $G(R)$ the wall shear rate ($=4\bar{U}/R$ in Poiseuille flow). If diffusion is very rapid compared to the rate of arrival of cells at the surface, J may be equated to the rate of adhesion of cells per unit area.

Values of the rate of cell adhesion to collagen fibers on the wall of a glass tube, obtained in washed platelet suspensions at wall shear rates $<20\ \mathrm{s}^{-1}$, are in fair agreement with those predicted by equation **3.** However, it is known that platelets close to the vessel wall migrate laterally inward, and that one would expect their concentration there to be considerably depleted with a consequent reduction in cell-wall interactions. The above-mentioned agreement with theory may therefore be fortuitous; adhesion may have been the result of platelet interactions with collagen fibers protruding out from the glass wall.

There is no doubt that in dilute suspensions wall migration is important and leads to a significant depletion in corpuscular concentration at the vessel periphery. In the case of red cells, their deformation even at low tube Reynolds number,

$$\mathrm{Re} = \frac{2R\bar{U}\rho}{\eta}, \quad \textbf{(4)}$$

ρ being the suspending fluid density, leads to inward migration at a rate which increases with increasing deformation, flow rate, and ratio of particle : tube diameter,[1] similar to that previously found with fluid drops.[22] At higher Re, when inertial forces in the suspending plasma become appreciable, there is migration of rigid glutaraldehyde-fixed red cells away from the tube wall, as well as away from the tube axis towards an equilibrium radial position[1]: the tubular pinch effect.[32] The rate of migration increases with increasing Re and ratio of particle : tube diameter. Inward migration of the relatively rigid platelets[33,34] and leukocytes[33,35] has been documented. Migrations due to either particle deformation or inertia of the suspending fluid are characterized by a rapid decrease in radial velocity with increasing distance from the vessel wall.

Normal Hematocrit

Radial Dispersion

At hematocrits greater than 20%, effects due to the continual collisions between the red cells and their crowding in the suspension come into play. Here we are mainly concerned with the erratic displacements of cell paths in directions normal to that of the flow, as illustrated in FIGURE 1. The effect has been documented by using photo-optical techniques in which the suspensions are made transparent to light and a small quantity of visible particles then added to serve as tracers of the cell movements in the interior of the flowing system. In blood, transparency is achieved by use of

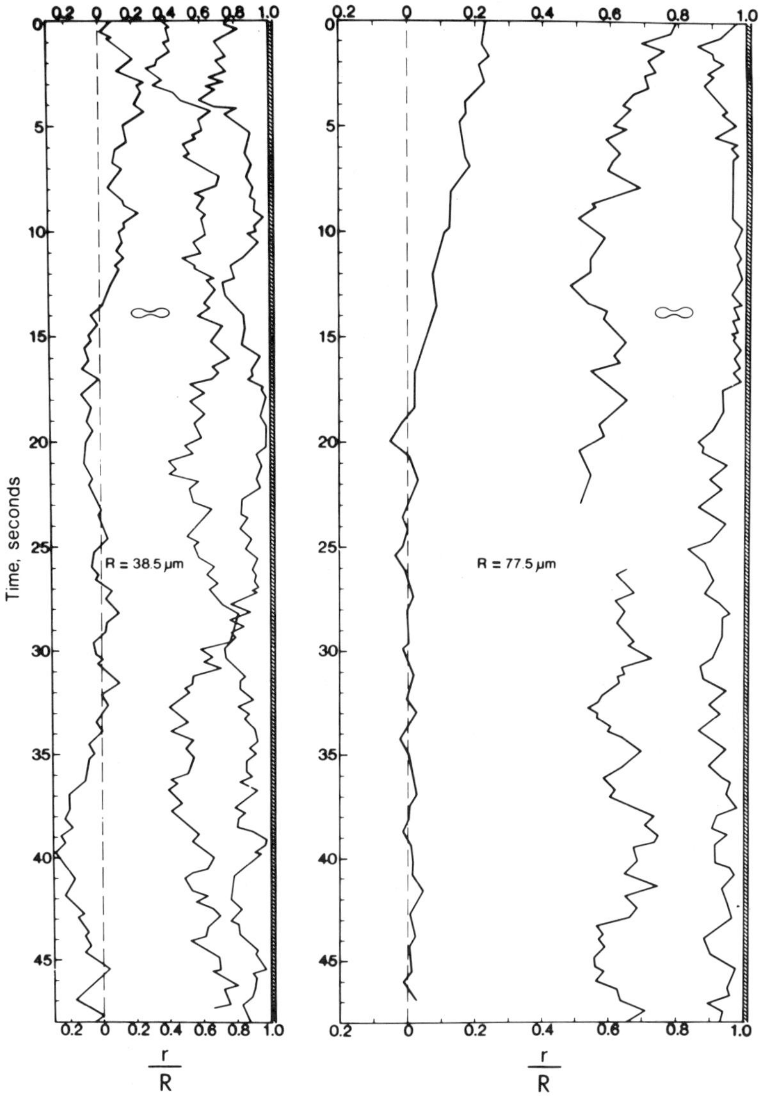

FIGURE 1. Radial displacements of tracer erythrocytes in a 40% ghost cell suspension in a 77-μm (*left*) and 155-μm (*right*) diameter tube. The cells situated in the region between $r = 0.4R$ and $0.8R$ appear to undergo the largest radial displacements. In the smaller tube, for the cell near the center at a mean $\bar{r}$ = 0.092R, the root mean square radial displacement $(\overline{\Delta r^2})^{1/2}$ = 2.0 μm; in the larger tube, for $\overline{\Delta r} = 0.076R$, $(\overline{\Delta r^2})^{1/2} = 1.62$ μm. The values of $\bar{r}/R$, and $(\overline{\Delta r^2})^{1/2}$ for the cells at the intermediate radial position were 0.583 and 3.32 μm, and 0.662 and 3.84 μm, in the 77 and 155 μm tubes, respectively. For the cells near the tube wall, the values were 0.830 and 2.96 μm, and 0.952 and 1.97 μm, respectively. (From Goldsmith and Marlow.[3] Reprinted with permission from the *Journal of Colloid and Interface Science*.)

reconstituted biconcave ghost cells in plasma with normal red cells, white cells, platelets or microspheres serving as tracers.[1,3]

One might have expected that in such a concentrated suspension the red cells would actually impede the diffusion of other cells and solutes. This is true when blood is stationary, but the opposite is observed in flow. The continued collisions between, and deformation of, the red cells in flowing blood actually lead to a continual radial displacement of their paths and an alternate method of solute mixing, similar on a macroscopic scale to the intermolecular collisions which result in Brownian motion.

By analogy with Brownian translational diffusion, a radial dispersion coefficient, D_r, obtained from the mean square radial distance $\overline{\Delta r^2}$ traveled by the particle in a time interval Δt can be calculated:

$$D_r = \frac{\overline{\Delta r^2}}{2\Delta t}. \tag{5}$$

This does not imply that the motions are considered to be random, as in Brownian diffusion, even though the paths in FIGURE 1 have the appearance of erratic random traces. The fluctuations in r are due to multibody collisions determined by the local velocity gradient, cell concentration, and deformation.

At local shear rates varying from 5 to 20 s^{-1} and ghostcrits from 20% to 70%, the values of the calculated radial dispersion coefficient ranged between 10^{-6} to 2×10^{-5} $mm^2 \cdot s^{-1}$ for red cells and 2-μm microspheres.[3] These values are one to two orders of magnitude greater than the translational Brownian diffusion coefficients for the blood cells.

FIGURE 2 shows calculated values of D_r for human red cells in 40–46% ghost cell suspensions as a function of the local shear rate, $G(\bar{r})$, the latter computed from the measured velocity distribution at the mean radial position, $\bar{r}$, of the sphere paths. Although there is appreciable scatter of the points, D_t is seen to increase markedly with $G(\bar{r})$. It appears that the paths of the cells situated at radial distances $0.4 < r/R < 0.8$ in the tube undergo the largest excursions (FIG. 1). Close to the wall, the excursions of the cell paths are smaller.

As a consequence of the radial dispersion of the red cells, white cells, and platelets, the frequency of wall encounters of the corpuscles increases with increasing hematocrit. In the case of the platelet, this has been correlated with the observed increased adhesion to subendothelium using denuded rabbit vessels in an annular perfusion chamber,[15,16] and to other surfaces using a spinning glass disk[17] and a Couette device[18] as the hematocrit is increased. The measured increase in diffusivity of platelets in blood as compared with that in plasma,[14] and the resulting increased cell-wall interactions, are of considerable importance in thrombotic processes as discussed in the succeeding section. Values of the dispersion, or effective platelet diffusion constant in whole blood, have been estimated to range from 3×10^{-5} to 8.6×10^{-4} $mm^2 \cdot s^{-1}$, *i.e.*, from 270 to 7700 times the Brownian diffusion constant, as the shear rate is increased from 50 to 10^4 s^{-1}.[16] According to equation **3**, these values would correspond to increases of 34 to 390 times in the diffusion-controlled adhesion of platelets. An even more striking increase in platelet adhesion to subendothelium with increasing hematocrit has been noted at the highest shear rate.[36] The extent to which erythrocyte deformation or size may affect the increase in the effective diffusion constant of cells and solute has also been studied. The transport of a molecular solute was found to increase slightly with both cell size and rigidity,[37] and the wall adhesion of platelets was observed to increase substantially with erythocyte size.[38]

Two other factors contribute to the enhancement of cell-wall encounters in flow through straight vessels.

Blunting of Velocity Profile

At hematocrits greater than 20%, the velocity distribution in vessels smaller than 200 μm diameter is no longer parabolic but blunted with a region of partial plug flow in the center where all the cells move with the same maximum velocity, u_M, which is less than the centerline velocity in Poiseuille flow, $u(0)$, at the same volume flow rate.[1,3] Near the wall, cell velocities are greater than those in Poiseuille flow, and the wall shear rate, G_W, is greater than that, $G(R)$, in Poiseuille flow. As shown in TABLE 1, model experiments with ghost cell suspensions reveal that the ratio $G_W/G(R)$ increases with increasing hematocrit, and with decreasing tube radius and flow rate. Such

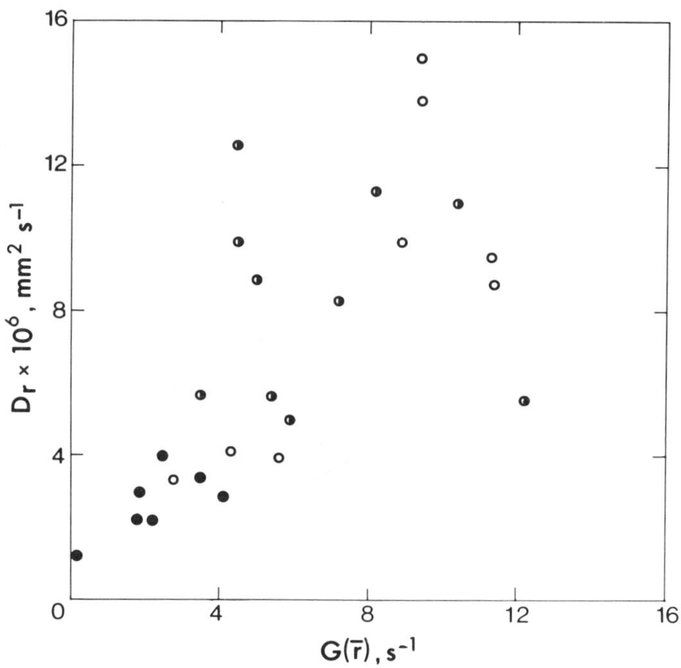

FIGURE 2. Radial dispersion coefficient, D_r, of tracer red blood cells in various ghost cell suspensions as a function of the shear rate, $G(\bar{r})$, at the mean radial position of the cell path. The ghost cell volume concentrations are: ○ = 47%; ● = 46%; ◑ = 40%. (From Goldsmith and Marlow.[3] Reprinted with permission from the *Journal of Colloid and Interface Science.*)

increases in the wall shear rate would only occur in the smallest arteries and only result in a 10–30% increase in the wall flux of platelets (equation **3**).

Redistribution of Platelets and White Cells

In addition to disturbing the motion of the other formed elements in blood, red cells appear to affect the distribution of white cells and platelets because of their more rapid radial migration away from the wall and aggregation in the core of the vessel where

TABLE 1. Centerline Velocities and Wall Shear Rates in Ghost Cell Suspensions

R (μm)	Ghostcrit (%)	u_M[a] ($mm \cdot s^{-1}$)	$u_M/u(0)$[b]	G_W[c] (s^{-1})	$G_W/G(R)$
41.8	73.0	0.213	0.679	65	4.3
41.8	48.7	0.279	0.777	28	1.6
41.8	24.3	0.251	0.815	15	1.1
75.4	74.5	0.063	0.719	7.5	3.2
75.4	49.7	0.061	0.736	5.0	2.2
75.4	24.8	0.074	0.870	3.0	1.3
77.5	64.2	0.189	0.723	20	3.0
42.6	64.7	0.236	0.748	60	4.1
42.6	64.7	0.236	0.748	60	4.1
42.6	64.7	3.465	0.787	505	2.4
75.4	49.7	0.061	0.736	5.0	2.2
75.4	49.7	4.025	0.832	180	1.4

[a]Measured tracer red cell centerline velocity.
[b]Ratio of measured centerline velocity to that in Poiseuille flow at the same volume flow rate.
[c]Measured wall shear rate.

shear rates are very low. The redistribution of platelets in whole blood occurs toward the vessel periphery: their concentration at a radial distance $r > 0.7R$ in 25 μm diameter arterioles is found to be twice that at the vessel center.[39] Similar results have been obtained in 100-μm glass tubes[34,40] and in a parallel flow chamber of 250 μm thickness.[41] Here platelet wall concentrations up to five times those in the bulk blood have been reported. This would lead to a fivefold increase in platelet wall flux (equation **3**). The extent to which such platelet redistribution occurs in larger vessels is not known.

The redistribution of white cells toward the vessel periphery, the so-called margination, is associated with low blood-flow states such as occur in shock and inflammation. At high flow rates in whole blood, white cells are found to have migrated away from the vessel wall.[35,42,43] However, when the red cells are caused to aggregate by addition of fibrinogen[42] or high molecular weight dextran,[43] or by reducing the flow rate,[35,43] white cells accumulate at the vessel periphery. This effect has been shown to be due to the outward displacement to the periphery of white cells by the inwardly migrating network of packed red cell rouleaux, which exclude plasma containing both white cells and platelets.[35]

CONVECTIVE TRANSPORT TO THE WALL

Investigators from the biomedical as well as the physical and engineering sciences have long been aware of the connection between the occurrence of localized arterial wall injury, especially at bifurcations, T-junctions, and curved segments, and the disturbed patterns of flow at such sites.[44] Rapid changes in the rate and/or direction of fluid motion in branching and curved vessels have been held responsible for bringing about alterations and injury, not only to the endothelium[45–47] and the media,[48] but also the corpuscles.[49] This, in turn, could lead to the aggregation and adhesion of the cells to the injured vessel wall. The question here is whether disturbed patterns of flow lead to increased, localized interactions of blood cells with the vessel wall. To obtain answers to this question, we were motivated to embark on a series of microrheological studies of the flow behavior of blood cells in idealized models of stenoses[4–6] and T-junctions[7,8] as well as in fixed transparent segments of natural arteries and veins.[9–12]

Disturbed Flow

We use the term "disturbed flow" to describe a flow regime that is neither laminar nor turbulent, such as is encountered at stenoses, branches, and curved segments of vessels. In these regions secondary fluid motions develop in directions away from that of the primary flow, and often there is separation of the streamlines from the vessel wall, with the formation of a vortex or a recirculation zone between the forward flowing mainstream and the wall.

A good example of such flow is provided by the annular vortex at a sudden tubular expansion, which we have used to study the flow behavior and wall interactions of blood cells.

Model Studies in an Annular Vortex

An example of the flow pattern observed in steady flow through a tubular expansion of a 150-μm into a 500-μm glass tube at a Reynolds number of 12 (based on upstream tube diameter and mean velocity) is shown in FIGURE 3. During a single orbit, the measured paths and velocities of the red cells in a dilute suspension within the vortex were in good agreement with those predicted by theory applicable to the fluid.[4,50] However, over longer periods of time, some interesting phenomena not predicted by

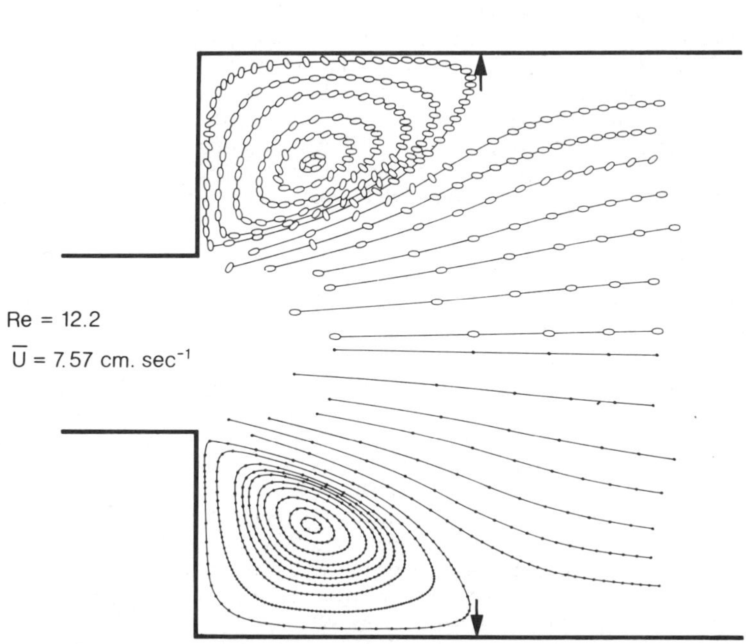

FIGURE 3. Flow separation as a dilute suspension of glutaraldehyde-fixed red cells enters a sudden concentric expansion of vessel lumen from 150 to 500 μm at an inflow Reynolds number, Re = 12.2, based on the mean upstream velocity, $\bar{U}$. The region of flow separation is an annular vortex. The streamlines traced out by the red cells and the cell orientations in the orbits of the vortex are shown in the lower and upper halves respectively. The *arrows* indicate the reattachment points of the flow. (From Karino and Goldsmith.[4] Reprinted with permission from the *Philosophical Transactions of the Royal Society of London.*)

theory were observed. Thus, single red cells and platelets, as well as aggregates $<20\ \mu m$ in diameter migrated outward across the closed streamlines of the vortex predicted by theory, and eventually rejoined the mainstream. Aggregates of cells $>30\ \mu m$ diameter, however, remained trapped within the vortex. In the case of citrated or heparinized platelet-rich plasma (PRP), shear-induced collisions between cells circulating in the orbits of the vortex resulted in the spontaneous formation and growth of aggregates which then became trapped.[5] In a given suspension, the formation and growth of platelet aggregates could only be observed in a narrow range of Reynolds numbers (based on upstream linear velocity and tube diameter), which varied from suspension to suspension. Thus, in heparinized platelet-rich plasma containing many sphered platelets with pseudopods and some microaggregates of 2–6 cells, the rate and extent of aggregation were the highest, large elongated, freely suspended aggregates $>100\ \mu m$ in length being observed to form in less than 1 min and within the widest range of Re, between 4.5 and 17. In citrated PRP and washed platelet suspensions, in which no microaggregates were seen prior to flow, the degree of aggregation was much reduced. However, when platelets in these suspensions were activated with subthreshold concentrations of ADP or thrombin, the large aggregates seen in heparinized PRP were again formed. When the above suspensions were subjected to pulsatile flow in the expansion tube, there was a marked decrease in the number and size of the aggregates. Presumably this was due to the continuously changing orbits of particles during the alternate expansion and contraction of the vortex, which shortened their residence times, as well as to the large variation in the shear rate in each cycle beyond the range favorable for platelet aggregation.

In red cell suspensions, at hematocrits from 15% to 45%, migration of single red cells out of the vortex still occurred and resulted in the lowering of the hematocrit in the vortex both in steady and pulsatile flow. In heparinized whole blood it was evident that, after the vortex had partially emptied of red cells, several large platelet thrombi, 50–150 μm diameter, had formed and were circulating in the vortex while others had adhered to the tube wall, a phenomenon never seen in PRP.[5] In citrated whole blood large thrombi were not observed, but platelets and smaller platelet aggregates adhered to the wall.

That wall adhesion of platelets is localized in the vortex was subsequently shown in a study of the initial adhesion of the cells to collagen fibers coating the inner wall of a larger expansion flow tube (0.92 into 3.0 mm diameter).[6] As illustrated in FIGURE 4, it was convincingly shown that platelet adhesion was localized within the vortex and downstream on either side of the reattachment point with a local minimum at the reattachment point itself. Furthermore, platelet adhesion increased, and both adhesion peaks became more pronounced, as the hematocrit increased. There was a five-fold increase in platelet adhesion density at the two peaks, as well as in the total number of platelets adhering in the vortex as the hematocrit increased from 11.5% to 50%. Surprisingly, however, as illustrated in FIGURE 5, the adhesion peak in the vortex decreased and flattened out as the Reynolds number increased. These results are inconsistent with a diffusion-controlled platelet adhesion (equation **3**), which should show an increase in adhesion number density with increasing shear rate. It appears that the particular flow pattern within the vortex is responsible for this localization. Thus, as illustrated in the upper panel of FIGURE 6, only those cells carried by the curved streamlines to within one particle radius of the surface interact with the vessel wall and adhere to it on both sides of the reattachment point, which is also a stagnation point.[6] It should be noted that here the two mechanisms of cell wall interactions reinforce each other. The increase in localized platelet adhesion with increasing hematocrit is due to the fact that the number of cells carried by the curved streamlines to within one particle radius of the surface increases with the hematocrit as the enhanced radial motion of the platelets permits collisions of cells with the surface at distances greater than one particle radius.

It follows from this that platelet adhesion onto the vessel wall, whether it be the natural endothelium or an artificial surface, will be localized wherever there is a stagnation point (or a reattachment point if it is a result of flow separation) where blood cells are carried by the flow toward the vessel wall along curved streamlines having a pronounced radial velocity component. If this mechanism operates in the circulation a relatively higher adhesion of platelets, and hence a higher risk of thrombus formation, is predictable, not only in regions of disturbed flow (adhesion peaks on either side of the reattachment point) such as downstream of aortic and

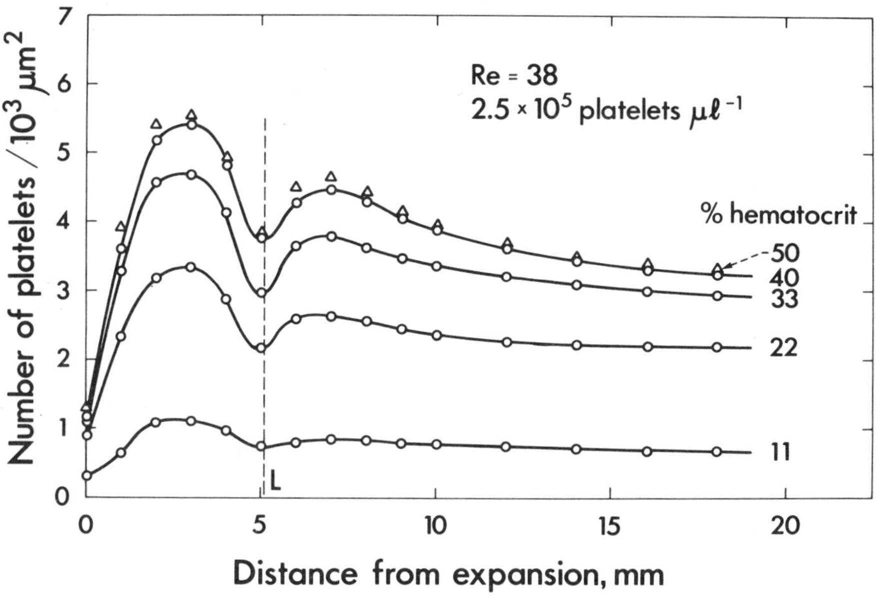

FIGURE 4. Plot of the measured number density of adhering platelets as a function of axial distance from the origin of an expansion of an 0.92-mm into a 3.0-mm glass tube. The figure shows the localized enhanced adhesion of platelets on either side of the reattachment point at *L*, indicated by the *vertical dashed line,* and the effect of hematocrit on the phenomenon. (From Karino and Goldsmith.[6] Reprinted with permission from *Microvascular Research.*)

venous valves, mural thrombi, and stenoses, but also in all the branching arteries at the flow divider where there is a stagnation point.

One example of such flow is given below; others will be found in the paper by Karino *et al.* in this volume.[51]

Model Studies in T-Junctions

Flow patterns and distributions of fluid velocity and shear rate were studied in 3-mm diameter glass models of T-junctions with branching angles from 30° to 135°

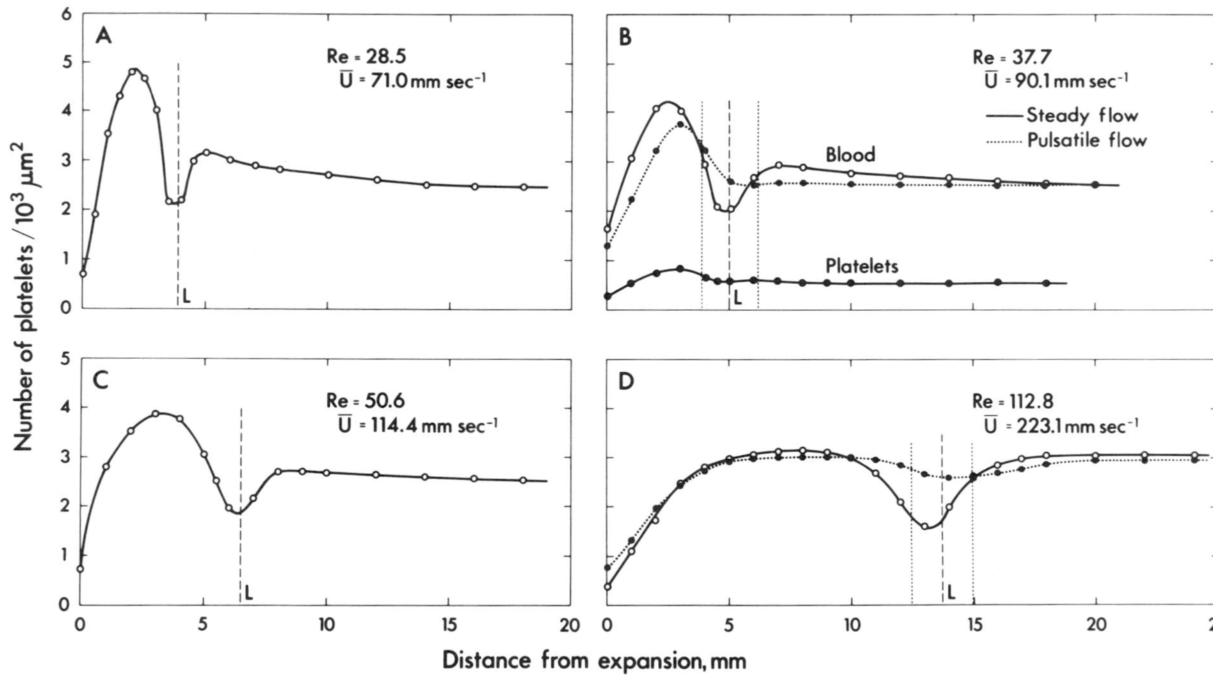

FIGURE 5. Plot, as in FIGURE 4, of the measured number density of platelets for blood of 20% hematocrit at increasing Reynolds number Re (based on upstream mean velocity $\overline{U}$) in steady as well as in pulsatile flow. Note that the adhesion peaks on either side of the reattachment point, *L*, decrease with increasing Re, and that, at a given Re in steady flow, the secondary peak levels off as an oscillatory flow is superimposed and the reattachment point oscillates between the positions shown by the dotted lines. (From Karino and Goldsmith.[6] Reprinted by permission from *Microvascular Research*.)

and side to main tube diameter ratios from 0.33 to 1.0, over a wide range of inflow Reynolds numbers Re_0 and branch to parent tube flow ratios, Q_1/Q_0.[7,8] FIGURE 7 shows the flow pattern obtained by photographing and then tracing the motions of 50 μm diameter latex spheres in a 60° uniform diameter T-junction with flow equally divided between main and side branch. A large recirculation zone, consisting of a pair of spiral secondary flows on both sides of the common median plane of the T-junction, was

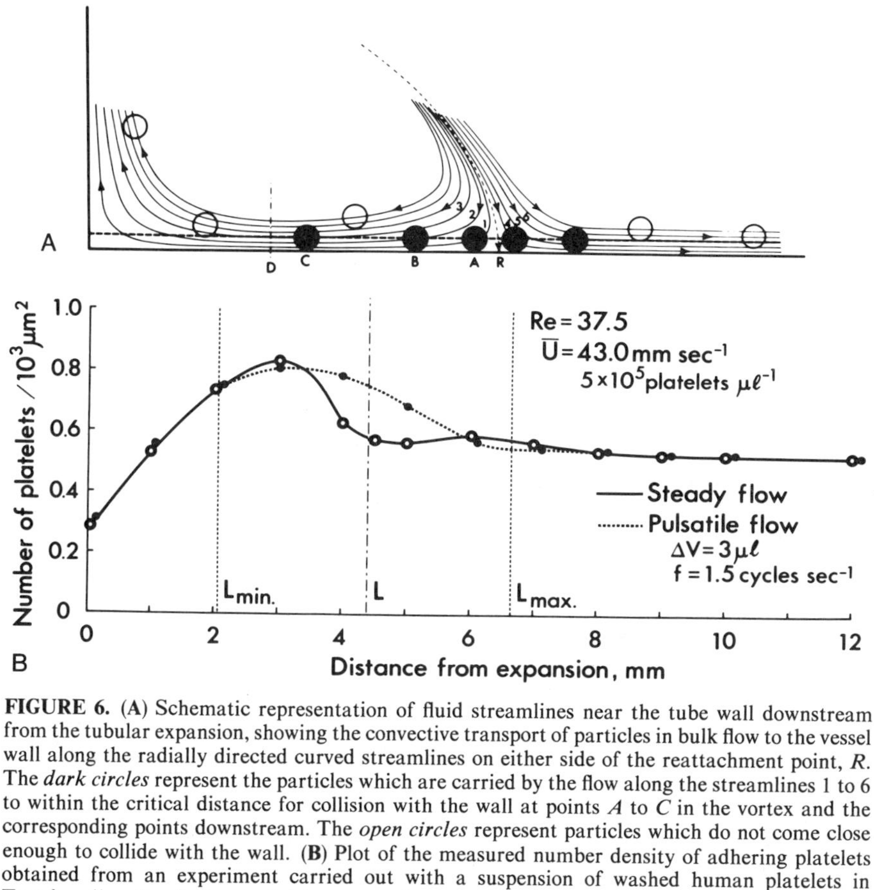

FIGURE 6. (**A**) Schematic representation of fluid streamlines near the tube wall downstream from the tubular expansion, showing the convective transport of particles in bulk flow to the vessel wall along the radially directed curved streamlines on either side of the reattachment point, *R*. The *dark circles* represent the particles which are carried by the flow along the streamlines 1 to 6 to within the critical distance for collision with the wall at points *A* to *C* in the vortex and the corresponding points downstream. The *open circles* represent particles which do not come close enough to collide with the wall. (**B**) Plot of the measured number density of adhering platelets obtained from an experiment carried out with a suspension of washed human platelets in Tyrodes-albumin solution containing no erythrocytes. The figure shows the relationship between the flow pattern and the degree of platelet adhesion in, and downstream from, the vortex in steady and in pulsatile flow when the reattachment point oscillates between the position L_{min} and L_{max}. (From Karino and Goldsmith.[52] Reprinted with permission from *Biorheology*.)

formed in the main tube (due to the sudden deceleration of fluid velocity as a portion of the flow is drawn off into the side tube) and a small, secondary recirculation zone was formed in the side tube (due to the sudden change in direction of the fluid which continues to move to the outside of the 60° corner, toward the flow divider). Particles entering the large recirculation zone described orbits in which the spheres circulated once. Some rejoined the flow through the main tube and others entered the side branch in a paired, spiral secondary flow with pronounced radial components; some of these circulated through the secondary recirculation zone. When the main tube was gradually occluded, the depth and size of the main vortex increased. When the flow rate ratio was reversed so that 80% of the flow left through the main tube, the main vortex disappeared, and a sizeable vortex formed in the side tube.

By varying the branching angle it was shown that the critical Re_0 for the formation of the main recirculation zone was lowest at 90° for all Q_1/Q_0, whereas for the side recirculation zone it decreased as the branching angle increased from 45° to 135°.

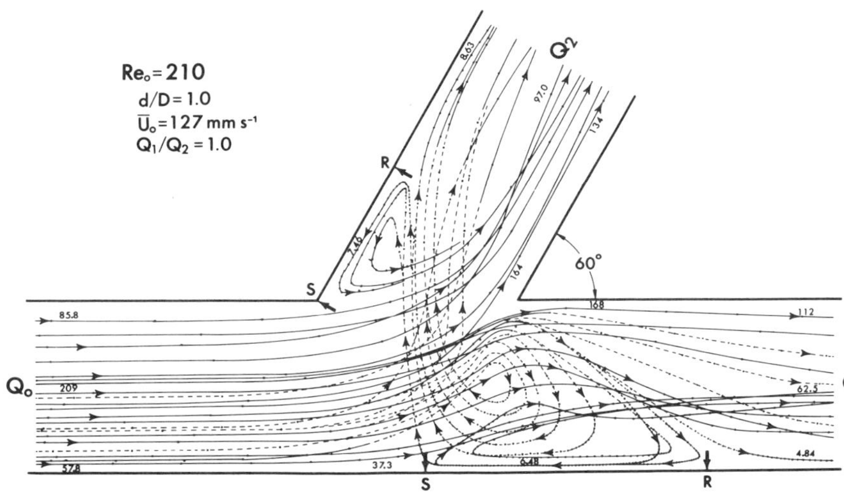

FIGURE 7. Flow patterns in the common median plane of a model 3-mm diameter 60° glass T-junction, as indicated by the paths of tracer 50-μm polystyrene spheres in aqueous glycerol. The suspension enters at the left with a mean velocity $\bar{U}_0$ (tube Reynolds number = Re_0), and flow is equally divided between main and side branches. The T-junction, made by fitting and gluing together two pieces of glass tubing, has a very low radius of curvature at the corner opposite the flow divider, as well as at the flow divider. This results in a small recirculation zone at the corner at the entry of the side tube filled with fluid from the main large recirculation zone in the parent vessel. The points are measured particle positions at intervals of 22 ms; the numbers indicate velocities in mm · s^{-1}. The *solid lines* represent particles traveling in, or close to, the median plane, the *dashed lines* those closer to the tube wall. The arrows at *S* and *R* indicate the respective points where flow first separates and then reattaches to the wall (From Karino and Goldsmith.[8] Reprinted with permission from *Biorheology*.)

When the diameter of the side tube was decreased, the paired spiral secondary flows of the main recirculation zone became smaller and were confined to a thin layer adjacent to the tube wall, wrapped around the mainstream.[8]

The effect of radius of curvature of the walls at the junction was studied by comparing the critical inflow Reynolds numbers and size of the recirculation zones in a square T-junction (radii of curvature <2% of tube radius) with that in a rounded T-junction (radii of curvature ~ tube radius).[7] It was found that the recirculation zone in the side tube formed at a much lower Re_0 in the square than in the rounded junction, and that at a given Re_0 and Q_1/Q_0, a larger main recirculation zone existed in the rounded junction. It appears that the formation of the side recirculation zone is largely affected by curvature of the wall at the bend opposite to the flow divider, while that of the main recirculation zone is largely affected by the curvature at the flow divider.

Results of studies of flow patterns in dog aortic T-junctions[9,10] have shown that the characteristic flow patterns described above in the model T-junctions will occur *in vivo* under physiologically representative conditions. However, instead of a large main standing recirculation zone, as in the glass models, there is only a pair of small recirculation zones confined to a thin layer close to the wall surrounding the mainstream. This is due to the sharp curvature of the bend at the flow divider and a reduction in the diameter of the aorta distal to each of the junctions. There is no side recirculation zone, no doubt due to the gentle curvature of the bend opposite the flow divider. These characteristics were shared by all the aortic T-junctions studied, and from the results obtained in the glass model T-junctions, represent the optimum condition for minimizing the size of both regions of separated flow. Nevertheless, the curved streamlines of the recirculation zone and the secondary flows will bring blood cells towards the vessel wall in a region around the flow divider and in the side branch on the outer wall.

Thus, the flow patterns described above would lead one to expect increased platelet flux to, and deposition on the wall of, the parent vessel around the reattachment point and on either side of the flow divider in 90° and acute angle T-junctions. Of the preferential areas for atherosclerosis and thrombosis clinically found in man and experimental animals,[19,20] the vessel wall around the flow divider is clearly implicated, and to a lesser extent the outer wall (hip) of the side branch.

ACKNOWLEDGMENTS

We thank Diane Chajczyk and Samira Spain for their excellent technical assistance and Pamela Lilley for typing the manuscript.

REFERENCES

1. GOLDSMITH, H. L. 1971. Red cell motions and wall interactions in tube flow. Fed. Proc. **30:** 1578–1588.
2. GOLDSMITH, H. L. & J. MARLOW. 1972. Flow behaviour of erythrocytes. I. Rotation and deformation in dilute suspensions. Proc. R. Soc. Ser. B. **182:** 351–384.
3. GOLDSMITH, H. L. & J. MARLOW. 1979. Flow behavior of erythrocytes. II. Particle motions in concentrated suspensions of ghost cells. J. Colloid Interface Sci. **71:** 383–407.
4. KARINO, T. & H. L. GOLDSMITH. 1977. Flow behaviour of blood cells and rigid spheres in an annular vortex. Phil. Trans. R. Soc. Ser. B. **279:** 413–445.
5. KARINO, T. & H. L. GOLDSMITH. 1979. Aggregation of human platelets in an annular vortex distal to a tubular expansion. Microvasc. Res. **17:** 217–237.
6. KARINO, T. & H. L. GOLDSMITH. 1979. Adhesion of human platelets to collagen on the wall distal to a tubular expansion. Microvasc. Res. **17:** 238–262.
7. KARINO, T., H. M. KWONG & H. L. GOLDSMITH. 1979. Particle flow behavior in models of branching vessels. I. Vortices in 90° T-junctions. Biorheology **16:** 231–248.
8. KARINO, T. & H. L. GOLDSMITH. 1984. Particle flow behavior in models of branching vessels. II. Effects of branching angle and diameter ratio on flow patterns. Biorheology **22:** 87–102.
9. KARINO, T. & M. MOTOMIYA. 1983. Flow visualization in isolated transparent natural blood vessels. Biorheology **20:** 119–127.
10. KARINO, T., M. MOTOMIYA & H. L. GOLDSMITH. 1982. Flow patterns in model and natural

vessels. *In* Biologic and Synthetic Vascular Prostheses. J. C. Stanley, Ed.: 153–178. Grune & Stratton. New York.

11. MOTOMIYA, M. & T. KARINO. 1984. Flow patterns in the human carotid artery bifurcation. Stroke **15:** 50–56.
12. KARINO, T. & M. MOTOMIYA. 1984. Flow through a venous valve and its implication in thrombogenesis. Thromb. Res. **36:** 245–257.
13. GOLDSMITH, H. L. & S. G. MASON. 1975. Some model experiments in hemodynamics. V. Microrheological techniques. Biorheology **12:** 181–192.
14. TURITTO, V. T., A. M. BENIS & E. F. LEONARD. 1972. Platelet diffusion in flowing blood. Ind. Eng. Chem. Fund. **11:** 216–223.
15. TURITTO, V. T. & H. BAUMGARTNER. 1975. Platelet interaction with subendothelium in a perfusion system: Physical role of red cells. Microvasc. Res. **9:** 335–344.
16. TURITTO, V. T. & H. J. WEISS. 1980. Red cells: Their dual role in thrombus formation. Science **207:** 541–543.
17. GRABOWSKI, E. F., L. I. FRIEDMAN & E. F. LEONARD. 1972. Effects of shear rate on the diffusion and adhesion of blood platelets to a foreign surface. Ind. Eng. Chem. Fund. **11:** 224–232.
18. BRASH, J. L., J. M. BROPHY & I. A. FEUERSTEIN. 1976. Adhesion of platelets to artificial surfaces: Effects of red cells. J. Biomed. Res. **10:** 429–443.
19. FLAHERTY, J. T., V. J. FERRANS, J. E. PIERCE, T. E. CAREN & D. L. FRY. 1972. Localization factors in experimental atherosclerosis. *In* Atherosclerosis and Coronary Heart Disease. W. Likoff, B. E. Segal, W. Insule & J. H. Moyer, Eds.: 40–104. Grune & Stratton. New York.
20. CORNHILL, J. F. & M. R. ROACH. 1976. A quantitative study of the localization of atherosclerotic lesions in the rabbit aorta. Atherosclerosis **23:** 489–501.
21. ZARINS, C. K., D. P. GIDDENS, B. K. BHARADVAJ, V. S. SCOTTIURAI, R. F. MABON & S. GLAGOV. 1983. Carotid bifurcation atherosclerosis: Quantitative correlation of plaque localization with flow velocity profiles and shear stresses. Circ. Res. **53:** 502–514.
22. GOLDSMITH, H. L. & S. G. MASON. 1962. The flow of suspensions through tubes. I. Single spheres, rods and discs. J. Colloid. Sci. **17:** 448–476.
23. MCDONALD, D. A. 1974. *In* Blood Flow in Arteries. 2nd edit. Williams & Wilkins. Baltimore.
24. GOLDSMITH, H. L. & V. T. TURITTO. 1986. Rheological aspects of thrombosis and haemostasis: Basic principles and applications. Thromb. Haemostas. **55:** 415–435.
25. EINSTEIN, A. 1956. The Theory of the Brownian Movement. Dover Publications. New York.
26. BRENNER, H. 1974. Rheology of a dilute suspension of axi-symmetric Brownian particles. Int. J. Multiphase Flow **1:** 195–341.
27. FROJMOVIC, M. M., M. NEWTON & H. L. GOLDSMITH. 1976. The microrheology of mammalian platelets: Studies of rheological transients and flow in tubes. Microvasc. Res. **11:** 203–215.
28. MALYSA, K. & T. G. M. VAN DE VEN. 1986. Rotational and translational motion of a sphere parallel to a wall. Int. J. Multiphase Flow **12:** 459–468.
29. LEVICH, V. G. 1962. *In* Physiocochemical Hydrodynamics. Prentice-Hall. Englewood Cliffs, NJ. pp. 112–116.
30. FRIEDMAN, L. I. & E. F. LEONARD. 1971. Platelet adhesion to artificial surfaces: Consequences of flow, exposure time, blood condition, and surface nature. Fed. Proc. **30:** 1641–1646.
31. TURITTO, V. T. & H. R. BAUMGARTNER. 1975. Platelet deposition on subendothelium exposed to flowing blood: Mathematical analysis of physical parameters. Trans. Am. Soc. Artif. Intern. Organs **21:** 593–600.
32. SEGRÉ, S. & A. SILBERBERG. 1962. Behaviour of macroscopic rigid spheres in Poiseuille flow. II. Experimental results and interpretation. J. Fluid Mech. **14:** 136–157.
33. PALMER, A. A. 1967. Platelet and leukocyte skimming. Bibliotheca Anat. **9:** 300–303.
34. BECK, M. R. & E. C. ECKSTEIN. 1980. Preliminary report on platelet concentration in capillary tube flows of whole blood. Biorheology **17:** 455–464.
35. GOLDSMITH, H. L. & S. SPAIN. 1984. Margination of leucocytes in blood flow through small tubes. Microvasc. Res. **28:** 204–222.

36. TURITTO, V. T. 1982. Viscosity, transport and thrombogenesis. *In* Progress in Hemostasis and Thrombosis, Vol. 6. T. H. Spaet, Ed.: 139–201. Grune & Stratton. New York.
37. WANG, N. H. & K. H. KELLER. 1979. Solute transport induced by erythrocyte motions in shear flow. Trans. Am. Soc. Artif. Intern. Organs **25:** 14–17.
38. AARTS, P. A., P. A. BOLHUIS, K. S. SAKARIASSEN, R. M. HEETHAR & J. J. SIXMA. 1983. Red blood cell size is important for adhesion of blood platelets to artery subendothelium. Blood **62:** 214–217.
39. TANGELDER, G. J., D. W. SLAAF, H. C. TEIRLINCK, R. ALWEIJNSE & R. S. RENEMAN. 1982. Localization within thin optical sections of fluorescent blood platelets flowing in a microvessel. Microvasc. Res. **23:** 214–230.
40. CORATTIYL, V. & E. C. ECKSTEIN. 1986. Regional platelet concentration in blood flow through capillary tubes. Microvasc. Res. **32:** 261–270.
41. BLACKSHEAR, P. L., K. W. BARTELT & R. J. FORSTROM. 1977. Fluid dynamic factors affecting particle capture and retention. Ann. N.Y. Acad. Sci. **283:** 270–279.
42. VEJLENS, G. 1938. The distribution of leukocytes in the vascular system. Acta Pathol. Microbiol. Scand. Suppl. **33:** 11–239.
43. NOBIS, V., A. R. FRIES & P. GÄHTGENS. 1982. Rheological mechanisms contributing to WBC-margination. *In* White Blood Cells: Morphology and Rheology Related to Function. U. Bagge, G. V. R. Born & P. Gähtgens, Eds.: 57–65. Martinus Nijhoff. The Hague, Boston.
44. GOLDSMITH, H. L. & T. KARINO. 1978. Mechanically induced thromboemboli. *In* Quantitative Cardiovascular Studies: Clinical and Research Applications. N. H. C. Hwang, D. R. Gross & D. J. Patel, Eds.: 289–351. University Park Press. Baltimore.
45. REIDY, M. A. & D. E. BOWYER. 1977. Scanning electron microscopy of arteries: The morphology of aortic endothelium in hemodynamically stressed areas associated with branches. Atherosclerosis **26:** 181–194.
46. GLAGOV, S. 1972. Hemodynamic risk factors: Mechanical stress, mural architecture, medial nutrition and the vulnerability of arteries to atherosclerosis, Chap. 6. *In* The Pathogenesis of Atherosclerosis. R. W. Wissler & J. C. Geer, Eds.: Williams & Wilkins. Baltimore.
47. FRY, D. L. 1977. Hemodynamic forces in atherogenesis. *In* Cardiovascular Diseases. P. Scheinberg, Ed.: 77–95. Raven. New York.
48. ROACH, M. R. 1977. The effect of bifurcation and stenosis on arterial disease. *In* Cardiovascular Flow Dynamics and Measurements. N. H. C. Hwang & N. A. Normann, Eds.: 489–541. University Park Press. Baltimore.
49. MUSTARD, J. F. & M. A. PACKHAM. 1975. The role of blood and platelets in atherosclerosis and the complications of atherosclerosis. Thromb. Diath. Haemorrh. **33:** 444–456.
50. MACAGNO, E. O. & T. K. HUNG. 1967. Computational and experimental study of a captive annular eddy. J. Fluid Mech. **28:** 43–64.
51. KARINO, T., H. L. GOLDSMITH, M. MOTOMIYA, S. MABUCHI & Y. SOHARA. 1986. Flow patterns in vessels of simple and complex geometries. This volume.
52. KARINO, T. & H. L. GOLDSMITH. 1984. Role of blood-cell wall interactions in thrombogenesis and atherogenesis: A microrheological study. Biorheology **21:** 587–601.

Video Microscopic and Immunochemical Evaluation of Cells at Surfaces[a]

IRWIN A. FEUERSTEIN

Departments of Chemical Engineering and Pathology
McMaster University
Hamilton, Ontario, Canada L8S 4L7

INTRODUCTION

Blood contact with nonbiological surfaces has been studied in various ways with both *in vitro* and *in vivo* protocols.[1,2] Early experimentation frequently dealt with measurements of thrombus mass and time spans for occlusion of conduits to occur. These results circumscribed the magnitude of the problem and indicated that material properties and flow parameters were important features of the process.

It was recognized that protein adsorption occurred before cell contact and that fibrin formation was both surface dependent and flow dependent.[1,2] High flow rates resulted in low fibrin deposition. Workers then focused on the several components of blood contact independently and in controlled ways. Several large bodies of work emerged that fall into a number of well-defined categories: (1) adsorption of single plasma proteins to solid substrates; (2) adhesion of single cell types, mainly platelets; and (3) plasma interaction with solids where an indication of clotting time was sought. Continuing efforts with proteins have led to studies of protein mixtures, exchange of proteins between the surface-bound and solution states, and the dependence of adsorbed protein molecule type on surface chemistry.[3]

The importance of flow conditions as key variables to control came out of several studies that pointed out the role of transport phenomena (diffusion and convection) in blood contact.[4-6] The role of the red cell as a physical mover of platelets and proteins to surfaces was elucidated along with the idea of a dispersion coefficient (same units as a diffusion coefficient) to characterize such transport.[7-9] Thus, the meaningfulness of experiments dealing with adsorption of proteins and adhesion of cells done in the absence of flow and red cells could be questioned.

The protein coating, the cells on the surface, and the moving fluid adjacent to the surface may be viewed as a system of interacting components. A number of time-dependent dynamic events may occur with this system. Of these, the adhesion and detachment of platelets is one such important event since detached platelets are likely to be altered from their normal, unstimulated state. Also, those cells remaining for longer times may alter or remove the protein between them and the solid surface and that protein adjacent to the cell. These topics form the subject of this paper.

PLATELET-SURFACE DYNAMICS SEEN WITH FLUORESCENT VIDEO MICROSCOPY

Microscopic observations of cell-surface contacts in the presence of physiological hematocrit, 35–45%, are not feasible with transmitted light. To overcome this problem,

[a]This work was supported by grants from the Heart and Stroke Foundation of Ontario and the Natural Sciences and Engineering Research Council of Canada.

a system utilizing video microscopy of fluorescently labeled platelets was developed. This required the inclusion of a video camera capable of low light level detection. Platelet adhesion to protein-coated substrates has been studied using whole blood, whole blood with anticoagulant and with suspensions of washed platelets, and red cells in a physiological medium. In order to maintain the surface concentration integrity of a precoated protein substrate and avoid the difficult-to-control action of thrombin on the substrate and platelets, washed cells in a solution containing Ca^{2+} and Mg^{2+} offer a good experimental alternative. The presence of Ca^{2+} and Mg^{2+} at physiological concentrations is an important condition for optimal physiological platelet function.[10] Washed suspension systems also provide a means for minimizing the presence of background fluorescence in the fluid phase. Anticoagulants that sequester divalent cations and heparin, which often has unpredictable effects on platelets, are other alternatives.

The measurements made with fluorescent video microscopy result from a microscope objective focused on the inner surface of a glass tube having a wall thickness approximating that of a coverslip. Fluorescently labeled platelets may be viewed only when they are attached to the surface of the glass tube. The small depth of field of the objective, the lack of resolution of the video camera with respect to time, and the ability of red cells to block incident and emitted fluorescent light are responsible for this finding. Two fluorescent dyes have been used; these are (1) mepacrine which is actively taken up and stored in the dense granules of platelets, and (2) carboxyfluorescein diacetate which is lipophilic promoting its passage into the cytosol where it is enzymatically converted to a polar compound. Both dyes are compatible with the optical components used for fluorescein. Platelets are labeled in suspension after separation from plasma and other cells and washed after labeling. Aggregation tests with low concentrations of ADP and thrombin show these platelets, labeled with either dye, to be as responsive as control suspensions.[11,12] The flow system used is one in which a stagnant suspension of platelets and red cells is drawn through a vertically mounted tube by a syringe pump. The measurement region is located 0.5 cm downstream from the glass tube's entrance (1.3 mm i.d.).

A video camera with a silicon intensifier target (SIT) tube was used to prepare video tapes, which were analyzed one frame at a time (the time between frames is 33 ms). The location and arrival and detachment time of each cell were recorded. Notations were made of the movement of cells to new positions on the surface and a record was made of unoccupied grid spaces that had previously contained cells. The surfaces examined were albumin- and fibrinogen-precoated glass. Exposure times to flow were kept short, 1–4 min, in order to minimize the effects of protein desorption and exchange.

Studies on fibrinogen-coated glass were done at wall shear rates of 40 s^{-1}, 80 s^{-1}, and 944 s^{-1}.[13] Data were reduced in order to give absolute rates of arrival and detachment and a net rate of adhesion as well as adhesion efficiencies, which are normalized quantities based on 100 platelets. Comparisons of the platelet arrival rates and net rates of adhesion among the three flow rates studied show a three- to fourfold increase even over the shear rate range. This phenomena is likely to be at least in part a result of the nonlinear increase in the transfer of platelets through the motions of rotating and translating red cells. The detachment rate of cells from the measurement region is greater at 944 s^{-1} than at 40 or 80 s^{-1}. Although these rates are small relative to the convective input of platelets into the glass tube, they may be important if they represent the rates of damaged cells returning to the circulation.

The efficiency for permanent adhesion on first contact is maximum at 80 s^{-1} (comparison with 40 s^{-1} and 944 s^{-1}) while the percentages of arriving cells moving to new positions and departing from the measurement region are minimum at 80 s^{-1}. An overall balance, which includes movement of cells and adhesion at new sites, indicates a maximum in the efficiency for permanent adhesion at 80 s^{-1} and a minimum in the *percentage* of arriving platelets departing from the measurement region at that wall shear rate. The overall picture is thus one of 40–60% of platelets adhering on arrival with an additional 30% permanently adhering after several moves along the surface. It is possible to think of these data in terms of forces promoting adhesion and forces promoting cell removal. The "sum" of these forces appears to change with increasing shear rate such that adhesion is favored up to a point, while departure is favored as the flow rate is increased.[13]

Additional experiments were performed to compare fibrinogen- and albumin-coated glass with respect to the details of the platelet adhesion process.[14] Using purified forms of fibrinogen and albumin it was demonstrated with ^{51}Cr-labeled platelets that the net rates of adhesion of platelets to these proteins are equal. The next task was to determine if the pathways leading to this were the same. Using video microscopy of mepacrine-labeled platelets, we found a difference in the pathways. At a wall shear rate of 80 s^{-1}, the percentage of platelets that adhere permanently on first contact is less on albumin than on fibrinogen, whereas the percentage of platelets that move to new positions is greater for albumin than for fibrinogen. The overall percentage of cells permanently adhering is the same for both surface types. At a shear rate of 456 s^{-1} these differences are absent and the adhesion efficiency on initial contact and overall adhesion efficiency are less than corresponding values for each protein coating at 80 s^{-1}. The mechanism of detachment and reattachment of surface-bound platelets is flow dependent and can lead to an equality of overall adhesion efficiency even when initial adhesion efficiencies are not equal.

Experiments with fluorescent video microscopy have also been used to focus on the adhesion of the platelets to unaltered fibrinogen and albumin and to regions on these protein substrates where platelets have detached, platelet-primed protein. On fibrinogen, no difference was found at low shear rates; at 944 s^{-1}, it was shown that the adhesion efficiency was greater on the platelet-primed protein.[13] On albumin, the platelet-primed protein was stickier at 80 s^{-1} and 456 s^{-1}.[14] A complete definition of the substrate protein remaining after detachment of platelets is not yet available. Evidence from experiments with fluorescein-conjugated antibody labeled fibrinogen and albumin and with fluroescein isothiocyanate-labeled fibrinogen and albumin do not show visible removal of these proteins for exposure times, to platelets and red cells, up to 2 min. This would not preclude partial removal of protein not detectable with our fluorescent labeling methods. More likely, however, is the deposition of protein secreted from the α-granules of platelets. Possibilities are fibrinogen (which could add to that already on the surface), fibronectin, thrombospondin, and von Willebrand factor. Another possibility is the deposition of platelet membrane components.

Another approach to describe the effects of protein coating and flow on platelet-surface contact is to consider the effects of these variables on platelet residence times. What is meant here is the time during which a cell will move from place to place along a surface before permanently adhering within the measurement region. During this period it can adhere and detach several times. In FIGURES 1 and 2 residence time information for fibrinogen and albumin coatings, respectively, are presented. In both cases, the effect of flow is to reduce residence time. At 80 s^{-1}, the residence time for most platelets is less than 60 s; at 456 s^{-1}, the residence time is less than 30 s. This information indicates that the time span associated with adhesion and detachment ranges from 0 to 60 s. This then is the time scale necessary for surface-bound protein to be made more adhesive due to the attachment and detachment of platelets.

Another question area probed was that of whether or not detached platelets were more sticky when they contacted a surface for the second timc. This question was asked

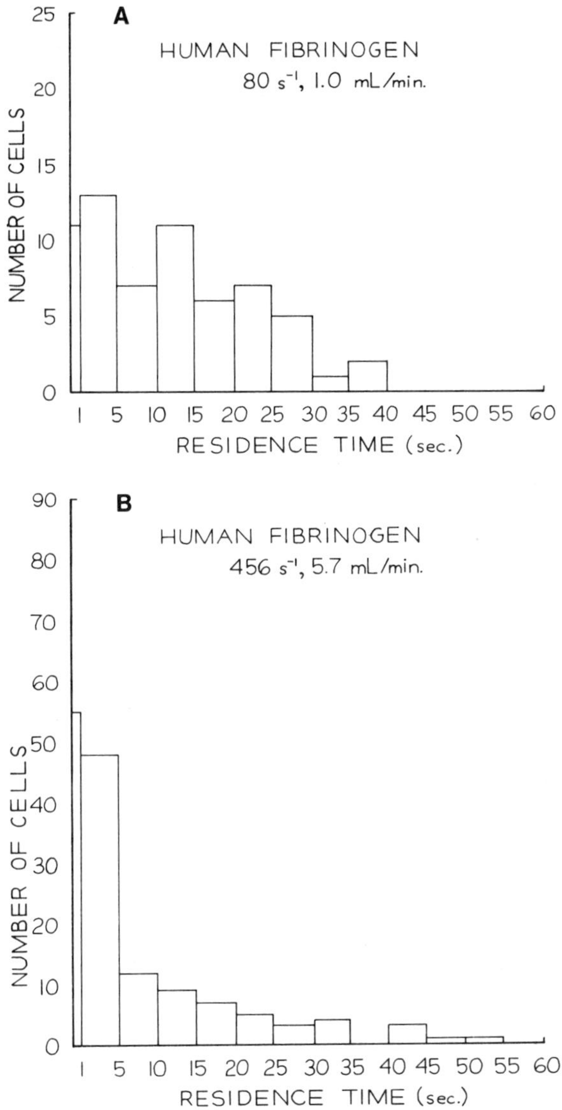

FIGURE 1. Residence time histogram for fibrinogen-coated glass at (**A**) 1 ml/min (80 s^{-1}) and (**B**) 5.7 ml/min (456 s^{-1}) for 1-min exposure to flow (see ref. 14 for experimental details of flow system and platelet preparation). "Residence time" refers to the time during which movement occurs before permanent adhesion. "Number of cells" refers to platelets contacting and moving within an area of 1370 μm^2 (entries are for the sums of 10 experiments).

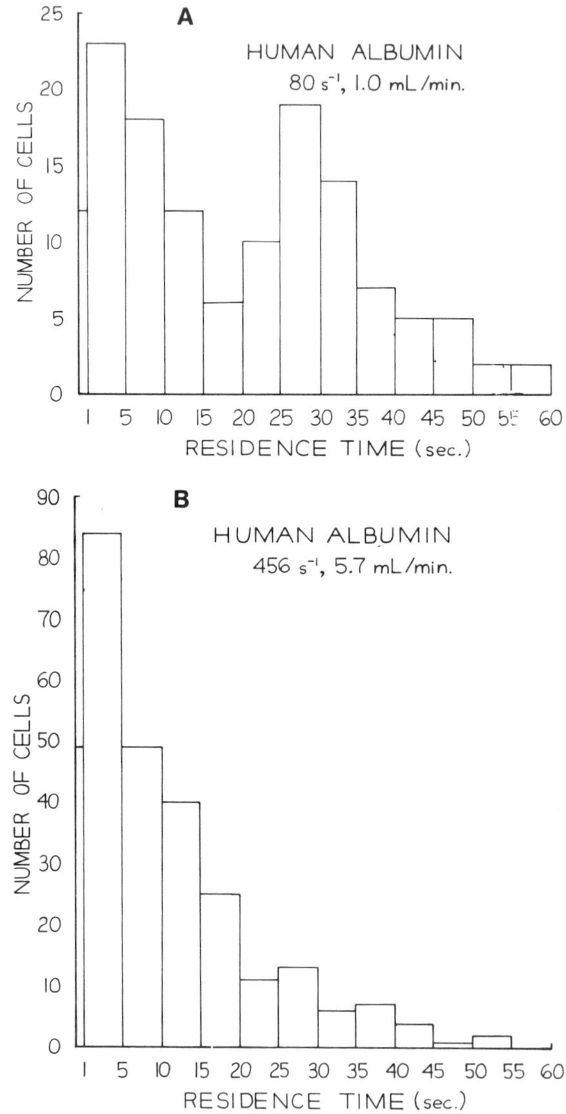

FIGURE 2. Residence time histogram for fibrinogen-coated glass at (**A**) 1 ml/min and (**B**) 5.7 ml/min for 1-min exposure to flow (see FIG. 1 for additional information).

by making observations on unaltered fibrinogen and albumin. Here it was demonstrated that second contacts are more efficient than first contacts.[13,14] Possible explanations may be an alteration of the platelet's membrane resulting from detachment, which makes it more adhesive, or that the mechanical features of a cell moving along a surface to a nearby spot, 1–5 μm away, favors adhesion to a greater extent than for a cell contacting from the bulk suspension.

LONG-TERM EFFECT OF ADHERENT PLATELETS ON SURFACE-BOUND PROTEIN

There are a number of potential mechanisms for the removal or alteration of surface-bound protein by cells:

- Enzymatic degradation by secreted or leaked enzyme. Platelets contain a number of enzymes. Amongst these are: (1) acid hydroloses,[15] which are granule-bound; (2) calcium-dependent neutral protease[16]; (3) an elastase[17]; and (4) a collagenase.[18]
- Exchange of surface-bound protein with secreted protein from the α-granules of platelets. Platelets contain a number of proteins that are secreted upon stimulation. These are: fibronectin, thrombospondin, von Willebrand factor, fibrinogen, albumin, and high molecular weight kininogen. High molecular weight kininogen is known to exchange with surface-bound fibrinogen.[19] Von Willebrand factor, which has a series of high molecular weight multimers above 10^6 daltons, would be a second important candidate protein with fibronectin, thrombospondin, and fibrinogen following.
- A capping-like phenomena is also possible. Surface-bound protein may move within the cell's membrane, causing a redistribution of the surface-bound protein. Such a redistribution has been demonstrated for the platelet's fibrinogen receptor, glycoprotein IIb-IIIa.[20] In this case surface-bound spread platelets were used to show changes in the distribution of the receptor with time on the side of the cell not contacting the solid surface.

The removal, alteration, or degradation of surface-bound protein by adherent cells, other than platelets, has been demonstrated with fluorescently labeled protein by others.[21,22] In my laboratory, we have chosen to label fibrinogen in the adsorbed state as opposed to solution labeling. Two methods have been utilized: (1) reaction with antifibrinogen followed by a secondary antibody conjugated with fluorescein isothiocyanate (FITC),[23] and (2) conjugation with FITC directly at pH 7.4 with several changes of FITC solution (2–4 changes with 10-min incubation between changes). Siliconized glass tubes prepared in these ways were exposed to flowing suspensions of platelets and red cells (80 s^{-1} for 2 min with unlabeled platelets), rinsed, and then incubated at 37°C for up to 2 hours. Observations were made of the lumenal fluorescent coating with our fluorescent video microscopy system.

Initially a uniform fluorescence was observed; platelets were not distinguishable since they were unlabeled. After approximately 30 min of incubation, dark regions surrounding a region of fluorescence brighter than adjacent areas were observed. This observation was made with both protein labeling methods and is shown in FIGURE 3. The presence of increased and localized fluorescence is consistent with manipulation of the surface-bound protein by adherent platelets. A capping-like phenomenon is possible with these observations, as is endocytosis of fibrinogen. What is clearly demonstrated is a distinct contribution of adherent platelets to the control of the surface concentration of adsorbed fibrinogen. This phenomenon and that of exchange with fluid phase plasma proteins are distinct mechanisms contributing to the time-dependent picture of protein at surfaces.

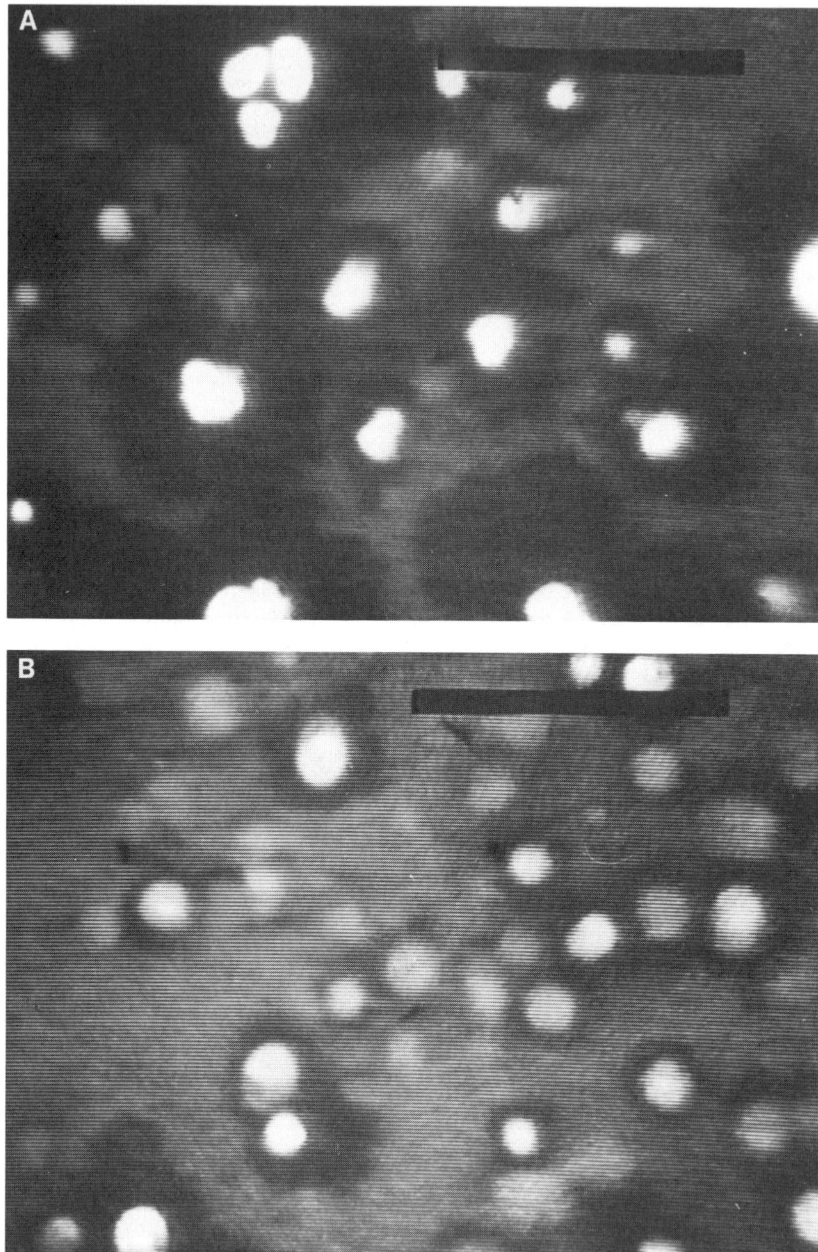

FIGURE 3. Photomicrographs showing fluorescently labeled fibrinogen on siliconized glass which has been exposed to platelets for 2 min at 1 ml/min (80 s^{-1}; see ref. 14 for experimental details of flow system and platelet preparation). (**A**) Adsorbed fibrinogen labeled using antifibrinogen and a fluorescently labeled secondary antibody; incubation time with adherent platelets is 36 min. (**B**) Adsorbed fibrinogen conjugated directly with fluorescein isothiocyanate; incubation time with adherent platelets is 34 min. The length markers represent 30 μm.

REFERENCES

1. Mechanical Surface and Gas Layer Effects on Moving Blood. 1971. Fed. Proc. **30:** 1485–1711.
2. Vroman, L. & E. F. Leonard, Eds. 1977. Ann. N.Y. Acad. Sci. **283:** 1–560.
3. Andrade, J. E., Ed. 1985. Surface and Interfacial Aspects of Biomedical Polymers, Vol. 2. Protein Adsorption. Plenum. New York.
4. Grabowski, E. F., L. I. Friedman & E. F. Leonard. 1972. Effects of shear rate on the diffusion and adhesion of blood platelets to a foreign surface. Ind. Eng. Chem. Fund. **11:** 224–232.
5. Baumgartner, H. R., R. Muggli, T. B. Tschopp & V. T. Turitto. 1976. Platelet adhesion, release and aggregation in flowing blood: Effects of surface properties and platelet function. Thromb. Haemostas. **35:** 124–138.
6. Adams, G. A. & I. A. Feuerstein. 1983. Platelet adhesion and release: Maximum fluid concentrations of materials released from platelets. Am. J. Physiol. **244:** H109–114.
7. Goldsmith, H. L. 1971. Red cell motions and wall interactions in tube flow. Fed. Proc. **30:** 1578–1588.
8. Turitto, V. T., A. M. Benis & E. F. Leonard. 1972. Platelet diffusion in flowing blood. Ind. Eng. Chem. Fund. **11:** 216–223.
9. Wang, N.-H. & K. H. Keller. 1979. Solute transport induced by erythrocyte motions in shear flow. Trans. Am. Soc. Artif. Intern. Organs **25:** 14–18.
10. Kinlough-Rathbone, R. L., J. F. Mustard, M. A. Packham, P. W. Perry, H.-J. Reimers & J.-P. Cazenave. 1977. Properties of washed human platelets. Thromb. Haemostas. **37:** 291–308.
11. Feuerstein, I. A. & L. E. Skupny-Garnham. 1986. Adhesion and aggregation of thrombin prestimulated human platelets: Evaluation of surface-bound fibrinogen and surface-bound albumin. Thromb. Res. **43:** 497–505.
12. Feuerstein, I. A. & J. Kush. 1983. Measurements of platelet adhesion efficiency upon virgin and platelet-primed (foot-printed) fibrinogen with fluorescent videomicroscopy. Trans. Am. Soc. Artif. Intern. Organs **29:** 430–434.
13. Feuerstein, I. A. & J. Kush. 1986. Blood platelet surface interactions on fibrinogen under flow as viewed with fluorescent video-microscopy. Trans. ASME J. Biomech. Eng. **108:** 49–53.
14. Feuerstein, I. A. & J. Kush. 1986. Platelet adherence and detachment: In what ways is surface-bound albumin different from surface-bound fibrinogen? Thromb. Haemostas. **55:** 184–188.
15. Holmsen, H. & H. J. Weiss. 1979. Secretable storage pools in platelets. Ann. Rev. Med. **30:** 119–134.
16. Kunicki, T. J., M. W. Mosesson & D. Pidard. 1984. Cleavage of fibrinogen by human platelet calcium-activated protease. Thromb. Res. **35:** 169–182.
17. James, H. L. 1985. A unique elastase in human blood platelets. J. Clin. Invest. **76:** 2330–2337.
18. Chesney, C. McI., E. Harper & R. W. Colman. 1974. Human platelet collagenase. J. Clin. Invest. **53:** 1647–1654.
19. Schmaier, A. H., L. Silver, A. L. Adams, G. C. Fischer, P. C. Munoz, L. Vroman & R. W. Colman. 1983. The effect of high molecular weight kininogen on surface-adsorbed fibrinogen. Thromb. Res. **33:** 51–67.
20. Albrecht, R. M. & J. C. Loftus. 1984. Redistribution of the fibrinogen receptor of human platelets after surface activation. J. Cell Biol. **99:** 822–829.
21. Avnur, Z. & B. Geiger. 1981. The removal of extracellular fibronectin from areas of cell-substrate contact. Cell **25:** 121–132.
22. Chen, W.-T., K. Olden, B. A. Bernard & F.-F. Chu. 1984. Expression of transformation-associated protease(s) that degrade fibronectin at cell contact sites. J. Cell Biol. **98:** 1546–155.
23. Feuerstein, I. A. & J. Kush. 1985. Platelets modify surface-bound fibrinogen Trans. Am. Soc. Artif. Intern. Organs **31:** 270–275.

Interaction of Transport Phenomena and Surface Reactions

PETER D. RICHARDSON

Division of Engineering
Brown University
Providence, Rhode Island 02912

INTRODUCTION

Transport phenomena in a fluid stream can be analyzed in terms of three equations and appropriate boundary conditions for them. The first equation of interest is the continuity equation: this is a very simple equation and has no peculiar features in its application to blood flow. The second equation of concern is the equation of motion. In this, the variables which are sought in solution are the velocity components throughout the physical space of interest, and solution requires information about the constitutive relation for the fluid which relates the stress tensor to the rate-of-deformation tensor. It is this latter information which is known rather imperfectly still for blood. It is well known that blood is a non-Newtonian fluid, with a raised effective viscosity at lower shear rates associated with the effects of formation of rouleaux of red cells. The information available is entirely empirical because no theory relating the macroscopic behavior to the microrheological events in suspensions of cells of the high suspended-fraction densities typical of blood is available, nor does it seem a likely prospect soon. When the concern is broadened to include the unsteady flow case, it has to be recognized that even empirical information is lacking concerning the effects of the rate of disaggregation of red cell rouleaux during an episode of increasing shear rate, and of the re-establishment of red cell rouleaux by aggregation during an episode of reduced shear rate. While some theories for the aggregation process have been initiated,[1,2] no results are available in real-time coordinates. Another factor that often intrudes to some degree in the solution of the equation of motion is the fact that the walls over which blood flows frequently have a significant compliance so that there is an interaction between the geometry of flow passages and the pressures and wall shear stresses developed within them.

The third equation of concern is the diffusion equation. For solution of this equation it is generally necessary to have already available the solution for the equation of motion, because the velocity components determined through the equation of motion provide coefficients for terms in the diffusion equation. In addition, there is a persistent lack of assurance that the coefficient of diffusion is adequately described for all circumstances. It is well known that in a blood flow many of the species and even the suspended cells exhibit effective diffusivities far higher than one would expect from the thermal random walk processes that commonly underlie diffusion in simple solutions. Through studies in the laboratories of Goldsmith and Leonard amongst others, it is now well appreciated that flows induced (and observable) on the microrheological scale typical of cells have a profound effect on the effective diffusivity, a kind of localized stirring motion being able to enhance diffusivity for some small cells or large molecules 100-fold or more compared with Brownian motion.

Over the past decade, as illustrated by other papers in this volume, there has been a growing realization that there is an intimate coupling between the macrorheological description of motion and transport and microrheological details within the flow. For example, it has become recognized increasingly that it is not just the red cells which have a nonuniform concentration distribution across flow in a duct or channel (in which it is usually found that the red cell concentration near the wall is less than in the center of the stream, and in which the flexibility of the red cells themselves is an important factor), but that the distribution of platelets across a flow can evolve so that there are considerable differences in concentrations in those parts of the flow near walls (where the concentrations can become relatively high) and in the center of the flow. Something similar can occur also with white cells. These concentration nonuniformities vary with the Reynolds number of the flow and to some degree with the upstream history of the flow. There are aspects to the development of the nonuniform distribution which remind one of the situation that can develop in the presence of nonuniform restricted random walks, a point which is brought out in the paper in this volume by Eugene Eckstein.[3] This information, while enlightening, is also somewhat dismaying, because it implies that making accurate predictions of the concentration distribution of various species in a blood flow is more difficult in the neighborhood of a surface than one finds in flows of simpler fluids (nonsuspensions), for which so much is already known in the literature on convective heat and mass transfer. The estimation of the convective transport is therefore more difficult for species of higher molecular weight in blood than of lower molecular weight (such as oxygen), because transport of the latter is less influenced by these local microrheological phenomena that become so important at the platelet scale. We now recognize that a computational approach to determination of transport in a bloodstream that will yield a degree of accuracy for high molecular weight species comparable to that for low molecular weight species is going to require more information and more computational effort. This means that at present we can, with a given level of expenditure, somewhat more confidently study transport by experimental methods (which do not require intimate knowledge of cell concentration distributions across the flow) than by an entirely analytical approach.

The analysis of convective transport within blood flow is important when the surface reaction is not the limiting step in transport. Initially there was a perception that surface reactions between the constituents of blood and any surface are fairly orderly. Because most devices built with foreign surfaces first have to be primed with a crystalline solution, which is then displaced by a proteinaceous solution or by whole blood, it was perceived that there is plenty of opportunity to assure that plasma proteins are the first macromolecular species to interact with the surface. It became clear fairly early that there is competition among these for adhesion on the surface and that different conformations of the proteins can arise depending upon the density of their adhesion upon the surface. Before about 10 years ago, the common method for investigating platelet adhesion at short times was to expose the surface to a platelet suspension, PRP, or whole blood for a fixed period of time, to wash it with a physiological solution, and then to observe the number-density of adherent platelets. This approach of taking single "snapshots" at fixed intervals of time did not lend itself to investigating the dynamics of the adhesion process. Within the past decade it has been demonstrated and confirmed, by using techniques where surfaces are continuously monitored, that platelets themselves vacate sites to which they have adhered, and other platelets can come and occupy the same sites later, only to repeat the process of subsequent departure.[4–6] In the course of this, it has been shown that the adhesion rate (in terms of new sites for adhesion being occupied) and the platelet turnover rate are affected by the local shear rate in the flow, and can be altered by administration of drugs to the donor or incubation of the drawn blood with drugs. The variations in behavior between specific donors and their response to changes in diet are discussed in a later section.

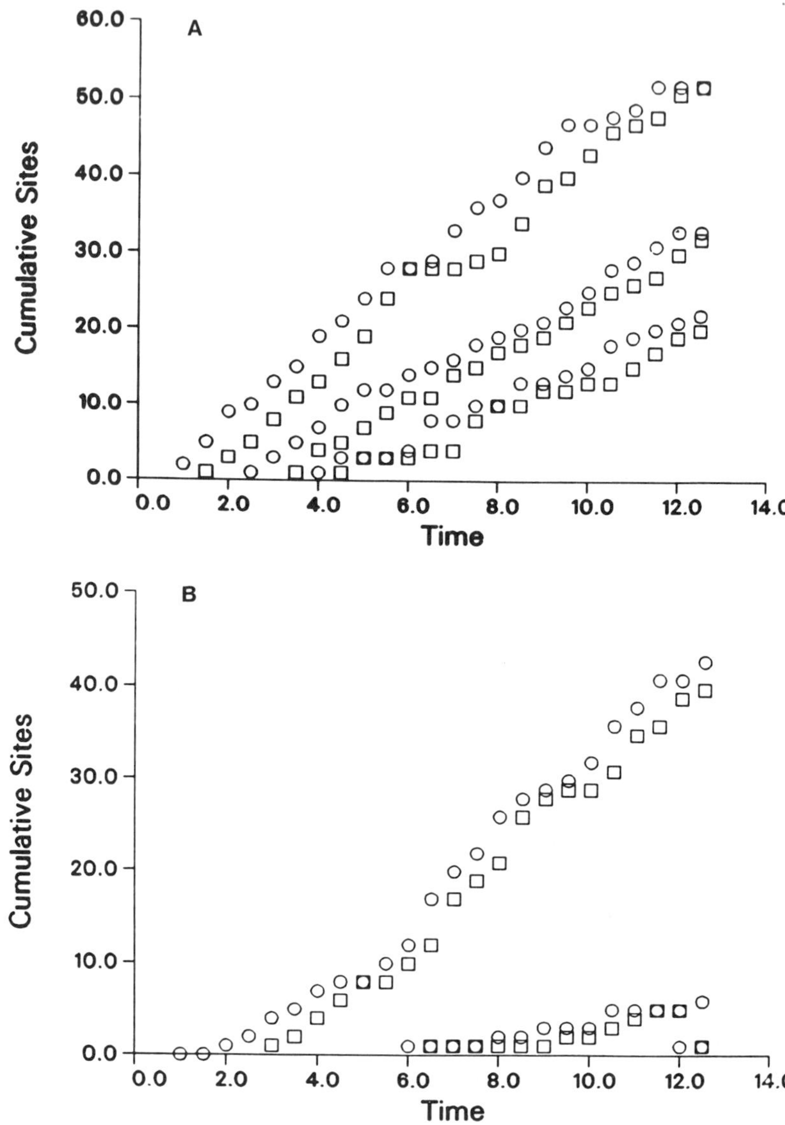

FIGURE 1. Adhesion and turnover of platelets drawn from donor (MF) as a function of time in minutes. At any time, the uppermost circle indicates the cumulative number of fresh sites that have been occupied by adherent platelets at least once; the uppermost square indicates the number of those sites that have been vacated by the first platelet occupant. The next circle down indicates the cumulative number of sites that have been reoccupied once, and the next square down indicates the number of those that have been vacated by the second platelet occupant, and so on. (**A**) Baseline results for adhesion to a slide coated with collagen I. (**B**) Results for adhesion to a similar slide after the donor had consumed 400 U vitamin A daily for 2 weeks; note the slightly reduced primary adhesion and much reduced readhesion.

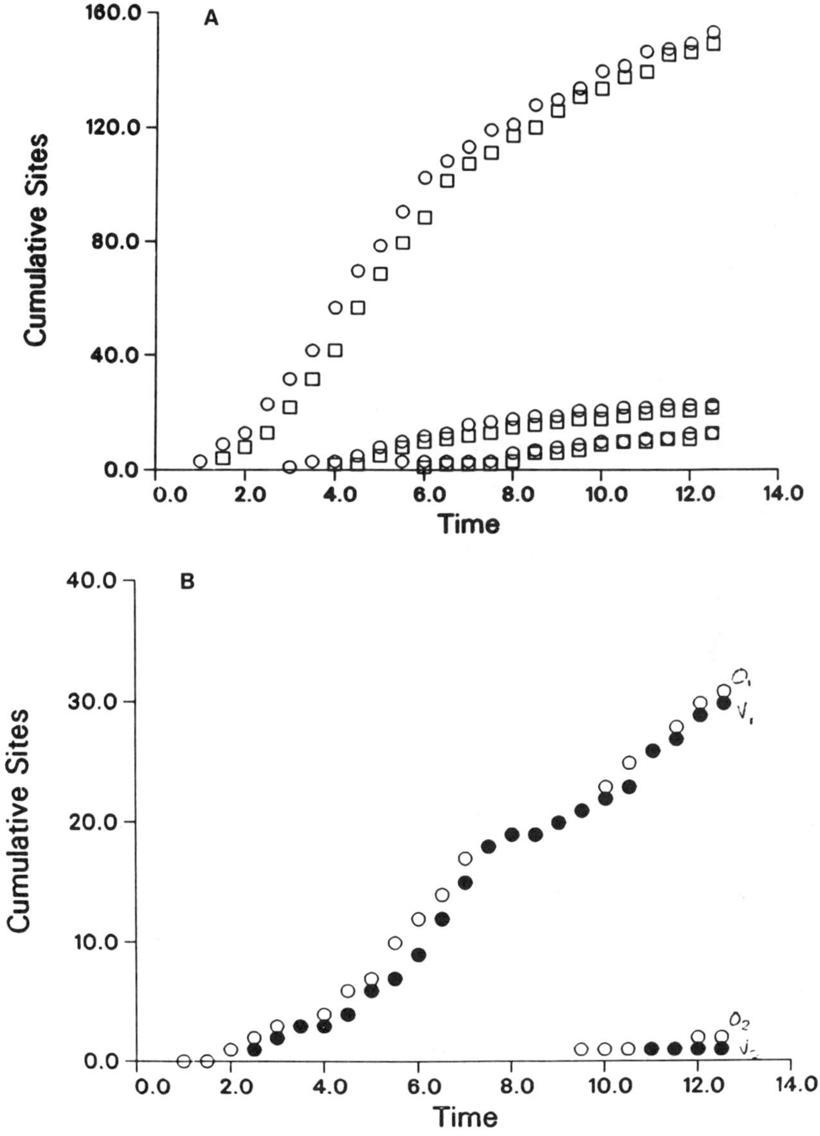

FIGURE 2. Adhesion and turnover of platelets, similar to FIGURE 1 except that the adhesive substrate was glass coated with fibronectin, and in **B** squares have been replaced by black circles. Note that both adhesion and turnover were down with vitamin E.

SOME PHENOMENOLOGICAL QUESTIONS

The basic approach in an engineering study in fluid mechanics and transport phenomena is to take the appropriate equations of motion and boundary conditions and then seek solutions. From the discussion in the INTRODUCTION, it should be clear that there are a number of phenomenological questions related to the interaction between phenomena on the microrheological scale of the individual cells and the macrorheological formulation that are generally appropriate on beginning to tackle specific problems. It needs to be pointed out that we have failed so far to determine much of the phenomenology surrounding processes at surfaces exposed to blood, and we have not grasped entirely what processes we should try to analyze in detail. For example, as thrombi on a surface mature (and that in itself is a concept something we do not yet fully understand) they deform and avalanche in the downstream direction while retaining integrity as a thrombus in most cases. This has been observed repeatedly *in vitro* and *in vivo* and yet it has not been subject to any systematic investigation. Avalanching is a phenomenon in the microscale of sedimentary geology, and those active in that field have even pointed out that clays (which form some of the geological sediment) have fixed surface charges themselves that can interact in processes. Geologists have performed extensive research on sedimentary mounds (dunes). They have described their morphology at length and investigated their kinematics and dynamics (see, for example, Allen[7]). On many occasions one can observe that thrombi exist on a surface rather like a chain of islands, with the chain axis in the direction of flow, and sometimes with bare patches between the thrombi. Some have observed that the gaps between relatively fixed "islands" (*i.e.,* individual thrombi) become filled with thrombotic material which grows to a certain size and them embolizes, and that this process repeats itself many times. Thus the island chains of attached thrombus, even when the individual thrombi do not grow themselves significantly in time, may be a major source of thromboembolism because of the material that accretes between them and embolizes. This process does not seem to have been the subject of systematic investigation.

Thrombi can attach at small points. In our flow chamber we have observed thrombi that have roughly the shape of kites with attachment to the surface on a very short string or tether. When the flow is made slightly pulsatile, such thrombi can be seen to oscillate on the tethers. We have no systematic knowledge of elastic behavior in thrombi and their attachment to surfaces, but we can join the perception of the physicist that the thrombus can then be essentially a mass on a spring, and the mass may grow by aggregation of platelets to the thrombus. In the latter circumstance, we would expect the natural frequency to continue to change, and in this process it might be able to reach a point of resonance with a pulsatile flow and then encounter increased probability of detachment.

EFFECT OF VITAMIN E ON PLATELET ADHESION AND TURNOVER

We have made measurements of platelet adhesion in a specially designed flow chamber first described about ten years ago.[3] In this chamber platelet-rich plasma or whole blood can flow in a geometry which determines the distribution of local shear stress with respect to position in the chamber. The adhesion of platelets to a local region of the surface, typically 67,000 μm^2, is observed with a microscope and recorded on videotape. The recorded images are examined at fixed time intervals using a computerized image analysis system. With this it is possible to identify the location of each adherent platelet in a coordinate system fixed relative to the chamber. Data on

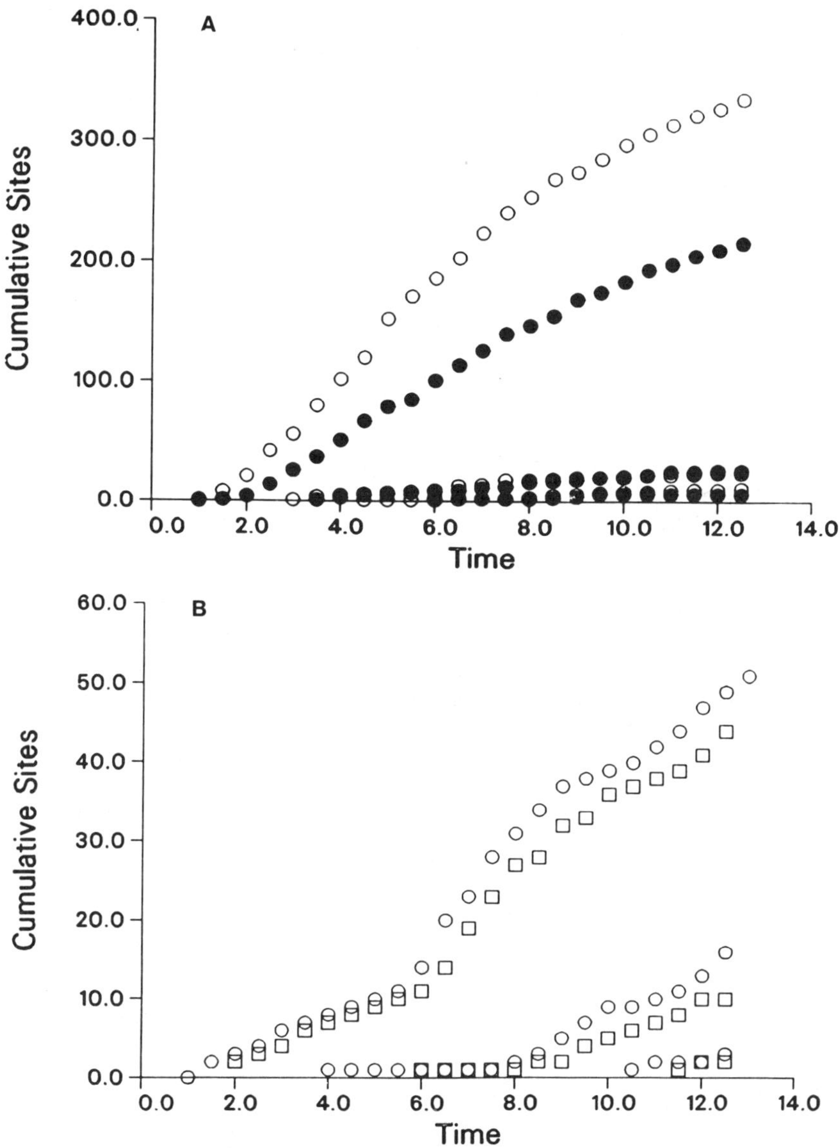

FIGURE 3. Adhesion and turnover of platelets, similar to FIGURE 1 except that the adhesive substrate was glass coated with fibrinogen. The primary adhesion rate was reduced by a factor of about 7 with vitamin E; the reuse of sites index increased slightly.

platelet adhesion sites are recorded for each time interval and the data are processed to determine various statistical features. These include the cumulative number of sites that has been occupied as a function of time (this is roughly linear with time after an initial period) and the times at which sites that have been occupied once are vacated, reoccupied a second time, revacated a second time, and so on, so that the number of sites which have been occupied at various totals over the period of a fifteen-minute run

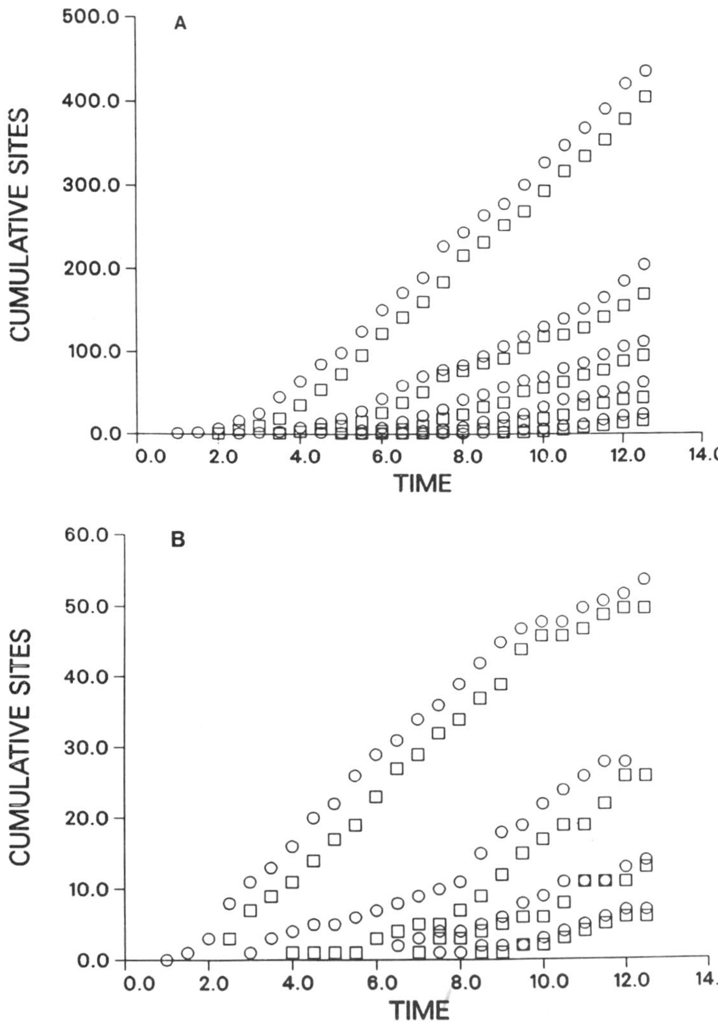

FIGURE 4. Adhesion and turnover of platelets, similar to FIGURE 1 except that the donor (JS) was different and, as in FIGURE 3, the adhesive substrate was glass coated with fibrinogen. The primary adhesion rate was again reduced by a factor of about 7 with vitamin E, and the reuse of sites index was little changed.

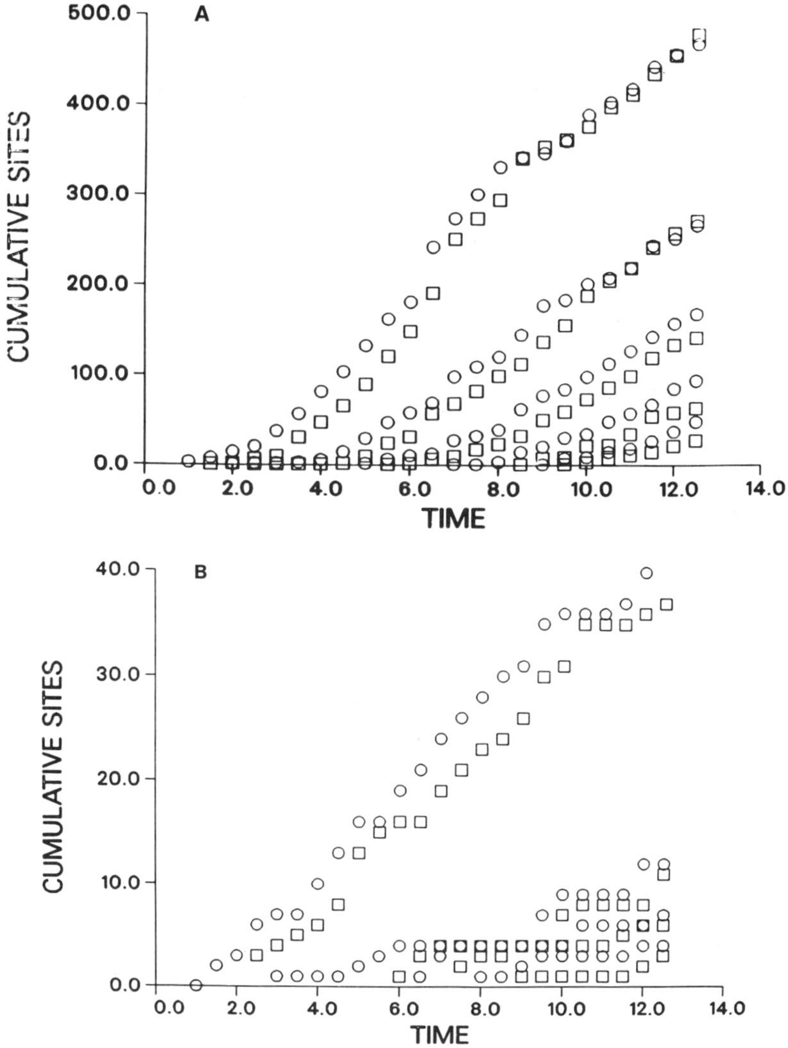

FIGURE 5. Adhesion and turnover of platelets, similar to FIGURE 1 except that the donor (JJ) was different from those for previous figures and, as in FIGURES 3 and 4, the adhesive substrate was glass coated with fibrinogen. The primary adhesion rate was reduced by an order of magnitude with vitamin E, and the reuse of sites index was also reduced.

can be examined. It has been found that there is a good correlation between the logarithm of the number of sites as a function of the times occupied. Clearly the largest number of sites were only occupied once, and the smallest number of sites was occupied the largest number of times, so that the regression line on the semilogarithmic scale has a negative slope. This slope is taken as the reuse of sites index (RUSI). Bodziak and Richardson[6] remarked that there are variations in platelet adhesion between (volunteer) donors; however, platelet turnover as measured by the reuse of sites index may be fairly constant for an individual. A preliminary review of statistics for repeat donors showed a tendency for a RUSI to be relatively constant for each donor. This was based on observations made with blood donated at intervals of several weeks. In the experiments reported previously it had been shown that the platelet adhesion rate and RUSI both could be modified by drugs[5]; all the experiments were based on exposure of the platelets to the drugs by incubation *in vitro*. We report now some results on the effects of introducing vitamin E daily into the diet of volunteer donors, with control data taken before the introduction of the vitamin E at 400 U per day, and with data taken subsequently after the donors had been on the diet for two weeks. Results are illustrated in FIGURES 1–5. The chamber walls on which the platelet adhesion was observed had been precoated with various substrates, identified in the figures. Both male and female donors were used with the donors reporting that they were free of recent consumption of platelet-active drugs. The figures here illustrate a subset of the data obtained, but demonstrate that independent of the adhesion substrate used, the adhesion rate and/or RUSI was reduced by the vitamin E diet. In other words, the rate at which platelets adhered per unit surface area was diminished, and/or the frequency at which vacated sites were reoccupied was diminished.

DISCUSSION

In the past decade much has been learned regarding transport phenomena in blood and interactions with surfaces. Long ago it had been suspected that the phenomena involved were complex. In the past decade it has become increasingly obvious that the suspicions were correct. The phenomenology involved has become much clearer qualitatively. It is recognized that it will require significant effort to establish firmly a quantitative analysis sufficiently accurate to make comparisons with experimental measurements meaningful. In the past decade there has been also a growth of understanding of the phenomenology at the surface itself, but the understanding is far from complete and in large measure is inadequate even at a qualitative level. The need for far better understanding of thrombotic and (particularly) embolic processes has been underscored by the recent experiences with implanted total artificial hearts in humans. The turnover of adherent platelets, the formation and slumping of mural thrombi under shear flows, and the processes of embolization all deserve further study.

SUMMARY

Phenomena that occur when blood contacts a foreign surface are controlled by transport processes in the bloodstream immediately above the surface and by reactions at the surface itself. All constituents of blood that attach to a surface may leave the surface and be replaced by other constituents. Some of the constituents may attach in superposition. This turnover of constituents at the surface is influenced by the nature of the substrate and the shear stress between the blood and the surface. The turnover process is easy to demonstrate with platelets. When platelets depart from a surface, the site they vacate has a higher attractiveness for adhesion of other platelets than the surrounding surface that has not had a cell attached to it, but this enhanced attractiveness diminishes in a few minutes if a new occupant does not occupy the site. As data accumulate, it is beginning to appear that platelet turnover differs between different blood donors but remains relatively constant for each individual unless dietary or pharmacological changes that affect the turnover rate are introduced.

ACKNOWLEDGMENT

The experimental results reported here were obtained by Ms. Jennifer Jandak, engineering graduate student, in collaboration with Manfred Steiner of the Memorial Hospital, Pawtucket, RI.

REFERENCES

1. SAMSEL, R. W. & A. S. PERELSON. 1982. Kinetics of rouleau formation. I. A mass action approach with geometric features. Biophys. J. **37:** 493–514.
2. SAMSEL, R. W. & A. S. PERELSON. 1984. Kinetics of rouleau formation. II. Reversible reactions. Biophys. J. **45:** 805–824.
3. ECKSTEIN, E. C., D. L. BILSKER, C. M. WATERS, J. S. KIPPENHAN & A. W. TILLES. 1987. Transport of platelets in flowing blood.
4. RICHARDSON, P. D., S. F. MOHAMMAD & R. G. MASON. 1977. Flow chamber studies of platelet adhesion at controlled, spatially varied flow rates. Eur. Soc. Artif. Organs **4:** 177–188.
5. RICHARDSON, P. D., R. KANE & K. AGARWAL. 1981. Effects of drugs on adhesion of human platelets. Trans. Am. Soc. Artif. Int. Organs **27:** 203–207.
6. BODZIAK, K. & P. D. RICHARDSON. 1982. Turnover of adherent platelets: Some effects of shear rate, ASA and reduced anticoagulation. Trans. Am. Soc. Artif. Int. Organs **28:** 426–429.
7. ALLEN, J. R. L. 1968. Current Ripples: Their Relation to Patterns of Water and Sediment Motion. North-Holland. Amsterdam.

The Close Approach of Cells to Surfaces

EDWARD F. LEONARD,[b] IRAJ RAHMIM,[b]
JANA K. ANGARSKA,[c] CHRISTIAN S. VASSILIEFF,[d]
AND IVAN B. IVANOV[d]

[b]*Artificial Organs Research Laboratory*
Department of Chemical Engineering
Columbia University
New York, New York 10027

[c]*Higher Pedagogical Institute*
Shoumen, Bulgaria

[d]*Faculty of Chemistry*
University of Sofia
Sofia, Bulgaria

INTRODUCTION

The attachment of cells to other cells and noncellular surfaces, commonly referred to as aggregation and adhesion, respectively, have come to be recognized as playing an important role in most biological and biotechnical processes. A number of examples can be cited. Tissue-specific adhesion plays a primary role in the generation of form during development.[1] Most microbial infections have specific or nonspecific adhesion as a step. Also, cell-cell adhesion is an integral part of the immune response to these infections. It has been shown that altered adhesion is a fundamental property of cancer cells.[2] Of greatest pertinence in the present context are the facts that adhesion is a major factor in thrombus formation, endothelial repair, and the response of blood to artificial surfaces.

Although the importance of adhesion and its prevalence in nature is appreciated, its fundamental physiological aspects are far from well understood. It is now known that the physics of aggregation and adhesion is very complex, involving a number of interacting factors that affect the process of approach in various ranges of separation.[3,4] From the point of view of the researcher, this process is difficult fully to comprehend, simulate, and control and measure experimentally. The first theory to be applied to cell interactions was that of lyophobic colloids.[5] Physical theories such as this have been gaining sophistication so as to include characteristics particular to cell adhesion,[4,6–8] although no model seems yet to be both physically and biologically satisfactory. The experimental techniques that make possible detailed studies of cell-cell and cell-surface interactions, in particular methods allowing direct visualization, are relatively new.[9–11]

The purpose of this article is twofold: to review current understanding of adhesion and aggregation, particularly as these processes might apply to blood cells, and to describe a possible experimental arrangement and procedure for a kinetic study of the behavior of a cell at certain critical separations from a target surface.

A BRIEF REVIEW OF RELEVANT ISSUES

One can *define* the process of approach to take place in three basic regimes. One regime comprises "far" distances, where cell movement is due to either fluid dynamical forces or chemotaxis. Another regime comprises very close distances where direct molecular attachment can take place. The third regime is that intermediate to the "far" and the "close" regimes; here fluid dynamical forces lose their influence as the opposing surfaces begin to sense and be affected by each other. The thickness of this regime, for which only vague boundaries can be drawn, is believed to be on the order of 100 nanometers.

Before further discussion, we remark upon the often used concept of distance. Distance can be formally defined as the linear extent of space between two points or objects, a definition that conforms to the vernacular usage. It appears to be the natural independent parameter when considering the problem of approach leading to adhesion. This concept is particularly useful at distances of separation of an order of magnitude equal to or greater than the maximum distance separating the parts of one cell, for then irregularities in shape of an approaching cell are negligible when compared to the separation. On the other hand, at small separations, where hills and valleys in the cell surface are of the same order of magnitude as some definition of mean separation, it becomes difficult to talk about cell-cell or cell-surface separation in a way that is both intuitive and adequate. Different parts of the cell can be at markedly different separations from another surface and can be responding to a different combination of forces. In fact, while portions of the two opposing surfaces could hardly be sensing one another, other parts could be in direct molecular contact caused by cellular extensions. The formal solution to this dilemma is to define and follow more than one point on the cell. The number of these points to be analyzed must be large enough to detail the cell contour. Mege *et al.*[12] have recently developed a simple method for quantifying cell surface irregularity, although their method has not yet been applied to the analysis of cells adhered to other cells or surfaces. Equivalently, one could follow the appearance and disappearance of certain configurations on the cell surface that would be of interest in such a study. These configurations could include pseudopods, wrinkles, bubbles, and indentations.

The "far" regime has been studied in detail.[13–16] Although the fluid dynamical forces in the "far" range are necessary for, and play an important role in, initially bringing a cell close to a surface, fluid dynamic juxtaposition does not guarantee adhesion. At separations of hundreds of nanometers (c.f. typical cell diameters of a few thousand nanometers), the fluid dynamical forces perpendicular to the wall (which are of interest in the case of approach) must compete with long-range molecular forces and are mediated by geometric details of the wall and the cell surface. Approximate calculations by Bongrand and Bell[4] show that in simple sedimentation the overall downward force (due to cell weight minus the buoyancy force) on one cell is about 10^{-13} N, whereas those for intercellular electrostatic repulsion and steric stabilization at a separation of 20 nm are on the order of 10^{-8} and 10^{-7} N, respectively, postulating an apposition area of one square micrometer. Even if the contact area is much less, as is probable, the combined repulsive force (to be discussed further in the following pages) would be several orders of magnitude larger than the downward fluid dynamical force. While one might attempt to extend the "far separation" range downward to encompass these distances, there already exists a discipline and a set of tools for dealing with interactions between surfaces at such separations, and it is thus fruitful to define a separate range.

The attachment in the "close" range can be nonspecific (*e.g.*, ionic) or specific (*e.g.*, immunochemical). It can include local cytoplasmic membrane separations as great as perhaps 20 nm, since a number of specific reacting molecules are known to project such distances out of the cell membrane. Furthermore, there is evidence suggesting that direct molecular contact between a surface and the outer coating of a cell, which in human erythrocytes is on the order of 10 nanometers thick, can result in adhesion.[17]

The chemical bonds in such interactions are individually weak and can counteract repulsive and shear forces only when numerous. The force of one antibody-antigen bond is estimated[18] to be about 10^{-10} N. If a cell is adherent to a surface so as to present a circular surface with a diameter of 3 μm to a fluid flowing over it at a shear rate of 100 s^{-1}, the flow will exert a force on the cell surface of 3×10^{-6} N, equivalent to about 30,000 bonds. Between 100 and 1000 of these bonds would be necessary per square micrometer of apposition area to counteract simple electrostatic repulsion at a distance of 10 nm. Even this is an underestimation of the bonds needed, since antibody-antigen bond lengths are much less than 10 nm and the electrostatic repulsion increases rapidly as separation decreases. Capo *et al.*[19] studied concanavalin-A-mediated thymocyte agglutination using electron microscopic techniques and estimated that at least 1000 ConA bonds are involved in the cross-linking of two bound cells, a number comparable to those given above.

We return to a further consideration of the intermediate regime, which holds greatest interest for us. The forces important in this region include not only those caused by "local" fluid dynamical phenomena (such as squeezing out of thin liquid layers)[46] but also steric and long-range molecular forces. The intermediate region, as we have defined it, is the least studied of the three, mainly because it is one to be passed through and not usually an end point in itself. It has not been conclusively demonstrated that a quasi-static approach can reveal the changes the cell surface would undergo in time as the opposing surfaces approach one another. Because of the inherent complexity of the system, equilibrium cell profiles at different separations (obtained by using different, fixed ionic strengths) cannot be assumed to be the same as those a cell obtains as it approaches another surface. Also, the rapid rates at which pseudopods, which we consider to be instrumental in primary adhesion, can form and change make the applicability of the quasi-static methods questionable.

Nevertheless, it is in the intermediate region that the processes of adhesion and aggregation are either confirmed or abrogated. At close distances, after the formation of a sufficient number of chemical bonds, one can consider the commitment of the cell to the surface to be complete. A number of detachment studies support this view.[19,20] For example, Trommler *et al.*[11] used the method of internal reflection microscopy to study the detachment of unfixed red blood cells from a glass surface. They found that when the ionic strength is lowered drastically after the cells are attached, decreasing the ionic strength from 157 and 10 mM, respectively, to 3 mM did not cause any cells to be removed. It is mainly in the intermediate region, where the cell is not yet completely "trapped," that alteration of some factors can have a significant impact on the outcome of the approach process. These alterations should be most apparent in flow systems where reaction time is limited and outcomes are determined by kinetics rather than by equilibrium.

Within the intermediate and close regions, several elements are considered important in adhesion and have been examined to various degrees. These include van der Waals attraction, electrostatic repulsion, ionic composition of the medium, glycocalyx effects, receptor mobility, and cell deformability. Less extensively studied are those resulting from the metabolic processes of the cell such as formation of pseudopods and microvilli, mainly because of the difficulty caused by the relatively high speeds with which these elements form and change. In what is to follow, a short description of some of these studies will be given. The reader will notice that the cited literature is drawn from two areas: biological studies using different experimental techniques and theoretical works modeling the cell-cell and cell-surface interaction as a physicochemical process of varying complexity.

The two forces that were first considered with respect to cell adhesion are electrostatic repulsion and van der Waals (electrodynamic) attraction, both of which operate over a relatively long range. The electrostatic force depends upon like charges on the two opposing surfaces, almost all cell membranes being negatively charged. The van der Waals attraction (whose range is greater than that of the electrostatic force) is the result of induced-dipole–induced-dipole interaction.[6,45] The idea that the long-range van der Waals attraction and long-range electrostatic repulsion would be in balance at a finite cell separation was first developed by Parsegian and Gingell.[21] This concept corresponds to the so-called secondary minimum (which is based on the classical DLVO theory borrowed from colloid chemistry). This theory has been verified in several studies including those of bimolecular lipid layers,[22] liposomes,[23] and glutaraldehyde-fixed erythrocytes in contact with artificial surfaces.[20,24]

The balance between electrodynamic and electrostatic forces is modulated by the ionic strength of the medium. The ions in the solution screen negative charges on the opposing surfaces, making close approach possible. Gingell and Todd,[10] using the method of interference reflection microscopy, studied the adhesion of glutaraldehyde-fixed red blood cells to a saline-oil interface, with the cells suspended in saline. At near-physiological salt concentrations (145 mM NaCl), the equilibrium separation was seen to be quite small, while in dilute salt concentrations (0.4 mM NaCl), the cells equilibrated in juxtaposition to the interface at a separation of about 100 nanometers. The latter distance is too great for any direct chemical interaction when glutaraldehyde-fixed cells are involved, distances of 5–20 nm being necessary for chemical binding to take place.

A different long-range force is exerted between two hydrophobic surfaces in water. Israelachvili[25] demonstrated that this very strong attractive interaction is not the result of hydrophobic bonds as previously believed, but rather is due to reconfiguration of water molecules in the vicinity of a hydrophobic surface. However, it has been demonstrated that when both hydrophobic and hydrophilic groups are present on the surfaces, the DLVO theory explains the attractive forces,[26] suggesting that such reconfiguration of water molecules does not reach far from the surface.

Nonidealities in Charge Interaction

Much attention has been paid recently to the fact that the "cell boundary" and the distribution of charges within it are not really two-dimensional.[7,27,28] The phospholipid bilayer has a finite thickness. Further, most mammalian cells are surrounded with a loosely bound, relatively thick gel-like coating (glycocalyx) that is charged.[29] In human erythrocytes under *in vivo* conditions, glycocalyx consists of glycoproteins, glycolipids, and serum proteins adsorbed from plasma.[27] Its charge, usually negative, is often due to the dissociation of carboxyl groups in sialic acid located at the outer edge of glycocalyx. The DLVO theory must be generalized to take such a three-dimensional, "deep" charge distribution into account. Furthermore, because the cell membrane is believed to behave like a two-dimensional fluid mosaic,[30] allowing the migration of individual molecules within it, one must consider that the charge distribution in the membrane near a point of adhesion may change as adhesion occurs. In two separate studies, Lerche[27] and Voigt *et al.*[7] simulated the energy interactions of two cells at close distance, including the effects of charge-carrying glycocalyx. Voigt *et al.* examined three different assumptions of the charge distribution in glycocalyx: flat, linear, and exponential. They not only found that the charge distribution profile influences the electrostatic repulsion energy, but also that the existence of distributed space charges can increase by several orders of magnitude the energy of repulsion at close distances. Lerche obtained similar results.

Other Effects of Glycocalyx

Glycocalyx further impedes close approach of cell membranes through steric stabilization. This effect depends on the resistance of the polymer chains composing the glycocalyx to deformation and lateral movement, and the osmotic tendency of the water that is trapped in glycocalyx to remain in the contact region. The classical DLVO theory would suggest that at near-physiological salt concentrations cells could get as close as 2 or 3 nm to each other. However, as calculations by Bongrand and Bell[4] demonstrate, glycocalyx interpenetration (at distances of less that twice the coat thickness) and compression (separations of less than the cell coat thickness, on the order of 10 nm) could prevent very close approach. In fact, in the interpenetration region, the repulsive force due to steric stabilization can be more than one order of magnitude greater than that due to electrostatic repulsion. This effect might cause one to believe that the major role of glycocalyx is to deter adhesion.

However, more recent experimental studies have suggested otherwise. Wolf and Gingell[17] and Trommler *et al.*,[11] in works to which previous reference has been made, studied the adhesion of red blood cells to a glass surface. The first study showed that for untreated red blood cells and ionic strengths down to 5 mM (corresponding to a separation at about 70 nm), the lateral movement of adhered cells is restricted. Since no molecules embedded in the cytoplasmic membrane are known to extend so far into the medium, and since lateral cell motion is not restricted by adhesion related to the secondary minimum, it is very likely that glycocalyx is involved in direct molecular contact with the substrate at least at part of the range of ionic strengths studied, with attachment at the largest distances (lowest ionic strengths) being mediated by pseudopods. The increased separations found at intermediate ionic strengths appear to depend also on swelling of the glycocalyx under electrostatic forces. In the latter study, the same cell-glass system was used to study the detachment of adhered cells from the surface with progressively decreasing ionic strengths. Results pointing to the same conclusions were obtained. Although an increase in separation was observed when the ionic strength was lowered (for example from 157 mM to 3 mM), this decrease failed to remove any cells. It thus appears that although glycocalyx interferes with the close approach of the membranes, it does not simply impede adhesion since it can take part in direct molecular contact that results in primary adhesion.

Cell Deformability

Most cells in their normal state are quite flaccid. Shape change may occur at the subcellular level (*e.g.*, formation and movement of microvilli) and also on the scale of the whole cell, as exemplified by widely reported deformations of red blood cells passing through small capillaries. The formation of "hills," "valleys," and pseudopods as well as their variation with time can be a significant factor in the adhesion process. It has been shown that cells near other cells advance microvilli towards each other.[31] Because at small separations the repulsion force is quite large, it appears reasonable that initial molecular contact involves pseudopods that have a small area (about 0.01 μm^2) and extend outside of the range of intercellular forces.[17,19] Bell *et al.*,[8] in an equilibrium simulation study of specific cell-cell adhesion using a model that included the effects of electrostatic repulsion, steric stabilization, diffusional mobility of receptors, cell deformability, and others, found that the initial contact area must be quite small, and that the final equilibrium state is a balance between maximizing the number of bonds and minimizing the surface area of the two cells in apposition to each other. This balance, their calculations suggest, is dependent on cell flexibility and the ability of molecules to migrate laterally within the membrane.

Many of the experimental studies on adhesion have been performed on modified cells and at subphysiologic ionic strengths. However, certain tentative conclusions about adhesion dynamics under physiological conditions can be drawn. To initiate the process, it appears that the opposing surfaces must be brought within the reach of long-range molecular forces by fluid dynamic forces or chemotaxis. If net fluid force allows the surfaces to stay in proximity for a sufficient amount of time, the long-range van der Waals force can act to draw the two surfaces as close to each other as the combined effect of the steric and repulsive forces permit. During this "final approach," direct molecular contact with either the glycocalyx or protrusions from the surfaces can occur. The opposing surfaces will be committed to one another if this direct molecular contact results in chemical bond formation and the number of bonds is increased to a point at which they can counteract repulsive and possible dynamical forces.

EXPERIMENTAL APPROACH

This brief review reflects a biophysical literature that emphasizes a thermodynamic and by extension, as noted above, a quasi-static, response of cells to the proximity of other surfaces. It represents largely a theoretical viewpoint that has been little challenged by available results from quantitative, dynamic experiments. The more comprehensive and interesting view involves measurement and analysis of responses that are intrinsically dynamic and involve very large changes in cell surface area and shape, such as those undergone by the blood platelet in the neighborhood of a growing thrombus. A dynamic, direct visualization method needs to be developed for such a study. One approach to this goal that interests us involves interference reflection microscopy, pioneered in biology by Curtis,[32] who used it to estimate the separation between fibroblasts and a glass surface under a variety of experimental conditions. This method has subsequently become a popular tool in cell biology. Gingell and Todd[10,33] quantified this approach by rigorous interpretation of the interference image obtained in monochromatic light reflected from interfaces associated with a cell surface and from a nearby, transparent surface. According to their theory, the thickness of the gap between cell and substratum can be estimated from interference colors or from experimentally measured relative irradiance for up to ten orders of interference. The processed experimental results show that the calculation of the gap generally depends upon an unknown cytoplasmic thickness. However, at a high value of the illuminating numerical aperture (ca. 1.20) it is possible to show theoretically that this dependence is markedly decreased.

The method suffers from insensitivity to the determination of gap widths much less than 100 nm, corresponding to the first interference minima. These nearly inaccessible distances constitute much of the range of interest to us. However, the weakest point of this highly quantitative approach is that the measured value of the irradiance gives information only about the closest approach of the cell to the surface. Thus, for example, it does not permit studying how the profile relates to the distribution of charge over the cell surface. More generally, the method can be used to evaluate experimental data in terms of physical forces of attraction and repulsion only by assuming a geometrical simplification of the cell shape.[24] This simplification is limiting because it requires that the interaction between cell and interface be dominated only by the parts of the cell nearest the wall. A different experimental methodology more appropriate to physiologically significant separations is needed.

It may be possible to convert another approach, total internal reflection fluorescence microscopy (TIRFM), to a quantitative method. This method, explored extensively by Axelrod,[34,35] is an application of total internal fluorescence (TIRF) to cellular microscopy and is an extension of the total internal reflection microscope illumination system introduced by Ambrose.[36] While the theory of total internal reflection was first laid out by Newton, its modern development largely follows from Harrick's book.[37] A brief summary, pertinent to what is proposed here, follows.

When light propagates through a transparent medium of high refractive index to impinge on an interface with a medium of lower index of refraction at an angle exceeding a "critical" angle ($\theta_c = \sin^{-1} n_2/n_1$, where θ_c is the critical angle of incidence and n_1 and n_2 are the refractive indices of media 1 and 2, respectively), all the incident light is reflected; one obtains *total reflection.* Nevertheless, the electromagnetic field establishes a shallow, standing, "evanescent" wave in the second medium. Its intensity decays exponentially with perpendicular distance Z from the interface:

$$I(Z) = I_o e^{-Z/d}.$$

I_o is the evanescent electric field intensity at the interface ($Z = 0$) and is on the order of the incident light intensity except for angles of incidence (θ) close to θ_c. The symbol d represents the effective wave penetration depth:

$$d = \frac{\lambda}{4\pi n_2}\left(\frac{\sin^2\theta}{\sin^2\theta_c} - 1\right)^{-1/2},$$

where λ is the wavelength of the incident light. The effective wave penetration depth, which depends on the wavelength of the incident light and the refractive indices of media one and two, normally varies from several tens to several hundreds of nanometers. The intensity of the evanescent wave is proportional to the square of the amplitude of the evanescent electric field E. This evanescent wave is capable of exciting fluorescent molecules that are within it.

In recent years, this method has been used to establish adsorption isotherms and measure adsorption rates and surface diffusivities.[38–40] This method has also been used to examine the cell-substratum contact region of primary cultured rat myotubes with acetylcholine receptors labeled by fluorescent α-bungarotoxin[35] and human skin fibroblasts labeled with a 3,3′-dioctadecylindocarbocyanine iodate.[34] The sharp, bright pictures obtained show that the rat myotube adheres to the substratum in a thin band around its periphery and in one small region at the center. These images have been compared with those obtained by epifluorescence and phase contrast illumination by Axelrod *et al.*[35]; they concluded that TIRFM was superior for examining specific fluorescent probes in the contact region. They also showed that this technique dramatically reduces background from cell autofluorescence and debris. Very recently, Gingell's group has begun to apply TIRFM to map the shape of the region between glass and the lower surface of spread, living cells.[41] The intensity of light from a fluorescent volume marker incapable of penetrating into the cell was used to obtain the topography of the cell-glass apposition.

These studies establish the qualitative use of TIRFM for studying cells in close apposition to a transparent, reflecting surface. They are not, however, quantitative, do not attack the problem of relating the intensity of fluorescence produced by the evanescent wave to the distance, Z, of the fluorescent material from the reflecting surface, and do not consider the kinetic problem of how cells approach the surface.

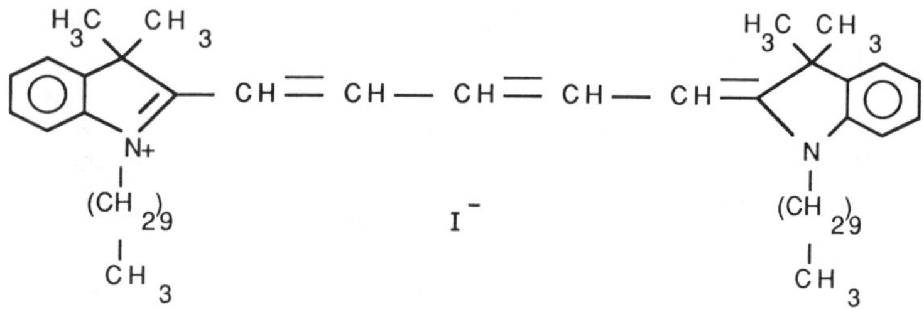

FIGURE 1. The structure of DiI-C_{10}-(5). The acyl chains will be embedded in the bilayer parallel to the phospholipid acyl chains.

We intend to quantify TIRFM and to use it for measuring $Z(x, y, t)$ between the red blood cell and a clean glass surface in order to obtain information about the cell substratum profile during the approach of the cell as well as the changes in approach and final position with alterations in cell surface and interface properties. The proposed study is to be concerned with all human blood cells, with ultimate interest directed especially toward white cells and platelets. However, the detailed study of the erythrocyte is considered essential for qualifying the method for use on these other cells, which are substantially more difficult to handle.

This experiment has several requirements: first, one must properly label the erythrocyte. The choice of a dye depends on many parameters. The dye must selectively interact with the cell membrane, it must have an excitation maximum close to the wavelength of the available light source, and its emission maximum must be at a wavelength to which the image aquisition device is sufficiently sensitive. We have

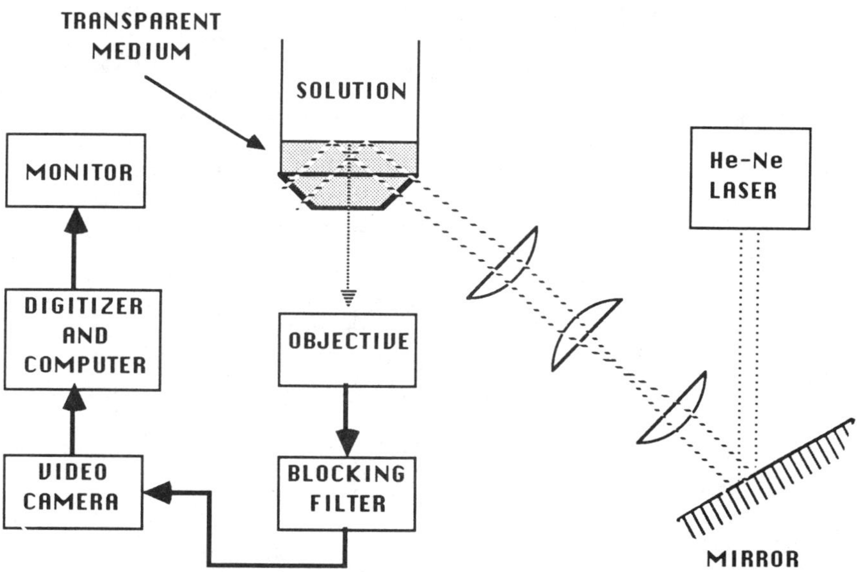

FIGURE 2. Schematic of a TIRFM arrangement for the study of cells in close apposition to a glass surface.

chosen a particular dye from the indocarbocyanine family, 1,1′-bidecyl-3,3,3′3′-tetramethyl indocarbocyanine iodide (DiI-C_{10}-(5), FIG. 1). Members of this family have been used as probes for monitoring of the membrane potentials in red blood cell membranes.[42] Axelrod[43] has shown these dyes to be oriented with the acyl chains embedded in the bilayer parallel to the phosopholipid acyl chains and the bridge chromophore lying parallel to the surface of the cell, a configuration appropriate for the studies proposed here. A preliminary examination of the fluorescence characteristics of this dye has shown that when excited at 620 nm, it has emission maxima of 658 and 668 nm in Tris buffer and cell suspension, respectively. The difference shows that red blood cells quench the emission, as Sims *et al.* have suggested.[42] The members of this dye family cover a large range of excitation and emission maxima. However, DiI-C_{10}-(5) was selected because of constraints imposed by the available excitation source (see below).

After the choice of dye, the second requirement for the proposed experiment is an excitation source and a focusing and optical system that permits TIR to occur and the dye to fluoresce. For the preliminary studies, a He-Ne laser (632.8 nm) is mounted on a compact optical bench attached to the observing microscope (FIG. 2). The beam leaves the laser, is reflected by a front-surface mirror, and passes through a system of three convex lenses. Two of these serve as a Gallilean telescope, enlarging the beam before it passes through the third lens, which focuses it. The optical path contains a spatial filter at the focal point of the first lens of the telescope and a shutter that prevents unwanted bleaching of dye. The laser beam reaches the interface between a microscope cover glass and the solution at an angle which is a chosen excess over the critical value for TIR, pasing through a small prism made of BK-7 glass with $n = 1.52$. This prism is kept in optical contact with the cover glass with oil of the same refractive index.

After the choice of the TIR illumination system, the third requirement is observation and analysis of the fluorescent image emitted from the cell surface. In the preliminary experiments a venerable Bausch & Lomb inverted metallographic microscope is used. The image is observed with considerable enhancement over what could be seen with the naked eye, using a Dage-MTI video camera with an RCA Silicon Intensifier Target (SIT) tube and a standard monitor. The RCA SIT tube is maximally sensitive at a wavelength of about 440 nm, with nearly a 70% reduction in sensitivity at 650 nm.[44] However, even with such a reduction, it is much more suitable than other, less sensitive tubes that demonstrate maximum sensitivity in the range of 600 to 700 nm. The obtained image is then digitized, enhanced, and stored.

A crude and preliminary apparatus that was built based on this principle has demonstrated the suitability of TIRFM for the dynamic study of the cell-surface adhesion process. An improved version that would allow visualizing more detail is now being prepared. Depending upon the particulars of the arrangement, many of which can be varied, a vertical resolution of down to two orders of magnitude less than the wavelength of the incident light can be expected. We expect to be able to achieve sufficient sensitivity and resolution (lateral as well as vertical) for a detailed analysis of the cell surface.

REFERENCES

1. HAM, R. G. & M. J. VEOMETT. 1979. Mechanisms of Development. Mosby. St. Louis. pp. 505–527.
2. MCCUTCHEON, M., D. R. COMAN & F. B. MOORE. 1948. Studies on invasiveness of cancer: Adhesiveness of malignant cells in various human adenocarcinomas. Cancer **1:** 460–467.

3. GINGELL, D. & S. VINCE. 1980. Long-range forces and adhesion: An analysis of cell-substratum studies. *In* Cell Adhesion and Motility. A. S. G. Curtis & J. D. Pitts, Eds.: 1–37. Cambridge Univ. Press. London and New York.
4. BONGRAND, P. & G. I. BELL. 1984. Cell-cell adhesions: Parameters and possible mechanism. *In* Cell Surface Dynamics: Concepts and Models. C. DeLisi, A. Perelson & F. Wiegel, Eds.: 459–493. Marcel Dekker. New York.
5. CURTIS, A. S. G. 1960. Cell contacts: Some physical considerations. American Naturalist **94:** 37–56.
6. DOLOWY, K. 1980. A physical theory of cell-cell and cell-substratum interactions. *In* Cell Adhesion and Motility. A. S. G. Curtis & J. D. Pitts, Eds.: 39–63. Cambridge Univ. Press. London and New York.
7. VOIGT, A., E. DONATH & R. HEINRICH. 1982. Free energy of the electrostatic interaction of cells with adjacent charged glycoprotein layer: A theoretical approach. J. Theor. Biol. **98:** 269–282.
8. BELL, G. I., M. DEMBO & P. BONGRAND. 1984. Cell adhesion: Competition between nonspecific repulsion and specific bonding. Biophys. J. **45:** 1051–1064.
9. IZZARD, C. S. & L. R. LOCHNER. 1976. Cell-to-substrate contacts in living fibroblasts: An interference reflection study with an evaluation of the technique. J. Cell Sci. **21:** 129–159.
10. GINGELL, D. & I. TODD. 1980. Red blood cell adhesion. II. Interferometric examination of the interaction with hydrocarbon oil and glass. J. Cell Sci. **41:** 135–149.
11. TROMMLER, A., D. GINGELL & H. WOLF. 1985. Red blood cells experience electrostatic repulsion but make molecular adhesions with glass. Biophys. J. **48:** 835–841.
12. MEGE, J., C. CAPO, A. BENOLIEL, C. FOA, R. GALINDO & P. BONGRAND. 1986. Quantification of cell surface roughness; A method for studying cell mechanical and adhesive properties. J. Theor. Biol. **119:** 147–160.
13. BRENNER, H. & P. M. BUNGAY. 1971. Rigid-particle and liquid droplet models of red cell motion in capillary tubes. Fed. Proc. **30:** 1565–1577.
14. GOLDSMITH, H. L. 1971. Red cell motions and wall interactions in tube flow. Fed. Proc. **30:** 1578–1590.
15. BLACKSHEAR, P. L., R. J. FORSTROM, F. D. DORMAN & G. O. VOSS. 1971. Effects of flow on cells near walls. Fed. Proc. **30:** 1600–1611.
16. GOLDSMITH, H. L. & V. T TURITTO. 1986. Rheological aspects of thrombosis and haemostasis: Basic principles and applications. Thromb. Haemostas. **55:** 415–443.
17. WOLF, H. & D. GINGELL. 1983. Conformational response of the glycocalyx to ionic strength and interaction with modified glass surfaces: Study of live red cells by interferometry. J. Cell Sci. **63:** 101–112.
18. BELL, G. I. 1978. Models for the specific adhesion of cells to cells. Science **200:** 618–627.
19. CAPO, C., F. GARROUSTE, A. BENOLIEL, P. BONGRAND, A. RYTER & G. I. BELL. 1982. Concanavalin-A-mediated thymocyte agglutination: A model for a quantitative study of cell adhesion. J. Cell Sci. **56:** 21–48.
20. PARSEGIAN, V. A., D. GINGELL & I. TODD. 1977. Long-range attraction between red cells and a hydrocarbon surface. Nature **268:** 767–769.
21. PARSEGIAN, V. A. & D. GINGELL. 1973. A physical force model of biological membrane interaction. *In* Recent Advances in Adhesion. L. H. Lee, Ed.: 153–192. Gordon and Breach. London.
22. PREVOST, M. & D. GALLEZ. 1984. The role of repulsive hydration forces on the stability of aqueous black films. J. Chem. Soc. Faraday Trans. **80:** 517–533.
23. MARGOLIS, L. B. 1984. Cell interaction with model membranes: Probing, modification and simulation of cell surface functions. Biochem. Biophys. Acta **779:** 161–189.
24. PARSEGIAN, V. A. & D. GINGELL. 1980. Red blood cell adhesion. III. Analysis of forces. J Cell Sci. **41:** 151–157.
25. ISRAELACHVILI, J. & R. PASHLEY. 1982. The hydrophobic interaction is long range, decaying exponentially with distance. Nature **300:** 341–342.
26. PARSEGIAN, V. A., N. FULLER & R. P. RAND. 1979. Measured work of deformation and repulsion of lecithin bilayers. Proc. Natl. Acad. Sci. U.S.A. **76:** 2750–2754.
27. LERCHE, D. 1983. A biophysical model for interaction of cells with a surface coat (glycocalyx). I. Electrostatic interaction profile. J. Theor. Biol. **104:** 231–248.

28. DONATH, E. & A. VOIGT. 1983. Charge distribution within cell surface coats of single and interacting surfaces—a minimum free electrostatic energy approach. Conclusions for electrophoretic mobility measurements. J. Theor. Biol. **101:** 569–584.
29. WINZLER, R. 1970. Carbohydrates in cell surface. Int. Rev. Cytol. **29:** 77–125.
30. SINGER, S. J. & G. L. NICOLSON. 1972. The fluid mosaic model of the structure of cell membranes: Cell membranes are viewed as two-dimensional solutions of oriented globular proteins and lipids. Science **175:** 720–731.
31. LOOR F. 1978. Structure and dynamics of lymphocyte surface. *In* B and T Cells in Immune Recognition. F. Loor & G. E. Roelants, Eds.: 153–189. Wiley. New York.
32. CURTIS, A. S. G. 1964. The adhesion of cells to glass: A study by interference reflection microscopy. J. Cell Biol. **19:** 199–215.
33. GINGELL, D. & I. TODD. 1979. Interference reflection microscopy: A quantitative theory for image interpretation and its application to cell-substratum separation measurement. Biophys. J. **26:** 507–526.
34. AXELROD, D. 1981. Cell-substrate contacts illuminated by total internal reflection fluorescence. J. Cell Biol. **89:** 141–145.
35. AXELROD, D., N. L. THOMPSON & T. P. BURGHARDT. 1983. Total internal reflection fluorescence microscopy. J. Microsc. **129:** 19–28.
36. AMBROSE, E. J. 1961. The movement of fibrocytes. Exp. Cell Res. **8** (Suppl.): 54–73.
37. HARRICK, N. J. 1967. Internal Reflection Spectroscopy. Wiley. New York.
38. VAN WAGENEN, R. A., S. ROCKHOLD & J. D. ANDRADE. 1982. Probing protein adsorption: Total internal reflection intrinsic fluorescence. *In* Biomaterials: Interfacial Phenomena and Applications. Advances in Chemistry Series, Vol. 199. S. L. Cooper & N. A. Peppas, Eds.: 351–370. American Chemical Society. Washington, D.C.
39. ROCKHOLD, S. A., R. D. QUINN, R. A. VAN WAGENEN, J. D. ANDRADE & M. REICHERT. 1983. Total internal reflection fluorescence (TIRF) as a quantitative probe of protein adsorption. Elsevier Sequoia **150:** 262–275.
40. AXELROD, D. 1984. Total internal reflection fluorescence. Ann. Rev. Biophys. Bioengr. **13:** 247–268.
41. GINGELL, D., I. TODD & J. BAILEY. 1985. Topography of cell-glass apposition revealed by total internal reflection fluorescence of volume markers. J. Cell Biol. **100:** 1334–1338.
42. SIMS, P. J., A. S. WAGGONER, C. WANG & J. F. HOFFMAN. 1974. Studies on the mechanism by which cyanine dyes measure membrane potential in red blood cells and phosphatidylcholine vesicles. Biochemistry **13:** 3315–3330.
43. AXELROD, D. 1979. Carbocyanine dye orientation in red cell membrane studied by microscopic fluorescence polarization. Biophys. J. **26:** 557–574.
44. INOUE, S. 1986. Video Microscopy. Plenum. New York. p. 211.
45. MILLER, C. A. & P. NEOGI. 1985. Interfacial Phenomena: Equilibrium and Dynamic Effects. Marcel Dekker. New York. p. 93.
46. CHEN, J. & J. C. SLATTERY. 1982. Effects of London-van der Waals forces on the thinning of a dimpled liquid film as a small drop or bubble approaches a horizontal solid plane. AIChE J. **28:** 955–963.

The Effect of Fluid Mechanical Stress on Cellular Arachidonic Acid Metabolism[a]

L. V. McINTIRE,[b] J. A. FRANGOS,[b] B. G. RHEE,[b]
S. G. ESKIN,[c] AND E. R. HALL[d]

[b]*Biomedical Engineering Laboratory*
Rice University
Houston, Texas 77251

[c]*Department of Surgery*
Baylor College of Medicine
Houston, Texas 77030

[d]*Department of Medicine*
University of Texas Medical School
Houston, Texas 77225

INTRODUCTION

High levels of fluid mechanical stresses can cause lysis of red blood cells, platelets, and leukocytes.[1–10] FIGURE 1 gives an estimate of the combination of stress magnitude and exposure time that can cause lysis for each cell type. The curves shown divide the lytic and sublytic regions. Lower stress levels and/or shorter exposure times can lead to cell-cell aggregation.[11-15] Mechanical stresses can also damage anchorage-dependent cells such as endothelial cells.[16-19] Other fluid stress effects on endothelial cells include orientation and alignment of the microtubule network parallel to the direction of fluid flow.[20–24]

The purpose of this paper is to examine the hypothesis that some sublytic levels of mechanical perturbations of cells can stimulate cell metabolism. We have chosen arachidonic acid as a marker metabolite. Metabolites of this 20 carbon chain fatty acid vary significantly depending on the cell type and the stimulus. Principal metabolites for platelets include the cyclooxygenase product thromboxane A_2 (TXA_2) and the lipoxygenase product 12-hydroperoxy-eicosatetraenoic acid (12-HPETE). Polymorphonuclear leukocytes (PMNLs) initially produce principally 5-HPETE, sometimes leading to the formation of leukotrienes, though many other metabolites of arachidonic acid have been isolated from activated neutrophils. Human umbilical vein endothelial cells utilize arachidonic acid to produce mainly prostaglandin I_2 (PGI_2). All of these metabolites are biologically active and modulate cell function, sometimes in quite contrasting ways. We will show that levels of sublytic mechanical stress exposure can stimulate arachidonic acid metabolism in all three of the cell types mentioned above. The biological implications of this stress-metabolism coupling may be quite far-reaching.

[a]This work was partially supported by National Institutes of Health grants nos. HL–18672, HL17437, and NS 23327, and grant no. C–938 from the Robert A. Welch Foundation.

MATERIALS AND METHODS

Preparation of Human PMNLs

Venous blood from normal healthy donors was drawn by venipuncture into heparin (10 U/ml, final concentration) in conical tubes. PMNLs were purified using standard techniques of dextran sedimentation, centrifugation on Ficoll-Hypaque, and hypotonic lysis of erythrocytes. Final cell suspensions contained a minimum of 95% PMNLs. Viability of the PMNLs was always greater than 95% as determined by trypan blue exclusion. PMNLs were labeled with 5.5 μmol/l of [1-^{14}C] arachidonate added during the first wash.

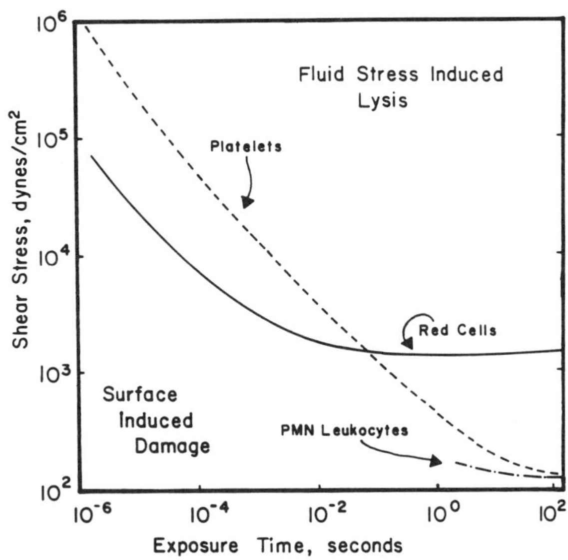

FIGURE 1. Effects of stress and exposure time on shear-related damage to blood cellular elements. Regions above and to the right of each line (high stress: long exposure time) would generate significant cell lysis for the given cell type. The curve for PMN leukocytes terminates at 1-s exposure times because the very short time experiments have not been done as yet.

Preparation of Platelet-Rich Plasma (PRP)

Blood was obtained by venipuncture of healthy volunteers. Ten milliliters of blood was quickly and gently mixed with 1.1 ml of heparin (100 U/ml) in siliconized glass tubes. The heparinized blood was centrifuged for 10 minutes at 150 $\times$g. The supernatant PRP was drawn off with a Pasteur pipette and transferred to a clean siliconized glass or plastic test tube. The remaining fractions were centrifuged for 5 minutes at 150 g to retrieve more PRP. Finally, the red blood cell fraction was centrifuged for 10 minutes at 1000 $\times$g. The resultant supernatant was platelet-poor plasma (PPP), which was transferred to a separate test tube. Platelet counts in all PRP samples were adjusted to 3×10^8/ml final concentration by dilution with PPP. For some experiments, platelets were also labeled with [1-^{14}C] arachidonate after washing.

Endothelial Cell Cultures

Human umbilical vein endothelial cells were harvested from umbilical cords by means of culture procedures adapted from Gimbrone.[26] For removal of the endothelial cells, the veins were cannulated, rinsed with 100 ml of phosphate-buffered saline (PBS), filled with 0.03% collagenase in medium 199 (Gibco), and incubated for 30 minutes at room temperature. After incubation the enzyme solution was flushed through the cord with 100 ml of PBS, and the effluent was collected and centrifuged at 100 $\times$g for 10 minutes. The cell pellet was resuspended in medium 199 supplemented with 20% fetal bovine serum (Hyclone), 100 units of penicillin per milliliter, and 100 mg of streptomycin per milliliter. The cell suspension was seeded onto glass slides (75 $\times$ 38 mm; Fisher) that had been treated earlier with 0.5 M NaOH for 2 to 3 hours and rinsed. Two slides were seeded per cord (5.0 $\times$ 10^4 to 1.0 $\times$ 10^5 cells per slide). Cultures became confluent after 3 or 4 days, and experiments were run 3 days after the cultures reached confluency.

Reagents

[1-^{14}C] Arachidonate (52.0 mCi/mmol, specific activity), [^{3}H]6-keto-PGF$_1\alpha$, thromboxane B_2, [^{3}H]PGF$_2\alpha$, [^{3}H]PGE$_1$, [^{3}H]PGE$_2$, and [^{3}H]PGD$_2$ were all purchased from New England Nuclear (Boston).

High-Performance Liquid Chromatography (HPLC) Analysis of Eicosanoids

In preparation for reversed-phase HPLC (RP-HPLC), cell suspensions were extracted by using Sep-PAK C18 cartridges and 90% methanol eluates were evaporated under nitrogen. Residues were dissolved in 100 μl of methanol, and 10 μl was injected onto the HPLC column. RP-HPLC was carried out on a 4-mm i.d. μ-PAK C18 (5 μm) column (Varian Assoc. Instrument, Palo Alto, CA) with water-methanol-acetonitrile as the eluting solvent. Fractions were collected, and the radiolabel content of each was determined in Hydrofluor by liquid scintillation counting. Identification of the peaks was done by comparison with standards. Under these conditions, stable cyclooxygenase products 6-keto-prostaglandin $F_1\alpha$ (6-keto-PGF$_1\alpha$), thromboxane B_2 (TXB$_2$), PGF$_2\alpha$, PGE$_1$, PGE$_2$, and PGD$_2$ were eluted at 4 to 10 minutes, leukotriene B_4 (LTB$_4$) at 20 to 22 minutes, mono-HETEs at 40 to 52 minutes, and unreacted arachidonate at 55 to 60 minutes.

Bulk Shear Stress Application

Leukocyte suspensions and PRP were subjected to shear stress in a specially modified Ferranti-Shirley Viscometer. The platens used gave a cone and plate geometry. Thus, the entire sample experienced the same constant shear stress. After shearing PRP for 1 minute at 150 dynes/cm^2, the sample was removed and rapidly centrifuged to produce a platelet-free supernatant. In some experiments, this superna-

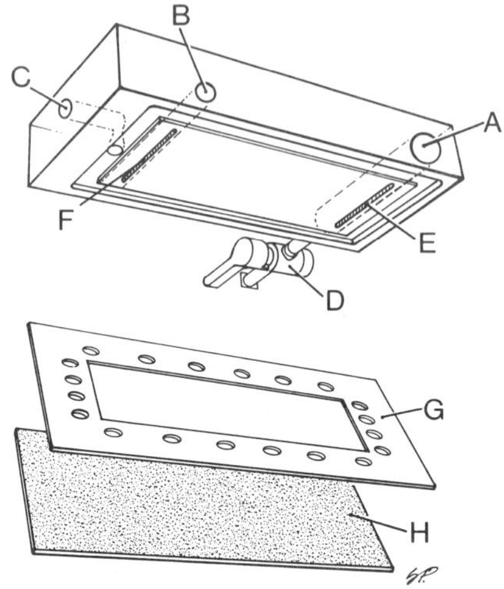

FIGURE 2. Parallel plate flow chamber. The polycarbonate plate, the gasket (*G*), and the glass slide (*H*) with the attached cells are held together by a vacuum (*C*), forming a channel of parallel plate geometry. Medium enters at entry port (*A*), through slit (*E*), into the channel, and exits through slit (*F*) and exit port (*B*). Entry port *A* also serves as a trap for bubbles, which can be removed through valve (*D*).

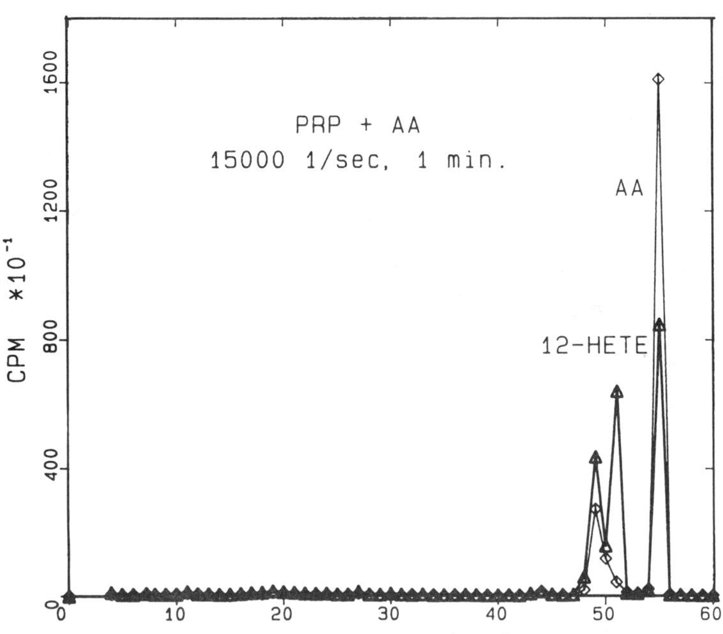

FIGURE 3. RP-HPLC chromatogram of the metabolites of arachidonic acid formed in PRP incubated with 5.5 μmol/l [1-^{14}C] arachidonic acid: ◇ = control; △ = after shearing at 150 dynes/cm^2 for 1 minute.

tant plasma was added to PMNL suspensions within 30 seconds. Labeled PMNL suspensions were also sheared for 1 minute at 150 dynes/cm^2. Supernatants were extracted for HPLC analysis as described above.

Flow Chamber for Endothelial Cells

The flow apparatus utilized is capable of subjecting cultured cells to a range of steady and pulsatile shear stresses. Briefly, it consists of two reservoirs situated one above the other with a parallel-plate flow chamber positioned between them. The flow

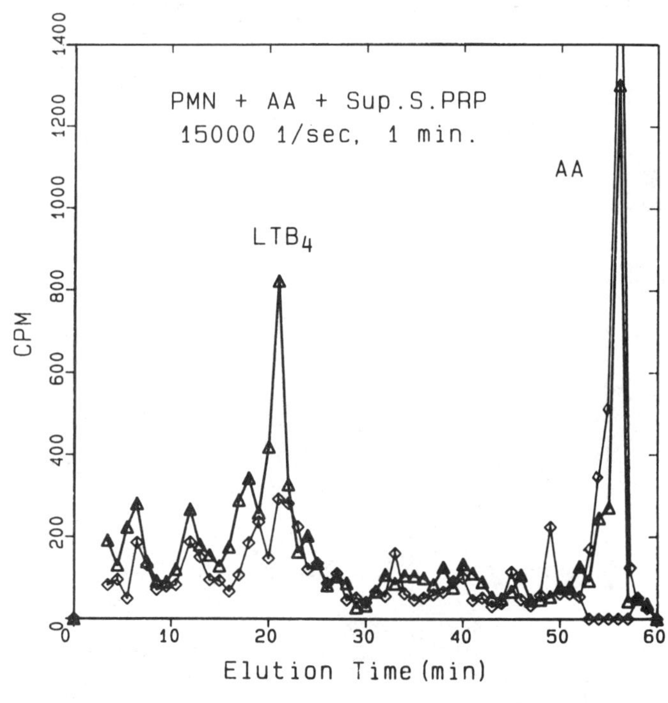

FIGURE 4. RP-HPLC chromatogram of the metabolites of arachidonic acid formed in human PMNL incubated with 5.5 μmol/l of [1-^{14}C] arachidonic acid in the presence of 1:1 by volume supernatant of sheared PRP: ◇ = control; △ = after shearing at 150 dynes/cm^2 for 1 minute.

through the chamber is driven by the hydrostatic pressure head created by the vertical distance between the two reservoirs. Pulsatile flow is introduced by a cam-drive clamp flow oscillator near the chamber. The flow oscillator was used to generate a pulsatile flow that produced maximum and minimum shear stresses of 12 and 8 dynes/cm^2, respectively, at a frequency of 1 Hz. The resulting waveform approximates a square wave. In addition, a range of steady flows producing wall shear stresses of between 0 and 24 dynes/cm^2 was employed. The flow chamber, shown in FIGURE 2, consisted of a machined polycarbonate plate, a rectangular Silastic (Dow Corning) gasket, and the glass slide with the attached endothelial cell monolayer. These were held together by a vacuum maintained at the periphery of the slide, forming a channel of parallel plate geometry. The polycarbonate plate has two slits through which medium enters and exits the channel. The flow rate was controlled by either adjusting the relative distance between the two reservoirs or via a hemodialysis clamp (Harvard Apparatus) upstream of the chamber. The flow rate was monitored by an electromagnetic flow probe. The tissue culture medium was recirculated from the lower reservoir to the upper reservoir by a roller pump. The channel depth was 220 μm, and the area of cells exposed to flow was 16 cm^2. The entire circuit was kept at 37°C by an air curtain incubator. The pH

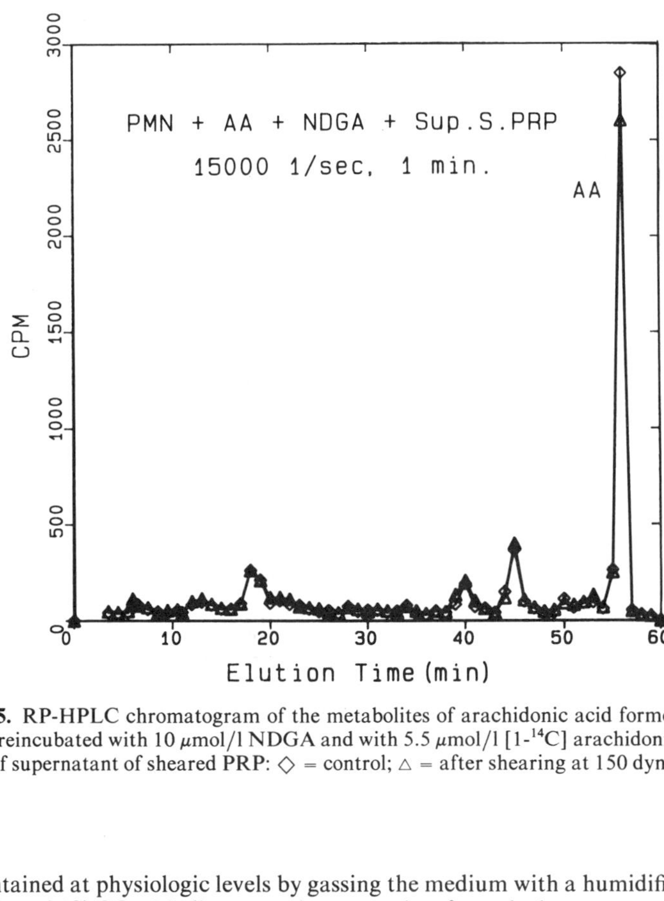

FIGURE 5. RP-HPLC chromatogram of the metabolites of arachidonic acid formed in human PMNLs preincubated with 10 μmol/l NDGA and with 5.5 μmol/l [1-^{14}C] arachidonic acid in the presence of supernatant of sheared PRP: ◇ = control; △ = after shearing at 150 dynes/cm^2 for 1 minute.

was maintained at physiologic levels by gassing the medium with a humidified mixture of 95% air and 5% CO_2. Medium samples were taken from the lower reservoir, thereby avoiding any disturbance of the flow field. From most experiments reported below, medium 199 (Gibco) supplemented with antibiotics and 20% fetal bovine serum was utilized as the circulating fluid above the endothelium monolayers.

Samples were drawn every 3 to 30 minutes, and the flow circuit was simultaneously replenished with fresh medium to maintain a constant circulating volume of 20 ml. Sample and replenishing volumes were both 1 ml. PGI_2 was assayed by radioimmunoassay of the stable nonenzymatic breakdown product, 6-keto-$PGF_1\alpha$.

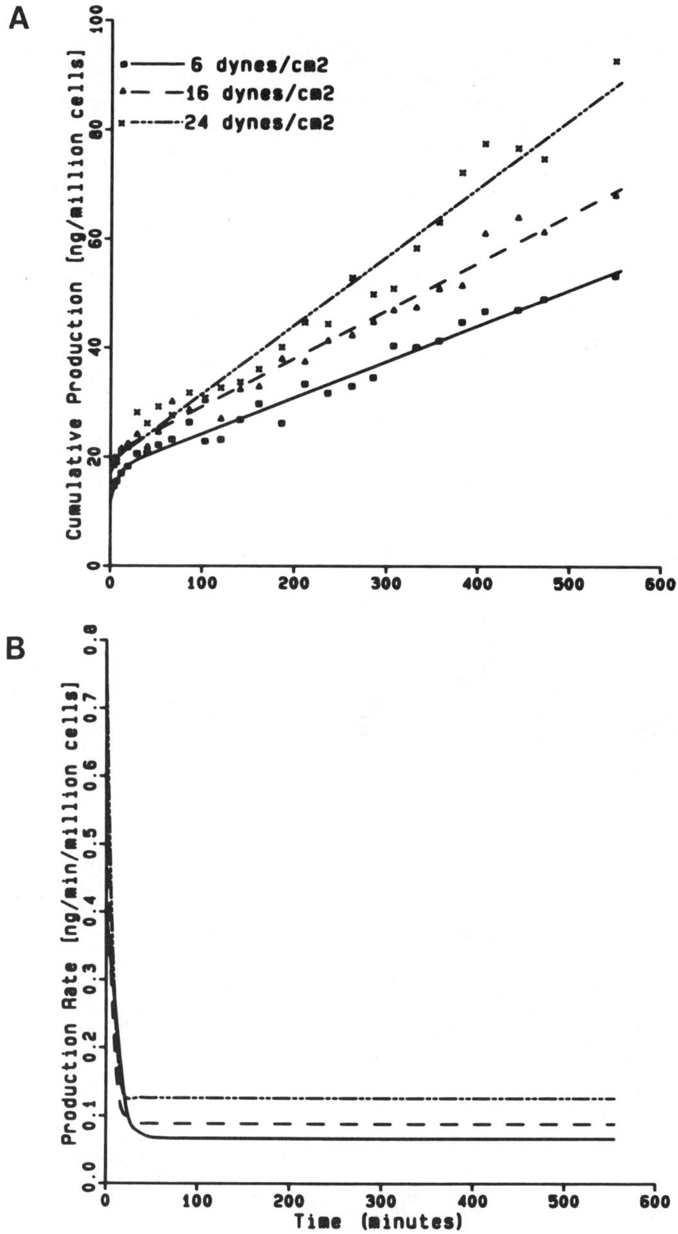

FIGURE 6. Effect of steady shear stress on prostacyclin production (representative set of experiments). Replicate cell monolayers were exposed to shear stresses of 6, 16, and 24 dynes/cm^2. (**A**) Cumulative production of prostacyclin. (**B**) Production rate computed as the derivative of the fitted curves in **A**.

Data Analysis

Cumulative production of PGI_2 was determined by performing a mass balance over the flow loop, taking into account samples withdrawn and medium replenished. By means of a Marquardt nonlinear regression analysis, measurements of cumulative production of PGI_2 were fitted to a four-parameter equation:

$$P_c = A + B(1 - \exp(-CT)) + DT, \tag{1}$$

where P_c is the cumulative production of PGI_2, T is time, and A, B, C, and D are the

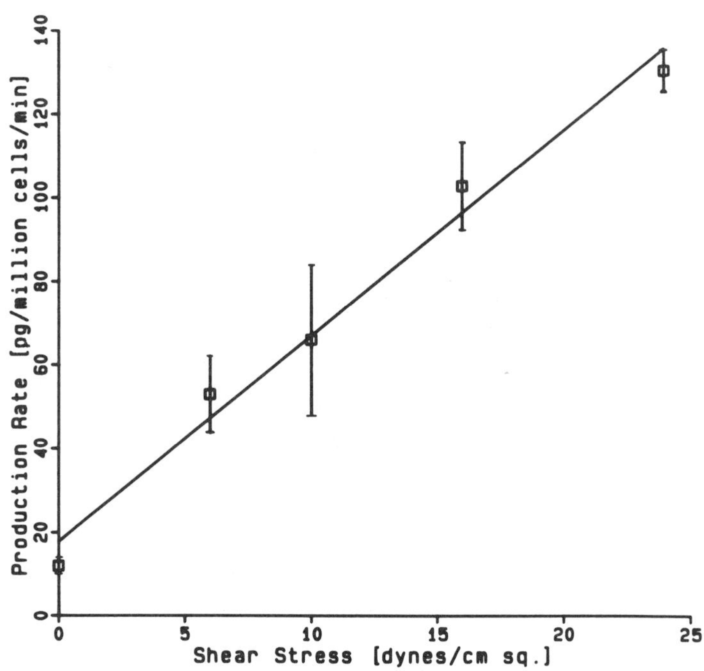

FIGURE 7. Effect of steady shear stress on prostacyclin production. The steady-state production rates are plotted against steady shear stress. The values 6, 16, and 24 dynes/cm^2 represent averaged values of three replicate sets of experiments. The values for 0.016 and 10 dynes/cm^2 were obtained from earlier work.[27] Errors represent the SEM.

parameters to be determined. By taking the time derivative of equation **1**, a smooth expression for the rate of production (P) as a function of time is obtained:

$$P = BC\exp(-CT) + D. \tag{2}$$

The parameters calculated by the regression analysis are related to the kinetics of the rate of production. The parameter, D, represents the steady-state or long-term production rate (SSR), and C was a measure of the rapidity of decay of the initial burst in production of PGI_2. Furthermore, the peak production rate can be expressed as the rate of production at time zero ($BC + D$).

RESULTS

Studies of platelet and/or PMNL arachidonate metabolites, identified by HPLC, were used to examine the effect of shear stress on arachidonic acid metabolism. When [^{14}C] arachidonate-labeled platelets were sheared at 150 dynes/cm^2 for 1 minute, the principal metabolite formed was 12-HETE (FIGURE 3). Very little cyclooxygenase products were detected after shear stress stimulation of platelets. PMNL suspensions sheared for 1 minute at 150 dynes/cm^2 in PBS buffer produced some 5-HETE, but the level was barely detectable using RP-HPLC. When supernatant from sheared PRP (see above) was combined one to one with the PMNL suspension and the mixture sheared at 150 dynes/cm^2 for 1 minute, significant amounts of the lipoxygenase product LTB_4 were produced (FIGURE 4). When the PMNL suspensions were preincubated with nordihydroguaiaretic acid (NDGA), an inhibitor of the lipoxygenase pathway, there was no detectable increase in LTB_4 production after stress exposure of the supernatant of sheared PRP/PMNL suspension mixture (FIGURE 5).

Primary human umbilical vein endothelial cells subjected to a mean shear stress of up to 24 dynes/cm^2 for eight hours remained adherent and viable. Comparison of light micrographs of the cell monolayers, before and after each experiment, revealed no significant changes in cell number or morphology.

The onset of flow led to a sudden increase in the production of PGI_2 that decreased to a constant or steady-state rate (SSR), corresponding to the parameter D in the data fitting algorithm, within several minutes (FIGURE 6). The SSR of endothelial cells subjected to steady flow of 10 dynes/cm^2 was 66 ± 18 pg per 10^6 cells per minute (mean ± SEM; $n = 3$), and cells subjected to pulsatile flow at 1 Hz with the same mean stress produced 161 ± 56 pg per 10^6 cells per minute.[27] The SSR of cells exposed to this pulsatile shear stress was thus 2.4 times greater than that for cells exposed to the same mean steady shear stress ($p < 0.05$). The ratio of peak production rate of pulsatile versus steady shear stress was not significantly different from unity. FIGURE 7 shows the SSR of cells exposed to steady shear stresses of near-zero, 6, 10, 16, and 24 dynes/cm^2. The response was essentially linear in this range of shear stress, with a slope of 4.9 ng/10^6 cells/min/dyne/cm^2.

The rate of basal release of PGI_2 from human umbilical vein endothelial cells under quiescent culture conditions was 10 pg per 10^6 cells per minute. Cell monolayers perfused at near-zero shear stresses of 0.016 dyne/cm^2 produced 11 ± 0.5 pg of PGI_2 per 10^6 cells per minute.

DISCUSSION

Human platelets, leukocytes, and endothelial cells all appear to be sensitive to mechanical stress-induced activation of arachidonic acid metabolism. Sheared PRP exhibited greatly increased synthesis of 12-HETE and surprisingly little thromboxane B_2 production (FIGURE 3). This indicates that shear stress stimulation of platelets may produce arachidonic acid metabolism quite different from that seen with many direct chemical stimuli, such as thrombin or collagen.

Our data demonstrate that a substance derived from shear-induced platelet activation may activate the C-5 lipoxygenase of human PMNL under stress, leading to the production of LTB_4 (FIGURE 4). We hypothesize that this substance may be 12-HPETE.[14,15,28] LTB_4 is known to be a very potent chemotactic factor and to induce PMNL aggregation and degranulation. Our studies provide further evidence that lipoxygenase products of one cell type can modulate production of lipoxygenase products in a second cell type, and that shear stress can initiate cell activation.[28–30] This kind of coupling could have far-reaching implications for our understanding of cell-cell interaction in flowing systems, such as in acute inflammation, artifical organ implantation, and tumor metastasis.

The data on PGI_2 production by endothelial cells demonstrate that physiological levels of shear stress can dramatically increase arachidonic acid metabolism. Step increases in shear stress led to a burst in production of PGI_2 which decayed to a

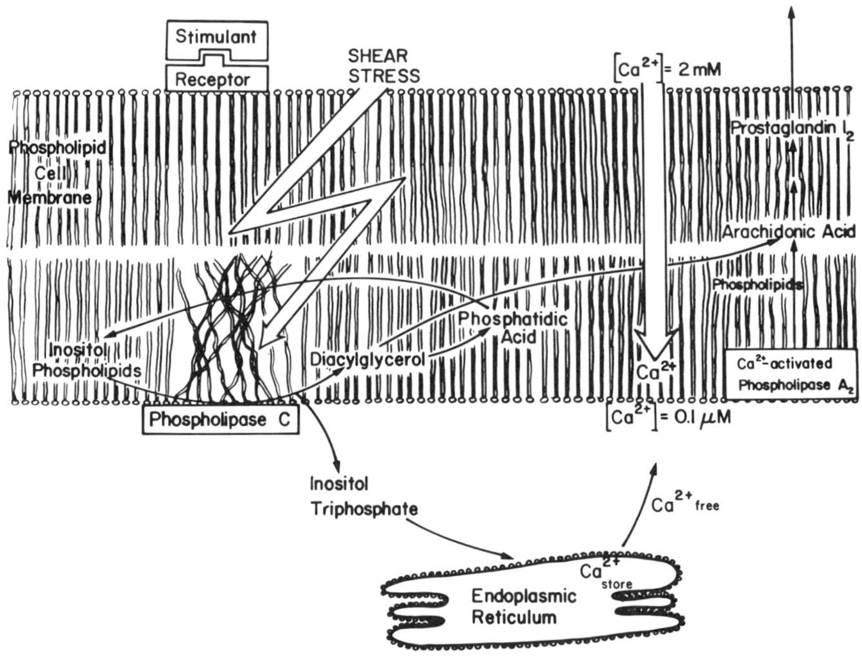

FIGURE 8. Diagram of a possible mechanism for transduction of shear-stress-induced membrane perturbations to intracellular reactions. Biochemical receptor binding can, in some cases, lead to activation of phospholipase C and production of diacylglycerol and inositol trisphosphate from inositol phospholipids. The net effect of these second messengers is an increase in intracellular calcium from both intracellular stores and from increased membrane permeability. Increased calcium can activate the calcium-sensitive phospholipase A_2, leading to PGI_2 synthesis or other arachidonic acid metabolites depending on the cell type. Shear stress, by inducing membrane perturbations or directly altering membrane fluidity, may bypass the receptor requirement and lead to increased phospholipase C activity, eventually resulting in increased synthesis of arachidonic acid metabolites via the cyclooxygenase or lipoxygenase pathways (experimental testing of this hypothesis is currently underway).

steady-state value in several minutes. This longer-term stimulation of prostacyclin production rate increased linearly with shear stress over the range of 0–24 dynes/cm^2. In addition, pulsatile flow of physiological frequency and amplitude caused approximately 2.4 times the PGI_2 production rate as steady flow with the same mean stress. Although only PGI_2 was measured, it is likely that other arachidonic acid metabolites of endothelial cells are also affected by shear stress.

The ability of cells to respond to external stimuli involves the transduction of a signal across the plasma membrane. One such external stimulus appears to be fluid shear stress. Steady shear flow induces cell rotation in suspended cells, leading to a periodic membrane loading, with the peak stress proportional to the bulk shear stress. On anchorage-dependent cells, such as endothelial cells, steady shear stress may act by amplifying the natural thermal or Brownian fluttering or rippling of the membrane.[31]

There are several possible mechanisms by which shear stress induced membrane perturbation could mimic a hormone-receptor interaction, leading to increased intracellular metabolism. One hypothesis is shown in FIGURE 8. Shear stress may induce increased phospholipase C activity, caused by translocation of the enzyme, increased substrate (arachidonic acid) pool availability to phospholipase C (particularly from that stored in phosphoinositols) due to shear-induced membrane movements or changes in membrane fluidity, direct activation of calcium-activated phospholipase A_2 by increased membrane calcium ion permeability, or most probably by a combination of these mechanisms. If stress activates cell metabolism via the mechanisms shown in FIGURE 8, it will have important implications not only regarding arachidonic acid metabolism, but also regarding the effect of mechanical stress on intracellular protein synthesis and cell growth.

REFERENCES

1. McCALLUM, R. N., E. C. LYNCH & J. D. HELLUMS. 1975. J. Lab. Clin. Med. **85:** 67–74.
2. BROWN, C. H., L. B. LEVERETT, C. W. LEWIS, C. P. ALFREY & J. D. HELLUMS. 1975. J. Lab. Clin. Med. **86:** 452–471.
3. HARDWICK, R. A., J. D. HELLUMS, D. M. PETERSON & J. L. MOAKE. 1981. Blood **58:** 678–681.
4. O'REAR, E. A., M. M. UDDEN, L. V. McINTIRE & E. C. LYNCH. 1982. Biochim. Biophys. Acta **691:** 274–280.
5. SUTERA, S. P. & M. H. MEHRJARDI. 1975. Biophys. J. **15:** 1–10.
6. SUTERA, S. P., P. A. CROCE & M. MEHRJARDI. 1972. Trans. Am. Soc. Artif. Intern. Organs **18:** 335–341.
7. DEWITZ, T. S., R. R. MARTIN, T. C. HUNG & L. V. McINTIRE. 1977. J. Lab. Clin. Med. **90:** 728–736.
8. DEWITZ, T. S., L. V. McINTIRE, R. R. MARTIN & H. D. SYBERS. 1979. Blood Cells **5:** 499–510.
9. DEWITZ, T. S., L. V. McINTIRE & R. R. MARTIN. 1980. Artif. Organs **4:** 311–316.
10. McINTIRE, L. V., D. J. STOCKWELL, R. R. MARTIN & H. D. SYBERS. 1980. Trans. Am. Soc. Artif. Intern. Organs **26:** 289–293.
11. DEWITZ, T. S., R. R. MARTIN, R. T. SOLIS, J. D. HELLUMS & L. V. McINTIRE. 1978. Microvasc. Res. **16:** 263–271.
12. MORITZ, M. W., R. C. REIMERS, R. K. BAKER, S. P. SUTERA & J. H. JOIST. 1983. J. Lab. Clin. Med. **101:** 537–544.
13. JEN, C. J. & L. V. McINTIRE. 1984. J. Lab. Clin. Med. **103:** 115–124.
14. RHEE, B. J., E. R. HALL & L. V. McINTIRE. 1986. Blood **67:** 240–246.
15. RHEE, B. G. & L. V. McINTIRE. 1986. Chem. Eng. Commun. **47:** 147–161.
16. FRY, D. L. 1968. Circ. Res. **22:** 165–197.
17. NEREM, R. M. & J. F. CORNHILL. 1980. J. Biomech. Eng. **102:** 181–189.
18. ROSS, R. 1981. Atherosclerosis **1:** 293–311.
19. ROACH, M. R. & N. B. SMITH. 1983. Perspect. Biol. Med. **26:** 287–303.
20. IVES, C. L., S. G. ESKIN, L. V. McINTIRE & M. E. DEBAKEY. 1983. Trans. Am. Soc. Artif. Intern. Organs **29:** 269–274.
21. DEWEY, C. F. 1984. J. Biomech. Eng. **106:** 31–35.
22. ESKIN, S. G., C. L. IVES, L. V. McINTIRE & L. T. NAVARRO. 1984. Microvasc. Res. **28:** 87–94.

23. Levesque, M. J. & R. M. Nerem. 1985. J. Biomech. Eng. **107:** 341–347.
24. Eskin, S. G., C. L. Ives, J. A. Frangos & L. V. McIntire. 1985. asaio J. **8:** 109–112.
25. Ives, C. L., S. G. Eskin & L. V. McIntire. 1986. In Vitro **22:** 500–507.
26. Gimbrone, M. A., Jr. 1976. Prog. Hemostas. Thromb. **3:** 1–28.
27. Frangos, J. A., S. G. Eskin, L. V. McIntire & C. L. Ives. 1985. Science **227:** 1477–1479.
28. Redl, H., D. E. Hammerschmidt & G. Schlag. 1984. Blood **61:** 125–131.
29. Marcus, A. J., M. J. Broekman, L. B. Satier, H. L. Ullman & N. Islam. 1982. Biochem. Biophys. Res. Commun. **109:** 130–137.
30. Marcus, A. J., L. B. Satier, H. L. Ullman, M. J. Broekman, N. Islam, T. D. Oglesby & R. R. Gorman. 1984. Proc. Natl. Acad. Sci. **81:** 903–907.
31. Schneider, M. B., J. T. Jenkins & W. W. Webb. 1984. Biophys. J. **45:** 891–898.

Summary

Flow in Simple and Complex Shapes

J. DAVID HELLUMS

George R. Brown School of Engineering
Rice University
Houston, Texas 77251

The papers in this part by Drs. Goldsmith and Karino concerned the influence of flow patterns on blood cell reactions with the vessel walls and on the patterns of arterial disease. Experimental observations in actual segments of the arterial tree, made transparent, were particularly impressive. They have been successful in placing this information on a quantitative basis that extends even to details of the flow and stress distribution in zones of detachment and recirculation. It was shown that blood cell transport to the wall is enhanced in recirculating flows and in secondary flows with a radial velocity component. Evidence was presented that these zones, which tend to be of low shear rate and longer retention time, tend to be sites of vascular disease.

Gene Eckstein gave us more information on his finding that platelets tend to be concentrated near the wall even in flow in straight cylindrical conduits, an important effect. In fact, under physiological conditions the concentration of platelets in the vicinity of the wall can be five times that near the centerline. The effect depends strongly on hematocrit, shear rate, and red cell deformability. It is, for example, negligible at low hematocrits outside the physiologic range.

Four papers (those by Turitto, Feuerstein, Richardson, and Leonard) considered the rates and mechanisms of platelet approach to the surface, surface contact, movement along the surface, adhesion, detachment, spreading, and aggregation.

Turitto gave an overall review of the factors that affect thrombus growth and stabilization, broken down into three categories: (1) fluid mechanical factors such as flow patterns and local shear rate; (2) blood-related factors such as cellular elements, including the membrane glycoproteins; and (3) vascular factors including, for example, procoagulant proteins and prostacyclin.

Feuerstein and Richardson discussed quantitative observations of platelet interaction with artificial coated surfaces in *ex vivo* flow chambers. Platelet contact followed by detachment leaves a "footprint," which increases the activity of the site toward platelets subsequently arriving at the site. Similarly, the detached platelet is activated and more likely to adhere in subsequent surface contact. Albumin and fibrinogen coatings give the same degree of permanent adherence of platelet, though the albumin coating results in more moves by platelets prior to permanent adherence. Feuerstein presents some interesting results using fluorescent proteins, which seem to show extensive effects of platelets on the coating in the vicinity of the platelet.

There are interesting questions pertaining to the relationship of these "short time" studies, which seem to give results contrary to the findings of several longer time studies. We need to tie the studies together with an improved understanding of surface activation and passivation effects. We also need to relate these findings to the long-term chronic implant studies of Harker and colleagues. Those studies revealed little influence of fluid mechanical factors because the slow surface reaction dominated the resistance.

Ed Leonard brought out the need for the use of the methods of colloidal and surface science in more basic studies. Such studies would bring the tools of these areas to bear on problems of cell approach and reaction with surfaces. He discussed some interesting preliminary studies on the use of certain photoprobes that can be placed in the cell bilipid membrane layer and can mark cell-cell contact.

Larry McIntire's paper focused on the influence of flow parameters on metabolic processes. He presented evidence that increasing shear rate results in increased rates of prostacylin production from endothelial cells. These increases are significant: they can be more than an order of magnitude. The shear rate itself is also important. A change in shear rate yields a burst of metabolic activity, and pulsatile flow yields much more production than steady flow. He also showed that leukocyte metabolism is stimulated and altered by the combination of shear stress and interaction with platelets.

THEME IV. THE STUDY OF PHENOMENA IN VIVO *AND* EX VIVO
PART I. METHODS OF ASSESSING THROMBOSIS

Thrombosis: Studies under Flow Conditions

LINA BADIMON, JUAN JOSÉ BADIMON,
VINCENT T. TURITTO, AND VALENTIN FUSTER

Division of Cardiology
The Mount Sinai Medical Center
New York, New York 10029

INTRODUCTION

Thrombosis is a process that involves various blood cells and proteins, the nature of the blood flow, and surface characteristics, either vascular or prosthetic. All blood-surface interactions *in vivo* are dynamic in nature; that is, they occur in the presence of flowing blood. Therefore, blood elements are exposed to fluid transport rates and local shear forces that differ substantially from those that occur in stagnant or tube reaction systems. Various studies have demonstrated that flow conditions can affect both qualitatively and quantitatively the deposition of cells[1,2] and proteins on surfaces.

There is increasing evidence that the acute clinical and manifestations of coronary atherosclerosis are due to plaque fissuring or rupture and although there has been considerable controversy regarding the causal role of coronary thrombosis in acute myocardial infarction, angiographic studies and the successful application of thrombolytic therapy make it certain that most cases of acute myocardial infarction are caused by coronary thrombosis.[3,4] The rheological changes in the coronary circulation due to coronary artery disease are probably factors contributing to the acute coronary syndromes. The present understanding of the influence of both vascular and rheological factors in thrombosis *in vivo* is limited. Additional investigation into the basic mechanisms by which platelets and coagulation proteins interact with the vessel wall is certainly required. In this article a summary of our recent work on the role of platelets in thrombus formation under defined flow conditions will be presented.

STUDIES WITH A TUBULAR PERFUSION CHAMBER

Various hemodynamic parameters of blood flow, such as diffusion, convection, velocity, shear rate, and shear stress, determine the interaction of cells with the vessel wall and prosthetic implants in the cardiovascular system.[5] The substrate itself also may act as a stimulus for the activation of cellular and proteinaceous components of blood, and may play an important role in the final outcome of the platelet response. For example, in an experimental model of carotid angioplasty, we have shown that mural thrombus formation is directly related to medial tear; the exposed media stimulates platelet aggregation and thrombus formation, even in fully heparinized animals.[6] Conversely, in areas of de-endothelialization without medial rupture, only discrete monolayers or bilayers of platelets are seen.[6] Deeper rupture of vascular surfaces exposes collagen fibrils normally not present on subendothelial surfaces; thus the major distinction in this model was related to the surface stimulation.

There are few techniques available for investigating the exposure of both prosthetic and biological material to blood under controlled blood flow conditions. A perfusion system which has become widely adopted for the exposure of vascular materials is the annular perfusion chamber first developed by Baumgartner,[7] which has been modified more recently in various ways.[8,9] However, the annular perfusion chamber is not easily amenable to the use of nonvascular materials and requires the preselection of vessels for appropriate dimensional characteristics. Therefore, we developed a perfusion chamber that retains the cylindrical shape of the vascular system and is flexible enough to accept a variety of biological and prosthetic materials, and to stimulate a broad range of physiological flow conditions in either *in vivo, ex vivo,* or in *in vitro* perfusion systems[1] (FIGURE 1). The perfusion chamber is placed within a carotid artery and jugular vein extracorporeal system in a heparinized pig. The substrates are mounted in the chamber and perfused with Vassar saline at 37°C for 60 seconds; blood is perfused through the chamber at a preselected flow rate for times ranging from 1 to 30 minutes. At the termination of the perfusion time, buffer is again passed for 30 seconds under identical flow conditions. The changes from buffer to blood and vice versa are achieved by a switch (three-way) valve without introduction of stasis in the chamber. In nonanticoagulated blood perfusions, blood derived from the catheterized vessel is perfused through the chamber and discarded. The selected flow rates are 5, 10, and 20 ml/min in the small (0.1 cm diameter) and large chamber (0.2 cm diameter). These

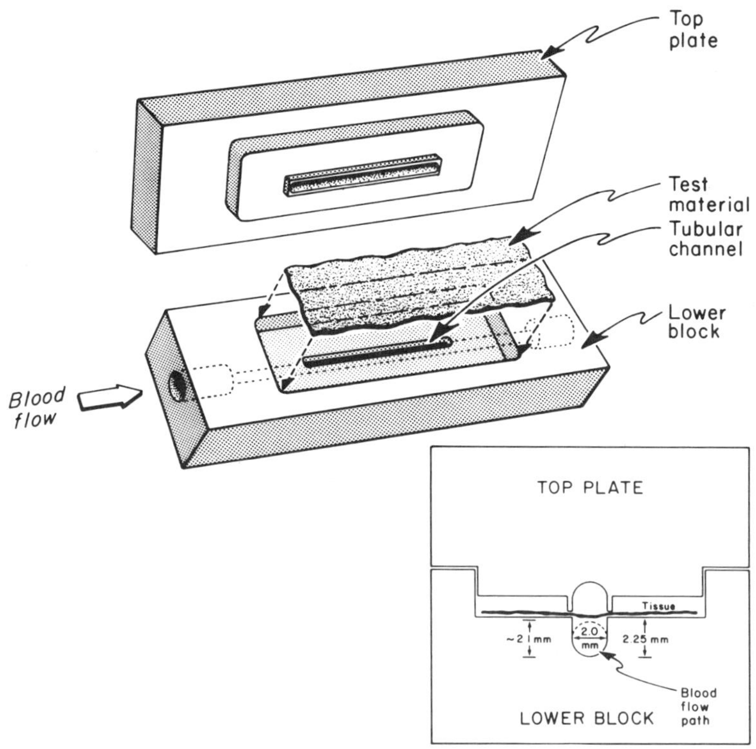

FIGURE 1. Sketch of Plexiglas perfusion chamber used to expose material to flowing blood. Entire chamber is placed in water bath at 37°C during perfusion experiments.

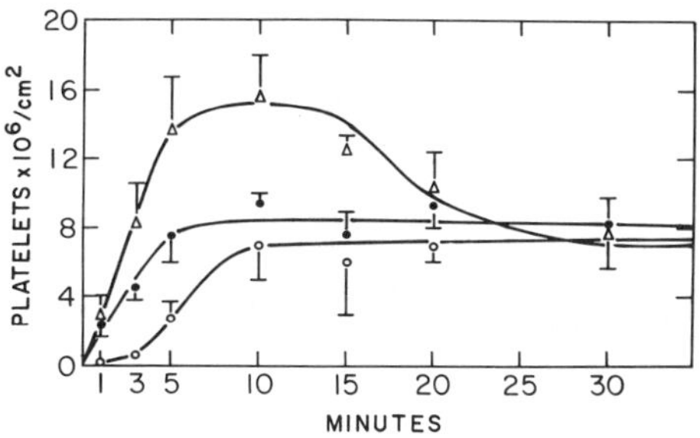

FIGURE 2. Platelet deposition on de-endothelialized vessel wall versus exposure time at different wall shear rates. Wall shear rates (s^{-1}): △ = 1690; ● = 212; and ○ = 106. (From Badimon *et al.*[1])

flows give theoretically calculated local wall shear rates from 106 to 3380 s^{-1}; these shear rates correspond to values ranging from those for large healthy (unobstructed) arteries (106 to 500 s^{-1}), to values typical of the developing flow regions of branched vessels, to values that can be reached at the stenotic areas of the atherosclerotic vessels and the microcirculation (1680 and 3380 s^{-1}).[2,10-12] Clinical and experimental studies have indicated that coronary arterial stenosis may be dynamic, and therefore the coronary lesions could be influenced by aortic pressure, distal coronary arteriolar resistance, and proximal coronary artery vasoconstriction. The interaction of these variables ultimately determines myocardial blood flow.[13] In some instances, the coronary arteriolar resistance bed dilates to compensate for the stenosis resistance and coronary blood flow is maintained at a normal level.[14] In this specific situation local shear rate conditions at the stenotic site may be considerably increased over those of a healthy and unobstructed coronary vessel, since local shear rate is directly related to the flow and inversely related to the cubic power of the patent lumen diameter. At these shear rates, blood may be considered to have Newtonian fluid properties with constant viscosity.[15,16] Shear rate conditions at the wall were calculated from the expression for shear rate given for a Newtonian fluid in tube flow.[17]

Platelet deposition was quantified by ^{111}In labeling of autologous platelets in plasma[1,18,19] and qualitatively analyzed by electron microscopy of selected areas.

Studies on Biological Substrates Using Heparinized Blood

We studied the effect of blood flow on platelet deposition on mildly injured vessel wall, as may occur in the early phases of arterial disease, and on collagen type I fibers, which may be exposed in severe arterial injury such as in a disrupted advanced atherosclerotic plaque. In *in vivo* heparinized blood studies, the perfusion chambers were placed within an extracorporeal system.

The exposure of de-endothelialized vessel wall to blood flow at shear rates of 106 to 424 s^{-1} resulted in platelet deposition on the exposed vessel that reached a maximum within 5 to 10 minutes of exposure, after which platelet accumulation remained relatively constant (FIGURE 2). At maximal deposition, the number of platelets on the vessel ranged from $7 \times 10^6/cm^2$ to $10 \times 10^6/cm^2$ (FIGURE 3). When wall shear rate was increased to 1690 s^{-1}, initial platelet deposition rate and maximal extent of deposition was higher than at the lower shear rate. The highest deposition was also observed at 5 to 10 minutes of perfusion (16×10^6 platelets/cm^2), but at longer

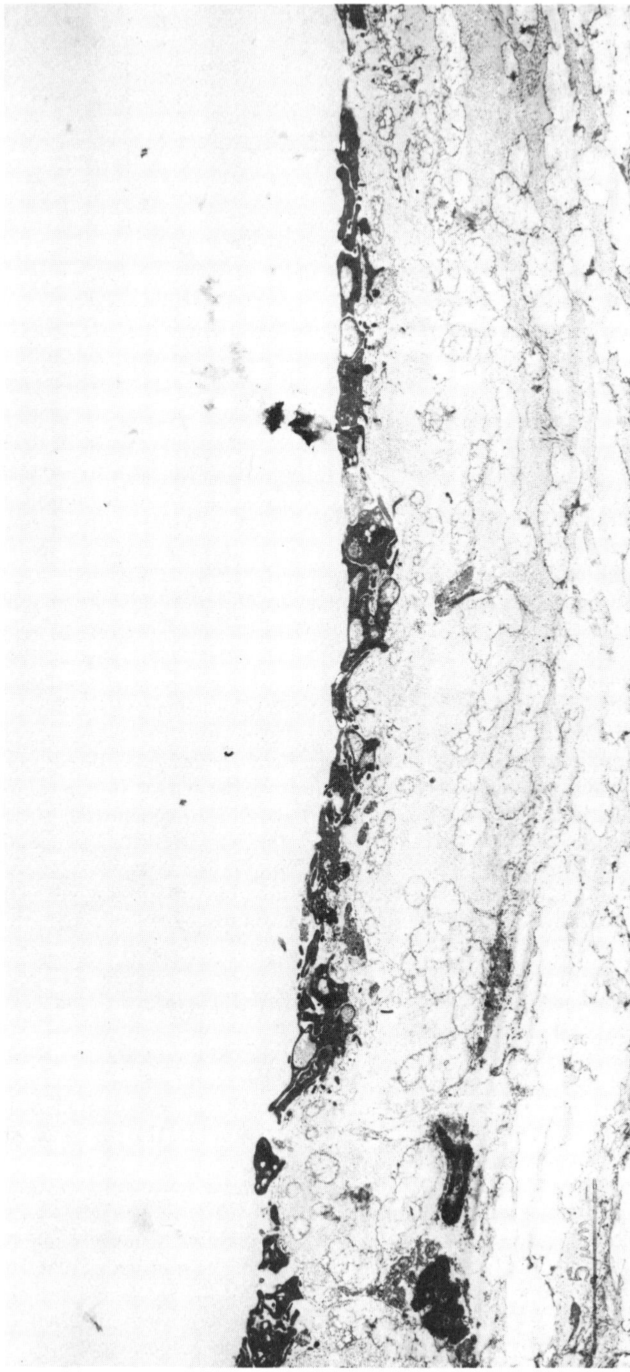

FIGURE 3. Transmission electron micrograph of normal pig platelets deposited on de-endothelialized normal pig thoracic aorta. Blood was perfused for 5 minutes at a shear rate (424 s^{-1}) typical of medium-size healthy arteries. (Magnification: 5000×).

exposure times platelet deposition decreased to values not significantly different from those at the lower shear rate for the same perfusion times (FIGURES 3–5).

Platelet deposition on collagen fibers was considerably higher than that on the vessel wall (FIGURE 6). Platelet deposition was two orders of magnitude greater than on subendothelium, and even at the highest shear rate studied, 3380 s^{-1}, platelet thrombi remained adherent to the surface without apparent dislodgement by the flow forces (FIGURE 7). These results indicate that collagen is much more reactive than subendothelium with respect to the growth and stability of platelet aggregates on the surface, and moreover suggest that flow mechanisms for depositing platelets on the two surfaces may be substantially different (FIGURE 8).

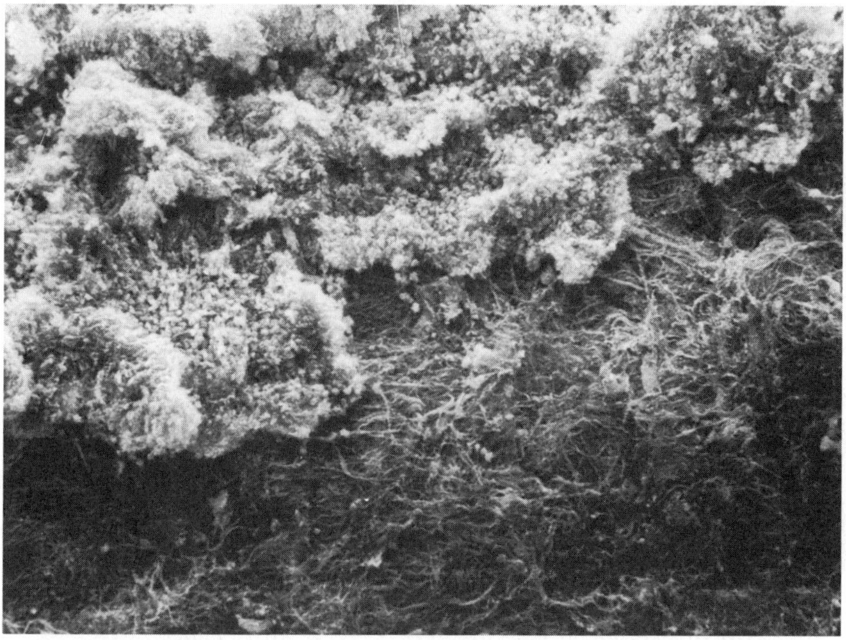

FIGURE 4. Scanning electron micrograph of normal pig platelets deposited on de-endothelialized normal pig thoracic aorta. Blood was perfused for 10 minutes at high shear rate (1690 s^{-1}). (Magnification: 500×).

Platelet deposition, and consequently the growth of platelet thrombi, may be regulated by the exposure of the fibrillar collagen, which will irreversibly aggregate platelets, and the patent luminal cross-sectional area of the vessel, which will regulate the local wall shear rate conditions. Both factors may play an important role in certain clinical conditions. When an atherosclerotic plaque ruptures, fibrillar collagen and connective tissue are exposed to the circulating blood. In addition, the luminal cross-sectional area patent to the blood flow depending on the extent of vascular disease or residual stenosis will be variable, but reduced from normal. The same events might occur after angioplasty. It appears from our studies that the nature of the surface will determine the overall stability of the thrombus, whereas the local flow conditions will influence the rate of growth of the platelet deposits. In any case, it can

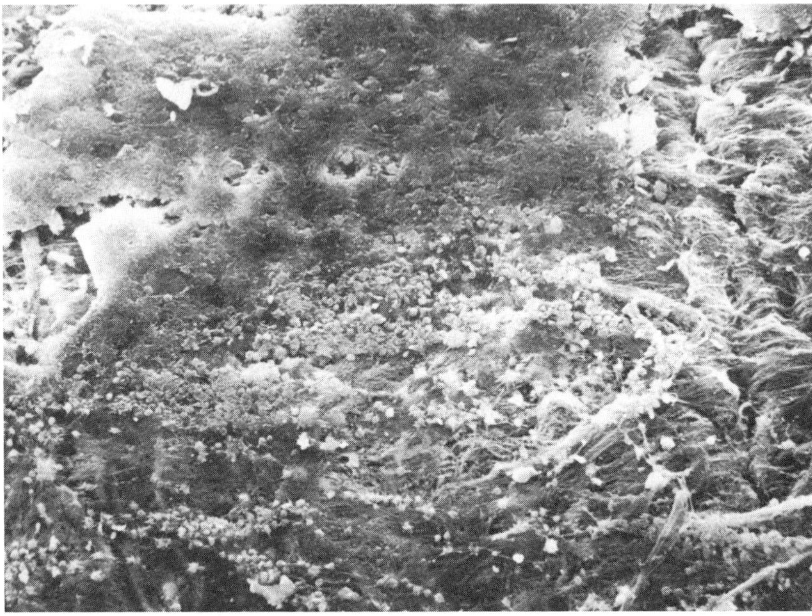

FIGURE 5. Scanning electron micrograph of normal pig platelets deposited on de-endothelialized pig thoracic aorta. Blood was perfused for 30 minutes at high shear rate (1690 s^{-1}). Comparison with FIGURE 4 clearly reproduces the effect evidenced in FIGURE 2; at exposure time longer than 15 minutes, fewer platelets remain attached onto the surface although those deposited appear more spread than at shorter perfusion times. (Magnification: 500×).

be expected that a layer of platelets will remain firmly adherent to any injured area. These platelets, either directly or through release of growth factors, may be responsible for the accelerated rate of restenosis observed in certain angioplasty studies.[20]

Studies on Biological Material Using Nonanticoagulated Blood

Thrombogenesis takes place *in vivo* in the presence of both platelets and the entire spectrum of coagulation zymogens and enzymes. Platelets accelerate clotting and act as membrane sites for the localization of proteins; conversely, thrombin generation dramatically influences platelet aggregation and secretion of granular contents. Intravascularly, untreated native blood circulates over damaged vascular surfaces, ruptured and unruptured atherosclerotic plaques, or implanted prosthetic materials; under such conditions all of the circulating molecular species and cells are available to trigger, or contribute to, the thrombotic process. It is therefore desirable to study the interaction of platelets and vessel wall when nonanticoagulated blood, directly derived from the donor, is perfused over the substrates.

On vascular subendothelium, at high local shear rate (1690 s^{-1}), the rate of platelet deposition from 1 to 5 minutes was much higher in native than in heparinized blood, indicating that thrombus growth was more rapid in native blood than in heparinized blood (platelets × 10^6 per cm^2 per min, mean ± SE: 8 ± 2 in heparinized vs. 16 ± 8 in native blood). The difference in platelet deposition was evident as early as 1 minute after beginning perfusion. In contrast, we have also studied shear rates similar to those of medium-size arteries (212 s^{-1}) and no difference was detected between native and heparinized blood. These findings suggest that under conditions of relatively low thrombogenicity (where few thrombi are formed) the presence of anticoagulation may be less important. Similar observations at high shear rates have been reported when studying citrated and native rabbit blood.[21] We have studied heparin as an anticoagulant because we are using an *in vivo* system of perfusion and also because it is more appropriate to our study since it is commonly used clinically in patients who are susceptible to developing thrombosis, in interventional procedures, and also in patients with prosthetic devices.

When the perfused substrate was the highly thrombogenic collagen type I, the study was performed for perfusion times of up to 3 minutes and the results were similar to those obtained with subendothelium but the extent of deposition was of higher order of magnitude. At a shear rate typical of medium-size arteries (212 s^{-1}) there was little difference in deposition using either heparinized or native blood; however, at the high shear rate of 1690 s^{-1} a statistically significant difference in total deposition was observed ($p < 0.005$). Under these conditions the rates of platelet deposition were 58 ± 12 in heparinized blood versus 85 ± 7 in native blood (platelets 10^6 per cm^2 per min, mean ± SE). These studies emphasize the importance of shear rate in thrombus growth. In spontaneous atherosclerotic plaque rupture, if the patent residual cross section is small an increased wall shear rate will develop which together with a possible nonanticoagulated condition of the blood might induce a rapid growth of a thrombus adhered on top of the lesion. A factor of importance is the exposure to the blood flow of the plaque components, as fibrillar collagen is significantly more active than de-

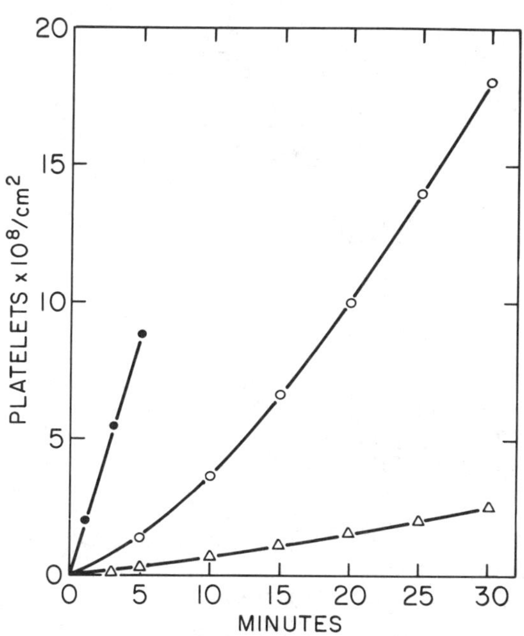

FIGURE 6. Platelet deposition on type I collagen strips of pig-tendon versus time at different shear rates. Shear rates (s^{-1}): ● = 3380; ○ = 1690, and △ = 212. (From Badimon *et al.*[1])

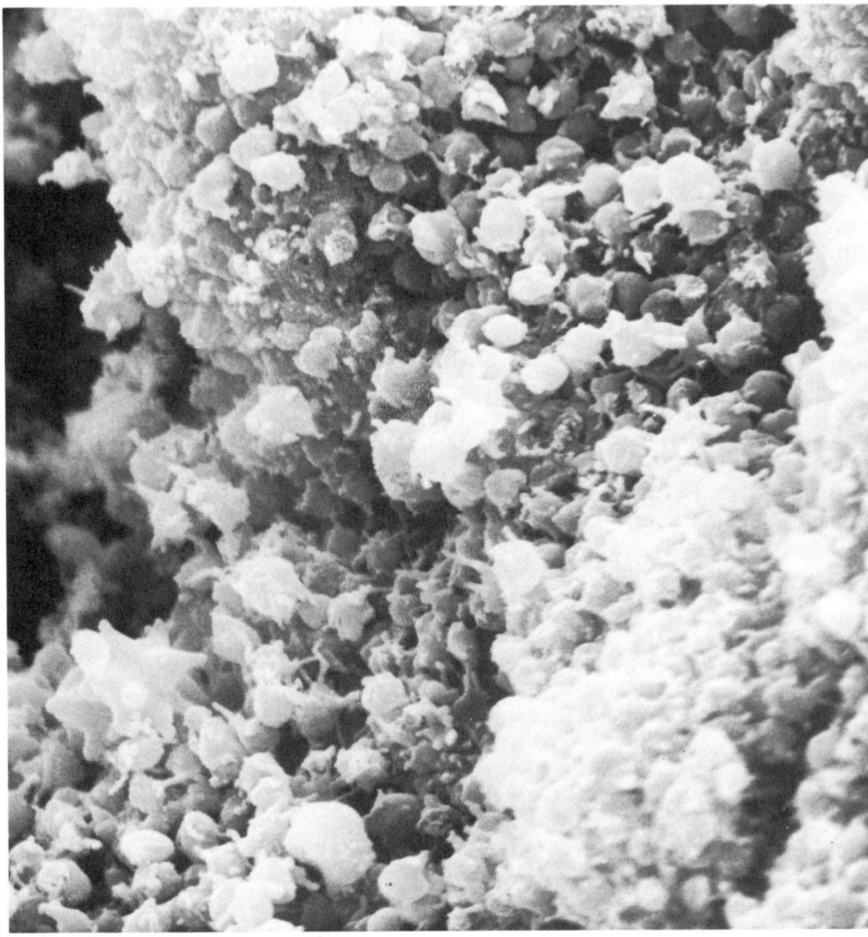

FIGURE 7. Scanning electron micrograph of platelet deposition on collagen after 10-min exposure at a shear rate of 212 s^{-1}. (Magnification: 2500×).

endothelialized vessel wall in the rate of thrombus growth. Exposure of the plaque matrix may stimulate platelets biochemically and, in addition, present a topologically rough surface with the consequent induction of local flow disturbances and recirculation zones (low shear rates). It has been recently reported in laminar flow conditions perfusing rabbit de-endothelialized aorta with nonanticoagulated blood that low shear rates enhance fibrin formation.[22]

With regard to the fluid dynamics at the stenotic areas, it should be emphasized that blood flowing through a vessel at a certain pressure in the axial direction is suddenly accelerated as it passes by the stenosis, and then is immediately decelerated. This deceleration induces flow separations, recirculation zones (vortexes) with a sudden decrease in pressure downstream of the stenosis. The combination of low shear rate areas (poststenotic recirculation zones) with high shear rate areas (stenotic luminal narrowing) may induce activation of both platelets and fibrin-dependent mechanisms simultaneously, and in this way it may contribute to the sudden thrombotic occlusion syndromes.

Studies on a Prosthetic Material Using Heparinized Blood

Gore-Tex® expanded polytetrafluoroethylene (PTFE) used for vascular surgery, was exposed in the perfusion chambers to blood recirculating at 10 ml/min (210 s^{-1}) for 1, 3, 5, and 10 minutes. The deposition of platelets increased linearly with increasing exposure time; the levels of platelet deposition were comparable to but somewhat less than that observed on subendothelium. At these exposure times platelet deposition did not reach the level of saturation seen on subendothelium. The average maximal deposition at 10 minutes of perfusion was 8×10^6 platelets/cm^2.

This surface was compared with subendothelium for de-endothelialized pig aorta and collagen type I bundles from rabbit Achilles tendon (FIGURE 6) with regard to rate of platelet deposition at wall shear rates 105–850 s^{-1}, in the largest perfusion chamber (i.d. 0.2 cm), and the platelet deposition rates were correlated with a theory for describing the mass transport of platelets to the test surface. The deposition of platelets on subendothelium was strongly dependent on the local flow conditions. Values of deposition on Gore-Tex obtained at a single flow condition (212 s^{-1}) were comparable to that observed on subendothelium. In contrast, deposition of platelets on collagen was more than an order of magnitude greater than on subendothelium and showed a dependence on flow only at the lowest flow rate studied (10 ml/min; shear rate, 212 s^{-1}).

Gore-Tex was also exposed in the small chamber (1960 s^{-1}) for 1, 3, and 5 minutes and the deposition of platelet increased linearly with increasing time. The rate of platelet deposition from 1 to 5 minutes of exposure calculated for both local shear rate conditions was 1.9 ± 0.2 at 212 s^{-1} and 4.8 ± 1.0 at 1690 s^{-1} (calculated as surface: blood radioactivity radio multiplied by 10^3 per cm^2 per min).

Studies on Prosthetic Material Using Nonanticoagulated Blood

Gore-Tex was exposed in both perfusion chambers to nonanticoagulated blood derived from the catheterized swine. Exposure times varied from 1 to 5 minutes and the

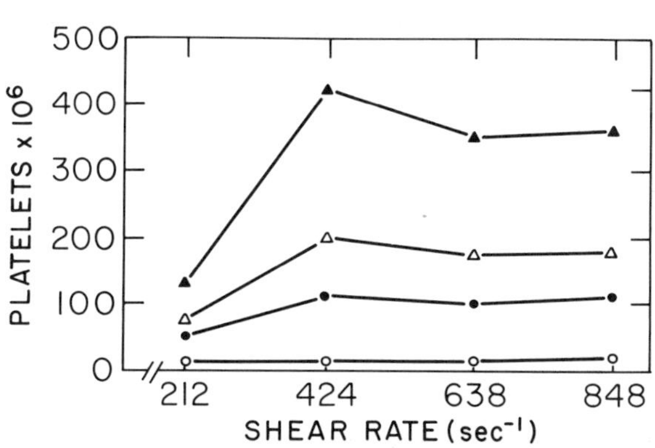

FIGURE 8. Platelet deposition on 50-mm^2 rabbit tendon collagen versus blood shear rate: ○ = 1 minute, ● = 3 minutes, △ = 5 minutes, and ▲ = 10 minutes of perfusion.

local shear conditions studies were 212 s^{-1} and 1690 s^{-1}. The rate of platelet deposition was calculated, as in the heparinized animals, as the ratio of substrate radioactivity to blood radioactivity normalized by exposed surface and perfusion times. At the local shear conditions of large arteries (212 s^{-1}) the rate of platelet deposition was 1.5 ± 0.3, whereas at the high shear rate studied the rate was 4.9 ± 1.0. When comparing these preliminary results with those obtained with heparinized blood, it is interesting to observe that there is no significant difference in rates of platelet deposition at either low (212 s^{-1}) or high (1690 s^{-1}) local shear rates between nonanticoagulated or heparinized blood perfusions. When biological substrates were perfused a significant difference was observed at high shear between heparinized and nonanticoagulated blood. The mechanisms of the different response in the prosthetic material warrants further investigation.

Effect of Blood Proteins in Stabilization and Control of Thrombus Growth

At high shear rate conditions platelet adhesion is independent of flow and more dependent on biochemical factors that influence the platelet-surface interaction. Such factors include glycoproteins in the platelet membrane, calcium levels in plasma, and components of the storage granules of the platelet.[23] The component most extensively investigated is the von Willebrand factor (vWF), a multimeric glycoprotein of high molecular weight. We have studied the role of vWF in platelet deposition in swine with von Willebrand disease. These pigs have a homozygous deficiency in vWF and have been described in detail elsewhere.[24-28]

Heparinized blood from swine with von Willebrand disease was perfused on either subendothelium of normal swine, collagen type I bundles, or Gore-Tex at shear rates from 212 s^{-1} to 3380 s^{-1}. We have observed that not only adhesion but also thrombus formation is reduced in the absence of vWF. Platelet-to-platelet interactions are less

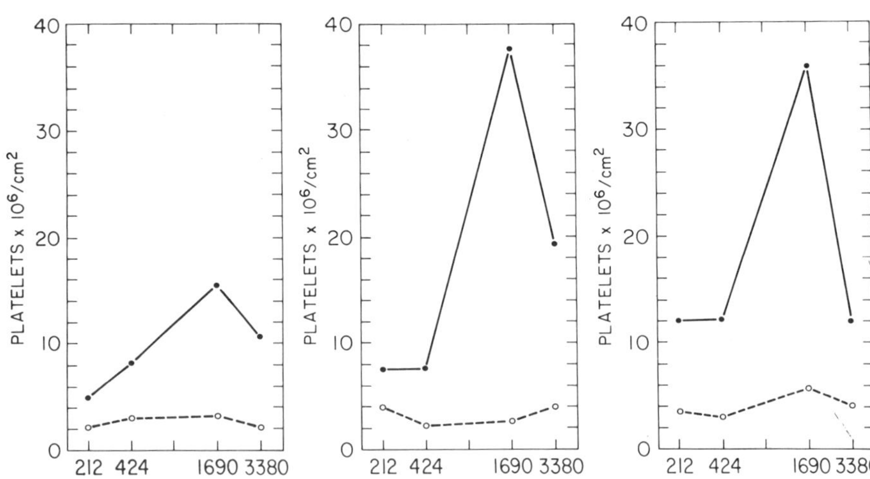

FIGURE 9. Shear rate dependence of platelet deposition on de-endothelialized pig thoracic aorta. Heparinized blood from normal (●) or von Willebrand (O) swine was perfused over the substrate for exposure times of 3 minutes (*left*), 5 minutes (*center*), and 10 minutes (*right*).

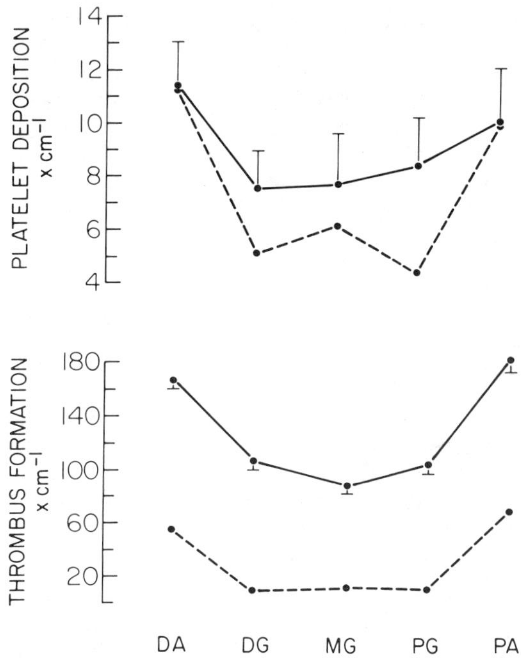

FIGURE 10. Platelet deposition (platelet number × 10^6 per cm^2) and thrombus formation (mg per cm) measured in five different areas of 1 hour implanted PTFE grafts: *DA*, distal anastomosis; *DG*, distal graft; *MG*, middle graft; *PG*, proximal graft; and *PA*, proximal anastomosis. In thrombus determinations the weights of the grafts have been substracted. *Continuous line* shows $\bar{x} \pm$ SE of experiments with nonanticoagulated blood ($n = 17$); *dashed line* shows one experiment using heparin perioperatively.

stable in the absence of this glycoprotein (FIGURE 9). When studies were performed with native blood, similar abnormalities in platelet deposition took place but higher shear rates were required to manifest the defect.

Interestingly, platelet interaction with Gore-Tex was also reduced in a manner dependent on the local flow conditions in von Willebrand disease, suggesting that vWF may also play a role in the attachment of platelets and growth of platelet aggregates on this prosthetic surface. The role of vWF in mediating thrombotic deposits on prosthetic surfaces and its potential dependence on blood flow has not been extensively studied.[29]

STUDIES WITH *IN VIVO* IMPLANTS

Platelets begin to accumulate immediately after blood flow is established through a damaged vascular area (postangioplasty or after the rupturing of an atherosclerotic plaque) or an artificial surface (after implantation), although the sequence of events may be different on these surfaces. We have previously reported the effect of antiplatelet drugs and calcium antagonists *in vivo* in preventing the deposition of platelets and thrombus development in polytetrafluoroethylene vascular graft material

(Gore-Tex) surgically placed in both femoral arteries in mongrel dogs for 3 hours under perioperative heparinization.[29] More recently, we have studied platelet deposition in Gore-Tex implants of the same dimensions (4 mm diameter × 5 cm length) placed in both carotid arteries in normal swine without perioperative heparinization. These were acute studies in which grafts were removed 1 hour postimplantation. Platelet thrombus was quantified by autologous ^{111}In-labeled platelets which were injected 24 hours before surgery. The processing of the grafts involved sectioning into five equal segments and analysis of the different areas in two ways. Formation of complex thrombus (platelets, fibrin, and other cells) was estimated from the weights of the graft sections and platelet deposition was calculated from radioactive measurements.

Interestingly, platelet deposition correlated closely with the weights of the graft segments, that is, in a flow system thrombus formation and platelet deposition occurred in the same areas on the graft. The areas of maximal activity were the anastomotic sites. Within the graft itself, deposition was reduced compared to the anastomotic areas, and no significant axial dependence in thrombus formation, as indicated either by platelet deposits or by thrombus weight, was found (FIGURE 10).

The interaction of blood with the suture line and the tissue-material junction is consequently an area of high risk for acute thrombotic events that may lead to occlusion. The rheological conditions of the area may play a major role in this specific situation. From *in vitro* and *ex vivo* studies it has been recognized that platelet-surface interactions are sensitive to the velocity of blood.[30-31] Low flows (less than 70 ml/min) have been associated, both clinically and experimentally, with early thrombosis whereas higher flows have resulted in greater patency rates.[31] In the swine carotid vascular bed, blood flow averaged 100 ± 20 ml/min (by electromagnetic flowmeter detection). In addition, the average local wall shear rate at the graft site is approximately 260 s^{-1}, and *ex vivo* perfusion studies in the cylindrical perfusion chamber (laminar streamline flow) under such shear conditions have shown that platelet deposition does not progress to occlusive thrombus formation. Both factors, therefore, flow and local shear rate conditions, favor graft patency. It is consequently the anomalous presence of the anastomosis, its induction of local flow recirculations (low shear rates), and areas of some lumen narrowing (high shear rates), together with the exposure of the thrombogenic subendothelial matrix, that increases platelet activation and stimulates the observed high platelet accretion to the implant.

CONCLUSION

In this article we have emphasized that flow, and specifically the local shear rate conditions, can mediate the attachment, growth, and stability of platelet masses on injured vessel walls and biomaterials. Indeed, rheology affects the biochemical mechanisms involved in interaction of platelets and vessel walls. Additionally, we have shown that blood coagulation enhances platelet deposition rate (native blood experiments). In an *in vivo* model of graft implantation we have shown that in an area of expected low platelet activation, flow and surface characteristics may operate synergistically and result in mural thrombosis and even occlusion. Since stenotic regions, or areas around partially occluding lesions, may induce the development of high shear rate conditions, attention should be given to the latent high potential risk of platelet activation and sudden thrombotic occlusion, mainly in those situations in which the coagulation enzymes and zymogens are freely available.

ACKNOWLEDGMENT

The authors thank James A. Rosemark, MCS, for his invaluable collaboration.

REFERENCES

1. BADIMON, L., J. J. BADIMON, A. GALVEZ, J. H. CHESEBRO & V. FUSTER. 1986. Arteriosclerosis **6:** 312–320.
2. TURITTO, V. T. & H. R. BAUMGARTNER. 1982. Platelet surface interaction. *In* Hemostasis and Thrombosis. R. H. Colman, J. Hirsch, V. J. Marder & E. M. Salzman, Eds.: 364–379. Lippincott. Philadelphia.
3. GORLIN, R., V. FUSTER & J. A. AMBROSE. 1986. Circulation **74:** 6–9.
4. DAVIES, M. J. & A. C. THOMAS. 1985. Br. Heart J. **53:** 363–375.
5. GOLDSMITH, H. L. 1972. The flow of model particles and blood cells and its relation to thrombogenesis. *In* Progress in Hemostasis and Thrombosis. T. H. Spaet, Ed.: 97–139. Grune & Stratton. New York.
6. STEELE, P. M., J. H. CHESEBRO, D. R. HOLMES, D. W. STANSON, L. BADIMON & V. FUSTER. 1985. Circ. Res. **57:** 105–112.
7. BAUMGARTNER, H. R. 1973. Microvasc. Res. **5:** 167–179.
8. TURITTO, V. T. & H. R. BAUMGARTNER. 1974. Thromb. Diath. Haemorrh. **60** (Suppl.): 17–24.
9. BAUMGARTNER, H. R. 1976. Schweiz. Med. Wochenschr. **106:** 1367–1368.
10. GOLDSMITH, H. L. & V. T. TURITTO. 1986. Thromb. Haemostas. **55:** 415–435.
11. EL MASRY, O. A. & I. A. FEUERSTEIN. 1982. J. Biomech. Eng. **104:** 290–295.
12. NEREM, R. M. 1981. Arterial fluid dynamics and interactions with the vessel wall. *In* Structure and Function of the Circulation, Vol. 2. C. J. Schwartz & N. T. Werthessen, Eds.: 719–835. Plenum. New York.
13. SANTAMORE, W. P. & A. A. BOVE. 1982. Alterations in the severity of coronary stenosis. *In* Coronary Artery Disease. W. P. Santamore & A. A. Bove, Eds: 157–172. Urban & Schwarzenberg. Baltimore, Munich.
14. GOULD, K. L., K. LIPSCOMB & C. CALVERT. 1975. Circulation **51:** 1085–1094.
15. MERRILL, E. W. 1969. Physiol. Rev. **49:** 863–888.
16. COPLEY, A. L. 1973. Biorrheology **10:** 87–105.
17. BIRD, R. B., W. E. STEWART & E. N. LIGHTFOOT. 1960. Transport Phenomena. John Wiley & Sons. New York.
18. BADIMON, L., V. FUSTER, J. H. CHESEBRO & M. K. DEWANJEE. 1983. Thromb. Haemostas. **50:** 639–644.
19. VALLABHAJOSULA, S., J. MACHAC, S. J. GOLDSMITH, H. LIPSZYC, L. BADIMON, J. RAND & V. FUSTER. 1986. J. Nucl. Med. **27:** 1669–1674.
20. FAXON, D. P., T. A. SANBORN & V. J. WEBER. 1984. Arteriosclerosis **4:** 189–195.
21. BAUMGARTNER, H. R. & K. S. SAKARIASSEN. 1985. Factors controlling thrombus formation on arterial lesions. Ann. N.Y. Acad. Sci. **1454:** 162-177.
22. WEISS, H. J., V. T. TURITTO & H. R. BAUMGARTNER. 1986. J. Clin. Invest. **78:** 1072–1082.
23. TURITTO, V. T., H. J. WEISS, H. R. BAUMGARTNER, L. BADIMON & V. FUSTER. 1987. Cells and aggregates at surfaces. This volume.
24. BOWIE, E. J. W., C. A. OWEN, P. E. COLLMAN, J. H. THOMPSON & D. N. FASS. 1973. Am. J. Vet. Res. **34:** 1405–1409.
25. FASS, D. N., W. J. BROCKAWAY, C. A. OWEN, & E. J. W. BOWIE. 1976. Thromb. Res. **8:** 319–327.
26. FUSTER, V., E. J. W. BOWIE, J. C. LEWIS, D. N. FASS, C. A. OWEN & A. L. BROWN. 1978. J Clin. Invest. **61:** 722–729.
27. FUSTER V., J. T. LIE, L. BADIMON, J. A. ROSEMARK, J. J. BADIMON & E. J. W. BOWIE. 1985. Arterioclerosis **5:** 67–73.

28. BADIMON, L., P. STEELE, J. J. BADIMON, E. J. W. BOWIE & V. FUSTER. 1985. ArteriscleroSis. **5:** 366–371.
29. FUSTER, V., C. W. PUMPHREY, J. H. CHESEBRO, L. BADIMON, P. M. STEELE & M. K. DEWANJEE. 1985. Antithrombotic action of calcium antagonists in the dog model. *In* Proceedings of the Tenth European Congress of Cardiology. P. R. Lichtlen, Ed.: 149–159. Schattaeur. Stuggart, New York.
30. GRABOWSKI, E. F., P. DIDISHEIM, J. C. LEWIS, J. T. FRANTA & J. Q. STROPP. 1977. Trans. Am. Soc Artif. Intern. Organs **23:** 141–144.
31. CHRISTENSON, J. T., J. MERGERMAN, K. C. HJANEL, G. J. L'ITALIEN, H. W. STRAUSS & W. M. ABBOTT. 1981. Trans. Am. Soc. Artif. Intern. Organs **27:** 188–191.

Methods of Assessment of Thrombosis *in Vivo*

MRINAL K. DEWANJEE[a]

Section of Nuclear Medicine
Mayo Clinic
Rochester, Minnesota 55905

The recognition of the various factors controlling the interaction between platelets and the vessel wall in normal hemostasis and the role of platelets, clotting factors, and prostaglandins in thromboembolic diseases, atherosclerosis, and postprosthesis implantation effects have stimulated interest in the evaluation of *in vivo* thrombus formation and the evaluation of various prophylactic and therapeutic interventions. *In vitro* studies of platelet adhesion to de-endothelialized vessel or biomaterials (catheters, synthetic vascular grafts, arterio-venous shunts, conduits, mechanical valves, ventricular assist devices, and artificial hearts) involve the use of light or electron microscopy and/or ^{51}Cr- or ^{111}In-labeled platelets and iodine-labeled clotting factors, mainly fibrinogen.[1–6] *In vivo* consumption of platelets has been measured with several tracers (FIGURES 1A–C), including ^{51}Cr- and ^{111}In-labeled platelets.[7–9] Chromium-51 appears to be a marker of platelet activation and ^{111}In a marker of platelet consumption. Although platelets have been labeled with technetium-99m, the radionuclide washes off from the platelets with time after administration. A platelet survival study representing global platelet consumption is not a sensitive technique, whereas an imaging study allows estimation of regional platelet consumption. Currently ^{123}I-labeled, ^{131}I-labeled, and ^{111}In-DTPA-coupled antibodies against platelet glycoproteins (IIb-IIIa) and fibrin are being evaluated in experimental animal models.[5,6] Due to faster blood clearance of these antibodies, early imaging could be carried out with these agents. The sensitivity of these latter techniques for detecting the sites of chronic low-grade thrombosis has not been tested. The techniques of labeling platelets with ^{111}In and fibrinogen with ^{125}I are shown in FIGURE 2.

The current techniques for diagnosis of thrombosis and atherosclerosis resulting in partial or total stenosis of vessel are based on the measurement of projected lumen diameter at the affected site or the resultant hemodynamic abnormalities. These techniques include impedance plethysmography, Doppler ultrasonography, phonoangiography, nuclear magnetic resonance, digital subtraction, and ^{111}In-labeled platelet scintigraphy.[10–12] The neutral complexes of indium-111, *i.e.*, ^{111}In-oxine, ^{111}In-acetylacetone, ^{111}In-tropolone, and ^{111}In-mercaptopurine-*N*-oxide penetrate the cell membrane because of their high lipid solubility (FIGURES 1A and 1C). After intracellular dissociation these tracers bind to soluble proteins and organelles, and also to a small extent to membrane proteins.[1,2] The more stable complexes of ^{111}In-tropolone and ^{111}In-mercaptopurine-*N*-oxide also permit cell labeling in plasma media, whereas ^{111}In-oxine permits cell labeling only in plasma-free media. Commercial preparation of ^{111}In-oxine also contains a surface-active agent (100 μg of Tween-80 per mCi of ^{111}In) to prevent adhesion of ^{111}In-oxine to the vial. ^{111}In, unlike ^{51}Cr, is released after

[a]Present address: Department of Radiology D-57, Jackson Memorial Hospital, P.O. Box 016960, Miami, FL 33101

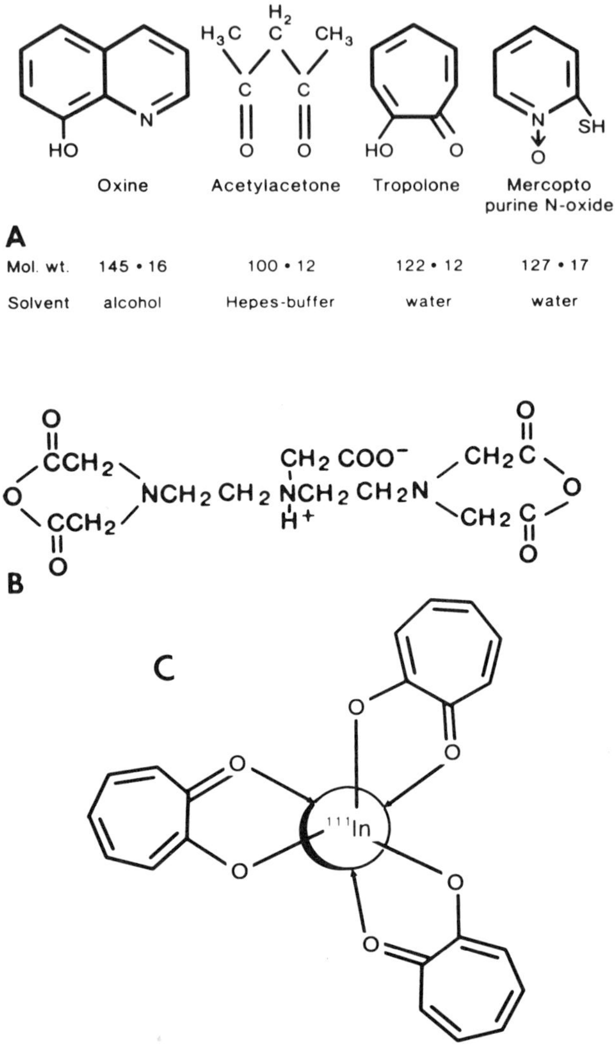

FIGURE 1. (**A**) Structures and physical properties of four chelating molecules used for formation of neutral and lipid-soluble ^{111}In complexes. ^{111}In-oxine and ^{111}In-tropolone are used frequently in cell-labeled studies. (**B**) Structure of bicyclic anhydride of DTPA. The DTPA-anhydride ligand is used as a coupling agent for binding metallic radionuclide via DTPA to the lysine group of soluble proteins, *e.g.*, labeled antibodies binding membrane glycoproteins of platelets and granulocytes. The blood clearance of ^{111}In-DTPA-coupled antibodies is faster than that of ^{111}In-labeled platelets, and the labeled antibody is stable *in vivo*. The rate of transchelation to transferrin is lower than dehalogenation. Dehalogenase action releases radioiodide from radioiodine-labeled antibody from adherent thrombus. In addition, ^{111}In radionuclide is more suitable for imaging than ^{123}I- and ^{131}I- radionuclides. ^{111}In chelation could be easily carried with DTPA-coupled protein available in kit form. For ^{111}In labeling of a protein, the DTPA-anhydride is mixed with protein in small volume and excess DTPA is removed by dialysis. This DTPA-conjugated protein could be maintained in freeze-dried form for future labeling with ^{111}In-citrate. The unbound ^{111}In-DTPA from ^{111}In-labeled protein is separated by gel filtration before use. In the current kit method of ^{111}In chelation, a small amount ($<10\%$) of unbound ^{111}In-DTPA is not separated before human administration. (**C**) Structure of ^{111}In-(tropolone)$_3$.

membrane lysis, and a major fraction of the ^{111}In then binds to transferrin present in plasma. Only a small percentage of the ^{111}In (less than 1%) is excreted in the urine in clinical evaluations. In addition, ^{111}In-labeled granulocytes or monocytes (where PMN granulocytes are separated by Ficoll-Hypaque or elutriation technique) and ^{111}In-

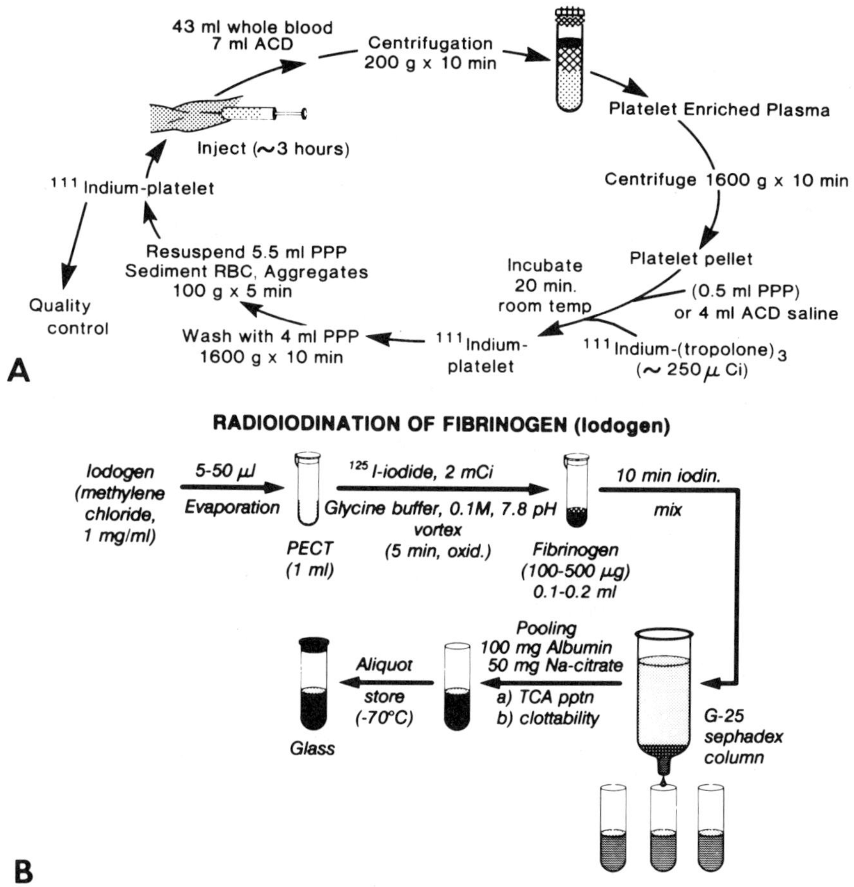

FIGURE 2. (**A**) Autologous platelet labeling with ^{111}In-tropolone. Harvested platelets resuspended in 0.5 ml of plasma were incubated with ^{111}In-tropolone. After removing unbound ^{111}In, labeled platelets are injected into the subject. (**B**) Radioiodination of fibrinogen with Iodogen transfer technique. In this method only oxidized radioiodide comes in contact with protein, thus reducing the probability of protein oxidation. After intravenous administration, denatured labeled fibrinogen is usually removed by the liver.

labeled lymphocytes might be ideal markers for quantification of granulocyte infiltration in inflammation, foreign body response, infection, abscess, and rejection.[16]

Thrombus imaging was possible in the case of large thrombi in the acute phase for vessels with deep injury or thrombogenic prosthetic surfaces. In the chronic phase, where platelets adhere to form a single layer, the deposition of the labeled platelet on the wall is relatively small with respect to the circulating radioactivity in the blood. In this situation, the imaging is not possible. Despite these limitations, the dynamic process of platelet deposition in most of the denuded atherosclerosed vessels and thrombogenic surfaces of the prosthesis in the circulatory system can be recorded. This ongoing thrombosis and embolization had been observed in 15-year-old vascular grafts of Teflon and Dacron biomaterials. These studies also permitted the evaluation of platelet-inhibitor drugs, for example, aspirin, persantine, sulfinpyrazone, motrin, several thromboxane inhibitors, anagrelide, prostacyclin, ticlopidine, and calcium-channel blockers. Decrease (minimal to moderate) in platelet deposition on prosthetic surfaces due to medical intervention had been observed by noninvasive imaging with ^{111}In-labeled platelets in animal models and patients. Subtraction of blood pool radioactivity with ^{99m}Tc-labeled autologous red blood cells and determination of thrombus-bound ^{111}In radioactivity on the wall of the prostheses have been made. The nature of the platelet deposition depends on the thrombogenicity of the surface, the amount of blood flow, the diameter and configuration of the prosthesis, and the time interval after prosthesis implantation. In the vascular prosthesis, platelet deposition as measured from ^{111}In radioactivity in the midsection of the graft is equal to, less than, or higher than the anastomotic site, giving rise to three types of platelet distribution, flat curved, concaved, or convexed. The nature of this platelet deposition also changes with time postimplantation. In at least two types of prostheses, we had the opportunity to quantify platelet thrombosis in the acute and chronic phases. For valvular prosthesis, similar techniques could be used for quantification of total number of adherent platelet deposition over a period of several hours. In addition, the effects of other medications were evaluated in the tissue valve and mechanical valve implanted in calves, dogs, and patients.

It has been suggested that in platelet adhesion the initial attachment and spreading occurs because of platelet glycoproteins (Ia and Ib) and in the latter phase of platelet aggregation and continuation of the thrombus formation, other glycoprotein complexes (IIb and IIIa) participate along with plasma proteins present in blood. The concentration of fibrinogen is about 3000 μg/ml, that of fibronectin about 300 μg/ml, von Willebrand factor (vWF) 7 μg/ml, and thrombospondin 0.02 μg/ml. Both vWF and fibronectin are synthesized by vascular endothelial cells and appear as glue between circulating platelets and vessel-wall components. The nature of the binding of vWF and fibronectin to platelet glycoproteins might be dependent on the shear rates, the types of surfaces, and the concentration of these adhesive proteins present at the site of interaction. With labeled platelets and proteins we were able to identify the molecular and cellular composition of thrombus in the arterial and venous system. Although the extent of activation of platelet and thrombus formation may be different, the platelet-fibrin organization in adherent thrombus on the de-endothelialized surface and prosthetic surface of grafts and valves implanted in calves and dogs at different sites appear similar; it is interesting to note that the composition of the thrombus calculated with the radioisotopic technique appears to be very similar for thrombus in the acute and chronic phases. In the *in vitro* model, because of the precipitation of some fibrinogen along with fibrin, the amount of fibrin per platelet tends to be higher. In addition, we have also evaluated the type of platelet damage, platelet consumption, and platelet release during open-heart surgery with bubble and membrane oxygenators. The labeled platelets and clotting factors thus provide very important markers for quantitative studies in animal models and for semiquantitative studies by imaging in animal models and patients.

^{111}In-labeled platelets provide a direct technique for quantification of regional platelet thrombus formation. This technique can also provide indirect information about the process of embolization. The embolization is usually indicated by the increase in the tissue:blood radioactivity ratio in the distal bed. In general, it has been thought that an increase in the amount of thrombus formation means the thrombus is further along in the sequence of events of embolization from prosthesis. The data on platelet thrombosis suggest that on most of the prostheses thrombus formation decreases with time postimplantation as the surfaces of the prostheses undergo organizational changes leading to passivation.

Numerous studies in our laboratory and others demonstrate that a mild injury that causes endothelial injury results in the adherence of a single layer of platelets, which is difficult to image. On the other hand, in the case of complex and deep injury, the large platelet aggregates formed at the site of injury could be imaged successfully with ^{111}In-labeled platelets.

Scintigraphy with ^{111}In-labeled Platelets

The half-life of 2.8 days, physical decay by electron capture process, and high photon abundance of ^{111}In radionuclide (90% of 171 keV ad 96% of 245 keV) make this radionuclide ideal for noninvasive imaging. The gamma camera head used for scintigraphic studies consists of a disk of thallium-doped sodium iodide crystal (25–54 cm in diameter, 6.4–12.7 mm in thickness) fitted with several photomultiplier tubes. The thinner disk (6.4 mm) in a portable gamma camera can be fitted with a specially designed collimator for bedside studies, although the detection efficiency is lower. In general, for most of the scintigraphic studies a large field of view gamma camera with a 12.7-mm-thick crystal fitted with a medium energy parallel hole collimator is used. The spectrometer windows (20% of photopeak energy) are adjusted to include the 171 and 245 keV peaks. Gamma rays of 320, 140, 159 and 364 keV are used for *in vitro* radioactivity measurements with a gamma counter of ^{51}Cr, ^{99m}Tc, ^{123}I and ^{131}I radionuclides, respectively. Attenuation and scatter of ^{111}In from platelet pool in the spleen and liver degrade the spatial resolution of the gamma camera images. The intrinsic spatial resolution of the gamma camera is 2–4 mm, but in practice is much higher. In spite of this limitation, the validation of *in vivo* distribution studies in animal models, the use of test objects with computerized gamma cameras, and *in vitro* measurements of isolated organs and components with gamma counters provide acceptable quantitative information of ^{111}In-labeled platelet distribution by scintigraphy. Since only a small percentage of labeled platelets participate in thrombosis on the wall of the injured vessel or prostheses, and platelet survival time is relatively long, a high blood background radioactivity is always present in the early phase. Ideal imaging time is usually 2 to 5 days postinjection of ^{111}In-labeled platelets. Several methods of measurement of thrombogenicity indices with ^{111}In-labeled platelets are shown in TABLE 1. The schematics of platelet labeling with ^{111}In-tropolone and radioiodination of fibrinogen with Iodogen transfer technique are shown in FIGURES 1A and 1B, respectively.

Platelet survival times with ^{51}Cr- and ^{111}In-labeled autologous platelets in healthy volunteers obtained in our laboratory[7] are shown in TABLE 2. Platelet clearance from blood was analyzed with linear, exponential, and multi-hit models. No significant difference in platelet survival values due to labeling in ACD-plasma and ACD-saline media was observed with ^{111}In-tropolone and ^{111}In-oxine. The linear platelet survival time in different species are as follows: human (10–11 days) > baboon, dog (5–7 days) > calf (5–6 days) > pig, rabbit, rat (3–4 days). The estimated radiation dose for 500 μCi of ^{111}In-labeled platelet administration is 1.13 rad to liver, 0.70 rad to lung, 16.75 rad to spleen, 1.16 rad to kidneys, 0.27 rad to red marrow, 0.17 rad to ovaries, 0.07 rad to testes, and 0.30 rad to the whole body. Adequate platelet survival studies can be

TABLE 1. Thrombogenicity Indices from Measurement of ^{111}In-labeled Platelet Radioactivity in Organs and Prostheses

I. Relative graft radioactivity (equal no. of pixels on graft and vessel) $= \dfrac{\text{cpm } ^{111}\text{In on graft}}{\text{cpm } ^{111}\text{In on normal vessel (contralateral)}}$

II. Relative thrombogenicity (equal no. of pixels on graft and soft tissue) $= \dfrac{\text{cpm } ^{111}\text{In on graft} - \text{cpm } ^{111}\text{In in soft tissue}}{^{111}\text{In activity } (\mu\text{Ci}) \times \text{no. of pixels}}$

III. Geometric mean method

A. Geometric mean cpm ^{111}In = (anterior cpm ^{111}In × posterior cpm ^{111}In)$^{1/2}$

B. Corrected organ cpm ^{111}In =

$$\frac{\text{Transmission coefficient}}{\text{sensitivity (cpm } ^{111}\text{In}/\mu\text{Ci)}} \times \text{geometric mean cpm } ^{111}\text{In},$$

where transmission coefficient and sensitivity of gamma camera are determined by measuring a known amount of ^{111}In radioactivity in a test object (phantom)

IV. Determination of focal-wall-adherent ^{111}In-labeled platelet radioactivity at region of interest (ROI) by subtraction of circulating ^{111}In-labeled platelet radioactivity in blood pool.

A. Excess cpm ^{111}In at focal thrombus = total cpm ^{111}In (ROI) − cpm ^{111}In (blood pool), assuming all counts from ^{99m}Tc-labeled RBC are in blood pool and only small cpm ^{111}In from wall-adherent thrombus

B. $\text{cpm } ^{111}\text{In (blood pool of ROI)} = \text{cpm } ^{99m}\text{Tc (ROI)} \times \dfrac{\text{cpm } ^{111}\text{In (reference region)}}{\text{cpm } ^{99m}\text{Tc (reference region)}}$,

where reference region refers to a region of blood pool with no thrombus

C. $\%\text{ Excess cpm } ^{111}\text{In of focal thrombus} = \dfrac{\text{excess cpm } ^{111}\text{In}}{\text{cpm } ^{111}\text{In (blood pool of ROI)}} \times 100$

performed with 100–150 μCi of ^{111}In-labeled platelets. The experimental and clinical studies carried out with ^{111}In-labeled platelets are summarized in TABLE 3. Due to high radiation dose to the spleen, most of the clinical studies with ^{111}In-labeled platelets were performed with 500 μCi, requiring longer imaging times (5–15 minutes per view of approximately 100,000 counts). During imaging, the motion of the patient or experimental animal should be reduced to a minimum. This is essential for blood pool subtraction with ^{99m}Tc-labeled RBCs (2 mCi of ^{99m}Tc for 0.5 mCi of ^{111}In). ^{111}In excess (%) had been determined for thrombus on atherosclerosed cartoid and aortic plaque in

TABLE 2. Platelet Survival Time in Days (Mean ± SD) of ^{111}In- and ^{51}Cr-labeled Autologous Platelets in Human Volunteers: Data Analyzed with Three Model Calculations

	^{51}Cr-labeled Platelets	^{111}In-labeled Platelets (Oxine-ACD-Saline)	^{111}In-labeled Platelets (Tropolone-Plasma)
Linear	10.1 ± 0.9	8.8 ± 0.6	10.2 ± 0.7
Exponential	6.8 ± 0.9	5.1 ± 0.6	5.4 ± 0.7
Multiple hit	9.1 ± 1.1 (men)	7.7 ± 0.9 (men)	8.9 ± 1.4 (men)
	9.8 + 1.6 (women)	8.1 ± 1.2 (women)	

TABLE 3. Qualitative and Quantitative Studies of Platelet Incorporation in Thrombus and Embolization with ^{111}In-labeled Platelets in Experimental and Clinical Studies

I. Arterial diseases
- A. Arterial grafts (internal mammary artery)
  1. Vein grafts (saphenous vein graft)
  2. Gore-Tex grafts
  3. Dacron grafts
  4. Polyurethane grafts (experimental)
  5. Endothelial cell seeded graft (experimental)
  6. Platelet inhibitors, prostacyclin, and other drugs
- B. Aneurysms
  1. Thoracic grafts
  2. Abdominal aneurysm
  3. Dissecting aneurysm
  4. Intracranial aneurysm
- C. Atherosclerosis (de-endothelialization and cholesterol feeding of animals), thrombosis, and embolization
  1. Carotid artery (ulcerating plaques)
- D. Endothelial damage
  1. Balloon angioplasty (rabbit, pig, human)
  2. Vein graft denudation (coronary and peripheral bypass)
  3. Renal artery thrombosis
  4. Coronary thrombosis and thrombolysis
  5. Homocystinuria, smoking, hypertension, hyperlipidemia
  6. Catheter damage during angioplasty
  7. Endarterectomy
- E. Vasculitis (temporal arteritis)

III. Venous diseases
- A. Venous thrombosis
- B. Renal vein thrombosis
- C. Sagittal sinus thrombosis
- D. Vena cava graft
- E. Pulmonary embolism
- F. Role of anticoagulants and thrombocytic agents

IV. Cardiac diseases
- A. Atrial thrombosis
- B. Ventricular thrombosis
- C. Bacterial endocarditis
- D. Valvular prostheses and vascular conduits (acquired and congenital defects)
- E. Myocardial hemorrhage

V. Microvascular injury (organ transplantation)
- A. Kidney
- B. Heart

VI. Miscellaneous prosthesis (temporary and semipermanent)
- A. Blood-biomaterial interactions
- B. Catheter-induced thrombosis and embolization
- C. Cardiopulmonary bypass (bubble and membrane oxygenator)
- D. Artery-vein shunts and other *ex vivo* circuits
- E. Left ventricular assist devices
- F. Artificial heart (four mechanical valves, two pumps; the most thrombogenic device)

primate, Gore-Tex grafts in dogs in acute and chronic phase, Gore-Tex grafts in patients, and thrombus in coronary artery and left ventricle. A graft undergoing thrombotic occlusion had two to three times more ^{111}In excess than a patent graft. ^{111}In excess values ranged from 3% to 80%; in experimental study a good correlation was obtained between ^{111}In excess and thrombus weight and platelet content. Blood-pool radioactivity in reference region is chosen at similar depth to that of region of interest; frequently blood pool in heart is used. We also determined the RBC:platelet ratio in thrombus by *in vitro* measurement. Several images in both anterior and posterior views are necessary for quantitative distribution of ^{111}In-labeled platelets in the whole body. From the geometric mean of the radioactivity in the anterior and posterior views, the percentage distribution of radioactivity in the liver, spleen, lungs, and the site of platelet thrombosis could be quantified more accurately. For most of the platelet deposition studies on injured vessel wall and cardiovascular prosthesis, the peak time of ^{111}In-labeled platelet deposition had been obtained in experimental and clinical studies. The time course of platelet deposition depends on the diameter of the vessel lumen, texture of surface, blood flow, shear rate, types of biomaterials used in prostheses, presence of drugs, and platelet reactivity.

The site of platelet thrombus formation could be imaged only for reasonably large thrombus in valvular prostheses, vascular grafts, ventricular assist devices, artificial heart, aneurysm, and ulcerating atherosclerosed plaque. An imaging technique is successful most of the time in the acute phase postinjury or after prosthesis implantation. Noninvasive imaging without background subtraction is not always a very sensitive technique for detection of platelet deposition in patients. We attempted to image platelet deposition on aortocoronary saphenous vein bypass grafts in ten control patients immediately postsurgery. Only the site of sternotomy incision was visualized, not the coronary bypass graft. In five control patients with carotid artery disease platelet deposition could not be imaged, although platelet deposition at the sites of endarterectomy was imaged. Six patients with bacterial endocarditis were scanned for the evaluation of platelet deposition without success. Three of these patients were treated with antibiotics. Platelet deposition on the sewing ring of mechanical and tissue valve prostheses could not be imaged in several patients at 1 to 5 years after-valve prosthesis implantation; during this period the sewing ring is covered with fibroblasts and most of the platelet thrombosis occurs on the disk of the leaflets. Our experimental study also indicates that the platelet thrombus provides a nucleation site for calcification in the tissue valve. Treatment with aspirin-persantine reduces both platelet thrombosis and calcification. The subtraction of blood-pool radioactivity with ^{99m}Tc-labeled RBC and calculation of ^{111}In excess factor[13] for the site of platelet thrombus formation increases the sensitivity of the diagnostic technique. The following sections will describe the applications of ^{111}In-labeled platelets for noninvasive imaging and quantification of platelet deposition on ulcerating plaque, aneurysm, venous thrombus, coronary bypass graft,[29] artery undergoing angioplasty,[43] synthetic vascular grafts, valvular prostheses, conduits, and artificial heart.

Semiquantitative Estimation of Platelet Deposition on Vascular Grafts with ^{111}In-labeled Platelet Scintigraphy

Platelet labeling with ^{111}In-oxine and ^{111}In-tropolone permits quantification of platelet thrombosis in atherosclerosis and thrombosis in the acute and chronic phase. About 600,000–700,000 vascular grafts are implanted annually in the United States; of these, 200,000–250,000 are autogenous vein grafts, 70,000–90,000 are vein bypass grafts, 200,000–225,000 are aortocoronary bypass grafts, and the rest are synthetic vascular grafts (greater than 5 mm in diameter). Most of the grafts in high blood flow and low-resistance regions of the aorta, iliac, and proximal femoral artery perform quite satisfactorily. The scheme of bilateral femoral graft implantation, the pattern of platelet and fibrin deposition, and possibilities of scintigraphy are shown in FIGURES 3–5. The change in the nature and extent of regional platelet deposition and effect of

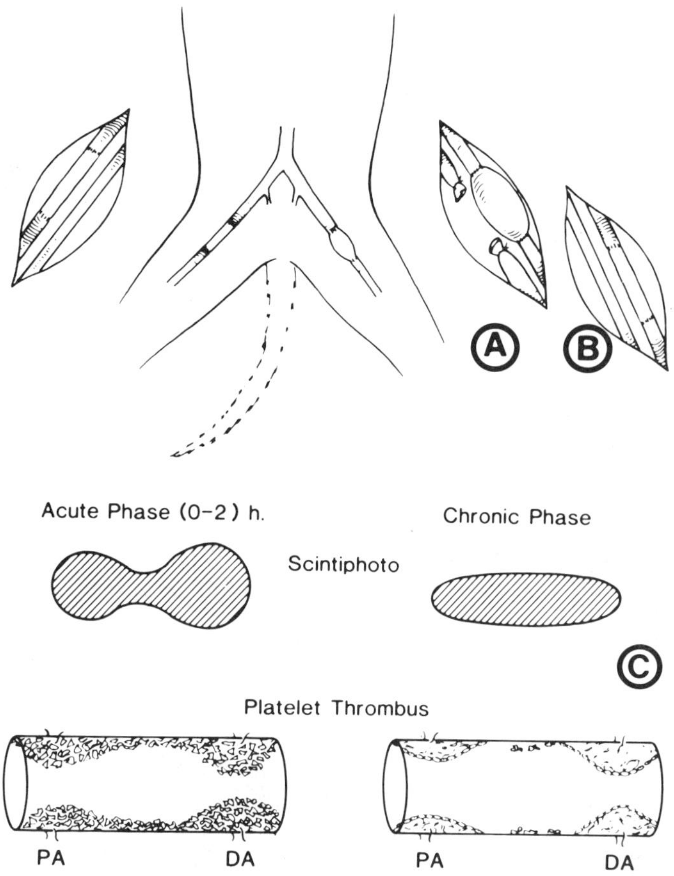

FIGURE 3. Scheme of bilateral femoral graft implantation in dogs. (**A**) EPTFE-vein graft. (**B**) EPTFE-EPTFE graft after 1 and 3 hours of perfusion. (**C**) ^{111}In-labeled platelets in vascular grafts. Schematics of platelet deposition in the acute and chronic phase. In the acute phase more platelets are deposited at the proximal and distal anastomoses and fewer in the middle. The converse is true for chronic phase. Scintiphoto indicates similar platelet distribution on vascular grafts in patients. Occasionally hot spots for focal thrombi were found in the mid region of the graft. (From Dewanjee.[16])

treatment on coronary bypass graft are shown in FIGURE 6. The amount of thrombus formation and embolization, and platelet survival time, could be measured simultaneously with ^{111}In-labeled platelets. For determination of platelet survival times, it is essential to subtract the plasma-bound ^{111}In activity from total radioactivity in blood.

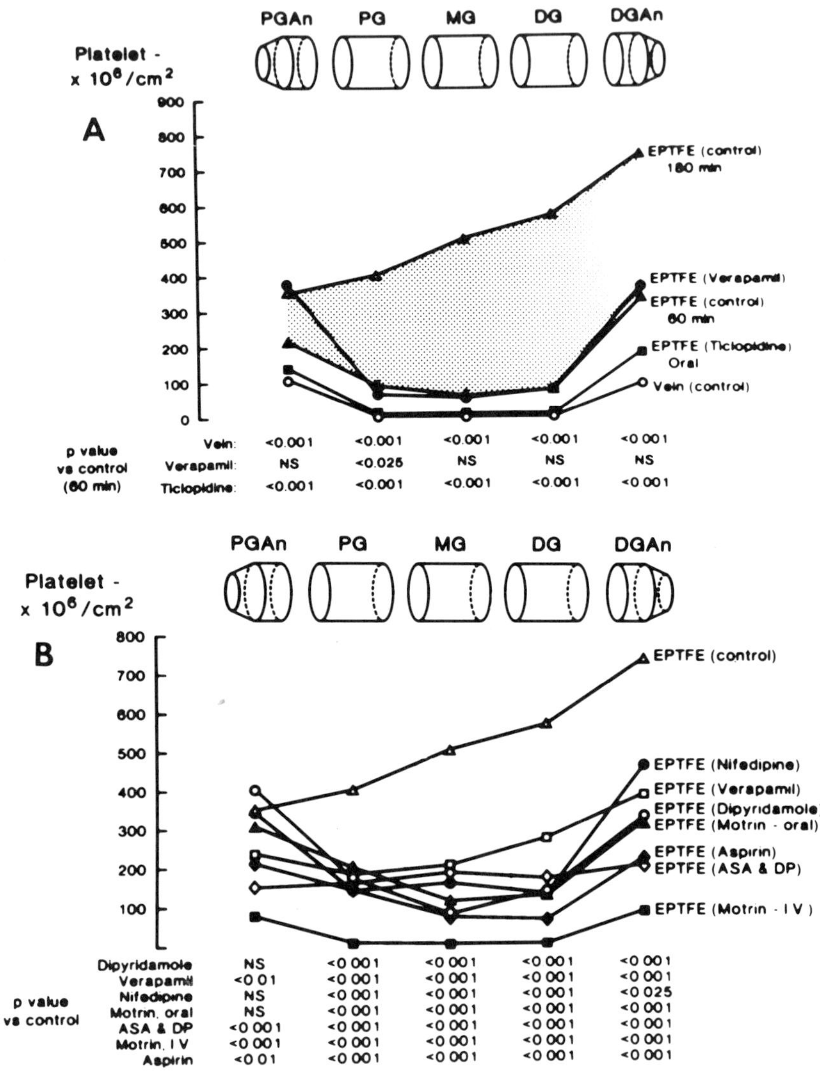

FIGURE 4. (**A**) Platelet deposition on vein and EPTFE graft at 60 minutes of perfusion in control and treated dogs. The shaded area represents different rate of regional platelet deposition during the 2-hour interval from 60 to 180 minutes of perfusion; platelet deposition rate is higher at distal anastomosis. (**B**) Platelet deposition on vein and EPTFE graft at 180 minutes of perfusion in control and treated dogs. Intravenous motrin reduces thrombogenicity of EPTFE graft to that of femoral vein graft. Aspirin, aspirin-persantine, and motrin are more effective than calcium-channel blockers in reducing platelet deposition. (From Dewanjee *et al.*[28])

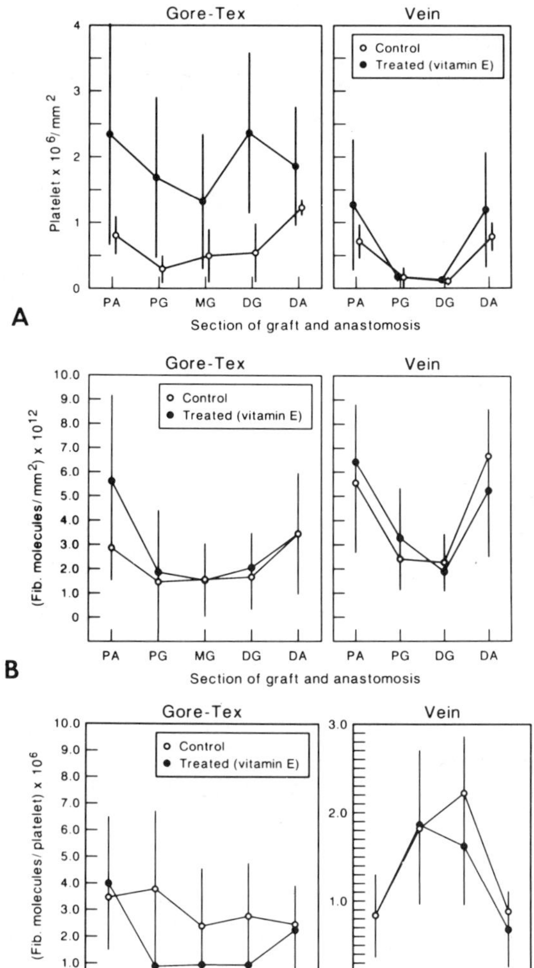

FIGURE 5. (**A**) Platelet density on anastomosis and midsections of Gore-Tex® and vein grafts after 1 hour of perfusion in control and vitamin-E-treated dogs. (**B**) Density of fibrin on sections of the same grafts. (**C**) Fibrin:platelet ratio on sections of the same grafts. (From Dewanjee *et al.*[47])

Several approaches have been made for measurement of platelet deposition on different types of prostheses, vascular grafts, and evaluation of the effect of drugs (FIGURES 7–20). Qualitative estimation of platelet thrombosis was made with a gamma camera at 12–120 hours after administration of ^{111}In-labeled platelets and 5–10 days after graft implantation. Subsequent follow-up of platelet consumption included measurement of platelet survival time and platelet deposition on the graft.

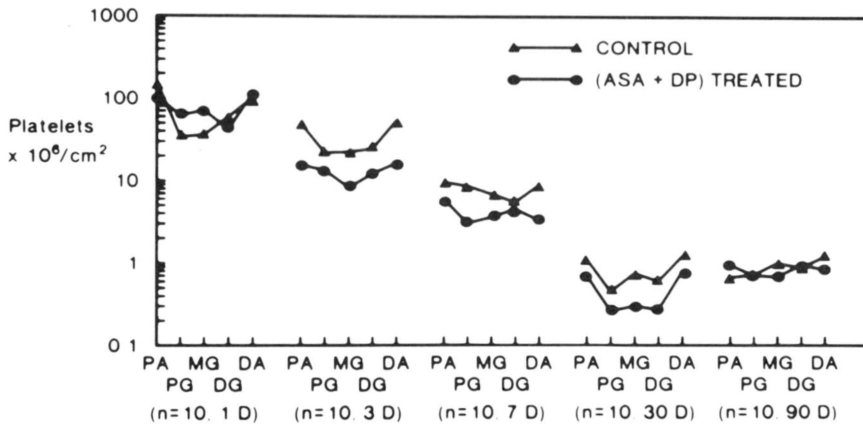

FIGURE 6. Time course of change in regional platelet deposition as represented by surface density of platelets on aortocoronary bypass graft in control and treated dogs. The number of platelets per cm^2 on graft surface (24 h postinjection) in untreated ("control") dogs and dogs treated orally with dipyridamole and aspirin was determined with ^{111}In-labeled platelets. Persantine (2.5 mg per kg per day) was administered 2 days prior to surgery and aspirin (15 mg per kg per day) immediately postoperation. Five dogs in each group were sacrificed at 1, 3, 7, 30, and 90 days after grafting. In each group of five joined points, points represent (from left to right) mean values from proximal anastomosis (*PA*), proximal graft segment (*PG*), midgraft segment (*MG*), distal graft segment (*DG*), and distal anastomosis (*DA*). Note lower platelet density in the treated group at 3, 7, and 30 days. (From Dewanjee.[29])

Unlike animal models, endothelial coverage occurs only at proximal and distal anastomosis in patients; the rest of the area is covered with fibrin-collagen matrix with a few fibroblasts scattered on the graft. This surface is thrombogenic and platelet deposition can be observed 5 to 15 years after graft implantation (FIGURE 10). High platelet deposition in the acute phase might lead to graft occlusion. Within 1 to 2 hours of perfusion, a dumbbell shape of platelet deposition is observed, with more deposition at anastomoses and less in the middle. The decline in ^{111}In-labeled platelet activity in the graft may be due to embolization of platelet aggregates. In the chronic phase, platelet deposition is observed in the midsection of the graft. In some studies, indium excess in graft was calculated after administration of ^{111}In-labeled platelets and ^{99m}Tc-labeled RBC. Incorporation of red cell in thrombus, presence of plasma-bound ^{111}In, proximity of vein, presence of ^{111}In in bone marrow, and motion artifacts make proper background subtraction difficult for calculation of excess ^{111}In.

In some studies, platelet deposition in the graft was compared with that in the contralateral femoral-popliteal vessel. Atherosclerosis, phlebosclerosis, varicosity in the contralateral vessel, and blood pool and marrow activity also led to error in estimating the radioactivity ratios. Stratton and Ritchie[32] evaluated graft thrombogenicity by measurement of graft ^{111}In activity with a gamma camera and blood radioactivity with a gamma counter. The graft:blood ratio is higher in a more thrombogenic surface. This vessel:blood ratio increases in normal vessels, and more so in the grafts and other thrombogenic surfaces, because of continuous platelet sequestration. In our studies[30] we have determined the number of ^{111}In counts per pixel per microcurie on the graft surface. A smaller number of counts per pixel necessitates longer imaging time. We have also evaluated platelet thrombosis on Dacron grafts and effect of medication.[30] As with other synthetic vascular grafts, higher platelet deposition occurs 2 to 3 days postadministration of labeled platelets.

Quantitation of Platelet Density on Vascular Grafts in Animals with ^{111}In-labeled Platelets

Thrombosis is a surface reaction. In quantitative studies, the most important parameters of thrombosis that should be obtained are the number of adherent platelets per unit area of atherosclerosed vessel or vascular graft and the analysis of the thrombus components (e.g., fibrin monomers per platelet). This is only possible in experimental animal studies on harvested grafts and tissue valves. Although we used meticulous tracer and surgical techniques in the measurement of platelet deposition, we observed a great deal of variation in platelet density.[47,48] This variation might be due to fibrinolysis, embolization, heterogenous degree of platelet activation due to differential synthesis of thromboxane by platelet and prostacylin by endothelial cells, and other rheological factors of blood flow. The equations describing the calculation of platelet and fibrin density and fibrin per platelet on the graft surface are shown in TABLE 4.

To understand the mechanism of occlusion in aortocoronary bypass (ACB) graft in patients, we have used a canine model and developed a treatment protocol with aspirin and persantine (FIGURE 6) to increase ACB graft patency in dogs.[29] This has also been shown to be useful in clinical studies in patients. *In vitro* studies of the interaction of platelet and coagulation factors with biomaterial surfaces provide incomplete informa-

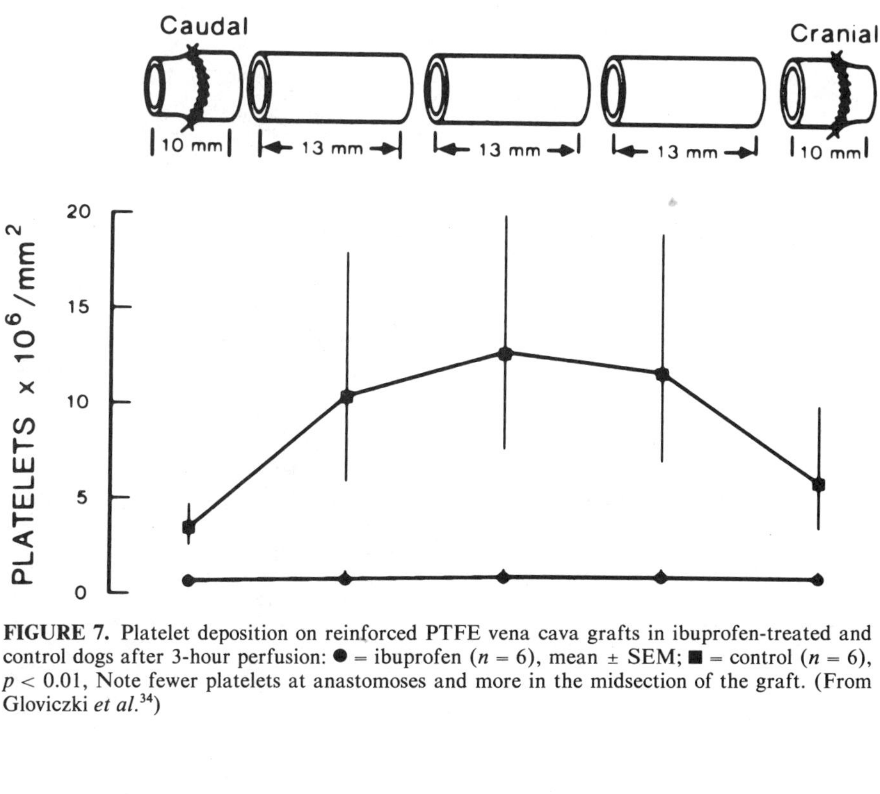

FIGURE 7. Platelet deposition on reinforced PTFE vena cava grafts in ibuprofen-treated and control dogs after 3-hour perfusion: ● = ibuprofen ($n = 6$), mean ± SEM; ■ = control ($n = 6$), $p < 0.01$, Note fewer platelets at anastomoses and more in the midsection of the graft. (From Gloviczki *et al.*[34])

TABLE 4

CALCULATION OF PLATELET DEPOSITION

$$\frac{\text{cpm platelet-bound } ^{111}\text{In}}{\text{ml blood}} = \frac{\text{cpm whole-blood } ^{111}\text{In}}{\text{ml blood}} \times \frac{(100 - \%\text{ free } ^{111}\text{In})}{100}$$

$$\frac{\text{no. platelets}}{\text{cpm } ^{111}\text{In}} = \frac{\text{no. platelets per ml blood}}{\text{cpm } ^{111}\text{In per ml blood}}$$

$$\frac{\text{no. platelets}}{\text{area (mm}^2)} = \frac{\text{cpm } ^{111}\text{In in specimen}}{\left(\dfrac{\text{cpm } ^{111}\text{In}}{\text{no. platelets}}\right) \times \text{area (mm}^2)}$$

CALCULATION OF FIBRINOGEN DEPOSITION

$$\frac{\text{cpm plasma } ^{125}\text{I}}{\text{volume (ml)}} = \frac{\text{cpm } ^{125}\text{I (plasma} - \text{background)}}{1.04 \times \text{plasma wt (g)}}$$

$$\frac{\text{fib. } (\mu\text{g})}{\text{cpm } ^{125}\text{I}} = \frac{\text{fib. (mg per dl)} \times 10}{\text{fib. bound } ^{125}\text{I (cpm per ml)}}$$

$$\frac{\text{fib. } (\mu\text{g})}{\text{area of specimen (mm}^2)} = \frac{\text{fib. } (\mu\text{g})}{\text{cpm } ^{125}\text{I}} \times \frac{\text{cpm } ^{125}\text{I (specimen)}}{\text{area (mm}^2)}$$

$$\text{total specimen fib. } (\mu\text{g}) = \frac{\text{fib. } (\mu\text{g})}{\text{mm}^2} \times \text{specimen area (mm}^2)$$

$$\frac{\text{molecules of fib.}}{\text{fib. } (\mu\text{g})} = 1.77 \times 10^{12}$$

CALCULATION OF FIBRINOGEN MOLECULES PER PLATELET IN SPECIMEN

$$\frac{\text{molecules of fib.}}{\text{single platelet}} = \frac{\text{fib. } (\mu\text{g}) \times 1.77 \times 10^{12} \text{ per mm}^2}{\text{no. of platelets per mm}^2}$$

tion in that only individual parts of this complex synergistic process can be studied at one time. In our laboratory, the *in vivo* deposition of platelets and the formation of thrombus on ACB graft and cardiovascular prostheses have been imaged and quantified with the use of ^{111}In-labeled platelets in several animal models and humans. We have also evaluated the effect of several platelet inhibitor drugs in reducing platelet thrombosis.

The dynamic process of buildup of platelet thrombus and embolization on the ulcerating atherosclerosed plaque, as well as thrombogenic surface, had been imaged noninvasively in animals models and human patients. The platelet activation due to higher shear rate, loss of endothelial cell, or ulceration of the plaque results in platelet thrombosis at this site. Powers *et al.*[13] evaluated platelet deposition on atherosclerosed plaque of aorta in cholesterol-fed primates after balloon injury. They have calculated ^{111}In excess factor for platelet deposition in plaques. The platelet uptake correlates with the severity of atherosclerotic lesion. The scintigraphic evidence of platelet deposition on arteriographically confirmed plaques in several series was quite variable and ranged from 0% to 78%. Powers *et al.*[17] recently reported results from 100 patients with suspected severe vascular diseases; scintigrams of platelet deposition on ulcerated carotid plaques are shown in FIGURE 8. Platelet deposition was observed at 41% of lesions shown in angiography and 13% in arteriography at the normal sites. The detection sensitivity as measured by test objects suggests that a carotid thrombus must contain at least 0.1% of injected dose of ^{111}In-labeled platelets for scintigraphic detection, and the same order of magnitude is required for successful imaging of venous thrombosis. Plaque could be imaged only when the plaque-to-blood radioactivity ratio was about 4.0–5.0. Due to the dynamic process of thrombus formation and embolization in the high-flow region of small diameter carotid artery, more frequent imaging might be necessary.

Evaluation of Platelet Thrombosis in Aneurysms

The turbulence of blood flow and stagnation in these cavities give rise to formation of thrombus of platelet, fibrin, and red cell, and continuous incorporation of platelet and fibrin on the uppermost layers of thrombus. ^{111}In-labeled platelets were used successfully for imaging these thrombus formations. The optimum time for imaging was 96–120 hours postinjection of ^{111}In-labeled platelets (FIGURE 9). Surgical repair of aneurysm and scintigrams of platelet deposition on Dacron grafts are shown in FIGURE 10. Patients with abdominal aortic aneurysms and bilateral femoral artery aneurysms had higher ^{111}In-labeled platelet activity at the site of aneurysm. No significant difference of platelet deposition was observed when the patients were medicated with aspirin and persantine, and sulfinpyrazone. Heyns *et al.*[24] observed 4.7 ± 3.6% of total administered ^{111}In radioactivity at 8 to 10 days postinjection in the aortic aneurysm.

^{111}In-labeled Platelet Scintigraphy in the Diseases of the Venous System

Thakur *et al.*[1] first imaged venous thrombi in the canine jugular veins induced by electric current injury. Knight *et al.*[3] studied the effect of aging of venous thrombus on platelet incorporation in dogs. All thrombi could be visualized 2 hours after ^{111}In-labeled platelet injection. The optimum time of imaging was 12 to 15 h postinjection.

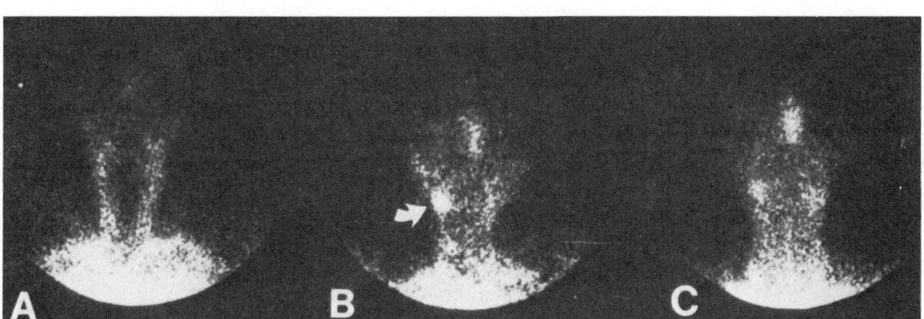

FIGURE 8. ^{111}In-labeled platelet scintigrams of the head and neck (anterior view of a 37-year-old woman). (**A**) Normal scintigram. (**B**) ^{111}In-labeled platelets in major vessels of carotid artery and jugular vein and nasopharyngeal blood pool are clearly outlined. A well-defined focus (*white arrow*) of increase in ^{111}In-labeled platelets at the right carotid bifurcation of a 42-year-old man who had an infarction of the ipsilateral cerebral hemisphere 5 days earlier can be seen. (**C**) A typical scintigram showing diffuse uptake at the carotid bifurcation of a 59-year-old man with right-sided amaurosis fugax. These thrombi could be followed by imaging with a gamma camera because of the transient nature of thrombosis and lack of embolization. (From Powers *et al.*[17])

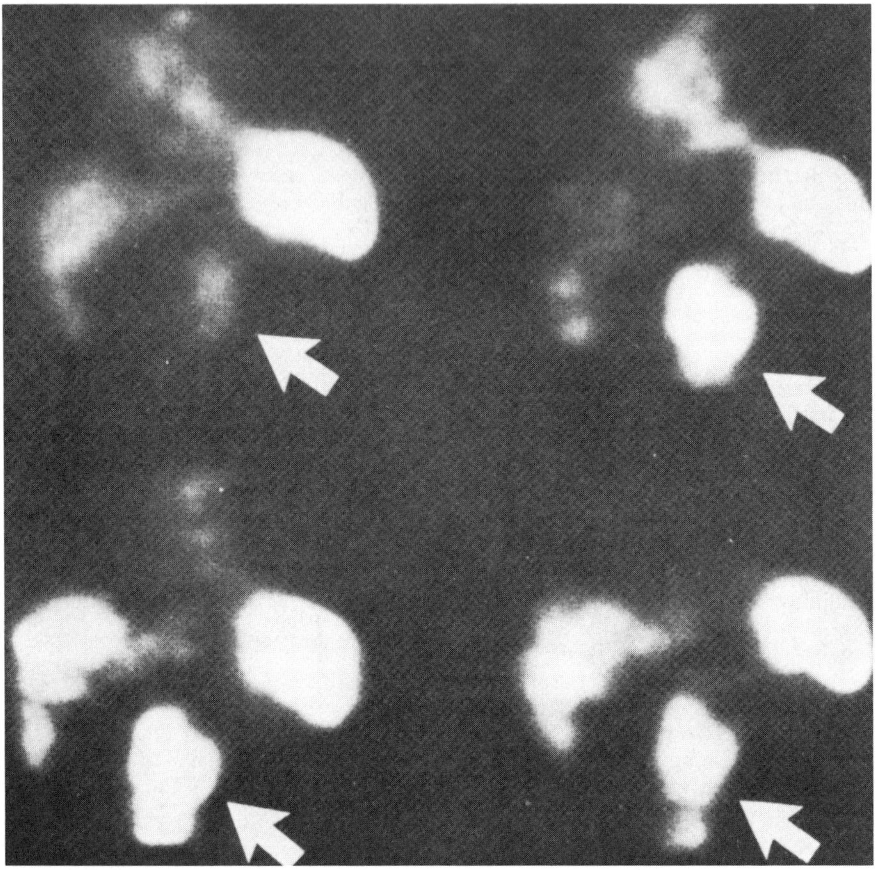

FIGURE 9. Scintigrams of a patient with abdominal aortic aneurysm (*arrows*) at 90 minutes (*top left*), 24 hours (*top right*), 48 hours (*bottom left*), and 144 hours (*bottom right*) postinjection of ^{111}In-labeled platelets. Optimum imaging time of accumulation of ^{111}In-labeled platelet in aneurysm is approximately 72–96 h; note the dynamic nature of platelet incorporation in the aneurysm. Splenic pooling and hepatic sequestration are visible in the anterior view image. (From Heyns *et al.*[24])

The thrombus-to-blood radioactivity ratio decreases from greater than 20 at 1–12 hours to 2–25 at 12–24 hours and 1–5 at 24–48 hours. Similar effects of aging and anticoagulant on ^{111}In-labeled platelet incorporation in thrombi and pulmonary emboli were also observed in the canine model by several investigators. Several clinical studies using venography, plethysmography, and ^{111}In-labeled platelet scintigraphy were utilized for diagnosis of venous thrombosis. In general, the thrombus could be visualized at 3 to 6 hours after injection of ^{111}In-labeled platelets (FIGURE. 12); therapy with anticoagulant, *i.e.*, heparin, decreases platelet incorporation in the thrombus.

Ezekowitz *et al.*[22] used ^{111}In-labeled platelets for imaging hematologically active thrombus in the left ventricle; in comparison with two-dimensional echocardiography, thrombus imaging was far more specific, although the former was more sensitive. False positive studies were quite common. The thrombus radioactivity measured at autopsy was 10–15 times higher than blood. FIGURE 13 demonstrates platelet deposition in ventricular thrombus obtained in our laboratory. No significant effect of anticoagulant and platelet inhibitor drug was observed in this study. The optimum time for imaging was 3 to 4 days postinjection of ^{111}In-labeled platelets.

Evaluation of Microvascular Injury and Platelet Thrombosis in Transplanted Organs and Vessels

The activation of T lymphocytes is the predominant factor for allograft rejection resulting in the loss of endothelial cells. Humoral antibodies also may dominate the

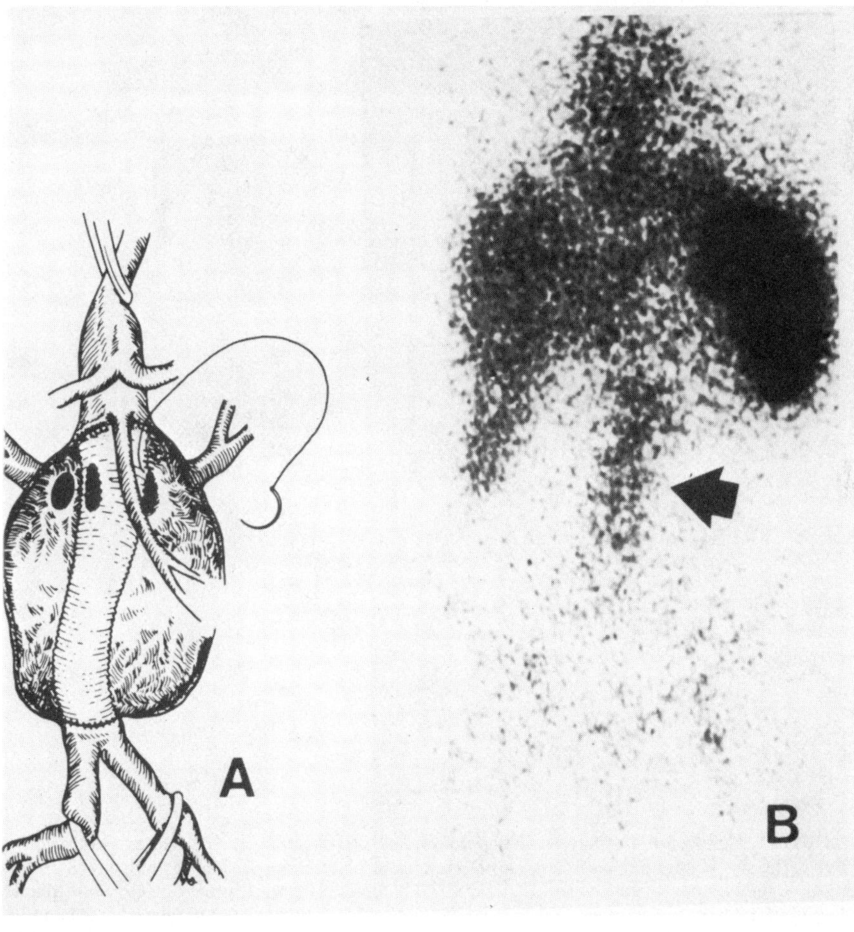

FIGURE 10. (**A**) Surgical repair of aneurysm, anastomosis to adjoining arteries, and Dacron graft. (**B**) Scintigrams of platelet thrombosis on Dacron graft (*arrow*) 24 hours after administration of ^{111}In-labeled platelets. Note diffuse distribution of platelet deposition in scintigram at 10 years postgrafting; most of the vascular grafts remain thrombogenic in the chronic phase. (From Robertson.[11])

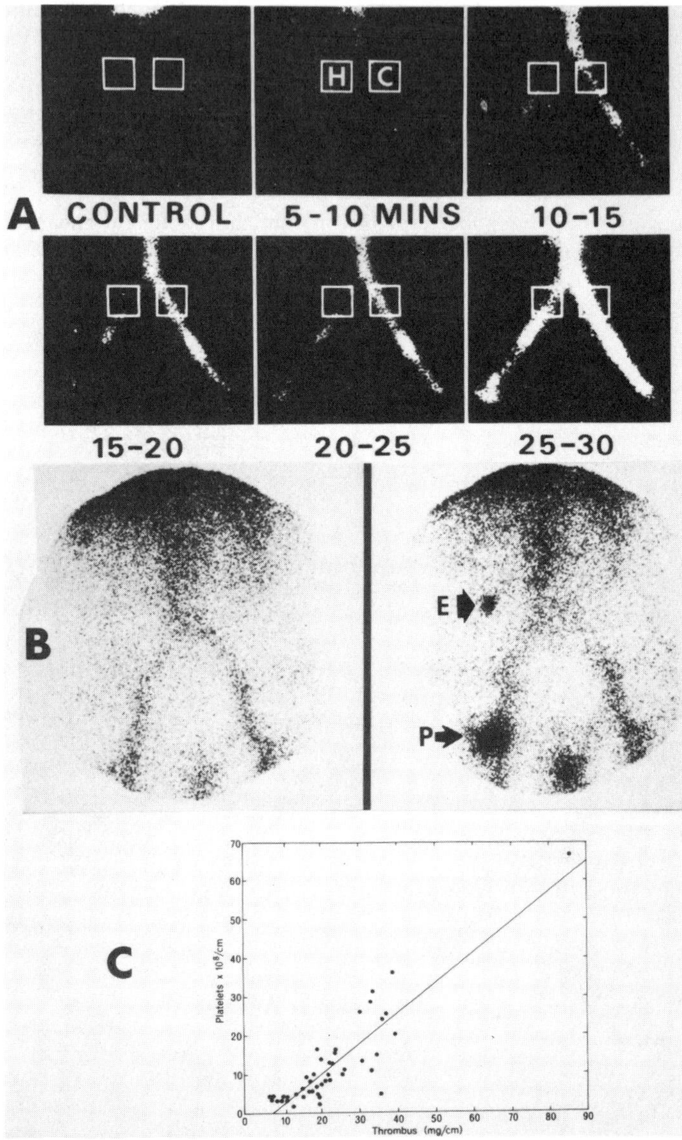

FIGURE 11. Scintiphoto of platelet deposition at the site of puncture (*P*) and extravasation of blood at the site of catheter insertion. (**A**) Dynamics of platelet deposition on control (*C*) and on heparin-immobilized polyethylene catheter (*H*) in dogs. (From Lipton.[44]) (**B**) Scintiphotos obtained in anterior view 1 hour pre- and postangiography in a patient. As the catheter is pulled out, the adherent emboli (*E*) are left in circulation. The emboli could be followed by imaging with a gamma camera. (From O'Connor.[46]) (**C**) Correlation of linear platelet density and adherent thrombus on polyethylene catheter inserted in carotid artery of goats. (From Rodvien.[45])

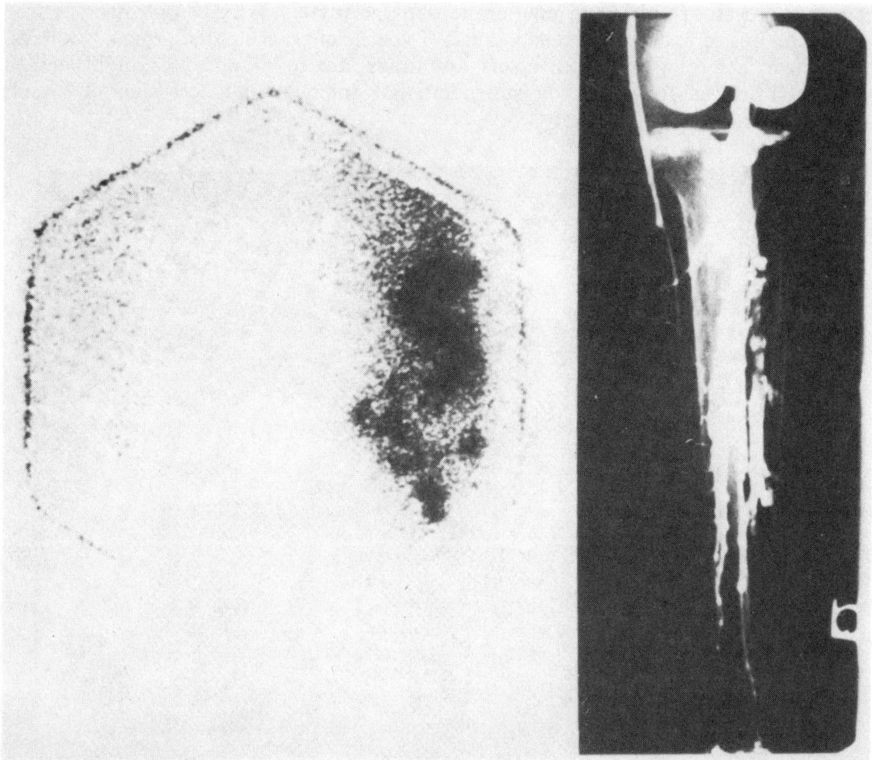

FIGURE 12. Scintiphoto (*left*) of platelet deposition (24 hours postinjection) in both calves in a patient with deep vein thrombosis. The tortuous area of increased activity represents a large venous thrombus. The corresponding venogram (*right*) shows filling defects in the areas where higher platelet deposition was observed. (From Ezekowitz *et al.*[23])

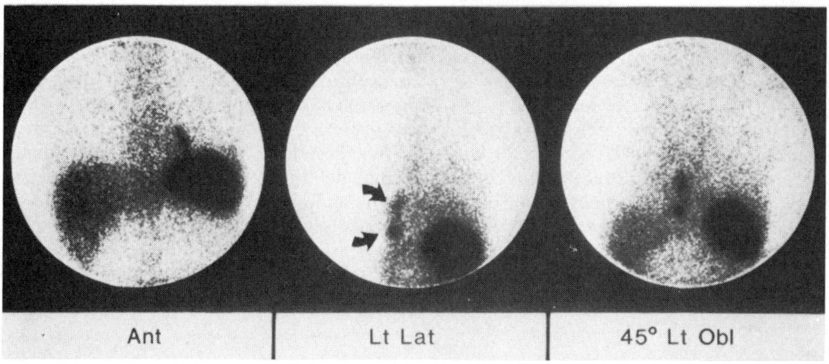

FIGURE 13. Scintiphoto of platelet deposition in left ventricular mural thrombus in a patient with anterolateral transmural infarct, 4 days after ^{111}In-labeled platelet injection. Note two focal spots of platelet thrombus in the anterior (*Ant*), left lateral (*Lt Lat*), and left anterior oblique view (*Lt Obl*). Proper positioning of gamma camera could identify the two thrombi in the lateral views.

rejection process, resulting in membrane damage (cytolysis by complement activation). The loss of endothelial cells in smaller vessels of transplanted organs (kidneys, heart, liver, heterologous blood vessels, and lungs) due to lymphocytes might lead to platelet thrombus formation on subendothelial collagen and occlusion of vessel,

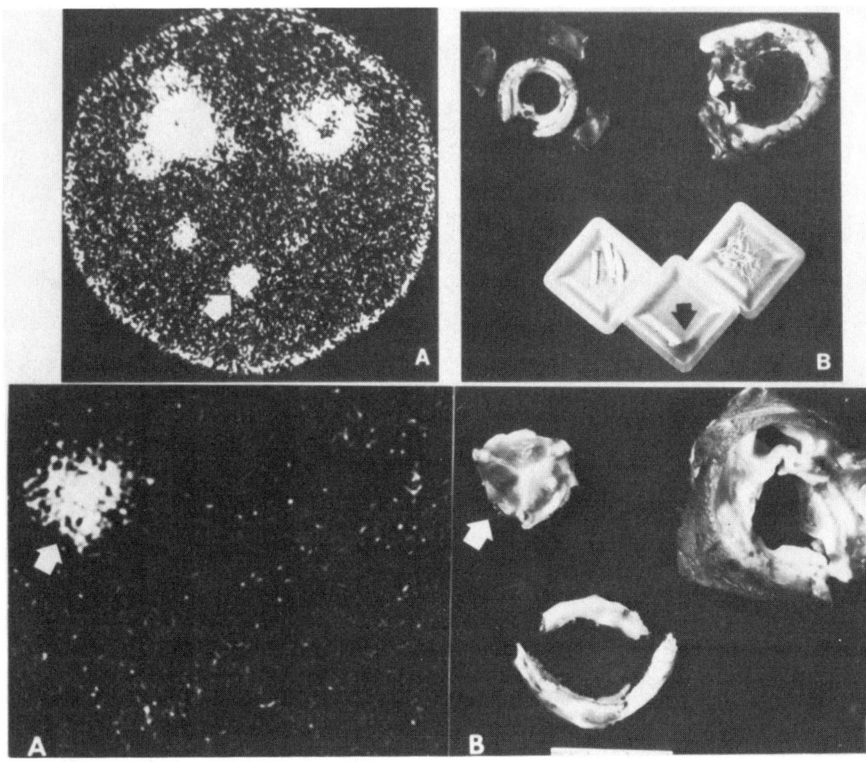

FIGURE 14. *Top:* (**A**) Scintiphoto (5000 counts) of isolated components of tissue valve prosthesis removed from a dog at 25 hours after implantation and 24 hours after administration of labeled platelets. *White arrow* indicates most intense radioactivity, which comes from platelet thrombus (*black arrow*) on sewing ring. (**B**) Photograph of same objects: sewing ring with three leaflets around it (*upper left*); perivalvular tissue (*upper right*); stent supports, thrombus from sewing ring, and suture (left to right) in trays (*below*). Thrombus from sewing ring amounted to 31.44 mg (wet wt). Our recent studies suggest that detergent treatment and diphosphonate immobilization reduce monocyte infiltration, expedite endothelial cell coverage of tissue valve, and inhibit calcification. *Bottom:* (**A**) In a similar scintiphoto at 30 days, most of the platelet deposition occurs in the leaflet and the sewing ring is covered with fibroblast and remains nonthrombogenic. (**B**) Photograph of components of the tissue valve explant at 30 days. (From Dewanjee *et al.*[39])

causing foci of microinfarcts. This platelet deposition could be imaged in the acute phase with ^{111}In-labeled platelets. Platelet deposition in the infarcted tissue is three to five times less than that in the normally perfused organ. However, French *et al.*[25] observed platelet deposition in the rejected kidney that was one to two times higher

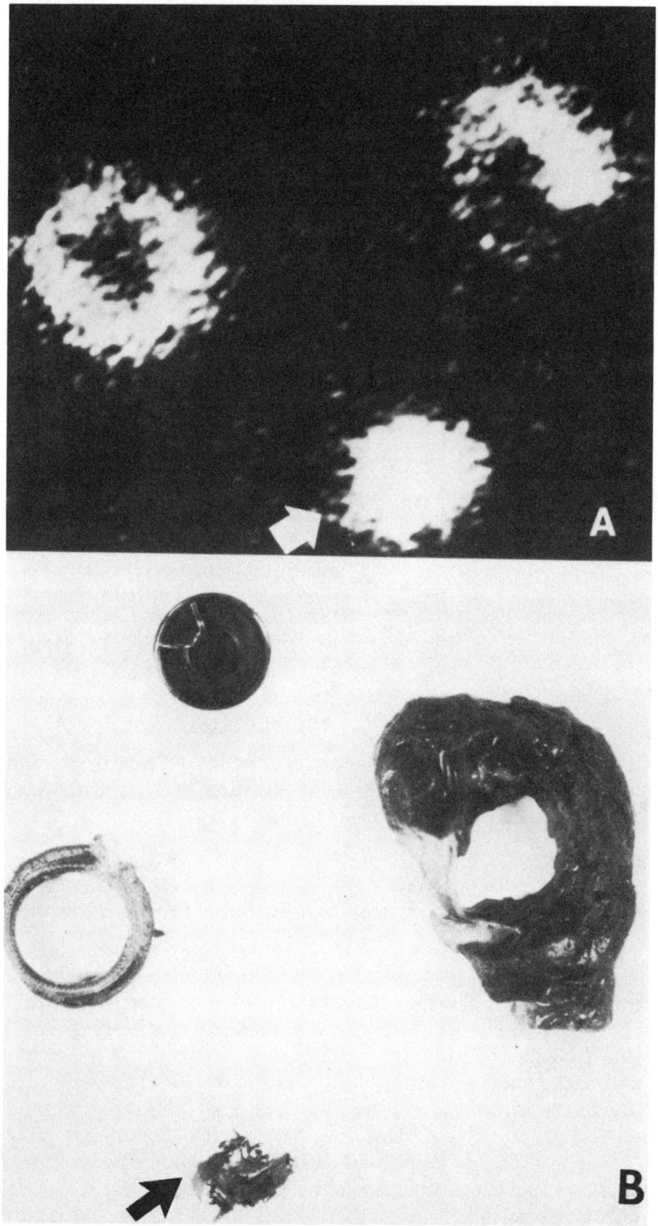

FIGURE 15. Scintiphoto of platelet deposition on components of mechanical valve prosthesis 24 hours postinjection of ^{111}In-labeled platelets and photographed in the same orientation. (**A**) Scintiphoto (25 hours after injection of ^{111}In-labeled platelets in a dog and 24 hours after implantation) of sewing ring (*left*), perivalvular tissue (*right*), and thrombus (*arrow, bottom*). The disk and housing of the valve had few adherent platelets (*top*). (**B**) Thrombogenicity of tissue and mechanical valve is identical in the acute phase. Photograph of the same components in the same orientation. (From Dewanjee *et al.*[40])

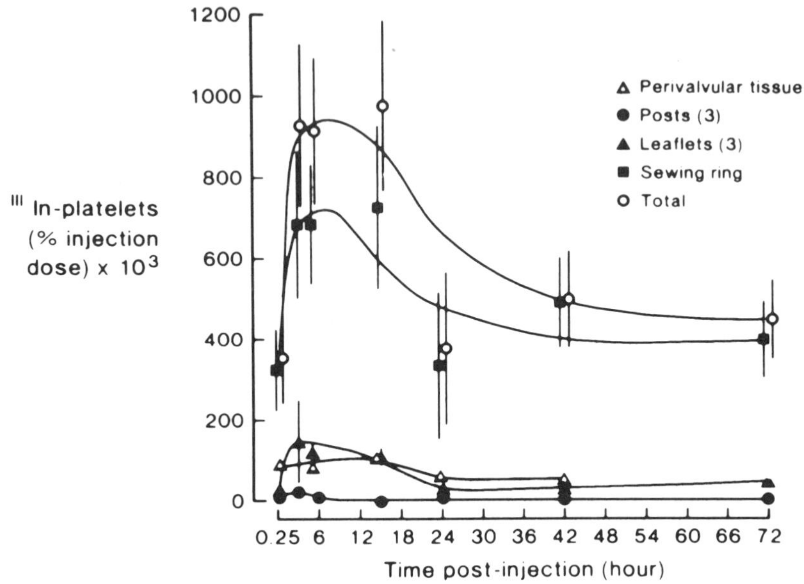

FIGURE 16. Quantification of platelet deposition on components of bovine pericardial tissue valve prosthesis implanted in calves. Note change in platelet deposition on all components with time, as observed with other vascular prostheses and conduits. (From Dewanjee *et al.*[41])

than in normal kidney. Prostacyclin infusion resulted in decrease of platelet incorporation and prolonged platelet survival time. Medication with aspirin, persantine, and sulfinpyrazone tends to increase renal graft viability.

Quantitation of Platelet Thrombosis in Valvular Prostheses in Animals

A variety of mechanical and tissue prosthetic values are used in patients with diseases of cardiac valves.[38] The major limitation of the former is a propensity to form thrombi and emboli, and that of the latter is a tendency to calcify. With ^{111}In-labeled platelets we have been able to image platelet deposition in the acute phase on both mechanical and tissue valve prostheses implanted in dogs and calves.[39–42] These valves were implanted in the mitral annulus and platelet deposition was followed for a 1- to 3-month period. In addition, *in vitro* studies with a gamma counter permitted quantitation of the number of adherent platelets on the components of the mitral valve prostheses. Higher tissue-to-blood radioactivity ratio in skeletal muscle and kidneys due to embolization was also observed. FIGURE 15 shows the dynamic process of platelet incorporation in the mitral annulus of bovine pericardial tissue valve prostheses in calves. The 24-hour platelet deposition showed a consistent decrease in all components of the tissue valve prostheses at 1, 14, 30, and 90 days postimplantation. The results of these quantitative studies of platelet density and total platelet deposition are shown in FIGURES 16–18.

Platelet Deposition on Extracardiac Conduits in Clinical Studies

The use of porcine-valved extracardiac conduits (Dacron tube 10–20 cm long, 1.2–2.6 cm external diameter, with or without porcine valve) in several congenital cardiac lesions, *e.g.*, pulmonary atresia, has permitted corrective surgery. We have

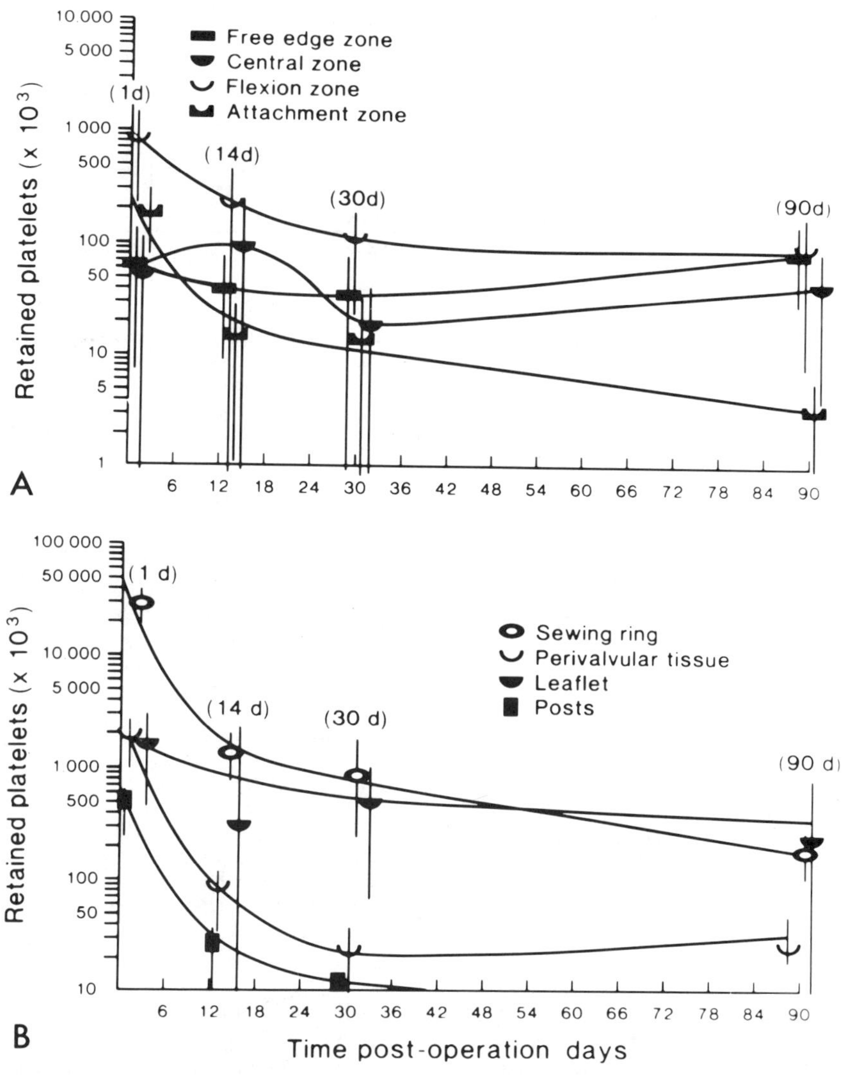

FIGURE 17. Time course of 24-hour platelet deposition expressed as total number of platelets (mean ± SD) on leaflet components at 1, 14, 30, and 90 days postimplantation of 25-mm tissue valves in calves. **(A)** Four zones of leaflets. **(B)** Components of tissue valve. (From Dewanjee *et al.*[42])

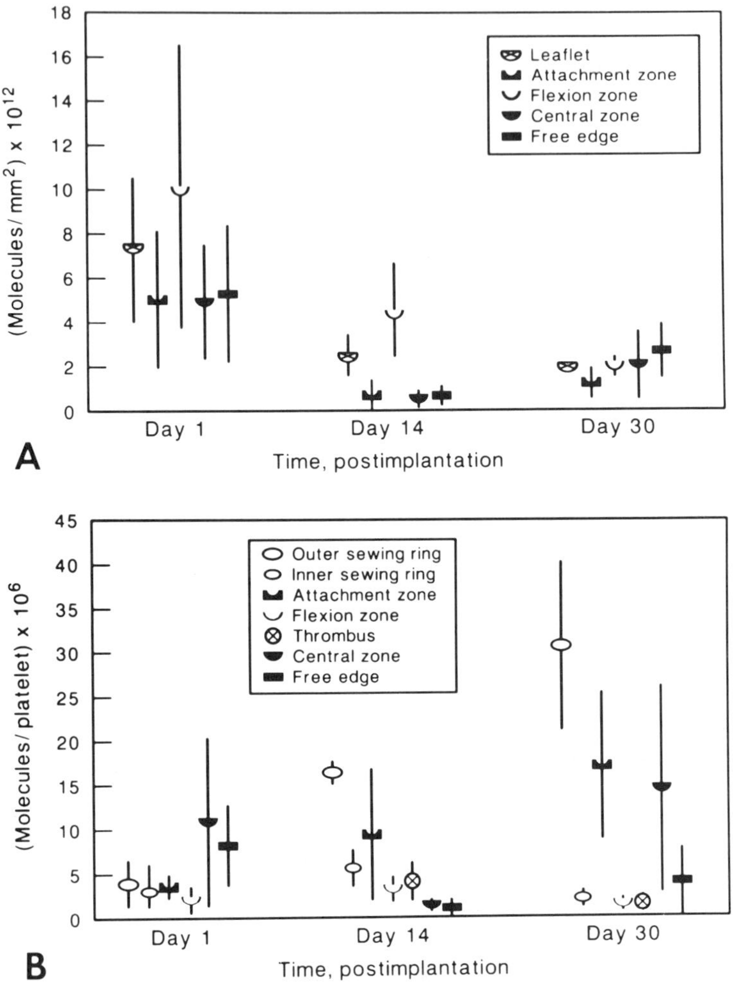

FIGURE 18. (**A**) Regional fibrin density on components of tissue valve at 1, 14, and 30 days postimplantation. (**B**) Regional distribution of fibrin monomer per platelet on components of prostheses. Although the fibrin density decreases, the fibrin:platelet ratio tends to increase for outer sewing ring, attachment, and central zone of tissue valve leaflet. (From Dewanjee *et al.*[48])

measured platelet deposition on conduits (six with valves and three without) with ^{111}In-labeled platelets in nine young patients.[37] In this study, ^{111}In-labeled platelets (290–483 μCi) were administered either immediately or on the fifth to eighth day postoperative, and imaging was performed between 1 and 6 days. Highest platelet deposition on conduit was observed at 3 to 4 days postinjection (FIGURE 19). Treatment with aspirin (75 to 325 mg) administered orally three times a day caused no recognizable changes. Three patterns of platelet deposition (no uptake, diffuse uptake, and focal uptakes at anastomoses and valves) were observed in the scintiphotos.

Platelet Deposition in Angioplasty

Angioplasty of the partially occluded artery by balloon dilation causes endothelial cell loss, cracking of internal elastic lamina, hemorrhage under the plaque, medial necrosis, and exposure of blood to subendothelial thrombogenic contents of plaque.[42] Platelet deposition at the site of deep injury could be imaged with ^{111}In-labeled platelets. Occasionally platelet deposition could also be observed in the embolus of cerebral artery and femoral artery. The site of arterial puncture for catherization, hematoma at the site of biopsy, and site of inflammation and infection also accumulate platelets. As the vessel undergoes partial re-endothelization, the platelet density (platelets per cm^2 for 1- and 24-h depositions) decreases from 45×10^6 at 1 day, to 1.2×10^6 at 1 week, to 0.1×10^6 at 2 months postangioplasty.[43]

Platelet Deposition on Catheters in Animal and Clinical Studies

Lipton *et al.*[44] studied platelet deposition on polyethylene catheters placed in the carotid artery of dogs for a period of 30 minutes to 24 hours. ^{111}In-labeled platelets were injected before and after catheter insertion. Direct correlation was obtained between thrombus weight on catheter and ^{111}In radioactivity. Highest activity in dogs was found at 40 minutes postinjection. At later periods, due to fibrinolysis, thrombus disaggregation, and embolization, the ^{111}In activity decreased. The heparin-bonded catheter accumulated fewer platelets than control catheters. Similar studies were carried out by O'Connell[46] in patients undergoing angiography; as catheters were pulled out, the adherent thrombus embolized and this site of catheter insertion and embolus could be shown in the scintiphoto (FIGURE 11). The full width at half of maximum (FWHM) of the time for increase, peaking, and decrease of platelet deposition is much broader in a larger orifice or lumen than for a smaller lumen. This is particularly high in the case of a catheter study; because of the substantial decrease in

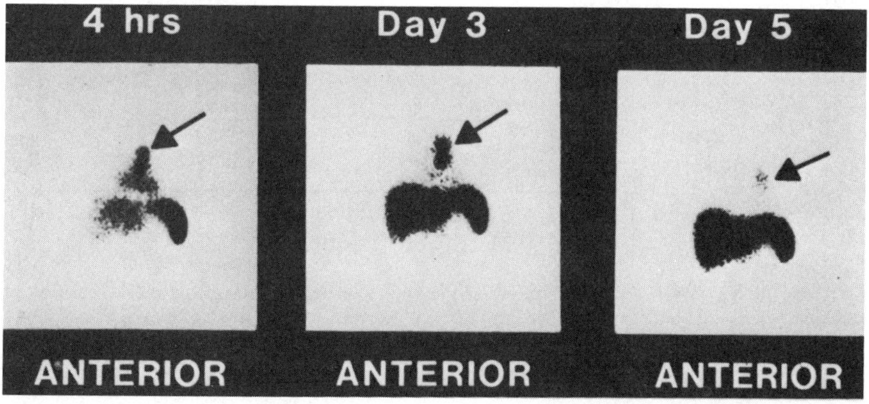

FIGURE 19. Scintiphoto of platelet accumulation in Hancock porcine-valved conduit at 4 hours to 5 days postinjection. Patient was treated wtih 75 mg of dipyridamole and 325 mg of aspirin (three times daily). Note uniform platelet deposition on conduit in the anterior view. Optimum time of imaging is approximately 72 hours. Note lower platelet deposition possibly due to fibrinolysis and embolization at 5 days. (From Agarwal *et al.*[37])

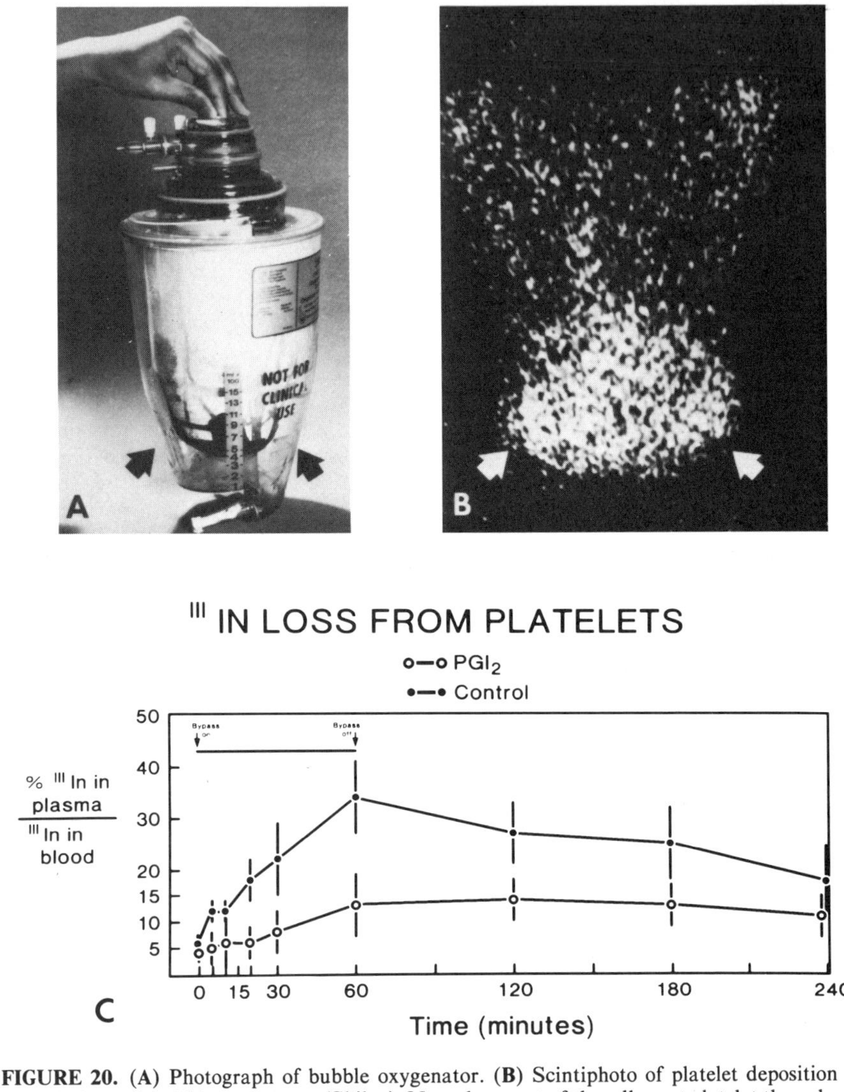

FIGURE 20. (**A**) Photograph of bubble oxygenator. (**B**) Scintiphoto of platelet deposition on (60-min bypass) bubble oxygenator (Shiley). Note that most of the adherent platelet thrombus is in the lower part of the oxygenator. (**C**) Quantitation of platelet lysis with ^{111}In-labeled platelets during cardiopulmonary bypass surgery with bubble oxygenator. Because of high shear rate effect on the platelet membrane of adherent thrombus, intraplatelet ^{111}In is released due to the stretching of platelet membrane. If we could estimate counts per platelet of ^{111}In this might be less for platelet in oxygenator-adherent thrombus than the circulating platelet. Note reduction of platelet lysis with PGI_2 infusion. (From Peterson.[51])

lumen diameter due to catheter insertion, the higher shear rate might increase platelet deposition on the catheter. Fortunately a lot of these platelet aggregates in acute adherent thrombus are not well organized. They may embolize or disintegrate because of fibrinolytic activity in the circulatory system, and thus may cause fewer complications after angiography. For a smaller lumen the FWHM is almost a spike function; either the lumen is patent (nonthrombogenic surface) or occluded (thrombogenic surface). For a large diameter graft, the rate of embolization of small-size platelet aggregates may be higher; patency might be maintained with the underlying risk of embolization.

Platelet Trauma during Cardiopulmonary Bypass Procedure in Platelet Consumption

Decreased platelet number and poor platelet function during cardiopulmonary bypass have been widely reported.[50,51] These changes have been linked to platelet activation by foreign surfaces in the extracorporeal circuit, especially that of air-blood interface in the oxygenator and cardiotomy suction component. With the cardiopulmonary bypass established between right atrium and femoral artery of dogs, we have quantified platelet consumption in the bubble and membrane oxygenator and evaluated the effect of several drugs.[51] In this study, autologous ^{111}In-labeled platelets were administered 20 hours before surgery. Platelet lysis was determined from the amount of free indium in the platelet-poor plasma by centrifugation of blood samples obtained sequentially after bypass procedure. Platelet lysis was found to be three times greater with the bubble oxygenator than with the membrane oxygenator. Prostacyclin infusion reduced platelet lysis from 30% to 18%. Platelet trapping in the bubble oxygenator was higher than that in the membrane oxygenator (FIGURES 20A–C). Scintiphotos demonstrate the uneven distribution of platelets in the bubble oxygenator, mainly in the blood contact area, and more uniform distribution in the membrane oxygenator.

In spite of limited clinical applications, we believe that tracer techniques will be essential for evaluation of platelet-active drugs in cardiovascular diseases and development of biocompatible prostheses, small vessel ($\leq$4mm) grafts, valves, and ventricular pumps.

SUMMARY

The contributions of platelets and clotting factors in thrombosis on injured vessel and cardiovascular prostheses have been quantified with several tracers. Thrombus formation *in vivo* could be measured semiquantitatively in animal models and humans with ^{111}In-labeled platelets, ^{123}I- and ^{131}I-labeled fibrinogen, ^{111}In-labeled antibody to the fibrinogen receptor on the platelet membrane and to fibrin. Thrombus localization by imaging was possible for large thrombus in vessel with deep injury of thrombogenic surface in the acute phase. A single layer of adherent platelet could not be imaged, due to the high background radioactivity present in blood.

Thrombogenicity of graft was compared with that of contralateral vessel. The dynamic process of platelet deposition could be followed accurately using the *in vivo* imaging technique. In addition, *in vitro* quantification permits determination of platelet and fibrin density and of the number of fibrin monomers per platelet in thrombus. The roles of prostacyclin, thromboxane inhibitors, and nonsteroidal antiinflammatory drugs have also been evaluated in animal models and humans. The tracer techniques thus provide invaluable information about platelet-fibrin deposition, its organization and dissolution, and for development of less thrombogenic surfaces for use in cardiovascular prostheses.

ACKNOWLEDGMENT

The author wishes to thank Ms. Randi Fravert for her assistance in typing the manuscript, and Dr. Jules Lam for reviewing the manuscript.

REFERENCES

1. THAKUR, M. L., M. J. WELCH, J. H. JOIST & R. E. COLEMAN. 1976. Indium-111 labeled platelets: Studies on preparation and evaluation of in vitro and in vivo functions. Thromb. Res. **9:** 345–357.
2. DEWANJEE, M. K., S. A. RAO & P. DIDISHEIM. 1981. Indium-111 tropolone, a new high-affinity platelet label: Preparation and evaluation of labeling parameters. J. Nucl. Med. **22:** 981–987.
3. KNIGHT, L. C., J. L. PRIMEAU, B. A. SIEGEL & M. J. WELCH. 1978. Comparison of In-111-labeled platelets and iodinated fibrinogen for the detection of deep vein thrombosis. J. Nucl. Med. **19:** 891–894.
4. DEWANJEE, M. K. 1988. Radioiodination: Theory, Practice and Biomedical Applications. CRC Press. Boca Raton, FL.
5. OSTER, Z. H., S. C. SRIVASTAVA, P. SOM, G. E. MEINKEN, L. E. SCUDDER, K. YAMAMOTO, H. L. ATKINS, A. B. BRILL & B. S. COLLER. 1985. Thrombus radioimmunoscintigraphy: An approach using monoclonal antiplatelet antibody. Proc. Natl. Acad. Sci. **82:** 3465–3468.
6. ROSEBROUGH, S. F., B. KUDRYK, Z. D. GROSSMAN, J. G. MCAFEE, G. SUBRAMANIAN, C. A. RITTER-HRNCIRIK, L. S. WITANOWSKI & G. TILLAPAUGH-FAY. 1985. Radioimmunoimaging of venous thrombi using iodine-131 monoconal antibody. Radiology **156:** 515–517.
7. DEWANJEE, M. K., H. W. WAHNER, W. L. DUNN, J. S. ROBERTSON, V. D. FUSTER & J. H. CHESEBRO. 1986. Comparison of three platelet markers for measurement of platelet survival time in healthy volunteers. Mayo Clin. Proc. **61:** 327–336.
8. MUSTARD, J. F., M. A. PACKHAM & R. L. KINLOUGH-RATHBONE. 1981. Platelets, atherosclerosis and clinical complications in vascular injury and atherosclerosis. *In* Biochemistry of Disease, Vol. 9. S. Moore, Ed.: 79. Dekker. New York.
9. HARKER, L. A. 1986. Antiplatelet drugs in the management of patients with thrombotic disorders. Semin. Thromb. Hemostas. **12:** 134–155.
10. SCHEFFEL, U., M-F. TSAN, T. G. MITCHELL, E. E. CAMARGO, H. BRAINE, M. D. EZEKOWITZ, E. L. NICKOLOFF, R. HILL-ZOBEL, E. MURPHY & P. A. MCINTYRE. 1982. Human platelets labeled with In-111 8-hydroxyquinoline: Kinetics, distribution, and estimates of radiation dose. J. Nucl. Med. **23:** 149–156.
11. ROBERTSON, J. S., M. K. DEWANJEE, M. L. BROWN, V. FUSTER & J. H. CHESEBRO. 1981. Distribution and dosimetry of ^{111}In-labeled platelets. Radiology **140:** 169–176.
12. PETERS, A. M. 1983. Splenic blood flow and blood cell kinetics. Clin. Haematol. **12:** 421–447.
13. POWERS, W. J., C. J. MATHIAS, M. J. WELCH, *et al.* 1982. Scintigraphic detection of platelet deposition in atherosclerotic macacques: A new technique for investigation of antithrombotic drugs. Thromb. Res. **25:** 137–143.
14. GUIDELINES FOR BLOOD-MATERIAL INTERACTIONS. Evaluation of cardiovascular devices and prostheses during in vivo function, Chap. 10. Report of the NHLBI Working Group. NIH Publication No. 85-2185. U.S. Department of Health and Human Services. Washington, D.C.
15. DEWANJEE, M. K. 1985. ^{111}In-platelets in bypass grafts: Experimental and clinical

applications. *In* Radiolabeled Cellular Elements of Blood. M. L. Thakur, M. Hardeman & M. D. Ezekowitz, Eds.: 229–263. Plenum.

16. DEWANJEE, M. K. 1984. Cardiac and vascular imaging with labeled platelets and leukocytes. Semin. Nucl. Med. **14(3):** 154–187.
17. POWERS, W. J., B. A. SIEGEL, H. H. DAVIS, C. J. MATHIAS, H. B. CLARK & M. J. WELCH. 1982. Indium-111 platelet scintigraphy in cerebrovascular disease. Neurology **32:** 938–943.
18. FEDULLO, P. F., K. M. MOSER, K. S. MOSER, R. KONOPKA & M. T. HARTMAN. 1982. Indium-111 labeled platelets: Effect of heparin on uptake by venous thrombi and relationship to the activated partial thromboplastin time. Circulation **66:** 632–637.
19. SOSTMAN, H. D., R. D. NEUMANN, S. S. ZOGHBI, P. F. LORD, M. L. THAKUR, P. CARBO, R. H. GREENSPAN & A. GOTTSCHALK. 1982. Experimental studies with 111-indium labeled platelets in pulmonary embolism. Invest. Radiol. **17:** 367–374.
20. DAVIS, H. H., W. A. HEATON, B. A. SIEGAL, C. J. MATHIAS, J. H. JOIST, L. A. SHERMAN & M. J. WELCH. 1978. Scintigraphic detection of atherosclerotic lesions and venous thrombi in man by indium-111 autologous platelets. Lancet **1:** 1185–1187.
21. FENECH, A., J. K. HUSSEY, F. W. SMITH, P. P. DENDY, B. BENNETT & A. S. DOUGLAS. 1981. Diagnosis of deep vein thrombosis using autologous indium-111-labeled platelets. Br. Med. J. **282:** 1020–1022.
22. EZEKOWITZ, M. D., D. A. WILSON, E. O. SMITH, R. D. BUROW, L. H. HARRISON, D. E. PARKER, R. C. ELKINS, M. PEYTON & F. B. TAYLOR. 1982. Comparison of indium-111-platelet scintigraphy and two-dimensional echocardiography in the diagnosis of left ventricular thrombi. N. Engl. J. Med. **306:** 1509–1513.
23. EZEKOWITZ, M. D., C. F. POPE, H. D. SOSTMAN, E. O. SMITH, M. GLICKMAN, S. RAPOPORT, K. W. SNIDERMAN, G. FRIEDLAENDER, R. R. PELKER, F. B. TAYLOR & B. L. ZARET. 1986. Indium-111 platelet scintigraphy for the diagnosis of acute venous thrombosis. Circulation **73:** 668–674.
24. HEYNS, A., M. G. LOTTER, P. N. BADENHORST, H. PIETERS, C. J. C. NEL & P. C. MINNAAR. 1982. Kinetics and fate of Indium-111 labeled platelets in patients with aortic aneurysms. Arch. Surg. **117:** 1170–1174.
25. FRENCH, A., A. NICHOLLS & F. W. SMITH. 1981. Indium (^{111}In)-labeled platelets in the diagnosis of renal transplant rejection: Preliminary findings. Br. J. Radiol. **54:** 325–327.
26. DEWANJEE, M. K., V. FUSTER, M. P. KAYE & M. JOSA. 1978. Imaging platelet deposition with ^{111}In-labeled platelets in coronary artery bypass grafts in dogs. Mayo Clin. Proc. **53:** 327–331.
27. HANSON, S. R., L. A. HARKER & B. D. RATNER. 1980. In vivo evaluation of artificial surfaces with a nonhuman primate model of arterial thrombosis. J. Lab. Clin. Med. **95:** 289–304.
28. DEWANJEE, M. K., C. W. PUMPHREY, K. P. MURPHY, V. D. FUSTER, M. P. KAYE, J. A. ROSEMARK & J. H. CHESEBRO. 1982. Evaluation of platelet-inhibitor drugs in a canine bilateral femoral graft implant model. Trans. Am. Soc. Artif. Intern. Organs **28:** 504–509.
29. DEWANJEE, M. K., M. TAGO, M. JOSA, V. FUSTER & M. P. KAYE. 1984. Quantification of platelet retention in aortocoronary femoral vein bypass graft in dogs treated with dipyridamole and aspirin. Circulation **69:** 350–356.
30. PUMPHREY, C. W., J. H. CHESEBRO, M. K. DEWANJEE, H. W. WAHNER, L. H. HOLLIER, P. C. PAIROLERO & V. FUSTER. 1983. In vivo quantititation of platelet deposition on human peripheral arterial bypass grafts using indium-111-labeled platelets: Effect of dipyridamole and aspirin. Am. J. Cardiol. **51:** 796–801.
31. CALLOW, A. D., R. CONNOLLY, T. F. O'DONNELL, R. GEMBAROWICZ, E. KEOUGH, K. RAMBERG-LASKARIS & R. VALERI. 1982. Platelet-arterial synthetic graft interaction and its modification. Arch. Surg. **117:** 1447–1455.
32. STRATTON, J. R. & J. L. RITCHIE. 1986. Reduction of indium-111 platelet deposition on Dacron vascular grafts in humans by aspirin plus dipyridamole. Circulation **73:** 325–330.
33. GOLDMAN, M. D., D. SIMPSON, R. J. HAWKER, H. C. NORCOTT & C. N. MCCOLLUM. 1983. Aspirin and dipyridamole reduce platelet deposition on prosthetic femoropopliteal grafts in man. Ann. Surg. **198:** 713–716.

34. Gloviczki, P., M. K. Dewanjee, V. F. Trastek, E. A. Hoffman & M. P. Kaye. 1984. Experimental replacement of the inferior vena cava: Factors affecting patency. Surgery **65:** 657–666.
35. Christenson, J. T., J. Megerman, K. C. Hanel, G. J. L'Italian, H. W. Strauss & W. M. Abbott. 1981. The effect of blood flow rates on platelet deposition in PTFE arterial bypass grafts. Trans. Am. Soc. Artif. Intern. Organs **27:** 188–191.
36. Didisheim, P., M. K. Dewanjee, C. S. Frisk & M. P. Kaye. 1984. Animal models for predicting clinical performance of biomaterials for cardiovascular use. *In* Contemporary Biomaterials: Material and Host Response, Clinical Applications, New Technology and Legal Aspects. J. W. Boretos, Ed.: 132–179. M. Eden Noyse Publications. Park Ridge, NJ.
37. Agarwal, K. C., H. W. Wahner, M. K. Dewanjee, V. Fuster, F. J. Puga, G. K. Danielson, J. H. Chesebro & R. H. Feldt. 1982. Imaging of platelets in right-sided extracardiac conduits in humans. J. Nucl. Med. **23:** 342–347.
38. Harker, L. A. & S. J. Slichter. 1970. Studies of platelet and fibrinogen kinetics in patients with prosthetic heart valves. N. Engl. J. Med. **283:** 1302–1305.
39. Dewanjee, M. K., V. F. Trastek, M. Tago, M. Torianni & M. P. Kaye. 1983. Noninvasive radioisotope technique for detection of platelet deposition on bovine pericardial mitral valve prosthesis and in vitro quantification of visceral microemboli in dogs. Trans. Am. Soc. Artif. Intern. Organs **29:** 188–193.
40. Dewanjee, M. K., V. Fuster, S. A. Rao, P. L. Forsham & M. P. Kaye. 1983. Noninvasive radioisotopic technique for detection of platelet deposition in mitral valve prostheses and quantitation of visceral microembolism in dogs. Mayo Clin. Proc. **58:** 307–314.
41. Dewanjee, M. K., P. Didisheim, M. P. Kaye, E. Solis, P. E. Zollman, M. D. Francis, M. Torianni, V. S. Trastek, M. Tago & W. D. Edwards. 1984. Platelet deposition on the calcification of bovine pericardial valve. Eur. Heart J. **5**(Suppl. D): 1–5.
42. Dewanjee, M. K., E. Solis, S. T. Mackey, J. Lenker, P. Didisheim, J. H. Chesebro, P. E. Zollman & M. P. Kaye. 1986. Quantification of regional platelet and calcium deposition on pericardial tissue valve prostheses in calves and effect of hydroxyethylene diphosphonate. J. Thorac. Cardiovasc. Surg. **92:** 337–348.
43. Steele, P. M., J. H. Chesebro, A. W. Stanson, D. R. Holmes, Jr, M. K. Dewanjee, L. Badimon & V. Fuster. 1985. Balloon angioplasty. Natural history of the pathophysiological response to injury in a pig model. Circ. Res. **57:** 105–112.
44. Lipton, M. J., P. W. Doherty, D. A. Goodwin, G. T. Bushberg, R. Prager & C. F. Meares. 1980. Evaluation of catheter thrombogenicity in vivo with indium-labeled platelets. Radiology **135:** 191–194.
45. Rodvien, R., R. Robinson, R. R. Mitchell, P. Litwak & D. C. Price. 1982. A new model for in vivo platelet and thrombus kinetics. *In* Biomaterials: Interfacial Phenomena and Applications, chap. 3. S. L. Cooper, N. A. Peppas, A. S. Hoffman & B. D. Ratner, Eds.:25–34. Washington, D.C. American Chemical Society. Washington, D.C.
46. O'Connor, M. K., S. S. Brennan & D. G. Shanik . 1986. Indium-111-labeled platelet deposition following transfemoral angiography. Radiology **158:** 191–194.
47. Dewanjee, M. K., E. Solis, S. T. Mackey, G. Gonzales, J. H. Chesebro & M. P. Kaye. 1986. Quantification of platelet and fibrinogen deposition on PTFE and vein grafts in dogs and the effect of vitamin E on graft thrombosis in the acute phase. Trans. Am. Soc. Artif. Intern. Organs. **32:** 187–192.
48. Dewanjee, M. K., E. Solis, J. Lenker, C. Tidwell, S. T. Mackey, P. Didisheim & M. P. Kaye. 1986. Quantification of platelet and fibrinogen-fibrin deposition on components of tissue valves (Ionescu-Shiley) in calves. Trans. Am. Soc. Artif. Intern. Organs. **32:** 591–596.
49. Badimon, L., V. Fuster, M. K. Dewanjee & J. C. Romero. 1982. A sensitive new method of ex vivo platelet deposition. Thromb. Res. **28:** 237–250.
50. Hope, A. F., A. Heyns, M. G. Lotter, O. R. V. Reenen, F. D. Kock, P. N. Badenhorst, H. Pieters, H. Kotze, J. M. Meyer & P. C. Minnaar. 1981. Kinetics and sites of sequestration of indium 111-labeled human platelets during cardiopulmonary bypass. J. Thorac. Cardiovasc. Surg. **81:** 880–886.

51. PETERSON, K. A., M. K. DEWANJEE & M. P. KAYE. 1982. Fate of indium-111-labeled platelets during cardiopulmonary bypass performed with membrane and bubble oxygenators. J. Thorac. Cardiovasc. Surg. **84:** 39–43.
52. HEYNS, A. D. P., P. N. BADENHORST & M. G. LOTTER. 1985. Platelet Kinetics and Imaging, Vol. 1: Techniques and Normal Platelet Kinetics. CRC Press, Boca Raton, FL.
53. HEYNS, A. D. P., P. N. BADENHORST & M. G. LOTTER. 1985. Platelets and Imaging, Vol. 2: Clinical Applications. CRC Press. Boca Raton, FL.

Methods of Assessment of Thrombosis *ex Vivo*[a]

STUART L. COOPER, DONNA J. FABRIZIUS, AND TIMOTHY G. GRASEL

Department of Chemical Engineering
University of Wisconsin
Madison, Wisconsin 53706

INTRODUCTION

Both *in vivo* and *ex vivo* techniques have been used as a means of evaluating the blood compatibility of polymeric biomaterials. This review compares the advantages and disadvantages of these two techniques and emphasizes the role *ex vivo* techniques have had in the analysis of blood-materials interactions. Several results from recent canine *ex vivo* studies will also be reviewed.

Ex vivo systems can be classified as being either "open" or "closed." In closed systems, the blood returns to the animal after it has passed through the test chamber or shunt. In open systems, the blood is either analyzed further or discarded without being returned to the animal. Open *ex vivo* systems are typically based upon either the Dudley clotting time test or upon flow through a test chamber under controlled conditions. The most common closed system configurations are arterio-venous (A-V) shunts or test chambers.

OPEN *EX VIVO* SYSTEMS

A summary of open *ex vivo* systems is given in TABLE 1. The Dudley clotting test[1–3] involves the insertion of a tube, via a catheter, into the vein of the test subject. The time required for the blood to stop dripping from the open end of the tubing is known as the Dudley clotting time. The clotting times obtained from different materials can be compared as long as the inner diameter of the tubing is kept constant. This test method is limited to materials that can be uniformly coated in a tubing with a diameter of about 0.02 inches, but the same subject may be used repetitively for the experiment over a period of time.

Stagnation flow experiments[5–8] are also open *ex vivo* systems. Blood flows perpendicularly onto a transparent flat plate. In stagnation point flow it flows radially, with a linearly decreasing shear rate, outward along the test plate and into a collecting trough. The adherence of formed blood elements can be directly observed with optical microscopy. This system has been used to observe how the wall shear rate affects cell adhesion and the sequence of events leading to thrombosis.

Grabowski *et al.*[9] developed an open *ex vivo* chamber for the study of ADP-induced platelet aggregation, which was quantified using a videodensitometer. By direct and

[a]The authors acknowledge the support of the National Institutes of Health through grant nos. HL-21001 and HL-24046.

continuous measurement of aggregate mean thickness, it was possible to observe frequent and repetitive detachment (embolization) of platelet aggregates as a function of shear rate. Other test chambers that have been reported include the Lyman flow cell,[11–13] the U-shaped cell,[14–16] and the T cell.[17] The blood exposure time of these open *ex vivo* experiments was typically less than 30 minutes and was limited by the blood loss from the animal during the experiment. Biocompatibility was primarily measured by platelet adhesion, which could be quantified by means of radiolabeled platelets or photomicroscopy.

CLOSED *EX VIVO* SYSTEMS

As seen in TABLE 2, most closed *ex vivo* systems are either A-V shunt or flow chamber configurations. The novel rotating shaft system of Schultz and coworkers[44–46]

TABLE 1. Open *ex Vivo* Systems

Configuration	Species	Exposure Time (min)	Measured Variable	Ref.
Open tube	dog	—	Dudley clotting time	Dudley *et al.*[1] Williams *et al.*[2] Fischer *et al.*[3]
Open tube	pig	3	platelet adhesion	Ward and Forest[4]
Stagnation point	dog	2–120	cell adhesion	Petschek *et al.*[5] Madras *et al.*[6] Nyilas *et al.*[7] Morton and Cumming[8]
Flat plate	dog	30	platelet adhesion thrombus formation	Grabowski *et al.*[9]
Relaminarization flow cell	dog	4	platelet adhesion	Zingg *et al.*[10]
Lyman flow cell	dog	0.5–4	platelet adhesion	Lyman *et al.*[11,12]
Lyman flow cell	sheep	3	platelet adhesion	Kim *et al.*[13]
U-shaped cell	dog	2.5–45	platelet adhesion	Friedman and Leonard [14] Leonard *et al.*[15] Grabowski *et al.*[16]
T cell	dog	2–15	platelet adhesion	Dutton *et al.*[17]

imposed a Couette-type flow upon blood flowing along the shaft, which was coated with the test material. Flow rate and shear could be controlled independently by separate control of flow rate through the chamber and the rotation of the central rod. Better control of flow was maintained in this system than in most other *ex vivo* flow chambers. Under their experimental conditions, Schultz *et al.*[46] have found that a uniform deposition of platelets was built along the rotating rod, suggesting that under the conditions used thrombus formation was not diffusion-limited.

For most chamber systems, the typical procedure is to flow blood through the chamber for a period of time, flush the blood out, and remove the sheet of test material for later analysis of platelet deposition. The assembling and dissembling of flow chambers may be tedious, however. Another disadvantage of test chambers is that the nonphysiological flow within the chamber is often not easily characterized. Pulsatile blood flow and changes in blood pressure can cause the mean flow rate to change during the experiment.

TABLE 2. Closed *ex vivo* Systems

Configuration	Species	Exposure Time (min)	Measured Variable	Ref.
A-V shunt	rabbit	30	thrombus formation	Rowntree and Shionoya[18]
A-V shunt	dog	2–120	radiolabeled platelet, fibrinogen deposition, platelet morphology	Barber *et al.*[19] Ihlenfeld *et al.*[20,21] Young *et al.*[22–24] Lelah *et al.*[25,26]
A-V shunt	dog	0.2–50	radiolabeled fibrinogen, platelet, and albumin	Baquey *et al.*[27] Basse-Cathalinat *et al.*[28]
A-V shunt	dog	5–60	platelet adhesion	Vale and Greer[29]
A-V series shunt	dog	0.5–60	radiolabeled platelet and fibrinogen platelet morphology	Lelah *et al.*[31,32]
A-V series shunt	rhesus	0.5–60	radiolabeled platelet and fibrinogen platelet morphology	Lambrecht *et al.*[33]
A-V shunt	baboon	2 weeks	radiolabeled platelet consumption	Harker *et al.*[34] Hanson *et al.*[35]
A-V shunt	baboon	2 weeks	platelet consumption, thromboemboli	Hoffman *et al.*[36]
A-V shunt	dog	—	patency	Galletti *et al.*[37]
A-V shunt	dog	—	patency	Ip *et al.*[38]
A-V shunt	dog	5 days	platelet serotonin release	Cholakis *et al.*[39]
V-V shunt	rabbit	1–480	platelet count, thrombus formation, clotting time	Toomasian *et al.*[40]
V-V shunt	dog	5–120	platelet adhesion	Olijslager[41]
Bifurcation	pig	20	thrombus growth, radiolabeled platelet	Mustard *et al.*[42] Murphy *et al.*[43]
Rotating shaft	dog	60	radiolabled platelet, fibrinogen deposition	Schultz *et al.*[44–46] Reichert *et al.*[47]
Annular axial rod	rabbit	5–10	platelet and thrombus coverage	Baumgartner and Haudenschild[48]
U cell	dog	2.5–60	platelet adhesion	Friedman *et al.*[49]
Flat plate	dog	2–120	radiolabeled platelet, fibrinogen deposition	Wilson *et al.*[50]
Captured vortex	dog	10–30	thrombus weight	Benis *et al.*[51]

Most test chamber and arterio-venous shunt systems monitor platelet deposition as a measure for assessing the thrombogenicity of a material. Deposition is generally determined by radiolabeling platelets with ^{111}In or ^{51}Cr or by counting platelets on the surface using photomicroscopy. Often fibrinogen is simultaneously labeled with ^{125}I. The coupling of platelet and fibrinogen deposition provides a versatile tool for examining thrombosis. The conversion of fibrinogen during the clotting cascade to fibrin[52] reinforces the growing thrombus.[53] Another useful parameter often studied in *ex vivo* systems is the change in platelet morphology on the test surface using scanning electron microscopy (SEM). This technique provides complementary information about platelet deposition, activation, aggregation, and thrombus formation on polymeric biomaterials.

Arterio-venous shunt experiments have also been used to measure the extent to which platelet consumption is accelerated by the shunt material. Harker *et al.*[34,36] used a baboon model to show that platelet consumption was directly related to the shunt surface area and was dependent on the shunt material. These investigators directly observed embolization from the shunt surface using a light-scattering technique.

Ex vivo experiments generally examine short-term interactions, and the experimental animal is usually sacrificed at the end of a set of experiments. To avoid animal-to-animal variability, chronic implants of exteriorized A-V shunts have been attempted. Galletti *et al.*[37] kept exteriorized A-V shunts patent for up to 7 weeks in beagles. Cell culture devices can be attached to the extracorporeal portion of the A-V shunt for evaluation of their activation of the immune system. Sefton and coworkers[38] showed that a chronic shunt could be inserted between the iliac artery and vein of a dog and be reused many times over a period greater than 6 months. Materials to be tested for short time periods were inserted in parallel with the exteriorized portion of the chronic shunt and were compared on the basis of their patency times. This same chronic configuration was used to test blood-material interactions for up to five days by inserting a test segment in series with the shunt.[39] These successful chronic implants eliminate the need for frequent surgery and reduce interanimal variability, while also providing the opportunity to obtain a long-term evaluation of test materials.

A CLOSED *EX VIVO* CANINE MODEL: SOME EXPERIMENTAL RESULTS

The studies described below represent our own efforts to develop a canine *ex vivo* protocol to evaluate thrombus formation on polymeric biomaterials.

Experimental

Adult mongrel dogs were screened for platelet aggregability to ADP and epinephrine, platelet count, fibrinogen level, and hematocrit. Platelets, radiolabeled with either ^{51}Cr or ^{111}In, and purified fibrinogen, radiolabeled with ^{125}I, were infused into the nonheparinized subject prior to the experiment.

The animal was anesthetized and respirated. The femoral artery and vein in one leg were exposed and ligated as shown in FIGURES 1–3. The artery and vein were then

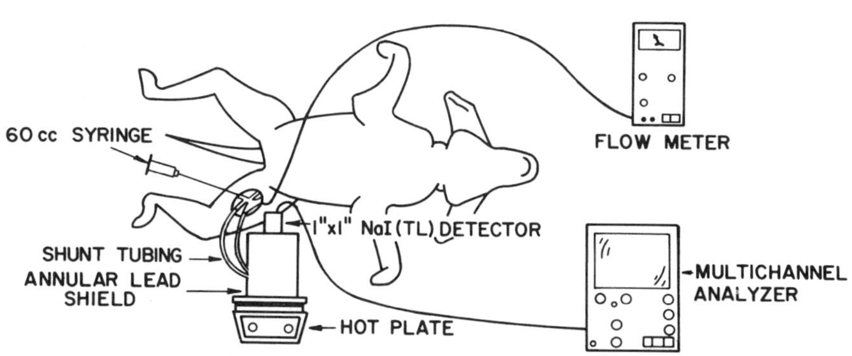

FIGURE 1. Schematic diagram of single shunt experiment. (From Ihlenfeld *et al.*[21])

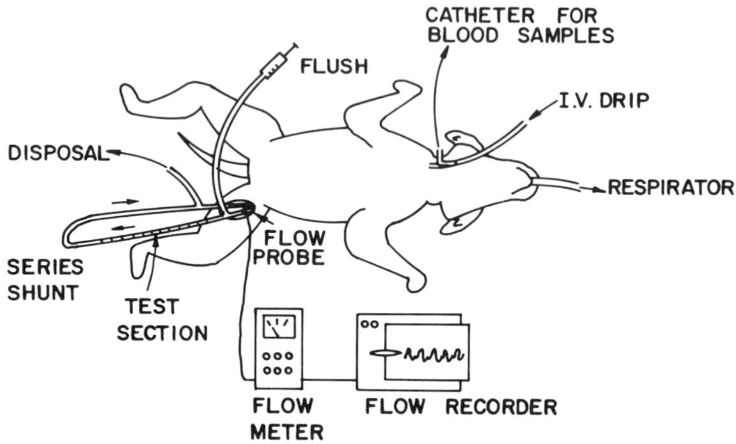

FIGURE 2. Schematic diagram of series shunt experiment. (From Lelah *et al.*[30])

cannulated with polyethylene entrance and exit sections connected to the shunt, which had been initially filled with a degassed divalent cation-free Tyrodes solution to prevent blood-air contact. A branch artery proximal to the shunt was cannulated with a 16-gauge catheter and connected to a flushing syringe containing Tyrodes solution. Thus, the blood could be flushed from the shunt following a predetermined interval of blood contact. The flushing step was necessary in order to detect the radioactivity associated with adherent blood elements.

Two possible configurations of the canine *ex vivo* shunt experiment are shown in FIGURES 1–3. The single shunt technique shown in FIGURE 1 was originally developed by Ihlenfeld *et al.*[21] Blood flow was initiated, and at each sample time point (from 2 to 120 minutes of blood contact) the artery was clamped and the blood was flushed from the shunt with Tyrodes solution. After flushing, the shunt was sampled for adherent radiolabeled species using a NaI (Tl doped) crystal detector connected to a multichannel analyzer. At each time point a 1.5-cm sample of tubing was removed from the venous end of the shunt and was fixed in 2% glutaraldehyde for later preparation for SEM examination. After counting for radioactivity, blood flow in the shunt was resumed until completion of the next sample time point.

In the series shunt technique[30] shown in FIGURES 2 and 3, a new set of identical test surfaces joined as a shunt section was inserted for each time period. Blood contact times for typical animal surgery ranged from 0.5 to 60 minutes. At the end of the time interval for blood exposure, the series was flushed with Tyrodes solution. Immediately following flushing, the joined test section was removed and fixed with 2% glutaraldehyde. A portion of each test surface was counted in a multichannel gamma counter. Small sections of each segment were prepared for examination by SEM.

Blood flow was continuously monitored in both single and series shunt experiments using an electromagnetic flow transducer connected to a chart recorder. Blood flow rates could be controlled by clamping the shunt downstream from the test surfaces.

At hourly time intervals, blood samples were removed through an indwelling jugular catheter to determine whole blood radioactivity, platelet count, fibrinogen level, hematocrit, activated thromboplastin time, thrombin time, plasma protamine paracoagulation, and euglobulin lysis time. Platelet aggregability to ADP, collagen, and epinephrine were monitored at the start and end of each experiment. Fibrinogen clottability was determined periodically throughout the experiment. Each animal was sacrified after a single surgery.

Results and Discussion

Ihlenfeld *et al.*[21,67] examined five biomedically important polymer surfaces: Extruded Grade Biomer® polyurethaneurea (Ethicon, Somerville, NJ), Silastic® silicone rubber (SIL) (Dow Corning, Midland, MI), polyacrylamide (PAM) and poly(hydroxyethyl methacrylate) (PHEMA) grafted onto silicone rubber, and Tygon® plasticized poly(vinyl chloride) (PVC) (Norton Plastics) in the nonheparinized canine single shunt configuration. As shown in FIGURE 4 for Biomer and Tygon, distinct patterns of transient thrombus formation were seen for each material. A time-dependent phase of thrombus deposition followed by thromboembolization was observed on the Tygon and Silastic surfaces, and was much less severe on the Biomer surface. Platelet deposition profiles obtained using radiolabeling were consistent with morphological analysis by SEM.

The adsorption of albumin, gamma globulin, and fibrinogen were measured on plasticized poly(vinyl chloride), silicone rubber, and polyurethaneurea in subsequent experiments in heparinized animals.[67] For PVC and SIL, fibrinogen adsorption was found to predominate initially, although that protein subsequently partially desorbed

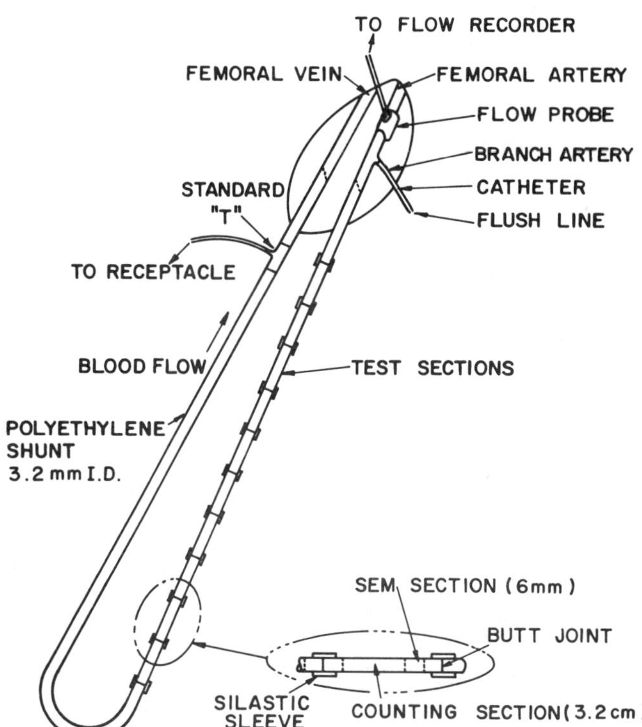

FIGURE 3. Cannulation site and details of series shunt experiment. (From Lelah *et al.*[30])

and was replaced by albumin and gamma globulin. On the Biomer polyurethaneurea, fibrinogen was less prominent initially; however, the adsorption of all three proteins increased with time following initial blood contact. After 60 minutes of exposure to flowing heparinized blood, a higher fraction of albumin was present on the surface of PVC compared to that at earlier blood contact times. These results indicate that displacement of adsorbed proteins occurs with time on polymer surfaces exposed to flowing blood *ex vivo*. Displacement of fibrinogen adsorbed from plasma has also been observed by other investigators.[70]

Solution Grade and Extruded Grade Biomer are polyetherurethanes that have been suggested for use in biomedical applications. A study by Lelah *et al.*[25] used the canine single shunt experiment to relate the distinct chemical and surface compositions of the different Biomers to canine *ex vivo* platelet and fibrinogen deposition. In this study, blood compatibility was correlated with increasing concentration of polyether soft segments on the surface.

The effect of proteins precoated onto blood-contacting biomaterials has been studied using the *ex vivo* canine single shunt experiment.[20,22–23,25,71] In early experiments[20,22,71] it was shown that preadsorption of several human proteins, including fibronectin, von Willebrand factor (vWF), thrombospondin, fibrinogen, α_2-macroglobulin (α_2M), and gamma globulin enhanced platelet and fibrinogen deposition, while albumin preadsorption passivated the surface. Later studies using homologous canine proteins indicated that preadsorption of canine vWF, fibronectin, partially purified fibrinogen, or purified fibrinogen enhanced platelet and fibrinogen deposition when compared to uncoated silicone rubber or PVC surfaces.[23] In recent studies, the effects of competitive and sequential preadsorption of a "thrombogenic" protein (canine

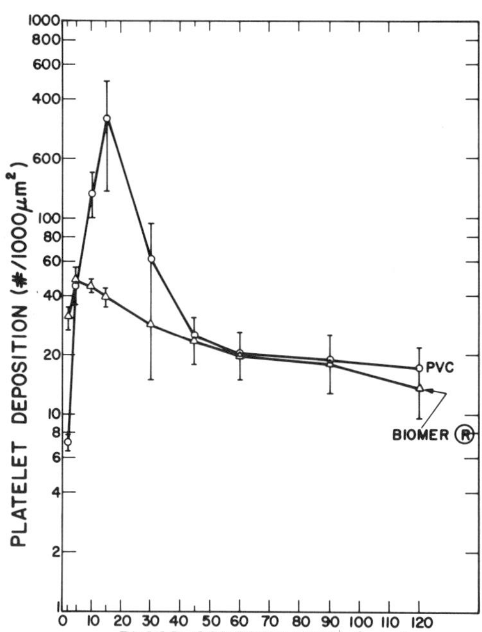

FIGURE 4. Transient platelet deposition on polymer surfaces Biomer polyurethaneurea and Tygon plasticized poly(vinyl chloride) (*PVC*). (From Ihlenfeld *et al.*[21])

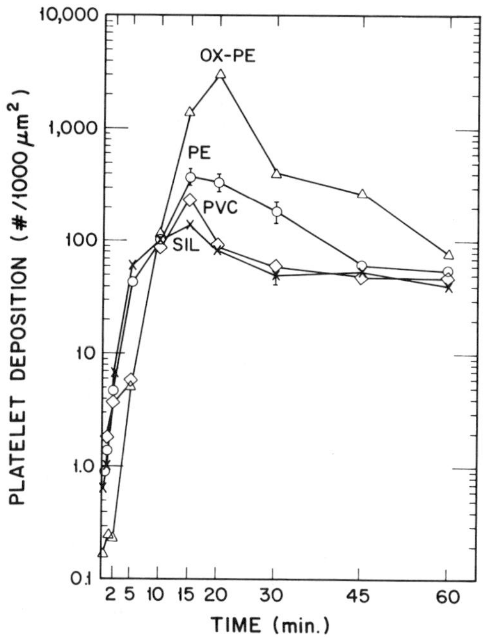

FIGURE 5. Transient platelet deposition obtained using series shunt experiment on polymer surfaces Intramedic polyethylene (*PE*), chromic-acid-etched PE (*OX-PE*), Silastic silicone rubber (*SIL*), and *PVC*. (From Lelah *et al.*[30])

fibrinogen) and a "nonthrombogenic" protein (canine albumin) on platelet deposition have been investigated.[72] It was found that the thrombogenic response of the surface was determined by the composition of the initially preadsorbed protein layer rather than the total concentration of protein on the polymer surface. The protein layer composition was found to determine the extent of platelet activation and the adhesive strength between platelets and the polymer surface. These examples show that the *ex vivo* canine single shunt model can be used to study the mechanisms of surface-induced thrombosis.

The previously discussed method of Ihlenfeld *et al.* was modified by Lelah *et al.*[30] to allow the evaluation of a series of polymer surfaces in the canine *ex vivo* arterio-venous shunt experiment. The series shunt technique was used to examine platelet and fibrinogen deposition on Intramedic® polyethylene (PE) Clay-Adams, Parsippany, NJ), SIL, PVC, and chromic-acid-etched PE (OX-PE). After an initial period of minimal deposition, platelet deposition on all surfaces increased to a peak at about 15–20 minutes of blood contact on all surfaces studied. The amount of adsorbed fibrinogen fell from initial levels to a minimum at approximately 5 to 10 minutes of blood contact and then increased to a peak at about the same time as observed for the platelet response. The peaks in platelet and fibrinogen deposition were attributed to the competition between thrombus formation and embolization. Peak platelet and fibrinogen deposition levels for PE were found to be inversely related to flow rate over the range studied. The chromic-acid-oxidized polyethylene showed the most platelet and fibrinogen deposition of the polymers studied, followed by PE, PVC, and SIL, as shown by the transient platelet deposition profile in FIGURE 5.

A prerequisite for a series arrangement is the independence of the position and thrombogenic nature of any surface on the thrombogenic nature of another section in the same shunt. At the relatively high flow rates used, no effect of segment position or any downstream effects were observed in the series shunt experiments.[30] It has been shown in this experiment that as the average blood shear rate increases, the role of the surface in thrombus formation assumes greater importance.[73]

Recent efforts using the series shunt experiment have concentrated on the study of the relationships between the surface properties and blood compatibility of polyetherurethanes,[74] polyether and polysiloxane urethaneureas,[75] and polyurethane ionomers.[76]

ASSESSMENT OF *EX VIVO* TECHNIQUES

The *ex vivo* canine shunt model that has just been described is a useful tool in the study of blood-materials interactions. Deposition of platelets, fibrinogen, or leukocytes, as well as other blood components, may be quantified using radiolabeling techniques. The processes of platelet and cell adhesion, spreading, and activation may be visualized using scanning electron microscopy. The use of preadsorbed proteins allows the study of some of the mechanisms of artificial-surface-induced thrombosis in the canine model. The series shunt is useful for examining the interactions of several surfaces under identical conditions and for comparing the blood responses of a number of different candidate biomaterials. By studying several materials simultaneously, the time, animal-to-animal variations, and expense associated with testing materials in nonanticoagulated flow systems can be reduced.

As opposed to *in vitro* systems, *ex vivo* and *in vivo* systems allow test materials to be assessed under more clinically relevant situations. Materials are tested under non-physiological conditions during *in vitro* experiments, since blood is totally separated from the body. *In vitro* systems also require that the blood be anticoagulated and are often performed at room temperature. Anticoagulants such as heparin and sodium citrate are used to block the activation of the coagulation pathways,[54,55] but these anticoagulants have been observed to affect platelet-surface interactions.[44,56–58] Experimental temperature also has been observed to affect platelet deposition.[59–60] *Ex vivo* systems are also more likely to allow the test material to be examined in the form that it will be clinically used.

Ex vivo systems typically examine short-term interactions during time periods of less than 4 hours of blood contact, whereas most *in vivo* experiments only measure long-term interactions. The unique element of most *ex vivo* systems, however, is that they enable dynamic quantification of platelet and protein deposition to be obtained. Fresh material can be exposed for each time point of observation in one experiment. This procedure allows different materials to be tested in the same animal under similar physiological conditions.

An important difference between *in vivo* and *ex vivo* techniques arises from the fact that in *in vivo* systems the most common measurement of blood compatibility is the assessment of patency. A vascular graft or intravascular ring is implanted into an animal for a certain period of time or until occlusion. The material is removed from the animal, and the degree of occlusion is determined. This qualitative measurement may be significantly affected by the variability between test subjects.[61] Since this type of measurement looks at an endpoint determination, the final patency evaluation may be misleading. A ring which was removed may have been thrombus-free throughout blood contact or thrombosis may have occured, followed by a period of embolization or fibrinolysis.[61] *Ex vivo* methods enable a more dynamic picture of thrombosis and embolization to be made through a series of end-point determinations on the same materials at different time points of blood exposure.

The primary disadvantage of *in vivo* and *ex vivo* experiments is that nonhuman subjects must be used. Studies have shown that platelet deposition on biomaterials is highly dependent upon animal species,[33,56] Other studies have shown that platelet aggregation characteristics are also species dependent, as is the sensitivity of red blood cells to hemolysis.[62,63] Blood from primates is hematologically very similar to human blood[64]; however the cost and shortage of primates make their use difficult. The dog is the most commonly used animal model. Canines have a low susceptibility to cardiovascular disease and pulmonary embolism. They also have a hyperplastic vascular response and have very active hemostatic and fibrinolytic systems.[64] These characteristics may favor the use of dogs as an animal model, because in some respects, the canine represents a worst-case situation for comparison with human blood-material responses.

Unfortunately, *ex vivo* systems are generally more expensive than *in vitro* systems. However, *ex vivo* methods tend to be less costly than *in vivo* techniques. Additionally, since *ex vivo* and *in vivo* experiments involve live animals, it may be difficult to control many of the experimental variables involved, expecially pulsatile blood flow. Another factor which must be considered is the variability of results obtained from *ex vivo* and *in vivo* systems due to variability between individual animals. When possible, materials should be compared by testing in the same animal. It has been widely observed that there are animal-to-animal differences that may greatly affect experimental results. This variability necessitates the repetition of experiments in order to obtain statistically valid results.

Ex vivo systems have primarily been used to measure platelet coverage on the surface. It must be emphasized that this parameter is only a partial assessment of thrombosis and may provide misleading results. Platelet adhesion is affected by many parameters not related to the test material. In addition to the chemical and physical nature of the surface, the rate of platelet deposition depends on the flow rate,[65] animal species,[56] anticoagulants,[44,56–58] and anesthetic used.[66] Studies of platelet morphological changes, embolization, and protein interactions should also be performed in addition to the measurement of platelet adhesion. Since thrombosis is a complex process, the monitoring of as many variables as possible may provide clues to the mechanisms of thrombosis and allow a more complete evaluation of the blood compatability of a material.

REFERENCES

1. DUDLEY, B., J. L. WILLIAMS, K. ABLE & B. MULLER. 1976. Synthesis and characterization of blood compatible surfaces. I. Dynamic tube test applied to heparinized surfaces. Trans. Am. Soc. Artif. Intern. Organs. **22:** 538–544.
2. WILLIAMS, J. L., A. RUMAKS & J. P. O'CONNELL. 1983. Development of non-thrombogenic materials. Polym. Prepr. **24:** 8.
3. FISCHER, J. P., P. FUGHE, K. BURG & N. HEIMBURGER. 1982. Methoden zur Herstellung und Charakterisierung von Kunststoffen mit verbesserter Blutvertraglichkeit. Angew. Makromol. Chem. **105:** 131–165.
4. WARD, C. A. & T. W. FOREST. 1976. On the relation between platelet adhesion and the roughness of a synthetic biomaterial. Ann. Biomed. Eng. **4:** 184–207.
5. PETSCHEK, H., D. ADAMIS & A. R. KANTROWITZ. 1968. Stagnation flow thrombus formation. Trans. Am. Soc. Artif. Intern. Organs **14:** 256–260.
6. MADRAS, P. N., W. A. MORTON & H. E. PETSCHEK. 1971. Dynamics of thrombus formation. Fed. Proc. **30:** 1665–1676.

7. NYILAS, E., W. A. MORTON, D. M. LEDERMAN, T. H. CHIU & R. D. CUMMING. 1975. Interdependence of hemodynamic and surface parameters in thrombosis. Trans. Am. Soc. Artif. Intern. Organs **21:** 55–69.
8. MORTON, W. A. & R. D. CUMMING. 1977. A technique for the elucidation of Virchow's triad. Ann. N.Y. Acad. Sci. **283:** 477–493.
9. GRABOWSKI, E. F., K. K. HERTHER & P. DIDISHEIM. 1974. Platelet aggregation quantified in an *ex vivo* chamber by means of videodensitometry. Thromb. Diath. Haemorrh. **60** (Suppl.): 127–134.
10. ZINGG, W., A. W. NEUMANN, A. B. STRONG, O. S. HUM & D. R. ABSOLOM. 1982. Effect of surface roughness on platelet adhesion under static and under flow conditions. Can. J. Surg. **25:** 16–19.
11. LYMAN, D. J., J. L. BRASH, S. W. CHAIKIN, K. G. KLEIN & M. CARINI. 1968. The effect of chemical structure and surface properties of synthetic polymers on the coagulation of blood. II. Protein and platelet interaction with polymer surfaces. Trans. Am. Soc. Artif. Intern. Organs **14:** 250–255.
12. LYMAN, D. J., K. G. KLEIN, J. L. BRASH & B. K. FRITZINGER. 1970. The interaction of platelets with polymer surfaces. I. Uncharged hydrophobic polymer surfaces. Thromb. Diath. Haemorrh. **23:** 120–128.
13. KIM, S. W., R. G. LEE, H. OSTER, D. COLEMAN, J. D. ANDRADE, D. J. LENTZ & D. OLSEN. 1974. Platelet adhesion to polymer surfaces. Trans. Am. Soc. Artif. Intern. Organs **20:** 449–455.
14. FRIEDMAN, L. I. & E. F. LEONARD. 1971. Platelet adhesion to artificial surfaces: Consequences of flow, exposure time, blood condition, and surface nature. Fed. Proc. **30:** 1641–1646.
15. LEONARD, E. F., E. F. GRABOWSKI & V. T. TURITTO. 1972. The role of convection and diffusion on platelet adhesion and aggregation. Ann. N.Y. Acad. Sci. **201:** 329–342.
16. GRABOWSKI, E. F., L. I. FRIEDMAN & E. F. LEONARD. 1972. Effects of shear rate on the diffusion and adhesion of blood platelets to a foreign surface. Ind. Eng. Chem. Fundam. **11:** 224–232.
17. DUTTON, R. C., R. E. BAIER, R. L. DEDRICK & R. L. BOWMAN. 1968. Initial thrombus formation on foreign surfaces. Trans. Am. Soc. Artif. Intern. Organs **14:** 57–62.
18. ROWNTREE, L. G. & T. SHIONOYA. 1927. Studies in experimental extracorporeal thrombosis. I. A method for the direct observation of extracorporeal thrombus formation. II. Thrombosis formation in normal blood in the extracorporeal vascular loop. III. Effects of certain anticoagulants (heparin and hirudin) on extracorporeal thrombosis and on the mechanism of thrombus formation. J. Exp. Med. **46:** 7–26.
19. BARBER, T. A., T. R. MATHIS, J. V. IHLENFELD, S. L. COOPER & D. F. MOSHER. 1978. Short-term interactions of blood with polymeric vascular graft materials: Protein adsorption, thrombus formation and leukocyte deposition. Scanning Electron Microsc. **2:** 431–440.
20. IHLENFELD, J. V., T. R. MATHIS, T. A. BARBER, D. F. MOSHER, L. M. RIDDLE, A. P. HART, S. J. UPDIKE & S. L. COOPER. 1978. Transient *in vivo* thrombus deposition onto polymeric biomaterials: Role of plasma fibronectin. Trans. Am. Soc. Artif. Intern. Organs **24:** 727–734.
21. IHLENFELD, J. V., T. R. MATHIS, L. M. RIDDLE & S. L. COOPER. 1979. Measurement of transient thrombus deposition on polymeric materials. Thromb. Res. **14:** 953–967.
22. YOUNG, B. R., L. K. LAMBECHT, S. L. COOPER & D. F. MOSHER. 1982. Plasma proteins: Their role in initiating platelet and fibrin deposition on biomaterials. Adv. Chem. Ser. **199:** 317–350.
23. LAMBRECHT, L. K., B. R. YOUNG, R. E. STAFFORD, R. M. ALBRECHT, D. F. MOSHER & S. L. COOPER. 1986. The influence of preabsorbed canine von Willebrand factor, fibronectin and fibrinogen on *in-vivo* surface-induced thrombosis. Thromb. Res. **41:** 99–117.
24. YOUNG, B. R., L. K. LAMBRECHT, R. M. ALBRECHT, D. F. MOSHER & S. L. COOPER. 1983. Platelet-protein interactions at blood-polymer interfaces in the canine test model. Trans. Am. Soc. Artif. Intern. Organs **29:** 442–447.
25. LELAH, M. D., L. K. LAMBRECHT, B. R. YOUNG & S. L. COOPER. 1983. Physicochemical

characterization and *in vivo* blood tolerability of cast and extruded Biomer. J. Biomed. Mater. Res. **17:** 1–22.
26. LELAH, M. D., R. J. STAFFORD, L. K. LAMBRECHT, B. R. YOUNG & S. L. COOPER. 1981. Cast vs. extruded Biomer for biomedical applications. Trans. Am. Soc. Artif. Intern. Organs **27:** 504–510.
27. BAQUEY, C., B. BASSE-CATHALINAT, B. MASSON, R. TORRIELLI, P. HOURDILLE, D. DUCASSOU & P. BLANQUET. 1980. An attempt to evaluate *in vivo,* by radioactive tracer techniques, the haemocompatibility of materials for vascular prosthesis. Adv. Biomater. **1:** 497–503.
28. BASSE-CATHALINAT, B., C. BAQUEY, Y. LLABADOR & A. FLEURY. 1980. Direct *in vivo* study of flowing blood-artificial surface interactions: An original application of dynamic isotopic techniques. Int. J. Appl. Radiat. Isot. **31:** 747–751.
29. VALE, B. H. & R. T. GREER. 1982. *Ex vivo* shunt testing of hydrogen-silicone rubber composite materials. J. Biomed. Mater. Res. **16:** 471–499.
30. LELAH, M. D., L. K. LAMBRECHT & S. L. COOPER. 1984. A canine *ex-vivo* series shunt for evaluating thrombus deposition on polymer surfaces. J. Biomed. Mater. Res. **18:** 475–496.
31. LELAH, M. D., C. A. JORDAN, M. E. PARISO, L. K. LAMBRECHT, S. L. COOPER & R. M. ALBRECHT. 1983. Morphological changes occurring during thrombogenesis and embolization on biomaterials in a canine *ex-vivo* series shunt. Scanning Electron Microsc. **4:** 1983–1994.
32. LELAH, M. D., C. A. JORDAN, M. E. PARISO, L. K. LAMBRECHT, R. M. ALBRECHT & S. L. COOPER. 1984. Blood compatibility of polyethylene and oxidized polyethylene in a canine A-V series shunt: Relationship to surface properties. *In* Polymers as Biomaterials. S. W. Shalaby, A. S. Hoffman, B. D. Ratner & T. A. Horbett, Eds.: 257–277. Plenum. New York.
33. LAMBRECHT, L. K., M. D. LELAH, C. A. JORDAN, M. E. PARISO, R. M. ALBRECHT & S. L. COOPER. 1983. Evaluation of thrombus deposition onto polymeric biomaterials in a new subhuman primate *ex vivo* series shunt model. Trans. Am. Soc. Artif. Intern. Organs **29:** 194–199.
34. HARKER, L. A., S. R. HANSON & A. S. HOFFMAN. 1977. Platelet kinetic evaluation of prosthetic material *in vivo*. Ann. N.Y. Acad. Sci. **283:** 317–331.
35. HANSON, S. R., L. A. HARKER, B. D. RATNER & A. S. HOFFMAN. 1979. Factors influencing platelet consumption by polyacrylamide hydrogels. Ann. Biomed. Eng. **7:** 357–367.
36. HOFFMAN, A. S., S. R. HANSON, L. A. HARKER, T. A. HORBETT, B. D. RATNER & L. O. REYNOLDS. 1982. Thrombotic events on grafted polyacrylamide-Silastic surfaces as studied in a baboon. Adv. Chem. Ser. **199:** 59–80.
37. GALLETTI, P. M., L. A. TRUDELL, D. PANOL, P. D. RICHARDSON & A. WHITTEMORE. 1976. Feasibility of small bore AV shunts for hybrid artificial organs in nonheparinized beagle dogs. Trans. Am. Soc. Artif. Intern. Organs **22:** 538–544.
38. IP, W. F., W. ZINGG & M. V. SEFTON. 1985. Parallel flow arteriovenous shunt for the *ex vivo* evaluation of heparinized materials. J. Biomed. Mater. Res. **19:** 161–178.
39. CHOLAKIS, C. H., G. R. LLANOS & M. V. SEFTON. 1986. The platelet compatibility of a heparin-polyvinyl alcohol hydrogel. Trans. Soc. Biomater. **12:** 44.
40. TOOMASIAN, J. M., G. A. HELMER, M. I. ZEME, J. N. OLTEAN, A. D. ORAN & R. H. BARTLETT. 1983. Control of thrombosis in extracorporeal circulation: Variations of anticoagulation. Trans. Am. Soc. Artif. Intern. Organs **29:** 194.
41. OLIJSLAGER, J. 1982. The Development of Test Devices for the Study of Blood-Material Interactions. Ph.D. thesis, Delft University, The Netherlands.
42. MUSTARD, J. F., E. A. MURPHY, H. C. ROWSELL & H. G. DOWNIE. 1962. Factors influencing thrombus formation *in vivo*. Am. J. Med. **33:** 621–647.
43. MURPHY, E. A., H. C. ROWSELL, H. G. DOWNIE, G. A. ROBINSON & J. F. MUSTARD. 1962. Encrustation and arteriosclerosis: The analogy between early *in vivo* lesions and deposits which occur in extracorporeal circulations. Can. Med. Assoc. J. **87:** 259–274.
44. SCHULTZ, J. S., A. CIARKOWSKI, J. D. GODDARD, S. M. LINDENAUER & J. A. PENNER. 1976. Kinetics of thrombus formation. Trans. Am. Soc. Artif. Intern. Organs **22:** 269–277.

45. SCHULTZ, J. S., J. D. GODDARD, A. CIARKOWSKI, J. A. PENNER & S. M. LINDENAUER. 1977. An *ex-vivo* method for the evaluation of biomaterials in contact with blood. Ann N.Y. Acad. Sci. **283:** 494–523.
46. SCHULTZ, J. S., S. M. LINDENAUER & J. A. PENNER. 1982. Thrombus formation on surfaces in contact with blood. Adv. Chem Ser. **199:** 43–58.
47. REICHERT, W. M., F. E. FILISKO & S. A. BARENBERG. 1982. Hemocompatibility: Effect of molecular motions of the polymer interface. Adv. Chem. Ser. **199:** 177–194.
48. BAUMGARTNER, H. R. & C. HAUDENSCHILD. 1972. Adhesion of platelets to subendothelium. Ann. N.Y. Acad. Sci. **201:** 22–36.
49. FRIEDMAN, L. I., H. LIEM, E. F. GRABOWSKI, E. F. LEONARD & C. W. MCCORD. 1970. Inconsequentiality of surface properties for initial platelet adhesion. Trans. Am. Soc. Artif. Intern. Organs **16:** 63–76.
50. WILSON, R. S., M. G. GOODE, M. D. LELAH & S. L. COOPER. 1982. An *ex vivo* narrow-slit flow device for evaluation of blood-material interactions. Trans. Am. Soc. Artif. Intern. Organs **28:** 420–425.
51. BENIS, A. M., H. L. NOSSEL, L. M. ALEDORT, R. M. KOFFSLY, J. F. STEVENSON, E. F. LEONARD, H. SHIANG & R. S. LITWAK. 1975. Extracorporeal model for study of factors affecting thrombus formation. Thromb. Diath. Haemorrh. **34:** 127–144.
52. MACFARLANE, R. G. 1972. The theory of blood coagulation. *In* Human Blood Coagulation, Hemostasis and Thrombosis, Vol. 1. R. Biggs, Ed. Blackwell Scientific. Oxford.
53. DAY, H. J. 1978. Platelet and endothelial cell participation in hemostasis and thrombosis. *In* Mechanisms of Hemostasis and Thrombosis, C. H. Mielke & R. Rodvien, Eds.: 1–18. Symposia Specialists. Miami.
54. HERMANS, J. & J. MCDONAGH. 1982. Fibrin: Structure and interactions. Semin. Thromb. Haemostas. **8(1):** 11–24.
55. ROSENBERG, R. 1977. Biologic actions of heparin. Semin. Hematol. **14:** 427–440.
56. DIDISHEIM, P., J. Q. STROPP, J. H. BOROWICK & E. F. GRABOWSKI. 1979. Species differences in platelet adhesion to biomaterials: Investigation by a new two-stage technique. asaio J. **2:** 124–132.
57. MOOLTEN, S. E., L. VROMAN, G. M. S. VROMAN & E. GOODMAN. 1949. Role of blood platelets in thromboembolism. Arch. Intern. Med. **84:** 667–710.
58. BOWIE, W. J., C. A. OWEN, J. H. THOMPSON & P. DIDISHEIM. 1969. A test of platelet adhesiveness. Mayo Clin. Proc. **44:** 306–308.
59. TURITTO, V. T. & H. R. BAUMGARTNER. 1974. Effect of temperature on platelet interaction with subendothelium exposed to flowing blood. Haemostasis **3:** 224–236.
60. ABSOLOM, D. R., Z. POLICOVA, A. W. NEUMANN & W. ZINGG. 1983. The effect of temperature on the extent of platelet adhesion to foreign surfaces. Trans. Amer. Soc. Artif. Organs **29:** 425–429.
61. LITWAK, R. S., G. SILVAY, H. SHIANG & E. F. LEONARD. 1977. Evaluation of artificial interfaces with *in vivo* systems. Ann. N.Y. Acad. Sci. **283:** 542–549.
62. SINAKOS, Z. & J. P. CAEN. 1967. Platelet aggregation in mammalians (human, rat, rabbit, guinea-pig, horse, dog): A comparative study. Thromb. Diath. Haemorrh. **17:** 99–111.
63. WURZINGER, L. J. & H. SCHMID-SCHONBEIN. 1981. Species differences in platelet aggregation and the influence of citrate and heparin in anticoagulation thereon. asaio J. **4:** 149–156.
64. MASON, R. G. *et al.* 1981. Guidelines for Blood-Material Interactions. NIH Publication No. 80-2185. Washington, D.C.
65. TURITTO, V. T., H. J. WEISS & H. R. BAUMGARTNER. 1979. Rheological factors influencing platelet interaction with vessel surfaces. J. Rheol. **23:** 735–749.
66. JOIST, J. H., J. P. CAZENAVE & J. F. MUSTARD. 1973. The effect of barbituric acid derivatives on platelet function *in vitro* and *in vivo*. Thromb. Diath. Haemorrh. **30:** 315–326.
67. IHLENFELD, J. V. & S. L. COOPER. 1979. Transient *in vivo* protein adsorption onto polymeric biomaterials. J. Biomed. Mater. Res. **13:** 577–591.
68. IHLENFELD, J. V. 1978. PhD. Dissertation, University of Wisconsin, Madison, WI.
69. DEWANJEE, M. K. 1984. Cardiac and vascular imaging with labeled platelets and leukocytes. Semin. Nucl. Med. **14:** 154–187.
70. VROMAN, L., A. L. ADAMS, G. C. FISCHER & P. C. MUNOZ. 1980. Interaction of high

molecular weight kininogen, factor XII and fibrinogen in plasma at interfaces. Blood **55:** 156–159.

71. YOUNG, B. R., M. J. DOYLE, W. E. COLLINS, L. K. LAMBRECHT, C. A. JORDAN, R. M. ALBRECHT & S. L. COOPER. 1982. Effect of thrombospondin and other platelet alpha-granule proteins on artificial surface-induced thrombosis. Trans. Am. Soc. Artif. Intern. Organs **28:** 498–503.
72. PARK, K., D. F. MOSHER & S. L. COOPER. 1986. Acute surface-induced thrombosis in the canine *ex vivo* model: Importance of the initial monolayer and platelet activation. J. Biomed. Mater. Res. **7:** 589–612.
73. GRASEL, T. G., R. S. WILSON, M. D. LELAH, H. W. BIELICH & S. L. COOPER. 1986. Blood flow and surface-induced thrombosis. Trans. Am. Soc. Artif. Intern. Organs. **32:** 515–520.
74. LELAH, M. D., T. G. GRASEL, J. A. PIERCE & S. L. COOPER. 1986. *Ex vivo* interactions and surface property relationships of polyurethanes. J. Biomed. Mater. Res. **20:** 433–468.
75. GRASEL, T. G. & S. L. COOPER. 1986. Surface properties and blood compatibility of polyurethaneureas. Biomaterials. **7:** 315–328.
76. LELAH, M. D., J. A. PIERCE, L. K. LAMBRECHT & S. L. COOPER. 1985. Polyether-polyurethane ionomers: Surface property/*ex vivo* blood compatibility relationships. J. Colloid Interface Sci. **104:** 422–439.

Evolution of Thrombosis

J. HIRSH, M. R. BUCHANAN, F. A. OFOSU,
AND J. WEITZ

Departments of Medicine and Pathology
McMaster University
Hamilton, Ontario L8N 3Z5, Canada

Both the composition of thrombi and their evolution differ in the arterial and venous circulation and are strongly influenced by hemodynamic factors.[1,2] Arterial thrombi form under conditions of high flow and are mainly composed of platelet aggregates consolidated by fibrin strands.[3–5] Venous thrombi form in areas of reduced flow and are composed of red cells with a large amount of interspersed fibrin and relatively fewer platelets. When thrombi form in regions of slow-to-moderate flow, for example, in cardiac chambers, they are composed of a mixture of red cells, platelets, and fibrin and are known as mixed platelet-fibrin thrombi.[4,5] Thrombi undergo constant structural change as they age.[6] Leukocytes are attracted by chemotactic factors released from fibrin and from aggregated platelets[2] and become incorporated into the thrombi. The aggregated platelets swell and undergo autolysis, and are gradually replaced by fibrin. Eventually, the fibrin is digested by plasma fibrinolytic enzymes[7] and by proteolytic enzymes released from leukocytes.[8]

VENOUS THROMBOSIS

Venous thrombi usually form in regions of slow or disturbed flow and begin as small deposits that frequently arise in large venous sinuses in the calf, in valve cusp pockets either in the deep veins of the calf or thigh,[9,10] or in venous segments that have been exposed to direct trauma.[11] The formation, growth, and dissolution of venous thrombi and pulmonary emboli reflect a balance between the effects of thrombogenic stimuli and a series of protective mechanisms.[12–14]

Venous thrombosis can be produced experimentally by a combination of stasis and an increase in blood coagulability, or by a combination of stasis and endothelial damage.[13,15] Clinically, the major predisposing factors to venous thrombosis are activation of blood coagulation and venous stasis.[12–14] Vascular wall damage is less important in the pathogenesis of venous thrombosis than arterial thrombosis but may predispose to venous thrombosis in special circumstances, *e.g.*, following hip surgery.[11,12,14,16] Venous thrombosis may occur when blood coagulation is activated by intravascular stimuli which are released at a remote site[17–19] (*e.g.*, the release of tissue thromboplastin from injured or infarcted tissue) or when blood coagulation is activated locally by vessel wall damage[11,14] (*e.g.*, damage to the femoral vein during hip surgery). Venous stasis predisposes to thrombosis by impairing the clearance of activated coagulation factors that rapidly increase in concentration through the autocatalytic activity of thrombin on the coagulation system.[13,20]

Most thrombi arise in the venous sinuses, which communicate directly with the deep veins of the calf. These thrombi are usually asymptomatic and most undergo spontaneous lysis. The same is true of most thrombi that extend into the deep venous system of the calf. Although thrombi confined to the calf may embolize to the lungs, the emboli are usually small and asymptomatic. Approximately 20% of calf vein thrombi extend into the proximal venous segment.[9] Proximal vein thrombi may also develop in the absence of calf vein thrombosis or may be noncontinuous with calf vein thrombi, particularly following hip surgery, during pregnancy and in women taking estrogen-containing birth control pills. Proximal vein thrombi produce clinical symptoms locally and embolize more frequently than calf vein thrombi.[9]

ARTERIAL THROMBOSIS

Arterial thrombi usually form in regions of disturbed flow where there is narrowing or irregularity caused by atheromata or stenosed arterial grafts.[21] The events leading to arterial thrombosis are controversial. There is evidence that rupture of atherosclerotic plaques with subsequent exposure of blood substances in the depths of the plaques is an important initiating event.[22] Arterial spasm may also be a contributing factor. When the thrombi only partially obstruct a vessel and blood flow is rapid, they tend to remain as mural thrombi or to embolize. In contrast, if the stimulus to thrombosis is strong or if flow is markedly compromised by severe stenosis or by vessel spasm, the thrombi may become totally occlusive. Mural thrombi may act as a nidus for further clot deposition and may eventually be incorporated into the vessel wall to form part of an atherosclerotic plaque.[21,23,24] Distal embolization of mural thrombi may cause a variety of clinical complications (depending on the site at which these emboli lodge) including cerebral and retinal ischemia, cardiac arrhythmias with sudden death, or limb or intestinal ischemia.

Factors that predispose to thrombosis are:

1. Damage to the vessel wall.
2. Stimulation of platelet adhesion and aggregation.
3. Activation of blood coagulation.
4. Stasis.

Protective mechanisms are:

1. Maintenance of the nonthrombogenic properties of endothelium.
2. Neutralization of activated coagulation factors by naturally occurring protease inhibitors.
3. Clearance of activated coagulation factors by the liver.
4. The fibrinolytic system.

THROMBOGENIC FACTORS

Damage to the Vessel Wall

The normal intact endothelium is nonthrombogenic and does not react with platelets or blood components.[25] The factors which contribute to the nonreactivity[2,21] are described in detail below under PROTECTIVE MECHANISMS.

Damage to a blood vessel results in denudation of the endothelial cell lining with subsequent exposure of the subendothelial structures to platelets and blood coagulation factors.[21,26–30] Vessel damage may result from direct injury or be mediated by immune complexes, viruses, hemodynamic stress, tobacco products, high blood cholesterol, or enzymes released from the platelets and leukocytes which accumulate at inflammatory sites.[2,21,27,31–35] Vascular damage and turbulent blood flow, two important factors predisposing to arterial thrombosis, are mutually reinforcing since each contributes to the genesis of the other.[21,27,33–37]

When the endothelial lining of an artery is removed experimentally by mechanical trauma, a monolayer of platelet covers the exposed subendothelium. However, large platelet aggregates and mural thrombi do not form as long as that blood flow remains essentially nonturbulent,[28,30,33,38] because in linear flow formed blood elements are concentrated in the central axial stream, which is separated from the luminal surface of the vessel by a zone of cell-free plasma. In addition, the luminal surface of the vessel wall is exposed to high shear forces which rapidly wash away adherent cells[3,39] with altered blood flow. However, in regions of disturbed flow, platelets interact with exposed subendothelium, adhere, aggregate, and form small platelet thrombi that are then stabilized by fibrin. These mural thrombi can produce major complications if they occlude an artery or if they embolize and lodge in the distal microcirculation, resulting in foscal tissue damage[2,21,26–31]

Stimulation of Platelet Adhesion and Aggregation

When platelets are exposed to a variety of stimuli they participate in reactions that are fundamental to thrombogenesis.[2,21] They adhere to a variety of surfaces, *the platelet adhesion reaction.* They undergo shape change and release their granular contents, *the platelet release reaction.* They aggregate to form clumps, *platelet aggregation,* and they also undergo surface changes that facilitate blood coagulation, *platelet coagulant activity.*

Platelet Adhesion

Platelets do not interact with intact endothelium but adhere to basement membrane and collagen, which is exposed when there is a break in the endothelial lining of blood vessels.[40–42] At physiological shear rates,[43] platelet adhesion to subendothelial collagen requires von Willebrand factor, which promotes adhesion by binding to a glycoprotein receptor (glycoprotein Ib) on the platelet surface.[39,44–46] Absence of this receptor leads to defective platelet adhesion (which occurs, for example, in a rare platelet disorder known as Bernard-Soulier syndrome).[47] If von Willebrand factor is defective or deficient in the plasma, which occurs in von Willebrand's disease,[39,44,47] platelet adhesion is also impaired.

Platelet adhesion to collagen is dependent on the primary structure of collagen and the extent of its polymerization. Recently, the adhesion of platelets to types I and III collagen has been shown to require a specific amino acid sequence.[48–50]

Platelet Release Reaction

A number of aggregating agents (including collagen, thrombin, epinephrine, and thromboxane A_2) cause platelets to release their granular contents.[51–58] With relatively weak stimuli, only the contents of the dense granules are released while stronger stimuli also cause release of alpha granule contents.[51,59,60] The dense granules contain serotonin and adenosine disphosphate while the alpha granules contain the platelet-specific proteins (platelet factor 4, β-thromboglobulin), platelet-derived growth factor, and other proteins including fibrinogen, factor V, and von Willebrand factor.[60] These release-inducing agents also activate the prostaglandin synthetic pathway of platelets[51,52,53,60] and induce platelet aggregation by various mechanisms, some of which depend on the platelet release mechanism, and others of which are independent of it.[61,62]

Platelet Aggregation

At lease four mediators of platelet aggregation have been identified. These are ADP, thromboxane A_2, thrombin, and the fatty acid known as platelet-activating factor (PAF)[54,56,58,62,63] Platelet aggregation is preceded by a change in platelet shape from discoid to spiny spheres. This shape change is mediated by the contractile microtubular system.

Platelet aggregation requires a platelet membrane glycoprotein receptor (glycoprotein IIb-IIIa) which is lacking in the rare congenital disorder known as Glanzman's thrombosthenia.[64] This glycoprotein is thought to be the receptor for fibrinogen, and fibrinogen interaction with platelets is of fundamental importance in platelet interaction.[65–67] Platelet-platelet bridging may also involve the platelet alpha granule proteins fibronectin and thrombospondin.[68,69]

Platelet activation by a variety of stimuli (including thrombin, collagen, and epinephrine)[58,60,70,71] results in the formation of thromboxane A_2, the major product of platelet prostaglandin synthesis. These stimuli activate a platelet membrane enzyme, phospholipase, which in turn releases arachidonic acid from platelet membrane phospholipid.[72] Arachidonic acid is oxidized by the enzyme cyclooxygenase to form the unstable cyclic endoperoxide PPG_2, which is then converted to PGH_2. PGH_2 is then transformed by the enzyme thromboxane synthetase to thromboxane A_2, which acts as potent vasoconstrictor and activator of platelet aggregation. Thromboxane A_2 is then converted into a stable breakdown product, thromboxane B_2. Although the endoperoxides (PGG_2 and PGH_2) also stimulate platelet aggregation, they are much less potent than thromboxane A_2.

Collagen induces platelet aggregation by stimulating both the synthesis of thromboxane A_2 and by releasing ADP through a prostaglandin-independent mechanism.[62] Thrombin induces platelet aggregation by stimulating the release of adenosine diphosphate, by activating the platelet prostaglandin pathway with resultant thromboxane A_2 formation, and by a third mechanism still poorly understood.[58,62,74] Platelet-activating factor is released from leukocytes and macrophages. It is chemotactic for leukocytes and also induces platelet aggregation. Its role in thrombogenesis is uncertain.[63]

All agonists that induce platelet aggregation probably act through a common pathway involving the mobilization of calcium from the cytoplasmic dense tubular system.[75–77] The mechanism responsible for calcium mobilization is uncertain, but calcium reuptake into the dense tubular system is cyclic AMP dependent. For example, prostacyclin stimulates adenylate cyclase, thereby increasing cyclic AMP levels.[73,78,79] An increase in cyclic AMP reduces calcium mobilization, and therefore inhibits platelet aggregation.

Agents that raise platelet cyclic AMP levels also inhibit the platelet release reaction.[73,77,78,79]

Platelet Coagulant Activity

Thrombin generation in plasma is greatly accelerated in the presence of platelets.[80,81] Stimulated platelets have an enhanced capacity to facilitate the interactions between coagulation factors. This platelet coagulant capacity is probably a manifestation of a rearrangement of the platelet surface lipoprotein which accompanies platelet shape change. The interaction between activated factor IX and activated factor VIII, which results in factor X activation, and the interaction of activated factor X with activated factor V, which results in prothrombin activation, occurs on the platelet surface. The rates of these surface-dependent activation reactions are greatly enhanced by platelets.[80,81] The vitamin-K-dependent clotting factors (prothrombin, factors VII, IX, and X) bind to the platelet membrane phospholipid through their calcium binding amino-terminal, glutamic acid residues. Specific receptors for von Willebrand factor (and thus presumably factor VIII) and for factor Xa have also been identified on the platelet surface.[82–84] The receptor for von Willebrand factor is glycoprotein IIb-IIIa,[85] while the specific receptor for factor Xa on activated platelets is factor Va.[82,83] Binding of factor Xa, thrombin, and activated factor VIII to platelets appears to protect the clotting factors from inhibition.[86,87] Platelets that have been exposed to ADP and collagen have been shown to activate factors XII and XI.[88,89]

Activation of Blood Coagulation

The process of blood coagulation involves a series of complex reactions, which results in the formation of a fibrin clot.[90–93] Blood coagulation can be initiated either by activation of the intrinsic pathway or activation of the extrinsic pathway.

The coagulation factors, with the exception of factors V and VIII, circulate in the form of inactive precursors or zymogens.[91] The activated forms of factors VIII and V are not enzymes but rather are cofactors for activated factors IX and X, respectively. When a coagulation zymogen is converted into the activated coagulation factor (enzyme), the enzyme activates the next zymogen in the coagulation sequence. With each step in the coagulation sequence, the system is amplified to produce increasing numbers of activated coagulation molecules and culminates in the generation of thrombin, the enzyme that converts fibrinogen to fibrin.[91] Thrombin is also a potent stimulator of platelet aggregation and activates factor XIII, which then serves to cross-link covalently and stabilize the fibrin clot.[94,95] Finally, feedback activation of factors V and VIII by thrombin results in further prothrombin activation and thrombin generation.

Intrinsic Pathway

The intrinsic pathway is initiated when blood comes in contact with a nonendothelialized vascular surface, which serves to convert the proenzyme factor XII to the enzyme factor XIIa.[96] Activated Factor XII in turn converts the zymogen factor XI to the enzyme XIa. Two other plasma proteins, prekallikrein and high molecular weight kininogen, are also involved in the contact activation reactions but the physiologic roles of these factors are uncertain. Although these contact reactions are calcium independent, all subsequent blood coagulation reactions require calcium and occur on a coagulant (phospholipid) surface.[97] Activated platelets provide an efficient surface for thrombin generation, as do endothelial cells[98] and probably monocytes.[99] Factor XIa activates factor IX, and factor IXa catalyzes the conversion of factor X to Xa in the presence of activated factor VIII, calcium, and negatively charged phospholipids. The rate of this reaction is greatly increased by the presence of an appropriate phospholipid surface and by the prior exposure of factor VIII to either of its activators (thrombin or factor Xa).[97,100]

Extrinsic Pathway

Factor X can also be activated by the extrinsic pathway.[101] This is achieved by exposing blood to tissue thromboplastin, a phospholipoprotein, in the presence of factor VIIa and calcium.

Common Pathway

The common pathway involves factor-Xa-mediated conversion of prothrombin to thrombin. This reaction is markedly enhanced by calcium phospholipid and factor Va. Platelets provide a phospholipid surface for prothrombin activation by binding factors Va and Xa in the presence of calcium. Factor Va serves as the factor Xa receptor on the platelet surface. In addition to platelets, endothelial cells and monocytes fulfil the requirements for surface assembly of the prothrombinase complex. Thrombin converts soluble fibrinogen to fibrin monomer in the plasma. The fibrin monomers spontaneously polymerize into an insoluble fibrin network. Initially the fibrin monomers are linked by electrostatic and hydrogen bonds, but are eventually stabilized by covalent cross-linking through a transamidation reaction catalyzed by activated factor XIII.[94] Factor XIII is activated by thrombin in a calcium-dependent reaction.

Blood coagulation is modulated by a number of positive and negative feedback loops and by interactions between constituents of the intrinsic and extrinsic pathway. Thus, thrombin and factor Xa provide positive feedback by activating factors VIII and V. Initially, factor Xa also provides positive feedback by activating factor VII. However, factor Xa then further suppresses factor X activation by inactivating factor VIIa.[101,103] Factor VII is also activated by factors XIIa and IXa.[104] Factor VIIa can also activate factor IX, thereby linking the extrinsic and intrinsic pathways.[102,103,105]

A variety of mechanisms exist for the initiation of the intrinsic and extrinsic pathways *in vivo*.[2] Factor XII is activated when blood comes in contact with nonendothelialized surfaces such as a damaged vessel wall or a prosthetic device. Factor VII is activated when endothelial cell damage exposes tissue thromboplastin[106] or when tissue thromboplastin is released into the blood stream as a result of extensive tissue damage.[107] Platelets exposed to ADP or collagen activate factors XII and XI directly,[89] while extracts of some malignant tissues can directly activate factor X.[108–110]

Venous Stasis

Stasis predisposes to venous thrombosis by preventing activated coagulation factors from being diluted by unactivated blood, by preventing clearance of activated coagulation factors, and by preventing mixing of activated coagulation factors with their inhibitors.[111,112]

Venous return from the legs is enhanced by contraction of calf muscles, which propels blood from the calf in the direction of the heart.[113–115] Venous stasis is produced by immobility, by venous obstruction, raised venous pressure, by venous dilatation, and by increased blood viscosity. Immobility is a common cause of venous stasis in the leg veins and an important risk factor for venous thrombosis. Immobility predisposes to venous thrombosis because it promotes blood pooling in the intramuscular sinuses of the calf,[113,115,116] which are dilated with blood, during recumbancy.[117,118] The prevalence of venous thrombosis found at autopsy rises steeply in patients who were confined to bed for more than a week before death.[113] Preoperative immobility is also associated with a higher frequency of preoperative venous thrombosis.[119,120] Postoperative patients remain at risk during the entire period of immobility, and late postoperative thrombosis is not prevented in patients who have prophylaxis in the first postoperative week (either with low dose heparin or with intermittent pneumatic compression) if they remain immobile beyond the period of prophylaxis.[121,122] Immobility contributes to the higher incidence of postoperative venous thrombosis reported in patients who undergo hysterectomy or prostectomy via the abdominal route as compared to those who have vaginal hysterectomy or transurethral prostatectomy.[123–127] The high frequency of thrombosis after hip or knee surgery[128–134] or in patients with hip fractures is also a result, at least in part, of immobility. The effect of immobility on thrombosis is well illustrated by comparing the location of thrombosis in stroke patients[135,136] with its location in paraplegic patients.[137] Venous thrombosis is a common complication in both groups, but the frequency of thrombosis is four to nine times greater in the paralyzed than in the nonaffected limb in patients with stroke, whereas it occurs with equal frequency in both legs in paraplegic patients.[135,137] Immobility also contributes to the high prevalence of thrombus in patients with cardiac failure and other serious medical illnesses.

PROTECTIVE MECHANISMS

Thrombogenesis is normally modulated by a number of efficient protective mechanisms. These include the normal intact endothelium, the inhibitors of activated coagulation factors, hepatic clearance of activated coagulation factors, and the fibrinolytic system.[2]

Nonthrombogenic Properties of Endothelial Cells

The fluidity of blood *in vivo* is enhanced by thromboresistant properties of normal vascular endothelium.[25] Endothelial cells synthesize prostaglandin I_2 or prostacyclin (a powerful inhibitor of platelet aggregation),[138–142] synthesize a lipoxygenase product 13-HODE, which inhibits platelet adhesion,[143] and synthesize glycosaminoglycans, which inhibit blood coagulation by enhancing the activities of antithrombin III and heparin cofactor II.[144–150]

Two classes of endothelial cofactors have been identified that contribute to thromboresistance of endothelial cells by inhibiting the action of thrombin.[151,152] One of these cofactors, designated thrombomodulin, is a thrombin receptor on the surface of the endothelium,[151] and the second class consists of the glycosaminoglycans heparan sulfate (which activates antithrombin III) and dermatan sulfate (which activates heparin cofactor II).[146,153,154]

The substrate specificity for thrombin changes markedly when it complexes with thrombomodulin. On binding with thrombomodulin, thrombin loses its ability to clot fibrinogen and to aggregate platelets. However, the complexed thrombin is still enzymatically active since it acquires an enhanced ability to activate protein C in the presence of calcium. Activated protein C is a powerful anticoagulant by virtue of its ability to inactivate proteolytically factors Va and VIIIa. Activated protein C has also been reported to stimulate the release of tissue plasminogen activator.[155] The inactivation of factors Va and VIIIa is greatly accelerated by calcium and phospholipids. Further, another vitamin-K-dependent protein, protein S, serves as a cofactor in this process. Thus, the binding of thrombin to thrombomodulin results in loss of its coagulant effects and an enhancement of its ability to activate protein C, and therefore, to inhibit thrombogenesis. Thrombin also binds to other receptors (such as heparan sulfate) on the endothelial surface where it is inactivated by antithrombin III.[156,157] Thrombin binding to endothelial cell provides a potent induction of endothelial cell prostaglandin synthesis and results in the generation of PGI_2, an inhibitor of platelet aggregation. The synthesis of PGI_2 is also induced by a variety of other stimuli, including epinephrine and trauma.[158]

Circulating Inhibitors

Four plasma proteins have been identified as important modulators of activation of blood coagulation. These are antithrombin III, heparin cofactor II, protein C and protein S.

Antithrombin III

Antithrombin III is an important coagulation inhibitor.[159,160] It inhibits thrombin and activated factors X, IX, XI, and XII (although inhibition of factors IXa, XIa, and XIIa in blood appears to be relatively minor).[161–163] The rates of reaction of antithrombin III with these enzymes are markedly increased by heparin.[160–164]

Thrombin binds to heparan sulfate and other glycosaminoglycans on the endothelial cell surface, where it is inactivated by antithrombin III.[145,165] Thrombin bound to thrombomodulin may also be susceptible to inhibition by antithrombin III.[166] Although thrombin bound to endothelium is rapidly inactivated in the presence of plasma, free thrombin is slowly inactivated by purified antithrombin III alone or by antithrombin-III-depleted plasma.[166] Thus, potentiation of the inhibition of endothelial cell-bound thrombin by glycosaminoglycans appears to be dependent not only on the presence of antithrombin III, but also on additional plasma factor.

Recent studies by Bauer and associates have provided new insights into the importance of the antithrombin-III–heparin system in modulating coagulation and thrombosis *in vivo*. These investigators measured the concentration of the activation peptide of prothrombin, prothrombin fragments (F_{1+2}), in patients with antithrombin III deficiency and in patients with α_1-proteinase inhibitor deficiency.[167] The basal concentrations of prothrombin fragments were higher in subjects with antithrombin III deficiency than in normal subjects, but were normal in subjects with α_1-proteinase inhibitor deficiency. These observations provide evidence that endogenous heparin-antithrombin–III is fundamental to inhibition of factor Xa in the circulation of humans. There is evidence[145,165,168] that heparin-like proteoglycans associated with vascular endothelium accelerate the formation of antithrombin-III–enzyme complexes.

There have been a number of reports of idiopathic and secondary venous thrombosis occurring in families with antithrombin III deficiency.[169–174] The trait is inherited in an autosomal-dominant manner and the affected patients have antithrombin III levels of 40% to 60% of normal. Although it is difficult to obtain exact figures on the risk of thrombosis in affected individuals because of the likelihood of reporting bias, review of the literature indicates that over 50% of affected individuals develop thromboembolic events before the age of 50 years. Thrombosis usually manifests as deep vein thrombosis in the lower extremities or as pulmonary embolism, but there are reports of thrombosis occurring in unusual sites, such as the mesenteric veins.

Decreased antithrombin III levels also occur in liver disease, during heparin therapy, and with disseminated intravascular coagulation. In patients with liver disease it may contribute to the increased risk of thrombosis that has been reported in these patients following infusions of concentrates containing factor II, VII, IX, and X.[175] There is no evidence that the mild reduction of antithrombin III that occurs during heparin therapy is clinically important.

Protein C

Protein C is a vitamin-K-dependent serine protease zymogen.[175] Like other vitamin-K-dependent coagulation factors, protein C contains glutamic acid residues.[177] The amino acid sequence of both bovine[178] and human protein C have recently been determined.[178]

Although protein C is slowly activated by thrombin,[179] the activation process is greatly enhanced by an endothelial cell surface factor known as thrombomodulin.[180] Activated protein C is a potent anticoagulant;[181] it exerts its anticoagulant properties by proteolytically inactivating activated factors V and VIII. The degradation of these factors is greatly accelerated by phospholipids and calcium. Activation of protein C also stimulates fibrinolysis[182,183] through the release of tissue plasminogen activation from endothelial cells. Walker and associates reported that another vitamin-K-dependent protein, protein S, functions as a cofactor for activated protein C in its degradation of factors V and VIII.[184]

Deficiency of protein C is associated with familial venous thrombosis.[185–187] Like antithrombin III deficiency, protein C deficiency is also inherited in an autosomal-dominant manner. The level of protein C in affected members is 40–60% of normal, similar to that seen in patients with antithrombin III deficiency. Most patients present with venous thromboembolism. Mesenteric vein thrombosis has also been described and there have been isolated reports of stroke or myocardial infarction occurring at a relatively early age. However, there is no convincing evidence that protein C predisposed to arterial thrombosis. Homozygous protein C deficiency presents in the neonatal period as purpura fulminans or recurrent thrombosis.

Protein S

Protein S is a vitamin-K-dependent plasma protein that acts as a cofactor for activated protein C and is required for the maximal expression of the anticoagulant effect of protein C.[188–190] Despite its relatively recent discovery, protein S deficiency has already been reported in over 50 patients with recurrent venous thrombosis.[188,191–194] Venous thromboembolism resulting from protein C deficiency is often idiopathic and may be familial. Venous thromboembolism in these cases frequently occurs before the age of 30 years. The clinical disorder affects both sexes equally and is expressed in heterozygotes whose levels of functional protein S are in the range of 15% to 50% of normal.[188,191] Preliminary reports suggest that patients with either protein S or protein C deficiency can be treated effectively with long-term oral anticoagulant therapy.

Heparin Cofactor II

Heparin cofactor II is a plasma protein that inactivates thrombin by forming a covalent complex with the enzyme. The reaction between thrombin and heparin cofactor II is an order of magnitude slower than that between thrombin and antithrombin III.[195] The formation of the thrombin and heparin cofactor II complex is catalyzed by heparin and dermatan sulfate. There have been two reports of thrombosis associated with heparin II cofactor deficiency, but a definite causal relationship has not been established.[196] In most conditions where thrombin–antithrombin-III complexes can be demonstrated in plasma (such as in disseminated intravascular coagulation) complexes of thrombin and heparin cofactor II are also present.

Hepatic Inactivation of Activated Coagulation Factors

The liver removes activated coagulation factors from the blood.[2] Thrombosis has been reported in patients with liver disease following the infusion of factor IX concentrates which also contain prothrombin, factors VII, IX and X, and protein C and protein S. These concentrates contain small amounts of activated coagulation factors that may not be adequately cleared by the reticuloendothelial system in patients with liver disease, thus leading to thrombosis.[197–199] The circulating levels of antithrombin III may also be lower in patients with liver disease due to impaired hepatic synthesis.

Fibrinolytic System

There are two components of the fibrinolytic system: a plasma component and a cellular component.

Plasma Fibrinolytic System

The basic reaction of the plasma fibrinolytic system is the conversion of a β-globulin, plasminogen, to the active proteolytic enzyme plasmin. This is effected through limited proteolytic cleavage mediated by a variety of plasminogen activators.[200] These plasminogen activators are synthesized by and released from endothelial cells and other tissues. Recently it has been demonstrated that endothelial cells produce two distinct classes of activators (tissue-type and urokinase-like) as well as a fast-acting plasminogen activator inhibitor.[201,202] Once plasminogen is activated to plasmin it has the capacity to hydrolyze fibrin (the desired physiological substrate) and various plasma coagulation proteins, including fibrinogen.[2,7] Like the coagulation system, the activity of the fibrinolytic system is modulated by inhibitors that serve to regulate both the activation of plasminogen and the proteolytic effect of plasmin.[203]

Physiological fibrinolysis occurs predominantly in the solid phase. During fibrin formation, plasminogen binds to fibrin and is incorporated into the consolidating thrombus.[7] Tissue plasminogen activator (TPA), which is derived from intact adjacent endothelium, also specifically binds to fibrin.[204,205] The activation of plasminogen by TPA occurs more efficiently when both enzyme and substrate are bound to fibrin.[206]

The main plasma inhibitor of plasmin is α_2-antiplasmin. Other but less important plasmin inhibitors include α_2-macroglobulin, antithrombin III, and α_1-proteinase inhibitor.[207] Factor XIIIa incorporates α_2-antiplasmin into the cross-linked fibrin. This modulates the rate of fibrinolysis. Inherited deficiency of α_2-antiplasmin results in a hemorrhagic tendency caused by the unopposed lysis of fibrin in hemostatic plugs.[208]

When plasmin is formed in plasma (in the absence of fibrin) by the interaction of plasminogen activators with plasminogen, it is rapidly inactivated by α_2-antiplasmin. Excess plasmin is inactivated by α_2-macroglobulin. If both of these inhibitors are overwhelmed (for example, during the course of thrombolytic therapy with TPA, urokinase, or streptokinase) then hydrolysis of plasma fibrinogen and other coagulation factors occurs.[7]

Cellular Fibrinolysis

There is considerable evidence that some fibrinolytic activity is derived from proteolytic enzymes released from neutrophils.[209] These inflammatory cells are attracted to the hemostatic plug by chemotactic products of platelets and fibrin. Proteolytic enzymes capable of degrading fibrin(ogen) are released when the neutrophils are stimulated or when they undergo autolysis.

REFERENCES

1. FREIMAN, D. G. 1982. The structure of thrombi. *In* Thrombosis and Hemostasis: Basic Principles and Clinical Practice. R. W. Coleman, J. Hirsh, V. Marder & E. W. Salzman, Eds. J. B. Lippincott. Philadelphia, PA.
2. HIRSH, J. & E. GENTON. 1974. Thrombogenesis. *In* Physiological Pharmacology. Academic. New York. p. 99.
3. BAUMGARTNER, H. R. 1973. The role of blood flow in platelet adhesion, fibrin deposition and formation of mural thrombi. Microvasc. Res. **5:** 167.
4. CHANDLER, A. B. 1969. The anatomy of a thrombus. *In* Thrombosis. S. Sherry, K. M. Brinkhous, E. Genton & J. M. Stengle, Eds.: 279. National Academy of Sciences. Washington, D.C.
5. JORGENSEN, L. 1964. Experimental platelet and coagulation thrombi: A histological study of arterial and venous thrombi of varying age in untreated and heparinized rabbits. Acta Pathol. Microbiol. Scand. A **62:** 189.
6. JORGENSEN, L., H. C. ROWSELL, T. HOVIG, J. F. MUSTARD. 1967. Resolution and organization of platelet-rich mural thrombi in carotid arteries of swine. Am. J. Pathol. **51:** 681.
7. COLLEN, D. 1980. On the regulation and control of fibrinolysis. Thromb. Haemostas. **43:** 77.
8. PLOW, E. F. & T. S. EDINGTON. 1975. An alternative pathway of fibrinolysis. I. The cleavage of fibrinogen by leukocyte proteases at physiologic pH. J. Clin. Invest. **56:** 30.
9. KAKKAR, V. V., C. FLANC, C. T. HOWE & M. B. CLARKE. 1969. Natural history of postoperative deep vein thrombosis. Lancet **2:** 230.
10. NICOLAIDES, A. N., V. V. KAKKAR, E. S. FIELD & J. T. RENNEY. 1971. The origin of deep vein thrombosis: A venographic study. Br. J. Radiol. **44:** 653.
11. STAMATAKIS, J. D., V. V. KAKKAR, S. SAGAR, *et al.* 1977. Femoral vein thrombosis and total hip replacement. Br. Med. J. **2:** 213.
12. HIRSH, J., E. GENTON & R. HULL. 1981. Venous thrombosis. *In* Venous Thromboembolism. J. Hirsh, E. Genton & R. Hull, Eds.: 42. Grune & Stratton. New York.
13. WESSLER, S. & E. T. YIN. 1969. On the mechanism of thrombosis. *In* Progress in Hematology. E. B. Brown & C. V. Moore, Eds. Grune & Stratton. New York.
14. DAVIES, G. S. & E. W. SALZMAN. 1979. The pathogenesis of deep vein thrombosis. *In* Venous and Arterial Thrombosis. H. J. Joist & L. A. Sherman, Eds.: 1. Grune & Stratton. New York.
15. HENRY, R. L. 1962. Methods for inducing experimental thrombosis. Angiology **13:** 544.
16. HIRSH, J., E. GENTON & R. HULL. 1981. Pathogenesis of venous thromboembolism. *In* Venous Thromboembolism. J. Hirsh, E. Genton & R. Hull, Eds.: 5. Grune & Stratton. New York.
17. BORGSTROM, S., L. E. GELIN & B. ZENDERFELD. 1959. The formation of vein thrombi following tissue injury. Acta Chir. Scand. Suppl. **247:** 1.
18. MOSCHOS, C. B., M. I. KHAN & T. J. REGAN. 1971. Thrombogenic properties of blood during early ischemic and non-ischemic injury. Am. J. Physiol. **220:** 1882.

19. Bjorklid, E., K. E. Giercksy & H. Prydz. 1978. An immunoradiometric assay for factor III (tissue thromboplastin). Br. J. Haematol. **39:** 445.
20. Davie, E. W., K. Fujikawa, K. Kurachi & W. Kisiel. 1979. The role of serine protease in the blood coagulation cascade. Adv. Enzymol. **48:** 277.
21. Mustard, J. F., R. L. Kinlough-Rathbone & M. A. Packham. 1982. The vessel wall in thrombosis. *In* R. W. Coleman, J. Hirsh, V. Marder & E. W. Salzman, Eds. Thrombosis and Hemostasis: Basic Principles and Clinical Practice. J. B. Lippincott. Philadelphia, PA.
22. Davies, M. J. & A. Thomas. 1984. Thrombosis and acute coronary-artery lesions in sudden cardiac ischemic death. N. Engl. J. Med. **310:** 1137.
23. Moore, S. 1973. Thromboatherosclerosis in normolipemic rabbits: A result of continued endothelial damage. Lab. Invest. **29:** 478.
24. E. A. Murphy, H. C. Roswell, H. G. Downie, G. A. Robinson & J. F. Mustard. 1962. Encrustation and atherosclerosis: The analogy between early *in vivo* lesions and deposits which occur in extracorporeal circulations. Can. Med. Assoc. J. **87:** 259.
25. Vasiliev, J. M. & I. M. Gelfand. 1978. Mechanism of non-adhesiveness of endothelial and epithelial surfaces. Nature **274:** 710.
26. Mason, R. G., S. F. Mohammad, H. Y. Chuang, *et al.* 1976. The adhesion of platelets to subendothelium, collagen and artifical surfaces. Semin. Thromb. Hemostas. **3:** 98.
27. Stemerman, M. B. 1982. Relationship of Thrombosis to Atheroslerosis. *In* Thrombosis and Hemostasis: Basic Principles and Clinical Practice. R. W. Coleman, J. Hirsh, V. Marder & E. W. Salzman, Eds. J. B. Lippincott. Philadelphia, PA.
28. Tschopp, Th. B., H. R. Baumgartner, K. Silberbauer, *et al.* 1979. Platelet adhesion and platelet thrombus formation on subendothelium of human arteries and veins exposed to flowing blood *in vitro:* A comparison with rabbit aorta. Haemostasis **8:** 19.
29. Tschopp, Th. B. 1977. Aspirin inhibits platelet aggregation on, but not adhesion to, collagen fibrils: An assessment of platelet adhesion and deposited platelet mass by morphometry and ^{51}Cr-labelling. Thromb. Res. **11:** 619.
30. Turitto, V. T. & H. R. Baumgartner. 1979. Platelet interaction with subendothelium in flowing rabbit blood: Effect of blood shear rate. Microvasc. Res. **17:** 38.
31. Harker, L. A. & S. M. Schwartz & R. Ross. 1981. Endothelium and atherosclerosis. Clin. Haematol. **10:** 283.
32. Majno, G. & L. Joris. 1978. Endothelium 1977: A review. Adv. Exp. Med. Biol. **104:** 169.
33. Ross, R. & J. A. Gomset. 1981. Atherosclerosis: A problem of the biology of arterial wall cells and their interactions with blood components. Arteriosclerosis **1:** 293.
34. Ross, R. & J. A. Gomset. 1976. The pathogenesis of atherosclerosis. N. Engl. J. Med. **295:** 369, 420.
35. Ross, R. & L. Harker. 1976. Hyperlipidemia and atherosclerosis. Science **193:** 1094.
36. Goldsmith, H. L. & T. Karino. 1977. Platelets in a region of disturbed flow. Trans. Am. Soc. Artif. Intern. Organs **23:** 632.
37. Karino, T. & H. L. Goldsmith. 1979. Adhesion of human platelets to collagen on the walls distal to a tubular expansion. Microvasc. Res. **17:** 238.
38. Turitto, V. T. & H. R. Baumgartner. 1982. Platelet surface interactions. *In* Thrombosis and Hemostasis: Basic Principles and Clinical Practice. J. B. Lippincott. Philadelphia, PA.
39. Weiss, H. J., V. T. Turitto & H. R. Baumgartner. 1978. Effect of shear rate on platelet interaction with subendothelium in citrated and native blood. I. Shear rate-dependent decrease of adhesion in von Willebrand's disease and the Bernard-Soulier syndrome. J. Lab. Clin. Med. **92:** 750.
40. Baumgartner, H. R., M. B. Stemerman & T. H. Spaet. 1971. Adhesion of blood platelets to the subendothelial surface: Distinct from adhesion to collagen. Experientia **27(3):** 282.
41. Cazenave, J.-P., D. Blondowska, M. Richardson, *et al.* 1979. Quantitative radioisotopic measurement and scanning electron microscopic study of platelet adherence to a collagen-coated surface and to subendothelium with rotating probe device. J. Lab. Clin. Med. **93:** 60.

42. MUSTARD, J. F. 1978. Platelet adherence to the vessel wall and to collagen-coated surfaces. Adv. Exp. Med. Biol. **102:** 31.
43. TURITTO, V. T., R. MUGGLI & H. R. BAUMGARTNER. 1977. Physical factors influencing platelet deposition on subendothelium: Importance of blood shear rate. Ann. N.Y. Acad. Sci. **283:** 284.
44. CAEN, J. P., H. MICHEL, G. TOBELEM, *et al.* 1976. Adhesion and aggregation of human platelets to rabbit subendothelium. A new approach for investigation: Specific antibodies. Experientia **33(1):** 91.
45. NURDEN, A. T. & J. P. CAEN. 1975. Specific roles for platelet surface glycoproteins in platelet function. Nature **255:** 720.
46. SAKARIASSEN, K. S., P. A. BOLHUIS & J. J. SIXMA. 1979. Human blood platelet adhesion to artery subendothelium is mediated by factor VIII-vWF bound to the subendothelium. Nature **279:** 636.
47. GEORGE, J. N. & T. A. REIMANN. 1981. Inherited disorders of the platelet membrane: Glanzmann's thrombasthenia and Bernard-Soulier disease. *In* Platelet Function and Disorders. p. 496. Churchill-Livingstone. Edinburgh.
48. BALLEISEN, L., S. GAY, R. MARX, *et al.* 1975. Comparative investigations on the influence of human bovine collagens type I, II, III on the aggregation of human platelets. Klin. Wochenschr. **53:** 903.
49. BARNES, M. J., A. J. BAILEY, J. L. GORDON, *et al.* 1980. Platelet aggregation by basement membrane-associated collagens. Thromb. Res. **18:** 375.
50. WANG, C. L., T. MIYATA, B. WEKSLER, *et al.* 1978. Collagen induced platelet aggregation and release. II Critical size and structural requirements of collagen. Biochim. Biophys. Acta **544:** 568.
51. HOLMSEN, H. 1982. Platelet secretion. *In* Thrombosis and Hemostasis: Basic Principles and Clinical Practice. R. W. Coleman, J. Hirsh, V. Marder & E. W. Salzman, Eds. J. B. Lippincott. Philadelphia, PA.
52. HOLMSEN, H. & H. J. DAY. 1970. The selectivity of the thrombin-induced platelet release reaction. Subcellular localization of released and retained substances. J. Lab. Clin. Med. **75:** 840.
53. KAPLAN, K. L., M. J. BROEKMAN, A. CHERNOFF, *et al.* 1979. Platelet alpha-granule proteins: Studies on release and subcellular localization. Blood **53:** 604.
54. KINLOUGH-RATHBONE, R. L., J. J. REIMERS & J. F. MUSTARD. 1976. Sodium arachidonate can induce platelet shape change and aggregation which are independent of the release reaction. Science **192:** 1011.
55. MUSTARD, J. F. & M. A. PACKHAM. 1970. Factors influencing platelet function: Adhesion, release and aggregation. Pharm. Rev. **22(2):** 97.
56. PACKHAM, M. A. 1976. Stages in the interaction of platelets with collagen. Thromb. Haemostas. **36:** 269.
57. PACKHAM, M. A., M. A. GUCCIONE, P. L. CHANG & J. F. MUSTARD. 1973. Platelet aggregation and release: Effects of low concentrations of thrombin or collagen. Am. J. Physiol. **225:** 38.
58. PACKHAM, M. A., R. L. KINLOUGH-RATHBONE, H.-J. REIMERS, *et al.* 1977. Mechanisms of platelet aggregation independent of adenosine diphosphate. *In* Prostaglandins in Hematology. M. J. Silver, J. B. Smith & J. J. Kocsis, Eds.: 247. Spectrum. New York.
59. HOLMSEN, H. 1978. Platelet secretion (release reaction): Mechanism and pharmacology. Adv. Pharmacol. Ther. **4:** 97.
60. HOLMSEN, H. 1977. Prostaglandin endoperoxide-thromboxane synthesis and dense granule secretion as positive feedback loops in the propagation of platelet responses during "the basic platelet reaction." Thromb. Haemostas. (Stutt.) **38(4):** 1030.
61. KINLOUGH-RATHBONE, R. L., M. A. PACKHAM & J. F. MUSTARD. 1977. Synergism between platelet-aggregating agents: The role of the arachidonate pathway. Thromb. Res. **11:** 567.
62. MUSTARD, J. F., D. W. PERRY, R. L. KINLOUGH-RATHBONE, *et al.* 1975. Factors responsible for ADP-induced release reaction of human platelets. Am. J. Physiol. **228(6):** 1757.
63. BENVENISTE, J., M. CHIGNARD, J. P. LE COUEDIC, *et al.* 1982. Biosynthesis of platelet-activating factor (PAF-ACETHER):II Involvement of phospholipase A_2 in the forma-

tion of PAF-ACETHER and lyso-PAF-ACETHER from rabbit platelets. Thromb. Res. **25:** 375.
64. Coller, B. S. 1980. Interaction of normal, thrombasthenic, and Bernard-Soulier platelets with immobilized fibrinogen: Defective platelet-fibrinogen interaction in thrombasthenia. Blood **55:** 169.
65. Bennett, J. S. & G. Vilaire. 1979. Exposure of platelet fibrinogen receptors by ADP and epinephrine. J. Clin. Invest. **64:** 1393.
66. Bennett, J. S., G. Vilaire & J. W. Burch. 1981. A role for prostaglandins and thromboxanes in the exposure of platelet fibrinogen receptors. J. Clin. Invest. **68:** 981.
67. Marguerie, G. A. & E. F. Plow. 1981. Interaction of fibrinogen with its platelet receptor: Kinetics and effect of pH and temperature. Biochemistry **20:** 1074.
68. Ginsberg, M. H., R. G. Painter, J. Forsyth, *et al.* 1980. Thrombin increases expression of fibronectin antigen on the platelet surface. Proc. Natl. Acad. Sci. U.S.A. **77:** 1049.
69. Jaffe, E. A., L. L. K. Leung, R. L. Nachman, *et al.* 1982. Thrombospondin in the endogenous lectin of human platelets. Nature **295:** 246.
70. Gorman, R. R. 1979. Modulation of human platelet function by prostacyclin and thromboxane A_2. Fed. Proc. **38(1):** 83.
71. Smith, J. B. 1980. The prostanoids in hemostasis and thrombosis: A review. Am. J. Pathol. **99:** 743.
72. Schoene, N. W. & J. M. Iacono. 1975. Stimulation of platelet phospholipase A_2 activity by aggregating agents (abstract). Fed. Proc. **34:** 257.
73. Needleman, P., M. O. Whitaker, A. Wyche, K. Watters, H. Sprecher & A. Ras. 1980. Manipulation of platelet aggregation by prostaglandins and their fatty acid precursors: Pharmacological basis for a therapeutic approach. Prostaglandins **19:** 165.
74. Packham, M. A. & J. F. Mustard. 1977. Clinical pharmacology of platelets. Blood **50:** 555.
75. Detwiler, T. C. 1978. Evidence that calcium regulates platelet function. Thromb. Haematol. **40:** 107.
76. LeBreton, G. C., R. J. Dinerstein, L. J. Roth & H. Feinberg. 1976. Direct evidence for intracellular divalent cation redistribution associated with platelet shape change. Biochem. Biophys. Res. Commun. **71:** 362.
77. Steel, M. L. & E. W. Salzman. 1982. *In* Thrombosis and Hemostasis: Basic Principles and Clinical Practice. R. W. Coleman, J. Hirsh, V. Marder & E. W. Salzman, Eds. J. B. Lippincott. Philadelphia, PA.
78. Gorman, R. R., S. Bunting & O. V. Miller. 1977. Modulation of human platelet adenylate cyclase by prostacyclin (PGX). Prostaglandins **13:** 337.
79. Salzman, E. W. 1972. Cyclic AMP and platelet function. N. Engl. J. Med. **286:** 358.
80. Majerus, P. W. & J. P. Miletich. 1978. Relationships between platelets and coagulation factors in haemostasis. Ann. Rev. Med. **29:** 41.
81. Walsh, P. N. 1982. Platelet-coagulant protein interactions. *In* Thrombosis and Hemostasis: Basic Principles and Clinical Practice. R. W. Coleman, J. Hirsh, V. Marder & E. W. Salzman, Eds. J. B. Lippincott. Philadelphia, PA.
82. Miletich, J., C. M. Jackson & P. W. Majerus. 1978. Properties of the factor X binding site on human platelets. J. Biol. Chem. **253:** 6908.
83. Miletich, J. P., W. H. Kane, S. L. Hofmann, *et al.* 1979. Deficiency of factor X-factor V binding sites on the platelets of a patient with a bleeding disorder. Blood **54(5):** 1015.
84. Suttie, J. W. 1977. Oral anticoagulant therapy: The biosynthetic basis. Semin. Hematol. **14:** 365.
85. Kao, K.-J., S. V. Pizzo, & P. A. McKee. 1979. Demonstration and characterization of specific binding sites for factor VIII/von Willebrand factor on human platelets. J. Clin. Invest. **63:** 656.
86. Ofosu, F. A., A. L. Cerskus, J. Hirsh, *et al.* 1984. The inhibition of the anticoagulant activity of heparin by platelets, brain phospholipids and tissue factor. Br. J. Haematol. **57:** 229.
87. Rick, M. E. & D. M. Krizek. 1986. Platelets modulate the proteolysis of factor VIII: C protein by plasmin. Blood **67:** 1649.
88. Walsh, P. N. 1974. Platelet coagulant activities and hemostasis: A hypothesis. Blood **43:** 597.

89. WALSH, P. N. & J. H. GRIFFIN. 1981. Contributions of human platelets to the proteolytic activation of blood coagulation factors XII and XI. Blood **57:** 106.
90. DAVIE, E. W. & K. FUJIKAWA. 1975. Basic mechanisms in blood coagulation. Ann. Rev. Biochem. **44:** 799.
91. DAVIE, E. W., K. FUJIKAWA, K. KURACHI & W. KISIEL. 1979. The role of serine protease in the blood coagulation cascade. Adv. Enzymol. **48:** 277.
92. FUJIDAWA, K., M. H. COAN, M. E. LEGAZ & E. W. DAVIE. 1974. The mechanism of activation of bovine factor X (Stuart factor) by intrinsic and extrinsic pathways. Biochemistry **13:** 5290.
93. ROSENBERG, R. D. 1977. Chemistry of the hemostatic mechanism and its relationship to the action of heparin. Fed. Proc. **36:** 10.
94. LORAND, L. & K. KONISHI. 1964. Activation of the fibrin-stabilizing factor of plasma by thrombin. Arch. Biochem. Biophys. **105:** 58.
95. MCKEE, P. A., M. L. SCHWARTZ, S. V. PIZZO & R. L. HILL. 1972. Cross-linking of fibrin by fibrin-stabilizing factor. Ann. N.Y. Acad. Sci. **202:** 127.
96. KAPLAN, A. P., H. L. MEIER & R. MANDLE, JR. 1976. The Hageman factor-dependent pathways of coagulation, fibrinolysis, and kinin generation. Semin. Thromb. Hemostas. **3:** 1.
97. HEMKER, C., M. J. LINDOUT & C. VERMEER. 1977. Blood coagulating factors at phospholipid surfaces. Ann. N.Y. Acad. Sci. **283:** 104.
98. STERN, D. M., P. P. NAWROTH, W. KISIEL, *et al.* 1984. A coagulation pathway or bovine aortic segment leading to generation of factor Xa and thrombin. J. Clin. Invest. **74:** 1910.
99. TRACY, P. B., M. S. ROHRBACH & K. G. MANN. 1983. Functional prothrombinase complex assembly on isolated monocytes and lymphocytes. J. Biol. Chem. **258:** 7264.
100. OSTERUD, B., S. I. RAPAPORT, S. SCHIFFMAN, *et al.* 1971. Formation of intrinsic factor-X-activator activity, with special reference to the role of thrombin. Br. J. Haematol. **21:** 643.
101. JESTY, J., A. K. SPENCER & Y. NEMERSON. 1974. The mechanism of action of factor X. Kinetic control of alternative pathways leading to the formation of activated factor X. J. Biol. Chem. **249:** 5614.
102. RAPAPORT, S. I., S. SCHIFFMAN, M. J. PATCH, *et al.* 1963. The importance of activation and antihemophilic globulin and proaccelerin by traces of thrombin in the generation of intrinsic prothrombinase activity. Blood **21:** 221.
103. JESTY, J. & S. A. SILVERBERG. 1979. Kinetics of tissue factor-dependent activation of coagulation factors IX and X in a bovine plasma system. J. Biol. Chem. **254:** 12337.
104. KISIEL, W., K. FUJIKAWA & E. W. DAVIE. 1977. Activation of bovine factor VII (proconvertin) by factor XIIa (activated Hageman factor). Biochemistry **16:** 4189.
105. OSTERUD, B. & S. I. RAPAPORT. 1977. Activation of factor IX by the reaction product of tissue factor and factor VII: Additional pathway for initiating blood coagulation. Proc. Natl. Acad. Sci. U.S.A. **74:** 5260.
106. ZELDES, S. M., Y. NEMERSON, F. PITLICK & T. LENTZ. 1972. Tissue factor (thromboplastin): Localization to plasma membrane by peroxidase-conjugated antibodies. Science **175:** 766.
107. BORGSTROM, S., L. E. GELIN & B. ZENDERFELDX. 1959. The formation of vein thrombi following tissue injury. Acta Chir. Scand. Suppl. **247:** 1.
108. GORDON, S. G., C. FRANKS & B. LEWIS. 1975. Cancer procoagulant A: A factor X activating procoagulant from malignant tissue. Thromb. Res. **6:** 127.
109. PINEO. G. F., E. REGOECZI & M. W. C. HATTON. 1973. The activation of coagulation by extract of mucus: A possible pathway of intravascular coagulation accompanying adenocarcinomas. J. Lab. Clin. Med. **82:** 225.
110. SLICHTER, S. J. & L. A. HARKER. 1974. Hemostasis in malignancy. Ann. N.Y. Acad. Sci. **230:** 252.
111. HIRSH, J. & E. GENTON. 1974. Thrombogenesis. *In* Physiological Pharmacology. W. S. Root & F. G. Hoffman, Eds. Academic. New York.
112. WESSLER, S. & E. T. YIN. 1969. On the mechanism of thrombosis. *In* Progress in Hematology. E. B. Brown & C. V. Moore, Eds.: 201. Grune & Stratton. New York.

113. GIBBS, N. M. 1957. Venous thrombosis of the lower limb with particular reference to bedrest. Br. J. Surg. **45:** 209.
114. MCLACHLIN, A. D., J. A. MCLACHLIN, T. A. JORY & E. G. RAWLING. 1960. Venous stasis in the lower extremities. Ann. Surg. **152:** 678.
115. ALMEN, T. & G. BYLANDER. 1962. Serial phlebography of the normal lower leg during muscular contraction and relaxation. Acta Radiol. **57:** 264.
116. KAKKAR, V. V., C. FLANC, C. T. HOWE & M. B. CLARKE. 1969. Natural history of postoperative deep vein thrombosis. Lancet **2:** 230.
117. NICOLAIDES, A. N., V. V. KAKKAR, E. S. FIELD & J. T. G. RENNEY. 1971. The origin of deep vein thrombosis: A venographic study. Br. J. Radiol. **44:** 653.
118. KAKKAR, V. V., C. T. HOWE, A. N. NICOLAIDES, *et al.* 1970. Deep vein thrombosis of the leg: Is there a "high-risk" group? Am. J. Surg. **120:** 527.
119. NICOLAIDES, A. N., Ed. 1975. Thromboembolism Aetiology: Advances in Prevention and Management. Medical and Technical Publishing Company. Lancaster, England. p. 193.
120. HEATLEY, R. V., L. E. HUGHES, A. MORGAN, *et al.* 1976. Preoperative or postoperative deep-vein thrombosis. Lancet **1:** 437.
121. TURPIE, A. G. G., A. GALLUS, W. S. BEATTIE, *et al.* 1977. Prevention of venous thrombosis in patients with intracranial disease by intermittent pneumatic compression of the calf. Neurology **27:** 435.
122. GALLUS, A. S., J. HIRSH, S. E. O'BRIEN, *et al.* 1976. Prevention of venous thrombosis with small subcutaneous doses of heparin. J. Am. Med. Assoc. **235:** 1980.
123. KAKKAR. V V., C. T. HOWE, A. N. NICOLAIDES, *et al.* 1970. Deep vein thrombosis of the leg. Is there a "high-risk" group? Am. J. Surg. **120:** 527.
124. NICOLAIDES, A. N., E. S. FIELD, V. V. KAKKAR, *et al.* 1972. Prostatectomy and deep vein thrombosis. Br. J. Surg. **59:** 487.
125. MAYO, M., T. HALIL & N. L. BROWSE. 1971. The incidence of deep vein thrombosis after prostatectomy. Br. J. Urol. **43:** 738.
126. NICOLAIDES, A. N., E. S. FIELD, V. V. KAKKAR, *et al.* 1972. Prostatectomy and deep vein thrombosis. Br. J. Surg. **59:** 487.
127. WALSH, J. J., J. BONNAR & F. W. WRIGHT. 1974. A study of pulmonary embolism and deep leg vein thrombosis after major gynaecologic surgery using labelled fibrinogen: Phlebography and lung scanning. J. Obstet. Gynaecol. Br. Commonwealth **81:** 311.
128. STAMATAKIS, J. D., V. V. KAKKAR, S. SAGAR, *et al.* 1977. Femoral vein thrombosis and total hip replacement. Br. Med. J. **2:** 213.
129. HAMILTON, H. W., J. S. CRAWFORD, J. H. GARDINER, *et al.* 1970. Venous thrombosis in patients with fracture of the upper end of the femur. J. Bone Joint Surg. **52B:** 268.
130. HARRIS, W. H., E. W. SALZMAN, C. A. ATHANSOULIS, *et al.* 1977. Aspirin prophylaxis of venous thromboembolism after total hip replacement. N. Engl. J. Med. **297(23):** 1246.
131. HUME, M., R. H. TURNER, T. X. KURIAKOSE & J. SURPRENANT. 1976. Venous thrombosis after total hip replacement. J. Bone Joint Surg. **58:** 933.
132. HAMPSON, W. G. J., F. C. HARRIS, H. K. LUCAS, *et al.* 1974. Failure of low-dose heparin to prevent deep vein thrombosis after hip replacement arthroplasty. Lancet **ii:** 795.
133. HULL, R., T. DELMORE, J. HIRSH, *et al.* 1979. Effectiveness of an intermittent pulsatile elastic stocking for the prevention of calf and thigh vein thrombosis in patients undergoing elective knee surgery. Thromb. Res. **16:** 37.
134. COHEN, S. H., G. E. EHRLICH, M. S. KAUFFMAN, *et al.* 1973. Thrombophlebitis after knee surgery. J. Bone Joint Surg. **55(1):** 106.
135. WARLOW, C., D. OGSTON & A. S. DOUGLAS. 1976. Deep venous thrombosis of the legs after strokes. Br. Med. J. **2:** 1178.
136. COPE, C., T. M. REYES & N. J. SKVERSKY. 1973. Phlebographic analysis of the incidence of thrombosis in hemiplegia. Diag. Radiol. **109:** 581.
137. BORS, E., C. A. CONRAD & T. B. MASSELL. 1954. Venous occlusion of lower extremities in paraplegic patients. Surg. Gynecol. Obstet. **99:** 451.
138. BURCH, J. W. & P. W. MAJERUS. 1979. The role of prostaglandins in platelet function. Semin. Hematol. **16:** 196.
139. MARCUS, A. J., B. B. WEKSLER & E. A. JAFFE. 1978. Enzymatic conversion of

prostaglandin endoperoxide H_2 and arachidonic acid to prostacyclin by cultured human endothelial cells. J. Biol. Chem. **253:** 7138.
140. Moncada, S. & J. R. Vane. 1979. The role of prostacyclin in vascular tissue. Fed. Proc. **38:** 66.
141. Weiss, H. J. & V. T. Turitto. 1979. Prostacyclin (prostaglandin I_2, PGI_2) inhibits platelet adhesion and thrombus formation on subendothelium. Blood **53:** 244.
142. Weksler, B. B., A. S. Marcus & E. A. Jaffe. 1977. Synthesis of prostaglandin I_2 (prostacyclin) by cultured human and bovine endothelial cells. Proc. Natl. Acad. Sci. U.S.A. **74:** 3922.
143. Buchanan, M. R., R. W. Butt, J. Hirsh, *et al.* 1986. Role of lipoxygenase metabolism in platelet function: Effect of aspirin and salicylate. Prostagl. Leukotr. Med. **21:**157.
144. Charonis, A. S., P. C. Tsilibary, R. H. Kramer, *et al.* 1983. Localization of heparin sulfate proteoglycan in the basement membrane of continuous capillaries. Microvasc. Res. **26(1):** 108.
145. Colburn, P. & V. Buonassisi. 1982. Anti-clotting activity of endothelial cell cultures and heparin sulfate proteoglycans. Biochem. Biophys. Res. Commun. **104(1)** :220.
146. Hatton, M. W. C., L. R. Berry & E. Regoeczi. 1978. Inhibition of thrombin by antithrombin III in the presence of certain glycosaminoglycans found in the mammalian aorta. Thromb. Res. **13:** 655.
147. Wang-Iverson, P. & M. V. Brown. 1982. Interaction of lipoprotein lipase with cultured endothelial cells. Ann. N.Y. Acad. Sci. **401:** 92.
148. Wight-Ross, R. 1975. Proteoglycans in primate arteries. II. Synthesis and secretion of glycosaminoglycans by arterial smooth muscle cells in culture. J. Cell Biol. **67:** 675.
149. Williams, M. P., H. B. Streeter, F. S. Wusteman, *et al.* 1983. Heparan sulphate and the binding of lipoprotein lipase to pocine thoracic aorta endothelium. Biochim. Biophys. Acta **756(1):** :83.
150. Winterbourne, D. J., A. M. Schor & J. T. Gallagher. 1983. Synthesis of glycosaminoglycans by cloned bovine endothelial cells cultured on collagen gels. Eur. J. Biochem. **135:** 271.
151. Esmon, C. T. & W. G. Owen. 1981. Identification of endothelial cell cofactors for thrombin catalyzed activation of protein C. Proc. Natl. Acad. Sci. U.S.A. **78:** 249.
152. Lollar, P. & W. G. Owen. 1980. Clearance of thrombin from circulation in rabbits by high affinity binding sites on endothelium: Possible role in the inactivation of thrombin by antithrombin III. J. Clin. Invest. **66:** 1222.
153. Busch, C. & W. G. Owen. 1982. Identification *in vitro* of an endothelial cell surface cofactor for antithrombin III. J. Clin. Invest. **69:** 726.
154. Teien, A. N., U. Abildgaard & M. Hook. 1976. The anticoagulant effect of heparan sulfate and dermatan sulfate. Thromb. Res. **8:** 859.
155. Esmon, N. L., W. G. Owen & C. T. Esmon. 1982. Isolation of a membrane-bound cofactor for thrombin-catalyzed activation of protein C. J. Biol. Chem. **257:** 859.
156. Lollar, P., S. C. McIntosh & W. G. Owen. 1984. Reaction of antithrombin III with thrombin bound to the vascular endothelium. J. Biol. Chem. **259:** 4535.
157. Hatton, M. W. C. & S. L. Moar. 1985. A role of pericullar proteoglycan in the binding of thrombin or antithrombin III by the blood vessel endothelium? Thromb. Hemostas. **53:** 238.
158. MacIntyre, D. E., J. D. Pearson & J. L. Gordon. 1978. Localization and stimulation of prostacyclin production in vascular cells. Nature **271:** 549.
159. Harpel, P. C., 1982. Blood proteolytic enzyme inhibitors: Their role in modulating blood coagulation and fibrinolytic enzyme pathways. *In* Thrombosis and Hemostasis: Basic Principles and Clinical Practice. R. W. Coleman, J. Hirsh, V. J. Marder & E. W. Salzman, Eds. J. B. Lippincott. Philadelphia, PA.
160. Rosenberg, R. D. 1982. Heparin-antithrombin system. *In* Thrombosis and Hemostasis: Basic Principles and Clinical Practice. R. W. Coleman, J. Hirsh, V. Marder & E. W. Salzman, Eds. J. B. Lippincott. Philadelphia, PA.
161. Pixley, R. A., M. Schapira & R. W. Colman. 1985. Effect of heparin on the inactivation rate of human activated factor XII by antithrombin III. Blood **66:** 198.
162. Scott, C. F., M. Schapira & R. W. Colman. 1982. Effect of heparin on the inactivation rate of human factor XIa by antithrombin-III. Blood **60:** 941.

163. McNEELY, T. B. & M. J. GRIFFITH. 1985. The anticoagulant mechanism of action of heparin in contact-activated plasma: Inhibition of factor X activation. Blood **65:** 1226.
164. ROSENBERG, R. D. 1976. Actions and interactions of antithrombin and heparin. N. Engl. J. Med. **292:** 146.
165. HATTON, M. W. C., L. R. BERRY & E. REGOECZI. 1978. Inhibition of thrombin by antithrombin III in the presence of certain glycosaminoglycans found in the mammalian aorta. Thromb. Res. **13:** 655.
166. LOLLAR, P. & W. G. OWEN. 1980. Clearance of thrombin from circulation in rabbits by high affinity binding sites on endothelium: possible role in the inactivation of thrombin by antithrombin III. J. Clin. Invest. **66:** 1222.
167. BAUER, K. A., T. L. GOODMAN, B. L. KASS, R. D. ROSENBERG. 1985. Elevated factor Xa activity in the blood of asymptomatic patients with congenital antithrombin deficiency. J. Clin. Invest. **76:** 826.
168. DRYJSKI, M., R. LARSSON, P. OLSSON, *et al.* 1983. Effect of glycosaminoglycans and antithrombin III on uptake and inhibition of thrombin by the vascular wall. Thromb. Res. **32(4):** 355.
169. EGEBERG, O. 1965. Inherited antithrombin deficiency causing thrombophilia. Thromb. Diath. Haemorrh. **13:** 516.
170. GRUENBERG, J. C., R. C. SMALLRIDGE & R. D. ROSENBERG. 1975. Inherited antithrombin III deficiency causing mesenteric venous infarction. Ann. Surg. **181:** 791.
171. MARCINIAK, E., C. H. FARLEY & P. A. DE SIMONE. 1974. Familial thrombosis due to antithrombin III deficiency. Blood **43:** 219.
172. VAN DER MEER, J., E. A. STOEPMAN-VAN DALEN & J. M. S. JANSEN. 1973. Antithrombin III deficiency in a Dutch family. J. Clin. Pathol. **26:** 532.
173. SAS, G., D. S. PEPPER & J. D. CASH. 1975. Plasma and serum antithrombin III: Differentiation by crossed immunoelectrophoresis. Thromb. Res. **6:** 87.
174. VON KAULLA, E. & K. N. VON KAULLA. 1972. Deficiency of antithrombin III activity associated with hereditary thrombosis tendency. J. Med. (Basel) **3:** 349.
175. KASPER, C. K. 1975. Thromboembolic complications. Thromb. Haemostas. **33:** 640.
176. STENFLO, J. 1976. A new vitamin-K dependent protein. Purification from bovine plasma and preliminary characterization. J. Biol. Chem. **251:** 355.
177. FERNLUND, P., J. STENFLO, P. ROEPSTORFF & J. THOMSEN. 1975. Vitamin K and the biosynthesis of prothrombin. V. Gamma-carboxyglutamic acids, the vitamin K-dependent structures in prothrombin. J. Biol. Chem. **250:** 6125.
178. FERNLUND, P. & J. STENFLO. 1979. Amino acid sequence of bovine protein C. *In* Vitamin K dependent proteins. J. W. Suttie, Ed.: 84. University Park Press. Baltimore, MD.
179. KISIEL, W., W. M. CANFIELD, L. G. ERICSSON & E. W. DAVIE. 1977. Anticoagulant properties of bovine plasma protein C following activation by thrombin. Biochemistry **16:** 5824.
180. ESMON, C. T. & W. G. OWEN. 1981. Identification of an endothelial cell cofactor for thrombin-catalyzed activation of protein C. Proc. Natl. Acad. Sci. U.S.A. **78:** 2245.
181. SEEGERS, W. H., R. A. MARLAR & D. WALZ. 1978. Anticoagulant effects of autothrombin-III-A and prothrombin fragment 1. Thromb. Res. **13:** 233.
182. MARLAR, R. A., A. J. KLEISS & J. G. GRIFFIN. 1981. Human protein C: inactivation of factor V and VIII in plasma by the activated molecule. Ann. N.Y. Acad. Sci. **370:** 303.
183. COMP, P. C. & C. T. ESMON. 1980. Evidence for multiple roles for activated protein C in fibrinolysis. *In* Regulation of Coagulation. K. G. Mann & F. B. Taylor, Eds.: 583. Elsevier. New York.
184. WALKER, F. J. 1981. Regulation of activated protein C by a new protein. A possible function for bovine protein. J. Biol. Chem. **256:** 11128.
185. GRIFFIN, J. H., B. EVATT, T. S. ZIMMERMAN, *et al.* 1982. Deficiency of protein C in congenital thrombotic disease. Thromb. Haemostas. **48:** 1.
186. BROEKMANS, A. W., J. J. VELTKAMP, I. K. VAN DER LINDEN & K. MERTENS. 1982. Protein C deficiency in a Dutch family with thrombotic disease. Thromb. Haemostas. **48:** 1.
187. BROEKMANS. A. W., J. J. VELTKAMP & R. M. BERTINA. 1983. Congenital protein C deficiency and venous thromboembolism. A study of three Dutch families. N. Engl. J. Med. **309:** 340.

188. Comp, P. C. & C. T. Esmon. 1984. Recurrent venous thromboembolism in patients with a partial deficiency of protein S. N. Engl. J. Med. **311:** 1525.
189. Walker, F. J. 1980. Regulation of activated protein C by a new protein. J. Biol. Chem. **255:** 5521.
190. Walker, F. J. 1981. Regulation of activated protein C by protein S: the role of phospholipid in factor Va inactivation. J. Biol. Chem. **256:** 11128.
191. Comp, P. C., R. R. Nixon, M. R. Cooper & C. T. Esmon. 1984. Familial protein S deficiency is associated with recurrent thrombosis. J. Clin. Invest. **74:** 2082.
192. Kamiya, T., T. Sugihara, K. Ogata, *et al.* 1986. Inherited deficiency of protein S in a Japanese family with recurrent venous thrombosis: A study of three generations. Blood **67:** 406.
193. Schwarz, H. P., M. Fischer, P. Hopmeier, *et al.* 1984. Plasma protein S deficiency in familial thrombotic disease. Blood **64:** 1297.
194. Comp, P. C., D. Doray, D. Patton & C. T. Esmon. 1986. An abnormal plasma distribution of protein S occurs in functional protein S deficiency. Blood **67:** 504.
195. Tollefsen, D. M. 1984. Activation of heparin cofactor II by dermatan sulfate. Nouv. Rev. Fr. Hematol. **26:** 233.
196. Sie, P., J. Pichon, D. Dupouy & B. Boneu. 1985. Constitutional heparin co-factor II deficiency associated with recurrent thrombosis. Lancet **I:** 414.
197. Kingdon, H. S., R. L. Lundblad, J. J. Veltkamp, *et al.* 1975. Potentially thrombogenic materials in factor IX concentrates. Thromb. Diath. Haemorrh. **33:** 617.
198. Pepper, D. S., D. Banhegyi, A. Howie, *et al.* 1977. *In vitro* thrombogenicity tests of factor IX concentrates. Br. J. Haematol. **36:** 573.
199. Blatt, P. M., R. L. Lundblad, H. S. Kingdon, *et al.* Thrombogenic materials in prothrombin complex concentrates. Ann. Intern. Med. **81:** 766. 1974.
200. Castellino, F. J. & B. N. Violand. 1979. The fibrinolytic system—basic considerations. Prog. Cardiovasc. Dis. **21:** 241.
201. Levin, E. G. & D. J. Loskutoff. 1982. Cultured bovine endothelial cells produce both urokinase and tissue-type plasminogen activators. J. Cell Biol. **94:** 631.
202. Van Mourik, J. A., D. A. Lawrence & D. J. Loskutoff. 1984. Purification of an inhibitor of plasminogen activator (antiactivator) synthesized by endothelial cells. J. Biol. Chem. **259:** 14914.
203. Wiman, B. & D. Collen. 1979. On the mechanism of the reaction between human alpha-2-antiplasmin and plasmin. J. Biol. Chem. **254:** 9291.
204. Matsuo, O., D. C. Rijken & D. Collen. 1981. Comparison of the relative fibrinogenolytic, fibrinolytic and thrombolytic properties of tissue plasminogen activator and urokinase *in vivo.* Thromb. Haemostas. **45:** 225.
205. Rijken, D. C. & D. Collen. 1981. Purification and characterization of the plasminogen activator secreted by human melanoma cells in culture. J. Biol. Chem. **256:** 7035.
206. Hoylaerts, M., D. C. Rijken, M. R. Lijnen & D. Collen. 1982. Kinetics of the activation of plasminogen by human tissue plasminogen activator. Role of fibrin. J. Biol. Chem. **257:** 2912.
207. Wiman, B. & D. Collen. 1978. On the kinetics of the reaction between human antiplasmin and plasmin. Eur. J. Biochem. **84:** 573.
208. Sakata, Y. & N. Aoki. 1980. Cross-linking an alpha-2-plasmin inhibitor to fibrin by fibrin-stabilizing factor. J. Clin. Invest. **65:** 290.
209. Moroz, L. A. 1977. Increased blood fibrinolytic activity after aspirin ingestion. N. Engl. J. Med. **296(10):** 525.

Interactions of Platelets and Vessel Wall in the Development of Restenosis after Coronary Angioplasty[a]

PHILIP C. ADAMS,[b] JULES Y.T. LAM,[c] LINA BADIMON,[b] JAMES H. CHESEBRO,[c] AND VALENTIN FUSTER[b]

[b]*Mount Sinai Medical School of the City University of New York New York, New York 10029*

[c]*Mayo Clinic Rochester, Minnesota 55905*

Coronary angioplasty has become a successful and popular treatment for coronary disease since its first clinical application in 1976.[1] Its use has been extended from the initial indication of refractory but stable angina, with single vessel disease, to cases of unstable angina,[2] multivessel disease,[3] and even acute myocardial infarction.[4] Despite this increase in the complexity of cases treated, primary success rates have improved and the rate of acute complications has decreased.[5] However, occlusion of the dilated artery (usually thrombotic) may occur acutely, while restenosis occurs more commonly and has been called the "Achilles heel" of angioplasty.

The reported incidence of restenosis varies with the definition used, but most studies suggest that it occurs in about one third of patients. The National Heart, Lung, and Blood Institute (NHLBI) registry reports restenosis in 33.6% of a selected population of 557 patients.[6] Review of several series[7] reveals that the rate is between 19% and 40% (TABLE 1). Most cases occur early, certainly in the first 6 months,[12] and there is increasing evidence that the vast majority occur within the first 3 months. Wijns *et al.*[13] showed that thallium scintigraphy 4 weeks after angioplasty can detect 74% of patients who have restenosis according to angiography at 6 months. Similarly, DePuey *et al.*[14] used exercise-gated radionuclide ventriculography to detect evidence of ischemia as early as 4 days after the percutaneous coronary angioplasty. Patients with ischemia had a higher restenosis rate than patients without such findings, and an abnormal radionuclide ventriculogram had an accuracy of 73% in predicting 50% or greater restenosis at the time of follow-up angiography.

The mechanism of restenosis is unclear. However, considerable evidence suggests that it occurs as part of the response to arterial wall injury, which seems to be a necessary component of the mechanism of angioplasty.[7,15] This article summarizes the experimental work of our group in the context of published clinical experience and the laboratory studies of other workers.

VESSEL WALL INJURY IN ANGIOPLASTY

Clinical and experimental observations show that injury is produced by angioplasty, and that this is the mechanism of its effects in reducing stenosis of the dilated

[a]Dr. Adams is supported by a British-American Research Fellowship of the British Heart Foundation and the American Heart Association.

TABLE 1. Immediate and Chronic Results of Percutaneous Transluminal Coronary Angioplasty in Representative Series

Author Ref.	Number of Patients (% with MVD)	Immediate Success	Acute Complications	Restenosis: Number with Follow-up Angio	Restenosis: Duration of Follow-up (months)	% Patients with Restenosis
Grüntzig[1] (1979)	50 (12%)	64%	10%	32	<3	19%
Vlietstra[3] (1983)	100 (100%)	72%	8%	55	>6	40%
Holmes[6] (1984)	—	—	—	665	6 (median)	34%
Cowley[8] (1985)	100 (100%)	79%	11%	44	26	34%
Mabin[9] (1985)	229 (38%)	67%	12%	100	13	32%
Leimgruber[10] (1985)	1880 (0%)	—	88%	986	7	29%
Vandormael[11] (1985)	113 (100%)	80%	7%	66	>6	20%

vessel.[15] The injury produced involves plaque fracture and distention of the media, with expansion of the external diameter of the artery. Thus, angiography immediately after angioplasty in man shows an increase in vessel diameter. However, other changes are also seen. Dissection, with a linear opacity reflecting contrast medium entering the false lumen of the vessel, is a relatively infrequent finding, reported in only 135 of 3079 cases in the National Heart and Blood Institute registry of percutaneous transluminal coronary angioplasty (PTCA).[16] Other angiographic features may point to intimal disruption. The raising of intimal flaps is a relatively common observation, seen in 22% of cases in the registry. Intraluminal haziness, a description applied to reduced contrast density at the site of the successful dilatation, has been described in 17% of angioplasty cases (17 out of 82 arteries successfully dilated).[16] This appearance is unusual outside the context of angioplasty. It has been taken to represent small fissures in the plaque. Typically, the haziness resolves within a few weeks of dilatation. In most patients, however, dilatation occurs without striking angiographic evidence of arterial wall disruption. This is more likely to reflect the insensitivity of angiography in the detection of damage than a lack of trauma.

Pathological studies in man are relatively few, testimony to the safety of the technique of angioplasty. However, they confirm that injury is usually seen following an angioplasty. For example, Block *et al.* describe two patients who died after a PTCA and a third who died after dilatation of a femoral artery.[17] In each case, splitting of the intima extending into the media was observed, as well as endothelial desquamation. It is generally accepted that such damage is usual during clinical angioplasty.

Animal studies support the concept that intimal and medial disruption is a prerequisite for a successful angioplasty. Fatty atherosclerotic lesions may be induced in rabbits by a high cholesterol diet, combined with balloon de-endothelialization, while a fibro-fatty lesion is produced which is more similar to human atherosclerotic plaque if such a diet is combined with the use of an in-dwelling catheter. Such lesions were produced in the iliac vessels in one study[18] and the response to angioplasty studied. In animals with fatty lesions, angioplasty resulted in neointimal fracture and dissection, while in animals with more fibrous lesions the major finding was of thinning and stretching of the nonatheromatous section of the vessel wall, with no definite evidence of neointimal fracture, despite a greater than 20% increase (from a mild baseline stenosis) in the diameter of the lumen in most of the animals studied. Evidence of cell damage with necrosis and loss of smooth muscle cells was a frequent finding.

More limited balloon inflation produces de-endothelialization alone. Such limited injury is unlikely in clinical angioplasty, but occurs as a component of the more severe disruption seen in this context.

HEMOSTATIC RESPONSE TO INJURY

Injury to the vessel wall is always produced by angioplasty; the response of the hemostatic system to this injury, in the context of the immediate hemodynamic result, is the major determinant of the response to angioplasty.

After experimental removal of the endothelial lining of a normal blood vessel, by a mild or superficial injury, the subendothelium is coated by a layer of adherent platelets. The rate at which this occurs is limited by the delivery of platelets to the site of injury by blood flow and lateral diffusion into the boundary layer, *i.e.,* the layer of plasma in the most intimate contact with the vessel wall. If blood flow is rapid and laminar, thrombi, *i.e.,* aggregates of platelets, do not form on the adherent platelets deposited, whereas if flow is disturbed, with vortices and eddies, platelet-platelet interaction occurs with aggregation and thus platelet thrombus formation.

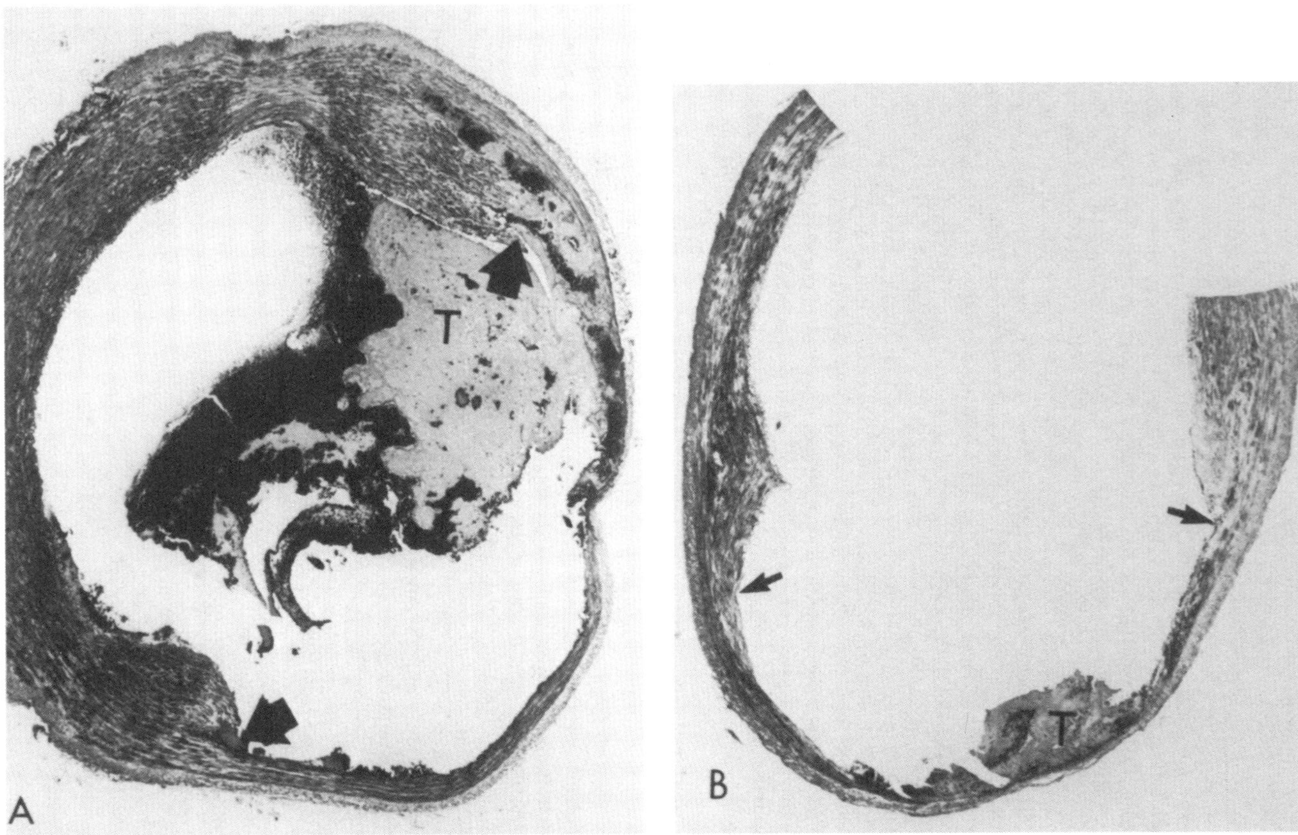

FIGURE 1. Section of carotid artery at the site of dilatation in the pig: normal vessel. A large thrombus (*T*) is seen in **A**, while in **B** a smaller thrombus (*T*), which would not have been visible at angiography, is seen in association with a tear into the media. In both frames the *arrows* indicate the site of medial tears. There is complete endothelial denudation at the site of the balloon dilatation. (From Lam *et al.*[27])

Adhesion, the process by which platelets attach to the exposed subendothelium, is dependent on platelet receptors, adhesive glycoproteins in the plasma, and exposure of activating sites in the subendothelium.[19] Glycoprotein Ib in the platelet membrane is necessary for normal initial contact of platelets with the subendothelial surface. Platelets from patients with Bernard-Soulier syndrome, which lack this glycoprotein, show impaired hemostasis clinically and impaired platelet adhesion in flow chambers.[20] Glycoprotein IIb-IIIa in the platelet membrane is the receptor for both fibrinogen and von Willebrand factor. This glycoprotein also plays an important role in the interaction of the platelet with the vessel wall.[21] This role can only be demonstrated at high shear rates, suggesting that other pathways of adhesion may be important at low shear rates. Von Willebrand factor is present, in man, in plasma, platelet alpha granules, and subendothelium, but the relative importance of the three locations is unknown. At these high shear rates, fibronectin is also important. Prior platelet activation with exposure of platelet membrane glycoproteins by a stereochemical change appears to enhance the interactions observed. A number of subendothelial components probably contribute to the reactivity of the subendothelium. Types I and III collagen are important platelet active components of the subendothelium,[22] while platelets are also detected adhering to the microfibrils around elastin. Von Willebrand factor, particularly the high molecular weight multimers, binds to collagen and to a noncollagenous material resembling elastin microfibrils, and this binding may be important in platelet adhesion. Thus platelet adhesion is dependent on platelet membrane glycoproteins, plasma constituents, and subendothelial constituents.

More severe injury exposes components of the arterial media, particularly fibrillar collagen (type III),[22] which is more thrombogenic than the collagens of the subendothelium. This exposure stimulates platelet aggregation and thrombus formation (FIGURE 1). Glycoprotein Ib is important in the initial attachment of the platelet, but exposure of glycoprotein IIb-IIIa by activation of the platelet in the presence of calcium allows fibrinogen and von Willebrand factor to form links between platelets and form aggregates. This process is stimulated by three processes[23]: (1) ADP released from platelet dense granules (and possibly also from erythrocytes by hemolysis) interacts with specific platelet membrane receptors to expose further glycoprotein IIb-IIIa receptors. (2) Arachidonic acid in the platelet membrane is converted into thromboxane A_2 by cyclooxygenase and thromboxane synthetase enzyme systems in the platelet. This prostanoid powerfully stimulates further platelet aggregation and is also a potent vasoconstrictor. (3) A further mechanism of platelet activation is by direct stimulation by collagen and thrombin,[23] the so-called "third pathway" perhaps mediated by the lipoxy ether, platelet-activating factor. However, as patients with a deficiency in platelet-activating factor synthesis maintain normal thrombin-induced aggregation,[22] this intermediary role has been questioned.

Not only does severe vessel wall injury stimulate platelet aggregation, but the coagulation cascade is also stimulated by exposure of negatively charged collagen groups and of tissue factor. Thrombin generation is a further stimulus to platelet aggregation.

During the above processes of platelet adhesion and aggregation the activated platelets release at least two mitogens,[25] epidermal growth factor and platelet-derived growth factor (PDGF), and also a growth factor (transforming growth factor β) which supports cell growth under some conditions and inhibits it under others. PDGF has both mitogenic and chemoattractant properties for smooth muscle cells, while other products of the platelet release reaction, platelet factor 4 and β-thromboglobulin, are chemoattractant for monocytes and perhaps to smooth muscle cells as well. These factors, as we shall see, may be important in the chronic reaction of the vessel wall to the type of injury produced during angioplasty.

EFFECTS OF EXPERIMENTAL ANGIOPLASTY

We have studied platelet deposition after experimental angioplasty consisting of dilatation of the normal carotid in the pig.[26] Platelet deposition has been quantified by the use of indium-111 labeled platelets, either by counting excised vessels in a well gamma counter, or by scintigraphy.[27]

In the first series of our experiments,[26] angioplasty was performed in 38 pigs and the effects were examined from 1 hour to 60 days later. In these experiments, the animals received a 100 USP U/kg heparin bolus immediately before the procedure. Balloon dilatation always produced complete endothelial denudation at the site. Four days after the procedure endothelial cells had partially regrown, while by 7 days most of the denuded area was recovered, except for areas where mural thrombus was still present. Additional changes included evidence of cell necrosis. Half of the arteries also showed a tear extending into the media (FIGURE 1). In the presence of such a tear, macroscopic mural thrombus was seen at 1 hour (FIGURE 2), while if there was no tear, mural thrombus was not apparent. There was a large excess of platelet deposition in arteries where a tear was seen.

A second technique was used in a series of experiments in which the relationship between degree of injury and the extent of thrombus deposition was further explored. Dual isotope subtraction scintigraphy was used to quantify platelet deposition in 12 animals, and the results validated by counting the excised vessels in a gamma well counter.[27] Using this imaging technique, at least 20 million platelets per cm^2 must be deposited for a 5-minute image to detect the thrombus. This number of platelets was also strongly associated with the presence of a medial tear (as seen in FIGURE 2). A positive scintigram was seen in 9 of the 12 arteries with macroscopic thrombus, all with more than 20 million platelets per cm^2 (FIGURE 3). Overall, complete thrombotic occlusion occurred in two arteries of a total of 32 with intimal tears, in which an extensive area of luminal surface was damaged.

These studies, using different techniques, clearly show that extensive platelet deposition with mural thrombus formation is strongly associated with damage which extends into the media, *i.e.,* with more severe injury. Mild damage, restricted to endothelial cell loss, was not associated with macroscopic thrombus formation. Similar findings have been reported in other experimental systems.[28] Furthermore, in the rabbit model studied by Faxon *et al.,*[18] thrombus formation was insignificant within 24 hours of angioplasty, while at 4 weeks[29] thrombus was seen in 4 out of 9 dilated vessels. The contribution of thrombosis to luminal narrowing in this study is not clear, but the investigators concluded that "intraluminal thrombosis plays a prominent role in reocclusion." Thus mural thrombus formation at the site of angioplasty is probably an important factor in acute thrombotic occlusion following coronary angioplasty and may contribute to the process of restenosis.

Over the hours and days following PTCA a reparative process occurred in the pig model. At 4 days after the procedure, connective tissue remodelling was seen which restored the luminal contour towards normal.[26] Platelet deposition decreased pari passu, coinciding with partial endothelial cell regrowth. By 7 days, there was no significant platelet deposition. Of the original 38 pigs, four progressed to thrombotic occlusion between 24 and 30 days after the procedure. Nonocclusive thrombi organized with fibrocellular infiltration to simulate a fibrous plaque, producing significant stenosis of the vessel in some cases. Intimal hyperplasia was also evident, intimal thickness increasing from 0.06 mm at 7 days to 0.08 to 0.09 mm from 14 to 60 days, much thicker than the control intima of 0.03 mm. Similar findings were made by Faxon and colleagues in the rabbit.[29] In addition to organizing thrombus as referred to above, fibrocellular tissue was seen in a pattern reminiscent of the original pattern of

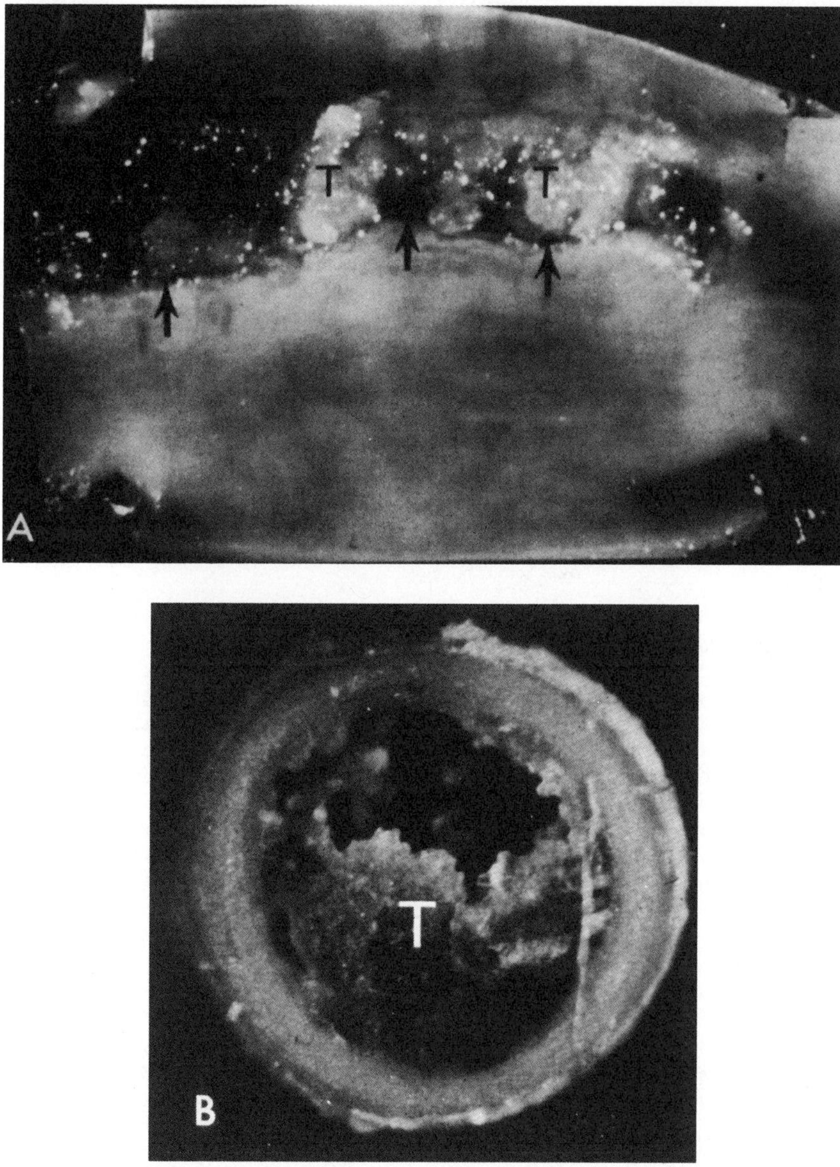

FIGURE 2. Endothelial surface of opened artery. (**A**) Clearly visible mural thombus lies over a longitudinal tear in the artery (shown by the arrows). (**B**) Cross section reveals that the thrombus occupies considerably more than 50% of the lumen of the artery. (From Lam *et al.*[27])

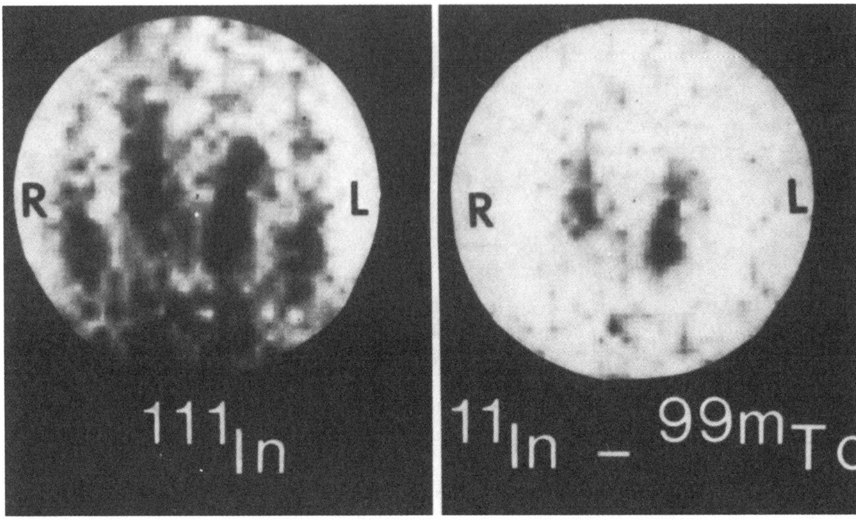

FIGURE 3. Platelet scintigram using platelets labeled with ^{111}In following bilateral carotid angioplasty. The image at *right* shows the effect of blood pool subtraction with ^{99m}Tc, which removes the component of the image due to the platelet label in the circulating blood. The lateral vessels, seen in the image to the *left* are the jugular veins. (*L*, left; *R*, right. From Lam *et al.*[27])

tearing. In some cases, a multilayered neointimal process with layers of loose connective tissue alternated with denser fibrocellular tissue. Thus two processes appear to have taken place: mural thrombus formation with subsequent organization, and intimal hyperplasia. The former is clearly related directly to acute platelet deposition, and probably to continuing platelet deposition, as the occlusions occurred late. The latter process is probably also stimulated by platelet deposition, although these experiments provide no direct evidence that this is the case.

When activated, platelets release a number of vasoconstrictor substances, including thromboxane A_2, serotonin, and PDGF. Spasm occasionally complicates coronary angioplasty acutely, and recurrent spasm has been associated with restenosis. For example, one report[30] documents the occurrence of troublesome recurrent spasms in the first two months after percutaneous coronary angioplasty in five patients. One patient finally died after coronary grafting, and the site of spasm was marked by the presence of a stenosis due to intimal smooth muscle cell proliferation.[31] We have investigated the relationship between vasospasm and platelet deposition in the carotid angioplasty model in the pig.[32]

Eighteen normal pigs underwent carotid angioplasty after three doses of aspirin, at a dose of 1 mg/kg, and the vessel response to angioplasty was compared to that of 24 untreated pigs. Angiography was used to quantitate the degree of vessel spasm produced and ^{111}In-labelled platelets were used to quantify platelet deposition by counting the excised arteries in a gamma well counter. Immediately proximal and distal to the dilated region of the vessel were areas of vasoconstriction of various degrees (FIGURE 4), while the dilated region itself showed evidence of the injury induced by the angioplasty, varying from mild damage with subendothelial exposure to tears extending into the media. There was a strong logarithmic correlation between platelet deposition on the whole artery and the degree of vasoconstriction. Similarly, there was a significant correlation between platelet deposition on to the area of vasoconstriction and the degree of constriction. As in the previous series of experiments, platelet deposition was greater where there was more damage. Similarly, vasoconstriction was more severe in these areas. Aspirin, which has no intrinsic vasoactive properties, decreased the degree of platelet deposition in the presence of severe vessel wall injury (FIGURE 5). A parallel decrease in the degree of vasospasm also occurred. These effects were not seen in the context of mild injury, the platelet response to which aspirin does not inhibit. Thus the effects of aspirin to reduce vasoconstriction were consistent with its action being entirely due to a reduction in platelet deposition. These findings strongly support the notion that platelet deposition can produce vasoconstriction *in vivo,* perhaps by release of humoral agents. This is further supported by the observation that the degree of vasoconstriction was greater distally than proximally, presumably due to blood flow carrying vasoactive compounds to the distal site.

The effects of other drugs have also been examined in this model. Ibuprofen has similar effects to aspirin, presumably due to cyclooxygenase inhibition. However, drugs with direct vasodilating properties (*e.g.,* prostacyclin), or those that block the effects of agents released from platelets reduce vasoconstriction, without effecting platelet deposition.

These studies suggest that the immediate consequence of angioplasty is platelet deposition in all cases, with frank thrombus formation if the injury is severe. Coronary spasm is an acute response to the platelet deposition, due to the release of vasoactive substances by platelets. Chronic effects include organization of thrombus with stenosis if the thrombus is of sufficient size, and intimal hyperplasia, due to stimulation of medial smooth muscle cells by growth factors. It is clear that the interaction between platelet and vessel wall is important in each of these processes.

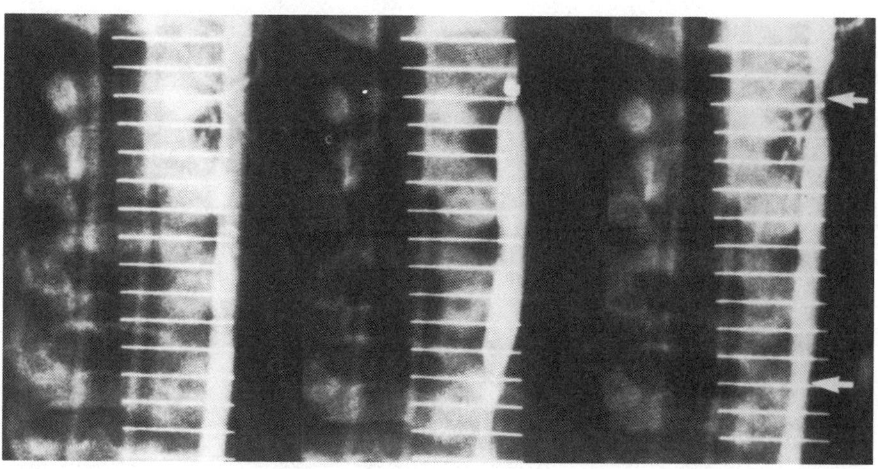

FIGURE 4. Angiogram frames showing the carotid before angioplasty (*left*), during balloon inflation (*center*), and after angioplasty (*right*). In the last frame there is a clearly visible constriction in the vessel, more marked distally, where the lumen is narrowed by approximately 75% of its diameter. Note that there is no vasoconstriction at the site of the balloon inflation itself. (From Lam *et al.*[27])

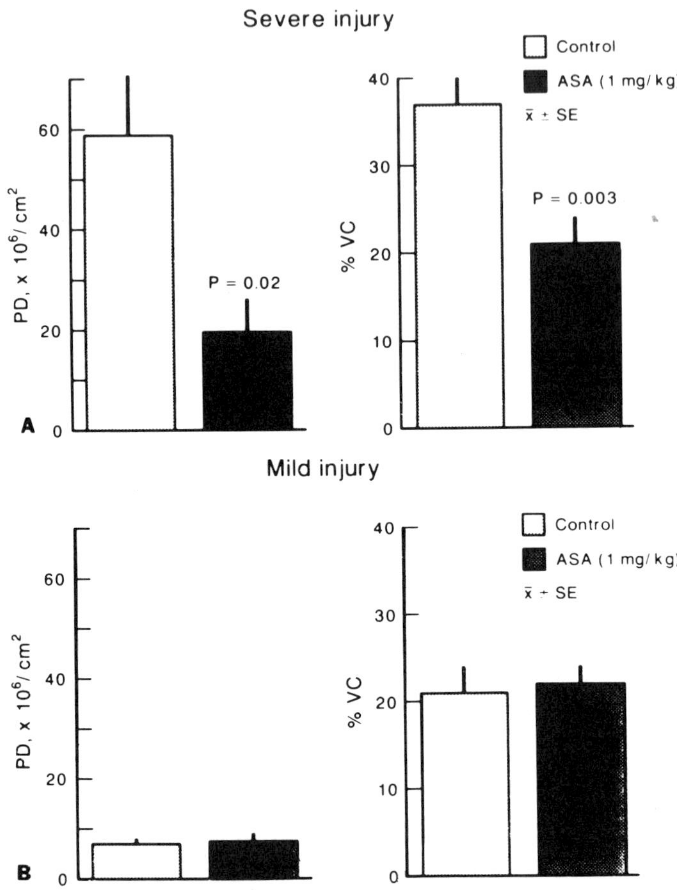

FIGURE 5. (**A**) In the presence of severe arterial wall injury, aspirin at a dose of 1 mg/kg decreased platelet deposition (*PD*) and vasoconstriction (*VC*) when compared to untreated animals. (**B**) With mild injury, however, aspirin in the same dose had no effect. This suggests that there is a component of the platelet response to injury of the arterial wall that is not amenable to prevention with aspirin. (From Lam *et al.*[32])

BLOOD FLOW AND PLATELET DEPOSITION

The foregoing discussion has highlighted the influences of biochemical and structural factors on the outcome of angioplasty, particularly by their effects on the hemostatic system. However, the flow characteristics of blood are also important determinants of the interaction between platelets and the vessel wall. The subject has been extensively reviewed in this volume (Badimon *et al.*[44]), and this section will thus address only those aspects directly related to the effects of angioplasty.

Platelet deposition onto a surface can be assessed using various flow chambers, in which flow conditions can be carefully controlled. Our studies have used an *ex vivo* system, in which the substrate for deposition can also be controlled, and the effect of (simulated) mild or severe injury can be determined. Mild injury has been reproduced by the use of de-endothelialized aorta, while severe injury is simulated by either exposure of tendon collagen or aorta from which the intima has been stripped. The former contains type I collagen in large bundles, similar to arterial media. When only subendothelial components are exposed, at shear rates of 106 to $424 s^{-1}$, platelet deposition reaches a maximum at 5–10 minutes at a number sufficient to produce a monolayer or bilayer of platelets. At higher shear rates initial deposition was more rapid, but the maximum reached at steady state was no more than with lower shear rates. However, if tendon collagen (type I) is used instead, platelet deposition was considerably greater, and continued to increase with increasing shear rates and with time, until, in some cases, occlusion of the flow chamber occurred after 30 minutes.[34] Similar findings have been made with exposed aortic media (platelet deposition between 5 and 100 times greater than with subendothelium). These observations underscore the greater reactivity of collagen of the type which would be exposed in severe injury to the arterial wall. Additionally, they demonstrate the increasing platelet deposition and greater likelihood of thrombus formation at high shear rates, when the type of substrate exposed resembles severe injury as it can occur in both experimental and therapeutic angioplasty. Thus two factors potentially or actually produced by angioplasty predispose to platelet deposition and thrombus formation: deep injury to the vessel wall with exposure of collagen and the presence of a residual stenosis with an increased local shear rate.

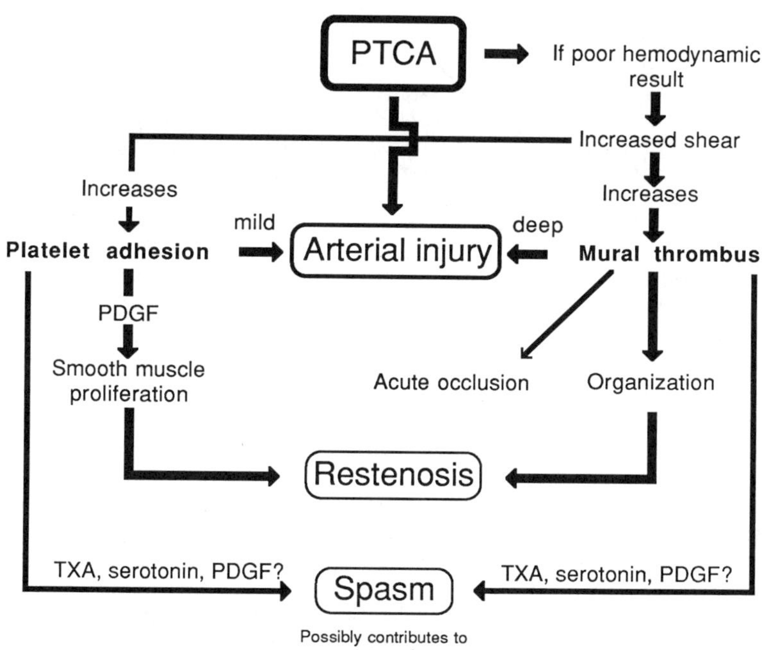

FIGURE 6. Schema showing factors which may contribute to restenosis. Platelet adhesion clearly contributes to mural thrombus formation. The relationship between spasm and restenosis is not clear.

Other changes in blood flow at the site of an angioplasty may increase the interaction of platelet and vessel wall or increase the activation of the coagulation cascade which also occurs. For example, if an intimal flap is produced, the disturbance of flow produced may be more severe than with the original lesion, with areas of high shear present to activate platelets and enhance the interaction of platelets and vessel wall, in addition to the greater area of exposed media resulting from the raising of the flap.

ACUTE AND SUBACUTE RESPONSE TO ANGIOPLASTY IN MAN

The experimental studies described above are very valuable in elucidating possible mechanisms in the response to angioplasty in man. However, the results obtained have to be seen in the light of the observations made in man. It must be emphasized that the arteries dilated in the experimental studies are not as severely stenosed as those dilated in man, while in many studies the arteries have not been atherosclerotic.

The acute effects of angioplasty in man (FIGURE 6) appear to be similar to those in the experimental animal. Block *et al.*[17] describe thrombus at the site of the dilatation in three cases who died soon after angioplasty. Essed and colleagues[35] describe a patient who died soon after a second angioplasty, restenosis having occurred after the first, which was complicated by dissection. The restenosis was due to medial disruption and dissection along the vessel, the dissection being filled with "fibrocellular proliferation" described as similar to that seen after aortic dissection when the media is disrupted.

Austin and colleagues[31] describe three patients who died 5, 17, and 62 days after angioplasty. Death was in no case felt to be associated with the angioplasty site itself, as all angioplasty procedures were apparently initially successful. In the case studied at 5 days, endothelial denudation, intimal splitting, focal intimal necrosis, and adventitial hemorrhage were seen, as described by other authors. Austin and colleagues emphasized the intimal smooth muscle proliferation at the site of previous damage, such that the patient dying at 62 days had circumferential stenosis of newly formed smooth muscle cells, containing no apolipoprotein A or B. The authors suggested that abnormalities of lipid metabolism were unlikely to have been important in the production of the stenosis.

Thus the animal evidence of acute thrombosis and of subacute medial proliferation is paralleled by human data.

CHRONIC RESPONSE TO ANGIOPLASTY IN MAN: RESTENOSIS

Any factors acting to reduce acute platelet deposition would, according to the above suggestions, be likely to reduce the likelihood of acute occlusion and the incidence of restenosis. Similarly, if such factors acted for some time after the procedure, interventions to reduce continuing platelet deposition would also be beneficial. The left side of FIGURE 6 presents a schema showing possible chronic effects of angioplasty in man.

In the report of Holmes *et al.*[6] from the NHLBI registry, a high rate of restenosis was associated with four variables. These were male sex, initial transstenotic gradient of 20 mm Hg or more, final postdilatation gradient of 20 mm Hg or more, and onset of angina in the 2 months before PTCA. Similarly, in the report of Leimgruber and colleagues from Emory,[10] the most important risk factor for restenosis was a high transstenotic gradient after dilatation. These data support our experimental observations suggesting a link between continuing high shear at the site of the angioplasty, produced by residual stenosis, and enhanced platelet deposition, resulting in a high rate of restenosis.

Our experimental findings suggest that the severity of injury to the vessel wall during angioplasty may be a determinant of restenosis. However, the Registry data[6] showed that arteriographic evidence of dissection, immediately after the procedure, was not predictive of restenosis after a mean follow-up of 7 months. This finding has not been confirmed by other workers,[36] who showed that early restenosis, detected by repeat angiography 2 days following PTCA, was more common in patients with arteriographic evidence of endothelial damage immediately after the procedure. The difficulty with all the human data is the unknown specificity of angiographic appearances for given pathological changes. Additionally, it is likely that all angioplasty sites are characterized by severe damage to the vessel wall, even where this is not angiographically evident.

THERAPY TO REDUCE RESTENOSIS

The data and hypotheses discussed above suggest that two factors are important in a reduction of the incidence of restenosis. These are: (1) a technically good result from the angioplasty procedure itself, which by reducing shear will reduce acute platelet deposition and also reduce platelet deposition in the interval after the procedure before re-endothelialization or passivation of the damaged area occurs; and (2) the use of appropriate drug therapy to reduce the hemostatic response to arterial wall injury, both thrombosis acutely and restenosis chronically. The former issue is beyond the scope of this article.

As discussed above, the response to angioplasty involves platelet deposition and stimulation of the coagulation system. As platelet deposition begins as soon as blood begins to flow over the area of damage, therapy to prevent acute thrombosis should ideally begin before the procedure. Various therapies have been tested in our pig carotid angioplasty model, and in other animal models. There are few clinical trials completed, although several are in progress.

Our studies in the pig have all been performed in the presence of heparin at the time of the angioplasty to inhibit the deposition of fibrin. Therapies that have been partially successful in reducing platelet deposition, when added to the heparin, have included the following: dipyridamole (2.5 mg/kg/day) plus aspirin (20 mg/kg/day), aspirin alone (1 mg/kg/day), an experimental platelet inhibitor drug, anagrelide, either used alone or with aspirin or aspirin and dipyridamole, and intravenous ibuprofen. Therapies that were ineffective in reducing platelet deposition, in the presence of heparin, included the following: low-molecular-weight dextran, prostaglandin E_1, prostacyclin, aspirin alone at a dose of 20 mg/kg/day, sulfinpyrazone, ticlopidine begun 4 days before the angioplasty, verapamil, nifedipine, ketanserin, and SQ 29,548 an experimental thromboxane A_2 receptor blocker.[37–39] In arteries with deep injury, mural thrombus was seen in some 80–90% of the cases in the presence of heparin alone, while the addition of platelet inhibitor therapy reduced this to 30–35% of the arteries. This reduction may only partially prevent restenosis, as it is likely that interaction of platelet and vessel wall without thrombus formation may be sufficient to stimulate the intimal hyperplasia, which is likely to be important in at least some of the cases. Thus other methods of preventing platelet deposition need to be tried. These might include the short-term use of monoclonal antibodies to block GPIb receptors or GPIIb-IIIa receptors that would inhibit platelet adhesion. Blockade of GPIIb-IIIa receptors certainly prevents platelet aggregation in dog coronary arteries stenosed by an external cuff (B. Coller, personal communication) although the effect on adhesion *in vivo* is not known. Other options could include the use of synthetic peptides to occupy receptor sites, for example the use of a peptide that occupies the GPIb receptor. It is likely that these strategies would be practical for short-term use only, as the hemorrhagic effects might well be too great for long-term use, as a condition simulating a bleeding diathesis would be produced. This would be so particularly for the blockade of GPIb or GPIIb-IIIa receptor sites. Blockade of receptors to PDGF might reduce the intimal hyperplasia without hemorrhagic effects, but other effects on the control of cell proliferation would have to be carefully sought.

In addition to studies of acute thrombosis, animal work has investigated the effect of antiplatelet therapy in retarding restenosis. In one study,[40] bilateral iliac stenoses were produced in rabbits by a combination of balloon de-endothelialization and a 2% cholesterol diet given over a 6-week period. Angioplasty was performed in one iliac in all rabbits. Following this, the animals received either aspirin (32 mg/day) plus dipyridamole 25 mg/day starting before the procedure, sulfinpyrazone (100 mg/day) starting after the procedure, or were untreated. Four weeks later the arteries were examined at autopsy. The combination of aspirin and dipyridamole and the use of sulfinpyrazone alone were effective in reducing the degree of restenosis when compared to the untreated animals. Thrombus was present in four out of nine control animals (in three of which it was occlusive) but in none of the treated animals. Both intraluminal thrombosis and intimal hyperplasia appeared to be decreased by therapy in this model. These studies suggest that a reduction in the degree of platelet deposition per se would be of some value.

Clinical studies have also been based on the evidence that platelet deposition and thrombosis are important in the pathogenesis of restenosis. Thornton *et al.* reported a randomized study[41] in which warfarin and aspirin (325 mg/day) were compared. There was no significant difference in the frequency of restenosis at 9 months of follow-up, although in patients with long standing angina the aspirin group appeared to benefit. Other workers have studied calcium channel blockers because of the association between spasm and restenosis in the small patient population described above. Neither nifedipine[42] nor diltiazem[43] have proven efficacious when added to platelet inhibitor therapy. However, the efficacy of platelet inhibitor therapy is not established in man. To this end, a trial currently in progress at the Mayo Clinic and at Mount Sinai Medical Center in New York is randomizing patients to platelet inhibitor therapy, beginning before PTCA and continuing therafter. The end point in this study is angiographic restenosis at 6 months. The results will be compared with a control group treated with placebo alone, while all patients in both limbs will receive intravenous heparin at the time of the procedure and for 24–48 hours thereafter. After the procedure a 2-week treatment with calcium channel blockers and nitrates will be given.

CONCLUSION

Angioplasty produces an increase in coronary luminal diameter by injury to both the vessel wall itself and the plaque. The response of the hemostatic system of this injury is a major determinant of the clinical outcome of angioplasty, and a clearer understanding of this response is needed to optimize strategies to prevent restenosis. The response is conditioned by both the exposure of hemostatically active components of the vessel wall (substrate) and by the flow conditions at the site of the damage (rheology). Animal studies have helped our understanding of the pathophysiology of interactions of platelets with the vessel wall, but further human studies are needed to define the value of the therapies currently available.

REFERENCES

1. GRÜNTZIG, A. R., A. SENNING & W. E. SIEGENTHALER. 1979. Nonoperative dilatation of coronary-artery stenosis: Percutaneous transluminal coronary angioplasty. N. Engl. J. Med. **301:** 61–68.
2. DE FEYTER, P. J., P. W. SERRUYS, M. VAN DEN BRAND, *et al.* 1985. Emergency coronary angioplasty in refractory unstable angina. N. Engl. J. Med. **313:** 1369–1375.
3. VLIETSTRA, R. E., D. R. HOLMES, JR., G. S. REEDER, *et al.* 1983. Balloon angioplasty in multivessel coronary artery disease. Mayo Clin. Proc. **58:** 563–567.
4. O'NEILL, W., G. C. TIMMIS, P. D. BOURDILLON, *et al.* 1986. A prospective randomized clinical trial of intracoronary streptokinase *versus* coronary angioplasty for acute myocardial infarction. N. Engl. J. Med. **314:** 812–818.
5. BLOCK, P. C. 1985. Percutaneous transluminal coronary angioplasty: Role in the treatment of coronary artery disease. Circulation, **72**(Suppl. V):161–165.
6. HOLMES, D. R., Jr., R. E. VLIETSTRA, H. C. SMITH, *et al.*, 1984. Restenosis after percutaneous transluminal coronary angioplasty (PTCA): A report from the PTCA registry of the National Heart, Lung and Blood Institute. Am. J. Cardiol. **53:** 77C–81C.
7. ADAMS, P. C., J.-J. BADIMON, L. BADIMON, J. H. CHESEBRO & V. FUSTER. 1987. Role of platelets in atherogenesis: relevance to coronary arterial restenosis after angioplasty. Cardiovasc. Clinics. *In* Cardiovascular Clinics: Thrombosis and Platelets in Myocardial Ischemia. A. N. Brest & J. L. Mehta. F. A. Davis. Philadelphia.
8. COWLEY, M. J., G. DORROS, S. F. KELSEY, M. VAN RODEN, K. M. DETRE. 1984. Acute coronary events associated with percutaneous coronary angioplasty. Am. J. Cardiol. **53:** 12C–16C.
9. MABIN, T. A., D. R. HOLMES, JR., H. C. SMITH, *et al.* Follow-up clinical results in patients undergoing percutaneous transluminal coronary angioplasty. Circulation **71:** 754–760.
10. LEIMGRUBER, P. P., G. S. ROUBIN, H. V. ANDERSON, *et al.*, 1985. Influence of intimal dissection on restenosis after successful coronary angioplasty. Circulation **72:** 530–535.
11. VANDORMAEL, M. G., B. R. CHAITMAN, T. ISCHINGER, *et al.* 1985. Immediate and short-term benefit of multilesion coronary angioplasty: Influence of degree of revascularization. J. Am. Coll. Cardiol. **6:** 983–991.
12. GRÜNTZIG, A. 1982. Results from coronary angioplasty and implications for the future. Am. Heart J. **103:** 779–783.
13. WIJNS, W., P. W. SERRUYS, J. H. C. REIBER, *et al.* 1985. Early detection of restenosis after successful percutaneous transluminal coronary angioplasty by exercise-redistribution thallium scintigraphy. Am. J. Cardiol. **55:** 357–361.
14. DEPUEY, E. G., L. L. LEATHERMAN, R. D. LEACHMAN, *et al.*, 1984. Restenosis after transluminal coronary angioplasty detected with exercise-gated radionuclide ventriculography. J. Am. Coll. Cardiol. **4:** 1103–1113.
15. CASTAÑEDA-ZUÑIGA, W. R., A. FORMANEK, M. TADAVARTHY, *et al.* 1980. The mechanism of balloon angioplasty. Radiology **135:** 565–571.
16. HOLMES, D. R., R. E. VLIETSTRA, M. B. MOCK, *et al.* 1983. Angiographic changes produced by percutaneous coronary angioplasty. Am. J. Cardiol. **51:** 676–683.
17. BLOCK, P. R., R. K. MYLER, S. STERTZER, & J. T. FALLON. 1981. Morphology after transluminal angioplasty in human beings. N. Engl. J. Med. **305:** 382–385.
18. FAXON, D. P., V. J. WEBER, C. C HAUDENSCHILD, *et al.* 1982. Acute effects of transluminal angioplasty in three experimental models of atherosclerosis. Arteriosclerosis. **2:** 125–133.
19. HAWIGER, J. 1987. Formation and regulation of platelet and fibrin hemostatic plug. Hum. Pathol. **18:** 111–122.
20. WEISS, H. J., V. T. TURITTO & H. R. BAUMGARTNER. 1986. Platelet adhesion and thrombus formation on subendothelium in platelets deficient in glycoproteins IIb-IIIa, Ib, and storage granules. Blood **67:** 322–330.
21. MOROOSE, R. & L. HOYER. 1986. Von Willebrand factor and platelet function. Ann. Rev. Med. **37:** 157–163.
22. MAYNE, R. 1986. Collagenous proteins of blood vessels. Arteriosclerosis **6:** 585–593.
23. VERMYLEN, J., M. VERSTRAETE & V. FUSTER. 1986. Role of platelet activation and fibrin formation in thrombogenesis. J. Am. Coll. Cardiol. **8:** 2B–9B.

24. STURK, A., M. C. L. SCHAAP, J. W. TEN CATE, *et al.* 1987. Platelet-activating factor: Mediator of the third pathway of platelet aggregation? J. Clin. Invest. **79:** 344–350.
25. ROSS, R. 1986. The pathogenesis of atherosclerosis: An update. N. Engl. J. Med. **314:** 488–500.
26. STEELE, P. M., J. H. CHESEBRO, A. W. STANSON, *et al.* 1985. Balloon angioplasty: Natural history of the pathophysiological response to injury in a pig model. Circ. Res. **57:** 105–112.
27. LAM, J. Y. T., J. H. CHESEBRO, P. M. STEELE, *et al.* 1986. Deep arterial injury during experimental angioplasty: Relation to a positive indium-111–labelled platelet scintigram, quantitative platelet deposition and mural thrombosis. J. Am. Coll. Cardiol. **8:** 1380–1386.
28. HONOUR, A. J., G. W. PICKERING & B. L. SHEPPARD. 1971. Ultrastructure and behaviour of platelet thrombi in injured arteries. Br. J. Exp. Pathol. **52:** 482–494.
29. FAXON, D. P., T. A. SANBORN, C. C. HAUDENSCHILD & T. J. RYAN. 1984. Effect of antiplatelet therapy on restenosis after experimental angioplasty. Am. J. Cardiol. **53:** 72C–76C.
30. HOLLMAN, J., G. E. AUSTIN, A. R. GRÜNTZIG, J. S. DOUGLAS, JR., S. B. KING III. 1983. Coronary artery spasm at the site of angioplasty in the first 2 months after successful percutaneous transluminal coronary angioplasty. J. Am. Coll. Cardiol. **2:** 1039–1045.
31. AUSTIN, C. E., N. B. RATLIFF, J. HOLLMAN, S. TABEI & D. F. PHILLIPS. Intimal proliferation of smooth muscle cells as an explanation for recurrent coronary artery stenosis after percutaneous transluminal coronary angioplasty. J. Am. Coll. Cardiol. **6:** 369–375.
32. LAM, J. Y. T., J. H. CHESEBRO, P. M. STEELE, *et al.* 1987. Is vasospasm related to platelet deposition? Relation in a porcine preparation of arterial injury in vivo. Circulation **75:** 243–248.
34. BADIMON, L., J. J. BADIMON, A. GALVEZ, *et al.* 1986. Influence of arterial wall damage and wall shear rate on platelet deposition: *ex vivo* study in a swine model. Arteriosclerosis **6:** 312–320.
35. ESSED, C. E., M. VAN DEN BRAND & A. E. BECKER. 1983. Transluminal coronary angioplasty and early restenosis: Fibrocellular occlusion after wall laceration. Br. Heart J. **49:** 393–396.
36. POWELSON, S., G. ROUBIN, H. WHITWORTH & A. GRÜNTZIG. 1986. Incidence of early restenosis after successful percutaneous transluminal coronary angioplasty (PTCA) (abstract). J. Am. Coll. Cardiol. **7:** 63A.
37. LAM, J. Y. T., J. H. CHESEBRO, L. BADIMON & V. FUSTER. Serotonin and thromboxane A_2 receptor blockade decrease vasoconstriction but not platelet deposition after deep arterial injury (abstract). Circulation **74**(Suppl. II): 97.
38. STEELE, P. M., J. H. CHESEBRO & V. FUSTER. 1984. The natural history of arterial balloon angioplasty in pigs and intervention with platelet-inhibitor therapy: Implications for clinical trials (abstract). Clin. Res. **32:** 209A.
39. STEELE, P. M., J. H. CHESEBRO, D. R. HOLMES, L. BADIMON & V. FUSTER. 1984. Balloon angioplasty in pigs: Comparative effects of platelet-inhibitor drugs (abstract). Circulation **70**(Suppl II): 361.
40. FAXON, D. P., T. A. SANBORN, C. C. HAUDENSCHILD & T. J. RYAN 1984. Effect of antiplatelet therapy on restenosis after experimental angioplasty. Am. J. Cardiol. **53:** 72C–76C.
41. THORNTON, M. A., A. R. GRÜNTZIG, J. HOLLMAN, S. B. KING III & J. S. DOUGLAS. 1984. Coumadin and aspirin in prevention of recurrence after transluminal coronary angioplasty: A randomized study. Circulation **69:** 721–727.
42. WHITWORTH, H. B., G. S. ROUBIN, J. HOLLMAN, *et al.* 1986. Effect of nifedipine on recurrent stenosis after percutaneous transluminal coronary angioplasty. J. Am. Coll. Cardiol. **8:** 1271–1276.
43. CORCOS, T., P. R. DAVID, P. G. VAL, *et al.* 1985. Failure of diltiazem to prevent restenosis after percutaneous transluminal coronary angioplasty. Am. Heart J. **109:** 926–931.
44. BADIMON, L., J. J. BADIMON, V. T. TURITTO & V. FUSTER. 1987. Thrombosis: Studies under flow conditions. This volume.

Blood Tests for the Detection of Thrombosis

Effects of Blood Flow and Location of the Sampling Site

JOHN OWEN AND KAREN L. KAPLAN

Department of Medicine
College of Physicians and Surgeons of Columbia University
New York, New York 10032

INTRODUCTION

In the clinical context of a patient suspected of having thrombosis, the physician's objective is to make or to exclude a specific diagnosis. This translates into changing the probability of thrombosis to a level that dictates a specific course of action. Such probabilistic reasoning does not require any knowledge of physiology nor indeed need there be any causal relationship between thrombosis and the blood test employed. The finding of an elevated white blood cell count would modify the probabilities of certain diseases, and so a simple blood count could qualify as a blood test for the diagnosis of thrombosis. Thus we readily accept clinical findings that we can relate to the site of thrombosis, or a measurement of a coagulation factor, as indicators for thrombosis. It is, however, an illusion that these are any less empirical than the white cell count, for the thrombus itself does not circulate nor can it be felt directly, much less seen with the naked eye.

Therefore if we are not to use an empirical approach, at least we should try to use tools that we can describe in pathophysiologic terms and that relate to specific processes. We have chosen to discuss the pitfalls of using blood tests to detect thrombosis, and will generally restrict ourselves to those tests that reflect activation of the various systems involved in hemostasis. These tests can be used in an investigative setting to address questions of the extent and time course of activation of the various pathways involved in thrombogenesis.

In order to select suitable blood tests we need to consider the details of the system under investigation. Three major points emerge all of which interact. These are location of the activating surface, the intrinsic sensitivity and specificity of the blood test, and last, but not least, the availability and dependability of the test system. Many considerations are common to the investigation of *in vivo* thrombosis occurring on native vascular surfaces or on an artificial surface. We have recently published a critical review of the available blood tests for the diagnosis of thrombosis,[1] with an emphasis on thrombosis occurring on natural surfaces. In this discussion we will focus on issues particularly pertinent to the diagnosis of thrombosis on artificial surfaces.

LOCATION OF THE ARTIFICIAL SURFACE

The problems encountered in demonstrating *in vivo* coagulation system activation are compounded in the case of artificial surfaces by the nature of the devices under investigation. The most important consideration is the relationship between the device

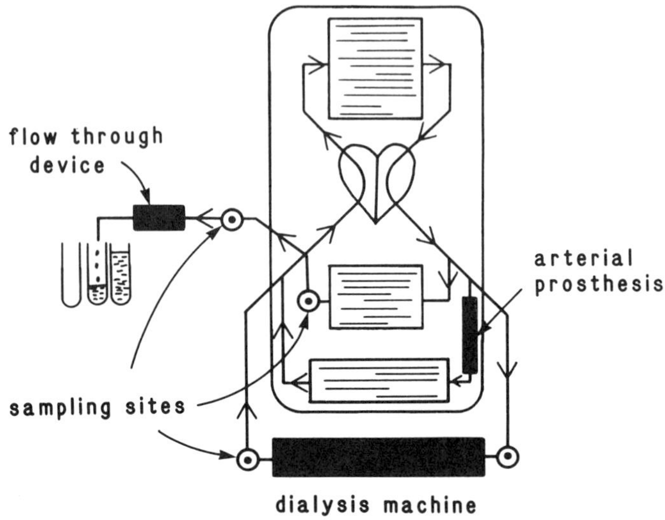

FIGURE 1. Diagrammatic view of different locations at which artificial surfaces come into contact with the circulation.

and the sampling port. Three distinct models can be envisaged and are shown diagrammatically in FIGURE 1.

In the first case, typified by arterial prostheses, the sampling point is removed from the device in such a way that dilution is significant and time delay as long as the recirculation time can be introduced. In general the sample will be collected from the antecubital fossa and will represent mixed venous blood. This sample will give steady state values that can be referred to the prosthesis by suitable allowance for dilution, recirculation, and clearance.

Single pass devices have been used to examine the effects of short-term exposure of artificial surfaces to flowing blood. The advantage to the investigator is that since the blood is not returned to the donor, only the venepuncture needle needs to be sterile. A second simplification follows: since there is no recirculation, the blood entering the device is usually presumed to be the same from start to finish. There is, however, a major trap inherent in this setup, which stems from the cascade nature of the coagulation system. In general, each stage in the coagulation pathway is characterized by the conversion of an inactive zymogen to an active serine protease. Each serine protease, in turn, becomes the activator for the next step. The activated clotting factors are inactivated by the action of circulating inhibitors such as antithrombin III.

A mathematical simulation of the coagulation cascade using the TUTSIM modeling program (APPLIED i, Palo Alto, CA 94306) was carried out to show the concentration of the active coagulation factors as a function time after activation (FIGURE 2). For simplicity, and without loss of generality, the model assumes that the rates of activation and clearance are the same for all clotting factors.

In this well-stirred system, a sample collected before 3 minutes would show little fibrin generation and we would conclude, erroneously, that there was no activation of coagulation if fibrin formation was our measure of activation. A similar error would be made if we measured the concentration of factor IXa at any time greater than 5 minutes. This model does not incorporate the added effects of flow, but the general principles are evident. One can see that the delay between exposing blood to the artifical surface and sample collection is critical to the experimental design. The temptation is to make this interval as short as possible to minimize artifact, a technique which should now be viewed with some skepticism.

In the third case, renal dialysis for example, blood can usually be sampled on the upstream and downstream sides of the device in addition to the usual site of sampling mixed venous blood. Interpretations are not straightforward. In this setting all of the problems outlined above come into play, with the additional consideration that the device is typically used episodically so that assumptions of steady state are not valid. Comparison of the values found at the three sites allows some inferences to be drawn concerning the extent of activation, though it may not be possible to define the site of activation. If all of the product is generated at the artificial surface, then sensitivity is maximized by sampling close to the device on the downstream side. However, if the product is generated in the fluid phase then the optimum sampling site will be somewhere downstream from the device. An example should make this clear. If we choose to use the fibrinopeptide A (FPA) level as an index of thrombin activity, then the optimum sampling point will depend on whether the thrombin is immobilized on the surface or released into the fluid phase where it could continue to act on circulating fibrinogen away from its site of generation. Thrombin released into plasma is inactivated by antithrombin III, and this reaction is markedly accelerated in the presence of heparin.[2] Thus, concomitant heparin administration might be expected to have a profound effect on the usefulness of tests for thrombin action as indices of thrombin generation.

In a simple experiment to determine the effect of heparin on thrombin action *in vitro,* we added thrombin to citrated plasma and observed the rate and extent of FPA release from fibrinogen. In the absence of heparin, and in keeping with the known kinetic constants for the interaction of thrombin with its principal inhibitor antithrombin III and the kinetics of FPA release from fibrinogen, we observed that thrombin was quickly inactivated, and that the concentration of FPA reached a plateau. The same pattern was observed over a wide range of added thrombin concentrations, and the data can be summarized by plotting the observed plateau concentrations against the amount

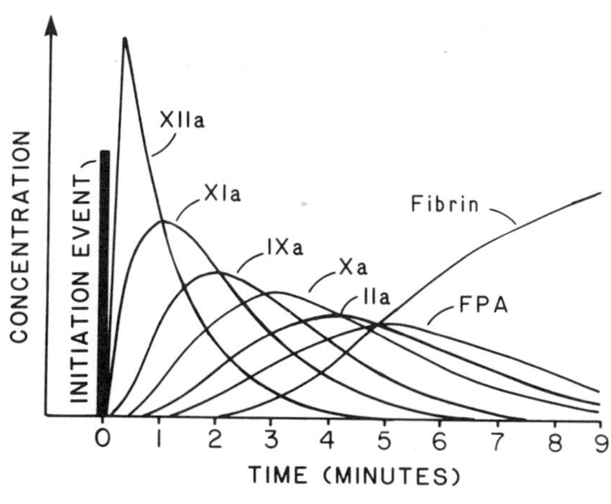

FIGURE 2. Simulation of the coagulation cascade showing the plasma concentration of the reactants as a function of time following initiation. For simplicity the reactions are assumed to occur in a well-stirred vessel, and the same kinetic constants were used for each reaction step.

of thrombin added. This plot (FIGURE 3) shows the expected relationship and implies that there is a constant relationship between the mass of thrombin released into the blood and the mass of FPA released. When the same experiment was carried out in the presence of heparin, one unit per ml of plasma, a close relationship between added thrombin and released FPA was again found. In the presence of heparin, however, at all concentrations of added thrombin the amount of FPA released was some 30 times less than that released in the absence of heparin.

The effect of heparin on *in vivo* plasma levels of FPA was well documented by Yudelman and colleagues in their study of patients with deep venous thrombosis.[3] They found that the infusion of heparin caused a prompt fall in the plasma FPA level, with a rate of decline equal to the half disappearance time of free FPA. This observation

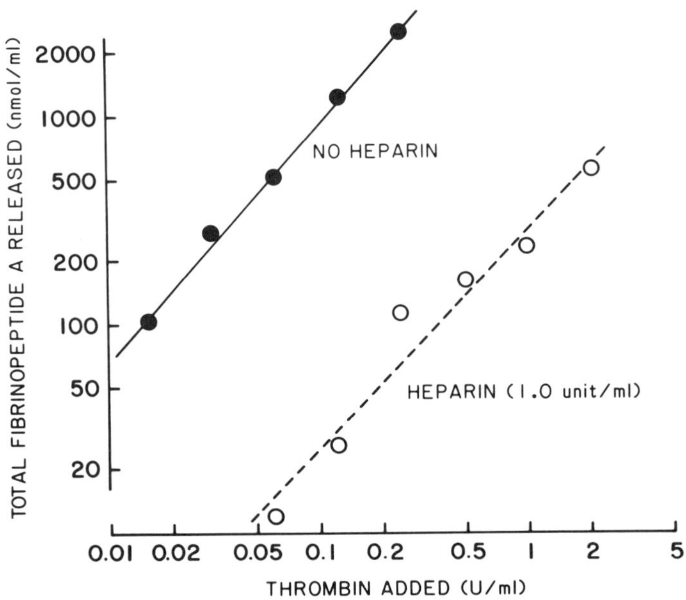

FIGURE 3. Total fibrinopeptide A cleaved from fibrinogen by added thrombin, before inactivation of the thrombin by plasma antithrombins. This experiment was carried out at 37°C with citrated plasma and in a separate experiment with added heparin.

suggested that heparin rapidly and completely abolished thrombin action. Interestingly, the FPA levels fell to the normal range but no lower. We have infused heparin into normal volunteers and found essentially no effect on the basal plasma FPA level. These data suggest that there is basal, heparin-insensitive thrombin activity. However, the administration of warfarin causes the plasma FPA to fall to extremely low values. Warfarin is an anticoagulant by virtue of its vitamin K antagonism, and possibly by direct interference with the synthesis of the vitamin-K-dependent coagulation zymogens. These data support the contention that the basal FPA reflects heparin-insensitive thrombin action.

This remained a curiosity until we began to study patients with acute myocardial infarction receiving tissue plasminogen activator (TPA). In those patients, in response to TPA infusion, we observed an increase in the plasma level of FPA. This increase was seen despite the prior administration of a large dose of heparin. These data are most easily interpreted as evidence that thrombin can exist in contact with the blood, but can be inaccessible to fluid-phase inactivators. Surface-bound thrombin may well be inhibited at a different rate than fluid-phase thrombin. There is no a priori reason to assume either an increased or a decreased rate, and arguments can easily be produced to support or to discredit either possibility. The idea of cell surface coagulant activity is now well established, and it would not be suprising if similar phenomena were to exist on artificial surfaces. Such activity presumably would not involve active participation by the artifical surface, but perhaps thrombin bound to fibrin deposits would be protected against inhibition, as previous studies in this laboratory have suggested.[4]

BIOCHEMICAL SENSITIVITY AND SPECIFICITY

The choice of a blood test to monitor a dynamic process is dependent on many factors. These factors can be controlled in some instances, such as training of personnel to perform specific tasks. In other instances the factors are intrinsic to the test system or to the dynamic process. The test of choice will usually be the one that exhibits the greatest reliability. In broad terms, reliability can be described as a signal-to-noise ratio in which the signal is determined by the dynamic process. The noise factor is influenced by biologic variation, the precision of the measurements, and by the pathophysiologic specificity of the test. An excellent and lucid discussion of reliability, and other relevant statistical issues, can be found in Fleiss's book *The Design and Analysis of Clinical Experiments.*[5] Two major areas of concern regarding blood tests for thrombosis are easily identified.

The first area of concern is sample preparation. This of course includes the technique used to perform the venipuncture and the subsequent processing up to the actual assay procedure. Stabilization of the level of the analyte in the sample is of paramount importance. Low-level activation of the coagulation cascade *ex vivo* can quickly swamp the relatively small signals typically seen in *in vivo* coagulation activation. Similarly, enzymatic cleavage by plasma enzymes such as the peptidase can cause rapid loss of analyte. Special considerations are necessary in such situations as the administration of tissue plasminogen activator.

The available assays of the highest sensitivity typically show some degree of cross-reactivity with other molecules present in plasma. For example, while assays for free fibrinopeptide A are quite discriminating, all show some degree of cross-reactivity with fibrinogen. The cross-reacting material is present at a concentration 10,000–20,000 times higher than free fibrinopeptide A. The complete removal of fibrinogen is thus important for accurate determination of FPA.

A similar problem exists with the presence of interfering substances. Assays developed for buffer systems usually need to be reformulated to be used on plasma samples. Likewise the application of tests developed for plasma systems will often not work on urine samples.

Sample storage presents special problems. Ultimate stability can be achieved by storage at $-135°C$, which is below the glass transition point of water. The period of freezing and thawing is still critical, and special attention must be given to the use of suitable enzyme inhibitors. Ongoing fibrinogen proteolysis in the cold is a particular problem. We have found that the only satisfactory way to ensure no storage-related increase in the level of fibrinopeptide $B\beta 1$–42 is to remove the fibrinogen prior to freezing. Removal of fibrinogen with 75% ethanol has proved a simple and satisfactory means of removing cross-reactivity material and of stabilizing samples for long-term storage. After ethanol precipitation we have found $-85°C$ to be suitable storage temperature, and even −20°C to be adequate for anything except very long-term storage.

The ultimate specificity of an immunoassay depends on the specificity of the antibody being used. Polyclonal antibodies are generally thought of as having only limited specificity, however it is clear that the rabbit can make some surprising distinctions. Antibodies to FPA show wide variation in their ability to distinguish free FPA from fibrinogen or even from small peptides containing FPA.[6]

Specificity can be improved by the use of monoclonal antibodies. By this method antibodies of exquisite specificity have been produced. Some of these antibodies have shown such specificity that removal of cross-reacting material is unnecessary. Unfortunately the price of increased specificity frequently is loss of sensitivity. In general monoclonal antibodies show lower affinity for their antigens than do polyclonal antibodies. This translates into loss of assay sensitivity. It is probable that better monoclonal antibodies will be produced in time, and we can look forward to new assay systems that exploit the characteristics of these antibodies. One such approach, using two complementary antibodies, is suggested by the work of Ehrlich and Moyle.[7]

A final point is the technology to be used. The choice is basically between radionuclide and enzymatic systems. In terms of specificity and sensitivity there is little to distinguish these systems overall. Capital equipment costs are a major factor in the choice, and consideration should be given to the ever-increasing problem of disposal of radioactive waste.

AVAILABILITY AND DEPENDABILITY

For any test to be of value it must be available. In general this translates into whether there is a commercial source for the reagents. In many instances the reagents can be purchased in kit form. Some kits are essentially complete and ready for use, others are more a collection of raw materials that allows an assay to be created. TABLES 1–3 give an indication of the availability of specific tests and in each case a representative reference is given as a point of departure for further reading. The assays are divided into groups according to the system being analyzed.

Assays reflecting activation of the coagulation system are shown in TABLE 1. The assay of fibrinopeptide A is by far the most widely used of this group. A measure of its popularity is that a computer search of the National Library of Medicine produced almost 500 publications. As would be expected, there is much less experience with the assays that are currently not commercially available. They hold such promise for the investigation of thrombosis that it is probable some enterprising manufacturer will soon market the necessary reagents. The inclusion of protein C activation peptide in

TABLE 1. Assays Reflecting Coagulation System Activity

Assay (ref.)	Reflects:	Commercial Availability
FPA[8]	fibrin I formation	yes
FPB[9]	fibrin II formation	yes
F1 + 2[10]	FXa activity	no
CAP[11]	protein C activation	no
Fibrin monomer[12]	fibrin formation	no
Thrombin-antithrombin complexes[13]	thrombin generation	no

TABLE 2. Assays Reflecting Fibrinolytic System Activity

Assay	Reflects:	Commercial Availability
FPBβ1–42[14]	fragment X formation	yes
FPBβ15–42[15]	fibrin II lysis by plasmin	yes
FDP total[16]	fibrin(ogen) proteolysis	yes
Fibrinogen antigen[17] by western blot	fibrin vs. fibrinogen proteolysis	no
D dimer[18]	lysis of cross-linked fibrin	yes
Fragment E[19]	fibrin(ogen) proteolysis	no
X oligomers[20]	lysis of cross-linked fibrin	no
Plasmin-antiplasmin complexes[21]	prior plasminogen activation	no

this group is appropriate even though the principal function of activated protein C is anticoagulant, since protein C activation is mediated by thrombin.

The prothrombin-derived F1+2 fragment, released when factor Xa converts prothrombin to thrombin, reflects factor Xa activity. This elegant and thus far unique technique allows the relationship between factor Xa and thrombin to be probed. At this time the assay is not widely available.

The principal inhibitor of thrombin is antithrombin III, and these proteins react to form a 1:1 inactive complex. Measurement of the circulating concentration of this complex would therefore allow an estimate to be made of the mass of thrombin formed in a given time period. Correlation of such data with levels of F1+2 and FPA measured simultaneously would give considerable information regarding the control of the terminal phase of coagulation.

Activation of the fibrinolytic system can be monitored by the plasma levels of a number of peptides or proteins, listed in TABLE 2. The assay of fibrinopeptide Bβ1–42 was originally accomplished by taking advantage of the increased immunoreactivity of this peptide, with an antibody raised against fibrinopeptide B (FPB) after thrombin cleavage of the Bβ14–15 Arg-Gly bond. The assay was made technically simpler by the introduction of antibodies, which requires an intact Bβ14–15 bond for full reactivity.[22,23] Fibrinogen has an intact Bβ14–15 bond and as expected cross-reacts fully in these assays. To obtain specificity it is therefore essential that all fibrinogen be removed. Larger peptides, containing the Bβ1–42 sequence, may not be removed along with the fibrinogen and could falsely elevate the result. To date we have not seen any evidence of such a peptide in clinical blood samples. Fibrinopeptide Bβ1–42 is cleared by the kidney, and very high plasma levels are found in individuals with renal failure. In such circumstances the plasma levels cannot be used to reflect plasmin activity. The introduction of an assay specific for Bβ chain peptides lacking FPB has led to the hope that measurement of this peptide in blood might be specific for thrombus dissolution. In practice the fibrinopeptide Bβ15–42 assay has not proved to be that specific, though more experience is needed before a complete picture can be drawn. Fibrinopeptide Bβ15–42, like FBPβ1–42, is cleared by the kidney and again its level in patients with renal failure does not reflect plasmin activity. The plasma concentration of D dimer can now be determined with a simple assay that does not require any pretreatment of the plasma sample. The level of this material should reflect thrombolysis, but it appears that the situation is more complex. In patients undergoing thrombolytic therapy with plasminogen activators, only a weak correlation is found between angiographically demonstrated thrombolysis and the plasma level of D dimer. Similarly, a high D dimer level is a poor index of successful thrombolysis. Also, D dimer levels are elevated in disseminated intravascular coagulation, where thrombosis does not necessarily occur. More experience is needed before such tests can be recommended for routine use.

Just as for thrombin-antithrombin complexes, the measurement of plasmin-antiplasmin complexes is attractive because it allows one, at least in principle, to determine the actual mass of plasmin released into the circulation. Such estimates coupled with estimates of plasmin action may be the key to determining whether the plasmin is in some way protected from inhibition. The measurement of fibrin(ogen) degradation products is the simplest method to determine *in vivo* plasmin action. In our hands the tanned RBC hemagglutination inhibition immunoassay is the method of choice for clinical diagnosis, but we find that technique to be too imprecise for investigational work. Instead we use a radioimmunoassay, which gives excellent sensitivity in the range of 50 to 5000 ng/ml. We have recently used western blotting in conjunction with radioimmunoassay to measure the total amount and the nature of the fibrinogen-derived material in a variety of subjects. This approach is relatively simple and easy to apply. It is of particular interest in situations where the available sample is severely limited, such as in the investigation of very small infants.[24]

Assays useful for monitoring platelet activation are listed in TABLE 3. The simplest

TABLE 3. Assays Reflecting Platelet Activation

Assay	Reflects:	Commercial Availability
Thromboxane B_2[25]	thromboxane A_2 production	yes
Platelet factor 4[26]	platelet release reaction	yes
β-thromboglobulin[26]	platelet release reaction	yes
Thrombospondin[27]	platelet release reaction	no
Circulating platelet aggregates[28]	platelet activation	no

assay, that for circulating platelet aggregates, is also the most difficult to interpret in pathophysiologic terms. There is little question that this test shows reproducible differences between individuals, but it is not so clear that aggregates of platelets actually circulate. Platelets generate and release thromboxane A_2 when they are stimulated. This thromboxane A_2 is rapidly degraded in plasma to its stable hydrolysis product thromboxane B_2. Immunoassays for this prostanoid appear to overestimate the amount present in plasma. Measurements by gas chromatography combined with mass spectrometry give levels an order of magnitude less than the levels found by immunoassay. In light of these data, it is difficult to recommend the immunoassay of thromboxane B_2 as an index of platelet activation.

The platelet alpha granules contain many proteins, and three of these, platelet factor 4, β-thromboglobulin, and thrombospondin, appear to be specific to the platelet. Heparin infusion markedly affects the clearance of platelet factor 4 from plasma, while bolus injections of heparin cause a rapid rise in plasma concentration. This rise is thought to be due to displacement of platelet factor 4 from endothelial cell surface heparin-like molecules. The kidney clears β-thromboglobulin from the circulation and its level is markedly increased in the plasma of patients with renal failure. Unlike platelet factor 4 however, it is not influenced by the administration of heparin. A degree of confusion surrounds the platelet alpha granule proteins since β-thromboglobulin is one of three closely related, immunologically cross-reacting proteins. These proteins are low affinity platelet factor 4, platelet basic protein, and β-thromboglobulin. Low affinity platelet factor 4 is not related to platelet factor 4. Thrombospondin is the platelet-specific alpha granule protein for which an assay has been developed most recently. Insufficient data has been accumulated to judge its usefulness as an index of platelet activation.

SUMMARY

Assays are available that allow the careful and wary investigator to use blood samples to derive useful information about hemostatic system activity. In practice the validity of the data will depend in very large part on the care which is taken in sample collection and processing. The particular system being studied profoundly influences the way in which the study should be performed. The details of the interacting issues are not yet resolved, and can only be dealt with as caveats. Finally and most importantly, these assays can not and should not be used to make the diagnosis of thrombosis. We believe that in general their use should be restricted to studies of pathophysiology. They are tools of exquisite sensitivity and specificity that allow us to probe the thrombotic process, and with care and imagination perhaps thrombogenesis itself.

REFERENCES

1. KAPLAN, K. L. & J. OWEN. 1986. Blood tests in the diagnosis of venous thrombosis. *In* Diagnosis and Treatment of Deep Venous Thrombosis. Methods in Hematology. J. Hirsh, Ed: 77–102. Livingstone. New York.
2. ROSENBERG, R. & P. DAMUS. 1973. The purification and mechanism of action of human antithrombin-heparin cofactor. J. Biol. Chem. **248:** 6490–6503.
3. YUDELMAN, I. M., H. L. NOSSEL, K. L. KAPLAN & J. HIRSH. 1978. Plasma fibrinopeptide A levels in symptomatic venous thromboembolism. Blood **51:** 1189–1195.
4. LIU, C. Y., H. L. NOSSEL & K. L. KAPLAN. 1979. The binding of thrombin by fibrin. J. Biol. Chem. **254:** 10421–10425.
5. FLEISS, J. L. 1986. The Design and Analysis of Clinical Experiments. Wiley. New York.
6. WILNER, G. D., H. L. NOSSEL, R. E. CANFIELD & V. P. BUTLER, JR. 1976. Immunochemical studies of human fibrinopeptide A using synthetic peptide homologues. Biochemistry **15:** 1209–1213.
7. EHRLICH, P. H. & W. R. MOYLE. 1983. Cooperative immunoassays: Ultrasensitive assays with mixed monoclonal antibodies. Science **221:** 279–281.
8. NOSSEL, H. L., I. YUDELMAN, R. E. CANFIELD, V. P. BUTLER JR, K. SPANONDIS, G. D. WILNER & G. D. QURESHI. 1974. Measurement of fibrinopeptide A in human blood. J. Clin. Invest. **54:** 43–53.
9. ECKARDT, T., H. L. NOSSEL, A. HURLET-JENSEN, K. S. LAGAMMA, J. OWEN & M. AUERBACH. 1981. Measurement of desarginine fibrinopeptide B in human blood. J. Clin. Invest. **67:** 809–816.
10. TEITEL, J. M., K. A. BAUER, H. K. LAU & R. D. ROSENBERG. 1982. Studies of the prothrombin activation pathway utilizing radioimmunoassays for the F2/F1+2 fragment and thrombin-antithrombin complex. Blood **59:** 1086–97.
11. BAUER, K. A., B. L. KASS, D. L. BEELER & R. D. ROSENBERG. 1984. Detection of protein C activation in humans. J. Clin. Invest. **74:** 2033–41.
12. SCHEEFERS-BORCHEL, U., G. MULLER BERGHAUS, P. FUGHE, R. EBERLE & N. HEIMBERGER. 1985. Discrimination between fibrin and fibrinogen by a monoclonal antibody against a synthetic peptide. Proc. Natl. Acad. Sci. U.S.A. **82:** 7091–7095.

13. COLLEN, D., F. DE COCK & M. VERSTRAETE. 1977. Quantitation of thrombin-antithrombin III complexes in human blood. Eur. J. Clin. Invest. **7:** 407–411.
14. NOSSEL, H. L., J. WASSER, K. L. KAPLAN, K. S. LAGAMMA, I. YUDELMAN & R. E. CANFIELD. 1979. Sequence of fibrinogen proteolysis and platelet release after intrauterine infusion by hypertonic saline. J. Clin. Invest. **64:** 1371–1378.
15. KUDRYK, B., D. ROBINSON, C. NETRE, B. HESSEL, M. BLOMBACK & B. BLOMBACK. 1982. Measurement in human blood of fibrinogen/fibrin fragments containing the Bβ15–42 sequence. Thromb. Res. **25:** 277–291.
16. MERSKY, C., G. J. KLEINER & A. J. JOHNSON. 1966. Quantitative estimation of split products of fibrinogen in human serum, relation to diagnosis and treatment. Blood **28:** 1–18.
17. VANDEWATER, L., J. M. CARR, D. ARONSON & J. MCDONAGH. 1986. Analysis of fibrin(ogen) degradation product levels in patients with liver disease. Blood **67:** 1468–1473.
18. WHITAKER, A. N., M. J. ELMS, P. P. MASCI, P. G. BUNDESEN & D. B. RYLATT. 1984. Measurement of cross linked fibrin derivatives in plasma. An immunoassay using monoclonal antibodies. J. Clin. Pathol. **37:** 882–887.
19. ZIELINSKI, A., J. HIRSH, G. STRAUMANIS, C. CARTER, M. GENT, D. L. SACKETT, R. HULL. *et al.* 1982. The diagnostic value of the fibrinogen/fibrin fragment E antigen assay in clinically suspected deep vein thrombosis. Blood **59:** 346–350.
20. GAFFNEY, P. J., F. JOE & M. MAHMOUD. 1980. Giant fibrin fragments derived from crosslinked fibrin: Structure and clinical implications. Thrombosis Research **20:** 647–662.
21. HARPEL, P. 1981. Alpha2-plasmin inhibitor and alpha2-macroglobulin-plasmin complexes in plasma. Quantitation by an enzyme-linked differential antibody immunosorbent assay. J. Clin. Invest. **68:** 46–55.
22. KUDRYK, B., A. ROHOZA, M. AHADI, J. CHIN & M. E. WIEBE. 1983. A monoclonal antibody with ability to distinguish between NH_2-terminal fragments derived from fibrinogen and fibrin. Mol. Immunol. **20:** 1191–200.
23. WEITZ, J. I., J. A. KOEHN, R. E. CANFIELD, S. L. LANDMAN & R. FRIEDMAN. 1986. Development of a radioimmunoassay for the fibrinogen-derived peptide B-beta1–42. Blood **67:** 1014–1022.
24. GREEN, N. S., K. D. FRIEDMAN & J. OWEN. 1985. Fibrinogen related antigen in the capillary blood of newborns (abstract). Thromb. Heamostas. **54:** 255.
25. GRANSTROM, E., H. KILDAHL & B. SAMUELSSON. 1976. Radioimmunoassay for thromboxane B2. Anal. Lett. **9:** 611–627.
26. KAPLAN, K. L. & J. OWEN. 1981. Plasma levels of beta-thromboglobulin and platelet factor 4 as indices of platelet activation in vivo. Blood **57:** 199–202.
27. DAWES, J., K. J. CLEMETSON, G. O. GOGSTAD, J. MCGREGOR, P. CLEZARDIN, C. V. PROWSE & D. S. PEPPER. 1983. A radiommunoassay for thrombospondin, used in a comparative study of thrombospondin, beta-thromboglobulin and platelet factor 4 in healthy volunteers. Thromb. Res. **29:** 569–81.
28. WU, K. K. & J. C. HOAK. 1974. A new method for the quantitative detection of platelet aggregates in patients with arterial insufficiency. Lancet **ii:** 924–926.

Animal Models for the Evolution of Thrombotic Disease[a]

W. JEAN DODDS

Wadsworth Center for Laboratories and Research
New York State Department of Health
Albany, New York 12201

The history of comparative studies utilizing animal models of the human hemorrhagic and thrombotic diseases goes back more than three decades.[1-3] Research with these models over the years has contributed much to our present knowledge of the pathophysiology and biochemistry of hemostasis and thrombosis as well as to the diagnosis, management, and treatment of disease.[2-5] Examples of naturally occurring acquired disease states that have served as models for studying thrombogenesis include: atrial thrombosis and consumption coagulopathy of aged hamsters; spontaneous hypertension and renal disease of fawn-hooded rats; disseminated intravascular coagulation from various causes in a variety of laboratory and domestic animals; parasite-mediated pulmonary thromboembolism secondary to canine heartworm disease; immune-mediated thrombocytopenia and/or hemolytic anemia of dogs, cats, and horses; and age- and sex-related spontaneous platelet aggregation of rats.[3] However, while such naturally occurring disease models often closely mimic analogous human conditions, they usually are difficult to obtain with reliability, consistency, or in sufficient numbers, and are expensive to maintain. As a result, the biomedical community for the most part has had to depend on experimentally induced disease models.[6] Their use, particularly when more invasive types of procedures are involved, presents two main disadvantages: relevancy to diseases of humans may be more difficult to establish or defend, and ethical considerations of the welfare of the animal subjects influence the cost-benefit equation of such research.[7]

Examples of successful experimentally induced thrombotic models are: numerous tumor models in rodents (benzopyrene fibrosarcoma, leukemias, lung carcinoma, sarcomas); the nephrotic syndrome of rats; mechanisms of inducing thrombosis in various laboratory and domestic animals (microembolism, arterial occlusion, venous stasis, diet, epinephrine, mechanical, laser or freezing injury, and homocystine); disseminated intravascular coagulation induced by bacterial sepsis, ADP, thrombin, thromboplastins, endotoxin, and Liquoid; arterio-venous shunts in the larger species; snake-venom-induced von Willebrand factor deficiency; platelet dysfunction induced by various drugs; and complement deficiency from cobra venom factor treatment in rabbits, guinea pigs, and rats.[3]

Three major factors contribute to the success and relevance of experimental models that use animals to define the evolution of thrombic disease in humans: species selected, experimental design, and presence or absence of anticoagulation.[4,6]

[a]This work was supported in part by NIH research grant no. HL09902, awarded by the National Heart, Lung, and Blood Institute, Public Health Service, Department of Health and Human Services.

SPECIES SELECTED

A large body of information is available pertaining to the various aspects of hemostasis in many species.[1,3] Much of this bibliography is obsolete, nonspecific, and contradictory, and few studies systematically compare platelet function, coagulation, and fibrinolysis among species. When species comparisons have been performed, differences in all stages of platelet function have been reported.[5,8,9] Similarly, with respect to coagulation, species differences begin with the earliest phases of coagulation fundamental to surface-plasma interactions, are evident throughout the coagulation cascade, and extend to the fibrinolytic and complement systems as well.[2,4,10] Finally, a virtually unexplored area involves the contribution of the vasculature to species variability.

Factors to be considered in defining and characterizing the species being selected include:

1. Age, sex, lifespan
2. Source, strain (outbred, inbred, random bred, closed colony)
3. Health and nutritional status (viral profile for small laboratory animals, presence of bacterial and parasitic diseases, incidence and type of diseases of aging, and tumor incidence)
4. Acclimated and/or conditioned laboratory animals versus farm, field, raw, or unconditioned animals
5. Environmental factors (housing and temperature requirements)
6. Cost of procurement and maintenance, including reutilization
7. Variability between and within stocks and strains

With respect to the choice of species, humans are preferred subjects whenever their use is possible and appropriate. Human blood is preferable for most *in vitro* testing, although animal blood is useful for some specific, well-defined test systems and conditions.[4,11,12]

Animals and animal bloods are employed for preclinical use testing models, including extracorporeal and *in vivo* systems. In general, the species selected should be relatively large (nonhuman primate, dog, calf, sheep, goat, or pig) so that if devices are intended to be used, they can eventually be tested in this species in the form of intended use. Smaller laboratory animal species (rabbits, cats, guinea pigs, rats) are also useful under special circumstances.[13,14]

Potential species problems exist as well. For example, small laboratory animal species have the advantages of being well-characterized, readily available, and less expensive, but are often too small to obtain sufficient volumes of blood for analysis or for testing of devices in configurational form. Larger species may be less well-defined and standardized, not as readily available, and more expensive to procure and maintain. However, they are preferred for short- and long-term preclinical use testing for reasons listed above.[15,16] Also, some expensive species of limited availability (nonhuman primates) can be effectively recycled for use in more than one project, provided humane considerations are addressed (*i.e.*, animals are not subjected to more than one major survival surgery).

Despite extensive use of the dog for both *in vitro* and *in vivo* studies of thrombogenesis and testing of biomaterials and cardiovascular devices, it may not be the species of choice. The following reasons pertain here: low susceptibility to cardiovascular disease and pulmonary embolism; very active hemostatic and fibrinolytic mechanisms; a hyperplastic vascular response to incitants causing rapid occlusion of vessels; the response of canine platelets to heparin, rendering this anticoagulant undesirable for comparative studies; and the societal pressure applied by public concern over the use of dogs for any type of research. On the other hand, the considerable literature available and experience with the dog as a test species argue persuasively for its continued use.[4,6,16]

EXPERIMENTAL DESIGN

The type and complexity of the test procedure to be used will influence selection of the model.[6-13] One of the most important considerations when working with animals or their blood is the method of handling them during procedures or for collecting and processing samples.[4] Selection of a more tractable species or a calm individual animal will minimize stress and anxiety that can adversely effect the results obtained. Preconditioning or "gentling" the animals to allow them to adapt to the handlers and procedure is clearly beneficial not only to the animals but also to the scientific outcome.[7] Proper collection technique is critical to minimize the activation or contamination of blood samples with thromboplastic materials. Thus, cardiac puncture (under anesthesia) is not a suitable alternative to careful, direct venipuncture or arterial puncture. Any use of anesthetics or tranquilizers should be noted and controlled, as these drugs may themselves alter the behavior of blood components. In small rodents blood is best collected by abdominal sampling from the vena cava or aorta of the anesthetized subject. When native blood is to be used, it is essential that collection techniques minimize tissue trauma. The preferred way to obtain anticoagulated specimens involves first placing the required amount of anticoagulant into the syringe and then withdrawing the appropriate volume of blood from the animal. Rapid blood flow is desirable, as is immediate mixing after collection.

TYPE AND NEED FOR ANTICOAGULATION

Most animal blood coagulates rapidly, a situation that usually precludes working with native whole blood or its components.[4,14,17] Despite this problem, it is preferable to use native blood test systems whenever possible in order to avoid the artifacts created by anticoagulation.[4-6] Basic studies of the mechanisms of thrombogenesis are best carried out in a normocalcemic environment to parallel the natural biological condition, whether the test system used involves *in vitro*, *ex vivo*, or *in vivo* methodologies. One such model developed in our laboratory utilizes native whole rabbit blood to assess blood-materials interactions.[12] This bioassay uses a standardized inbred strain of large rabbits, prelabels blood platelets *in vivo* with [^{14}C]serotonin prior to study (a very sensitive indicator of platelet-surface interaction which effects release of the radiolabel), and employs a standard column of glass beads to provide a large surface area for perturbation of the native arterial blood collected after a variety of known or potentially biocompatible or incompatible challenges.

While specialized systems like that described above have been developed and successfully exploited, most investigations are carried out for convenience, or by necessity, on anticoagulated blood or in anticoagulated animals. Nevertheless, the repsonse of different animal species to anticoagulants such as heparin and citrate varies widely.[4-6] For example, various heparins cause platelet aggregation or thrombocytopenia in many species, including man. Rabbits, dogs, cats, and guinea pigs are the most susceptible to the *in vitro* and *in vivo* effects of the anticoagulant. In contrast, mouse, rat and hamster platelets are relatively nonreactive to heparin. Problems related to species also exist with citrate, as the optimum concentration required to anticoagulate blood for platelet and coagulation studies varies. Citrate concentration is known to affect platelet reactivity, and most animal species require a high final concentration (0.32% to 0.38% is compatible with all species).

SUMMARY

Naturally occurring hemorrhagic and thrombotic diseases of animals closely parallel their human counterparts. While such models may be particularly useful in studying the pathogenesis of human disease, it is usually more realistic to depend upon experimentally induced disease models. The species selected for use is therefore of major importance in providing meaningful extrapolation to humans, as are the experimental design and type of procedure (*in vitro*, *ex vivo*, *in vivo*).

Regardless of the test system used when *in vitro* procedures are employed, these must be translated eventually to the *in vivo* situation. Information about the normal aging process of different species is important here and should influence selection of the species and test system. The ideal situation may not be feasible or pertain because of cost, availability, size, and investigator familiarity, or lack thereof, with the most suitable species or model.

REFERENCES

1. ROWSELL, H. C. 1968. The hemostatic mechanism of mammals and birds in health and disease. Adv. Vet. Sci. Comp. Med. **12:** 337–410.
2. DODDS, W. J. 1974. Hereditary and acquired hemorrhagic disorders in animals. *In* Progress in Hemostasis and Thrombosis, Vol. 2. T. H. Spaet, Ed.: 215–247. Grune & Stratton. New York.
3. DODDS, W. J. 1981. Second international registry of animal models of thrombosis and hemorrhagic diseases. ILAR News **24:** R3-R50. National Academy of Sciences. Washington, D.C.
4. DODDS, W. J. 1980. Species effects in testing materials and cardiovascular devices in experimental animals. *In* Guidelines for Blood-Materials Interactions. R. G. Mason, Ed.: 9–18. PHS/DHHS Publication No. 80-2185. National Institutes of Health. Bethesda, MD.
5. DODDS, W. J. 1977. Platelet function in animals: Species specificities. *In* Platelets: A Multi-disciplinary Approach. G. de Gaetano & S. Garattini, Eds.: 45–59. Raven. New York.
6. DODDS, W. J. 1982. Animal models for testing vascular prostheses. *In* Biologic and Synthetic Vascular Prostheses. J. C. Stanley, Ed.: 249–255. Grune & Stratton. New York.
7. DODDS, W. J. & F. B. ORLANS. 1982. Scientific Perspectives on Animal Welfare. Academic. New York.
8. ADDONIZIO, V. P., JR., L. H. EDMUNDS, JR. & R. W. COLMAN. 1978. The function of monkey (*M. mulatta*) platelets compared to platelets of pig, sheep, and man. J. Lab. Clin. Med. **91:** 989–997.
9. LEACH, C. M. & G. D. THORBURN. 1982. A comparative study of collagen induced thromboxane release from platelets of different species: Implications for human atherosclerosis models. Prostaglandins **24:** 47–59.
10. MASON, R. G. & M. S. READ. 1971. Some species differences in fibrinolysis and blood coagulation. J. Biomed. Mater. Res. **5:** 121–128.
11. TODD, M. E., E. MCDEVITT & E. I. GOLDSMITH. 1972. Blood clotting mechanisms of nonhuman primates: Choice of the baboon model to simulate man. J. Med. Primatol. **1:** 132–141.

12. Dodds, W. J., J. M. Dinovo & J. A. Bergeron. 1981. A native whole blood assay for blood-materials interaction. Thromb. Haemostas. **45:**122–127.
13. Bruck, S. D. 1977. Consideration of species-related hematological differences in the evaluation of biomaterials. Biomater. Med. Dev. Artif. Organs **5:** 97–113.
14. Saunders, R. N. 1982. Evaluation of platelet-inhibiting drugs in models of atherosclerosis. Ann. Rev. Pharmacol. Toxicol. **22:** 279–295.
15. Hanson, S. R., L. A. Harker, B. D. Ratner & A. S. Hoffman. 1980. In vivo evaluation of artificial surfaces with a nonhuman primate model of arterial thrombosis. J. Lab. Clin. Med. **95:** 289–304.
16. Dewanjee, M. K., M. P. Kaye, V. Fuster & S. A. Rao. 1980. Noninvasive radioisotopic technique for detection of platelet deposition in mitral valve prothesis and renal microembolism in dogs. Trans. Am. Soc. Artif. Intern. Organs **26:** 475–480.
17. Reyers, I., L. Mussoni, M. B. Donati & G. De Gaetano. 1981. Severe thrombocytopenia delays but does not prevent the occlusion of an arterial prosthesis in rats. Thromb. Haemostas. **46:** 558–560.

Appropriate Animal Models for Research on Blood in Contact with Artificial Surfaces

CHERYL F. SCOTT

Temple University
Thrombosis Research Center
Philadelphia, Pennsylvania 19140

In order to develop less thrombogenic biomaterials, it is essential to understand the mechanism of the interactions of blood with artificial surfaces. Furthermore, since there are quantitative and qualitative differences between species, it is important to select the most appropriate animal model so that the knowledge gained from these experiments can be successfully applied to human clinical situations. In this report, I will focus on the contact activation system.

Briefly, the contact system is composed of three zymogens (factor XII, factor XI, and prekallikrein) and the procofactor, high molecular weight kininogen (HMWK). When plasma contacts an artificial surface, the zymogen factor XII is converted to an active enzyme (FIGURE 1). Activated factor XII (XIIa) then activates prekallikrein and factor XI on the surface after they are transported there by HMWK.[1] Kallikrein can then generate additional XIIa by a positive feedback reaction.[1] Each of these reactions is strictly controlled by plasma protease inhibitors as well as by *in vivo* clearance mechanisms. For a more detailed description of contact activation, see Colman *et al.*[2] (this volume).

Contact activation occurs on every artificial surface that has been tested to date, although the rate of activation differs among surfaces. The surface itself may display a higher affinity for contact proteins than for protease inhibitors, thereby allowing a high degree of local surface activation to occur. The consequence of these reactions would be activation of intrinsic coagulation with eventual formation of fibrin, as well as stimulation of platelets and neutrophils by kallikrein and XIIa. These reactions all lead to thrombogenesis and/or activation of the complement system.

The contact activation system in dogs, rabbits, seals,[3] and cows[4] is markedly different from human, rat, monkey, and pig.[3] Activation of factor XII is slower in the former group and the reactions are incomplete, due to the greater efficiency of plasma protease inhibitors. Therefore, the effects of extensive contact activation that might occur in humans exposed to certain artificial surfaces could possibly be missed if dog, seal, rabbit, or cow were used as animal models. *In vitro* models, even if they employ human blood, lack *in vivo* clearance mechanisms and are artificially anticoagulated. Therefore, one must cautiously interpret results obtained with such a system.

The interchange of plasma proteins on artificial surfaces (the Vroman effect)[5] primarily involves the displacement of fibrinogen by HMWK.[6,7] Our recent evidence[8,9] indicates that HMWK must be activated to HMWKa[10] (which happens via factor-XII-dependent contact activation) before this displacement can occur. Therefore, differences between the contact system of humans and certain animals used in experiments could lead to erroneous conclusions concerning the efficacy and safety of the biomaterial in question. For example, in the dog, contact activation is slower and less complete than in humans and fibrinogen from dog blood remains on the surface longer than fibrinogen from human blood, because HMWK is activated more slowly in the former. Furthermore, since platelets only adhere to artificial surfaces on which a layer of fibrinogen has been adsorbed,[11] dog platelets would be expected to adhere to the surface longer, resulting in an interaction that would greatly differ from human blood exposed to the same surface. Moreover, human blood, when exposed to cuprophane, deposits leukocytes whereas canine blood does not.[12] This observation could also be the result of activation of leukocytes by active contact factors.

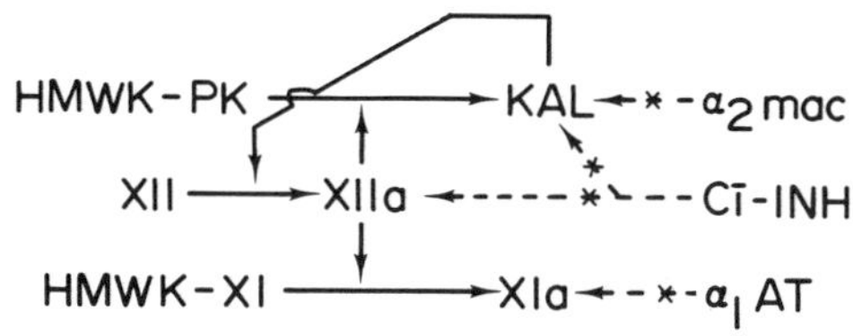

FIGURE 1. The contact activation system: *PK,* prekallikrein; *KAL,* kallikrein; *XII,* factor XII; *XIIa,* activated factor XII; *XI,* factor XI; *XIa,* activated factor XI; *C$\bar{1}$-INH,* C$\bar{1}$ inhibitor; α_2*mac,* α_2 macroglobulin; α_1 *AT,* α_1 antitrypsin; *HMWK,* high molecular weight kininogen. *Solid arrows* indicate activation, *dashed arrows (with cross)* denote inhibition.

In summary, the interaction of blood components with artificial surfaces exhibits species variation. Furthermore, *in vitro* systems, although they may utilize human blood components, do not possess clearance mechanisms. Therefore, care must be taken in selecting the appropriate animal model for each application, and caution must be exercised in interpreting results from animal or *in vitro* experiments before applying this information to clinical use in humans. Moreover, it is essential for all investigators involved in research on blood in contact with artificial surfaces (biochemists, biomedical engineers, physiologists, cardiovascular surgeons, hematologists, and others) to communicate on a regular basis in order to understand the strengths and pitfalls of each other's research.

REFERENCES

1. COLMAN, R. W. 1984. J. Clin. Invest. **73:** 1249–1253.
2. COLMAN, R. W., C. F. SCOTT, A. H. SCHMAIER, Y. T. WACHTFOGEL, R. A. PIXLEY & L. H. EDMUNDS, JR. 1987. This volume.
3. GREEN, J. G., R. C. TALAMO & R. W. COLMAN. 1974. Am. J. Physiol. **226:** 784–790.
4. SUGO, T., A. HAMAGUCHI, T. SHIMADA, H. KATO & S. IWANAGA. 1982. J. Biochem. **92:** 689–698.
5. VROMAN, L. 1964. Thromb. Diath. Haemorrh. **10:** 445–493.
6. VROMAN, L., A. L. ADAMS, G. C. FISCHER & P. C. MUNOZ. 1980. Blood **55:** 156–159.
7. SCHMAIER, A. H., L. SILVER, A. L. ADAMS, G. C. FISCHER, P. C. MUNOZ, L. VROMAN & R. W. COLMAN. 1983. Thromb. Res. **33:** 51–67.
8. BRASH, J. L., C. F. SCOTT, P. TEN HOVE & R. W. COLMAN. 1985. Abstract. Trans. Soc. Biomater. **8:** 105.
9. SCOTT, C. F., J. L. BRASH, P. TEN HOVE, P. WOJCIECHOWSKI & R. W. COLMAN. 1987. Thromb. Haemostas. **58(1):** 33 (abstract).
10. SCOTT, C. F., L. D. SILVER, M. SCHAPIRA & R. W. COLMAN. 1984. J. Clin. Invest. **73:** 954–962.
11. ZUCKER, M. B. & L. VROMAN. 1969. Proc. Soc. Exp. Biol. Med. **131:** 320.
12. SCHWARTZ, A., K. H. STENZEL, I. KOHNO, D. AST, T. MIYATA & A. L. RUBIN. 1975. J. Biomed. Mater. Res. **9:** 453.

Thromboembolic and Infectious Complications of Total Artificial Heart Implantation

RICHARD A. WARD,[a] SAMUEL R. WELLHAUSEN,[a]
JOANNE J. DOBBINS,[b] GEORGE S. JOHNSON,[c]
AND WILLIAM C. DEVRIES[d]

[a]Division of Nephrology
School of Medicine
University of Louisville
Louisville, Kentucky 40292
[b]Department of Biology
Bellarmine College
Louisville, Kentucky 40205
[c]Department of Pathology
[d]Humana Heart Institute International
Humana Hospital Audubon
Louisville, Kentucky 40217

INTRODUCTION

Treatment of end-stage heart disease presents a major therapeutic challenge. Although the advent of the immunosuppressive drug cyclosporin has given a major boost to cardiac transplantation, the number of donor hearts available continues to limit severely the number of patients who can be treated by this modality.[1] In the last 4 years use of a total artificial heart, both as a short-term bridge between failure of the patient's natural heart and transplantation and as a long-term replacement for cardiac function, has been attempted with increasing frequency in a number of centers. In the majority of cases, the total artificial heart has been used as a bridge to cardiac transplantation. However, in six cases it has been used for long-term replacement of cardiac function. In these six cases, patients were maintained for periods of time ranging from 112 to 620 days. The courses of most of these patients were complicated by thromboembolism and/or infection.[2-4] Indeed, sepsis was a contributing factor in the demise of five of the patients. In this paper, we review the thromboembolic and infectious complications that occurred in two of these patients. We discuss how the two problems may interrelate and some maneuvers that may ameliorate the problems in subsequent long-term implantation of an artificial heart.

PATIENTS

The following discussion is based on the cases of two patients who received permanent implants of a total artificial heart (Jarvik-7, 100 ml stroke volume, Symbion Inc., Salt Lake City, UT). At the time of implantation both patients were class IV according to the New York Heart Association classification and were deemed unsuitable for cardiac transplantation; death was imminent. A summary of the patients and key events in their postoperative courses are presented in TABLE 1. Detailed case histories have been presented elsewhere.[4]

THROMBOEMBOLIC COMPLICATIONS

Cerebrovascular accidents (CVAs) occurred in both patients (TABLE 1). Three of the CVAs were thromboembolic in nature as demonstrated by CT scan or arteriogram, a fourth was hemorrhagic, and the etiology of the fifth was uncertain. These findings were later confirmed at autopsy. Possible origins for the emboli were also evident at autopsy, when thrombi were found around the valves of the artificial heart and at the anastomoses between the heart and the patient's blood vessels; the chambers of the hearts were free of thrombi. With one exception, the pulmonary valve in patient 2, all valves and anastomotic junctions showed evidence of thrombus formation. A typical example is shown in FIGURE 1. Histological examination of the thrombi showed them to be of mixed coagulation type with lines of Zahn (FIG. 2) and in some cases evidence of organization, suggesting that they had been present in the device for some time.

TABLE 1. Demographic Data and Clinical Courses of Patients

	Patient 1	Patient 2
Sex	M	M
Age	54	58
Primary diagnosis	chronic ischemic heart disease	dilated congestive idiopathic cardiomyopathy
Secondary diagnoses	diabetes (type II) renal insufficiency (serum creatinine, 0.14 mmol/l) malnourished	chronic obstructive pulmonary disease renal insufficiency (serum creatinine, 0.18 mmol/l) malnourished
Length of implant	620 days	488 days
Complications	acute tubular necrosis (3–5)[a] cerebral vascular accidents: thromboembolic (19,352), hemorrhagic (163), etiology unknown (620) recurrent infections hemolysis (1–196) progressive decline in renal function	acute tubular necrosis (4–14) hemothorax (11–14) respiratory insufficiency (30–488) thromboembolic cerebral vascular accident (107) recurrent infections hemolysis (1–116)
Cause of death	respiratory failure sepsis	renal failure sepsis

[a]Numbers indicate days postimplantation.

Thrombus formation has been described in similar locations in other patients implanted with Jarvik-7 artificial hearts as bridges to transplantation[5,6] as well as in animal studies.[7] In one of these cases[5] the patient also developed a transient neurological deficit. In addition, a mild CVA has been reported in one other patient maintained with the Penn State total artificial heart.[8] Neurological damage is rarely reported as a significant complication in animal trials. However, the majority of these studies have been performed in calves and the anatomy of the calf differs from that of man. Blood flow to the brain of the calf passes through an anatomical structure, the rete mirabile, which may serve to filter out emboli before they reach the brain. On the other hand, renal infarction has been reported to occur commonly in calves following artificial heart implantation,[9] suggesting that thromboemboli do occur in these animals.

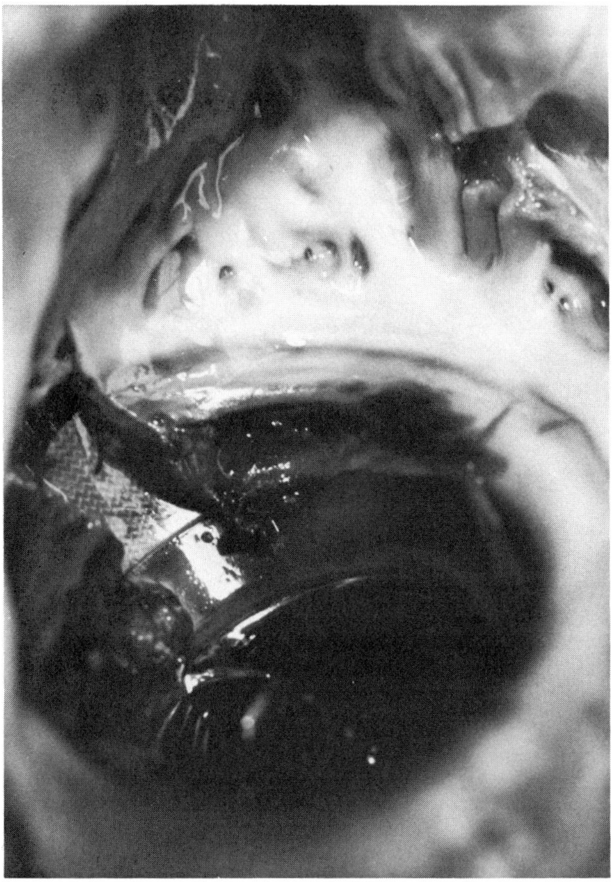

FIGURE 1. Superior view of the tricuspid valve from patient 1 at autopsy showing thrombus formation at the junction between the atrial cuff and the polycarbonate mounting ring of the valve.

The pathogenesis of thrombus formation in the artificial heart is undoubtedly multifactorial. Contributing factors may include the geometry and flow dynamics of the device, the anticoagulation regimen used, and concomitant medical problems such as infection. Crevices and other surface discontinuities can serve as nidi for thrombus formation. The present design of the Jarvik-7 contains a number of crevices and discontinuities associated with the four Medtronic-Hall valves and the manner in

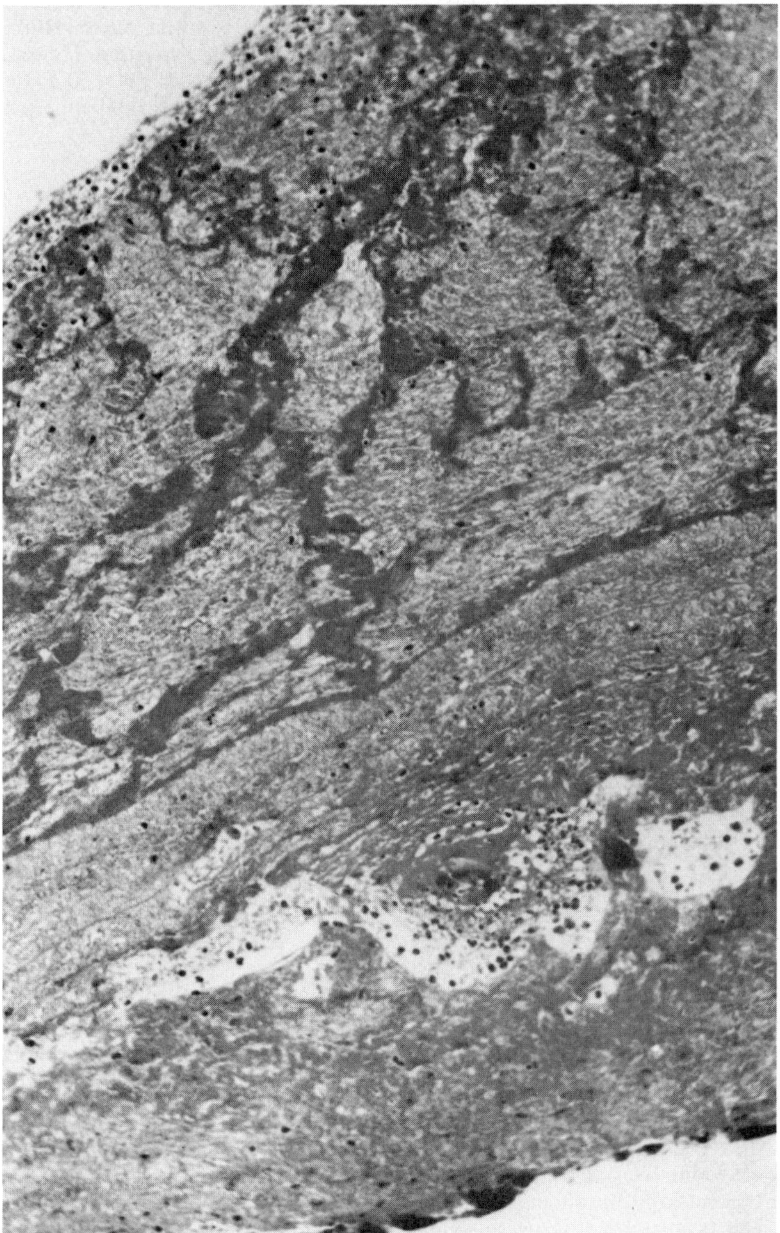

FIGURE 2. Photomicrograph of a mixed coagulation thrombus from the pulmonic valve from patient 1 showing lines of Zahn. Hematoxylin and eosin stain; magnification: 10×.

which they are incorporated into the Jarvik-7.[5] An analysis of flow through the device also demonstrates that these areas are associated with eddy formation and stagnant flow (FIG. 3), which may further predispose to thrombus formation. Indeed, these were the areas in which thrombi were observed in this (FIG. 1) and other[5] studies. Thromboembolism is also a complication of prosthetic valve implantation. However, the incidence with the Medtronic-Hall valve is low (2.1 episodes per 100 patient years[10]) compared with that experienced in our patients (5 episodes in 3 patient years), suggesting involvement of other factors.

In most artificial organs, the degree to which thrombus formation occurs is a

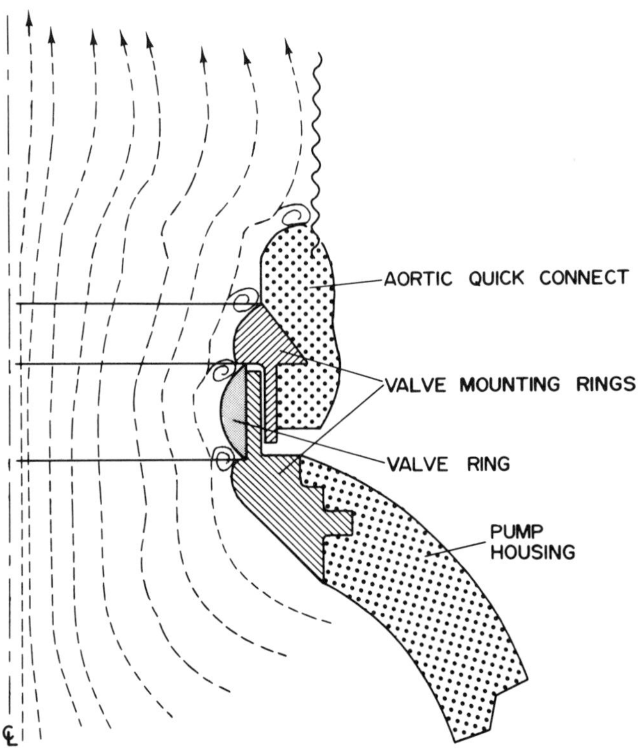

FIGURE 3. Schematic of valve housing showing streamlines and sites of eddy formation. (Courtesy of Symbion, Inc.)

function of the materials in contact with the blood and the anticoagulation regimen used. A well-defined anticoagulation regimen has yet to be developed for the total artificial heart. Our patients were treated with various combinations of warfarin, heparin, dipyridamole, and aspirin. The aim of anticoagulant therapy was to achieve a prolongation in the prothrombin and partial thromboplastin times 1.5 to 2 times that of control. The antiplatelet drugs were added as deemed necessary, based on changes in platelet count and plasma levels of platelet factor 4 and β-thromboglobulin. Details of the evolution of these regimens and their efficacy have been described in detail elsewhere.[11]

In the week prior to the initial CVA in patient 1, the partial thromboplastin time was not elevated above control (ratio of patient to control in the range 0.93 to 1.11). The partial thromboplastin time was also somewhat below the target range in patient 2 during the 2 weeks prior to his CVA, the average ratio of patient to control being 1.21. These data suggest that inadequate anticoagulation may have played a role in these events. The difficulty with long-term anticoagulation in these patients is that intercurrent events may adversely affect what was previously an adequate anticoagulation regimen. For example, initiation of Tegretol therapy for seizure control in patient 1 led to a precipitous decrease in platelet count (from 300,000 to 50,000 μl^{-1}). This, in turn, probably led to the hemorrhagic CVA that occurred in this patient. In addition, Levinson *et al.*[5] have described the development of a hypercoaguable state, possibly due to surgical stress, that may have led to the embolic CVA in their patient. These two events underscore the difficulty in maintaining the balance between insufficient anticoagulation, with the risk of thromboembolism, and excessive anticoagulation, with the risk of hemorrhage. Nevertheless, at the time of the other thromboembolic CVAs in patient 1, the prothrombin and partial thromboplastin times were within the target range. This suggests that other factors may also be involved in the thromboembolic process, among which may be the infectious complications described in the following section.

INFECTIOUS COMPLICATIONS

The courses of both patients were punctuated by repeated infections. Positive cultures were obtained on many occasions from multiple sites, including blood, tracheal secretions, urine, sputum, chest tube drainage, and from the drive line exit sites. The dominant organism in patient 1 was *Staphylococcus epidermidis*. In patient 2 *Pseudomonas* species, in particular *Pseudomonas aeruginosa* and *Pseudomonas maltophilia*, predominated. Details of these infections have been given elsewhere.[12] Significantly, all four CVAs in patient 1 were associated with clusters of positive blood cultures. The single CVA in patient 2 occurred at a time when blood cultures were negative; however, the sites of infection in this patient were predominantly extravascular.

These data suggest an association between infection and the thromboembolic events. Further evidence of this association was gained from cultures and histologic examination of thrombi obtained from both artificial hearts at autopsy. All cultures of thrombi taken from patient 1 were positive for *Staphylococcus epidermidis* and/or *Candida albicans*. The thrombi in the artificial heart from patient 2 were positive for *Pseudomonas* species, except for the thrombus superior to the pulmonary valve, which was culture negative. Histological examination of these thrombi confirmed the presence of the organisms. For example, FIGURE 4 shows the presence of bacterial colonies deep in the thrombus from the atrial anastomosis in patient 1 as revealed by a Brown and Brenn stain. These results demonstrate that both patients developed subacute bacterial endocarditis of their artificial hearts. Infected thrombi are also a frequent finding in animals implanted with total artificial hearts.[13] Once bacteria become enmeshed in a thrombus, they are less susceptible to attack by host defense mechanisms.[14] Further, such infections may exacerbate thrombus formation. There is some evidence that *Staphylococcus epidermidis* may secrete procoagulant enzymes,[15] and *Pseudomonas aeruginosa* secretes exotoxin A, which may promote platelet aggregation.[16]

Apart from the thrombi described above, two other areas associated with infection in both patients were the regions around the drive lines at their point of exit through the

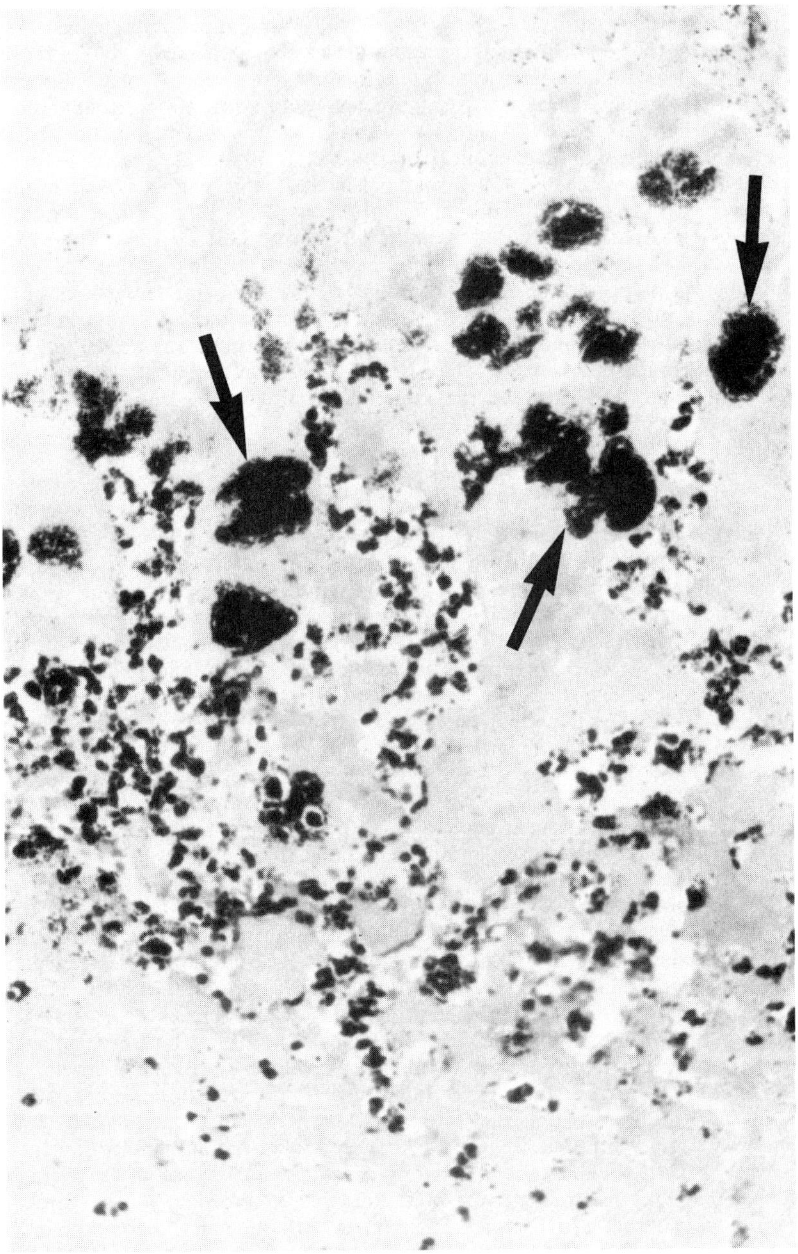

FIGURE 4. Photomicrograph of thrombus from the atrial anastomosis in patient 1. *Arrows* indicate examples of bacterial colonies as revealed by Brown and Brenn stain; magnification: 25×.

skin and the pseudopericardial sac that developed around the artificial heart. Infections of the drive line exit sites were evident in both patients at various times throughout their courses. A drive line abscess was noted in patient 1 on day 65. The abscess was subsequently drained and appeared to resolve; however, at autopsy, an abscess was found associated with the right drive line distal to the artificial heart. Patient 2 developed a drive line abscess about day 100, which was also subsequently drained. This abscess did not completely resolve and at autopsy abscesses were found around the distal portions of both drive lines. Similar drive line infections have been reported as a frequent complication in animal[13] and other clinical[3,17] studies.

Numerous CT scans throughout the courses of both patients failed to reveal the mediastinal infections in either patient. Nevertheless, widespread and apparently long-standing infection was found around the artificial heart in both patients. Deep-seated infection of the area around the artificial heart with *Staphylococcus aureus* was also found in another patient maintained with a Jarvik-7 total artificial heart for 247 days.[3] In contrast, another patient showed no signs of device-related infection after 112 days of implantation in spite of the occurrence of positive blood cultures.[2] The data, to date, suggest that infection of the external surface of the artificial heart will occur frequently, given a sufficiently long period of implantation.

Infection of the mediastinum is a significant complication that may limit the useful life of a total artificial heart. There are several possible routes by which this infection may have been introduced. One obvious route is the break in the mechanical barrier associated with the drive lines, particularly since both patients experienced abscesses around the drive line sites. Migration along the drive lines has been suggested as the mechanism of mediastinal infection in one patient,[3] as has migration along pressure monitoring lines in cases of mediastinal infection reported in animal studies.[13] To examine the role of the drive lines in the infectious process in our patients, the drive lines were carefully isolated and sectioned serially into 0.5-cm transverse sections at autopsy using sterile technique.[18] Each section was then cultured. While the sections of drive line adjacent to the artificial heart and at the skin exit site cultured positive, the midsection of both drive lines from each patient were essentially organism free. An example of the culture results for one drive line is shown in FIGURE 5. The other drive lines showed similar patterns.[18] Further, the biotypes of the organisms isolated from the proximal and distal sections of the drive lines were different. These data suggest that mediastinal infections did not arise from migration of organisms up the drive line.

Infection may also have developed via hematogenous, transpulmonary, or urinary tract routes. It is likely that all three played a role in our patients. There were several opportunities for the introduction of blood-borne infections; these included the use of central monitoring lines and multiple venipunctures for blood sampling. The transpulmonary route was probably an important pathway in patient 2. A small pneumothorax during the process of draining blood from the pleural cavity may have led to infection of this area. Finally, the first positive cultures of the *Candida* species found in both patients at autopsy were in the urine, suggesting that the urinary tract may have been the route of introduction of these organisms.

Why did these infections become so overwhelming that they ultimately became a major factor in the demise of the patients? Foreign bodies, such as the artificial heart, are considered to facilitate the development of infection. The exact mechanisms by which this occurs are not fully understood; however, a number of factors are thought to play a role.[19,20] These include encapsulation of the foreign body by fibrous tissue, adherence of bacteria to the implanted materials, and enhancement of bacterial growth and/or inhibition of host defense mechanisms by the implanted materials or their breakdown products. Considering that a major site of infection was the poorly

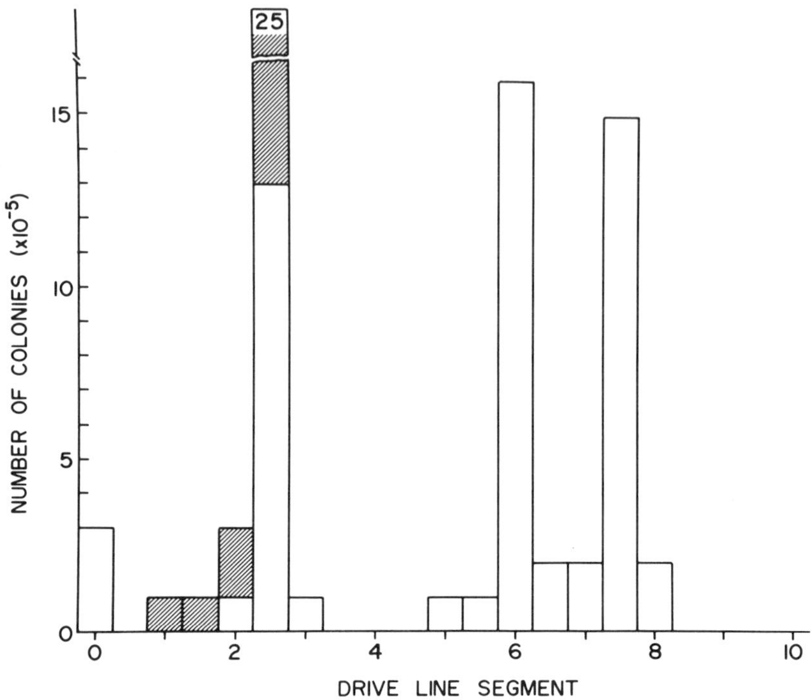

FIGURE 5. Distribution of organisms along the left drive line from patient 1. No anaerobic bacteria and essentially no fungi were cultured. The skin interface corresponds to segment 0 and the junction with the drive line to the artificial heart corresponds to segment 10. The *open bars* represent the drive line and the *hatched bars* the skin button.

vascularized area between the artificial heart and its surrounding fibrous capsule, it might be speculated that an inability of the body's host defense mechanisms to gain access to the organisms sequestered in this area may have been an important problem. Access to the device-associated infections may have been further compromised by the development of a protective biofilm over the organisms (particularly evident on the drive lines). The Velcro® snaps used to join the two halves of the Jarvik-7 were found to be substantially digested at autopsy, suggesting that the materials of the device may have served as substrate for bacterial adhesion and proliferation. Destruction of the Velcro may have been exacerbated by oxidants released by invading neutrophils.

Compromise of host defense mechanisms may also have contributed to the failure of the patients to adequately handle their infections. Indeed, decreased neutrophil phagocytic activity has been reported in animals following artificial heart implantation.[21] However, serum complement and polymorphonuclear leukocyte function remained intact in our patients.[22,23] In contrast, both patients did become B and T lymphopenic and demonstrated a decrease in their ratios of helper-inducer to suppressor-cytotoxic cells,[22] suggesting that there may have been suppression of the lymphoid elements of their immune systems. Further support for this was obtained at autopsy, when histologic examination of lymphoid tissues revealed reduced numbers of germinal centers and depletion of T-lymphocyte-containing areas.[23] Nevertheless, we were able to demonstrate, using an ELISA technique,[24] that patient 2 produced antibodies against the principal organism with which he was infected, *Pseudomonas aeruginosa* (FIG. 6). However, he was apparently unable to produce antibody against *Pseudomonas maltophilia*, with which he subsequently became infected,[23] suggesting that the ability to mount a response to an antigenic challenge may have decreased with time. We were unable to examine the ability to produce antibody in patient 1 using the ELISA technique because of nonspecific binding to protein A found on the surface of *Staphylococcus epidermidis*. Histologic examination of tissue obtained from both

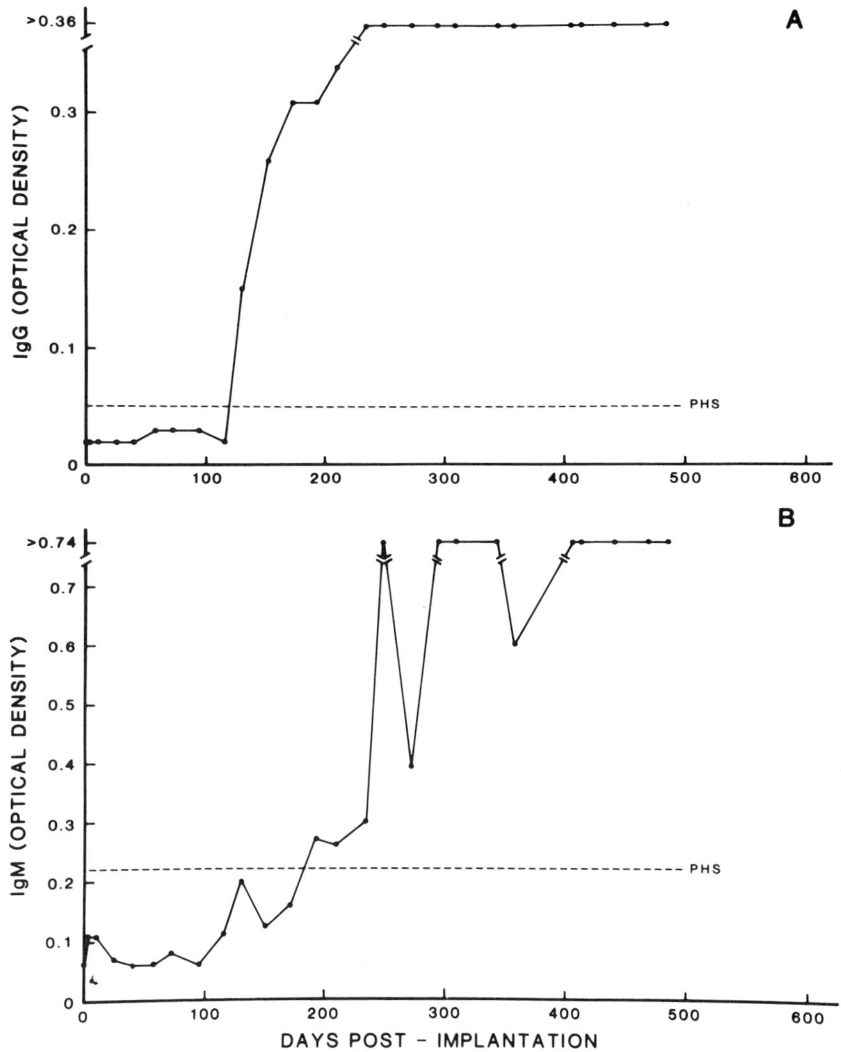

FIGURE 6. Serum concentrations of (**A**) IgG and (**B**) IgM antibodies against *Pseudomonas aeruginosa* in patient 2. Antibody levels in pooled human serum (PHS) are indicated by horizontal lines.

patients at autopsy showed significant hemosiderin deposits in their reticuloendothelial cells (that is, secondary hemochromatosis). These deposits were widespread, involving the lymph nodes, liver, spleen, bone marrow, lung, and brain. It seems likely that this hemochromatosis led to a blockade of the reticuloendothelial system (RES), resulting in the progressive loss of lymphoidal elements, and compromised the ability of the patient to respond to bacterial infections.[23]

Depression of RES function has previously been reported in animals following prolonged blood pumping,[25] and RES blockade in our patients may have been exacerbated, at least in part, by destruction of blood elements by the Jarvik-7. Impairment of RES function by blood transfusions[26] and hemolysis[27] has been well documented. In the initial period following implantation (days 1–196 and days 1–116 in patients 1 and 2, respectively) the dP/dt of the drive system of the artificial heart resulted in continued shear-related hemolysis, necessitating frequent blood transfusions.[22] The volume of blood transfused in the period was further increased by bleeding episodes in both patients.[4] RES blockade may have been exacerbated by complement activation associated with high dP/dt of the drive system[22] as well as by thrombogenic processes through the generation of microthrombi.[28]

SUMMARY

Thromboembolic and infectious events were found to be major complications of long-term total artificial heart implantation in two patients. Similar complications have been reported in other patients, as well as in animal studies. The thromboembolic events and the infectious complications appear to be interrelated. On the one hand, thrombi located on the valves and at the vascular anastomoses of the artificial heart were found to be infected at autopsy; such infections are known to exacerbate formation of thromboemboli. On the other hand, the generation of microthrombi may have contributed to the RES blockade seen in our patients. We hypothesize that this RES blockade led to a progressive decrease in lymphoid system function and impaired the patients' capacity to clear microorganisms from the circulation. These phenomena arose, in part, from the design of the artificial heart and were exacerbated by associated therapy, such as blood transfusions.

Our data suggest several measures that might be taken in order to reduce the severity of both the thrombogenic and infectious complications. Improved anticoagulation regimens, which increase the ability of the physician to maintain the proper balance between thrombotic and hemorrhagic potential, are needed. This may require not only improved methods of monitoring anticoagulation and predicting changes in the effectiveness of various agents as other events supervene, but also new anticoagulant and antithrombotic drugs, for example, low molecular weight heparins and prostacyclin derivatives. It is also clear that the design of the artificial heart should be modified in order to improve fluid dynamics so that they will approximate as closely as possible those of the natural heart. This includes redesigning the mounting of the valves to eliminate crevices and discontinuities that allow stagnant flow and predispose to thrombus formation as well as imposing a dP/dt that minimizes shear-related hemolysis, thereby minimizing the need for blood transfusions. Prevention of infections presents a more difficult problem. Transcutaneous lines (regardless of their use) are an obvious route for infection, and attention should be given to minimizing the number and length of use of monitoring lines. However, until a totally implantable drive system is available, the drive lines will remain a potential avenue for the introduction of infections. The risk may be minimized by rigorous attention to care of the exit sites and by improved designs that will provide a better mechanical barrier by, for example, enhancing epithelial ingrowth into the materials of the drive line. Materials such as Velcro®, which appear to serve as a substrate for bacterial proliferation, should also be eliminated.

Although these improvements will undoubtedly reduce the complications associated with use of the total artificial heart, the question of mediastinal infections remains. The artificial heart represents an extreme case of the implantation of a foreign body. If, as our data suggest, the pseudopericardial sac can become infected by routes other than transcutaneous lines, mediastinal infections will continue to be a major problem with long-term implantation of such devices. New and innovative approaches that will prevent seeding of this area with bacteria and at the same time permit ready access of host defense mechanisms to any infection that does arise are required before this problem can be minimized and eventually eliminated.

REFERENCES

1. EVANS, R. W., D. L. MANNINEN, L. P. GARRISON & A. M. MAIER. 1986. Donor availability as the primary determinant of the future of heart transplantation. J. Am. Med. Assoc. **255(14):** 1892–1898.
2. DEVRIES, W. C., J. L. ANDERSON, L. D. JOYCE, F. L. ANDERSON, E. H. HAMMOND, R. K. JARVIK & W. J. KOLFF. 1984. Clinical use of the total artificial heart. N. Engl. J. Med. **310(5):** 273–278.
3. LEVINSON, M. M., R. G. SMITH, R. CORK, J. GALLO, T. ICENOGLE, R. EMERY, R. OTT & J. G. COPELAND. 1986. Three recent cases of total artificial heart before transplantation. J. Heart Transplant. **5(3):** 215–228.
4. DEVRIES, W. C. A permanent artificial heart: Four case reports. J. Am. Med. Assoc. In press.
5. LEVINSON, M. M., R. G. SMITH, R. C. CORK, J. GALLO, R. W. EMERY, T. B. ICENOGLE, R. A. OTT, G. L. BURNS & J. G. COPELAND. 1986. Thromboembolic complications of the Jarvik-7 total artificial heart: Case report. Artif. Organs **10(3):** 236–244.
6. GRIFFITH, B. P., R. L. KORMOS, L. M. WEI, H. S. BOROVETZ, A. TRENTO & R. L. HARDESTY. 1986. Use of the total artificial heart as an interim device: Initial experience in Pittsburgh with four patients. J. Heart Transplant. **5(3):** 210–214.
7. KESSLER, T. R., A. B. PONS, R. K. JARVIK, J. H. LAWSON, K. J. RAZZECA & W. J. KOLFF. 1978. Elimination of predilection sites for thrombus formation in the total artificial heart: Before and after. Trans. Am. Soc. Artif. Intern. Organs **24:** 532–535.
8. MAGOVERN, J. A., J. L. PENNOCK, D. B. CAMPBELL, W. E. PAE, W. S. PIERCE & J. A. WALDHAUSEN. 1986. Bridge to heart transplantation: The Penn State experience. J. Heart Transplant. **5(3):** 196–202.
9. OLSEN, D. B., F. UNGER, H. OSTER, J. LAWSON, T. KESSLER, J. KOLFF & W. J. KOLFF. 1975. Thrombus generation within the artificial heart. J. Thorac. Cardiovasc. Surg. **70(2):** 248–255.
10. BEAUDET, R. L., N. L. POIRIER, D. DOYLE, G. NAKHLE & C. GAUVIN. 1986. The Medtronic-Hall cardiac valve: 7½ years clinical experience. Ann. Thorac. Surg. **42(6):** 644–650.
11. SCULLIN, D., G. S. JOHNSON, Y. LIU, L. HARKER & W. C. DEVRIES. Thromboembolic and hemorrhagic events associated with the use of the total artificial heart: Observations in four patients. J. Am. Med. Assoc. In press.
12. KUNIN, C. M., J. J. DOBBINS, J. C. MELO, M. N. LEVINSON, K. LOVE, L. D. JOYCE & W. C. DEVRIES. Pathogenesis of infection in long-term recipients of the Jarvik-7 artificial heart: Brief case reports and comments. J. Am. Med. Assoc. In press.
13. MURRAY, K. D., S. HUGHES, D. BEARNSON & D. B. OLSEN. 1983. Infection in total artificial heart recipients. Trans. Am. Soc. Artif. Intern. Organs **29:** 539–544.
14. FRIEDMAN, M., L. N. KATZ, K. HOWELL, E. LINDNER & M. MENDLOWITZ. 1938. Experimental endocarditis due to *Streptococcus viridans:* Biological factors in its development. Arch. Intern. Med. **61(1):** 95–118.

15. BADDOUR, L. M., G. D. CHRISTENSEN, M. G. HESTER & A. L. BISNO. 1984. Production of experimental endocarditis by coagulase-negative *Staphylococci:* Variability in species virulence. J. Infect. Dis. **150(5):** 721–727.
16. LIU, P. V. 1974. Extracellular toxins of *Pseudomonas aeruginosa.* J. Infect. Dis. **130**(Suppl.): S94–S99.
17. JOYCE, L. D., M. R. PRITZKER, J. C. KISER, D. M. NICOLOFF, T. E. KERSTEN, T. J. VON RUEDEN, F. EALES, K. E. JOHNSON, C. R. JORGENSEN, F. L. GOBEL & R. A. VAN TASSEL. 1986. Use of the mini Jarvik-7 total artificial heart as a bridge to transplantation. J. Heart Transplant. **5(3):** 203–209.
18. DOBBINS, J. J., C. M. KUNIN, B. GIAMMARA & W. C. DEVRIES. Post mortem microbiological findings of two long-lived total artificial heart recipients. Submitted.
19. DOUGHERTY, S. H. & R. L. SIMMONS. 1982. Infections in bionic man: The pathobiology of infections in prosthetic devices. Curr. Probl. Surg. **19(5):** 217–264.
20. SUGARMAN, B. 1986. Infections and prosthetic devices. Am. J. Med. **81**(Suppl. 1A): 78–84.
21. PAPING, R., L. R. WEBSTER, T. H. STANLEY, K. RAZECCA & W. J. KOLFF. 1978. White blood cell phagocytosis after artificial heart implantation. Trans. Am. Soc. Artif. Intern. Organs **24:** 578–580.
22. STELZER, G. T., R. A. WARD, S. R. WELLHAUSEN, K. R. MCLEISH, G. S. JOHNSON & W. C. DEVRIES. 1987. Alterations in select immunologic parameters following total artificial heart implantation. Artif. Organs. **11(1):** 52–62.
23. WELLHAUSEN, S. R., R. A. WARD, G. S. JOHNSON & W. C. DEVRIES. Immunologic complications of long-term implantation of a total artificial heart. Submitted.
24. COST, K. M., C. S. WEST, D. BRINSON & H. C. POLK. 1985. Measurement of human antibody activity against *Escherichia coli* and *Pseudomonas aeruginosa* using formalin treated whole organisms in an ELISA technique. J. Immunoassay **6(1,2):** 23–43.
25. KUSSEROW, B. K., R. W. LARROW & J. E. NICHOLS. 1975. Decreased reticuloendothelial phagocytic function following prolonged in vivo blood pumping: Preliminary observations. Trans. Am. Soc. Artif. Intern. Organs **21:** 388–394.
26. LOEGERING, D. J., G. J. GROVER & M. J. SCHNEIDKRAUT. 1984. Effect of red blood cells and red blood cell ghosts on reticuloendothelial system function. Exp. Mol. Pathol. **41(1):** 67–73.
27. SCHNEIDKRAUT, M. J. & D. J. LOEGERING. 1980. Reticuloendothelial system depression with hemolyzed blood. Adv. Shock Res. **3:** 273–282.
28. KAPLAN, J. E. 1979. Effect of reticuloendothelial blockade on the development of hypotension after trauma, sepsis, and intravascular coagulation. Adv. Shock Res. **2:** 73–81.

Summary

Methods of Assessing Thrombosis

LINA BADIMON

Division of Cardiology
The Mount Sinai Medical Center
New York, New York 10029

Since 1968, we have seen dramatic reductions in mortality rates from all cardiovascular disease. Despite this progress, heart and vascular diseases remain a leading cause of morbidity and mortality in the U. S. and other Western countries. The high mortality and morbidity of atherosclerosis (and its grave complications such as coronary heart disease, cerebrovascular disease, and peripheral vascular disease) are related to the fact that it is the underlying cause of arterial thrombosis. Thrombosis may occur in any part of the circulatory tree and develop silently until either local obstruction or distant obstruction by embolization produces clinical symptomatology. Thrombosis is a dynamic process; it occurs in flowing blood, and blood elements are exposed to fluid transport rates and local shear forces that differ substantially from those occuring in stagnant or tube reaction systems. Overt vessel wall disease does not appear to be an important factor in venous thrombosis, which tends to occur in the lower limbs and in areas of relative stasis. Arterial thrombosis, on the other hand, tends to occur in areas of higher flow and shear stress.

The importance of thrombosis is highlighted by its dramatic consequences, which are the concern of numerous studies aimed at improving both treatment and diagnosis. Ultimately these studies are based on the evolving research on the mechanism of thrombus formation. Blood factors, vessel wall factors, and cell-cell interactions in the context of fluid dynamics regulate thrombus formation and should be thoroughly investigated.

This very stimulating area of great pathophysiological importance was embraced by theme IV of the conference, the Study of Phenomena *in vivo* and *ex vivo*. Session VI, Methods of Assessing Thrombosis, began with an introductory note by me (the session chair) on the importance of studying thrombosis under well-characterized flow conditions, followed by methodological presentations. The assessment of thrombosis *in vivo* by radioactive tracers and scintigraphy was discussed comprehensively by Dr. Mrinal Dewanjee. His paper described human and animal studies using ^{111}In-labeled platelets, ^{123}I and ^{131}I-labeled fibrinogen, and ^{111}In-labeled antibody to the fibrinogen receptor.

The second paper, by Dr. Stuart L. Cooper, brought us data on methods of assessment of thrombosis *ex vivo*. His well-presented communication focused on experimental research using animal models, and described the thrombogenic responses consequent to blood-material interactions under controlled flow conditions.

The second part of the session dealt with the pathophysiology of thrombotic disease, which was addressed by Drs. J. Hirsh and Valentin Fuster. Their excellent presentations offered physiologically grounded clinical insights to an audience composed in large part of basic researchers. Dr. Hirsch described the evolution of thrombotic disease, highlighting venous thrombosis and advances in the study of low molecular weight heparin. Dr. Fuster discussed experimental and clinical findings on arterial thrombosis, vascular atherosclerotic disease, and interactions of platelets and vessel wall responsible for the development of restenosis after coronary angioplasty.

Dr. J. Owen's paper addressed the topic of blood tests as markers of thrombosis. Indices of the activity of the coagulation system for detection of the thrombotic and prethrombotic states are most needed. As Dr. Owen made clear to us, however, blood tests must be interpreted with caution.

In experimental animal research, species selection is of major importance if data is to be applied to humans. The paper by Dr. W. J. Dodds emphasized that regardless of the test system employed in *in vitro* procedures, results must eventually be corroborated in the *in vivo* situation.

Dr. Cheryl F. Scott contributed more information on the appropriate use of animal models for research on the interaction of blood and artificial surfaces. Data from her group has shown that the contact activation system in dog, rabbit, seal, and cow is markedly different from that of human, rat, monkey, and pig. She also made the point that even if *in vitro* systems utilize human blood components, they do not possess clearance mechanisms. Therefore, in accord with Dr. Dodds's comments, she concluded that care must be taken in interpreting results from animals or *in vitro* experiments.

The thromboembolic and infectious complications of total artifical heart implantation were discussed by Dr. Richard A. Ward. The artificial heart represents the ultimate example of the implantation of a foreign body. His group's data indicate that mediastinal infections are a major problem in long-term implantation of the device. He reviewed the thromboembolic and infectious complications that occurred in two patients.

The papers presented at this session help us develop a better understanding of the thrombotic process by bringing a multidisciplinary approach to bear on the problem. We have here the combined viewpoints of basic scientists, rheologists, clinicians, and laboratory hematologists. Our end purpose, of course, is to generate fundamental information that will lead to a better understanding of thrombus formation in the human being, and of how it might be prevented.

Vascular Graft Thrombus Formation[a]

STEPHEN R. HANSON AND LAURENCE A. HARKER

Roon Research Center for Arteriosclerosis and Thrombosis
Department of Basic and Clinical Research
Scripps Clinic and Research Foundation
La Jolla, California 92037

INTRODUCTION

Thrombosis and thromboembolism are the major deterrents to the use and further development of cardiovascular prosthetic devices.[1] For devices employed or implanted for short periods, important determinants include the device configuration, hematologic and hemodynamic variables, gross thrombus formation, and possibility of embolism. With chronic implants, emphasis has been placed on the time course of thrombosis, thromboembolism, and the consumption of circulating blood species. Thrombus formation may be greatly influenced by surgical technique, variable thrombolytic and embolic phenomena, and possible alterations in exposed surface, *e.g.*, endothelialization.

Exposure of prosthetic biomaterial surfaces to circulating blood initiates platelet and coagulation reactions that may result in thrombosis.[2] Initially, this process involves platelet adhesion and release of constituents to form enlarging platelet masses.[3,4] Arterial high shear conditions promote the formation of thrombus that is composed largely of platelets, whereas low shear venous flow conditions facilitate thrombin generation and fibrin formation with entrapment of erythrocytes. Arterial blood flow also disrupts the accumulating platelet mass into platelet microemboli. Because thrombosis represents a localized accumulation of hemostatic material, the nature of the process and rate of thrombus formation may be assessed kinetically *in vivo* by measurement of the relative consumption and deposition of platelets and fibrinogen in its genesis[5] together with determination of activation products appearing in plasma.

SELECTION OF ANIMAL MODELS

Animal models of acute arterial thrombosis have had limited usefulness because the assessment of vascular occlusion has usually involved the use of experimental animals of questionable relevance to humans observed at a single point in time after an initiating vascular insult.[2,6] Some of the uncontrolled variables that compromise the quantitative aspects of such approaches include: the type and extent of the initial vascular injury, loss of thrombus by embolization, loss of thrombus by thrombolysis, hemodynamic characteristics of the model, and the timing and type of observations at sacrifice.

To quantify continuously the overall rate of thrombus formation *in vivo* in a

[a]This work was supported in part by grants HL31950 and HL31469 from the National Institutes of Health, Division of Heart, Lung and Blood Diseases. This is publication number 4680BCR from the Research Institute of Scripps Clinic, La Jolla, CA.

manner that is free of uncontrolled variables, we have used a primate model of prosthetic device thrombosis.[7,8] The choice of the baboon for these studies was based on the baboon's hemostatic similarity to humans, together with its size, logistical ease of frequent blood sampling, and its long-term acceptance of chronically patent A-V cannulae. Although it is difficult to establish equivalent thrombogenicity among humans and other species, available evidence suggests that the baboon is a good animal for simulating arterial thrombotic processes in humans.[9,10] We have studied the hemostatic mechanism in the baboon and found it to resemble closely that of humans in a number of respects, including concentrations of coagulation factors and plasminogen, bleeding time, platelet count, platelet volume, platelet morphology, platelet aggregation and release *in vitro,* and plasma levels of platelet factor 4, β-thromboglobulin, fibrinopeptide A, factor V, protein C and S, von Willebrand factor, factor VIII:C, and tissue plasminogen activator (using human radioimmune assays).

EVALUATION OF BIOMATERIALS

In our system thrombosis is induced in the baboon by introducing the artificial surfaces as cannular segments into a chronic femoral A-V shunt. Thrombogenesis in this segment is measured as the rate of cannula platelet consumption.[7,8] It is a steady-state process of selective platelet consumption that does not involve measurable utilization of circulating fibrinogen and is unaffected by heparin anticoagulation. Whereas measurements of platelet survival time and overall platelet turnover (including senescent platelet removal) may be influenced by shunt geometry (as well as type) and the circulating platelet concentration, measurements of cannula platelet consumption per unit area have been found to be reproducible and strongly dependent on material properties, yet independent of total exposed surface area, cannula blood flow rate, and circulating platelet concentration over wide ranges of these variables. Such observations thus provide a more meaningful assessment of material performance and facilitate considerably the general usefulness of this model system.

Rates of platelet consumption by ten commercial polyurethane materials ranged from 2.2–23.3 $\times$ 10^8 platelets per cm^2 per day (FIGURE 1) and correlated inversely ($r = -0.767$) with measurements of the percentage of surface carbon atoms forming hydrocarbon (C-H) bonds as determined by electron spectroscopy for chemical analysis (ESCA).[11] Thus for these polyurethanes studied there was approximately a tenfold variation in the rate of platelet consumption per unit area, with the more polar materials being the most reactive. Further studies using ESCA may thus provide useful information regarding the relative importance of surface-chemical moieties present in a variety of polymeric materials.

In other studies, an excellent correlation was also found between the bulk water content of acrylic and methacrylic graft polymers and copolymers and the rate at which they consumed platelets *in vivo.*[8] Approximately an eightfold variation in the rate of platelet consumption per unit area was observed, with the more fully hydrated materials being the most thrombogenic. The extent of hydration of the grafted layer appeared to be the only significant independent variable, although materials tested included graft polymers prepared by both radiation and chemical initiation techniques, grafts on different substrates, and one graft copolymer with a net negative charge.

Four other materials, Teflon, Silastic, poly(vinyl chloride), and polyethylene, were all found to consume less than 2 $\times$ 10^8 platelets per cm^2 per day and were thus the least consumptive materials tested. Excluding poly(vinyl chloride), these materials exhibit relatively nonpolar surfaces to the flowing blood. However, spectroscopic analysis of poly(vinyl chloride) tubing indicated that the surface of this material is also nonpolar, possibly as a result of migration to the surface of plasticizers or other predominantly C-H type additives. Thus, in general, the results of all studies have suggested that polar surfaces, including surfaces that absorb water to a large extent, are consumptive towards platelets.

EVALUATION OF ANTITHROMBOTIC THERAPIES FOR SMOOTH VASCULAR PROSTHESES

In patients with older-style, caged-ball-type aortic, mitral, or combined aortic and mitral valve replacements, platelet consumption was found to be a steady-state process

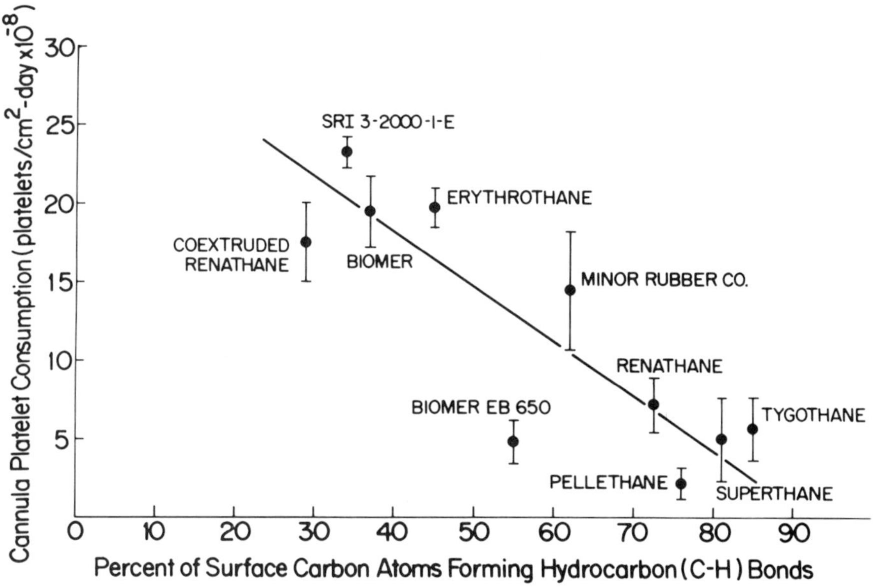

FIGURE 1. Platelet consumption by polyurethanes. Cannula platelet consumption per unit area is inversely related to the percentage of surface carbon atoms forming C-H bonds, as determined from ESCA of polyurethane shunts. Shown are mean values ± 1 SE. (From Hanson *et al.*[11] Reprinted with permission of John Wiley & Sons.)

that did not change appreciably with time,[12] presumably because the nonfabric artificial surfaces do not undergo significant endothelialization *in vivo*. Although these prosthetic heart valves were constructed of several different materials and are more complex from a geometric and hemodynamic standpoint, excellent correlations were found between valve platelet consumption and ball surface area ($r = 0.935$) or the number of valves replaced ($r = 0.907$). There was also a general correlation between the frequency of clinical thromboembolic complications and platelet consumption. Moreover, the capacity of dipyridamole to normalize platelet consumption correlated with the reduction in thromboembolic events produced by dipyridamole administration in clinical trials.[13]

To assess the relative antithrombotic efficacy of various clinically available drug regimens, we have used the model of steady-state arterial thromboembolism in baboons that involves selectively increased platelet destruction in the thrombotic process.[14] In this model, thrombogenic tubular polyurethane was inserted as an extension segment between chronic femoral cannulae to form an arterio-venous shunt. The overall rate of thrombus formation *in vivo* was quantified by measuring the consumption of circulating radiolabeled platelets induced by the thrombogenic segment. Cannula platelet consumption correlated directly with the surface area for the polyurethane segment and remained in the steady state for months. Despite increased rates of platelet consumption, the destruction of circulating fibrinogen was not measurably increased. Moreover, the rate of platelet consumption was independent of normal variations in cannula blood flow rate and platelet count, and was unaffected by heparin anticoagulation or ancrod defibrinogenation. ^{111}In-labeled platelet imaging of thrombogenic tubular segments of polyurethane demonstrated luminal accumulation and subsequent embolization of irregular platelet thromboemboli that were also directly demonstrable by laser light-scattering techniques,[15] or by trapping in blood filters or perfused kidneys.[7]

To resolve questions of drug actions, efficacy, and interactions for platelet-modifying agents used clinically, we have compared the relative capacities and mechanisms of aspirin, dipyridamole, sulfinpyrazone, and dazoxiben to prevent arterial thromboembolism in a baboon model. The antithrombotic efficacy of a given therapy was determined by its capacity to interrupt steady-state platelet utilization induced by thrombogenic arterio-venous cannulae. When given alone, oral dipyridamole and sulfinpyrazone reduced the rate at which platelets were utilized by thrombus formation in a dose-dependent manner with essentially complete interruption by dipyridamole at 10 mg per kg per day and sulfinpyrazone at 100 mg per kg per

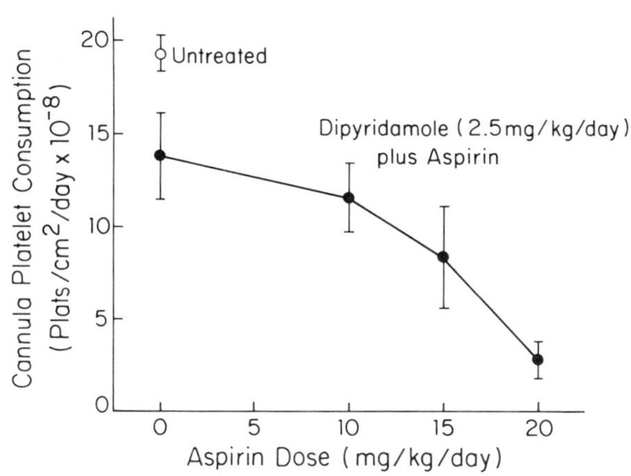

FIGURE 2. Potentiating effect of aspirin on dipyridamole. Baboons with consumptive cannulae received small constant doses of dipyridamole in combination with progressively increased doses of aspirin (*closed circles*). The effect is near maximal at 20 mg per kg per day aspirin. Untreated control value is represented by the *open circle*. Animals given aspirin (20 mg per kg per day) plus dipyridamole have significantly less platelet destruction than animals given dipyridamole only ($p < 0.001$). (From Hanson *et al.*[14] Reprinted with permission of the American Society for Clinical Investigation.)

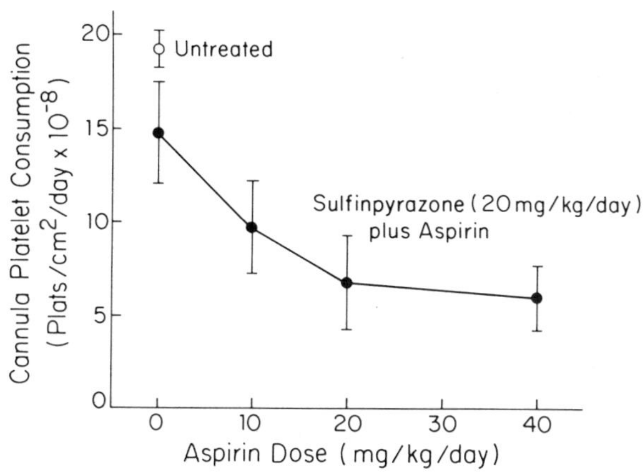

FIGURE 3. Effect of aspirin in combination with sulfinpyrazone. When aspirin is given at increasing doses in combination with a minimally effective dose of sulfinpyrazone (20 mg per kg per day), a modest enhancement is observed in the inhibition of cannula platelet consumption in baboons (*closed circles*). Untreated control value is represented by the *open circle*. Animals given aspirin (40 mg per kg per day) plus sulfinpyrazone had significantly less platelet destruction than animals given sulfinpyrazone only ($p < 0.05$). (From Hanson *et al.*[14] Reprinted with permission of the American Society for Clinical Investigation.)

day.[7,14] In contrast, neither aspirin (2–100 mg per kg per day) nor dazoxiben (20–100 mg per kg per day) decreased cannula platelet consumption detectably despite the striking reduction in the capacity of platelets to produce thromboxane B_2. However, aspirin, but not dazoxiben, potentiated the antithrombotic effects of dipyridamole and sulfinpyrazone in a dose-dependent fashion without changing the pharmacokinetics for any of the agents (FIGURES 2 and 3). Complete potentiation required aspirin at 20 mg per kg per day to be given with each dose of dipyridamole. Because dozoxiben's blockade of platelet thromboxane A_2 production was not associated with antithrombotic potentiation, and because complete potentiation by aspirin required a dose that fully inhibited vascular production of prostaglandin I_2 (PGI_2), we conclude that aspirin's potentiating effect on dipyridamole is independent of PGI_2 production or inhibition of thromboxane A_2 formation. In addition, because frequent repeated and synchronous dosing of aspirin was necessary, aspirin's potentiating effects appear to be produced by mechanism(s) unrelated to its potent, irreversible inhibition of platelet cyclooxygenase.

ACUTE ARTERIAL VASCULAR GRAFT THROMBOSIS

A model of acute Dacron graft thrombosis in baboons has been developed in which thrombus formation was initiated by Dacron vascular grafts inserted as extension segments into chronic arterio-venous Silastic shunts.[16] Following platelet labeling with ^{111}In-oxine, platelet deposition was measured for 1 hour following blood contact under arterial flow conditions using a scintillation camera. Graft platelet activity rapidly increased 40- to 50-fold, plateauing by 1 hour (FIGURE 4). All grafts produced equivalent reductions in circulating platelet count and blood ^{111}In-labeled platelet radioactivity, demonstrating that the labeled cells were functionally equivalent to the total platelet population. After graft placement, the remaining platelets survived normally. Acute platelet deposition was equivalent on grafts placed 1, 24, 48, and 72 hours following injection of the labeled cells, indicating that a variable delay between platelet labeling and graft imaging was without detectable consequence. This model was developed specifically to produce an acute, significant, and reproducible thrombotic challenge such that the relative importance of *in vivo* variables and therapies could be determined.

Dacron vascular grafts were chosen as the thrombogenic surface because these materials have direct application in man, and because platelet thrombus formed under well-defined conditions of flow and geometry. Thus, the graft length and period of exposure were selected to produce measurable platelet accumulation without causing a compromising change in the circulating platelet count. In contrast to the smooth cannular model of thromboembolism described earlier, acute platelet deposition onto thrombogenic Dacron grafts depends strongly upon circulating platelet concentration as well as upon flow and does not modify platelets that continue to circulate. Thrombosis involves both platelets and fibrin. This model of acute arterial thrombosis

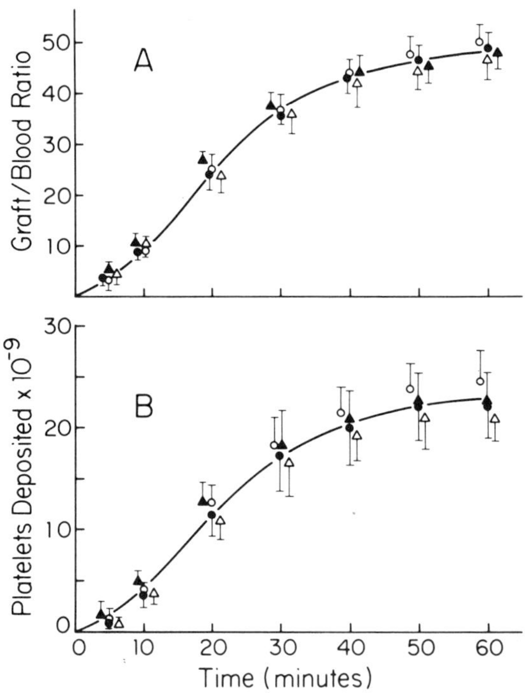

FIGURE 4. Platelet deposition on grafts placed sequentially. Identical grafts were placed for 1 hour daily in the following sequence: day 1 (*open circles*); day 2 (*closed circles*); day 3 (*open triangles*); day 4 (*closed triangles*). No significant variations ($p > 0.2$) were observed among the sequential studies performed over 4 days when results were expressed as (**A**) the graft:blood ratio of ^{111}In-labeled platelet activity or (**B**) total deposited platelets. Values are mean ± 1 SE in six animals (days 1, 2, 3) or four animals (day 4). (From Hanson *et al.*[16] Reprinted with permission of the American Heart Association.)

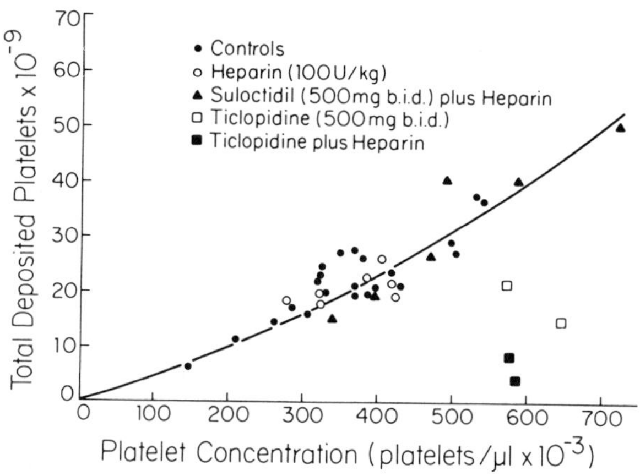

FIGURE 5. Correlation of total platelet deposition with platelet count. In control animals platelet deposition correlated directly with platelet count where total deposited platelets equaled 3290 × (platelets/μl).[16,17] Significant reduction in platelet deposition was observed in animals given ticlopidine but was unaffected by heparin or suloctidil. (From Hanson and Harker.[17] Reprinted by permission from *Thrombosis and Haemostasis.*)

presents a severe challenge for therapeutic interventions and simulates acute thrombosis associated with small caliber vascular grafts, and possibly occlusion following angioplasty or reocclusion following thrombolytic reperfusion in patients with acute myocardial infarction.

To determine the suitability of evaluating platelet-modifying drugs[17] using the vascular graft model of acute arterial thrombosis, we compared the effects of ticlopidine and suloctidil (FIGURE 5). We used ticlopidine because it is both global and potent in its antiplatelet actions.[18] Ticlopidine is chemically unrelated to other antiplatelet drugs and appears to have a unique, albeit unknown, mechanism of action. It is neither a prostaglandin synthesis inhibitor nor a cyclic AMP phosphodiesterase inhibitor. There are several reports which indicate that ticlopidine may act on the platelet membrane to alter its reactivity to activating stimuli. The broad spectrum of antiplatelet activity of ticlopidine and its apparently novel mechanism of action sets the drug apart from currently available antiplatelet agents. The fact that ticlopidine does not inhibit prostacyclin synthesis in the arterial wall but can still inhibit aggregation induced by thromboxane A_2 and prostaglandin endoperoxide is a theoretical advantage over other drugs. Suloctidil, on the other hand, is basically a peripheral vasodilator,[19] without a well-defined antithrombotic mechanism although it is reported to normalize platelet survival in patients with prosthetic heart valves. Since the mechanism of acute thrombus formation induced by Dacron vascular grafts is a thrombin-related process, heparin (in conventional anticoagulant doses) was also administered in the acute Dacron graft studies to block thrombin action without affecting platelet deposition, thereby enhancing the capacity of the system to detect platelet-mediated antithrombotic effects. Thus, with the addition of heparin anticoagulation this model of acute arterial thrombosis appears to detect platelet alterations with greater sensitivity.

Suloctidil at oral dose of 100 mg per kg per day had no effect on acute thrombus formation with or without heparin.[17] In contrast, ticlopidine alone in doses of 20 mg per kg per day produced substantial reduction in acute ^{111}In-labeled platelet deposition.

The effect of ticlopidine on platelet deposition was enhanced by the addition of heparin (FIGURE 5).

To assess the hemostatic consequences and antithrombotic effectiveness of blocking the platelet glycoprotein (GP) IIb-IIIa receptor for fibrinogen and other adhesive glycoproteins *in vivo,* well-characterized murine monoclonal antibodies against the platelet GPIIb-IIIa complex, AP-2 and LJCP-8, were infused intravenously into baboons.[20] Four animals each received doses of 0.2, 0.4, and 1.0 mg/kg of purified AP-2 IgG or 10 mg/kg of LJCP-8 followed by serial measurements of platelet count, bleeding time, platelet aggregation (induced by ADP, collagen, and gamma thrombin) and ^{111}In-labeled platelet deposition onto acutely placed Dacron vascular grafts. At the highest dose, radiolabeled antibody bound to an average of about 40,000 sites per platelet in circulation. Whereas the AP-2 antibody caused a dose-dependent reduction (20–40%) in the circulating platelet count over 24 hours, LJCP-8 had no effect on the platelet count. Although the lowest dose of antibody had no effect on bleeding time

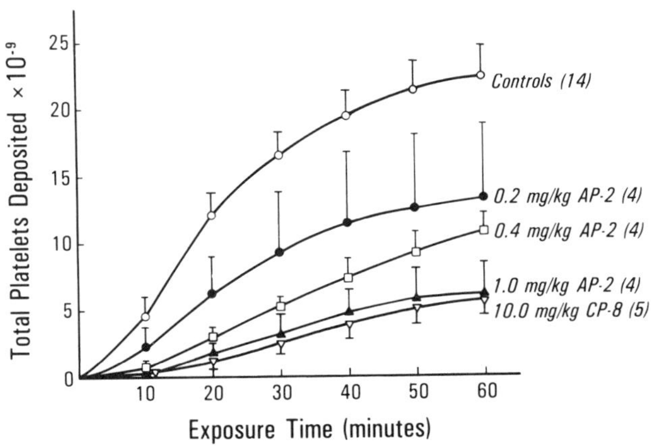

FIGURE 6. Effect of monoclonal antibodies on graft platelet deposition. Well-characterized murine monoclonal antibodies against the platelet GPIIb-IIIa complex, AP-2 and LJ-CP8, were infused intravenously into baboons. Four animals each received doses of 0.2, 0.4, and 1.0 mg/kg of purified AP-2 IgG. Five additional animals were given 10 mg/kg LJ-CP8. Platelet deposition onto Dacron vascular grafts was measured over a 1-h exposure period. (From Hanson *et al.*[20] Reprinted with permission of the American Society for Clinical Investigation.)

(5.2 ± 0.4 min) compared to control studies (4.7 ± 0.2 min), the highest dose markedly prolonged the bleeding time acutely (19.2 ± 3.4 min for AP-2 and >30 min for LJCP-8) with only partial normalization over 48 hours. Platelet aggregation in response to all three agonists was reduced or absent acutely, with subsequent normalization over 24 hours (0.2 mg/kg AP-2), 48 hours (0.4 mg/kg AP-2), or only partial normalization by 48 hours (1.0 mg/kg AP-2 or 10 mg/kg LJCP-8). Marked reductions in graft-associated platelet thrombus formation were observed, averaging 34%, 44%, and 73% of control values with increasing doses of AP-2, or with 10 mg/kg LJCP-8 (FIGURE 6). LJCP-8 also prevented occlusion of the vascular graft. In contrast, neither heparin (100 U/kg) nor aspirin (32.5 mg/kg b.i.d.) showed antithrombotic efficacy in this model. Thus antibodies that functionally alter the platelet GPIIb-IIIa complex may produce immediate, transient, and potent antihemostatic and antithrombotic effects.

REFERENCES

1. SALZMAN, E. W. 1982. Surgical treatment of arterial thromboembolic disease. *In* Hemostasis and Thrombosis: Basic Principles and Clinical Practice. R. W. Coleman *et al.*, Eds.: 1093. J. B. Lippincott. Philadelphia.
2. NHLBI WORKING GROUPS. 1985. Guidelines for Blood-Material Interactions. NIH Publication No. 85-2185. National Institutes of Health. Bethesda, MD.
3. ZUCKER, M. B. 1980. The functioning of blood platelets. Sci. Am. **242:** 86.
4. BAUMGARTNER, H. R., R. MUGGLI, T. B. TSCHOPP & V. T. TURRITTO. 1976. Platelet adhesion, release and aggregation in flowing blood: Effects of surface properties and platelet function. Thromb. Haemostas. **35:** 124.
5. HARKER, L. A. & S. J. SLICHTER. 1972. Platelet and fibrinogen consumption in man. N. Engl. J. Med. **287:** 999.
6. DIDISHEIM, P. 1972. Animal models useful in the study of thrombosis and antithrombotic agents. Prog. Hemostas. Thromb. **1:** 165.
7. HARKER, L. A. & S. R. HANSON. 1979. Experimental arterial thromboembolism in baboons: Mechanism, quantitation and pharmacologic prevention. J. Clin. Invest. **64:** 559.
8. HANSON, S. R., L. A. HARKER, B. D. RATNER & A. S. HOFFMAN. 1980. In vivo evaluation of artificial surfaces with a nonhuman primate model of arterial thrombosis. J. Lab. Clin. Med. **95:** 289.
9. HAMPTON, J. W. & C. MATTHEWS. 1966. Similarities between baboon and human blood clotting. J. Appl. Physiol. **21:** 1713.
10. TODD, M. E., E. L. MCDEVITT & E. I. GOLDSMITH. 1972. Blood-clotting mechanisms of nonhuman primates: Choice of the baboon model to simulate man. J. Med. Primatol. **1:** 132.
11. HANSON, S. R., L. A. HARKER, B. D. RATNER & A. S. HOFFMAN. 1982. Evaluation of artificial surfaces using a baboon arteriovenous shunt model. Adv. Biomater. **3:** 519.
12. HARKER, L. A. & S. J. SLICHTER. 1970. Studies of platelet and fibrinogen kinetics in patients with prosthetic heart valves. N. Engl. J. Med. **283:** 1302.
13. SULLIVAN, J. M., D. E. HARKEN & R. GORLIN. 1971. Pharmacologic control of thromboembolic complications of cardiac-valve replacement. N. Engl. J. Med. **284:** 1391.
14. HANSON, S. R., L. A. HARKER & T. D. BJORNSSON. 1985. Effects of platelet-modifying drugs on arterial thromboembolism in baboons. J. Clin. Invest. **75:** 1591.
15. HOFFMAN, A. S., D. COHN, S. R. HANSON, L. A. HARKER, T. A. HORBETT & L. O. REYNOLDS. 1983. Application of radiation-grafted hydrogels as blood-contacting biomaterials. Radiat. Phys. Chem. **22:** 267.
16. HANSON, S. R., H. F. KOTZE, B. SAVAGE & L. A. HARKER. 1985. Platelet interactions with Dacron vascular grafts. Arteriosclerosis **5:** 595.
17. HANSON, S. R. & L. A. HARKER. 1985. Studies of suloctidil in experimental thrombosis in baboons. Thromb. Haemostas. **53:** 423.
18. O'BRIEN, J. R. 1983. Ticlopidine: A promise for the prevention and treatment of thrombosis and its complications. Haemostasis **13:** 1.
19. ROBA, J., G. DEFREYN & G. BIAGI. 1983. Antithrombotic activity of suloctidil. Thromb. Res. **4:** 53.
20. HANSON, S. R., F. I. PARETI, Z. M. RUGGERI, T. J. KUNICKI, R. R. MONTGOMERY, T. S. ZIMMERMAN & L. A. HARKER. 1986. Effects of monoclonal antibodies against the platelet glycoprotein IIb/IIIa complex on thrombosis and hemostasis in the baboon. J. Clin. Invest. In press.

Thrombogenesis in and Contiguous with Pumping Chambers

G. L. BURNS AND D. B. OLSEN

Artificial Heart Research Laboratory
Institute for Biomedical Engineering
University of Utah
Salt Lake City, Utah 84103

Evaluation of total artificial hearts (TAH) in animal models has provided the basis for clinical use of the devices. During the developmental period many iterations of the designs, fabrication techniques, and materials have taken place. Serial improvements in the surgical implantation procedures and postoperative management of the device recipients have led to prolonged survival and enhanced quality of life. In general, mechanical reliability of electromechanical and pneumatically driven devices is relatively high and the fundamental designs have been well characterized.[1,2] Mechanical function has proven to be adequate to meet the normal physiologic needs of the recipients for extended periods of time. Several other aspects of the device-host interaction remain unresolved, however. Postoperative infections, activation of the coagulation and complement cascades, activation of platelets, thrombogenesis on blood-contacting surfaces, and thromboembolism remain as significant problems in both the experimental and clinical applications of the devices. We review several of these problem areas in this paper reporting TAH implantations in 35 calves.

STUDY GROUP

Thirty-five 3- to 4-month-old calves were implanted with pneumatically driven total artificial hearts in this study. Twenty-nine of the animals were Holstein, three were Hereford, and three Angus. The group was composed of 29 males and six females. The mean survival time was 44.9 days, with a range of 2 to 208 days. The animals received similar preoperative and postoperative care, including similar diets and housing.

Each animal was implanted with one of four models of a pneumatically powered polyurethane TAH. Component parts of the devices are depicted in FIGURE 1. The most frequently used devices were fabricated by solution casting over stainless steel molds. Included in ths group are eight Jarvik-5® (J-5) hearts, nine Jarvik-7® (J-7) hearts, and four Utah-100 (U100) hearts. Fourteen J-7 hearts manufactured by vacuum-forming methods are also included. The housings of the solution cast hearts were made from Biomer® with machined Isoplast 301® bases. Isoplast was also used for the valve-holding rings, which were coated with Biomer during assembly. Different durometer grades of Pellethane® were used to form the housing, base, and valve-holding rings of the vacuum-formed hearts. Medtronic-Hall valves were used in both inflow and outflow positions in all but one of the Biomer hearts. These valves utilize a tilting pyrolytic carbon disk in a titanium ring. The remaining heart had natural valves in the aortic and pulmonic positions and Medtronic-Hall valves in the inflow positions. Vacuum-formed hearts were equipped with a variety of valves including Medtronic Hall valves, St. Jude valves, Bjork Shiley valves, and experimental polyurethane valves. Low-porosity Cooley vascular grafts were bonded to cast Biomer rims to provide a connector system between the device and remnant portions of the aorta and pulmonary artery. A Biomer-coated, woven Dacron velour was bonded to a similar connector system for attachment to the right and left atria. The vascular graft materials were attached to the remnant tissue using polypropylene suture.

Devices were recovered from the animals at necropsy for examination and documentation of changes.

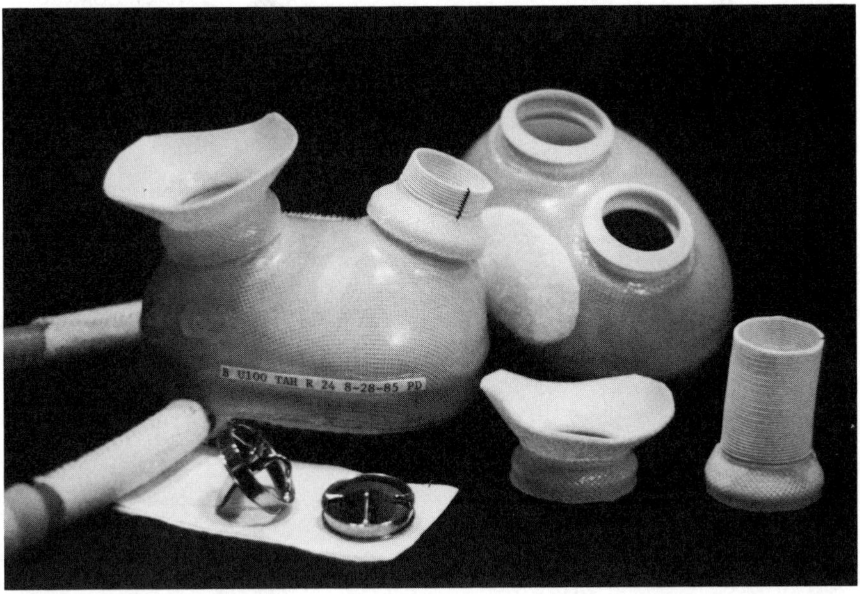

FIGURE 1. UTAH 100 pneumatic artificial ventricles (background). Medtronic Hall inflow and outflow valves are in the foreground at left. Inflow and outflow quick connectors with attached vascular grafts are in the foreground at right.

RESULTS

Evidence of thrombogenesis was present in 30 of the 35 retrieved devices (85%). Thrombus formation was present as early as 4 days postoperatively, but several devices from animals surviving over 60 days contained thrombi at only a single location.

Thrombus formation was present in 71% of the right inflow tracts of the devices, 46% of the right outflow tracts, 69% of the left inflows, and 51% of the left outflows. The inflow tracts were defined as all structures from the suture line between the atrium and atrial cuff to the subvalvular area of the inflow valve. The outflow tracts included all structures from the subvalvular areas of the outflow valves to the suture line between the vascular graft and the great vessels. Supravalvular and subvalvular thrombi originated from the junctions between the valve rings and the valve holding rings. The most common sites of thrombus formation in the inflow and outflow tracts are depicted in FIGURES 2 and 3. An additional site of thrombus formation occurred at the flexion line between the device housing and blood diaphragm, but this was a

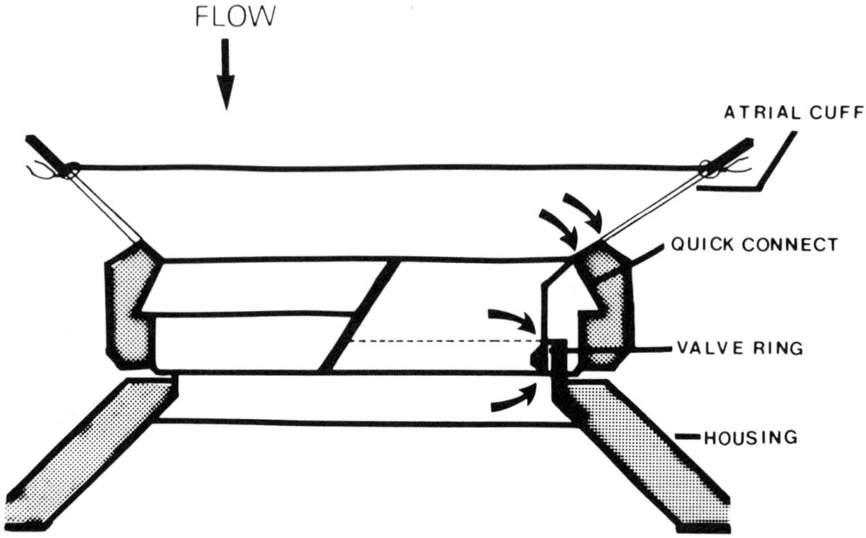

FIGURE 2. Schematic drawing of inflow tract from artificial heart. *Arrows* indicate points of thrombus formation.

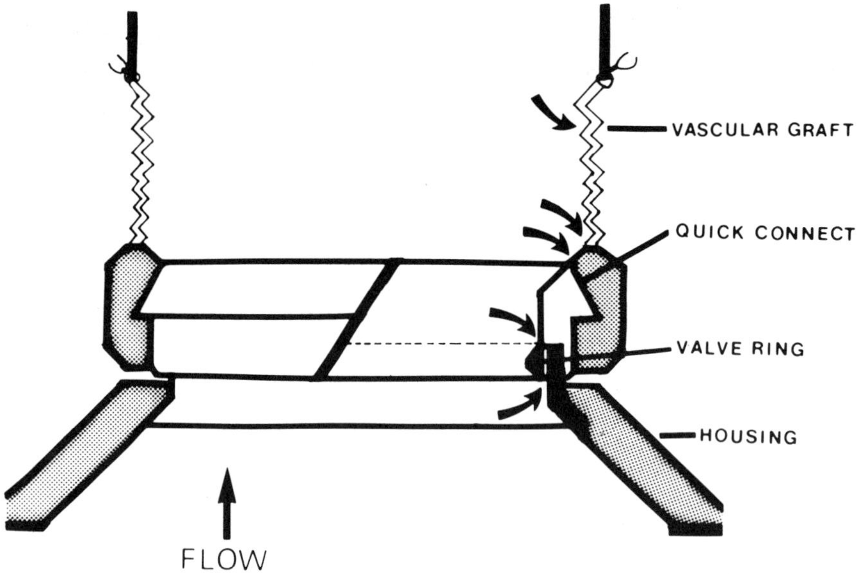

FIGURE 3. Schematic drawing of outflow tract from artificial heart. *Arrows* indicate points of thrombus formation.

relatively rare occurrence. Other thrombi were attached to the stents of the valve ring and at the junction between the graft material and connector.

A variety of changes were seen during histopathologic examination of the thrombi retrieved from the devices. Many of the thrombi associated with valves and valve rings were vegetative in character (FIGURES 4 and 5). Photomicroscopy demonstrated that these thrombi were composed of laminated layers of fibrin, whole or lysed red blood cells, and leukocytes (FIGURE 6). Platelets were often identifiable as major components of the thrombi. Bacterial colonies, accumulations of fungal hyphae, and focal areas of mineralization were also present in some vegetative lesions (FIGURES 6–8), particularly in those animals surviving for extended periods of time. Thrombi associated with the vascular graft materials tended to be flattened, with relatively smooth, endothelialized

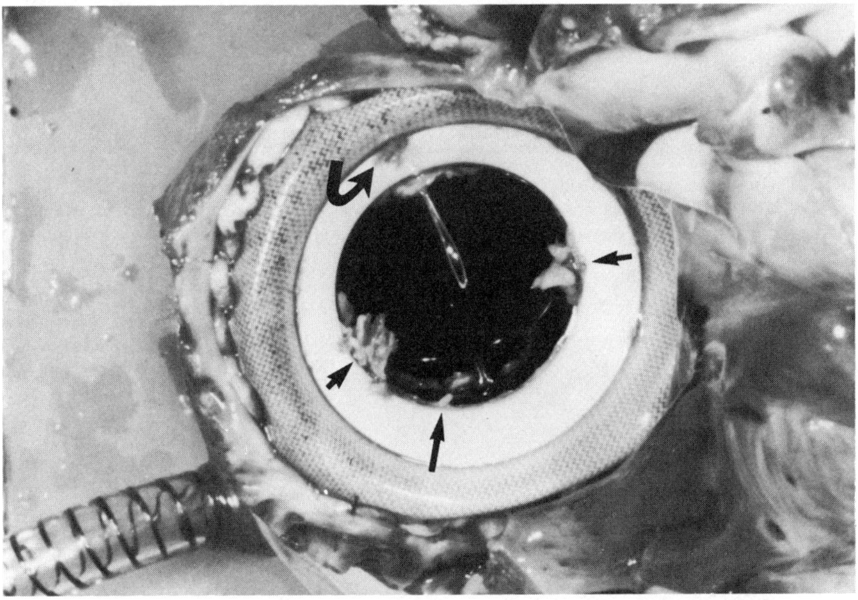

FIGURE 4. *Short straight arrows* indicate vegetative thrombi attached to valve stents. *Long straight arrow* indicates small thrombus originating from the gap between the valve ring and connector. *Curved arrow* indicates red thrombus at the junction between the atrial cuff and connector. The calf had survived 5 days following TAH implantation.

surfaces (FIGURE 9). Thrombi of this type, as well as those originating from suture lines, contained more active fibroplasia and evidence of fibroblastic penetration of the vegetative fibrin masses (FIGURE 10).

Samples for bacterial culture were taken from areas of thrombus formation in twenty of the devices at necropsy. Nineteen of the twenty samples (95%) produced bacterial growth. A summary of the organisms isolated from the devices is included in TABLES 1 and 2. In addition to the device cultures, 11 of 17 blood cultures (65%) obtained from animals at various intervals during the postoperative course were positive. Blood cultures were taken if the animals showed evidence of hyperthermia, cachexia, or other overt signs of infection. Results are based on a single blood sample

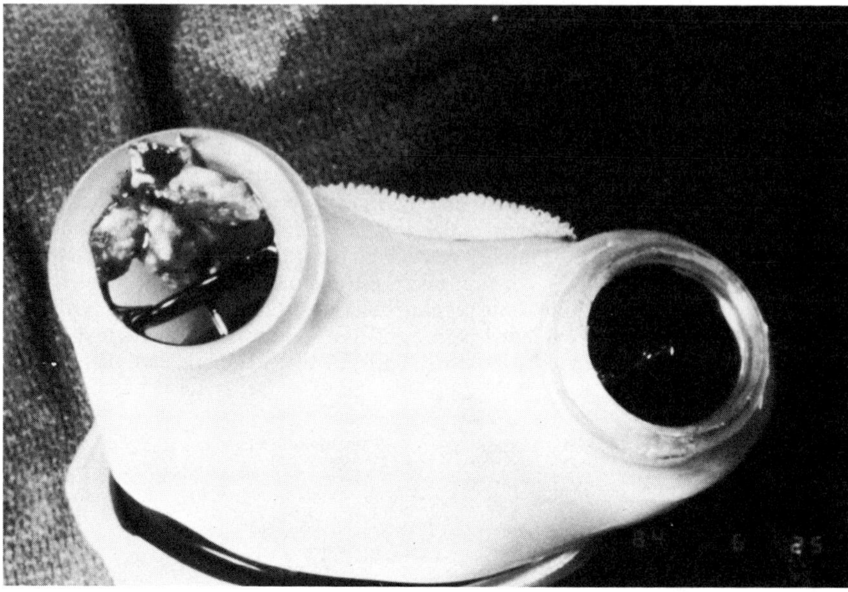

FIGURE 5. Inflow valve at left contains a large vegetative thrombus that interfered with valve function. Outflow valve at right was free of thrombus. This J-7 right ventricle was retrieved from a calf that had survived 131 days following TAH implantation. No postoperative anticoagulant therapy was given.

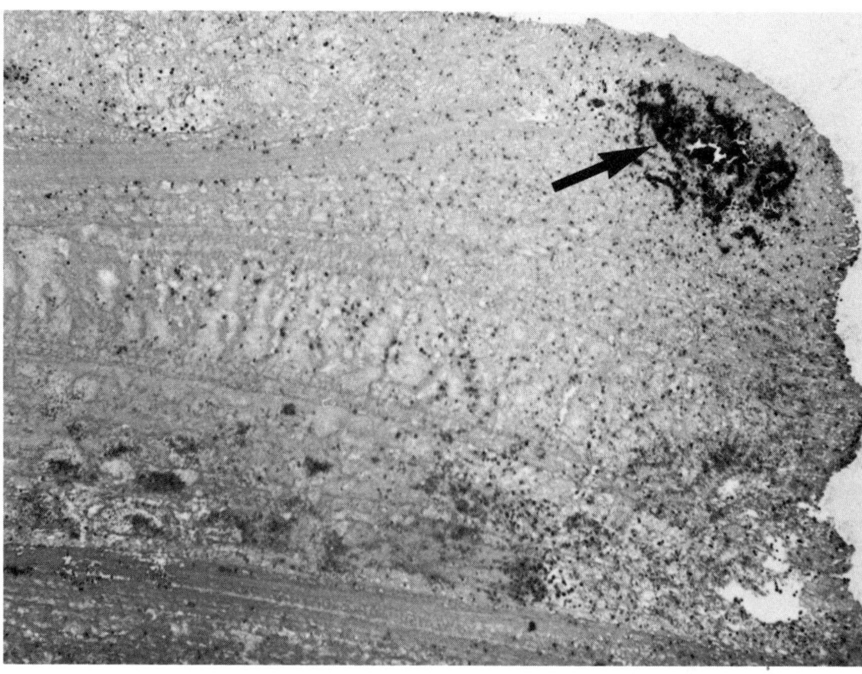

FIGURE 6. Photomicrograph of thrombus composed of multiple layers of fibrin and red blood cells with a mild diffuse infiltration of leukocytes. *Arrow* indicates area of mineralization. Sample was taken from a calf that had survived 13 days following TAH implantation. Magnification: 40×; hematoxylin and eosin stain.

drawn from the jugular vein using aseptic techniques. Blood and device cultures were not taken from some animals, in accordance with the specifications of the experimental protocols.

Antibiotic therapy for each animal followed a similar routine procedure. Cefazolin sodium (Ancef, 2 g, i.v., every 6 h) and gentamicin sulfate (160 mg, i.v., every 6 h) were given preoperatively and continued for 5 days postoperatively. Antibiotic therapy was reinstituted if body temperature remained above 40°C for more than 24 hours or if the animal was showing other overt signs of infection. Blood cultures were drawn before antibiotic therapy was reinstituted. Prolonged antibiotic therapy was based on results of antibiotic sensitivity evaluations.

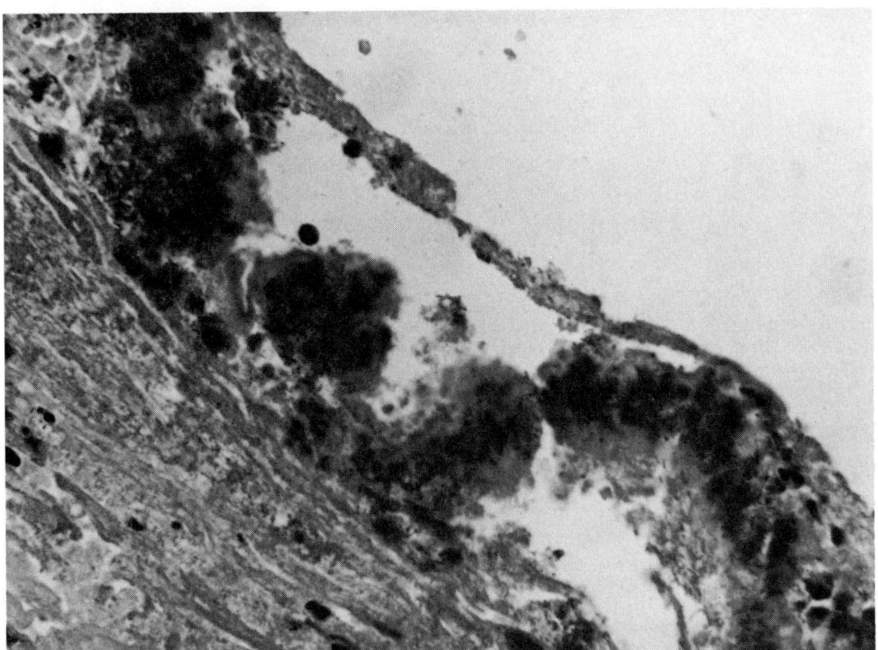

FIGURE 7. Photomicrograph of multiple bacterial colonies on the surface of a thrombus removed from a total artificial heart implanted in a calf for 63 days. Magnification: 400×; hematoxylin and eosin stain.

Anticoagulation therapy varied with the experimental protocols. Eleven of the 35 animals included in this study received no anticoagulation. Nine of the animals received warfarin sodium (Coumadin) and aspirin orally. Fifteen of the animals received only Coumadin. Coumadin dosage sufficient to maintain the prothrombin time (PT) at two to two and 9 half times normal was considered therapeutic. In general this resulted in a Coumadin dose of 5–20 mg per animal per day.

In our study group there was no clear-cut difference in the amount or location of thrombus formation between animals that received anticoagulation therapy and those that did not. A real difference may indeed exist, but could not be demonstrated from

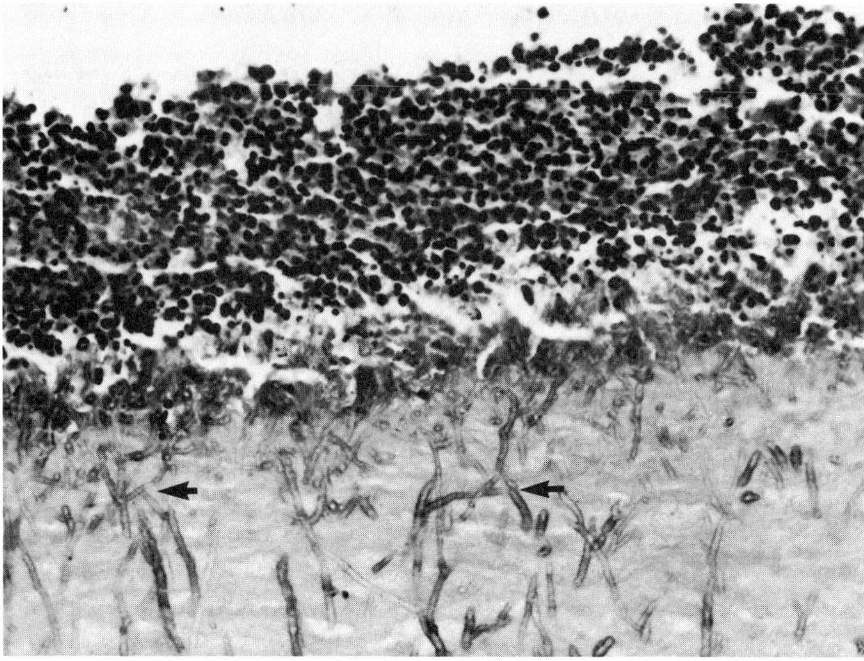

FIGURE 8. Photomicrograph of multiple fungal hyphae (*arrows*) within a fibrin thrombus. Surface accumulation of leukocytes and macrophages is also present. Samples from a calf surviving 63 days. Magnification: 400×; hematoxylin and eosin stain.

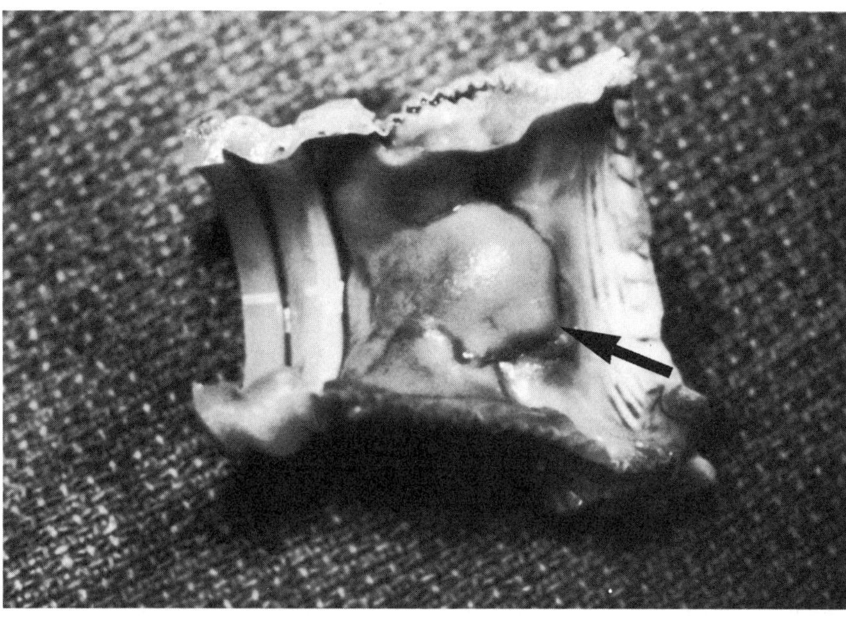

FIGURE 9. *Arrow* indicates endothelial-covered thrombus attached to the blood-contacting surface of an outflow vascular graft. Quick connect at the left end, suture line at right. The graft was removed after 97 days of implantation.

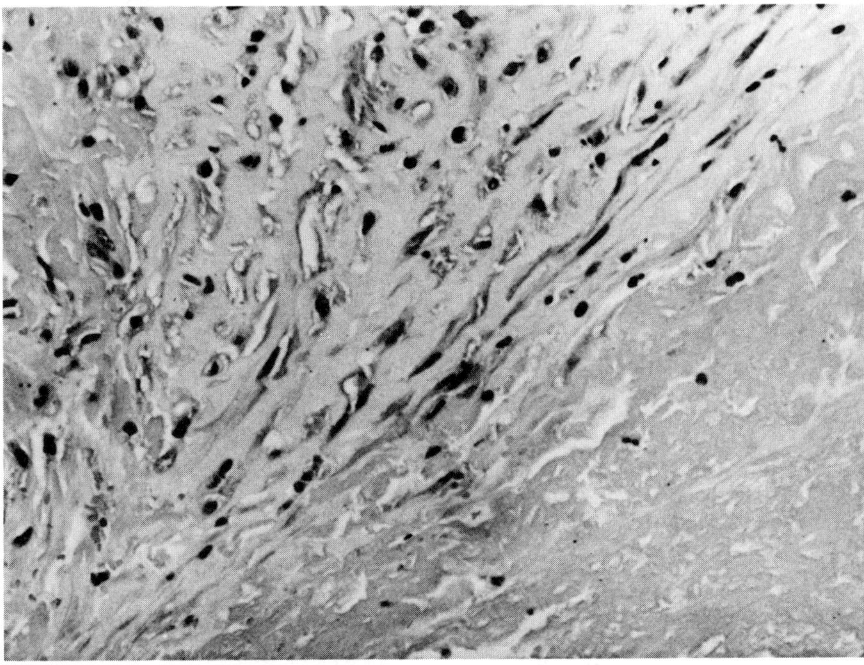

FIGURE 10. Photomicrograph of fibroplastic response at upper left that has penetrated fibrin mass at lower right. Sample originated from a graft suture line in a calf that had survived 63 days. Magnification: 250×; hematoxylin and eosin stain.

available data. Similarly there was no identifiable difference in infection rates between anticoagulated animals and those not receiving anticoagulants.

DISCUSSION

The presence of thrombi in pumping devices and associated structures retrieved from calves and sheep has been reported by several authors.[3–8] A recent report has also documented the location and severity of thrombi in a TAH that was implanted for nine days in a human patient awaiting transplantation.[9] These reports have identified numerous similarities between the lesions present in the human heart and the devices

TABLE 1. Blood Bacterial Culture Results: 11 of 17 (65%) Positive[a]

Coliforms	6/11 (55%)
Pseudomonas	3/11 (27%)
Corynebacteria	2/11 (18%)
Staphylococci	1/11 (10%)
Proteus	1/11 (10%)
Moraxella	1/11 (10%)

[a]Multiple organisms were isolated from some samples.

implanted in the animal models. Factors such as turbulent blood flow, deposition of platelet-fibrin masses, and bacteremia have been implicated in the pathogenesis of lesions in the TAH just as they have been in the pathogenesis of vegetative endocarditis in the natural heart.

Vegetative thrombi were frequently encountered at the junction between the valve-holding ring and the valve ring in devices explanted from our calves. Similar findings were reported to occur in a similar location in the device explanted from the human recipient.[9] In all cases, we have found blood behind the valve ring due to improper sealing of the two surfaces. The difficulty in obtaining a proper seal at this site is attributable in part to the shape of the valve ring itself. Originally designed for placement in the natural annulus of the heart, the ring has a rounded inner surface. For application in the TAH a flat inner surface would align more precisely with the holding ring. Such a valve is currently under development for this application. The availability of this valve will allow a redesign of the valve-holding apparatus in conjunction with a redesign of the quick connect system and may eliminate the preferential sites of thrombus formation in both the inflow and outflow tracts of the devices. Rheological considerations are also important in the valve areas. The prosthetic valves produce a certain amount of turbulence despite their sophisticated designs. In addition, the transitions from the natural tissues to the vascular graft material and from the graft to the smooth surface of the devices also provide numerous areas of disrupted flow. Thrombus formation was seen in the experimental implants in areas where there was

TABLE 2. Bacterial Device Cultures: 19 of 20 (95%) Positive[a]

Organism	Positive
Coliforms	15/19 (79%)
Pseudomonas	11/19 (58%)
Staphylococci	5/19 (26%)
Proteus	2/19 (11%)

[a]Multiple organisms were isolated from some samples.

kinking of the graft material, protrusion of sutures at graft-vessel interfaces, inversion of tissue margins into the vascular lumen with exposure of subendothelial tissues, or protrusion of material surrounding a pressure port orifice. These were common sites of thrombus formation, while surrounding structures of the same material were unaffected.

The incidence of infection in the implanted animals appears to be closely related to thrombus propagation in the devices.[10,11] This seems plausible in light of the myriad complications associated with other device-related infections, such as those occurring with prosthetic heart valves.[12,13] The presence of bacteria in a fibrin matrix at a blood surface interface triggers a complex array of leukocyte responses, complement activation, and coagulation cascades that enhance the vegetative proliferation. Postmortem cultures of thrombi found in devices retrieved from our animals were consistently positive, with Pseudomonas species and coliforms isolated most commonly. These same gram negative organisms were also the organisms most commonly isolated from antemortem blood cultures.

The precise progression of septic thrombus formation in the implanted devices has not been well defined. A likely source of contamination may be the intravascular catheters, which are left in place for several days postoperatively to allow pressure monitoring, and antibiotic and fluid administration. It has also been postulated that the infections may begin at the skin surface of the implanted calves. Penetration of bacteria around the percutaneous access device may be followed by bacteremia or bacterial migration along the drivelines and eventual localization in the thoracic cavity. Indeed, in some cases this appears to be true. Bacterial cultures of drainage surrounding drivelines have produced the same organisms as blood cultures or culture of the device at postmortem. In other cases, however, positive cultures can be obtained from the device when no overt signs of skin infection are present.

Transient bacteremia is known to occur in humans following manipulations of the skin, upper airway, mouth, and intestine.[14] A similar bacterial shower may occur in the calf during the intraoperative or postoperative periods. The likelihood of a bacteremia may be enhanced by the presence of large numbers of bacteria and other commensal microorganisms in the rumen of these animals.

The immune status of the recipient is an additional consideration in evaluation of the occurrence of infections. Several reports have suggested that there may be leukocyte dysfunction following device implantation.[15-17] The significance of this suppression is not known but may be an important factor in the initial stages of bacterial colonization. Even transient immunosuppression associated with cardiopulmonary bypass may allow pathogenic microorganisms to colonize the surfaces of the device.

Various anticoagulants and antiplatelet drugs have been used during the experimental implant studies. Coumadin is used alone or in combination with other drugs in the experimental animals because of the relative ease of administration over prolonged periods of time and a previous study which suggested that Coumadin reduces mineralization of TAH implanted in the calf.[18] There are, however, several drawbacks to the use of Coumadin. The 1–3 day lag period between initial administration of Coumadin and full therapeutic effect, combined with the standard postoperative period of 3–5 days before anticoagulation therapy is instituted, allows significant time for thrombogenesis to begin. Secondly, data on the use of Coumadin in the animal models does not transfer well to the human recipients since the agent is not commonly used for implanted patients. A completely satisfactory anticoagulation protocol has not yet been identified for either the animal or human TAH recipients.

Levinson[9] has reported the difficulties encountered in patient management following TAH implantation. As the patient's general condition improved and coagulation mechanisms began to function normally, frequent dosage adjustments had to be made to obtain adequate anticoagulation. We have encountered the reverse situation as the calves outgrow the devices. As these animals begin to undergo congestive heart failure, liver dysfunction, and loss of normal coagulation responses late in the course of the implantation, lower anticoagulant doses must be used to avoid hemorrhage.

CONCLUSION

The formation of thrombi in and adjacent to artificial pumping devices is a complex and frustrating problem. Improvements in the surface characteristics of the materials, elimination of surface irregularities exposed to the blood, reduction in the incidence of infection, refinements in the flow characteristics of the devices, and improvements in the anticoagulation regimens will all be required to lower the incidence of thrombosis. The use of a relatively large prosthetic device in the body requires a special set of circumstances. The long-term well-being of the recipients will be determined by optimization of the design, careful attention to detail at implantation, and enlightened postoperative management.

REFERENCES

1. PIERCE, W. S. 1986. The artificial heart, 1986: Partial fulfillment of a promise. Trans. Am. Soc. Artif. Intern. Organs **32:** 5–10.
2. MURRAY, K. D. & D. B. OLSEN. 1985. Design and functional characteristics of blood pumps. *In* New Developments in Cardiac Assist Devices. S. Attar, Ed.: 54–78. Praeger Scientific. New York.
3. OLSEN, D. B., F. UNGER, H. OSTER, J. LAWSON, T. KESSLER, J. KOLFF & W. J. KOLFF. 1975. Thrombus generation within the artificial heart. J. Thorac. Cardiovasc. Surg. **70(2):** 248–255.
4. UNGER, F., D. B. OLSEN, H. OSTER & W. J. KOLFF. 1976. Material and design factors in thromboembolization in total artificial heart recipients living 100–2000 hours. Eur. Surg. Res. **8:** 105–116.
5. KESSLER, T. R., A. B. PONS, R. K. JARVIK, J. H. LAWSON, K. J. RAZECCA & W. J. KOLFF. 1978. Elimination of predilection sites for thrombus formation in the total artificial heart: Before and after. Trans. Am. Soc. Artif. Intern. Organs **24:** 532–535.
6. JARVIK, R. K., T. R. KESSLER, L. D. MCGILL, D. B. OLSEN, W. C. DEVRIES, J. DENERIS, J. T. BLAYLOCK & W. J. KOLFF. 1981. Determinants of pannus formation in long-surviving artificial heart calves, and its prevention. Trans. Am. Soc. Artif. Intern. Organs **27:** 90–95.
7. HASTINGS, W. L., J. L. AARON, J. DENERIS, T. R. KESSLER, A. B. PONS, K. J. RAZZECA, D. B. OLSEN & W. J. KOLFF. 1981. A retrospective study of nine calves surviving five months on the pneumatic total artificial heart. Trans. Am. Soc. Artif. Intern. Organs **27:** 71–76.
8. WEIDEMANN, H., K. M. MULLER, E. HENNIG, M. MEIBLER, M. BUNZEL & E. S. BUCHERL. 1986. Infection and obstructive vegetative endocarditis after TAH replacement. Proc. Eur. Soc. Artif. Organs **13:** 29–31.
9. LEVINSON, M. M., R. G. SMITH, R. C. CORK, J. GALLO, R. W. EMERY, T. B. ICENOGLE, R. A. OTT, G. L. BURNS & J. G. COPELAND. 1986. Thromboembolic complications of the Jarvik-7 total artificial heart: Case report. Artif. Organs **10(3):** 236–244.
10. FIELDS, A., H. HARASAKI, D. SANDS & Y. NOSE. 1983. Infection in artificial blood pump implantation. Trans. Am. Soc. Artif. Intern. Organs **29:** 532–538.
11. MURRAY, K. D., S. D. HUGHES, D. BEARNSON & D. B. OLSEN. 1983. Infection in total artificial heart recipients. Trans. Am. Soc. Artif. Intern. Organs **29:** 539–544.
12. ZIMMERLI, W., P. D. LEW & F. A. WALDVOGEL. 1984. Pathogenesis of foreign body infection: Evidence of a local granulocyte defect. J. Clin. Invest. **73(4):** 1191–1200.
13. SUGARMAN, B. 1984. Infections associated with often-used surgical materials. *In* Infections Associated with Prosthetic Devices. B. Sugarman & E. J. Young, Eds.: 11–22. CRC Press. Boca Raton, FL.
14. EVERETT, E. D. & J. V. HIRSHMAN. 1977. Transient bacteremia and endocarditis prophylaxis: A review. Medicine **56:** 61–77.
15. KUSSEROW, B., R. LARROW & J. NICHOLS. 1969. Metabolic and morphological alterations in leukocytes following prolonged blood pumping. Trans. Am. Soc. Artif. Intern. Organs **15:** 40–44.
16. MCINTIRE, L. V., T. S. DEWITZ & R. R. MARTIN. 1976. Mechanical trauma effects on leukocytes. Trans. Am. Soc. Artif. Intern. Organs **22:** 444–447.
17. PAPING, R., L. R. WEBSTER, T. H. STANLEY, K. REZECCA & W. J. KOLFF. 1978. White blood cell phagocytosis after artificial heart implantation. Trans. Am. Soc. Artif. Int. Organs **24:** 578–580.
18. HUGHES, S. D., D. L. COLEMAN, P. A. DEW, G. L. BURNS, D. B. OLSEN & W. J. KOLFF. 1984. Effects of coumadin on thrombus and mineralization in total artificial hearts. Trans. Am. Soc. Artif. Intern. Organs **30:** 75–79.

Mechanisms of Arterial Graft Failure: The Role of Cellular Proliferation

ALEXANDER W. CLOWES[a] AND MICHAEL A. REIDY[b]

[a]*Department of Surgery*
[b]*Department of Pathology*
University of Washington School of Medicine
Seattle, Washington 98195

INTRODUCTION

During the last 80 years, vascular surgery has evolved as a specialty in large measure because of the development of prostheses for arterial reconstruction. In many circumstances, these grafts represent satisfactory and durable substitutes for diseased arteries, but under conditions of low flow and in reconstructions of small diameter vessels, only autogenous vein grafts are suitable since synthetic grafts develop spontaneous thrombosis, or at late times, luminal narrowing due to exuberant intimal thickening, particularly at anastomotic sites.[1] The relationship of this pathological intimal thickening to normal healing processes in grafts remains to be defined.

ENDOTHELIAL REPAIR IN SYNTHETIC GRAFTS

Early investigators demonstrated by means of silver staining that an endothelial-like covering develops over the luminal surface of Dacron graft.[2-4] This process was generally thought to be due to migration of cells from the cut edges of adjacent artery. Isolated observations of spontaneous patchy endothelial coverage were reported and were attributed to endothelial embolization and attachment.[5] As an alternative explanation, Florey and colleagues[3] suggested that capillaries traversing the matrix of Dacron grafts might also serve as sources of endothelium and thus produce patchy healing. They were unable to provide convincing proof of this intriguing hypothesis.

One of the problems encountered in studies of vascular grafts was the difficulty in unambiguously identifying the cells participating in the healing process. For example, most studies have relied upon scanning and transmission electron microscopy for the identification of endothelium. The cells exhibit a characteristic surface morphology and contain Weibel-Palade bodies. More recently, these cells have been shown to stain for factor-VIII-related antigen.

We undertook a reexamination of the healing process in synthetic grafts using a baboon polytetrafluoroethylene (PTFE) aortoiliac graft model. We addressed the hypothesis that the pathological development of anastomotic intimal thickening was the consequence of abnormal repair along the length of the graft. In conventional, low-porosity (30 μm internodal distance) PTFE grafts, we observed that the endothelium was derived from the cut edges of adjacent artery and that these cells migrated and proliferated as a continuous sheet toward the center of the graft.[6,7] In grafts ranging in length from 6–9 cm, we found that approximately 50% of them were healed by one year and that, in general, the shorter grafts were totally covered while the longer grafts remained denuded in the central portion. Although the limits of endothelial repair were not defined precisely, in this baboon model endothelial ingrowth seemed to cease approximately 2–3 cm from the heel of the graft. This finding was in keeping with previous results by Reidy and colleagues in rabbits and rats demonstrating a limit to endothelial ingrowth of between 5 and 10 mm.[8,9] In the baboon model, endothelial cells were unequivocally identified using antibody to human factor-VIII-related antigen on cross sections and en face preparations. As expected, endothelial proliferation was associated with the growing edge. Surprisingly, proliferation persisted in regions already covered by endothelium despite the fact that defects in the endothelial layer were not detected. We have found that this does not occur in regenerating endothelium over injured artery. We will come back to this point later on, since it may be of importance for the mechanism by which intimal thickening is regulated.

The possibility that capillaries could serve as sources of endothelium was examined using porous (60 μm internodal distance) PTFE grafts inserted into the baboon aortoiliac circulation.[10] Islands of endothelium appeared at intervals along the length of these grafts by 7 days and formed a confluent monolayer by 14 days. Numerous orifices were identified and shown to communicate to microvessels outside the graft in the surrounding granulation tissue. This was accomplished by infusing liquid latex rubber (Microfil) into the lumen of the grafts and demonstrating rubber in the lumina of vessels outside the grafts. The capillary endothelium was identified by immunostaining for factor-VIII-related antigen and appeared to shift from a tubular configuration to a monolayer upon reaching the luminal surface of the graft. This phenotypic switch has been described as a cell culture curiosity, but has not been identified in *in vivo* situations.[11–14] The mechanism of the phenotypic switch has not been determined. As in the case of the less porous 30-μm PTFE grafts, endothelial proliferation did not cease once the layer had been established on the surface of the 60-μm PTFE grafts.

The observation that endothelial proliferation persisted at late times despite complete coverage of the graft suggested that endothelial injury and repair might be an ongoing process in the synthetic grafts. A detailed morphological examination of the surface by scanning electron microscopy, however, failed to reveal endothelial loss. We tried to detect subtle forms of denudation by infusing indium-111-labeled platelets. We expected these labeled platelets to adhere to even the smallest defect. However, the amount of radioactivity accumulating in morphologically endothelialized intima was the same as in adjacent artery.[15] Based on these observations, we have concluded the endothelial replication must be in response to a chronic desquamating but nondenuding form of endothelial injury as described by Reidy in other vascular pathological situations.[9,16] It would appear from cell culture studies[17] that endothelial cells, when they die, do not simply fall off but are released slowly from the underlying matrix and are replaced by migration and proliferation of neighboring cells so as to keep the subendothelial layer covered. The reason for this ongoing endothelial injury is not obvious but might relate to the rigid structure of the underlying graft as well as the fragility of the newly synthesized subendothelium.

THE ROLE OF SMOOTH MUSCLE CELL PROLIFERATION IN THE DEVELOPMENT OF INTIMAL THICKENING

Intimal thickening in synthetic grafts appears to be the consequence of cellular proliferation and extracellular matrix accumulation. The type and source of connective tissue cell responsible for the intimal thickening has not been defined. In the past, investigators have identified fibroblasts, myofibroblasts, and smooth muscle cells in the intima. Because of the morphological similarities of proliferating fibroblasts and smooth muscle cells, an unequivocal identification of cell type was not possible.

By using the low-porosity and high-porosity PTFE grafts, we have found that smooth muscle cells appear in the intima of healing baboon grafts and can be identified by their expression of α-actin.[6] Fibroblasts identified morphologically and by the lack of staining with antibody to α-actin as well as the paucity of sulfated matrix about them appear to reside within the graft matrix and in the surrounding granulation tissue; they do not seem to participate in the formation of the intimal thickening. In healing low-porosity grafts, SMC are derived from the cut edges of adjacent artery and appear to migrate and to proliferate only underneath the endothelium and not where endothelium is absent. Once endothelial repair has progressed, SMC proliferation appears to slow down except in the region of the anastomosis. In consequence, intimal thickening in 30-μm PTFE grafts is greatest at the anastomoses and less toward the middle of the graft. By comparison, the formation of intimal thickening is quite different in 60-μm PTFE grafts.[10] In this circumstance, SMC accompany the capillary endothelium to the luminal side of the graft and appear to proliferate and accumulate only after the overlying endothelial layer is fully formed. Only rarely have we observed SMC proliferating in the absence of an overlying endothelial layer.

These observations suggest that a synthetic prosthesis inserted into the arterial circulation is incorporated in such a fashion as to recapitulate the structure of a normal artery. An endothelial layer is formed at the luminal surface and this overlies a compartment (neointima) containing SMC. Fibroblasts appear to reside only outside this layer in graft matrix or surrounding granulation tissue. Similar observations have been made in a variety of species. In man, it would appear from occasional clinical observations that intimal thickening and endothelial repair of the graft surface is limited to a region just adjacent to anastomoses despite the fact that many of the most commonly used synthetic grafts (*e.g.*, Dacron) are quite porous.[18] One possibility is that the Dacron grafts in some manner inhibit either migration of cells from the cut edges of adjacent artery or the invasion of capillaries from outside the graft. In preliminary studies of Dacron grafts inserted into the baboon aorotoiliac circulation, we have found that this is indeed the case. Ultimately, these grafts, like the porous PTFE grafts, are covered by endothelium but the process is markedly delayed.

MECHANISMS OF GROWTH CONTROL WITHIN THE NEOINTIMA

Much of our understanding of SMC and endothelial growth control comes from studies on injured arteries and cell culture. In injured vessels,[19,20] endothelial cells proliferate and migrate to regenerate the surface; once a region is covered proliferation ceases. At the same time, and only in denuded regions, SMC proliferate within the media and then migrate and continue to proliferate in the intima. Once an overlying layer of endothelium develops, intimal SMC proliferation ceases. Although this process is reliably demonstrated in models of massive denudation, the growth factors responsible for stimulating SMC proliferation have nevertheless not been identified. In culture, a variety of well-defined growth factors appear to regulate cell growth.

In striking contrast, endothelial cells covering grafts appear to continue to proliferate despite the presence of an intact and complete layer. As suggested earlier, this might be due to ongoing injury and compensatory repair. The other striking difference between healing grafts and healing injured arteries is the presence of SMC proliferation in the intima *only* when an overlying endothelium is present and not where endothelium is absent. These observations have suggested to us that at late times regulatory factors are unlikely to come from platelets adherent to the wall. Instead, we have speculated that these factors might come from the vascular wall cells themselves. (FIG. 1) This hypothesis is supported by the observation that endothelial cells and SMC in culture can, under some conditions, produce molecules similar to platelet-derived growth factor (PDGF). For example, Nilsson *et al.*,[21] Walker *et al.*,[22] and Seifert *et al.*[23] have demonstrated that rat SMC are capable of proliferation in the absence of serum and produce PDGF-like growth factor. Gajdusek *et al.*[24] have shown that endothelial cells produce mitogen for SMC, and DiCorleto and Bowen-Pope[25] have demonstrated that a portion of this mitogenic activity is PDGF-like. Barrett *et al.*[26] have shown that endothelial cells *in vivo* and *in vitro* express the proto-oncogene *sis*, and PDGF β-chain appears to be the product of *sis* expression.[27,28] Hence the possibility exists that vascular wall cells, in addition to other blood-borne cells such as macrophages and platelets, might be responsible for generating growth factor.

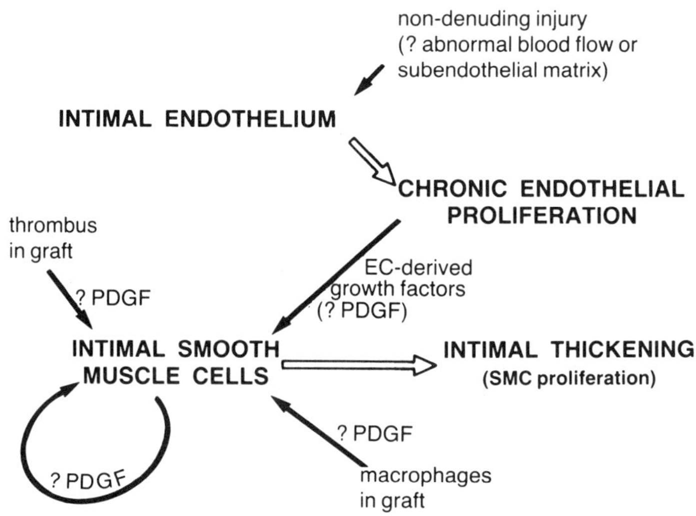

FIGURE 1. Endothelial and smooth muscle cells (SMC) enter graft intima by ingrowth from adjacent artery or from granulation tissue surrounding graft. Diagram suggests how chronically injured and proliferating endothelium might synthesize growth factors such as platelet-derived growth factor (PDGF) and regulate intimal SMC proliferation and intimal thickening. Alternatively, SMC growth factors could come from accumulated platelets, macrophages, or even SMC themselves.

IMPLICATIONS FOR THE CLINICAL USE OF SYNTHETIC GRAFTS

Two major problems remaining to be solved are spontaneous thrombosis and late luminal stenosis due to exuberant intimal thickening. The observations described above suggest that spontaneous thrombosis might be prevented by the rapid and early development of an endothelial covering. At present, it would appear that this might best be accomplished by either seeding endothelial cells directly onto the graft or by stimulating the development of an endothelial layer by increasing capillary migration onto the graft from surrounding granulation tissue. Control of intimal thickening must depend upon a detailed understanding of mechanisms of cellular proliferation within the neointima. As suggested above, one possibility is that the cells themselves secrete growth factor and regulate their own growth. The stimulus leading to continued endothelial damage and the release of growth factor, as suggested by Fox and DiCorleto,[29] has not been defined. Ultimately, the structure of the graft (for example, its elasticity or its diameter with respect to host vessel) might be of fundamental importance. These factors must be investigated in detail before a comprehensive picture can be developed.

REFERENCES

1. CLOWES, A. W. & M. C. ADAMS. 1986. Smooth muscle cell proliferation and arterial graft failure. *In* Reoperative Arterial Surgery. J. J. Bergan & J. S. T. Yao, Eds.: 3–13. Grune & Stratton. New York.
2. YONG, N. K., J. B. KINMONTH & G. W. TAYLOR. 1963. The endothelial lining of vascular grafts. Surg. Gynecol. Obstet. **117:** 305–310.
3. FLOREY, H. W., S. J. GREER, J. KISER, J. C. F. POOLE, R. TELANDER & N. T. WERTHESEN. 1962. The development of the pseudointima lining fabric grafts of the aorta. Br. J. Exp. Pathol. **43:** 655–660.
4. STEWART, G. J., N. ESSA, K. H. Y. CHANG & F. A. REICHLE. 1975. A scanning and transmission electron microscope study of the luminal coating on Dacron prostheses in the canine thoracic aorta. J. Lab. Clin. Med. **85:** 208–226.
5. HARKER, L. A., S. J. SLICHTER & L. R. SAUVAGE. 1977. Platelet consumption by arterial prostheses: The effects of endothelialization and pharmacologic inhibition of platelet function. Ann. Surg. **186:** 594–601.
6. CLOWES, A. W., A. M. GOWN, S. R. HANSON & M. A. REIDY. 1985. Mechanisms of arterial graft failure. I. Role of cellular proliferation in early healing of PTFE prostheses. Am. J. Pathol. **118:** 43–50.
7. CLOWES, A. W., T. R. KIRKMAN & M. M. CLOWES. 1986. Mechanisms of arterial graft failure. II. Chronic endothelial and smooth muscle cell proliferation in healing polytetrafluoroethylene prostheses. J. Vasc. Surg. **3:** 877–884.
8. REIDY, M. A., A. W. CLOWES & S. M. SCHWARTZ. 1983. Endothelial regeneration. V. Inhibition of endothelial regrowth in arteries of rat and rabbit. Lab. Invest. **49:** 569–575.
9. REIDY, M. A. 1985. A reassessment of endothelial injury and arterial lesion formation. Lab. Invest. **53:** 513–520.
10. CLOWES, A. W., T. R. KIRKMAN & M. A. REIDY. 1986. Mechanisms of arterial graft healing. Rapid transmural capillary ingrowth provides a source of intimal endothelium and smooth muscle in porous PTFE prostheses. Am. J. Pathol. **123:** 220–230.
11. SCHWARTZ, S. M. 1978. Selection and characterization of bovine endothelial cells. In Vitro **14:** 966–980.
12. FOLKMAN, J. & C. HAUDENSCHILD. 1980. Angiogenesis *in vitro*. Nature **288:** 551–556.
13. MCAUSLAN, B. R., G. N. HANNAN & W. REILLY. 1982. Signals causing change in morphological phenotype, growth mode, and gene expression of vascular endothelial cells. J. Cell. Physiol. **112:** 96–106.
14. MADRI, J. A. & S. K. WILLIAMS. 1983. Capillary endothelial cell cultures: Phenotypic modulation by matrix components. J. Cell Biol. **97:** 153–165.
15. REIDY, M. A., S. S. CHAO, T. R. KIRKMAN & A. W. CLOWES. 1986. Endothelial regeneration. VI. Chronic non-denuding injury in baboon vascular grafts. Am. J. Pathol. **123:** 432–439.
16. REIDY, M. A. & S. M. SCHWARTZ. 1983. Endothelial injury and regeneration. IV. Endotoxin: a non-denuding injury to aortic endothelium. Lab. Invest. **48:** 25–34.
17. HANSSON, G. K. & S. M. SCHWARTZ. 1983. Evidence for cell death in the vascular endothelium *in vivo* and *in vitro*. Am. J. Pathol. **112:** 278–286.
18. BERGER K., L. R. SAUVAGE, A. M. RAO & S. J. WOOD. 1972. Healing of arterial prostheses in man: Its incompleteness. Ann. Surg. **175:** 118–127.
19. SCHWARTZ, S. M., C. C. HAUDENSCHILD & E. M. EDDY. 1978. Endothelial regeneration. I. Quantitative analysis of initial stages of endothelial regeneration in rat aortic intima. Lab. Invest. **38:** 568–580.
20. CLOWES, A. W., M. A. REIDY & M. M. CLOWES. 1983. Kinetics of cellular proliferation after arterial injury. I. Smooth muscle growth in the absence of endothelium. Lab. Invest. **49:** 327–333.

21. NILSSON, J., M. SJOLUND, M. PALMBERG, J. THYBERG & C. H. HELDIN. 1985. Arterial smooth muscle cells in primary culture produce a platelet-derived growth factor-like protein. Proc. Natl. Acad. Sci. U.S.A. **82:** 4418–4422.
22. WALKER, L. N., D. F. BOWEN-POPE, R. ROSS & M. A. REIDY. 1986. Production of platelet-derived growth factor-like molecules by cultured arterial smooth muscle cells accompanies proliferation after arterial injury. Proc. Natl. Acad. Sci. U.S.A. **83:** 7311–7315.
23. SEIFERT, R. A., S. M. SCHWARTZ & D. F. BOWEN-POPE. 1984. Developmentally regulated production of platelet-derived growth factor-like molecules. Nature **311:** 669–671.
24. GAJDUSEK, C. M., P. DICORLETO, R. ROSS & S. M. SCHWARTZ. 1980. An endothelial cell derived growth factor. J. Cell. Biol. **85:** 467–472.
25. DICORLETO, P. E. & D. F. BOWEN-POPE. 1983. Cultured endothelial cells produce a platelet-derived growth factor-like protein. Proc. Natl. Acad. Sci. U.S.A. **80:** 1919–1923.
26. BARRETT, T. B., C. M. GAJDUSEK, S. M. SCHWARTZ, J. K. MCDOUGALL & E. P. BENDITT. 1984. Expression of the *sis* gene by endothelial cells in culture and *in vivo.* Proc. Natl. Acad. Sci. U.S.A. **81:** 6772–6774.
27. WATERFIELD, M. D., G. T. SCRACE, N. WHITTLE, P. STROOBANT, A. JOHNSON, A. WASTESON, B. WESTERMARK, C. H. HELDIN, J. S. HUANG & T. F. DEUEL. 1983. Platelet-derived growth factor is structurally related to the putative transforming protein $p28^{sis}$ of simian sarcoma virus. Nature **304:** 35–39.
28. DOOLITTLE, R. F., M. W. HUNKAPILLAR, L. E. HOOD, S. G. DEVARE, K. C. ROBBINS, S. A. AARONSON & H. N. ANTONIADES. 1983. Simian sarcoma virus oncogene, v-sis, is derived from the gene (or genes) encoding a platelet-derived growth factor. Science **221:** 275–277.
29. FOX, P. L. & P. E. DICORLETO. 1984. Regulation of production of a platelet-derived growth factor-like protein by cultured bovine aortic endothelial cells. J. Cell. Physiol. **121:** 298–308.

Thrombosis in Extracorporeal Devices

PIERRE M. GALLETTI

Division of Biology and Medicine
Brown University
Providence, Rhode Island 02912

When Ted Spaet, Ed Leonard, and Leo Vroman called the first conference on blood in contact with natural and artificial surfaces in 1976, following up the precursor meeting organized by Ed Varco in 1971 in San Diego,[1] we at Brown University were involved in a large-scale evaluation of multiple types of membrane lungs and pump-oxygenator circuits.[2-4] Thrombosis was not an uncommon phenomenon. In each particular case of genesis of mural thrombus formation we could speculate on, and occasionally provide evidence for, the relative weight of local flow conditions, material properties, and biological modifications in terms of topical and distant effects. There was little doubt at the time that thrombosis originating in an extracorporeal circuit would occasionally present a major barrier to surgical cardiopulmonary bypass. Thus it was not irrational to believe that this predicament could also be implicated in less dramatic circumstances, and that research should be pursued vigorously to analyze, understand, and eliminate the problem.

Research has been pursued vigorously for the past 15 years, and yet the clinical importance of thrombosis in extracorporeal circuits remains in dispute. Some wise and experienced investigators discount thrombosis as a significant impediment in the clinical use of blood-handling devices. Others see thrombus formation as a limiting factor for long-term treatment involving extracorporeal procedures, whether or not one uses pharmacologic anticoagulation.

Thus I find myself at the end of this conference asked to draw conclusions from the integrated experience, both in the research laboratory and the clinical setting. Should thrombosis in extracorporeal devices be qualified as a major unresolved problem, a second-order uncommon complication, a complex but irrelevant annoyance, or merely an esthetic defect? I was tempted for a moment to illustrate my answer with slides, but whether I selected a show of horrors or a display of beauties, the nagging question persisted: To what extent is any particular observation generally applicable to the clinical setting? Thus in an attempt to combine scientific wisdom with practicality, I will formulate global statements and attempt to document them by inferential evidence rather than anecdotes.

First, thrombosis in extracorporeal devices is not a widespread, limiting clinical problem at this time. I am talking here about cardiopulmonary bypass, hemodialysis, and extracorporeal ventricular assistance, procedures that are usually accompanied by systemic heparinization. The morbidity of these procedures, as far as one can distinguish from the medical conditions for which the devices are used, is minimal. Although not negligible, it is uncommon in experienced hands, and almost always treatable. Thrombosis is less common an issue than it was 10 years ago because of natural selection. The most trouble-prone devices have been weeded out by competition, there are fewer models in clinical use, and each benefits from a much longer experience. For standard procedures, the basic principles of flow patterns and material selection are now empirically, if not always analytically, understood. H. Schmid-Schönbein[5] has drawn our attention to the fact that artificial organs commonly involve blood flow in noncylindrical conduits, and that abnormal fluid dynamic conditions enhance a reactive cascade of biochemical events that occasionally reaches the stage of explosive amplification. Manufacturers of extracorporeal devices may not appreciate all the fine points of flow-related and material-induced thrombogenesis, but empirically they have corrected the most obvious defects of their blood circuits. Modes of assembly, connection, and priming have also been streamlined. There is more quality control, traceability of construction materials, and insistence on good manufacturing practices than were applied in the fabrication of devices in the artisanal days between 1960 and 1975. Gross device defects are now uncommon, and as a result, there is rarely the need to change devices during the course of an extracorporeal circulation procedure.

Clean room fabrication has also become the rule rather than the exception for clinical devices. Here I will hazard a second generalization. Once you invade the bloodstream, the human body is better equipped to deal with occasional breaches of sterility than with transgressions of cleanliness. The cleanliness of a device is not guaranteed by its sterility. Cleanliness always matters for thrombogenesis in extracorporeal circuits. Sterility matters sometimes. To respect both, we should avoid confusing them. The best illustration of the progress made possible by a mix of empirical appreciation of thrombogenesis and modern fabrication techniques stems from the history of hollow fiber oxygenators. At the time of our 1976 meeting, laboratory and clinical trials with the ancestors of these devices had shown an unacceptably high incidence of thrombus formation. Thus industrial production was postponed indefinitely. Yet in the past three years, a number of manufacturers have revitalized this product and brought it to widespread clinical application. Hollow fiber oxygenators are not yet problem free,[6] but they are certainly acceptable as a clinical tool because the quality control during production is measurably better than it was a decade ago.

Now that I have spoken positively about the low incidence of thrombosis and its roots in better quality control, and focused on the design and biomaterials aspects of the equation while playing down the biological modifications inherent to the use of extracorporeal circulation devices, let me take some of it back. Many observers of the extracorporeal circulation scene, experimental as well as clinical, have developed the nagging suspicion that our scientific method, which relies on averaging information collected from a statistically significant number of observations, may on occasion bury the biological reality rather than highlight it. One report at this conference[7] showed how some individuals consistently differ from others in the reactivity of their platelets to a particular flow-material environment. There are individuals, animals as well as humans, who display thrombotic phenomena of a magnitude considerably beyond others. We tend to exclude such individuals from a series in a scientific report, but we cannot ignore them as a clinical reality. Their reaction to an extracorporeal circuit is not predictable since we do not have a test to identify them in advance of the procedure. We do not know yet how to characterize these "outliers" and avoid the uncommon accident, but we are better equipped than in 1976 to deal with the accident when it occurs.

While I am on the issue of exceptions to the rules and negative results, let me comment on the early reports from the European experience with extracorporeal membrane oxygenation (ECMO). ECMO is instructive because it lasts longer than surgical cardiopulmonary bypass and requires a higher blood flow than hemodialysis, although the circuits are geometrically comparable. The longest ECMO procedure associated with patient survival is 28 days, which expressed in terms of the volume of blood processed corresponds to more than a year of intermittent hemodialysis. This is the good news. The bad news is that overall, 25% of ECMO procedures are marred by progressive deterioration of the gas exchange status that cannot be explained by simple concepts of hypoxia or hemodynamic instability.[8] One cannot say at this point whether the failures are associated with damaging blood-material interactions in the extracorporeal circuit, or a disseminated biological reaction (perhaps related to nonspecific activation of the complement alternative pathway), or toxic action of neutrophils that have migrated out of the bloodstream. Although the analysis is by no means complete, and the ECMO data will of necessity reflect the combined experience of several centers rather than the most experienced one, one cannot escape the impression that the extracorporeal device is in some fashion implicated in the occasional failures of this therapeutic modality.

This brings me to another group of considerations that apply to experimental as well as clinical perfusions, namely the threat of continuing or repeated infections. Earlier I downplayed the relative importance of sterility vs. cleanliness for preventing thrombosis in short-lasting extracorporeal circulation procedures. This should not be construed to mean that infection is not a factor. The association of bloodstream infection with thrombosis has long been established for cardiac valves and vascular grafts. The postmortem experience with the totally implantable heart, however limited in the number of patients involved, also suggests a much greater incidence of infection-associated thrombosis than had been suspected from clinical observations. Infection close to an implant that elicits a permanent foreign body reaction cannot be cured by antibiotics. Much as we moved in the 1970s from an obsession with hemolysis to an appreciation of the role of thrombocytes in blood-material interactions, we must now address the complex behavior of leukocytes in extracorporeal circuits and the perfused organisms, particularly when the duration of the extracorporeal blood circulation procedure becomes commensurate with the life cycle of these elements.

This brings me to a final consideration, which was anticipated by the prior comments of Paul Didisheim in this volume.[9] The time scale of most laboratory observations of thrombosis-related phenomena is on the order of seconds, minutes, or hours, much shorter than the time scale of clinically relevant problems, which become worrisome after days, weeks, or months. The question then becomes one of how to integrate the component phenomenology observed under short-lived, controlled conditions, and apply it to the chronic situation associated with long-term use of devices. Here I move beyond the immediate scope of my topic and shift from extracorporeal devices to permanent cardiovascular implants. Biomaterials assume a new importance, but because of their prolonged exposure to a warm, humid, and corrosive environment, they may no longer be the same materials as were characterized prior to implantation. Blood flow patterns are important, but they may well have been modified by tissue growth in response to the implant. Distant effects of thrombosis, whether they be embolization, activation, or depression of homeostatic phenomena, now have time to be fully expressed and even to become dominant. The concertation of nonspecific responses to a device, which H. Schmid-Schönbein found at the root of thrombogenesis in artificial organs, cannot reach full expression unless we introduce the corrective factors of convective dilution that underlie all natural defense mechanisms in the body.[5] At this point we are limited not only by the properties of materials, but also by inadequate instrumentation to monitor thrombus formation in a noninvasive manner over long periods of time. This is the next challenge for the study of blood-material interactions. I predict that some of you will meet again in 10 years to assess our advances in the analysis of *prolonged* blood-material interactions.

REFERENCES

1. GALLETTI, P. M. 1971. Blood interfacial phenomena: an overview. Fed. Proc. **30:** 1491.
2. GALLETTI, P. M., P. D. RICHARDSON & M. T. SNIDER. 1971. Blood Oxygenator Testing and

Evaluation. I. Evaluation Techniques. NIH Report No. 69-2047-1. National Institutes of Health. Bethesda, MD.
3. FRIEDMAN, L. I., P. D. RICHARDSON & P. M. GALLETTI. 1973. Blood Oxygenator Testing and Evaluation. II. Procedures and Results. NIH Report No. 69-2047-2.
4. RICHARDSON, P. D. & P. M. GALLETTI. 1976. Correlation of effects of blood flow rate, viscosity and design features on artificial lung performance. *In* Physiological and Clinical Aspects of Oxygenator Design, vol. 29. S. G. Dawids & H. C. Engell, Eds. Elsevier/North-Holland Biomedical Press. Luxembourg.
5. SCHMID-SCHONBEIN, H. 1987. Surface abnormalities and conduit characteristics as a cause of blood trauma in artificial internal organs: The interaction of fluid-dynamic, physico-chemical and cell biological reactions in thrombus formation. This volume.
6. BARTHELEMY, R., J. P. ESQUERRE & N. BOYER. Flow distribution in membrane oxygenators. Life Support Systems **4(1):** 18.
7. RICHARDSON, P. D. Interaction of transport phenomena and surface reactions. This volume.
8. GILLE, J. P. 1986. Editorial: Extracorporeal support for respiratory insufficiency, essential and workable. Life Support System **4:** 189.
9. DIDISHEIM, P. 1987. Summary: Plasma systems. This volume.

Summary

Thrombogenesis on Prosthetic Surfaces

SUZANNE G. ESKIN

Department of Surgery
Baylor College of Medicine
Houston, Texas 77030

The baboon shunt model described by Dr. Harker has provided a useful technique for demonstrating that although smooth surfaces may appear thrombus free, they may be very thrombogenic as evidenced by formation of systemic emboli. Drs. Burns and Olsen have studied the performance of polyurethane in pumping chambers implanted in calves and sheep for several months. They noted that thrombus formation was evidenced by renal infarction and was influenced by the health of the animal, complexities of flow patterns in the chambers, and infection.

By studying the performance of the PTFE graft in baboon arteries, Dr. Clowes has shown that the mode of healing (endothelialization) of these grafts is a function of graft porosity. Comparisons of graft healing to healing of injured arteries have led him to suggest that intimal thickening is regulated by cells within the vessel wall rather than blood-borne factors. Dr. Galletti stated that thrombogenesis on extracorporeal oxygenator systems is no longer a widespread clinical problem because of the long experience with them and quality control that has developed. However, individual patients may vary an order of magnitude in thrombotic potential. There are also infection problems. Foreign materials are thrombogenic, but the time scale of thrombogenesis is much shorter than observed clinical problems. Another problem is that the composition of implanted materials changes during long-term implantation.

Presentations on chronic implants reveal different problems and different levels of development. Extracorporeal membrane oxygenators used clinically are limited not by thrombogenesis but by infection. This is also the case with ventricular assist devices and total artificial hearts, clinically as well as in animal models. Thrombus formation is still a very real factor in the failure of small-diameter arterial grafts. Ongoing experimentation at the basic level is necessary to discern the relative roles of thrombogenesis, flow dynamics, and abnormal intimal proliferation in occlusion of these grafts. Perhaps immunologically controlled organ culture systems using biodegradable substrates will ultimately provide the vascular prosthetic replacements we seek.

Postscript

About Success and Failure

EDWARD F. LEONARD,[a] VINCENT T. TURITTO,[b]
AND LEO VROMAN[c]

[a]*Department of Chemical Engineering and Applied Chemistry
Columbia University School of Engineering
New York, New York 10027*

[b]*Department of Medicine
Mount Sinai School of Medicine
New York, New York 10029*

[c]*Interface Laboratory
Veterans Administration Medical Center
Brooklyn, New York 11209*

Basic research on blood-biomaterial interactions has been nurtured by the failures of its practical applications, so that our view of those interactions has both sharpened and expanded. Causal relationships, once thought simple, are proving more indirect and more branched each time we try to capture and domesticate them. A typical sequence is as follows. Basic researchers find that a broad range of surfaces adsorbs and activates a clotting factor A, which produces B, a dangerous enzyme. Industry first tries to avoid adsorption of factor A, but control experiments show that purified A is adsorbed on all surfaces. Then some basic researchers, generously supplied by industry with leftover A, show that A does not really form B but destroys its inhibitor C. Now industry wants to incorporate C into its materials and starts supporting basic research in C, from which the discovery is made that C is activated by B in the presence of D, which must be coadsorbed with C to render it active.

The greatest danger to basic research appears to be some kind of immediate success of its application. In the seventies, some thought the ultimate answer (*e.g.*, Biomer) had been found, so that funds for finding the matching ultimate answer ("Why does it work?") dwindled. Now, failure to create an everlasting artificial heart or permanently patent narrow vessels has rekindled the search for sounder foundations.

If the intensity and widening scope of this search is a measure of technical failure, it is also a measure of increasing scientific commitment—or at least of increasing dissatisfaction with the quality of our earlier knowledge. Our failures have certainly generated pessimism. We have at times begun to believe that clinical success will require a measure of perfection, and yet the basic properties of an ideal blood-compatible material cannot even be agreed upon in principle. All we can say with certainty is that perfectly blood-compatible materials should be able to last the natural lifetime of an otherwise healthy recipient.

A stream of peculiar substances is being generated for clinical use. The development of these substances has been based on the poorly understood theoretical work of others, marginally funded by a rapid succession of government individuals with poorly founded preferences, and brought to fruition by industrial companies with their own diverse views of cost-effectiveness.

One wonders, in the face of such chaos, how progress is made, and even more whether such devices will enhance significantly the survival rate and quality of life of patients. However, such pessimism does not hold up well in science, and it is unwise to emphasize negatives too strenuously. Many problems once considered "impossible" have yielded, with amazing speed, to the relentless onslaught of scientific investigation. The current volume is a testament to the magnitude of our recent efforts. As we were perhaps overly optimistic 10 years ago, let us not be overly pessimistic now. Ten years from now we may find that a postscript about success and failure will not be necessary.

Index of Contributors